Veterinary Hematology

A Diagnostic Guide and Color Atlas

John W. Harvey, DVM, PhD, DACVP
Professor and Executive Associate Dean
College of Veterinary Medicine
University of Florida
Gainesville, Florida

with 836 *illustrations*

ELSEVIER

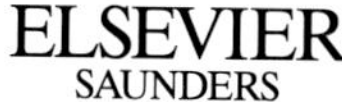

SAUNDERS

3251 Riverport Lane
St. Louis, Missouri 63043

Veterinary Hematology: A Diagnostic Guide and Color Atlas ISBN: 978-1-4377-0173-9

Notices

Knowledge and best practice in this field are constantly changing. As new research and experience broaden our understanding, changes in research methods, professional practices, or medical treatment may become necessary.

Practitioners and researchers must always rely on their own experience and knowledge in evaluating and using any information, methods, compounds, or experiments described herein. In using such information or methods they should be mindful of their own safety and the safety of others, including parties for whom they have a professional responsibility.

With respect to any drug or pharmaceutical products identified, readers are advised to check the most current information provided (i) on procedures featured or (ii) by the manufacturer of each product to be administered, to verify the recommended dose or formula, the method and duration of administration, and contraindications. It is the responsibility of practitioners, relying on their own experience and knowledge of their patients, to make diagnoses, to determine dosages and the best treatment for each individual patient, and to take all appropriate safety precautions.

To the fullest extent of the law, neither the Publisher nor the authors, contributors, or editors, assume any liability for any injury and/or damage to persons or property as a matter of products liability, negligence or otherwise, or from any use or operation of any methods, products, instructions, or ideas contained in the material herein.

Library of Congress Cataloging-in-Publication Data

Harvey, John W.
Veterinary hematology : a diagnostic guide and color atlas / John W. Harvey.
p. ; cm.
Includes bibliographical references and index.
ISBN 978-1-4377-0173-9 (pbk. : alk. paper)
I. Title.
[DNLM: 1. Hematologic Diseases–veterinary–Atlases. 2. Animals, Domestic–blood–Atlases.
3. Hematologic Tests–veterinary–Atlases. SF 769.5]
636.089'615–dc23

2011039099

Vice President and Publisher: Linda Duncan
Acquisitions Editor: Heidi Pohlman
Associate Developmental Editor: Brandi Graham
Publishing Services Manager: Catherine Jackson
Senior Project Manager: Carol O'Connell
Design Direction: Jessica Williams

Transferred to digital printing in 2015

This book is dedicated to the memory of Charles F. Simpson, DVM, PhD. Charlie trained as a veterinarian at Cornell University and as a pathologist at the University of Minnesota. He was a member of the University of Florida faculty for 33 years. Charlie's research focused on the cardiovascular system, including blood. When I joined the University of Florida faculty in 1974, he had already published hematology papers on babesiosis in horses, anaplasmosis in cattle, sickle cell formation in deer, the extrusion of the metarubricyte nucleus, the maturation of reticulocytes, and the formation of Heinz bodies in erythrocytes. His major research tool was the transmission electron microscope shown in the image below. As a mentor and friend, Charlie opened not only his laboratory, but also his home to me. During the years our careers overlapped, we published 11 papers together. Nineteen of his transmission electron microscope images are included in this book. To me and others who knew him, Charlie is remembered as a warm, generous person with an inquisitive mind and a wonderful sense of humor. His memory also lives on in the form of the Charles F. Simpson Memorial Scholarship that is given each year to a graduate student in the College of Veterinary Medicine at the University of Florida.

John Harvey

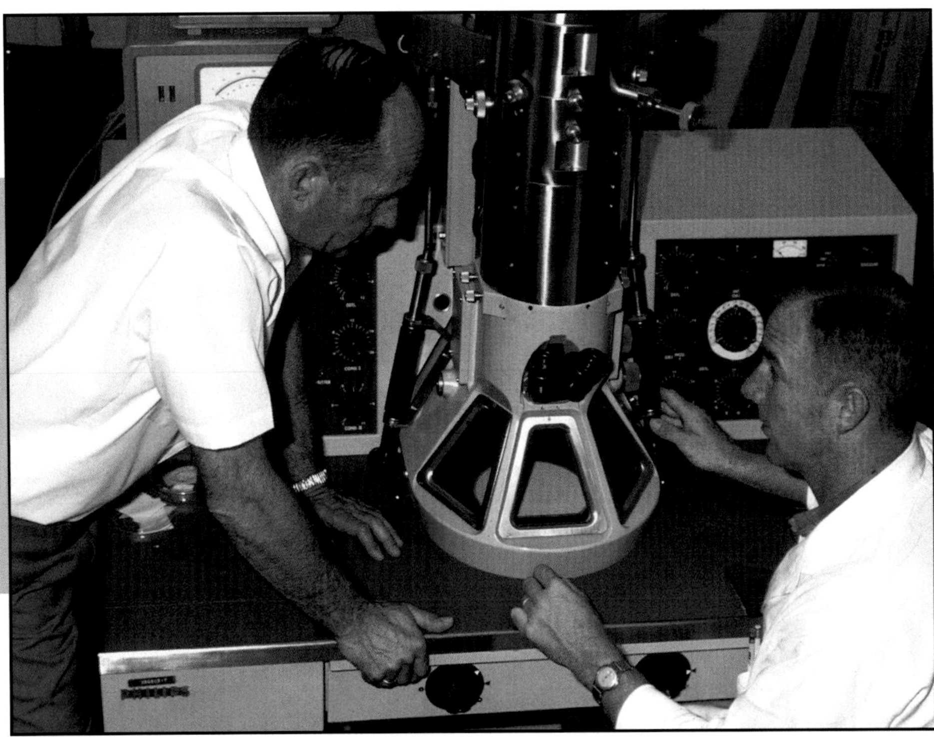

Dr. Charles F. Simpson *(left)* and his technologist J.W. Carlisle in front of their transmission electron microscope.

FOREWORD

Benefits for the Veterinarian and the Veterinary Clinical Pathologist

When the *Atlas of Veterinary Hematology* first appeared in 2001, it was an instant classic. The atlas was well-organized, concise, and extremely well-illustrated. The accompanying reference list was comprehensive. Furthermore, and perhaps most important, the atlas provided readers with the singular experience, insight, and perspective of one of the world's most well-known and well-respected veterinary hematologists, John Harvey. It quickly became a standard reference for veterinary clinical pathologists, pathology trainees, private practitioners, veterinary technicians, and veterinary students alike.

This long-awaited revision will do nothing but add to the original text's legacy of excellence. Under the new title *Veterinary Hematology: A Diagnostic Guide and Color Atlas,* this edition is significantly expanded and updated. The outstanding illustrations that made the original *Atlas of Veterinary Hematology* such a valuable contribution have been augmented by additional illustrations that even include electron micrographs of a number of significant hematologic disorders. The discussions of the physiology and pathophysiology of blood and bone marrow have been very significantly enhanced throughout the text, thereby making the new volume even more valuable to specialists and students at all levels. Of note, the bibliography, outstanding in the 2001 Atlas, has been comprehensively updated.

From cover to cover, *Veterinary Hematology: A Diagnostic Guide and Color Atlas* reflects the commitment to excellence, attention to detail, and dedication to the discipline of veterinary hematology that have made John Harvey such a credit to the specialty of veterinary clinical pathology. Although future updates will surely be needed, this new book serves as a timeless contribution to our knowledge and understanding of comparative hematology. As a contemporary colleague and friend of John's, I have personally had the privilege to learn from him directly through our numerous discussions, interactions, and case reviews. Through this, his new master work, his wisdom is preserved and made available for the ages.

Alan H. Rebar, DVM, PhD, DACVP
Senior Associate Vice President for Research
Executive Director of Discovery Park
Professor of Veterinary Clinical Pathology
School of Veterinary Medicine
Purdue University

FOREWORD

Benefits for the Veterinary Technician

Veterinary professionals and students alike need comprehensive medical reference texts that may better enable us to perform our jobs accurately and help our patients. Even the brightest minds are not walking encyclopedias. Therefore, *Veterinary Hematology: A Diagnostic Guide and Color Atlas* is a needed source of knowledge for both study and in practice.

I first met Dr. Harvey more than 30 years ago during an internship at the University of Florida, and I have attended many of his continuing education lectures through the years. Dr. Harvey has always been my 'go-to' specialist. If I am looking under the microscope, he's always just a 'flip of a page' away!

The original *Atlas of Veterinary Hematology: Blood and Bone Marrow of Domestic Animals* has for years been a valuable resource both as a bench-top reference for practicing veterinarians, veterinary students, and veterinary technicians and an aid to technician students in their quest for mastery of this complex topic. This exciting new book is a combination of the *Atlas* with *Veterinary Laboratory Medicine: Interpretation and Diagnosis.*

Veterinary Hematology: A Diagnostic Guide and Color Atlas provides additional information on techniques for performing hematology testing. Veterinary technicians and students will especially appreciate the logical organization of the material as well as the additional information included regarding clinical and diagnostic aspects of specific diseases.

Veterinary Hematology: A Diagnostic Guide and Color Atlas enhances understanding of the material and serves as a vital reference text for both veterinary technician students and practicing veterinary technicians. I am confident this reference atlas and guide will be a welcomed addition to every veterinary clinic and classroom throughout the veterinary world.

Elaine Anthony MA, CVT
Associate Professor
School of Veterinary Technology
St. Petersburg College

PREFACE

This reference presents images and information concerning the hematology of common domestic mammals including dogs, cats, horses, cattle, sheep, goats, pigs, and llamas. The hematology of nonmammalian species is presented superficially, primarily focusing on comparisons with mammals. This book updates and expands the material published in 2001 in the *Atlas of Veterinary Hematology: Blood and Bone Marrow of Domestic Animals* by John Harvey and combines its morphologic content with additional updated topics covered in the introduction and hematology chapters of *Veterinary Laboratory Medicine. Interpretation and Diagnosis*, 3rd edition, which was published in 2004 by Dennis Meyer and John Harvey. Even more information is provided concerning the clinical and hematologic appearance of specific disorders, and electron microscopy images have been added to provide ultrastructual detail of cell morphology.

This new text and atlas covers all aspects of hematology except therapy. It contains concise discussions of hematopoiesis and the physiology of erythrocytes, leukocytes, and hemostasis that provide the foundation needed to understand disorders of blood. These topics are presented in sufficient detail to be beneficial in the training of interns and residents, as well as veterinary students. The differential diagnoses of anemia, leukocyte disorders, and hemostatic disorders are presented in such a way as to emphasize the pathophysiology underlying these processes. The utilization and interpretation of both routine and specialized diagnostic tests are also discussed.

Veterinary technologists will likely find the techniques and blood cell morphology sections most useful. Attempts were made to include both common and rare morphologic findings in blood and bone marrow, including preparation and staining artifacts. Often, more than one example of a cell type, parasite, or abnormal condition is shown, because the morphology can be variable. The benefits and pitfalls of automated instrumentation are discussed, as is the importance of manual blood film review as an important quality control measure for hematology instrument-generated data and in the identification of morphologic abnormalities and parasites that cannot be detected using automated instruments.

Practicing veterinarians and veterinary students should benefit from this complete reference, even if they are not directly involved in bone marrow evaluation, because the bone marrow chapters provide the basis for understanding diseases that result in abnormalities in the peripheral blood. The electron microscopy images and bone marrow aspirate smear cytology and core biopsy histology chapters will be most useful to clinical pathologists, anatomic pathologists, and residents in training for these disciplines. Readers interested in learning more about a given topic will hopefully appreciate the extensive bibliography provided.

John Harvey

ACKNOWLEDGMENTS

I want to acknowledge those most responsible for my education as a clinical pathologist. Few people have the opportunity to receive training from the giants of their profession, but I was blessed in being trained by Jerry Kaneko, the father of veterinary clinical biochemistry, and Oscar Schalm, the father of veterinary hematology, during my graduate training at the University of California, Davis. Many other colleagues have contributed to my development as a hematologist, with Alan Rebar and Victor Perman being particularly noteworthy, as we challenged one another with unknown hematology slides in front of various national audiences. Past and present University of Florida faculty members, Charles Simpson, Dennis Meyer, Rose Raskin, Mary Christopher, Rick Alleman, Heather Wamsley, Roger Easley, Mark Dunbar, and many University of Florida residents have greatly advanced my understanding of veterinary hematology.

University of Florida clinical pathologists and technologists, most notably Melanie Pate, Lane Pritchard, and Tina Conrad, have also helped me by identifying and preparing material included in this text. I greatly appreciate all the colleagues who have submitted material to the annual American Society for Veterinary Clinical Pathology slide review sessions. Contributors are acknowledged in appropriate figure legends for photographs I have taken from these glass slides. Likewise, I am extremely grateful for images enthusiastically provided by colleagues that are also acknowledged in the figure legends.

Jennifer Owen, Heather Wamsley, and Chi-Chung Chou provided the conscientious reviews and helpful suggestions for which I will be forever grateful. Completion of text was only possible because Glen Hoffsis, Dana Zimmel, John Haven, and Rachel DiSesa assumed some of my job duties during the last year. I also appreciate the strong support from Elsevier staff members, most notably Brandi Graham and Carol O'Connell.

Finally, I especially want to thank my wife Liz for her patience, understanding, and support, not only during the many months required to produce this text, but during my entire academic career. Joseph Campbell urged everyone to "Follow your bliss." For me that has been teaching and research in veterinary hematology, and this pathway would not have been possible without Liz's many years of support.

John Harvey

CONTENTS

CHAPTER

1

INTRODUCTION TO VETERINARY HEMATOLOGY

Laboratory tests are done for a variety of reasons. Screening tests, such as a complete blood count (CBC), may be done on clinically normal animals when they are acquired to avoid a financial and/or emotional commitment to a diseased animal, to examine geriatric patients for subclinical disease, or to identify a condition that might make an animal an anesthetic or surgical risk. Screening tests are often done when an ill animal is first examined, especially if systemic signs of illness are present and a specific diagnosis is not apparent from the history and physical examination. Tests are also done to confirm a presumptive diagnosis. A test may be repeated or a different test may be done to confirm a test result that was previously reported to be abnormal. Tests may be done to assist in the determination of the severity of a disease, to help formulate a prognosis, and to monitor the response to therapy or progression of disease.

Decisions to request hematology tests in animals are largely based on the cost of the test versus the potential benefit of the result to the animal. A CBC is routinely done to establish a database for patient evaluation, while other hematology tests may be done in an attempt to evaluate a specific problem. Examples of more specific hematologic tests that focus on a problem identified during the diagnostic evaluation of an animal include coagulation tests, such as prothrombin time; bone marrow biopsy and interpretation; and immunologic tests, such as the direct Coombs' test. Although single tests may be done to address a specific problem (e.g., an erythrocyte phosphofructokinase assay), multiple tests are often utilized to provide a more comprehensive answer to a broader problem (e.g., a hemostasis panel is generally requested to evaluate a bleeding animal).

Stat is an abbreviation for *statim* (Latin meaning "immediately"). Stat tests are tests that are given high priority and begun immediately in situations where rapid results are needed for the medical management of critically ill patients. Additional fees may be charged for stat tests because they disrupt the flow of work in the laboratory and result in inefficiency.

INTERNAL VERSUS EXTERNAL LABORATORIES

A variety of factors should influence the decision of whether a test will be done in an in-house laboratory or be sent to an external laboratory. A major concern is whether the necessary personnel, equipment, and supplies are available to perform the test accurately. Considerations include personnel knowledge of species differences and a willingness to conduct quality-control tests to verify that the procedure is working properly. The costs per test (technician time, reagent costs, equipment costs) must be compared to determine which option is more economical. The stability of the test may determine whether it will be done internally. The time it takes to obtain results may be important, especially with critically ill patients. The hours of operation of the laboratories are important for test results that are needed at night or on the weekend. Commercial laboratories generally have better quality control than laboratories within private practices.

Commercial veterinary laboratories are preferred to commercial human laboratories because errors can occur if tests designed to evaluate human samples are used without modification to test samples from animals. Hematology analyzers must be calibrated for species differences to obtain accurate results. Technologists must be aware that blood cell morphology and blood parasites are different in various animal species. Antibody-dependent immunology tests designed for humans are generally not valid in animals. Veterinary laboratories are more likely to have established their own reference intervals for various animal species (as opposed to extracting them from the literature) than are human laboratories. A knowledge of specific animal diseases and training in veterinary laboratory medicine is essential for the evaluation of hematologic specimens and interpretation of laboratory data; consequently a veterinary clinical pathologist should be available to perform certain subjective tests and provide consultation concerning all test results.

REFERENCE INTERVALS

In order to be able to interpret laboratory data from ill animals, it is essential that appropriate reference intervals be established from apparently healthy animals drawn from the same general population as the ill animals to be examined. The term *reference interval* is preferred to the commonly used *normal range*. The latter term implies that it is the range of test results from all "normal" animals. In reality, a low percentage of apparently healthy "normal" animals will have test values outside the normal range, and, depending on the test, many abnormal (diseased) animals may have values within the normal range. Healthy animals may have transient increases or decreases in laboratory test results based on changes in environment, emotional status, diet, and so on, and a low percentage of healthy animals simply have values above or below the general population of healthy animals. Apparently healthy animals may also have occult disease that causes one or more abnormal laboratory test results, and sample collection, handling, and laboratory errors can result in artifactually high or low values from healthy animals. Consequently it is not appropriate simply to use the actual range of values from all apparently healthy animals assayed. To develop useful reference intervals, one must decide which animals will be assayed, how many animals need to be analyzed, and what method or methods will be used to remove high or low outliers that would otherwise render the interval of limited value as a reference.

Selection of Reference Animals

Specific reference intervals are needed for each species of animal being tested. Less often, a different reference interval is needed for an analyte from a specific breed of animal (e.g., hematocrit values in greyhound dogs are higher than those in most other dog breeds). Values may vary with the age of the animal, with major changes occurring prior to puberty (e.g., 3-week-old pups have lower hematocrits than adults). Consequently some analytes need different reference intervals for different age groups. Some analytes also vary with sex, pregnancy, emotional state, and activity level. The types of animals sampled and environmental conditions present during the establishment of a reference interval should be defined, along with the methods and equipment used, so that the user can make appropriate evaluations. Ideally, a reference interval should be established using a population of healthy animals with a composition (age, breed, sex, diet, etc.) like the population of ill animals being evaluated. Homogeneous populations generally have more narrow reference intervals than heterogenous populations. Establishing a reference interval for a blood analyte using a group of male foxhound dogs housed in a research colony, fed the same diet, and conditioned to phlebotomies would likely result in reference intervals too narrow for the population of dogs examined in a typical small-animal practice. Reference intervals are generally established for a species by utilizing samples from apparently healthy adult animals of both sexes and various breeds. Monogastric animals should have been fasted overnight prior to blood sample collection.

Determination of Reference Intervals

Specific reference intervals should be established for each instrument and each test evaluated. Ideally, each animal would have its own reference intervals established by multiple assays done over time when the animal was healthy. In some instances, limited numbers of baseline values are available for an animal that can be helpful, but rarely are analytes measured often enough to establish an accurate reference interval for an individual animal. Consequently population-based reference intervals are used.

When the frequency diagram of test results from a healthy population is examined, many analytes exhibit a Gaussian or bell-shaped distribution (Fig. 1-1). When a Gaussian distribution is present, a minimum of 40 individuals (100 or more is preferred) should be assayed for statistical validity.[2] In this case, the reference interval is calculated using the mean ±2 standard deviations (SD). This interval approximates the 95% confidence interval. In other words, about 95% of healthy animals have test values within this reference interval, with about 2.5% of healthy animals having values above and about 2.5% of healthy animals values below the reference interval. A common mistake made by novices is to calculate the reference interval from the mean ±1 SD. When this is done, about 32% of healthy animals will have values outside the calculated interval. If less than 40 healthy animals are available, the upper and lower values measured should be used to create an estimated reference interval.[5]

Some analytes do not exhibit a Gaussian distribution. Most commonly there is a skew toward the higher values. The use of mean ±2 SD to calculate reference intervals results in inappropriate reference intervals for skewed populations, as shown in Figure 1-2. Data may be manipulated (e.g., log or

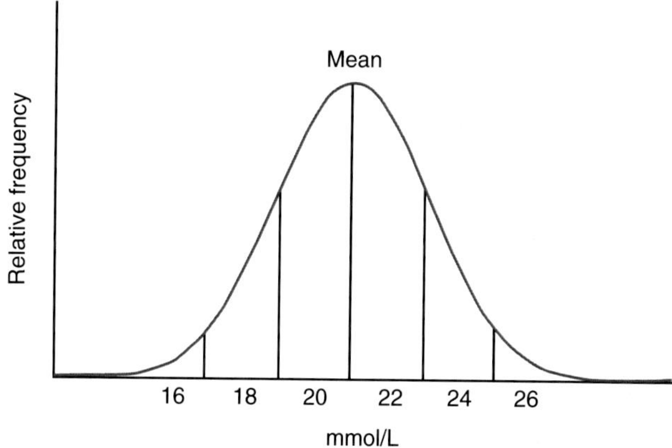

FIGURE 1-1

Frequency diagram of a hypothetical plasma analyte with Gaussian distribution. The central (tallest) vertical line denotes the mean. Each additional vertical line represents one standard deviation (SD) from the adjacent vertical line. The reference interval calculated using mean ±2 SD (21 ± 4 mmol/L) is 17 to 25 mmol/L.

square root transformation) so that the frequency distribution of the transformed data approximates a Gaussian distribution. The boundaries are determined as before and results are retransformed to determine the reference interval. Alternatively, one can use percentiles to determine upper and lower limits, especially if large numbers of healthy animals are evaluated. Values are listed in ascending order. The lower limit is determined by the formula $(n + 1) \times 0.025$, and the upper limit is determined by the formula $(n + 1) \times 0.975$, where n = the number of normal animals assayed.[2] If 119 animals were used, the value for the 3rd lowest animal would be used as the lower limit and the value from the 117th animal (3rd from the top) would be used as the upper limit.

Interpretation of Test Results Relative to Reference Intervals

The common usage of the 95% confidence interval to establish reference intervals means that 5% of healthy animals will be reported as abnormal for a given test. When multiple tests are done in laboratory medicine profiles, the probability of at least one test being abnormal increases with the number of tests done. For example, there is a 64% chance that at least one abnormal test result will be obtained when 20 analytes are measured from a healthy animal.[6] The degree to which a test result is above or below the reference interval is generally important in deciding whether a high or low value should be taken seriously.

Use of Published Reference Intervals

Routine hematology test results are usually similar between laboratories; consequently published reference intervals for values such as total leukocyte counts and hematocrits are often used to interpret results from a species (e.g., wallaby) when reference values have not been established in the laboratory conducting the test. Hematology indices such as the red cell distribution width (RDW) vary more between laboratories, making the use of published reference intervals less acceptable.

The units used in reporting values can vary by laboratory and a conversion factor may be needed to compare a measured value to a published reference interval. For example, blood iron might be reported as 100 μg/dL or 18 μmol/L. Most U.S. laboratories continue to use conventional units, such as mg/dL; Canadian and European laboratories use the International System of Units (SI units), such as mmol/L. Where possible, moles are used rather than weight (e.g., mg) for SI units. This cannot be done for analytes, such as serum protein concentration, where the molecular weight is variable and/or unknown. For enzymes, an SI enzyme unit is defined as 1 μmol/min of substrate utilized or product formed. SI units are reported per liter.

For many wild animal species, reference intervals may not be published for some or all tests. The simultaneous measurement of a healthy "control" animal from the same species, preferably a cohort, can be used as a rough guideline reference value and therefore can aid interpretation of the patient's results.

SENSITIVITY AND SPECIFICITY OF TESTS

Ideally analyte values obtained from a healthy animal population would not overlap with values obtained form a diseased animal population. Unfortunately there is almost always some overlap in the distribution of individual analyte test results between the two groups (Fig. 1-3). When the disease being considered has a major impact on an analyte, little overlap in

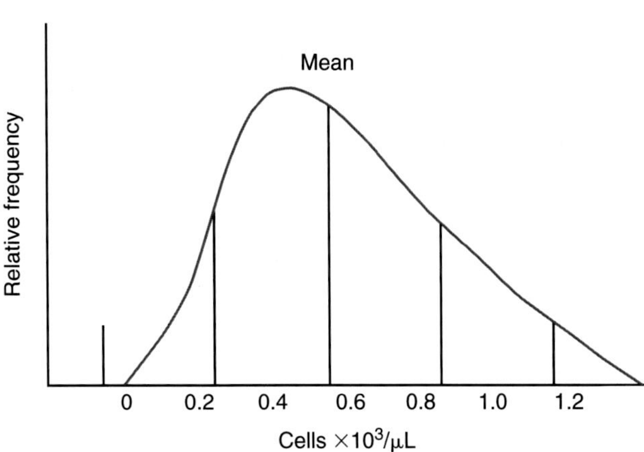

FIGURE 1-2

Frequency diagram of hypothetical absolute blood cell counts with a skewed population. The central (tallest) vertical line denotes the mean. Each additional vertical line represents one standard deviation (SD) from the adjacent vertical line. The use of mean ±2 SD to calculate the reference interval is inappropriate, as demonstrated by the lower limit being an impossible negative value.

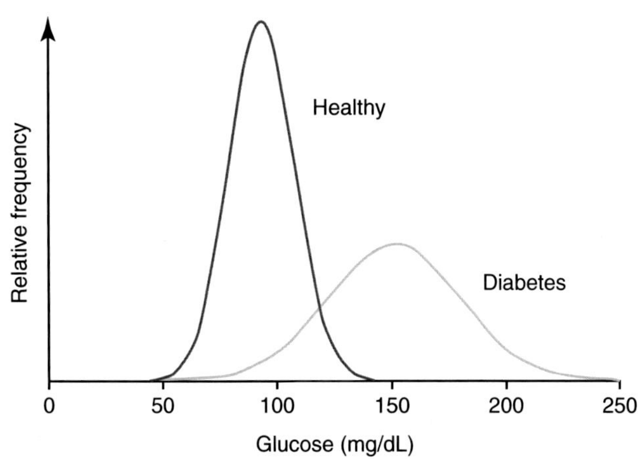

FIGURE 1-3

Overlapping Gaussian distributions of a healthy dog population compared with a population of dogs with type 2 diabetes mellitus.

The figure is redrawn from Farver TB. Concepts of normality in clinical biochemistry. In: Kaneko JJ, Harvey JW, Bruss ML, eds. Clinical Biochemistry of Domestic Animals. *6th ed. San Diego: Academic Press; 2008:1-25.*

values will occur; however, extensive overlap occurs if the analyte concentration is minimally altered by the disease being considered. True positives (TPs) are positive test results from animals *with* the disease for which they are being tested, false positives (FPs) are positive test results for animals *without* the disease for which they are being tested (Fig. 1-4), true negatives (TNs) are negative test results from animals *without* the disease for which they are being tested, and false negatives (FNs) are negative test results from animals *with* the disease for which they are being tested. As can be seen in Figure 1-4, if one increases the reference interval of the healthy population in order to minimize the FPs, the number of FNs increases.

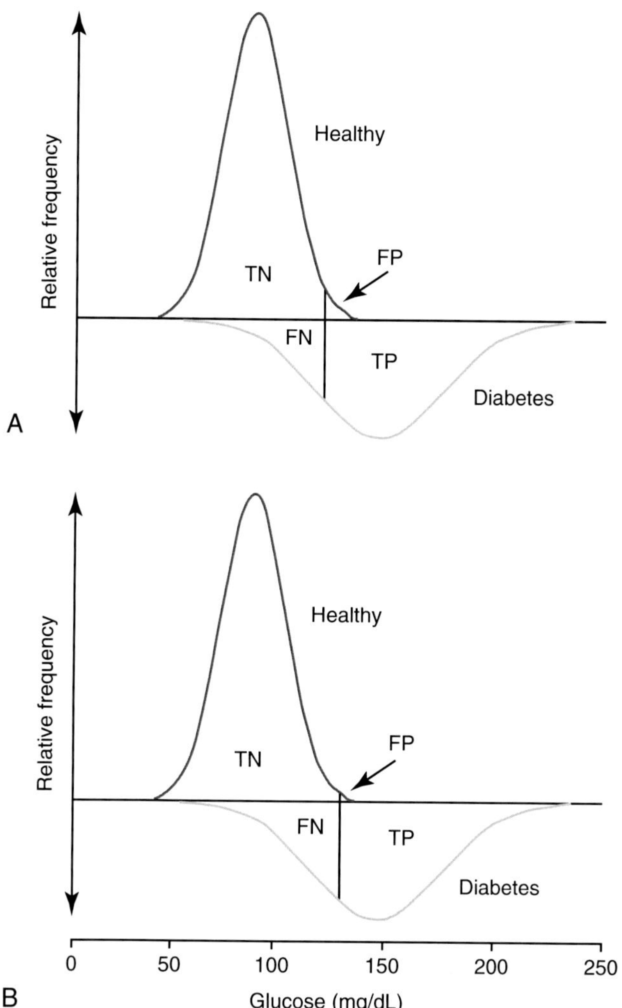

FIGURE 1-4
Frequency diagrams of a healthy dog population compared with a population of dogs with type 2 diabetes mellitus. Graphs are redrawn from Figure 1-3 to demonstrate true-negative (TN), false-negative (FN), true-positive (TP), and false-positive (FP) values used to calculate sensitivity, specificity, and predictive values. The top graph **(A)** demonstrates the effect of using the mean +2 standard deviations (SD) to set the upper limit of the reference interval. The lower graph **(B)** demonstrates the effect of using the mean +3 SD to set the upper limit. The number of FP tests are reduced but the number of FN tests are increased by using the higher reference limit.

The figure is redrawn from Farver TB. Concepts of normality in clinical biochemistry. In: Kaneko JJ, Harvey JW, Bruss ML, eds. Clinical Biochemistry of Domestic Animals. *6th ed. San Diego: Academic Press; 2008:1-25.*

A clinical test should be safe and practical, and should accurately indicate the presence or absence of a specific disease or pathology. Sensitivity, specificity, and predictive value constitute measures of a test's utility for ruling in or ruling out a given disease.

Sensitivity is the likelihood of a positive or abnormal test result occurring in animals with the disease being considered (Box 1-1). For example, if 23 of 28 cats with feline infectious peritonitis (FIP) are recognized to have a low absolute lymphocyte count in blood, the sensitivity of lymphopenia as a diagnostic test for cats with FIP is calculated to be 82% (Tables 1-1 and 1-2).[7]

Specificity is the likelihood of obtaining a negative or normal test result in nondiseased animals—that is, animals without the particular disease under consideration. In other words, specificity represents the proportion of animals without the disease in question that have normal tests. Specificity may be calculated in two distinctly different ways, either by assuming that all of the nondiseased animals are healthy or by assuming that although nondiseased animals do not have the particular disease for which the analysis is being performed, they may have other diseases.

Determining the specificity of a test in a group of healthy animals is of little value because reference intervals are generally established to include 95% of the total population of healthy animals, with 2.5% of healthy animals having values above and 2.5% of healthy animals having values below the reference interval. The specificity of a test is much more useful when the population of animals typically evaluated in a veterinary hospital setting is being used.[1] In this approach, the "nondiseased" group includes not only healthy animals presented for elective procedures but also animals with diseases other than the disease being considered.

PREDICTIVE VALUES AND DISEASE PREVALENCE

Predictive values demonstrate how well a test performs in a given population. In contrast to sensitivity determinations (which are made using only a population of animals with the disease in question) and specificity determinations (which are made using only a population of animals without the disease under consideration), predictive value determinations are made from populations that contain animal both with and without the disease in question.

The predictive value of a positive test (PVPT) considers only animals in the population being studied that have a positive test result and determines what percentage of animals actually have the disease being considered (see Box 1-1). It answers the question "How likely is it that an animal with a positive test will actually have the disease being considered?"

TABLE 1-1

Test Results from the Evaluation of 224 Cats with a History and Clinical Signs Consistent with Feline Infectious Peritonitis (FIP) Resulting in the Inclusion of FIP in the List of Differential Diagnoses[a]

	NUMBER OF CATS AFFECTED		
Test	**Have FIP (*N* = 28)**	**Do Not Have FIP (*N* = 196)**	**Total Cats (*N* = 224)**
Lymphopenia (<1.5 x 10^3 cells/μL)	23	43	66
Monocytosis (>0.9 x 10^3 cells/μL)	2	43	45
Hyperglobulinemia (>5.1 g/dL)	11	7	18
Coronavirus titer positive	22	84	106

N, Number of cats.

[a]Data from Sparkes AH, Gruffydd-Jones TJ, Harbour DA. An appraisal of the value of laboratory tests in the diagnosis of feline infectious peritonitis. *J Am Anim Hosp Assoc.* 1994;30:345-350.

BOX 1-1

Formulas for the Calculation of Sensitivity, Specificity, Predictive Value of a Positive Test, Predictive Value of a Negative Test, and Prevalence

$$\text{Sensitivity (\%)} = \frac{TP \times 100}{TP + FN}$$

$$\text{Specificity (\%)} = \frac{TN \times 100}{TN + FP}$$

$$\text{Predictive value of a positive test (\%)} = \frac{TP \times 100}{TP + FP}$$

$$\text{Predictive value of a negative test (\%)} = \frac{TN \times 100}{TN + FN}$$

$$\text{Prevalence (\%)} = \frac{(TP + FN) \times 100}{TP + TN + FP + FN}$$

TP, true positive (the number of animals with the disease being tested for that have a positive test result); FP, false positive (the number of animals without the disease being tested for that have a positive test result); TN, true negative (the number of animals without the disease being tested for that have a negative test result); and FN, false negative (the number of animals with the disease being tested for that have a negative test result).

TABLE 1-2

Examination of Lymphopenia as a Diagnostic Test for Feline Infectious Peritonitis (FIP)[a,b]

	NUMBER OF CATS AFFECTED		
Test	**Have FIP (*N* = 28)**	**Do Not Have FIP (*N* = 196)**	**Total Cats (*N* = 224)**
Lymphopenia	23 True positive	43 False positive	66 Total positive
No lymphopenia	5 False negative	153 True negative	158 Total negative

N, Number of cats.

[a]Cats with a history and clinical signs consistent with FIP were evaluated, resulting in FIP being included in the list of differential diagnoses. Lymphopenia was defined as <1.5 x 10^3 lymphocytes per microliter of blood.

[b]Data from Sparkes AH, Gruffydd-Jones TJ, Harbour DA. An appraisal of the value of laboratory tests in the diagnosis of feline infectious peritonitis. *J Am Anim Hosp Assoc.* 1994;30:345-350.

Based on the selected population of cats presented in Tables 1-1 and 1-2, there is a 23/66 or 35% chance that a cat with lymphopenia in this population will have FIP.[7]

The predictive value of a negative test (PVNT) considers only animals in the population being studied that have a negative or normal test result and determines what percentage of animals with negative test results do not have the disease being considered (see Box 1-1). It answers the question "How likely is that an animal with a negative or normal test result will be free of the disease being considered?" Based on the selected population of cats presented in Table 1-2, there is a 153/158 or 97% chance that a cat with a normal or increased blood lymphocyte count will not have FIP.

The prevalence of a disease in a population is simply the percentage of animals in a given population that have a certain disease (see Box 1-1). The prevalence of FIP in the selected population presented in Table 1-1 is 28/224 or 12.5%. The prevalence of a disease affects the predictive values of a test used to diagnose the disease but not its sensitivity or specificity. For most tests, the PVPT will be low and the PVNT will be high if the disease has a low prevalence in the population being studied. The PVPT will be low because low prevalence magnifies the number of false-positive results—that is, most positive test results are false positives because few animals actually have the disease (see Box 1-1). The exception would be a test where false-positive results occur infrequently (e.g., polymerase chain reaction tests for specific infectious agents or inherited blood cell defects). The PVNT will be high because few false-negative results are present in a population when the disease prevalence is low.

To improve diagnostic accuracy, the prevalence (likelihood) of the disease being considered can be increased by using the history, physical examination, and adjunctive diagnostic tests to restrict the population, as described for cats in Table 1-1. The prevalence of FIP in the general cat population is much lower than 12.5%. By ruling out one or more diseases that can give the same positive test result as the disease being considered, a clinician decreases the size of the population being studied, thereby increasing the prevalence of the disease in the population and increasing the positive predictive value of the test for the disease being considered.

Laboratory tests are used to help rule in or rule out a specific disease. When significant hazards are associated with treatment (e.g., amputation or high-risk chemotherapy) or euthanasia is being considered, it is necessary to be as certain as possible that the disease is actually present. Consequently tests with high positive predictive values are needed for a rule-in strategy. When the penalty for missing a diagnosis is high, as with a disease for which therapy is effective if begun quickly, tests with high negative predictive values are theoretically important as a rule-out strategy. A normal test result by virtue of its high negative predictive valuc would suggest that the disease is not present. Unfortunately many diseases have low prevalence, which by itself can result in a high negative predictive value. The best evidence for ruling out a disease is finding a negative test result for an assay that has a high sensitivity for recognizing the disease. Based on the selected population of cats presented in Tables 1-1 and 1-2, finding a normal or increased blood lymphocyte count is more reliable for ruling out FIP than is finding a low lymphocyte count for making a diagnosis of FIP.

Information is generally available concerning the sensitivity of routine tests for common diseases, but information is often lacking concerning all diseases that may have a positive test result and the frequency of these diseases in the population being evaluated. Consequently, the specificity of a test can vary when populations containing animals with other diseases are analyzed. PVPTs and PVNTs also vary considerably depending on the population analyzed. Although accurate values are not usually available for PVPTs and PVNTs, clinicians use their knowledge and experience, combined with the principles outlined above, to make informed judgments concerning the likelihood that a disease can be ruled in or ruled out of the differential diagnosis. These decisions are seldom based on a single test result; instead, information in the history is considered along with the clinical signs and results of the physical examination, diagnostic imaging, and other laboratory tests. The likelihood that a disease will be present increases if several findings are supportive of the diagnosis. For example, in the FIP study discussed above, the PVPT was 35% for cats with lymphopenia, 77% for cats with lymphopenia and hyperglobulinemia, and 89% for cats with lymphopenia, hyperglobulinemia, and a positive coronavirus titer. The PVNT increased from 97% when lymphopenia alone was absent to 99% when all three findings were absent. Minimal change occurs in the PVNT because the relatively low disease prevalence in the population is a major contributing factor to the high negative PVNT. This contribution is most clearly demonstrated by looking at blood monocyte data in the FIP study presented in Table 1-1. Only 7% of FIP cats have a monocytosis (sensitivity), and the PVPT for monocytosis is only 4%, yet the PVNT for a cat lacking a monocytosis is 88%.

CUTOFF VALUES

The PVPT may be increased by using a cutoff value above or below the standard reference interval, depending on whether the disease under consideration results in an increase or a decrease in the analyte being measured. For example, low mean cell volume (MCV) is a diagnostic test suggestive of chronic iron deficiency in dogs. If we use 64 fL as the lower limit of the reference interval to calculate its positive predictive value, the value would not be remarkably high because there are various other relatively common disorders that can result in low MCVs in dogs, most notably inflammatory conditions and portosystemic shunts. However, it is recognized that the other causes of microcytosis rarely result in MCV values below 52 fL. Consequently, if a dog has a MCV below 52 fL, chronic iron deficiency anemia is highly likely and the PVPT using this cutoff value would approach 100%. However, 52 fL is not routinely used as a cutoff value for a positive test because many cases of chronic iron deficiency would be missed. Nonetheless, it is important to realize that dogs with especially low MCV values almost certainly have chronic iron deficiency anemia.

The effects of varying the cutoff value of a test on sensitivity, specificity, and predictive values are demonstrated in Table 1-3, where plasma fibrinogen concentration was evaluated as a diagnostic test for *Rhodococcus equi* pneumonia in 165 foals from a single farm.[3] It is important to recognize that fibrinogen is an acute-phase protein that often increases in association with various causes of inflammation in horses and that the heat precipitation assay used to measure fibrinogen (while easily performed and clinically useful) is relatively imprecise. As the cutoff value for plasma fibrinogen concentration is increased, the specificity and PVPT increase, but the sensitivity and PVNT decrease (see Table 1-3). Results from this study also demonstrate that the PVPT increases and the PVNT decreases as the prevalence of disease in a population increases. In choosing the most appropriate cutoff value for a test, one must consider a number of factors including sensitivity and specificity of the test, prevalence of disease in the population being tested, and consequences of false-positive and false-negative tests. In the example above, failure to identify an infected foal (false-negative test) might result in the debilitation or death of the foal. Conversely, the treatment of healthy foals based on false-positive test findings could result in unnecessary financial losses and potential injury to healthy foals as a result of the adverse side effects of antimicrobial therapy.

ACCURACY VERSUS PRECISION

The accuracy of an analytical procedure is determined by how closely the result approaches the true value of the analyte being measured. An accurate test is one where the average of several assay results is close to the true value (Fig.

TABLE 1-3

Sensitivity, Specificity, and Predictive Values of Plasma Fibrinogen Concentrations at Selected Cutoff Values for the Early Identification of Foals with *Rhodococcus equi* Pneumonia, Assuming Two Different Prevalences of Disease[a]

			PREDICTIVE VALUES			
			PREVALENCE 10%		PREVALENCE 40%	
Cutoff value (mg/dL)	Sensitivity (%)	Specificity (%)	PVPT (%)	PVNT (%)	PVPT (%)	PVNT (%)
300	100	6	11	100	42	100
400	91	51	17	98	55	89
500	71	68	20	96	60	78
600	38	96	51	93	86	70
700	29	97	51	92	86	67
800	12	100	100	91	100	63

PVPT, Predictive value of a positive test; PVNT, predictive value of a negative test.

[a]Data from Giguère S, Hernandez J, Gaskin J, Miller C, Bowan JL. Evaluation of white blood cell concentration, plasma fibrinogen concentration, and an agar gel immunodiffusion test for the early identification of foals with *Rhodococcus equi* pneumonia. *J Am Vet Med Assoc.* 2003;222:775-781.

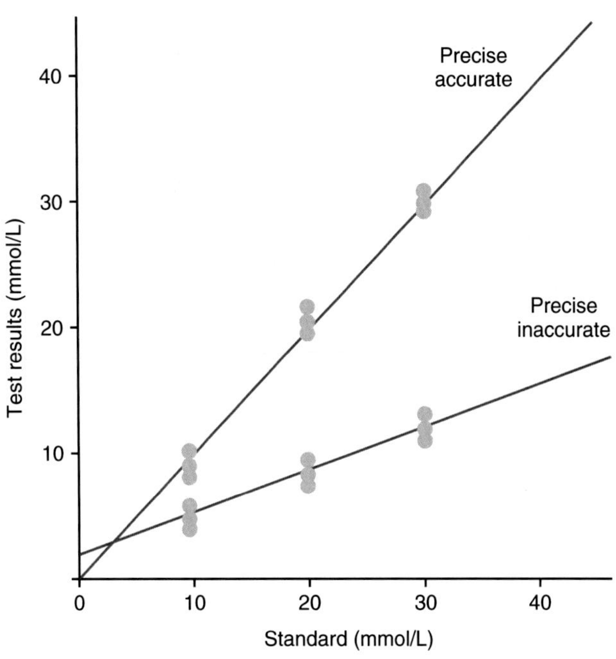

FIGURE 1-5

Plots comparing test results of triplicate assays of three standards (y-axis) to the known values of the standards (x-axis). The top plot is accurate with good precision. The bottom plot has good precision but is inaccurate.

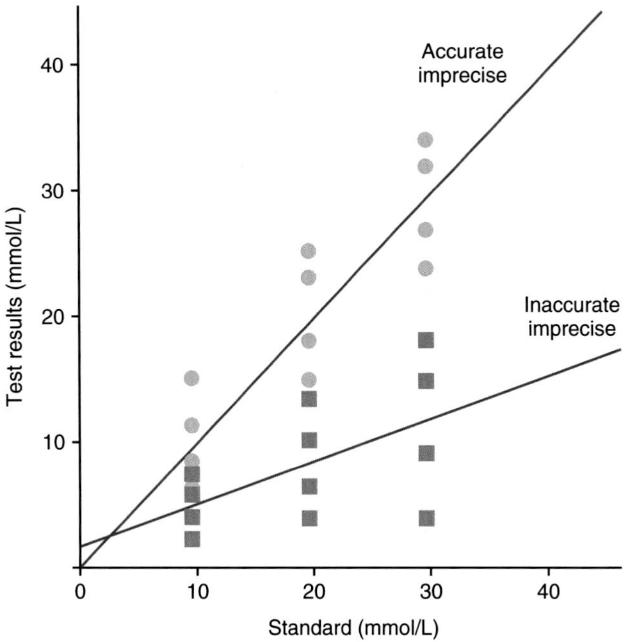

FIGURE 1-6

Plots comparing test results of four replicate assays of three standards (y-axis) to the known values of the standards (x-axis). The top plot is accurate but imprecise. The bottom plot is inaccurate and imprecise.

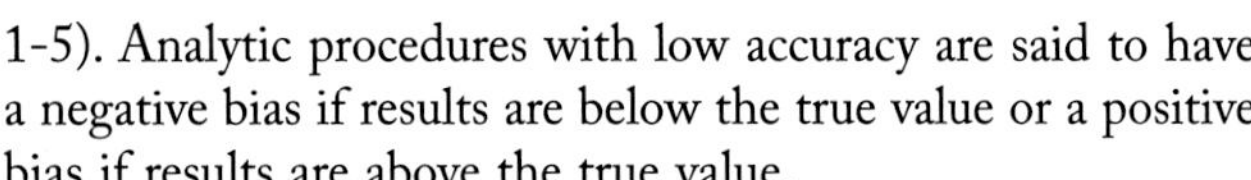

1-5). Analytic procedures with low accuracy are said to have a negative bias if results are below the true value or a positive bias if results are above the true value.

The precision of a test reflects how reproducible the test results are when the assay is replicated. Precision is independent of accuracy (Fig. 1-6); consequently test results can be highly reproducible but erroneous (see Fig. 1-5, lower plot). Precision or, more accurately, the amount of imprecision present in an assay, is determined by calculating the coefficient of variation (CV) for repeated measurements made on a single sample. The CV is the standard deviation (SD) of the repeated measurements expressed as a percent of the mean of the repeated measurements (SD/mean × 100). The CV indicates the amount of random error (imprecision) that is present in an assay. A high CV value (e.g., more than 10%) indicates that an assay lacks precision. A low CV value (e.g., less than 5%) indicates that assay results are reproducible, varying little with repeated measurement. The degree of imprecision of an assay can also be measured over time intervals to assess within-run, between-run, or between-day variation.

Automated versus Manual Methods

As can be seen in Figures 1-7 and 1-8, manual leukocyte and platelet counts are less precise (CV 15% and 13%, respectively) than automated leukocyte and platelet counts (CV 2% and 4%, respectively). These values do not indicate whether manual or automated methods are more accurate. In fact, the mean manual platelet count is probably more accurate (more near the true platelet count) than the mean automated platelet count because platelets in small platelet clumps can be visualized and counted separately in a hemacytometer chamber but would be counted as one platelet or not counted at all in an automated cell counter.

For manual differential leukocyte counts, the CV varies with the percentage of a given leukocyte type present in the blood film and the total number of leukocytes included in the differential leukocyte count. For example, 100 cell differential counts were performed by a single technologist on each of 80 stained coverslip blood films from a dog with a mild basophilia. CVs were calculated from results of 20 randomly selected blood films (100 cells per differential). CVs were also calculated from results from 20 pairs of randomly selected slides (200 cells per differential). Last, CVs were calculated from results from 20 quads of randomly selected slides (400 cells per differential). As expected, the CVs for leukocyte types that were numerous (e.g., neutrophils) were much lower than CVs for leukocyte types that were present in low numbers (e.g., basophils), and CVs decreased as the total number of cells counted in the differential increased (Figs. 1-9 and 1-10). The CVs for each of the five leukocyte types from this dog were plotted versus the mean percentage of each leukocyte type for 100-, 200-, and 400-cell manual differential counts and compared with a like plot with data determined by performing 20 automated differential counts on blood from a single dog using an Advia 120 (Siemens Healthcare Diagnostics, Inc., Tarrytown, NY) hematology analyzer (Fig. 1-11). Automated hematology analyzers have lower CVs for each percentage of leukocyte type present because they examine thousands of leukocytes (assuming a normal leukocyte count) in performing the differential leukocyte count.

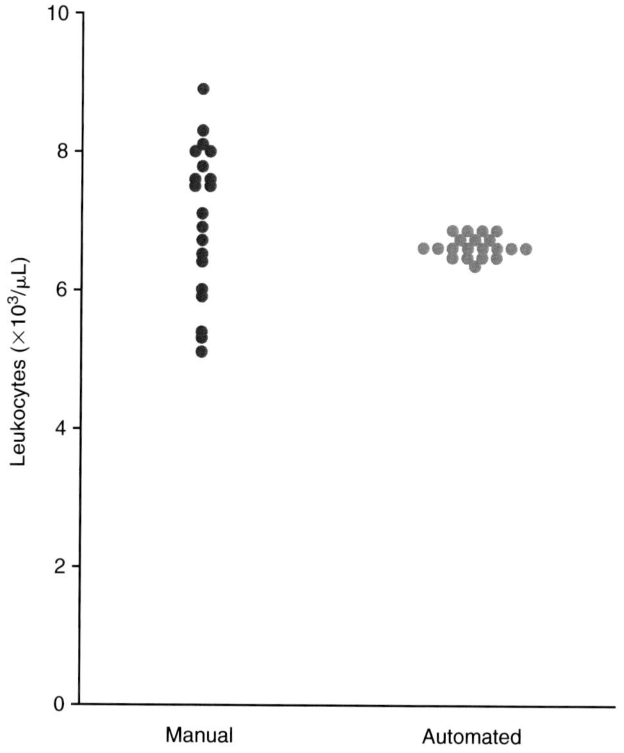

FIGURE 1-7
Individual plots of total leukocyte counts performed 20 times each using a manual method and an automated method on the same canine blood sample. The manual method utilized 20 separate dilutions (Unopette 365855, Becton Dickinson Co., Franklin Lakes, NJ), followed by the counting of all leukocytes in 1 µL of 1/100 diluted blood in a hemacytometer chamber. A Cell-Dyn 3500 (Abbott Laboratories, North Chicago, IL) calibrated for canine blood was used to perform the automated cell counts. The mean and coefficient of variation (CV) for the manual counts were $7.1 \times 10^3/\mu L$ and 15% respectively. The mean and CV for the automated counts were $6.7 \times 10^3/\mu L$ and 2% respectively.

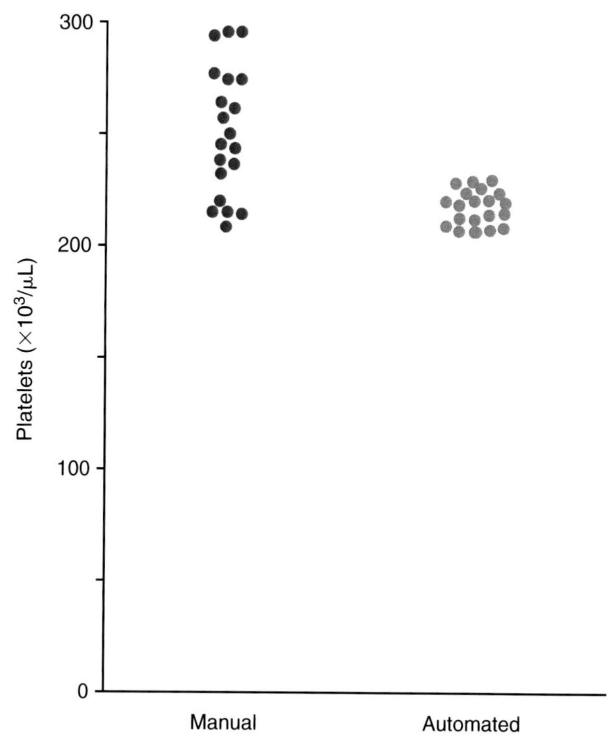

FIGURE 1-8
Individual plots of platelet counts performed 20 times each using a manual method and an automated method on the same canine blood sample. The manual method utilized 20 separate dilutions (Unopette 365855, Becton Dickinson Co., Franklin Lakes, NJ), followed by the counting of all platelets in 1/25 µL of 1/100 diluted blood in a hemacytometer chamber. A Cell-Dyn 3500 (Abbott Laboratories, North Chicago, IL) calibrated for canine blood was used to perform the automated cell counts. The mean and coefficient of variation (CV) for the manual counts were $240 \times 10^3/\mu L$ and 13% respectively. The mean and CV for the automated counts were $219 \times 10^3/\mu L$ and 4% respectively.

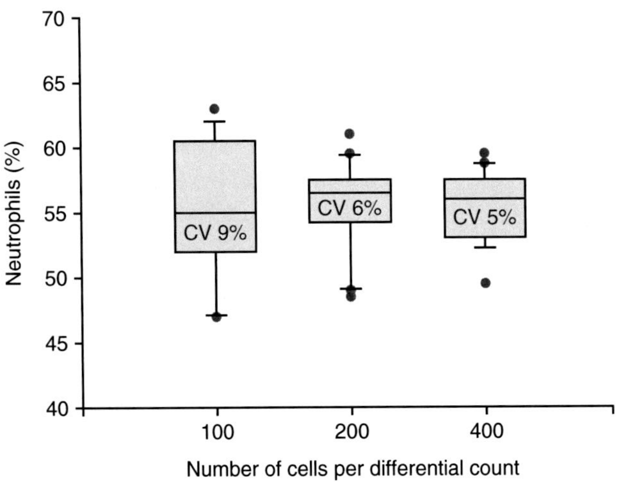

FIGURE 1-9
Box plots of neutrophil percentages and coefficients of variation (CVs) from manual differential counts from a single dog with 55.4% neutrophils. Values represent the results of 20 differential leukocyte counts each of 100, 200, and 400 nucleated cells. A median line is shown. Boxes include 25th to 75th percentiles and error bars include 10th to 90th percentiles.

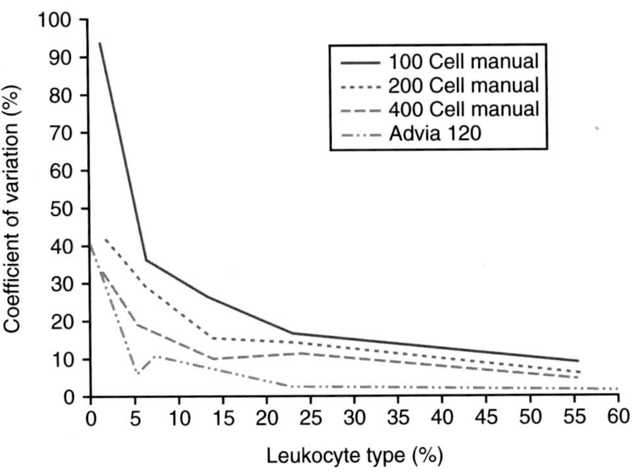

FIGURE 1-11
Mean coefficient of variation (CV) values for each of the five leukocyte types from a single dog are plotted versus the mean differential counts of each leukocyte type. Mean values were determined from 20 differential leukocyte counts each of 100, 200, and 400 nucleated cells. A like plot with data determined by performing 20 automated differential counts on blood from a single dog using an Advia 120 hematology analyzer is included for comparison.

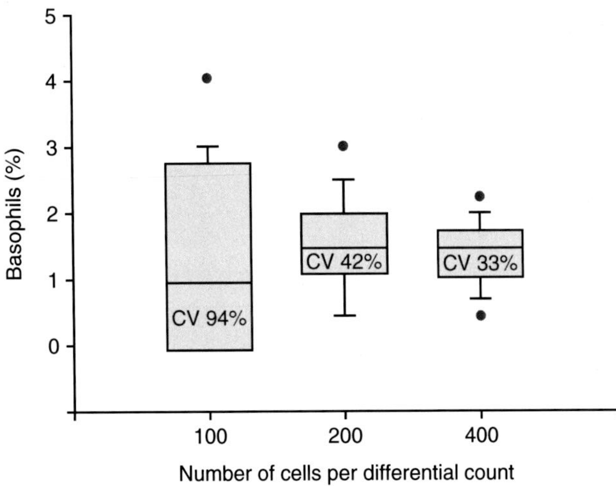

FIGURE 1-10
Box plots of neutrophil percentages and coefficients of variation (CVs) from manual differential counts from a single dog with 1.4% basophils. Values represent the results of 20 differential leukocyte counts each of 100, 200, and 400 nucleated cells. A median line is shown. Boxes include 25th to 75th percentiles and error bars include 10th to 90th percentiles.

However, they are not always more accurate. The inability to correctly identify certain cell types (especially basophils), abnormal cell morphology, or abnormal cell types can lead to the misclassifications of cell types. For example, the Advia 120 failed to identify any basophils in blood from a cat with 39% basophils or a dog with 14% basophils identified on manual differential leukocyte counts.

Critical Difference

The CV of an assay affects how the results are interpreted, especially if an assay is being repeated to determine whether a treatment is effective. For example, if the total leukocyte count for a dog is 4600/μL before treatment and 5800/μL after treatment, does this represent a real improvement or might it reflect imprecision in the measurement of the total leukocyte count? An additional confounding variable in this example is the biological variability of the animal itself. Jensen et al.[4] calculated the analytical CV for an automated total leukocyte count in healthy laboratory beagles to be 3.7%, while the CV for repeated total leukocyte counts from individual beagles (within dog CV) was 12.1%.[4] From these numbers, a critical difference of 35% was calculated. This means that the total leukocyte count would have to increase by more than 35% before the therapy could be assumed to have an influence on this analyte. In the example above, the automated total leukocyte count would have to exceed 4600/μL × 1.35, or 6200/μL, before a therapeutic effect might be assumed. A considerably greater difference would be required if total leukocyte counts were done using a manual method because of its higher analytical CV. A greater critical difference might also have been calculated in the above example had client-owned animals been used for this study rather than laboratory animals, because it is likely that the biological variation would be higher in client-owned animals that were not accustomed to the phlebotomy procedure, the individuals handling them, or the environment in which the phlebotomy was done.

Unfortunately, critical difference measurements have been done for few analytes in veterinary medicine, and values will vary depending on methods and instruments used and animal populations evaluated. Nonetheless, clinicians develop knowledge and intuition through study and experience that can help them to make informed judgments concerning the importance of changes in laboratory data.

REFERENCES

1. Braun JP, Concordet D, Lyazrhi M, et al. Overestimation of the predictive value of positives by the usual calculations of the specificity of diagnostic tests. *Vet Res Commun.* 2000;24:17-24.
2. Farver TB. Concepts of normality in clinical biochemistry. In: Kaneko JJ, Harvey JW, Bruss ML, eds. *Clinical Biochemistry of Domestic Animals.* 6th ed. San Diego: Academic Press; 2008:1-25.
3. Giguère S, Hernandez J, Gaskin J, et al. Evaluation of white blood cell concentration, plasma fibrinogen concentration, and an agar gel immunodiffusion test for the early identification of foal with *Rhodococcus equi* pneumonia. *J Am Vet Med Assoc.* 2003;222:775-781.
4. Jensen AL, Iversen L, Petersen TK. Study on biologic variability of haematological components in dogs. *Comp Haematol Int.* 1998;8:202-204.
5. Lumsden JH. Reference values. In: Feldman BF, Zinkl JG, Jain NC, eds. *Schalm's Veterinary Hematology.* 5th ed. Philadelphia: Lippincott Williams & Wilkins; 2000:12-15.
6. Marshall WJ. The interpretation of biochemical data. In: Marshall WJ, Bangert SK, eds. *Clinical Biochemistry. Metabolic and Clinical Aspects.* 2nd ed. New York: Churchill Livingstone Elsevier; 2008:17-27.
7. Sparkes AH, Gruffydd-Jones TJ, Harbour DA. An appraisal of the value of laboratory tests in the diagnosis of feline infectious peritonitis. *J Am Anim Hosp Assoc.* 1994;30:345-350.

CHAPTER

2

HEMATOLOGY PROCEDURES

COMPOSITION OF BLOOD

Blood is composed of cells (erythrocytes, leukocytes, and platelets) circulating within fluid called plasma (Fig. 2-1). Erythrocytes or red blood cells are most numerous, with several million erythrocytes per microliter of blood in mammals (Appendix Table 1). Depending on the species, erythrocytes typically account for one-fourth to one-half of the total blood volume as measured by determining the hematocrit. Platelets or thrombocytes are the next most numerous cell type in blood, with platelet counts as low as $100 \times 10^3/\mu L$ in healthy horses to several hundred thousand per microliter in other mammalian species. Total leukocyte or white blood cell counts are much lower than erythrocyte and platelet counts, with total leukocyte counts ranging from about $5 \times 10^3/\mu L$ to about $20 \times 10^3/\mu L$ in mammals. The proportion of leukocyte types present varies by species, with neutrophils being the most numerous leukocyte type present in the blood of carnivores and lymphocytes being the most numerous leukocyte type present in the blood of ruminants and rodents.

Plasma consists primarily of water that contains about 6 to 8 g/dL of plasma proteins and 1.5 to 2.0 g/dL of inorganic salts, lipids, carbohydrates, hormones, and vitamins.[19] Plasma is prepared in the laboratory by collecting blood with an anticoagulant, followed by centrifugation to remove the blood cells. If blood is collected without anticoagulant and allowed to clot, the fluid that is obtained following centrifugation is called serum. The protein concentration in serum is usually about 0.2 to 0.5 g/dL lower than that in plasma, primarily owing to the absence of fibrinogen—which is consumed during coagulation—in serum. Serum proteins may be separated by electrophoresis into albumin, α-globulins, β-globulins, and γ-globulins (Fig. 2-2). Albumin is a single protein that generally accounts for nearly half of the total plasma proteins present by weight. Each of the globulin classes is composed of many different proteins.[12]

CALCULATION OF BLOOD VOLUME

Total blood volume accounts for about 10% to 11% of body weight in hot-blooded horses; 8% to 9% in dogs; 6% to 7% in cats, ruminants, laboratory rodents, and cold-blooded (draft) horses; and 5% to 6% in pigs. The total blood volume of young growing animals often exceeds 10% of body weight.[33] It may be desirable to calculate the total blood volume of an animal in determining the size of a needed blood transfusion, or the amount of blood that can safely be removed for a series of diagnostic tests, or when an animal is to be used as a blood donor. For example, the total blood volume of a 4-kg cat is 0.07×4 kg = 0.28 kg = 280 mL, assuming that 7% of body weight is blood in cats and the specific gravity of blood is 1.0 (1 mL weighs 1 g). Since one can safely remove 20% of the blood volume from an animal, the calculated amount that can be removed from the cat in this example is $280 \times 0.2 = 56$ mL.

SAMPLE COLLECTION AND HANDLING

In monogastric animals, an overnight fast avoids postprandial lipemia, which can interfere with plasma protein, fibrinogen, and hemoglobin determinations. Ethylenediaminetetraacetic acid (EDTA) is the preferred anticoagulant for complete blood count (CBC) determination in most species, but blood from some birds and reptiles hemolyzes when collected into EDTA. In those species, heparin is often used as the anticoagulant. The disadvantage of heparin is that leukocytes do not stain as well (presumably because heparin binds to leukocytes),[24] and platelets generally clump more than they do in blood collected with EDTA. However, as discussed later, platelet aggregates and leukocyte aggregates may occur even in properly collected EDTA-anticoagulated blood

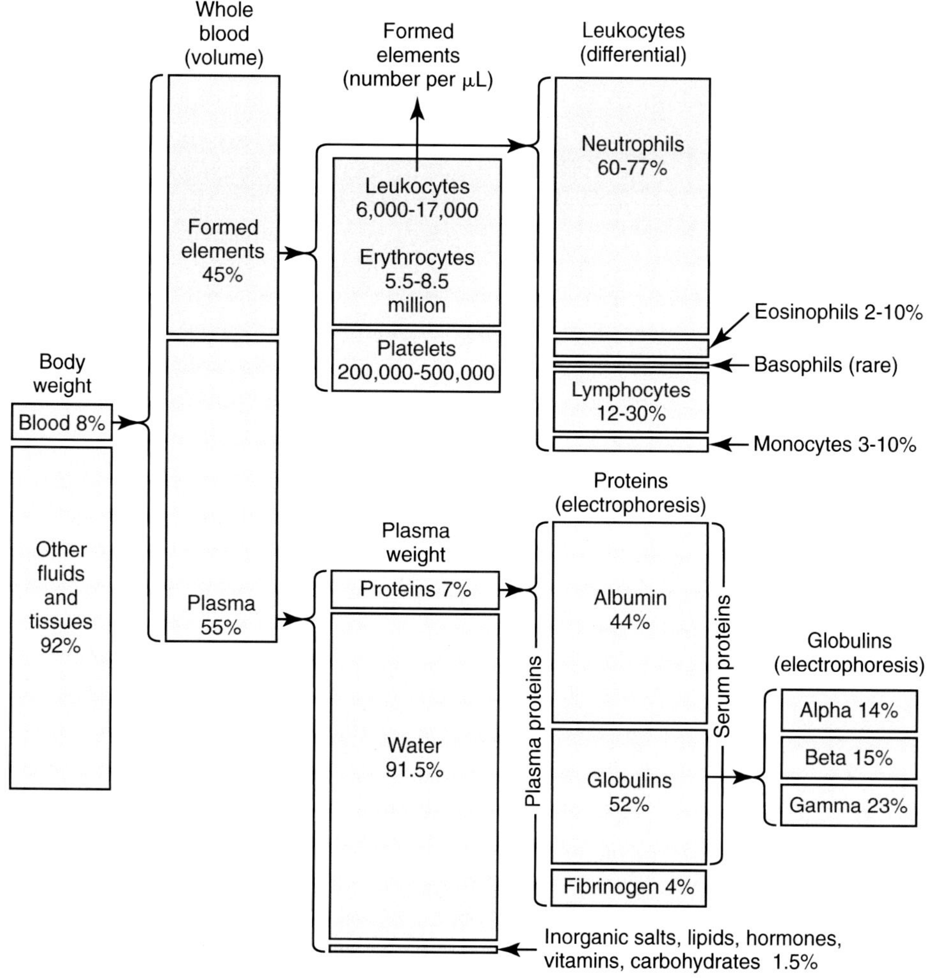

FIGURE 2-1
Approximate composition of normal dog blood.

samples.[10,29,41,49,53] In those cases, collection of blood using another anticoagulant (e.g., citrate) may prevent the formation of cell aggregates. Cell aggregation tends to be more pronounced as blood is cooled and stored; consequently processing samples as rapidly as possible after collection may minimize the formation of leukocyte and/or platelet aggregates.

Collection of blood directly into a vacuum tube is preferred to collection of blood by syringe and transfer to a vacuum tube. This method reduces platelet clumping and clot formation in samples for CBC determinations, as even small clots render a sample unusable. Platelet counts are markedly reduced, and a significant reduction can sometimes occur in hematocrit (HCT) and leukocyte counts as well. Also, when the tube is allowed to fill based on the vacuum within the tube, the proper sample-to-anticoagulant ratio will be present. Inadequate sample size results in decreased HCT due to excessive EDTA solution. Care should be taken to avoid iatrogenic hemolysis, which interferes with plasma protein, fibrinogen, and various erythrocyte measurements. Samples should be submitted to the laboratory as rapidly as possible, and blood films should be made as soon as possible and rapidly dried to minimize morphologic changes.

GROSS EXAMINATION OF BLOOD SAMPLES

Samples are checked for clots and mixed well (gently inverted 20 times) immediately before removing aliquots for hematology procedures. Horse erythrocytes settle especially rapidly because of rouleaux formation (adhesion of erythrocytes together like a stack of coins). Blood should be examined grossly for color and evidence of erythrocyte agglutination. The presence of marked lipemia may result in a blood sample with a milky red color resembling "tomato soup" when oxygenated.

Methemoglobinemia

Hemoglobin is a protein consisting of four polypeptide globin chains, each of which contains a heme prosthetic group within a hydrophobic pocket. Heme is composed of a tetrapyrrole

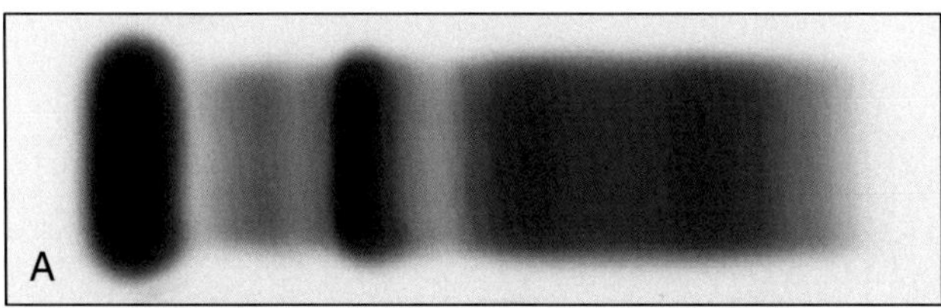

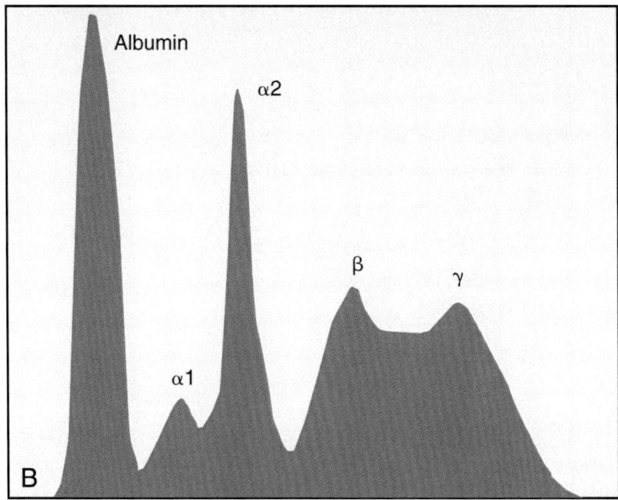

FIGURE 2-2

Serum protein electrophoresis from a dog with a polyclonal hyperglobulinemia, including increased α_2-globulin and β-γ bridging. **A,** Agarose gel stained with Coomassie blue for protein. Albumin *(band on the far left)* migrates more rapidly than other proteins. **B,** Densitometer tracing of the agarose gel used to determine the contribution of each protein type: total protein 7.7 g/dL, albumin 2.05 g/dL, α_1 0.42 g/dL, α_2 1.51 g/dL, β 1.86 g/dL, γ 1.86 g/dL.

with a central iron molecule that must be maintained in the ferrous (+2) state to reversibly bind oxygen. Methemoglobin differs from hemoglobin only in that the iron molecule of the heme group has been oxidized to the ferric (+3) state and is no longer able to bind oxygen.[28] The presence of large amounts of deoxyhemoglobin accounts for the dark bluish color of normal venous blood samples. Methemoglobinemia may not be recognized in venous blood samples because the brownish color of methemoglobin is not readily apparent when methemoglobin is mixed with deoxyhemoglobin (Fig. 2-3, *A*). When deoxyhemoglobin binds oxygen to form oxyhemoglobin, it becomes bright red; consequently the brownish coloration of methemoglobin becomes more apparent in the oxygenated samples (Fig. 2-3, *B*). A simple spot test provides a rapid way to oxygenate a venous blood sample and to determine whether clinically significant levels of methemoglobin are present. One drop of blood from the patient is placed on a piece of absorbent white paper and a drop of normal control blood is placed next to it. If the methemoglobin content is 10% or greater, the patient's blood will have a noticeably brown color compared with the bright red color of control blood (Fig. 2-4).[28] Accurate determination of methemoglobin content requires that blood be submitted to a laboratory that has this test available. Methemoglobinemia results from either increased production of methemoglobin by oxidants or decreased reduction of methemoglobin resulting from a hereditary deficiency in the erythrocyte cytochrome-b_5 reductase enzyme (see Chapter 4).[27]

Erythrocyte Agglutination

The appearance of red granules in a well-mixed blood sample (Fig. 2-5) suggests the presence of erythrocyte autoagglutination. However, it is important to differentiate agglutination

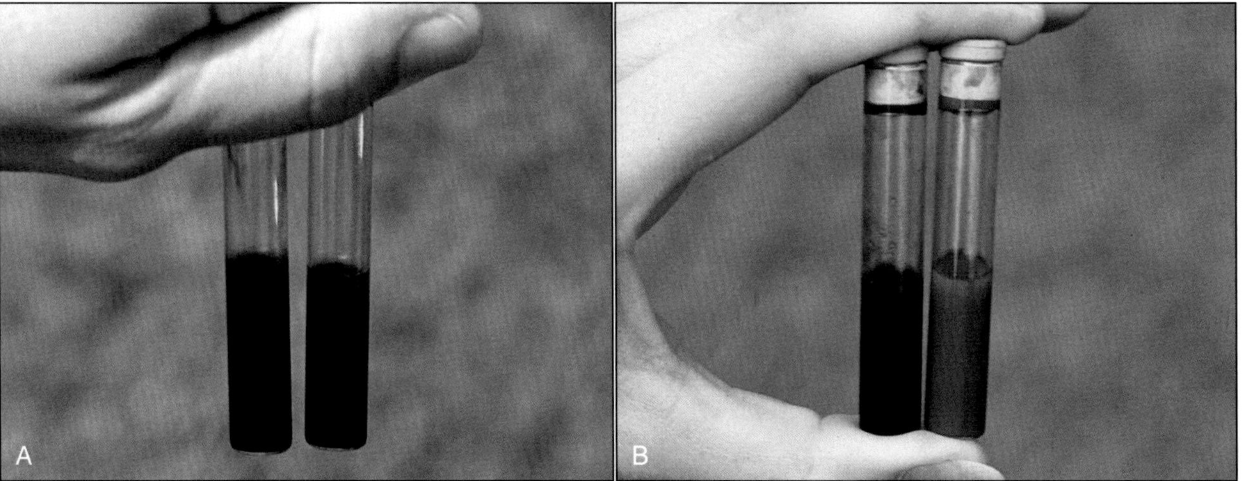

FIGURE 2-3

Gross appearance of mixtures of oxyhemoglobin, deoxyhemoglobin, and methemoglobin. **A,** Venous blood sample from a cat with 28% methemoglobin *(left sample)* compared with blood from a normal cat with less than 1% methemoglobin *(right sample)*. Both samples also contain a mixture of oxyhemoglobin and deoxyhemoglobin. **B,** Oxygenated blood sample from a cat with 28% methemoglobin *(left sample)* compared with blood from a normal cat with less than 1% methemoglobin *(right sample)*. The sample on the left contains a mixture of oxyhemoglobin and methemoglobin; the one on the right contains almost exclusively oxyhemoglobin.

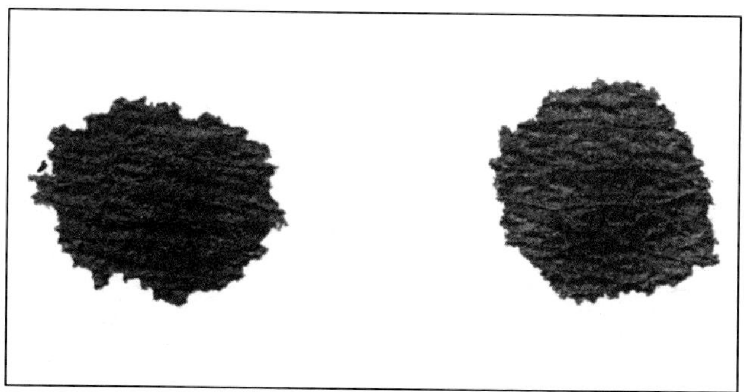

FIGURE 2-4
Methemoglobin spot test. A drop of blood from a methemoglobin reductase-deficient cat with 50% methemoglobin *(left)* is placed on absorbent white paper next to a drop of blood from a normal cat with less than 1% methemoglobin.

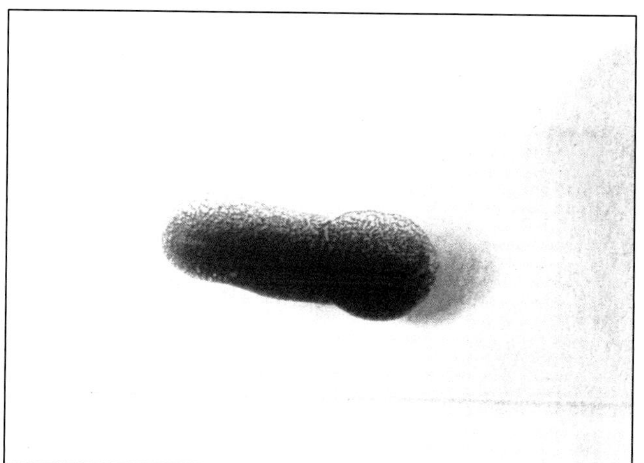

FIGURE 2-5
Grossly visible agglutination in blood from a dog with immune-mediated hemolytic anemia.

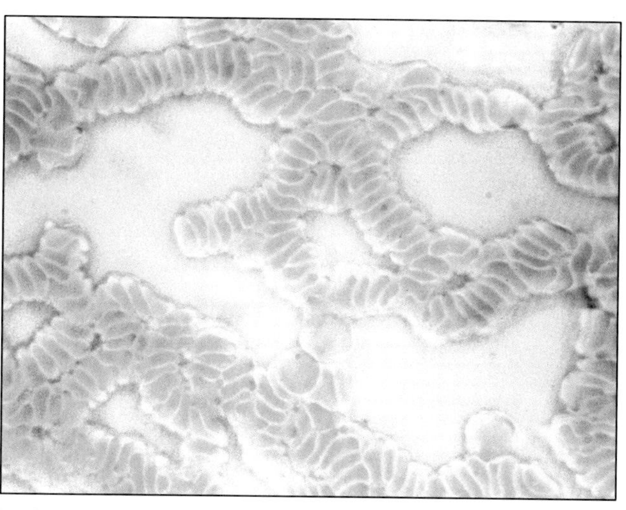

FIGURE 2-6
Microscopic rouleaux in an unstained wet mount preparation of normal cat blood.

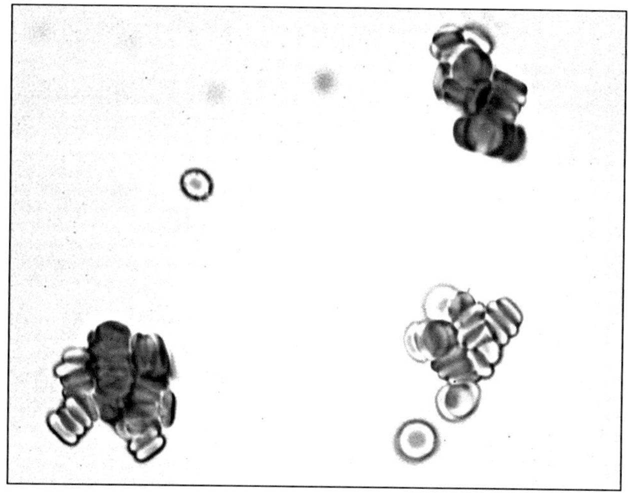

FIGURE 2-7
Microscopic agglutination in an unstained wet mount preparation of saline-washed erythrocytes from a foal with neonatal isoerythrolysis.

(aggregation of erythrocytes together in clusters) from rouleaux (adherence of erythrocytes together like a stack of coins), which can be seen in the blood from healthy horses and cats (Fig. 2-6). Rouleaux formation is eliminated by washing erythrocytes in physiologic saline, but agglutination is not. This differentiation requires centrifugation of blood, removal of plasma, and resuspension of erythrocytes in saline. A rapid way to differentiate rouleaux from agglutination is to mix five drops of physiologic saline with a drop of anticoagulated blood on a glass slide and examine it as a wet mount using a microscope. This dilution reduces rouleaux, but agglutination is not affected. The microscopic appearance of agglutination in a sample of washed erythrocytes is shown (Fig. 2-7). The presence of agglutination indicates that the erythrocytes have increased surface-bound immunoglobulins. These immunoglobulins are usually of the IgM type when agglutination is present, because the greater distance between binding sites on IgM molecules compared with IgG molecules makes it easier for IgM molecules to overcome normal repulsive forces between negatively charged erythrocytes.[67] In addition, there are 10 antigen-binding sites per IgM molecule compared with 2 binding sites per IgG molecule (Fig. 2-8). A direct antiglobulin test is not needed to identify the presence of immunoglobulin bound to erythrocytes if agglutination is present in saline solution-washed erythrocyte samples.

MICROHEMATOCRIT TUBE EVALUATION

A microhematocrit tube is filled to about 90% of capacity with well-mixed blood and sealed with clay at one end. The tube is then placed in a microhematocrit centrifuge with the clay plug oriented to the periphery of the centrifuge head and

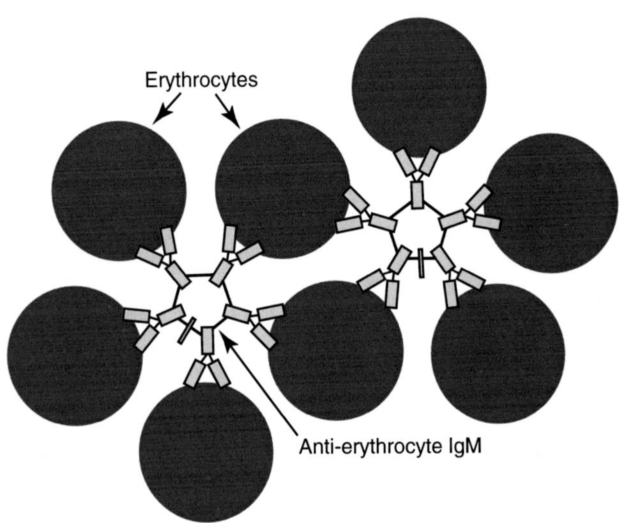

FIGURE 2-8
Antierythrocyte IgM antibodies causing erythrocyte agglutination.

centrifuged for 5 minutes. After centrifugation, the blood sample will be separated into three layers based on density, with packed erythrocytes located at the bottom. A white "buffy coat" is located above the erythrocyte layer, and the acellular plasma is located above the buffy coat.

When blood is submitted for a CBC, most commercial laboratories determine an electronic HCT rather than a packed cell volume (PCV) by centrifugation. This efficiency negates the need to centrifuge a microhematocrit tube filled with blood. Unfortunately useful information concerning the appearance of plasma is missed unless a serum or plasma sample is also prepared for clinical chemistry tests.

Packed Cells

The PCV is measured after centrifugation by determining the fraction of total blood volume in a microhematocrit tube that is occupied by erythrocytes. Leukocytes and platelets are primarily located within the buffy coat, although certain leukocyte types may be present in the top portion of the packed erythrocyte column in some species (e.g., neutrophils in cattle). The width of the buffy coat generally correlates directly with the total leukocyte count. A large buffy coat suggests leukocytosis (Fig. 2-9, *A*) or thrombocytosis, and a small buffy coat suggests that low numbers of these cells may be present. The buffy coat may appear reddish owing to the presence of a marked reticulocytosis.

The Appearance of Plasma

Plasma is normally clear in all species. It is nearly colorless in small animals, pigs, and sheep but light yellow in horses because they naturally have higher bilirubin concentrations. Plasma varies from colorless to light yellow (carotenoid pigments) in cattle, depending on their diet.[62] Increased yellow coloration usually indicates increased bilirubin concentration. This increase often occurs secondarily to anorexia (fasting hyperbilirubinemia) in horses owing to reduced removal of unconjugated bilirubin by the liver.[13] Failure of the liver to remove unconjugated bilirubin from blood has also been reported to cause hyperbilirubinemia in one-fourth of the sick (often anorectic) cattle in one study.[40] In other species, yellow plasma with a normal HCT suggests hyperbilirubinemia secondary to liver disease. Hyperbilirubinemia associated with a marked decrease in the HCT suggests an increased destruction of erythrocytes; however, the concomitant occurrence of liver disease and a nonhemolytic anemia could produce a similar finding (Fig. 2-9, *B*).

Red discoloration of plasma indicates the presence of free hemoglobin. This discoloration may represent either true hemoglobinemia, resulting from intravascular hemolysis, or hemolysis occurring after sample collection due to such causes as rough handling, fragile cells, lipemia, or prolonged storage (Fig. 2-9, *C,D*). The HCT value may help differentiate between these two possibilities, with red plasma and a normal HCT suggesting in vitro hemolysis. The concomitant occurrence of hemoglobinuria indicates that intravascular hemolysis has occurred. Plasma will also appear red following treatment with cross-linked hemoglobin blood substitute solutions.

Lipemia is recognized as a white opaque appearance caused by chylomicrons and very low density lipoproteins (VLDLs). The presence of chylomicrons may also result in a white layer at the top of the plasma column (Fig. 2-9, *E*). The presence of lipemia is frequently the result of a recent meal (postprandial lipemia), but diseases including diabetes mellitus, pancreatitis, hypothyroidism, hyperadrenocorticism, protein-losing nephropathy, cholestasis, obesity, and starvation may also contribute to the development of lipemia in dogs and cats.[23,72] Transient lipemia and accompanying anemia has been described as a syndrome in kittens, but a direct link between hyperlipidemia and anemia has not been clearly documented.[23] Hereditary causes of lipemia include lipoprotein lipase deficiency in cats and idiopathic hyperlipidemia in miniature schnauzer dogs.[20,73]

Equids of any age and either sex may develop lipemia, but obese ponies, miniature horses, and miniature donkeys are most susceptible. Lipemia has been associated with a broad range of diseases, but it is more prevalent in association with pregnancy, lactation, and/or anorexia.[65] Lipemia has also been reported in llamas and alpacas with severe systemic diseases. It is not associated with age, sex, or reproductive status in these camelids.[64] The pathogenesis of marked secondary hyperlipidemia is not always clear. It often appears to result from a mobilization of unesterified fatty acids from adipose tissue and the subsequent overproduction of VLDLs by the liver, but it may also result from ineffective clearance of VLDLs by tissues or a combination of both, as occurs in diabetes mellitus.

Plasma Protein Determination

After the PCV is measured and the appearance of the plasma and buffy coat is noted, the microhematocrit capillary tube is broken just above the buffy coat and the plasma is placed in

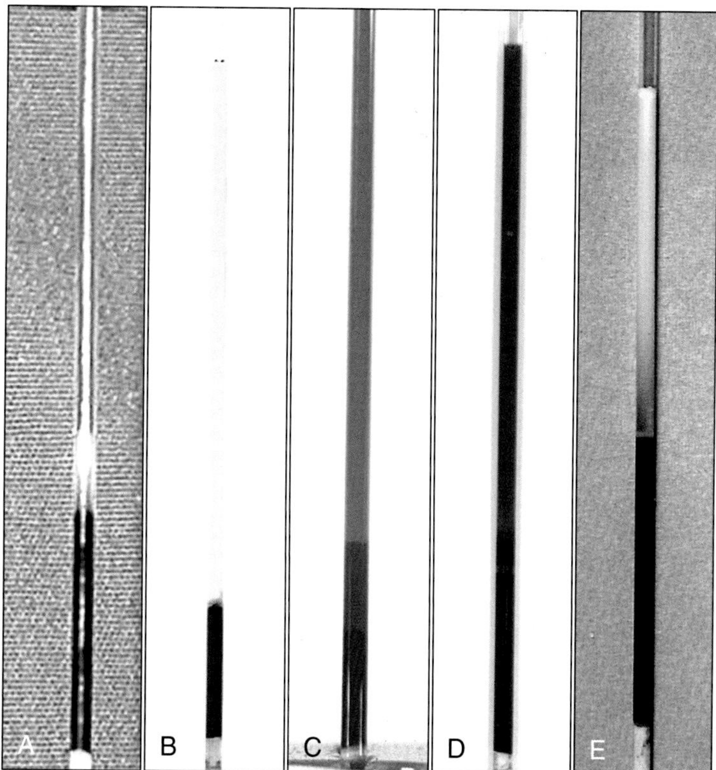

FIGURE 2-9

Gross appearance of microhematocrit tubes demonstrating leukocytosis, icterus, hemolysis, and lipemia. **A,** Microhematocrit tube from a cat with a large buffy coat resulting from a chronic lymphocytic leukemia. **B,** Microhematocrit tube from an anemic cat, with icteric plasma secondary to hepatic lipidosis. **C,** Microhematocrit tube with evidence of hemolysis in plasma from a cat with acetaminophen-induced Heinz body hemolytic anemia. Less dense erythrocyte ghosts can be seen above the packed intact erythrocytes. **D,** Microhematocrit tube with evidence of hemolysis in plasma from a horse with intravascular hemolysis induced by the inadvertent intravenous and intraperitoneal administration of hypotonic fluid. Less dense erythrocyte ghosts can be seen above the buffy coat. **E,** Microhematocrit tube with marked lipemia in plasma from a dog with hypothyroidism that was also being treated with prednisone for an allergic dermatitis. It was unclear from the medical record if this was a fasting blood sample.

A, *Courtesy of Heather Wamsley.*

a refractometer for plasma protein determination. Plasma protein concentrations in newborn animals (approximately 4.5 to 5.5 g/dL) are lower than adult values and increase to within the adult range by 3 to 4 months of age.[33] The presence of lipemia or hemolysis will falsely increase the measured plasma protein value. Maximum information can be gained by interpretation of the HCT and plasma protein concentrations simultaneously (see Chapter 4).

Fibrinogen Determination

Fibrinogen can be measured in a hematocrit tube because it readily precipitates from plasma when heated to 56°C to 58°C for 3 minutes. The difference between the total protein of the plasma and the total protein of the defibrinogenated (heated) plasma gives an estimate of the fibrinogen concentration in the plasma.[32] This method is useful in identifying high fibrinogen concentrations, but it is not accurate in identifying low fibrinogen concentrations.[4,11]

BLOOD CELL COUNTING AND SIZING

Total leukocyte counts, erythrocyte counts, and platelet counts in mammals may be determined using manual or automated techniques.

Manual Cell Counting

Manual erythrocyte counts are not accurate enough to be useful. Manual total leukocyte counts and platelet counts can be performed using commercially available reservoirs and pipettes to dilute the sample and lyse erythrocytes prior to the microscopic counting of leukocytes and platelets using a hemacytometer chamber. Manual leukocyte counts and platelet counts are done when errors are suspected in cell counts generated by automated cell counters. Manual cell counts may also be done in an emergency situation when automated cell counts are not available.

All blood cell types in birds and reptiles are nucleated, making accurate separation and counting difficult or impossible with automated cell counters. Consequently manual leukocyte counts are generally required in nonmammalian species. Thrombocytes can be estimated based on the number present in stained blood films.[47]

If properly maintained, automated blood cell counters are more precise and accurate than manual techniques in mammalian species. Various technologies—including quantitative buffy coat analysis, impedance measurements, laser flow cytometry, and cytochemistry—are utilized to generate these cell counts.

Automated Cell Counting

Quantitative buffy coat analysis (QBC VetAutoread Hematology System, IDEXX, Inc., Westbrook, ME) depends on variations in cell density to separate cell types. Cells are not actually counted; instead the widths of the various layers of cell types that form are measured and the cell "count" is generated assuming a standard cell size for the cell type in question.[35]

Impedance counters such as the Heska CBC-Diff (Heska Corporation, Loveland, CO) and Abaxis VetScan HMII (Abaxis, Union City, CA) depend on the principle that cells are poor electrical conductors. Blood is diluted in an electrically conductive solution and a precise volume of this diluted suspension is drawn through a small aperture between two electrodes. Each cell produces a change in electrical impedance, resulting in a change in voltage that is proportional to the size of the cell counted. Several thousand cells per second can be counted and sized. Erythrocytes and platelets can be differentiated by size alone in many species using impedance counters, but not in cats, because their platelets are large and their erythrocytes relatively small. Leukocytes are counted as free nuclei following lysis of erythrocytes and platelets.

The development of laser flow cytometry for use in instruments such as the CELL-DYN 3500R (Abbott Laboratories, Abbott Park, IL), the Advia 120 (Siemens Healthcare Diagnostics, Inc., Tarrytown, NY), the Sysmex XT-2000iV (Sysmex Corporation, Kobe, Japan), and the LaserCyte (IDEXX, Inc., Westbrook, ME) has allowed for cells to be characterized in greater detail. Individual cells pass through a laser beam, absorbing and scattering light. Interruptions in light are used to count cells and light scatter is used to determine size and internal complexity or density. The Advia 120 also utilizes a peroxidase channel to aid in determining specific leukocyte types. When properly calibrated, laser flow analysis allows for a more complete and accurate differential leukocyte count than can be done using cell size alone. Laser flow cytometry also permits the development of automated reticulocyte counts and reticulated platelet counts[36,44] as well as the development of new erythrocyte and reticulocyte parameters based on the simultaneous measurement of size and hemoglobin concentration within individual cells.[17]

Nucleated erythrocytes are counted as leukocytes in most electronic cell counters; consequently total leukocyte counts must usually be corrected for the presence of nucleated erythrocytes when present.

Errors in Blood Cell Counting and Sizing

The accuracy of blood cell counting depends on the quality and characteristics of the blood sample as well as the accuracy of the analytic methods used. Storage of blood samples for more than a few hours can result in sample deterioration and inaccurate cell counts. The presence of even small clots in the blood tube invalidates all cell counts. Even without clot formation, platelet aggregation may occur if platelets become activated during blood collection, as can happen when specimens are collected with a syringe and then transferred to an anticoagulant tube. Heparin is generally not used as an anticoagulant because it does not prevent platelet clumping, and leukocyte staining is poor on blood films. EDTA is the preferred anticoagulant for CBC determinations in most species, but EDTA may induce platelet, leukocyte, and erythrocyte aggregate formation in some individuals with antibodies bound to the surfaces of these respective cell types.[10,29,54,71,75] When this occurs, collection of blood into citrate may prevent the problem. Cell aggregation tends to be more pronounced as blood is cooled and stored; consequently processing samples as rapidly as possible after collection may minimize the formation of leukocyte and/or platelet aggregates. EDTA can cause marked hemolysis in some species of birds (ostriches, emus, and jays),[25,35] reptiles (turtles and tortoises),[25,42] and fish (carp and brown trout).[43,66] Heparin is used as an anticoagulant in these species. Both lysis and clumping can result in reduced cell counts of the cell types involved.

Platelet clumping can not only result in an erroneously decreased platelet count[59] but also in a falsely increased mean platelet volume (MPV) and occasionally a falsely increased total leukocyte count.[35,75] Autoagglutination of erythrocytes in the blood sample can result in a spuriously increased mean cell volume (MCV) and mean cell hemoglobin concentration (MCHC) and a decreased HCT and total erythrocyte count.[48] As indicated earlier, with the use of most hematology analyzers, the presence of nucleated erythrocytes can result in a falsely increased total leukocyte count. Residual erythrocyte stroma from inadequate lysing of erythrocytes may also result in spuriously increased total leukocyte counts.[35,76]

The presence of severe lipemia can result in spuriously increased hemoglobin and MCHC values and possibly even increased platelet and total leukocyte counts.[75] The presence of in vitro or in vivo hemolysis in the sample or prior treatment with a cross-linked hemoglobin solution can result in an erroneously increased MCHC value.[38] The presence of numerous Heinz bodies in erythrocytes can also result in spuriously increased hemoglobin and MCHC values, increased automated reticulocyte counts,[14,52] and sometimes increased total leukocyte counts.[69] The precipitation of an IgM paraprotein in blood from a dog by the lysing reagent used in the CELL-DYN 3500 falsely increased the spectrophotometric measurement of hemoglobin (Hb), which falsely increased the calculated MCHC.[8]

Laboratory errors may occur as a result of mistakes made by operators. These operator errors include a lack of knowledge or the skills for the test being done, improper labeling of samples, dilution errors, use of outdated reagents, inadequate quality control measures, or improper calibration of equipment. The instruments being used must be optimized and validated for the species being tested.

Erythrocytes and platelets vary considerably in volume among animal species, and instruments must be adjustable to accurately count and size these blood cells for the species being assayed. Cats naturally have large platelets and moderately small erythrocytes. The resultant overlap of erythrocyte and platelet size makes separation of cat platelets and erythrocytes unreliable with the use of impedance counters.[77] Consequently cat platelet counts are spuriously decreased when measured with impedance counters. This inclusion of platelets in the erythrocyte measurements can result in increased erythrocyte counts and HCT values and reduced MCV and MCHC values, but the ratio of platelets to erythrocytes is usually not large enough to have appreciable effects on these parameters (exceptions include cats with severe anemia and/or marked thrombocytosis).[76] Leukocytes are generally included in erythrocyte measurements, but the ratio of leukocytes to erythrocytes is usually not large enough to have appreciable effects on erythrocyte parameters (exceptions include animals with severe anemia and marked leukocytosis). In these instances the inclusion of leukocytes in erythrocyte measurements can result in increased erythrocyte counts, HCT and MCV values, and reduced MCHC values because leukocytes are larger than erythrocytes.[76] These errors resulting from difficulties in separating cell type by size alone should be minimized in automated cell counters that separate cells not only by size but also by internal complexity.

With the advent of new laser flow cytometry techniques, it is now possible to perform automated differential leukocyte counts; however, most instruments cannot accurately count basophils. For most instruments, a high basophil count is an error,[35] as has been noted in old blood samples.[63] These flow cytometers must be specifically calibrated for each species, and they work best when leukocyte morphology is normal. More reliable flags are needed to identify the presence of left shifts and neoplastic cells.[35]

The examination of a stained blood film is essential as a quality control measure regardless of the technology used to count blood cells. In addition to verifying the accuracy of leukocyte and platelet counts, a number of other evaluations are made. Examples include determining whether erythrocyte polychromasia, erythrocyte shape abnormalities, neutrophilic left shifts, neutrophil toxicity, reactive lymphocytes, blast cells, mast cells, and/or blood parasites are present.

Quality Control

Commercial control samples (preferably at two levels) approved by the instrument's manufacturer should be run each day; the values obtained should fall within the confidence intervals supplied with the control sample.[37] Proficiency testing programs provide external quality control. Samples are periodically sent to participating laboratories for analysis. Results are sent back to the agency supplying the samples and these values are compared with those from reference laboratories and other participating laboratories using the same methods. Proficiency testing programs provide valuable peer review of instruments and methods used, but the expense is beyond the means of most private practices.

Manual methods are also used as quality control measures for automated hematology instruments. A PCV can be measured following centrifugation of a blood sample for comparison to the HCT determined electronically. If values do not match within a couple of percentage points after adequate sample mixing, it suggests that the MCV or the RBC count is probably incorrect, because these two values are used to determine the HCT.

Stained blood films should be examined as a part of each CBC. The blood film is scanned to verify that the automated total leukocyte count and the platelet count appear to be correct. If the automated platelet count is low, it is especially important to examine for platelet clumps that could result in a spuriously low count. If an electronic differential leukocyte count is to be reported, one must review the blood film to verify that the percentages of each leukocyte type recorded appear to be correct and that there are no other cell types present that are not identified (e.g., basophils are not identified by most electronic cell counters). More details concerning the estimation of cell counts and the proper examination of stained blood films are given later in this chapter.

BLOOD-FILM PREPARATION

Blood films should be prepared within a couple of hours of blood sample collection to avoid artifactual changes that will distort the morphology of blood cells. Blood films are prepared in various ways including the slide (wedge) method, coverslip method, and automated slide spinner method. It is essential that a monolayer of intact cells is present on the slide so that accurate examination and differential leukocyte counts can be performed. If blood films are too thick, cells will be shrunken and may be difficult to identify. If blood films are too thin, erythrocytes will be flattened and lose their central pallor and some leukocytes (especially lymphocytes and blast cells) will be ruptured.[30]

Glass-Slide Blood-Film Method

A clean glass slide is placed on a flat surface and a small drop of well-mixed blood is placed on one end of the slide (Fig. 2-10). This slide is held in place with one hand and a second glass slide (spreader slide) is placed on the first slide and held between the thumb and forefinger with the other hand at about a 30- to 45-degree angle in front of the drop of blood. The spreader slide is then backed into the drop of blood, and as soon as the blood flows along the back side of the spreader slide, the spreader slide is rapidly pushed forward. The

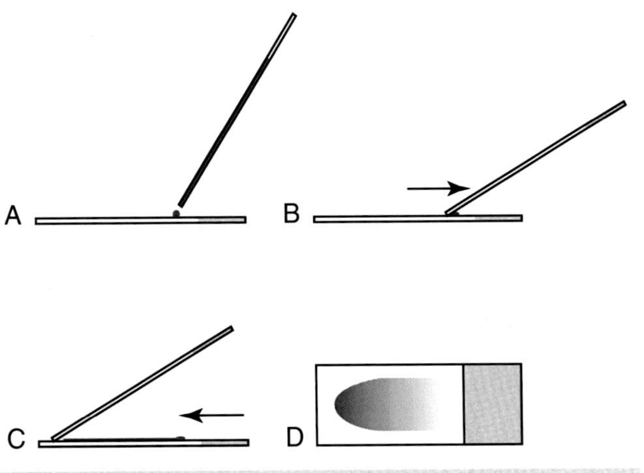

FIGURE 2-10

Slide blood-film preparation. **A,** A glass slide is placed on a flat surface and a small drop of well-mixed blood is placed on one end of the slide using a microhematocrit tube. **B,** A second glass slide (spreader slide) is placed on the first slide at about a 30-degree angle in front of the drop of blood. The spreader slide is then backed into the drop of blood. **C,** As soon as the blood flows along the back side of the spreader slide, the spreader slide is rapidly pushed forward. **D,** The blood film produced is thick at the back of the slide, where the drop of blood was placed, and thin at the front (feathered) edge of the slide.

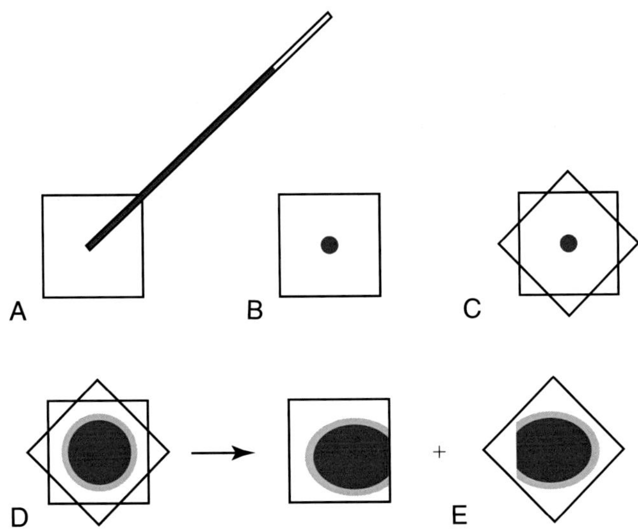

FIGURE 2-11

Coverslip blood film preparation. **A, B,** One clean coverslip is held between the thumb and index finger of one hand and a small drop of blood is placed in the middle of it using a microhematocrit tube. **C,** A second clean coverslip is dropped on top of the first in a crosswise position. **D,** Blood spreads evenly between the two coverslips and a feathered edge forms at the periphery. **E,** The coverslips are rapidly separated by grasping an exposed corner of the top coverslip with the other hand and pulling apart in a smooth, horizontal manner.

thickness of the smear is influenced by the size of the blood drop, the viscosity of the sample (HCT), the angle of the spreader slide, and the speed of spreading. The greater the angle (a more upright spreader slide) and faster the speed of spreading, the thicker and shorter the blood film will be. Thus the spreader slide should be held more upright in preparing smears from anemic patients so as to create a thicker blood film.[30]

If the drop of blood is the proper size, all of the blood will remain on the slide and a smear will be prepared that is thick at the back of the slide, where the drop of blood was placed, and thin at the front (feathered) edge of the slide. If the drop of blood is too large, some of the blood will be pushed off the end of the slide, causing potential problems. Often these blood films will be too thick for accurate evaluation. Second, clumps of cells tend to be pushed off the slide, making them unavailable for examination.

Once prepared, the slide is immediately dried by waving it in the air or holding it in front of a hair dryer set on a slightly warm-air setting. Holding the slide close to a dryer set on a hot-air setting can result in fragmentation of cells. Slow drying can cause cells to contract, making them difficult to identify.[30] Slides are identified by writing on the thick end of the smear or the frosted end of the slide with a graphite pencil or a pen containing ink that is not removed by alcohol fixation.

Coverslip Blood-Film Method

Two 22-mm square No. 1½ coverslips are required to make coverslip blood films (Fig. 2-11). A camel's hair brush is used to remove particles from the surfaces that will contact blood. One coverslip is held between the thumb and index finger of one hand and a small drop of blood is placed in the middle of the coverslip using a microhematocrit tube. The drop of blood should be as perfectly round as possible to produce even spreading between coverslips. The second coverslip is dropped on top of the first in a crosswise position. After the blood spreads evenly between the two coverslips and a feathered edge forms at the periphery, the coverslips are rapidly separated by grasping an exposed corner of the top coverslip with the other hand and pulling apart in a smooth, horizontal manner. Coverslips are immediately dried as described above and then identified by marking on the thick end of the smears with a graphite pencil or a pen containing ink that is not removed by alcohol fixation.

If the drop of blood used is too large, a feathered edge will not form and the blood film will be too thick. Multiple coverslip blood films may be stained in small slotted coplin jars or in ceramic staining baskets that are placed in beakers of fixative and stain.

BLOOD-FILM STAINING PROCEDURES

Romanowsky-Type Stains

Blood films are routinely stained with a Romanowsky-type stain (e.g., Wright or Wright-Giemsa) either manually or using an automatic slide stainer. Romanowsky-type stains are composed of a mixture of eosin and oxidized methylene blue (azure) dyes. The azure dyes stain acids, resulting in blue to

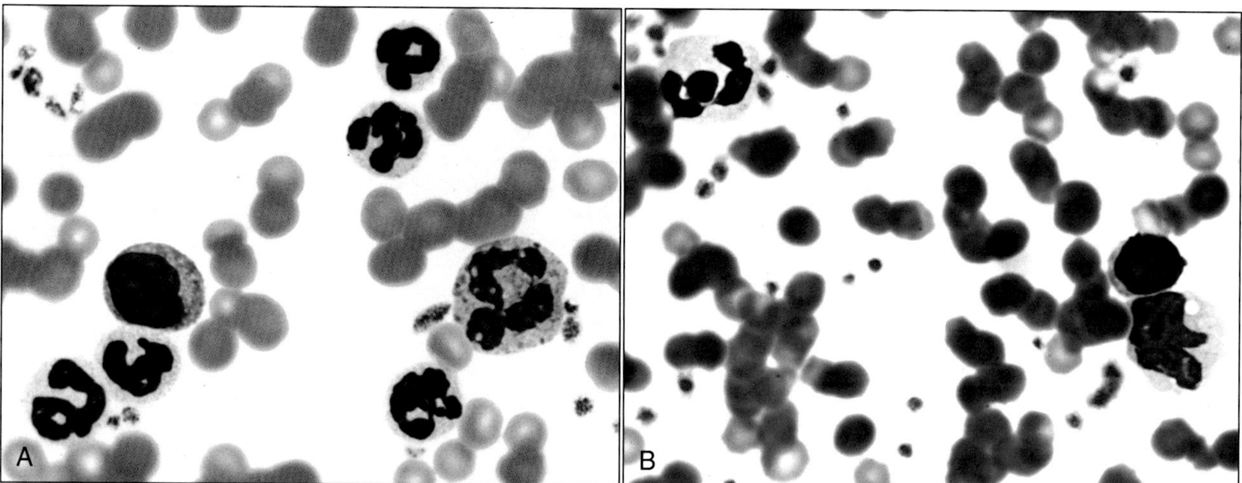

FIGURE 2-12

Appearance of blood films from a normal cat stained with Wright-Giemsa. **A,** Blood film was rinsed in distilled water. Five neutrophils, a basophil *(far right),* and a lymphocyte (round nucleus) are present. Erythrocytes exhibit rouleaux, a normal finding in cats. **B,** Blood film was rinsed in tap water. A neutrophil *(left),* monocyte *(bottom right),* and lymphocyte *(top right)* are present. The blue color of the erythrocytes results from using water with inappropriate pH.

purple colors, and eosin stains bases, resulting in red coloration (Fig. 2-12, *A*). These staining characteristics depend on the pH of the stains and the rinse water as well as the nature of the cells present (Fig. 2-12, *B*). Low pH, inadequate staining time, degraded stains, or excessive washing can result in excessively pink-staining blood films. High pH, prolonged staining, or insufficient washing can result in excessively blue-staining blood films.[30]

Blood films should be fixed in methanol within 4 hours (preferably within 1 hour) of preparation. If the methanol contains more than 3% water, morphologic artifacts including loss of cellular detail and vacuolation may be present.[30] Blood films may have an overall blue tint if stored unfixed for long periods before staining or if the unfixed blood films are exposed to formalin vapors, as occurs when blood films are shipped to the laboratory in a package that also contains formalin-fixed tissue. Blood films prepared from blood collected with heparin as the anticoagulant have an overall magenta tint owing to the mucopolysaccharides present.[30]

Drying or fixation problems can result in variably shaped refractile inclusions in the erythrocytes; these may be confused with erythrocyte parasites (Fig. 2-13). The presence of stain precipitation can make identification of leukocytes and blood parasites difficult (Fig. 2-14). Precipitated stain may be present because the stain or stains needed to be filtered, the staining procedure was too long, or the washing was not sufficient. Carboxymethylcellulose has been infused into the peritoneal cavity of horses and cattle in an attempt to prevent abdominal adhesions after surgery. This material can appear as a precipitate between cells in blood that resembles stain precipitation (Fig. 2-15).[6]

Various rapid stains, such as Diff-Quik (Dade Behring Inc., Newark, DE), are available. The quality of Diff-Quik-stained blood films is generally somewhat lower than that

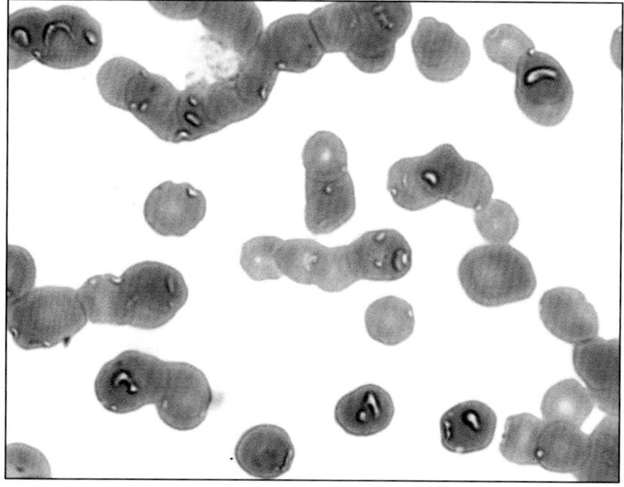

FIGURE 2-13

Refractile inclusions in erythrocytes from a horse are artifacts resulting from drying or fixation problems. Erythrocytes exhibit rouleaux, a normal finding in horses. Wright-Giemsa stain.

obtained by longer staining procedures, but staining quality is improved by allowing the blood film to remain in the fixative for several minutes. The Diff-Quik stain is classified as an aqueous stain, even though the fixation is done in methanol, because the component stains were prepared in water. A significant limitation of the Diff-Quik stain and other aqueous stains, such as Hema 3 (Fisher Scientific, Pittsburgh, PA) and the stain used in the automated stainer Aerospray 7120 (Westcore, Inc, Logan, UT), is that they do not stain basophil, mast cell, or large granular leukocyte granules well (Fig. 2-16).[1] However, these aqueous stains are superior to conventional methanolic Wright or Wright-Giemsa stains in the staining of distemper inclusions in canine blood cells.[1,26]

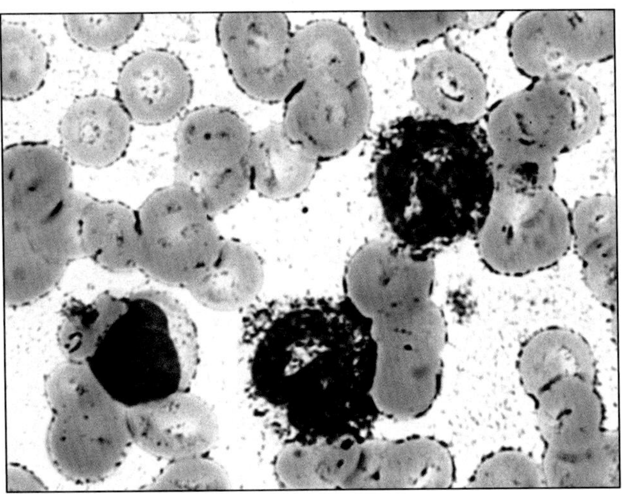

FIGURE 2-14

Stain precipitation in blood from a dog. The two neutrophils present might be mistaken for basophils because of the adherent precipitated stain. Wright-Giemsa stain.

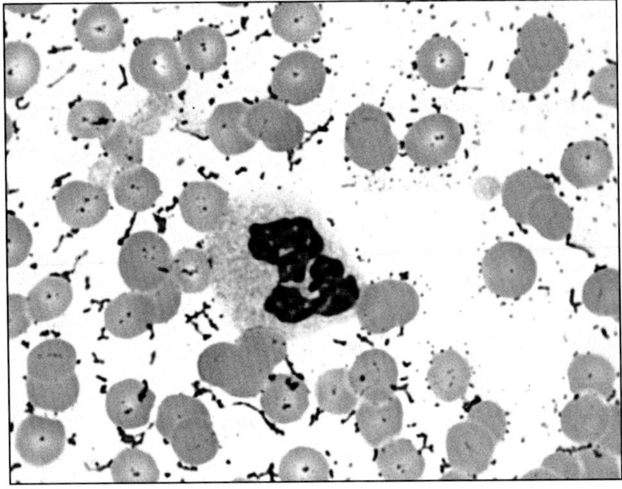

FIGURE 2-15

Carboxymethylcellulose precipitation. The blue-to-purple precipitate present between erythrocytes in this horse blood results from treatment with carboxymethylcellulose. Wright-Giemsa stain.

Photograph of a stained blood film from a 1994 ASVCP slide review case submitted by M.J. Burkhard, M.A. Thrall, and G. Weiser.

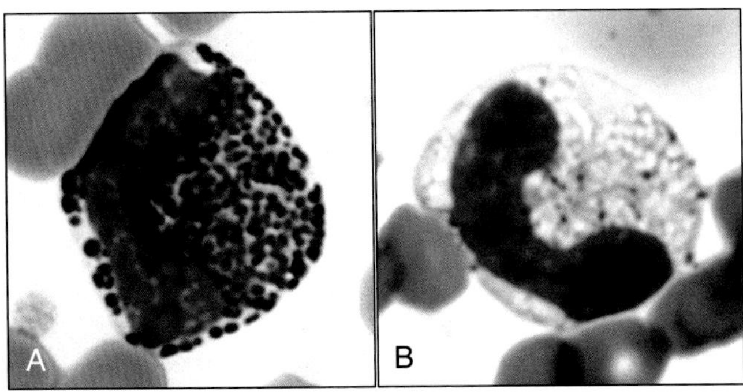

FIGURE 2-16

Band basophils in the blood of a horse. **A,** Granules stain well with Wright-Giemsa. **B,** Most granules are not stained with Diff-Quik stain.

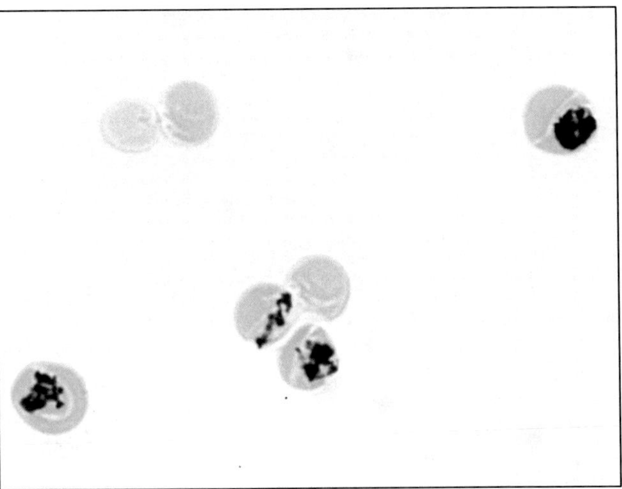

FIGURE 2-17

Reticulocytes in dog blood. Four reticulocytes (with blue-staining material) and three mature erythrocytes in blood from a dog with a regenerative anemia. New methylene blue reticulocyte stain.

Reticulocyte Stains

Reticulocyte stains are commercially available (N. Brecher, Harleco, EMD Chemicals). Those wishing to prepare their own stain can do so by dissolving 0.5 g of new methylene blue and 1.6 g of potassium oxalate in 100 mL of distilled water. Following filtration, equal volumes of blood and stain are mixed together in a test tube and incubated at room temperature for 10 to 20 minutes. After incubation, blood films are made and reticulocyte counts performed by examining 1000 erythrocytes and determining the percentage that are reticulocytes. The use of a Miller's disc in one of the microscope oculars saves time in performing the reticulocyte count.

The blue-staining aggregates or "reticulum" seen in reticulocytes (Fig. 2-17) does not occur as such in living cells but results from the precipitation of ribosomal ribonucleic acid (RNA; the same RNA that causes the bluish color seen in polychromatophilic erythrocytes) in immature erythrocytes during the staining process.[33] As a reticulocyte matures, the number of ribosomes decreases until only small punctate (dot-like) inclusions are observed in erythrocytes (punctate reticulocytes) stained with the reticulocyte stain (Fig. 2-18). To reduce the chance that a staining artifact would result in misclassifying a mature erythrocyte as a punctate reticulocyte when using a reticulocyte stain, the cell in question should have two or more discrete blue granules that are visible without requiring fine focus adjustment. These inclusions should be away from the cell margin to avoid confusion with hemotrophic mycoplasmas (formerly *Haemobartonella* organisms) or small Heinz bodies.

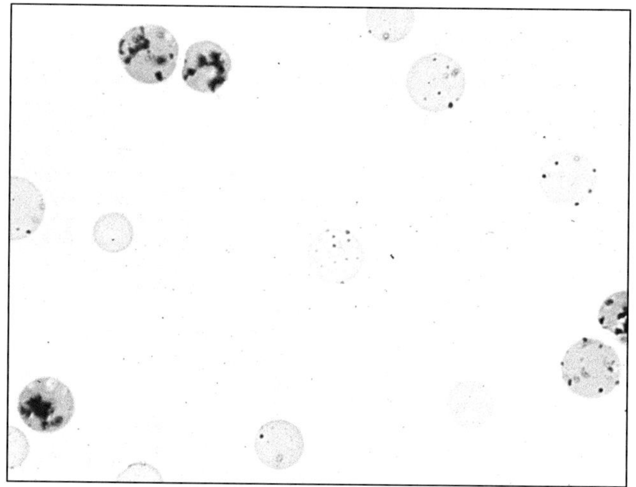

FIGURE 2-18
Reticulocytes in cat blood. Three whole aggregate reticulocytes (containing blue-staining aggregates of RNA) and half of an aggregate reticulocyte *(far right)* in blood from a cat with a markedly regenerative anemia. A majority of the remaining cells are punctate reticulocytes containing discrete dot-like inclusions. New methylene blue reticulocyte stain.

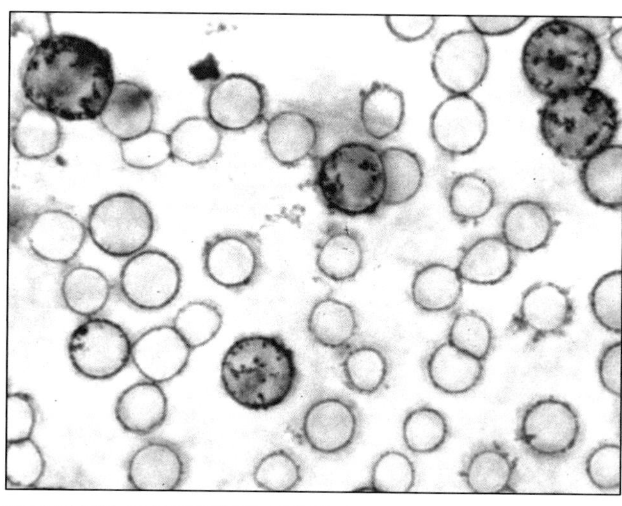

FIGURE 2-19
Reticulocytes in the blood of a dog. Five reticulocytes (with blue-staining material) in blood from a dog with a regenerative anemia in a new methylene blue-stained wet preparation. Note the difference in morphology compared with reticulocytes stained with a standard reticulocyte stain (see Figure 2-17). New methylene blue-stained wet preparation.

In normal cats as well as in cats with a regenerative anemia, the number of punctate reticulocytes is much greater than that seen in other species.[2] This apparently occurs because the maturation (loss of ribosomes) of reticulocytes in cats is slower than in other species. Consequently reticulocytes in cats are classified as aggregate (if coarse clumping is observed) or punctate (if small individual inclusions are present). Percentages of both types should be reported. Based on composite results from several authors, normal cats generally have from 0% to 0.5% aggregate and 1% to 10% punctate reticulocytes as determined by manual means. Higher punctate numbers of 2% to 17% have been reported using flow cytometry.[46]

The percentages of aggregate reticulocytes in cats directly correlate with the percentages of polychromatophilic erythrocytes observed in blood films stained with Wright-Giemsa.[2] Aggregate reticulocytes mature to punctate types in a day or less. Several more days are required for maturation (total disappearance of ribosomes) of punctate reticulocytes in cats.[9,15]

In contrast to those of the cat, most reticulocytes in other species are of the aggregate type. Consequently no attempts are made to differentiate the stages of reticulocytes in species other than the cat. In most species, the percentages of reticulocytes directly correlate with the percentages of polychromatophilic erythrocytes observed on routinely stained blood films.

In examining a reticulocyte-stained blood film, one should also be careful not to confuse precipitated RNA with Heinz bodies. Heinz bodies are composed of denatured precipitated hemoglobin. They are spherical, stain pale blue with reticulocyte stains, and are usually found at the periphery of the erythrocyte.

New Methylene Blue "Wet Mounts"

A new methylene blue "wet mount" preparation can be used for rapid information concerning the number of reticulocytes, platelets, and Heinz bodies present on a blood film. The stain consists of 0.5% new methylene blue dissolved in 0.85% NaCl. One milliliter of formalin is added per 100 mL of stain as a preservative. This stain is filtered after preparation and stored in dropper bottles. Alternatively, the stain may be stored in a plastic syringe with a 0.2-μm syringe filter attached so that the stain is filtered as it is used. Dry, unfixed blood films are stained by placing a drop of stain between the coverslip and a glass slide. This preparation is not permanent and does not stain mature erythrocytes or eosinophil granules. Punctate reticulocytes are not demonstrated, but aggregate reticulocytes appear as erythrocyte ghosts containing blue to purple granular material (Fig. 2-19). Platelets stain blue to purple, and Heinz bodies appear as refractile inclusions within erythrocyte ghosts. Although this staining method is not optimal for differential leukocyte counts, the number and type of leukocytes present can be appreciated.

Iron Stains

An iron stain such as the Prussian blue stain is used to verify the presence of iron-containing (siderotic) inclusions in blood and bone marrow cells and to evaluate bone marrow iron stores. Smears may be sent to a commercial laboratory for this stain, or a stain kit can be purchased and applied in house (Harleco Ferric Iron Histochemical Reaction Set, #6498693, EM Diagnostic Systems, Gibbstown, NJ). Iron-positive material stains blue, in contrast to the pink color of the cells and the background when this stain is applied.

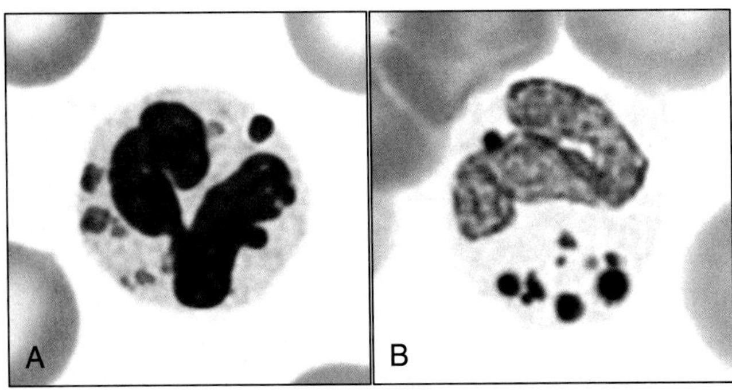

FIGURE 2-20
Neutrophils containing hemosiderin (sideroleukocytes) in blood from a dog with a hemolytic anemia. **A,** Wright-Giemsa stain. Hemosiderin inclusions stain gray or brownish. **B,** Prussian blue stain. Hemosiderin inclusions stain dark blue.

The presence of focal areas of basophilic stippling within erythrocytes stained with Romanowsky-type blood stains suggests that the stippling may contain iron. Iron-containing erythrocytes are referred to as siderocytes. Neutrophils and monocytes may also contain dark bluish-black or greenish iron-positive particles within their cytoplasm when they are stained with Romanowsky-type stains. Leukocytes containing iron-positive inclusions have been called sideroleukocytes (Fig. 2-20).

Prussian blue stain applied to bone marrow aspirate smears is a useful way to evaluate the amount of storage iron present in the marrow. Minimal or no iron is expected in iron deficiency anemia (although cats normally have no stainable iron in the marrow), whereas normal or excess iron may be observed in animals with hemolytic anemia and those with anemia resulting from decreased erythrocyte production.

Cytochemical Stains

A variety of cytochemical stains—such as peroxidase, chloroacetate esterase, alkaline phosphatase, and nonspecific esterase—are utilized to classify cells in animals with acute myeloid leukemias.[22,33,50] Reactions vary not only by cell type and stage of maturation but also by species.[50] These stains are done in a limited number of laboratories, and special training and/or experience is required to interpret the results. The appearance of positive reactions also varies depending on the reagents used. Because of the complexities of the staining procedures and interpretation of results, minimal information on cytochemical stains is presented in this book. As more antibodies become available for immunophenotyping acute myeloid leukemias, the need for cytochemical stains will decrease.[60]

EXAMINATION OF STAINED BLOOD FILMS

An overview and organized method of blood film examination are presented here. Descriptions and photographs of normal and abnormal blood cell morphologies, inclusions, and infectious agents are given in subsequent chapters.

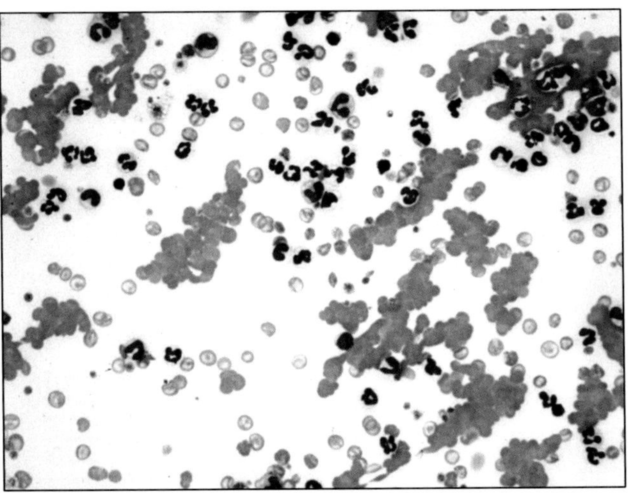

FIGURE 2-21
Autoagglutination of erythrocytes in blood from a dog with immune-mediated hemolytic anemia and marked leukocytosis. Wright-Giemsa stain.

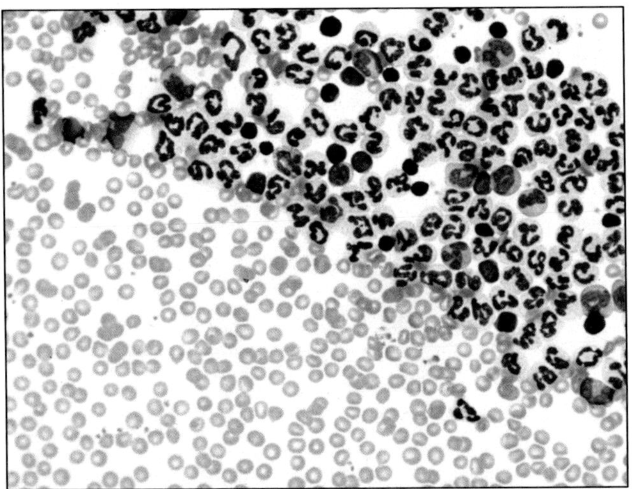

FIGURE 2-22
Leukocyte aggregate in blood from a dog. Leukocyte aggregates were present when EDTA was used as the anticoagulant but not when citrate was used as the anticoagulant. Wright-Giemsa stain.

Blood films are generally examined following staining with Romanowsky-type stains such as Wright or Wright-Giemsa. These stains allow for the examination of erythrocyte, leukocyte, and platelet morphology. Blood films should first be scanned using a low power objective to estimate the total leukocyte count and to look for the presence of erythrocyte autoagglutination (Fig. 2-21), leukocyte aggregates (Fig. 2-22), platelet aggregates (Fig. 2-23), microfilaria (Fig. 2-24), and abnormal cells that might be missed during the differential leukocyte count. It is particularly important that the feathered end of blood films made on glass slides be examined

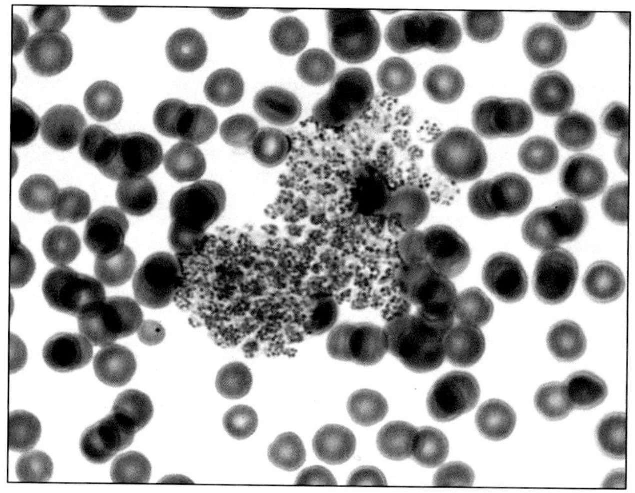

FIGURE 2-23
Platelet aggregate in blood from a cow. Wright-Giemsa stain.

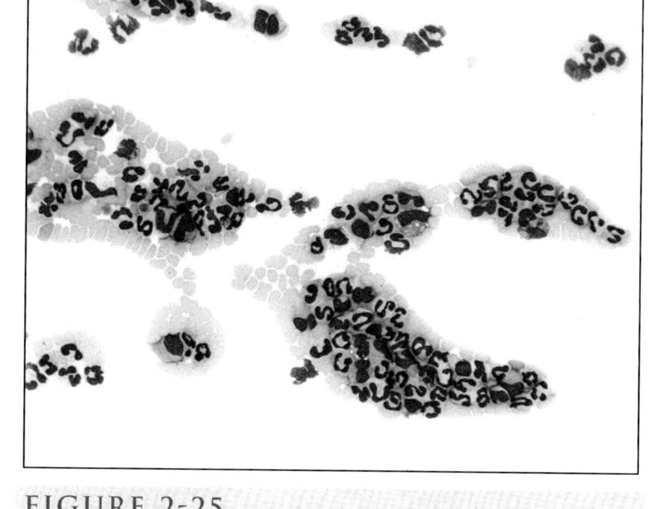

FIGURE 2-25
Leukocytes concentrated in the feathered edge of a blood film from a dog. The blood film was prepared using glass slides. Wright-Giemsa stain.

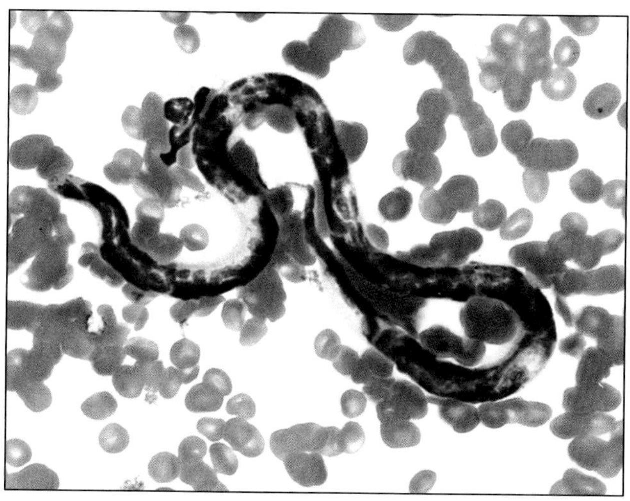

FIGURE 2-24
Dirofilaria immitis microfilaria in blood from a cat with heartworm disease. Wright-Giemsa stain.

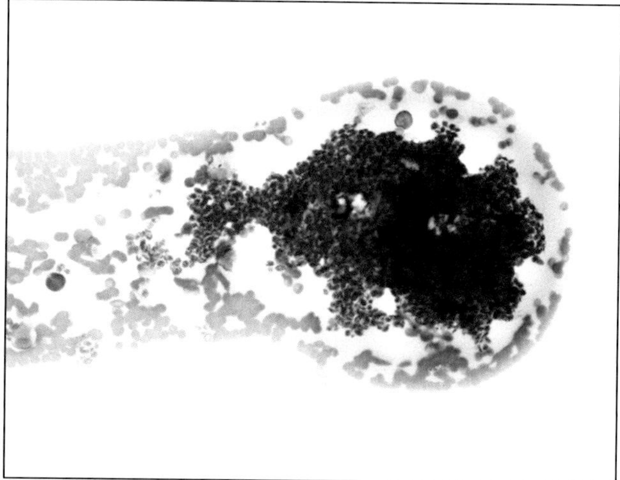

FIGURE 2-26
Platelet aggregate in the feathered edge of a blood film from a cat. The blood film was prepared using glass slides. Wright-Giemsa stain.

because leukocytes (Fig. 2-25) and platelet aggregates (Fig. 2-26) may be concentrated in this area. Conversely, aggregates of cells tend to be in the center of blood films rather than at the feathered edge when the coverslip blood-film method is used.

In examining a glass slide blood film, the blood film will be too thick to evaluate blood cell morphology at the back of the slide (Fig. 2-27, *A*) and too thin at the feathered edge, where cells are flattened (Fig. 2-27C). The optimal area for evaluation is generally in the front half of the smear behind the feathered edge (Fig. 2-27, *B*). This area should appear as a well-stained monolayer (a field in which erythrocytes are close together with approximately half of the cells touching each other).

Leukocyte Evaluation

As a quality control measure, the number of leukocytes present should be estimated to assure that the number present on the slide is consistent with the total leukocyte count measured. If 10× oculars and a 10× objective are used (100× magnification), the total leukocyte count in blood (cells per microliter) may be estimated by determining the average number of leukocytes present per field and multiplying by 100 to 150. If a 20× objective is used, the total leukocyte count may be estimated by multiplying the average number of leukocytes per field by 400 to 600. The correction factor used may vary, depending on the microscope used. Consequently the appropriate correction factors for the microscope being used should be determined by performing estimates on a number of blood films

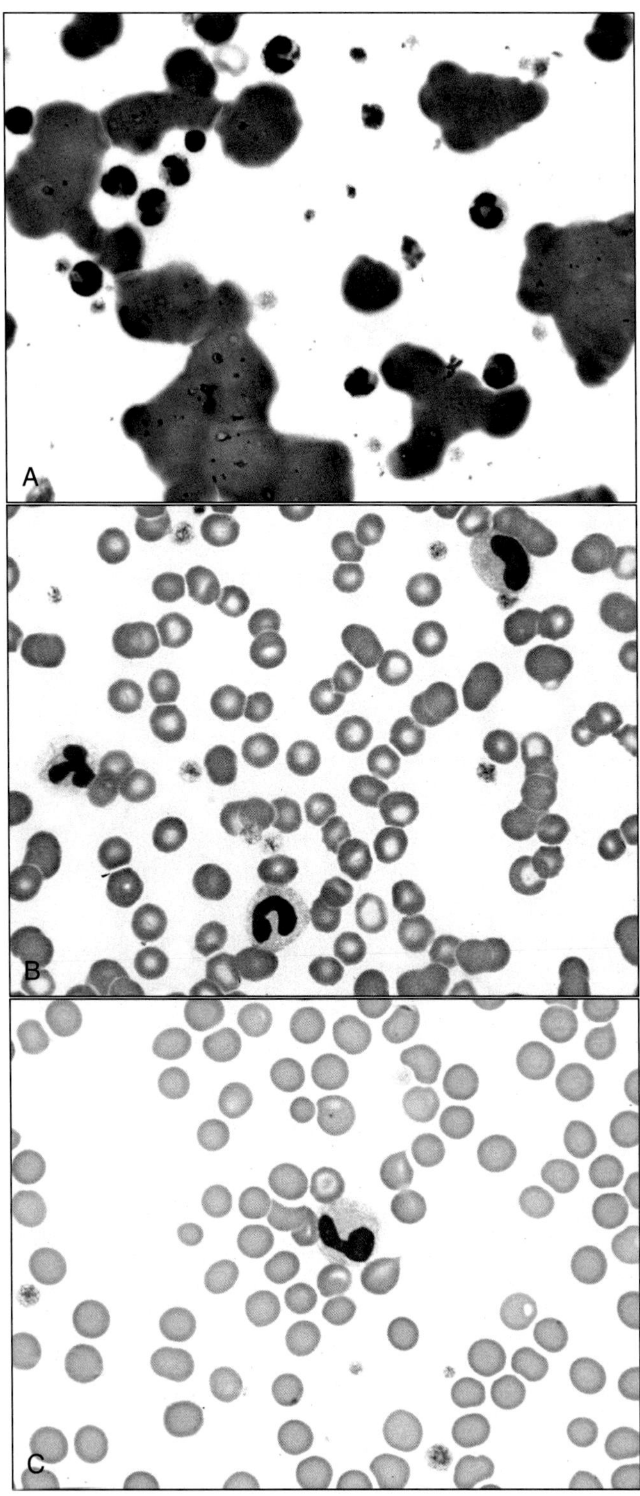

FIGURE 2-27

Selection of the appropriate area for microscopic examination of a slide blood film prepared from a dog. **A,** Thick area in the back end of a blood film. **B,** Optimal area for morphologic evaluation in the front half of the blood film. **C,** Thin area near the feathered edge of the blood film. Erythrocytes are flattened to the extent that central pallor is not readily apparent. Wright-Giemsa stain.

in which the total leukocyte counts have been accurately determined. Manual differential leukocyte counts are inherently imprecise, so it is also important to scan the blood film to gain an appreciation for the relative distribution of leukocyte types present prior to performing the differential leukocyte count.[34]

Leukocytes tend to smudge in samples with high hematocrits, making it difficult to perform a differential leukocyte count (Fig. 2-28, *A*). When this occurs, one can dilute a portion of the blood sample with equal parts of plasma or serum and make another blood film for examination (Fig. 2-28, *B*). Obviously estimated cell counts will be proportionally reduced in this dilute blood film.

A differential leukocyte count is done by identifying 200 consecutive leukocytes using a 40× or 50× objective. Because monocytes and other large leukocytes are pushed to the sides and ends of wedge-prepared blood films, differential counts are done by examining cells in a pattern that evaluates both

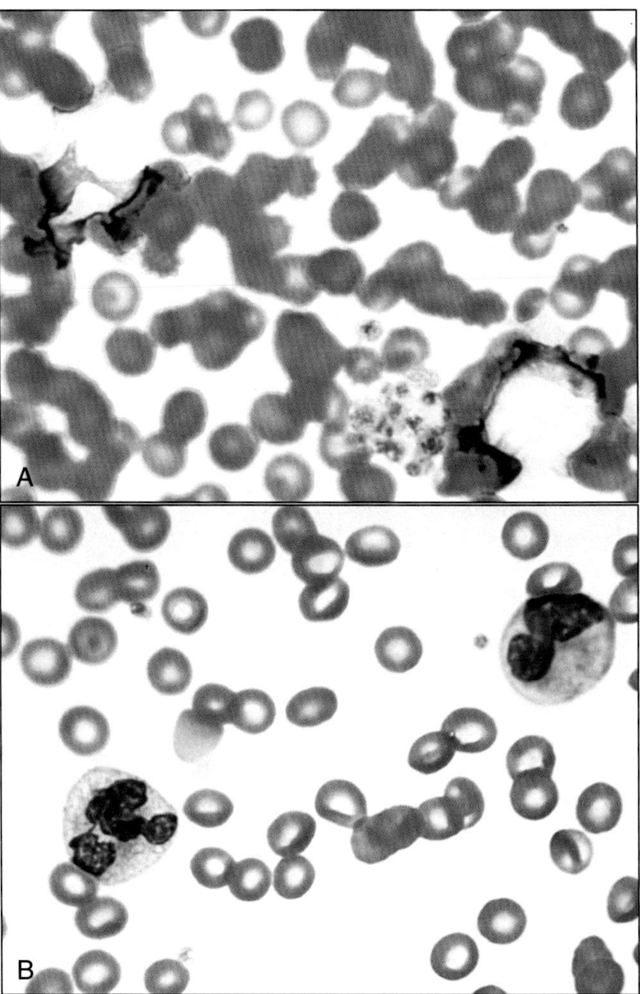

FIGURE 2-28

Blood films from a dog with a high hematocrit and toxic left shift prior to **(A)** and after **(B)** dilution of the blood sample with serum. Leukocytes are smudged and difficult to classify prior to blood sample dilution.

the edges and the center of the smear (Fig. 2-29).[30] After the count is complete, the percentage of each leukocyte type present is calculated and multiplied by the total leukocyte count to get the absolute number of each cell type present per microliter of blood.

It is the absolute number of each leukocyte type that is important. Relative values (percentages) can be misleading when the total leukocyte count is abnormal. Let us consider two dogs, one with 7% lymphocytes and a total leukocyte count of 40,000/µL and the other with 70% lymphocytes and a total leukocyte count of 4000/µL. The first would be said to have a "relative" lymphopenia and the second would be said to have a "relative" lymphocytosis, but they would both have the same normal absolute lymphocyte count (2800/µL).

Nucleated red blood cells (NRBCs) are counted along with the leukocytes when leukocyte counts are done using manual methods or automated impedance cell counters. As encountered during blood-film examination, the number of NRBCs per 100 leukocytes should be tabulated and the total leukocyte count corrected for the number of NRBCs present (see formula below) prior to calculating the absolute cell counts for each blood cell type.

$$\text{Corrected leukocyte count} = (\text{measured leukocyte count} \times 100)/(100 + \text{NRBC})$$

If leukocyte counts are performed with automated cell counters using technology that can differentiate NRBCs from leukocytes (e.g., morphologic characteristics of cells are determined by using a laser beam), the above calculation will not be necessary. However, the number of NRBCs present should still be recorded.

The presence of abnormal leukocyte morphology—such as toxic cytoplasm in neutrophils or increased reactive lymphocytes (e.g., more than 5% reactive lymphocytes)—should be recorded on the hematology report form. The frequency of toxic neutrophils is reported as few (5% to 10%), moderate (11% to 30%), or many (more than 30%) and the severity of toxic change is recorded as 1+ to 3+ (Box 2-1).[68]

Erythrocyte Morphology

Erythrocyte morphology should be examined and recorded as either normal or abnormal. Erythrocytes on blood films from normal horses, cats, and pigs often exhibit rouleaux formation; those from normal horses and cats may contain a low percentage of small, spherical nuclear remnants called Howell-Jolly bodies. Rouleaux and the presence of Howell-Jolly bodies should be recorded on the hematology form when they appear in blood films from species in which these are not normal findings.

Additional observations regarding erythrocyte morphology, such as the degree of polychromasia (presence of polychromatophilic erythrocytes), anisocytosis (variation in size), and poikilocytosis (abnormal shape) should also be made. Polychromatophilic erythrocytes are reticulocytes that stain bluish-red because of the combined presence of hemoglobin (red-staining) and ribosomes (blue-staining). Abnormal erythrocyte shapes should be classified as specifically as possible, because specific shape abnormalities can help to determine the nature of a disorder that may be present. Examples of abnormal erythrocyte morphology include echinocytes, acanthocytes, schistocytes, keratocytes, dacryocytes, elliptocytes, eccentrocytes, and spherocytes. The number of abnormal cells should be reported in a semiquantitative fashion, such as that shown in Table 2-1.[68]

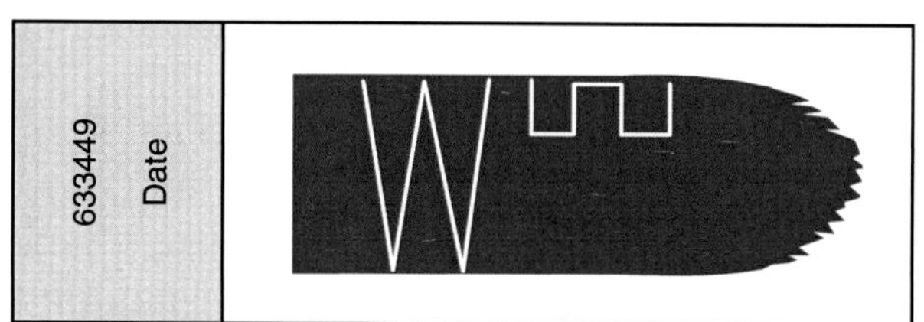

FIGURE 2-29
Patterns of slide blood film examination *(marked in white)* that may be used to improve the accuracy of differential leukocyte counts.

Platelets

Platelet numbers should be estimated as low, normal, or increased. Blood smears from most domestic animals normally average between 10 and 30 platelets per field examined under 10× oculars and the 100× objective (1000× magnification). As few as 6 platelets per 1000× field may be present in normal horse blood films.[68] Platelet numbers may be estimated by multiplying the average number per field by 15,000 to 20,000 to get the approximate number of platelets per microliter of blood.[61,68] While special attention will be given to the estimation of platelet numbers in animals with hemostatic diatheses, it is important to routinely estimate the platelet numbers on blood films, because many animals with thrombocytopenia exhibit no evidence or past history of

BOX 2-1 Semiquantitative Evaluation of Toxic Changes in the Cytoplasm of Neutrophils

Neutrophils with Toxic Change	
Few	5-10 (%)
Moderate	11-30 (%)
Many	>30 (%)
Severity of Toxic Change in Cytoplasm	
Döhle bodies[a]	1+
Mildly basophilic	1+
Moderately basophilic with Döhle bodies	2+
Moderately basophilic and foamy	2+
Dark blue-gray and foamy[b]	3+
Basophilic with toxic granules[b]	3+

[a]One or two Döhle bodies are sometimes seen in a few neutrophils from cats that do not exhibit signs of illness.
[b]May also contain Döhle bodies.

TABLE 2-1

Semiquantitative Evaluation of Erythrocyte Morphology Based on Average Number of Abnormal Cells per 1000× Microscopic Monolayer Field[a]

	1+	2+	3+	4+
Anisocytosis				
Dog	7-15	16-20	21-29	>30
Cat	5-8	9-15	16-20	>20
Cattle	10-20	21-30	31-40	>40
Horse	1-3	4-6	7-10	>10
Polychromasia				
Dog	2-7	8-14	15-29	>30
Cat	1-2	3-8	9-15	>15
Cattle	2-5	6-10	11-20	>20
Horse	Rarely observed	—	—	—
Hypochromasia and Shapes				
Hypochromasia[a]	1-10	11-50	51-200	>200
Poikilocytosis[a]	3-10	11-50	51-200	>200
Codocytes (dogs)	3-5	6-15	16-30	>30
Spherocytes[b]	5-10	11-50	51-150	>150
Echinocytes[b]	5-10	11-100	101-250	>250
Other shapes[c]	1-2	3-8	9-20	>20

[a]A monolayer field is defined as a field in which erythrocytes are close together with approximately half touching each other. In severely anemic animals, such monolayers may not be present. When erythrocytes are generally not touching (e.g., tend to be separated by the distance of one cell diameter), the number of erythrocytes with morphologic abnormalities are counted for two fields.
[b]The same parameters are used for all species.
[c]Parameters are used for acanthocytes, schistocytes, keratocytes, elliptocytes, dacrocytes, drepanocytes, and stomatocytes in all species.
From Weiss DJ. Uniform evaluation and semiquantitative reporting of hematologic data in veterinary medicine. *Vet Clin Pathol.* 184;13:27-31.

bleeding tendencies. If a thrombocytopenia is suspected, it should be confirmed with a platelet count. Dogs and cats have larger platelets than do horses and ruminants. Platelets contain magenta-staining granules, but these granules generally stain poorly in horses. The presence of abnormal platelet morphology (large or hypogranular platelets) should also be recorded on the hematology form.

Degenerative Changes in Blood Samples

Degenerative changes are apparent in blood samples within a few hours after collection; consequently blood films should be made and stained and blood cell counts performed as soon as possible after collection. Blood samples should be refrigerated if tests cannot be performed within a couple of hours. CBCs are often performed on day-old blood that has been kept refrigerated and submitted to a commercial laboratory, but some changes will already be present. Various progressive changes may be observed depending on the animal species and the time and temperature of storage of blood samples.[7,18,31] Erythrocytes can swell, which results in increased MCV and HCT and decreased MCHC within 12 hours. Platelets tend to aggregate and degranulate, resulting in lower automated platelet counts and higher MPV values.[18,45] Electronically determined differential counts become less accurate with blood storage.[7] Nuclear swelling may be present in leukocytes, a process that can result in an increased percentage of bands on microscopic examination.[35] Neutrophil cytoplasmic vacuolation develops, which may be confused with toxic changes.[21]

Leukocytes that undergo programmed cell death (apoptosis) exhibit pyknosis and karyorrhexis (Fig. 2-30). Pyknosis involves shrinkage or condensation of a cell with increased nuclear compactness or density. Karyorrhexis refers to the subsequent nuclear fragmentation. It may not be possible to determine the cell of origin. These abnormalities can occur in vivo but are more commonly associated with prolonged or inadequate sample storage before blood films are made.[30] With excessive storage, all blood cell types will lyse, resulting in cytopenias.

Infectious Agents or Inclusions of Blood Cells

Blood films are examined for the presence of infectious agents or intracellular inclusions using the 100× objective. Infectious agents or inclusions that may be seen in blood cells include Howell-Jolly bodies, Heinz bodies (unstained), basophilic stippling, canine distemper inclusions, siderotic inclusions, Döhle bodies, *Babesia* species, *Cytauxzoon felis*, hemotrophic *Mycoplasma* (formerly *Haemobartonella*) species, *Ehrlichia* species, *Anaplasma* species, *Hepatozoon* species, and *Theileria*

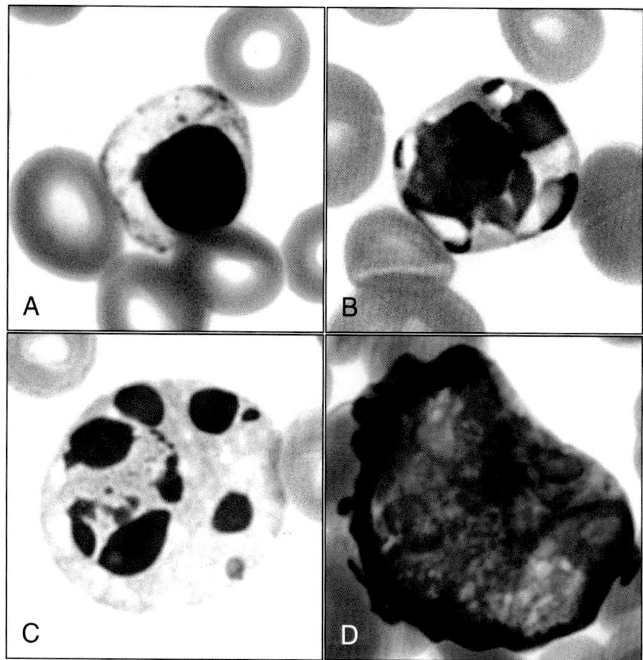

FIGURE 2-30
Pyknotic and karyorrhexic cells in blood. **A,** Pyknotic cell with condensed chromatin in blood from a dog with a toxic left shift. **B,** Pyknosis and karyorrhexis of a cell in blood from a dog with dirofilariasis. **C,** Pyknosis and karyorrhexis of a cell in blood from a dog with acute monocytic leukemia (AML-M5). **D,** Pyknosis and karyorrhexis of a cell in blood from a cow with leukemic lymphoma. Wright-Giemsa stain.

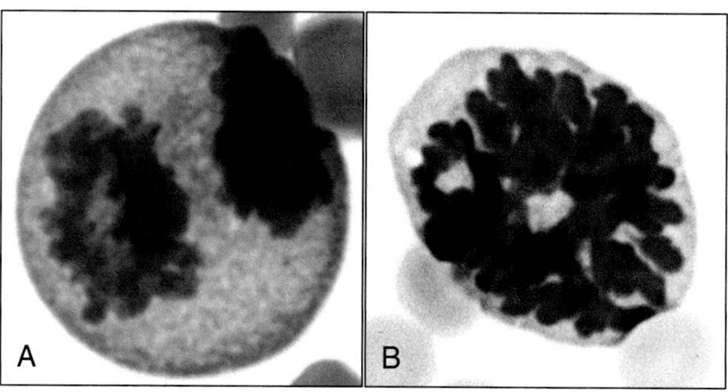

FIGURE 2-31
Mitotic cells in blood. **A,** Mitotic cell in anaphase in blood from a cat with erythroleukemia (AML-M6). **B,** Mitotic cell (presumably lymphoid) in prophase in blood from a horse with equine infectious anemia. Wright-Giemsa stain.

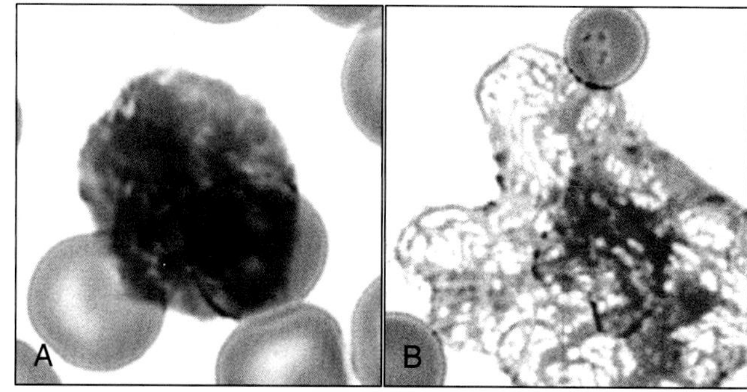

FIGURE 2-32
Free nuclei in blood. **A,** Free nucleus in blood from a dog with chronic lymphocytic leukemia. **B,** Free nucleus with a distorted net-like structure ("basket cell") in blood from a cat. Wright-Giemsa stain.

species. The appearance of these agents and inclusions is discussed in subsequent chapters.

Miscellaneous Cells and Parasites in Blood

Degenerative cells, mitotic cells, vascular lining cells, and other cells not typically seen in blood may occasionally be recognized during blood film examination. Parasites and bacteria that are not associated with blood cells may also be seen in blood. However, bacterial rods and cocci between cells are usually the result of contaminated stain.

Mitotic Cells

Mitotic cells may be present in the blood of animals with malignant neoplasia (Fig. 2-31, *A*), but they may also occur in nonneoplastic disorders, such as lymphocytes undergoing blast transformation (Fig. 2-31, *B*), nucleated erythroid precursors in regenerative anemia, and activated mononuclear phagocytes.

Free Nuclei

When cells are lysed during blood-film preparation, free nuclei (nuclei without cytoplasm) may be seen (Fig. 2-32, *A*). When a free nucleus is spread thin on the blood film, it appears as a net-like pinkish structure, which has been referred to as a "basket cell" (Fig. 2-32, *B*). This is a misnomer, because a basket cell is not truly a cell but only the distorted nucleus of a cell. Lymphocytes are the most likely blood cell type to lyse during blood-film preparation.

Endothelial Cells

Spindle-shaped endothelial cells with elongated nuclei may sometimes be seen in blood films (Fig. 2-33). Endothelial cells line vessels and may become dislodged as the needle enters the vein during blood sample collection.

Megakaryocytes

Megakaryocytes are multilobulated, platelet-producing giant cells that lie against the outside of vascular sinuses in bone marrow (see Thrombopoiesis section in Chapter 3 for more details). Cytoplasmic processes of mature megakaryocytes extend into the sinus lumen, where they develop into proplatelets and subsequently individual platelets. Sometimes whole megakaryocytes enter vascular sinuses, accounting for the rare recognition of these cells in blood films from animals (Fig. 2-34).[51] Megakaryocytes are more easily found by

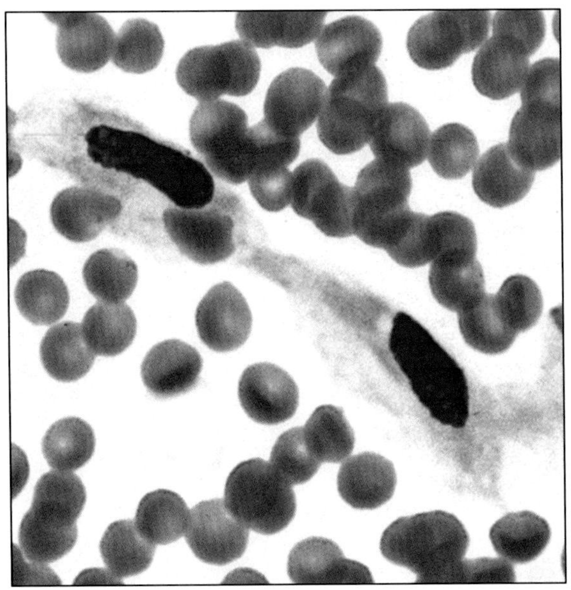

FIGURE 2-33
Two spindle-shaped endothelial cells with elongated nuclei in blood from a cow. These cells were likely dislodged from the vessel wall during blood sample collection. Wright-Giemsa stain.

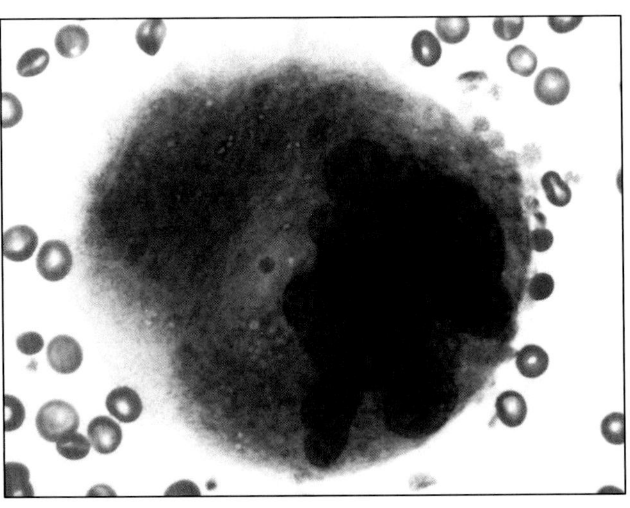

FIGURE 2-34
Mature megakaryocyte in blood from dog with an abscess and accompanying toxic left shift. Wright-Giemsa stain.

Courtesy of Heather Wamsley.

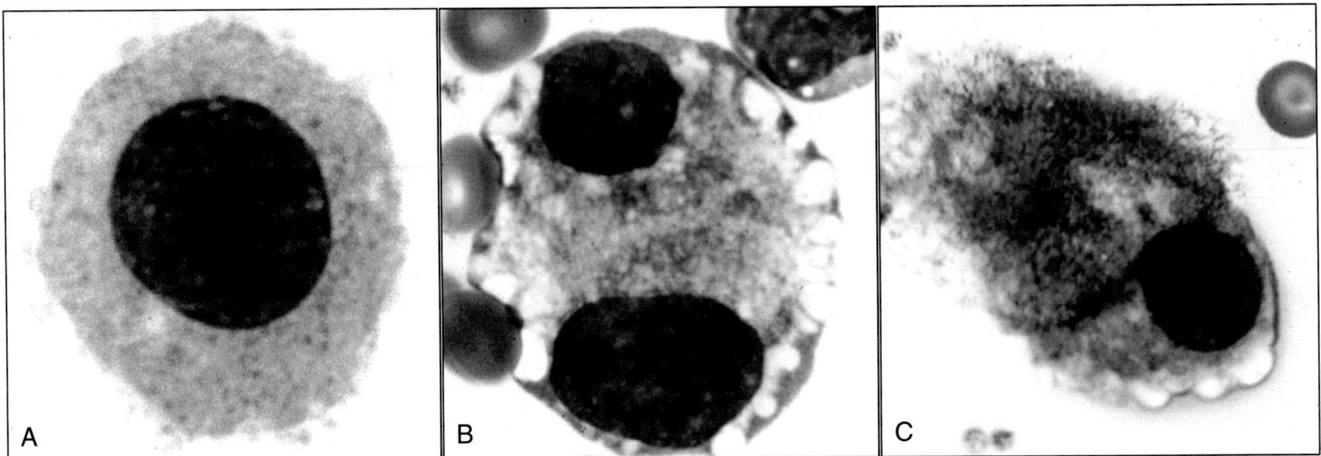

FIGURE 2-35
Dwarf megakaryocytes in blood from dogs with myeloid neoplasms. **A,** Dwarf megakaryocyte with single nucleus in blood from a dog with chronic myeloid leukemia (CML). **B,** Dwarf megakaryocyte with two nuclei in blood from a dog with CML. **C,** Dwarf megakaryocyte in blood from a dog with AML-M7. Wright-Giemsa stain.

examination of blood buffy coat smears. Those reaching the blood are quickly trapped in lung capillaries, where continued platelet production may occur.

Dwarf megakaryocytes are smaller than normal mature megakaryocytes and have decreased nuclear ploidy, but their cytoplasm generally contains granules and appears similar to that of blood platelets (Fig. 2-35). Dwarf megakaryocytes are common in the bone marrow of animals with myeloid neoplasms but are only rarely seen in blood.

Microfilaria

Microfilariae (nematode larvae) that might be observed include *Dirofilaria immitis* (see Fig. 2-24) and *Dirofilaria repens* in dogs, cats, and wild canids, *Dipetalonema reconditum* in dogs, and *Setaria* species in cattle and horses.[74]

Trypanosoma *Species*

Various *Trypanosoma* species may be seen in blood. These elongated, flagellated protozoa cause important diseases of

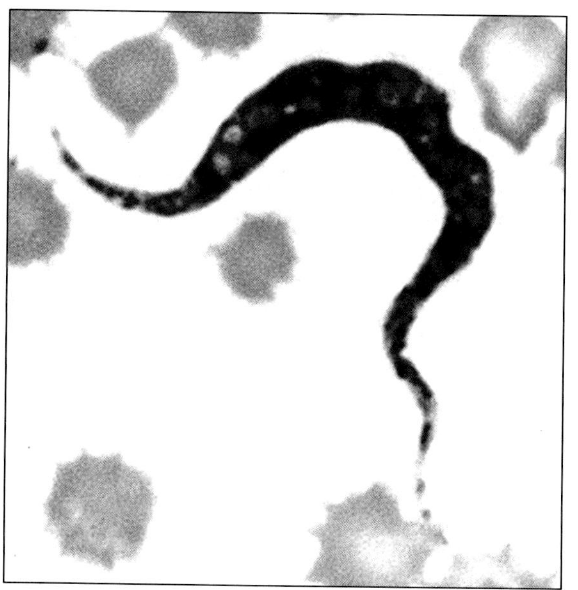

FIGURE 2-36
Trypanosoma theileri in blood from a 3-day-old female Angus calf. Wright stain.

Photograph of a stained blood film from a 1989 ASVCP slide review case submitted by H. Bender, A. Zajak, G. Moore, and G. Saunders.

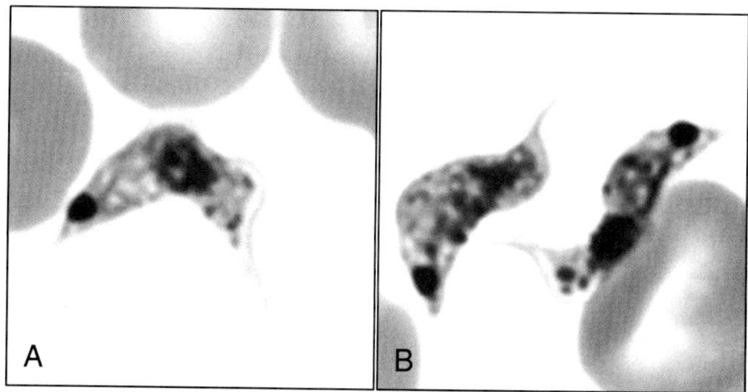

FIGURE 2-37
A, B, *Trypanosoma cruzi* organisms in blood from a dog. Wright stain.

Photographs of a stained blood film from a 2006 ASVCP slide review case submitted by P.K. Patten and J.M. Meinkoth.

livestock outside the United States,[74] but the species seen in cattle (*T. theileri*) in the United States is usually nonpathogenic (Fig. 2-36).[16,39] Many dogs are infected with *T. cruzi* in the United States, but organisms are rarely seen in blood and most cases are subclinical (Fig. 2-37). When present, clinical forms of disease have principally involved heart or neural dysfunction.[3]

Bacteria

Various bacterial species may be present in blood films. It is important to verify that these are not contaminants, especially during the staining procedure. The presence of phagocytized

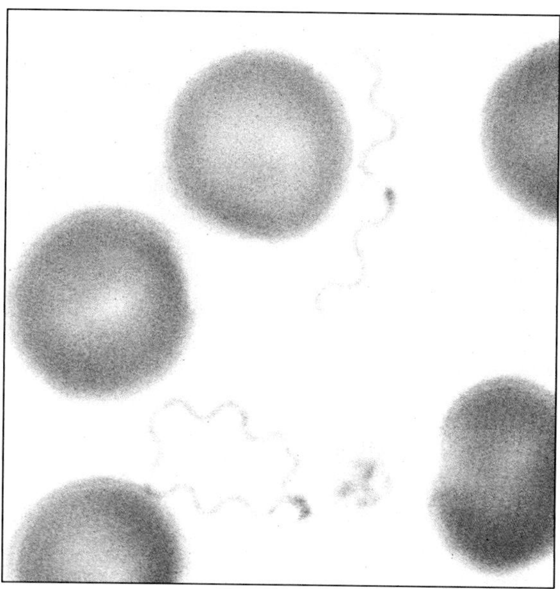

FIGURE 2-38
Two *Borrelia turicatae* spirochetes in blood from a North Central Florida dog. Wright-Giemsa stain.

bacteria within neutrophils indicates that the bacteria are likely of clinical significance. Spirochetes have been seen in blood from dogs with *Borrelia* infections.[55] *Borrelia burgdorferi* does not usually result in microscopically detectable spirochetemia.[56] However, relapsing fever spirochetes, *Borrelia turicatae* and *Borrelia hermsii*, have been readily identified in stained blood films from dogs in the United States (Fig. 2-38).[5,57,58,70]

REFERENCES

1. Allison RW, Velguth KE. Appearance of granulated cells in blood films stained by automated aqueous versus methanolic Romanowsky methods. *Vet Clin Pathol.* 2010;39:99-104.
2. Alsaker RD, Laber J, Stevens JB, et al. A comparison of polychromasia and reticulocyte counts in assessing erythrocyte regenerative response in the cat. *J Am Vet Med Assoc.* 1977;170:39-41.
3. Barr SC. American trypanosomiasis. In: Greene CE, ed. *Infectious Diseases of the Dog and Cat.* 3rd ed. St. Louis, MO: Saunders Elsevier; 2006:676-681.
4. Blaisdell FS, Dodds WJ. Evaluation of two microhematocrit methods for quantitating plasma fibrinogen. *J Am Vet Med Assoc.* 1977;171:340-342.
5. Breitschwerdt EB, Nicholson WL, Kiehl AR, et al. Natural infections with *Borrelia* spirochetes in two dogs in Florida. *J Clin Microbiol.* 1994;32:352-357.
6. Burkhard MJ, Baxter G, Thrall MA. Blood precipitate associated with intra-abdominal carboxymethylcellulose administration. *Vet Clin Pathol.* 1996;25:114-117.
7. Clark P, Mogg TD, Tvedten HW, et al. Artifactual changes in equine blood following storage, detected using the Advia 120 hematology analyzer. *Vet Clin Pathol.* 2002;31:90-94.
8. Corn SC, Wellman ML, Burkhard MJ, et al. IgM paraprotein interference with hemoglobin measurement using the CELL-DYN 3500. *Vet Clin Pathol.* 2008;37:61-65.
9. Cramer DV, Lewis RM. Reticulocyte response in the cat. *J Am Vet Med Assoc.* 1972;160:61-67.
10. Deol I, Hernandez AM, Pierre RV. Ethylenediamine tetraacetic acid-associated leuko agglutination. *Am J Clin Pathol.* 1995;103:338-340.
11. Dintenfass L, Kammer S. Re-evaluation of heat precipitation method for plasma fibrinogen estimation: effect of abnormal proteins and plasma viscosity. *J Clin Pathol.* 1976;29:130-134.

12. Eckersall PD. Proteins, proteomics, and the dysproteinemias. In: Kaneko JJ, Harvey JW, Bruss ML, eds. *Clinical Biochemistry of Domestic Animals.* 6th ed. San Diego: Academic Press; 2008:117-155.
13. Engelking LR. Evaluation of equine bilirubin and bile acid metabolism. *Comp Cont Ed Pract Vet.* 1989;11:328-336.
14. Espanol I, Pedro C, Remacha AF. Heinz bodies interfere with automated reticulocyte counts. *Haematologica.* 1999;84:373-374.
15. Fan LC, Dorner JL, Hoffman WE. Reticulocyte response and maturation in experimental acute blood loss anemia in the cat. *J Am Anim Hosp Assoc.* 1978;14:219-224.
16. Farrar RG, Klei TR. Prevalence of *Trypanosoma theileri* in Louisiana cattle. *J Parasitol.* 1990;76:734-736.
17. Fry MM, Kirk CA. Reticulocyte indices in a canine model of nutritional iron deficiency. *Vet Clin Pathol.* 2006;35:172-181.
18. Furlanello T, Tasca S, Caldin M, et al. Artifactual changes in canine blood following storage, detected using the ADVIA 120 hematology analyzer. *Vet Clin Pathol.* 2006;35:42-46.
19. George JW. The usefulness and limitations of hand-held refractometers in veterinary laboratory medicine: an historical and technical review. *Vet Clin Pathol.* 2001; 30:201-210.
20. Ginzinger DG, Clee SM, Dallongeville J, et al. Lipid and lipoprotein analysis of cats with lipoprotein lipase deficiency. *Eur J Clin Invest.* 1999;29:17-26.
21. Gossett KA, Carakostas MC. Effect of EDTA on morphology of neutrophils of healthy dogs and dogs with inflammation. *Vet Clin Pathol.* 1984;13:22-25.
22. Grindem CB. Blood cell markers. *Veterinary Clinics of North America, Small Animal Practice.* 1996;26:1043-1064.
23. Gunn-Moore DA, Watson TD, Dodkin SJ, et al. Transient hyperlipidaemia and anaemia in kittens. *Vet Rec.* 1997;140:355-359.
24. Harenberg J, Malsch R, Piazolo L, et al. Preferential binding of heparin to granulocytes of various species. *Am J Vet Res.* 1996;57:1016-1020.
25. Harr KE, Raskin RE, Heard DJ. Temporal effects of 3 commonly used anticoagulants on hematologic and biochemical variables in blood samples from macaws and Burmese pythons. *Vet Clin Pathol.* 2005;34:383-388.
26. Harvey JW. Hematology tip—stains for distemper inclusions. *Vet Clin Pathol.* 1982;11:12.
27. Harvey JW. Pathogenesis, laboratory diagnosis, and clinical implications of erythrocyte enzyme deficiencies in dogs, cats, and horses. *Vet Clin Pathol.* 2006;35: 144-156.
28. Harvey JW. The erythrocyte: physiology, metabolism and biochemical disorders. In: Kaneko JJ, Harvey JW, Bruss ML, eds. *Clinical Biochemistry of Domestic Animals.* 6th ed. San Diego: Academic Press; 2008:173-240.
29. Hinchcliff KW, Kociba GJ, Mitten LA. Diagnosis of EDTA-dependent pseudothrombocytopenia in a horse. *J Am Vet Med Assoc.* 1993;203:1715-1716.
30. Houwen B. Blood film preparation and staining procedures. *Lab Hematol.* 2000; 6:1-7.
31. Ihedioha JI, Onwubuche RC. Artifactual changes in PCV, hemoglobin concentration, and cell counts in bovine, caprine, and porcine blood stored at room and refrigerator temperatures. *Vet Clin Pathol.* 2007;36:60-63.
32. Jain NC. *Schalm's Veterinary Hematology.* 4th ed. Philadelphia: Lea & Febiger; 1986.
33. Jain NC. *Essentials of Veterinary Hematology.* Philadelphia: Lea & Febiger; 1993.
34. Kjelgaard-Hansen M, Jensen AL. Is the inherent imprecision of manual leukocyte differential counts acceptable for quantitative purposes? *Vet Clin Pathol.* 2006;35: 268-270.
35. Knoll JS. Clinical automated hematology systems. In: Feldman BF, Zinkl JG, Jain NC, eds. *Schalm's Veterinary Hematology.* 5th ed. Philadelphia: Lippincott Williams & Wilkins; 2000:3-11.
36. Lilliehook I, Tvedten H. Validation of the Sysmex XT-2000iV hematology system for dogs, cats, and horses. I. Erythrocytes, platelets, and total leukocyte counts. *Vet Clin Pathol.* 2009;38:163-174.
37. Lumsden JH. Quality control. In: Feldman BF, Zinkl JG, Jain NC, eds. *Schalm's Veterinary Hematology.* 5th ed. Philadelphia: Lippincott Williams & Wilkins; 2000: 16-19.
38. March H, Barger A, McCullough S, et al. Use of the ADVIA 120 for differentiating extracellular and intracellular hemoglobin. *Vet Clin Pathol.* 2005;34:106-109.
39. Matthews DM, Kingston N, Maki L, et al. *Trypanosoma theileri* Laveran, 1902, in Wyoming cattle. *Am J Vet Res.* 1979;40:623-629.
40. McSherry BJ, Lumsden JH, Baird JD. Hyperbilirubinemia in sick cattle. *Can Vet J.* 1984;48:237-240.
41. Moraglio D, Banfi G, Arnelli A. Association of pseudothrombocytopenia and pseudoleukopenia: evidence for different pathogenic mechanisms. *Scand J Clin Lab Invest.* 1994;54:257-265.
42. Muro J, Cuenca R, Pastor J, et al. Effects of lithium heparin and tripotassium EDTA on hematologic values of Hermann's tortoises *(Testudo hermanni). J Zoo Wildl Med.* 1998;29:40-44.
43. Orlov SN, Aksentsev SL, Kotelevtsev SV. Extracellular calcium is required for the maintenance of plasma membrane integrity in nucleated cells. *Cell Calcium.* 2005;38:53-57.
44. Pankraz A, Bauer N, Moritz A. Comparison of flow cytometry with the Sysmex XT2000iV automated analyzer for the detection of reticulated platelets in dogs. *Vet Clin Pathol.* 2009;38:30-38.
45. Pastor J, Cuenca R, Velarde R, et al. Evaluation of a hematology analyser with canine and feline blood. *Vet Clin Pathol.* 1997;26:138-147.
46. Perkins PC, Grindem CB, Cullins LD. Flow cytometric analysis of punctate and aggregate reticulocyte responses in phlebotomized cats. *Am J Vet Res.* 1995;56: 1564-1569.
47. Pierson FW. Laboratory techniques for avian hematology. In: Feldman BF, Zinkl JG, Jain NC, eds. *Schalm's Veterinary Hematology.* 5th ed. Philadelphia: Lippincott Williams & Wilkins; 2000:1145-1147.
48. Porter RE, Weiser MG. Effect of immune-mediated erythrocyte agglutination on analysis of canine blood using a multichannel blood cell counting system. *Vet Clin Pathol.* 1990;19:45-50.
49. Ragan HA. Platelet agglutination induced by ethylenediaminetetraacetic acid in blood samples from a miniature pig. *Am J Vet Res.* 1972;33:2601-2603.
50. Raskin RE. Cytochemical staining. In: Weiss DJ, Wardrop KJ, eds. *Schalm's Veterinary Hematology.* 6th ed. Ames, IA: Wiley-Blackwell; 2010:1141-1156.
51. Roszel J, Prier JE, Koprowska I. The occurrence of megakaryocytes in the peripheral blood of dogs. *J Am Vet Med Assoc.* 1965;147:133-137.
52. Sato S, Hirayama K, Koyama A, et al. Pseudoreticulocytosis in a patient with hemoglobin Koln due to autofluorescent erythrocytes enumerated as reticulocytes by the Cell-Dyn 4000. *Lab Hematol.* 2004;10:65-67.
53. Savage RA. Pseudoleukocytosis due to EDTA-induced platelet clumping. *Am J Clin Pathol.* 1984;81:317-322.
54. Schaefer DM, Priest H, Stokol T, et al. Anticoagulant-dependent in vitro hemagglutination in a cat. *Vet Clin Pathol.* 2009.
55. Schalm OW. Uncommon hematologic disorders: spirochetosis, trypanosomiasis, leishmaniasis, and Pelger-Huet anomaly. *Can Pract.* 1979;6:46-49.
56. Schwan TG, Burgdorfer W, Rosa PA. Borrelia. In: Murray PR, Baron EJ, Pfaller MA, et al, eds. *Manual of Clinical Microbiology.* 7th ed. Washington, DC: ASM Press; 1999:746-758.
57. Schwan TG, Raffel SJ, Schrumpf ME, et al. Phylogenetic analysis of the spirochetes *Borrelia parkeri* and *Borrelia turicatae* and the potential for tick-borne relapsing fever in Florida. *J Clin Microbiol.* 2005;43:3851-3859.
58. Stevenson C, Schwan T. *Borrelia hermsii* spirochetemia in a dog (abstract). *Proc XIVth Cong Int Soc Anim Clin Pathol.* 2010;18.
59. Stokol T, Erb HN. A comparison of platelet parameters in EDTA- and citrate-anticoagulated blood in dogs. *Vet Clin Pathol.* 2007;36:148-154.
60. Tasca S, Carli E, Caldin M, et al. Hematologic abnormalities and flow cytometric immunophenotyping results in dogs with hematopoietic neoplasia: 210 cases (2002-2006). *Vet Clin Pathol.* 2009;38:2-12.
61. Tasker S, Cripps PJ, Macklin AJ. Estimation of platelet counts on feline blood smears. *Vet Clin Pathol.* 1999;28:42-45.
62. Tennant BC, Center SA. Hepatic function. In: Kaneko JJ, Harvey JW, Bruss ML, eds. *Clinical Biochemistry of Domestic Animals.* 6th ed. San Diego, CA: Academic Press; 2008:379-412.
63. Tvedten H. Advanced hematology analyzers. Interpretation of results. *Vet Clin Pathol.* 1993;22:72-80.
64. Waitt LH, Cebra CK. Characterization of hypertriglyceridemia and response to treatment with insulin in llamas and alpacas: 31 cases (1995-2005). *J Am Vet Med Assoc.* 2008;232:1362-1367.
65. Waitt LH, Cebra CK. Characterization of hypertriglyceridemia and response to treatment with insulin in horses, ponies, and donkeys: 44 cases (1995-2005). *J Am Vet Med Assoc.* 2009;234:915-919.
66. Walencik J, Witeska M. The effects of anticoagulants on hematological indices and blood cell morphology of common carp (Cyprinus carpio L.). *Comp Biochem Physiol C Toxicol Pharmacol.* 2007;146:331-335.
67. Wardrop KJ. The Coombs' test in veterinary medicine: past, present, future. *Vet Clin Pathol.* 2005;34:325-334.
68. Weiss DJ. Uniform evaluation and semiquantitative reporting of hematologic data in veterinary laboratories. *Vet Clin Pathol.* 1984;13:27-31.
69. Werner LL, Christopher MM, Snipes J. Spurious leukocytosis and abnormal WBC histograms associated with Heinz bodies (abstract). *Vet Clin Pathol.* 1997;26: 20.
70. Whitney MS, Schwan TG, Sultemeier KB, et al. Spirochetemia caused by *Borrelia turicatae* infection in 3 dogs in Texas. *Vet Clin Pathol.* 2007;36:212-216.
71. Wills TB, Wardrop KJ. Pseudothrombocytopenia secondary to the effects of EDTA in a dog. *J Am Anim Hosp Assoc.* 2008;44:95-97.
72. Xenoulis PG, Steiner JM. Lipid metabolism and hyperlipidemia in dogs. *Vet J.* 2009.

73. Xenoulis PG, Suchodolski JS, Levinski MD, et al. Serum liver enzyme activities in healthy Miniature Schnauzers with and without hypertriglyceridemia. *J Am Vet Med Assoc.* 2008;232:63-67.
74. Zajac A, Conboy GA, Sloss MW. *Veterinary Clinical Parasitology.* 7th ed. Hoboken, NJ: Wiley-Blackwell; 2006.
75. Zandecki M, Genevieve F, Gerard J, et al. Spurious counts and spurious results on haematology analysers: a review. Part I: platelets. *Int J Lab Hematol.* 2007;29:4-20.
76. Zandecki M, Genevieve F, Gerard J, et al. Spurious counts and spurious results on haematology analysers: a review. Part II: white blood cells, red blood cells, haemoglobin, red cell indices and reticulocytes. *Int J Lab Hematol.* 2007;29:21-41.
77. Zelmanovic D, Hetherington EJ. Automated analysis of feline platelets in whole blood, including platelet count, mean platelet volume, and activation state. *Vet Clin Pathol.* 1998;27:2-9.

CHAPTER

3

HEMATOPOIESIS

OVERVIEW

Sites of Blood Cell Production

In mammals, primitive hematopoiesis begins outside the body of the embryo in the yolk sac and shortly thereafter within the aorta-gonad-mesonephros (AGM) region of the embryo.[42,130,139] Small clusters of hematopoietic stem cells (HSCs) have been identified attached to the endothelium of the yolk sac and the dorsal aorta. These HSCs and the associated endothelial cells are produced by common embryonic stem cells known as hemangioblasts.[34,74,150] In addition to HSCs, committed erythroid and megakaryocytic progenitor cells, primitive erythrocytes (large nucleated cells containing embryonal hemoglobin), large primitive reticulated platelets, and rare primitive macrophages are also produced in the yolk sacs of rodents and humans.[98,136] Notably, these primitive macrophages appear to develop directly from progenitor cells in the yolk sac without passing through a monocyte stage.[14] Definitive erythropoiesis, prominent megakaryocytopoiesis, and limited leukocyte production also occur in the yolk sacs of cats, with hematopoiesis persisting longer during gestation than it does in rodents and humans.[134] The AGM region transiently supports the development of HSCs and some committed hematopoietic progenitor cells (HPCs), but recognizable blood cells are not produced in the AGM.[93]

Sites of blood cell production shift during embryonic and fetal development as optimal microenvironments are produced in various tissues (Fig. 3-1).[102] The liver and, to a lesser extent, the spleen become the major hematopoietic organs by midgestation in the fetus.[129,134] Current evidence suggests that the AGM is more important than the yolk sack in providing HSCs to seed the liver and spleen, but the relative importance of each area in embryonic and fetal hematopoiesis remains to be clarified.[102] Blood cell production begins in bone marrow and lymphoid organs during midgestation in mammals, with nearly all blood cells being produced in these organs at the time of birth.[134] Blood cells are produced in the bone marrow of adult birds[20]; the bone marrow and sometimes the spleen of adult reptiles[30]; the kidney, liver, spleen, and/or bone marrow of amphibians[5,42]; and the kidney and/or spleen of fish.[42,48]

Organization of Bone Marrow

Bone marrow develops in mammals during the second trimester.[21] Rudimentary fetal bone is initially filled with cartilage. Chondrocytes hypertrophy and promote mineralization of the cartilage matrix in the center of the rudimentary bone. This is followed by the entry of progenitor cells, which develop into chondroclasts that partially degrade the mineralized cartilage and form bone marrow spaces colonized by incoming blood vessels.[23,131] Osteoblast progenitors enter the space created, adhere to remaining cartilage, develop into mature osteoblasts, and begin the formation of bony trabeculae. Vascular sinuses and extravascular mesenchymal cells subsequently form a connective tissue meshwork within which HSCs originating from the liver (and probably the spleen) bind, proliferate, and differentiate, ultimately producing circulating blood cells.[131] When these structures are fully developed, blood is supplied to the bone marrow by nutrient arteries and periosteal capillaries (Fig. 3-2).[7]

The stroma of the marrow is a connective tissue consisting of stromal cells (fibroblast-like cells, also called reticular cells), adipocytes, vascular elements (endothelial cells and myocytes), neural elements, and extracellular matrix (ECM), with the arrangement creating both intravascular and extravascular spaces (Figs. 3-3, 3-4).[146,147] In postnatal mammals, blood cells are continuously produced within the extravascular spaces of bone marrow. Leukocytes are also produced within the extravascular spaces of bone marrow in birds, but erythrocytes and thrombocytes are produced within the vascular spaces of the avian marrow.[20]

This specialized arrangement of the marrow vasculature is important in the organization of intramedullary hematopoietic microenvironments, as marrow endothelial cells are actively involved in the regulation of transendothelial (not interendothelial) movement of hematopoietic cells and blood cells between the extravascular hematopoietic space and peripheral blood.[92,114] Together, endothelial cells and stromal cells produce the ECM, which consists of collagen fibers, various macromolecules capable of binding cells, and basal laminae of the sinuses.[100,109] The marrow stromal cells have

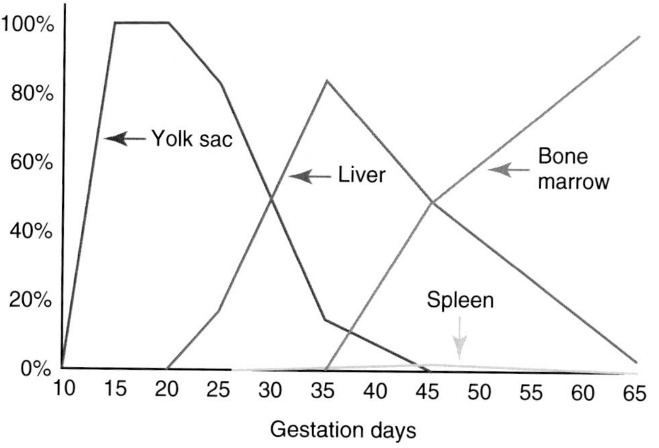

FIGURE 3-1
Sites of definitive hematopoiesis during prenatal development in cats. Percentages represent relative contributions of sites to definitive blood cell production. Lymphoid populations also develop in lymph nodes and thymus beginning in midgestation *(not shown)*.

Redrawn from Tiedemann K, van Ooyen B. Prenatal hematopoiesis and blood characteristics of the cat. Anat Embryol (Berl). *1978;153:243-267.*

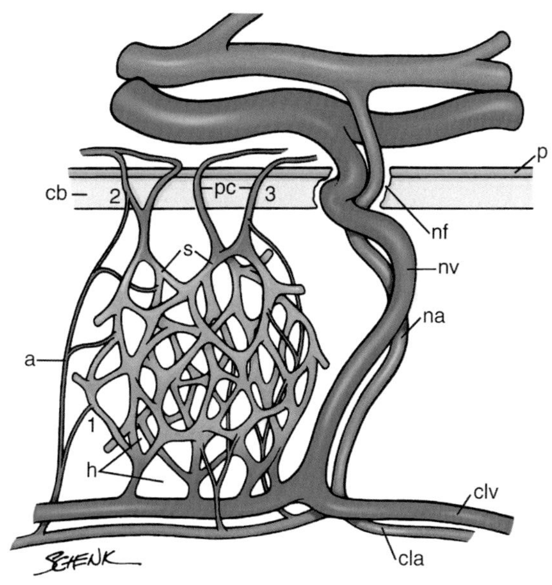

FIGURE 3-2
Anatomy and circulation of the bone marrow. Periosteum (p), cortical bone (cb), nutrient foramen (nf), nutrient artery (na), nutrient vein (nv), central longitudinal artery (cla), central longitudinal vein (clv), periosteal capillaries (pc), arteriole (a), sinuses (s), hematopoietic compartment (h), anastomosis of the nutrient capillaries and sinuses (1), anastomosis of the nutrient artery capillaries and periosteal capillaries (2), anastomosis of the periosteal capillaries and sinuses (3).

From Alsaker RD. The formation, emergence, and maturation of the reticulocyte: a review. Vet Clin Pathol. *1977;6(3):7-12.*

extensively branched cytoplasmic processes and, along with the fibers that they produce, provide structural support for the marrow (Fig. 3-5).[147] These stromal cells have generally been considered to be fibroblast-like, but they also display smooth muscle characteristics in culture and have been classified as myofibroblasts by some investigators.[122] The particular stromal cells that support the endothelium of the venous sinuses are termed adventitial stromal cells (Fig. 3-6).[147] Granulopoiesis also occurs primarily on the surface of stromal cells.[125] Adipocytes develop from mesenchymal stem cells and may share common hematopoietic functions with stromal cells.[47] Autonomic nerves occur in bone marrow. Their function is not clear, but direct and indirect effects of the sympathetic nervous system on hematopoietic stem cell and hematopoietic progenitor cell proliferation and motility have been described.[61]

In addition to hematopoietic cells and developing blood cells, a number of accessory cells involved in regulating hematopoiesis reside within the extravascular space of mammalian bone marrow. These accessory cells include macrophages, mature lymphocytes, and natural killer (NK) cells.[12,31,33,85] Erythrocyte development occurs in close association with marrow macrophages.[26]

In contrast to other organs such as skin and intestine, where continuous new cell production occurs throughout life, hematopoietic cells and their progeny in bone marrow are not arranged in stratified layers of progressively more differentiated cells. Although some segregation of cell types may be visualized by microscopic examination of stained bone marrow sections, the overall impression is that bone marrow contains an unstructured mixture of cells of different lineages and stages of maturation. Nonetheless, hematopoietic cells develop in specialized microenvironmental niches within the bone marrow.

Hematopoietic Stem Cells and Progenitor Cells

Beginning in midgestation and continuing throughout postnatal life, mammalian blood cells are produced continuously from HSCs within the extravascular spaces of the bone marrow. HSCs are capable of proliferation; they exhibit long-term self-renewal and differentiation. HSCs replicate only once every 8 to 10 weeks.[2] The term *hematopoietic progenitor cell* (HPC) refers to cells that form colonies in bone marrow culture like HSCs but do not have long-term self-renewal capacities. HSCs and HPCs are mononuclear cells that cannot be distinguished morphologically from lymphocytes. The presence of a transmembrane glycoprotein termed cluster of differentiation antigen 34 (CD34) has been used to identify HSCs and early HPCs, but some HSCs (possibly inactive ones) lack CD34.[43] In addition, CD34 is also present on the surface of nonhematopoietic stem cells and vascular endothelial cells.[72,149] CD34 is believed to play a role in cell adhesion.[43]

The most primitive HSC has the capacity to differentiate into HPCs of all blood cell lineages and several cell types in tissue. The frequency of HSCs in the marrow is estimated to be less than 0.01% of nucleated marrow cells in adult mice and less than 0.0001% of nucleated marrow cells in adult cats.[2] HSCs produce HPCs that can give rise to one or more blood cell types. Thus, HPCs are much more numerous in marrow

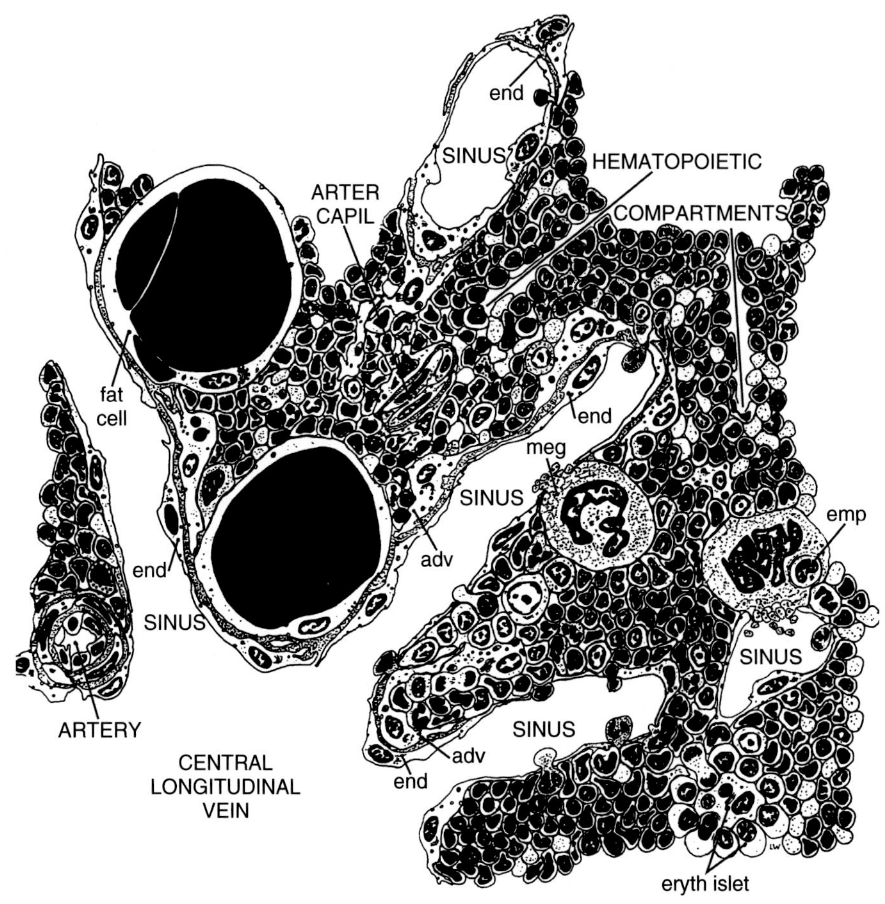

FIGURE 3-3

Schematic view of a cross section of bone marrow near the central longitudinal vein. Hematopoietic cells lie in the hematopoietic compartment between the vascular sinuses that drain into the central vein. The sinus wall consists of endothelial cells *(end)*, a basement membrane, and, in some areas, adventitial stromal cells *(adv)*. Megakaryocytes *(meg)* lie against the outside of the vascular sinus wall and discharge proplatelets directly into the vascular lumen through apertures in the sinus wall. Erythroid cells are shown developing in an erythroid islet *(eryth islet)* around a central macrophage. Emperipolesis *(emp)*, the entry of megakaryocyte cytoplasm by other cells, is occasionally observed.

From Weiss L. The Blood Cells and Hematopoietic Tissues. *New York: Elsevier; 1984.*

than are HSCs. Less than 2% of nucleated bone marrow cells in adult dogs are $CD34^+$, but up to 18% $CD34^+$ cells have been reported in neonatal pups.[38,128]

The HSC produces a common lymphoid progenitor (CLP) and a common myeloid progenitor (CMP), as shown in Figure 3-7. The CLP is believed to give rise to B lymphocytes, T lymphocytes, and NK cells.[16] The CMP is believed to give rise to all nonlymphoid blood cells (see Fig. 3-7) as well as macrophages, dendritic cells, osteoclasts, and mast cells.[66,89] HPCs proliferate with higher frequency than do HSCs, but the self-renewal capabilities of HPCs decrease as progressive differentiation and cell lineage restrictions occur. When measured in an in vitro cell culture assay, HPCs are referred to as colony-forming units (CFUs). HPCs that rapidly proliferate, retain their ability to migrate, and form multiple subcolonies around a larger central colony in culture are called burst-forming units (BFUs).

The CMP (also called a colony-forming unit-granulocyte-erythrocyte-monocyte-megakaryocyte [CFU-GEMM]) gives rise to the megakaryocyte-erythrocyte progenitor (MkEP) and the granulocyte-monocyte progenitor (GMP). The MkEP produces megakaryocyte progenitors (MkP) and erythrocyte progenitors (EP). The GMP produces the granulocyte progenitor (GP), the monocyte-dendritic cell progenitor (MDP), the basophil-mast cell progenitor (BMaP), and the eosinophil progenitor (EoP) in mice (see Fig. 3-7). However, in humans, the EoP may develop from the CMP, rather than the GMP.[89]

Mesenchymal Stem Cells

Mesenchymal stem cells (MSCs) are estimated to occur in bone marrow at a frequency of 0.001% to 0.0002% of nucleated marrow cells.[84] Evidence suggests that the MSC lineage differentiation pathways are less strictly delineated (exhibit

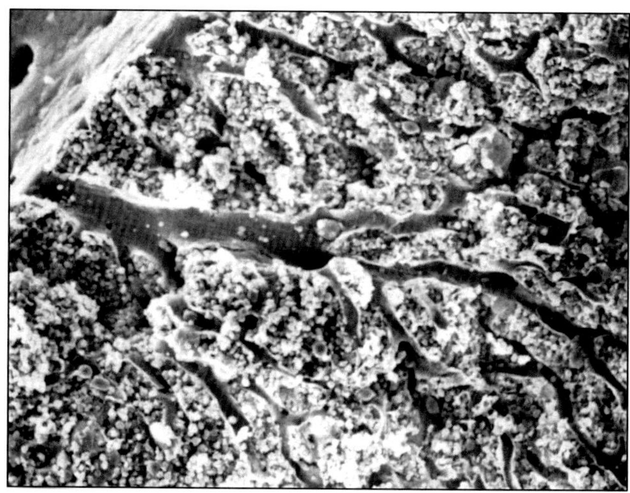

FIGURE 3-4

A scanning electron micrograph of the cut surface of bone marrow showing a system of vascular sinuses originating at the periphery of the marrow *(right side of field)* and draining into a large vein *(upper left corner)*. The large vein has several apertures in its wall, representing tributary venous sinuses. Hematopoietic tissue lies between the vascular sinuses.

From Weiss L. The hematopoietic microenvironment of the bone marrow: an ultrastructural study of the stroma of rats. Anat Rec. *1976;186:161-184.*

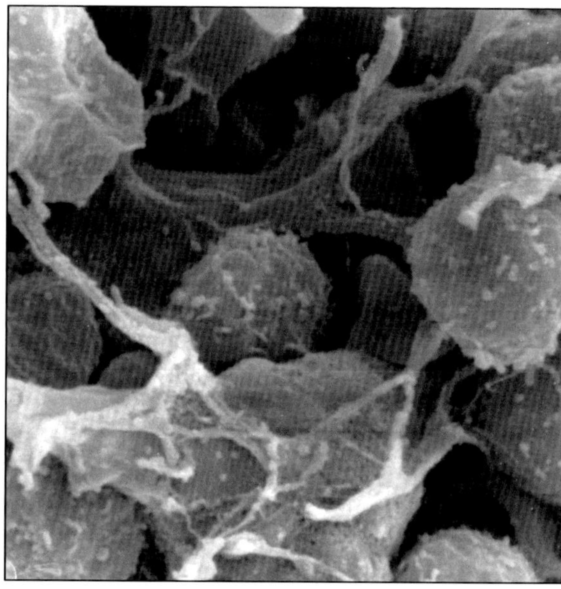

FIGURE 3-5

A scanning electron micrograph from the extravascular space in rat bone marrow. Spherical hematopoietic cells are shown developing in close association with marrow stromal cells and their cytoplasmic processes.

Courtesy of Ahmed Deldar.

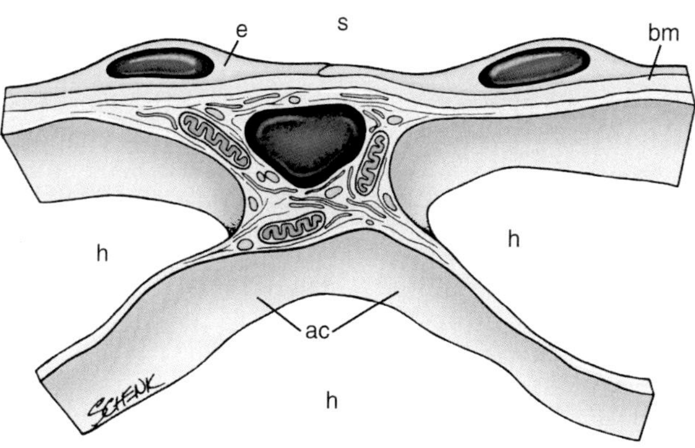

FIGURE 3-6

Structure of the bone marrow sinus wall. Sinus lumen (s), endothelial cell (e), basement membrane (bm), hematopoietic compartment (h), adventitial stromal cell with processes (ac).

From Alsaker RD. The formation, emergence, and maturation of the reticulocyte: a review. Vet Clin Pathol. *1977;6(3):7-12.*

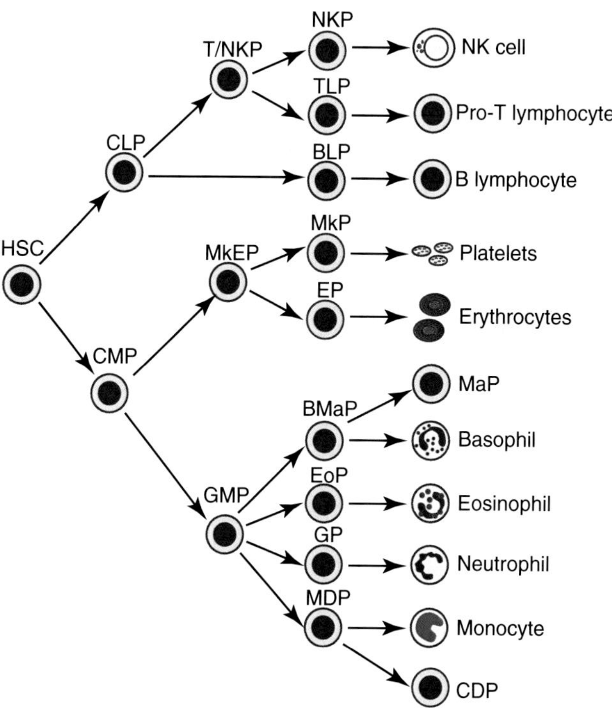

FIGURE 3-7

Simplified working model of hematopoiesis. HSC, hematopoietic stem cell; CLP, common lymphoid progenitor; CMP, common myeloid progenitor; T/NKP, T lymphocyte-natural killer cell progenitor; MkEP, megakaryocyte-erythroid progenitor; GMP, granulocyte-monocyte progenitor; NKP, natural killer cell progenitor; TLP, T lymphocyte progenitor; BLP, B lymphocyte progenitor; MkP, megakaryocyte progenitor; EP, erythroid progenitor; BMaP, basophil-mast cell progenitor; EoP, eosinophil progenitor, GP, granulocyte progenitor; MDP, monocyte-dendritic cell progenitor; NK, natural killer; MaP, mast cell progenitor; CDP, common dendritic progenitor.

greater plasticity) than the HSC pathways.[115] MSCs have the ability to differentiate into multiple lineages, including marrow stromal cells, adipocytes, osteoblasts, chondrocytes, fibroblasts, and myoblasts.[95] Progenitor cells for a variety of peripheral tissue cell types are also present in bone marrow. Some studies suggest that MSCs may also produce epithelial cells, hepatocytes, and neuronal cells.[81,115] Endothelial progenitor cells are present in bone marrow and blood; however, their origin remains to be clarified. Evidence has been presented suggesting an association with both MSCs and HSCs.[24,118]

Homing of Hematopoietic Stem Cells and Progenitor Cells to the Marrow

Homing is the process by which circulating HSCs and HPCs bind to the luminal surface of bone marrow endothelial cells, migrate through the endothelial cells, bind selectively to sites in the extravascular space, and begin the process of proliferation and differentiation. Homing of HSCs/HPCs is mediated by chemoattractants produced by endothelial cells and other cells in the microenvironment and by adhesion molecules expressed on the surfaces of HSCs/HPCs that bind to proteoglycans and glycoproteins on the surfaces of various marrow cells and the extracellular matrix.[27]

The chemokine (chemoattractant cytokine) CXCL12, also called stromal cell-derived factor-1 (SDF-1), is especially important in the homing of HSCs/HPCs, but other chemoattractants are also involved in this process. SDF-1 is produced by both marrow endothelial cells and stromal cells, and migration of HSCs/HPCs from blood to bone marrow occurs toward an SDF-1 gradient by virtue of an SDF-1 receptor CXCR4 expressed on these migrating cells. SDF-1 promotes the expression of CXCR4 and other adhesion molecules on the surface of HSCs/HPCs and induces transendothelial migration.[27]

HSCs/HPCs must be activated by locally produced factors (including SDF-1) for optimal transendothelial migration to occur. P- and E-selectin molecules (membrane-spanning, sugar-binding glycoproteins), expressed on bone marrow endothelial cells, bind to glycosylated ligands on HSCs/HPCs to promote an initial loose, rolling-type adhesion between HSCs/HPCs and endothelial cells in blood. Tight adhesion and migration through endothelial cells is dependent on integrin molecules—particularly the $\alpha_4\beta_1$-integrin (very late antigen-4, VLA-4) on the surfaces of migrating cells—binding to their counterreceptors, especially vascular cell adhesion molecule-1 (VCAM-1), on endothelial cells.[27]

The first successful bone marrow transplants were done experimentally in dogs in the late 1950s.[6] Because of the homing properties of HSCs, bone marrow transplants are performed by injecting bone marrow cells into the blood. In addition, HSCs/HPCs naturally circulate in blood. The physiologic mechanisms involved in the release of these hematopoietic cells from the bone marrow are not well defined, but HSC and HPC numbers can be increased markedly in blood following injection of growth factors such as granulocyte colony-stimulating factor (G-CSF).[113] In fact, intravenous injection of growth factors is one approach used to collect increased numbers of stem cells from blood for human bone marrow transplantation.[46]

Hematopoietic Microenvironment

Blood cell production occurs throughout life in the bone marrow of adult animals because of the unique microenvironment present there. The hematopoietic microenvironment is a complex meshwork composed of stromal cells, endothelial cells, adipocytes, macrophages, subsets of lymphocytes, NK cells, osteoblasts, ECM components, and glycoprotein growth factors that profoundly affect HSC and HPC engraftment, survival, proliferation, and differentiation.[1]

Stromal cells and endothelial cells produce components of the ECM, including collagen fibers, basement membranes of vessels and vascular sinuses, proteoglycans, and glycoproteins. In addition to providing structural support, the ECM is important in the binding of hematopoietic cells and soluble growth factors to stromal cells and other cells in the microenvironment so that optimal proliferation and differentiation can occur by virtue of these cell-cell interactions (Fig. 3-8).[1,106]

Collagen fibers produced by stromal cells may not have direct stimulatory effects on hematopoiesis but rather are permissive, promoting hematopoiesis by forming a scaffolding around which the other elements of the microenvironment are organized. Hematopoietic cells can adhere to collagen types I and VI.[22]

Adhesion molecules (most importantly β_1-integrins) on the surface of hematopoietic cells bind to ECM glycoproteins such as VCAM-1, hemonectin, fibronectin, laminin, vitronectin, and thrombospondin. The spectrum of the expression of adhesion molecules on hematopoietic cells that differentially bind to ECM glycoproteins varies with the type, maturity, and activation state of the hematopoietic cells. In addition to anchoring cells to a given microenvironmental niche, the binding of adhesion molecules on hematopoietic cells also

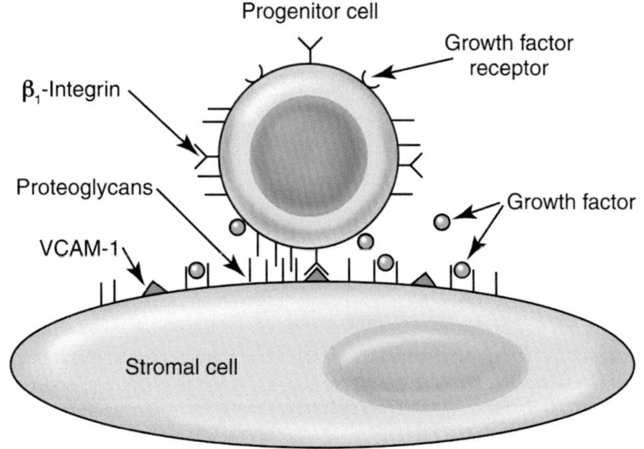

FIGURE 3-8
Interactions between a progenitor cell and a stromal cell in the extravascular microenvironment of the bone marrow. VCAM-1, vascular cell adhesion molecule-1.

plays a role in cell regulation directly by activating signal pathways for cell growth, survival, and differentiation or indirectly by modulating the responses to hematopoietic growth factors.[22]

A proteoglycan consists of a protein core with repeating carbohydrate glycosaminoglycans (GAGs) attached. Major proteoglycans in the marrow include heparan sulfate, chondroitin sulfate, hyaluronic acid, and dermatan sulfate. Proteoglycans enhance hematopoiesis by trapping soluble growth factors in the vicinity of hematopoietic cells and by strengthening the binding of hematopoietic cells to the stroma.[28]

Hematopoietic cells develop in specific niches within the marrow. During steady-state conditions, quiescent HSCs are concentrated near endosteal and trabecular bone, where osteoblasts help to regulate their numbers.[152] HSCs and HPCs are also located near vascular sinuses, where they appear more active. HSCs and HPCs in this vascular niche likely have homeostatic roles during steady-state conditions.[94] Erythroid cells develop around macrophages and megakaryocytes form adjacent to sinusoidal endothelial cells; granulocyte development is associated with stromal cells located away from the vascular sinuses.[1,63,66]

Hematopoietic Growth Factors

Proliferation of HSCs and HPCs cannot occur spontaneously but requires the presence of specific hematopoietic growth factors (HGFs); these may be produced locally in the bone marrow (paracrine or autocrine) or more remotely by peripheral tissues and transported to the marrow through the blood (endocrine). All cells in the hematopoietic microenvironment, including the hematopoietic cells themselves, produce HGFs and/or inhibitors of hematopoiesis.[69] Some HGFs have been called poietins (erythropoietin [EPO] and thrombopoietin [TPO]). Other growth factors have been classified as colony-stimulating factors (CSFs) based on in vitro culture studies. Finally, some HGFs have been described as interleukins (ILs).[67]

Hematopoietic cells express receptors for more than one HGF on their surfaces. The number of each receptor type present depends on the stage of cell activation and differentiation. Binding of an HGF to its receptor results in a series of enzymatic reactions that generate transcription factors; these promote the synthesis of molecules that inhibit apoptosis, the formation of cell-cycle regulators (cyclins), and the synthesis of additional HGFs and their receptors.[22,67] The pathways involved in generating lineage-restricted transcription factors is complex and beyond the scope of this text.[22]

HGFs vary in the type(s) of HSCs and/or HPCs that they can stimulate to proliferate. Factors are often synergistic in their effects on hematopoietic cells. In some instances, an HGF may not directly stimulate the proliferation of a given cell type, but may potentiate its proliferation by inducing the expression of membrane receptors for HGFs that do directly stimulate proliferation. Some glycoproteins, such as IL-1 and tumor necrosis factor-α (TNF-α), can modulate hematopoiesis indirectly by stimulating marrow stromal cells, endothelial cells, and T lymphocytes to produce HGFs. Different combinations of HGFs regulate the growth of different types of HSCs and/or HPCs.[66]

Early-acting HGFs are involved with triggering dormant (G_O) primitive HSCs to begin cycling. Stem cell factor (SCF), fms-like tyrosine kinase 3 ligand (Flt3L), and TPO are important early factors that act in combination with one or more other cytokines such as IL-3, IL-6, IL-11, and G-CSF.

Intermediate-acting HGFs have broad specificity. IL-3 (multi-CSF), granulocyte-macrophage-CSF (GM-CSF), and IL-4 support proliferation of multipotent HPCs. These factors also interact with late-acting factors to stimulate the proliferation of a wide variety of committed progenitor cells. Late-acting HGFs have restricted specificity. Macrophage-CSF (M-CSF), G-CSF, EPO, TPO, and IL-5 are more restrictive in their actions. They have their most potent effects on committed progenitor cells and on later stages of development when cell lines can be recognized morphologically.[67] TPO appears to be an exception. In addition to stimulating platelet production, it is important in maintaining a population of HSCs in their osteoblastic niche.[8]

ERYTHROPOIESIS

Primitive Erythropoiesis

Primitive erythropoiesis begins and predominates in the yolk sac but also occurs later in the liver. Primitive erythrocytes are large (more than 400 fL in humans), generally nucleated cells with high nuclear:cytoplasmic ratios. Their nuclei have open (noncondensed) chromatin and their cytoplasm contains predominantly embryonal hemoglobin (Hb) with a high oxygen affinity.[117,133,138] In mammals as in nonmammalian species, primitive RBCs enter the blood as nucleated cells, but in contrast to nonmammalian species, enucleation can eventually occur in the circulation.[70] These extruded nuclei circulate for a short time in the blood. They are surrounded by a small amount of cytoplasm and have been called pyrenocytes.[97]

A switch to definitive erythropoiesis occurs during fetal development. This results in the production of smaller cells that generally extrude their nuclei before entering the blood, produce fetal Hb (in some species) and adult Hb, and are highly dependent on EPO for proliferation.[138]

Hematopoietic Progenitor Cells and the Bone Marrow Microenvironment

The CMP gives rise to the MkEP, which can differentiate into megakaryocyte progenitors (MkPs) or erythroid progenitors (EPs). The production of EPs is stimulated by SCF, IL-3, GM-CSF, and TPO.[67,78] The earliest EP is the burst-forming-unit erythrocyte (BFU-E), which differentiates into the colony-forming-unit erythrocyte (CFU-E). EPO is the primary growth factor involved in the proliferation and differentiation of CFU-Es into rubriblasts, the first morphologically recognizable erythroid cells. CFU-Es are more responsive to EPO than BFU-E cells because CFU-Es exhibit greater numbers of surface receptors for EPO.[116]

Marrow macrophages are important components of the hematopoietic microenvironment involved with erythropoiesis. Both early and late stages of erythroid development occur with intimate membrane apposition to central macrophages in "erythroid islands." Several adhesion molecules on erythroid cells and macrophages, and extracellular matrix glycoproteins are important in forming these erythroid islands.[26] Direct contact with these macrophages enhances the proliferation of erythroid precursors under basal conditions. Central macrophages may promote basal erythrocyte production by producing positive growth factors, including EPO; however, they may inhibit erythropoiesis by producing negative factors such as IL-1, TNF-α, transforming growth factor-β (TGF-β), and interferons (IFNs)-α, -β, and -γ in inflammatory conditions.[25,145,154] The finding that EPO can also be produced by erythroid progenitors suggests that these cells may support erythropoiesis by autocrine stimulation.[126] Although some degree of basal regulation of erythropoiesis occurs within the marrow microenvironment, humoral regulation is also important, with EPO production occurring primarily within peritubular interstitial cells of the kidney and various inhibitory cytokines being produced at sites of inflammation throughout the body.

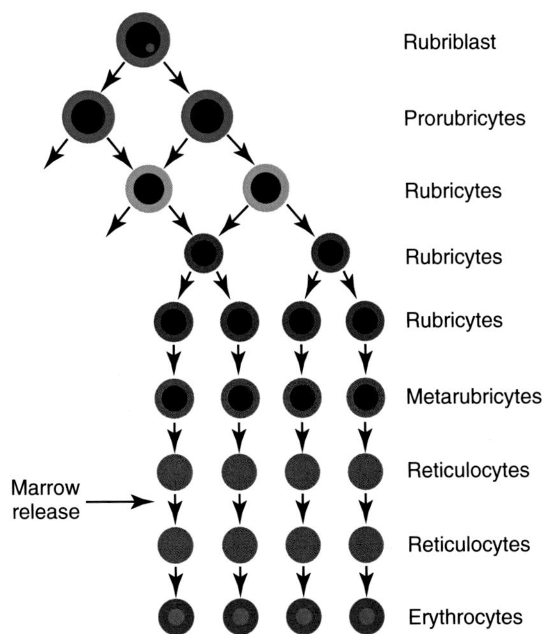

FIGURE 3-9
Diagram of erythropoiesis showing the release of reticulocytes into blood as it normally occurs in dogs.

Nutrients Needed for Erythropoiesis

In addition to amino acids and essential fatty acids, several metals and vitamins are required for normal erythropoiesis. Iron is needed for the synthesis of heme, an essential component of Hb and certain enzymes. Copper, in the form of ceruloplasmin, is important in the release of iron from tissue to plasma for transport to developing erythroid cells. Vitamin B_6 (pyridoxine) is needed as a cofactor in the first enzymatic step in heme synthesis.

Tetrahydrofolic acid, the active form of folic acid (a B vitamin), is needed for the transfer of single carbon-containing molecules in DNA and RNA synthesis. The physiologic mechanism of B_{12} involvement in erythrocyte production is not well understood, but it is related to folate metabolism. Cobalt is essential for the synthesis of B_{12} by ruminants.[51]

Maturation of Erythroid Cells

Rubriblasts are continuously generated from progenitor cells in the extravascular space of the bone marrow. The production of a rubriblast initiates a series of approximately four divisions over a period of 3 or 4 days to produce about 16 metarubricytes that are no longer capable of division (Fig. 3-9).[36] These divisions are called maturational divisions because there is a progressive maturation of the nucleus and cytoplasm concomitant with each division.

When they are stained with Romanowsky-type blood stains, early precursors have intensely blue cytoplasm owing to the presence of many basophilic ribosomes and polyribosomes that are actively synthesizing globin chains and smaller amounts of other proteins. As these cells divide and mature, overall cell size decreases, nuclear chromatin condensation increases, cytoplasmic basophilia decreases, and Hb progressively accumulates, imparting a red coloration to the cytoplasm (Fig. 3-10). Cells with both red and blue coloration are described as having polychromatophilic cytoplasm. An immature erythrocyte, termed a reticulocyte, is formed following extrusion of the metarubricyte nucleus. This generally occurs while cells are still bound to central macrophages.[26] Extruded nuclei are bound and phagocytosed by a novel receptor on the surface of bone marrow macrophages.[107] However, nuclei can be extruded in blood when metarubricytes are released from the bone marrow (Fig. 3-11).[119]

Early reticulocytes have polylobulated surfaces. Their cytoplasm contains ribosomes, polyribosomes, and mitochondria necessary for the completion of Hb synthesis.[15] Reticulocytes derive their name from a network or reticulum that appears when they are stained with basic dyes such as new methylene blue and brilliant cresyl green. That network is not preexisting but rather an artifact formed by the precipitation of ribosomal ribonucleic acids and proteins secondary to staining.[57] As reticulocytes mature, the amount of ribosomal material decreases until only a few basophilic specks can be visualized with reticulocyte staining procedures. These mature reticulocytes have been referred to as type IV reticulocytes[53] or punctate reticulocytes.[7,101]

The development of a reticulocyte into a mature erythrocyte is a gradual process that requires a variable number of days depending on the species involved. Consequently the morphologic and physiologic properties of reticulocytes vary with the stage of maturation. The cell surface undergoes extensive remodeling, with loss of membrane material and ultimately the formation of the biconcave shape of mature

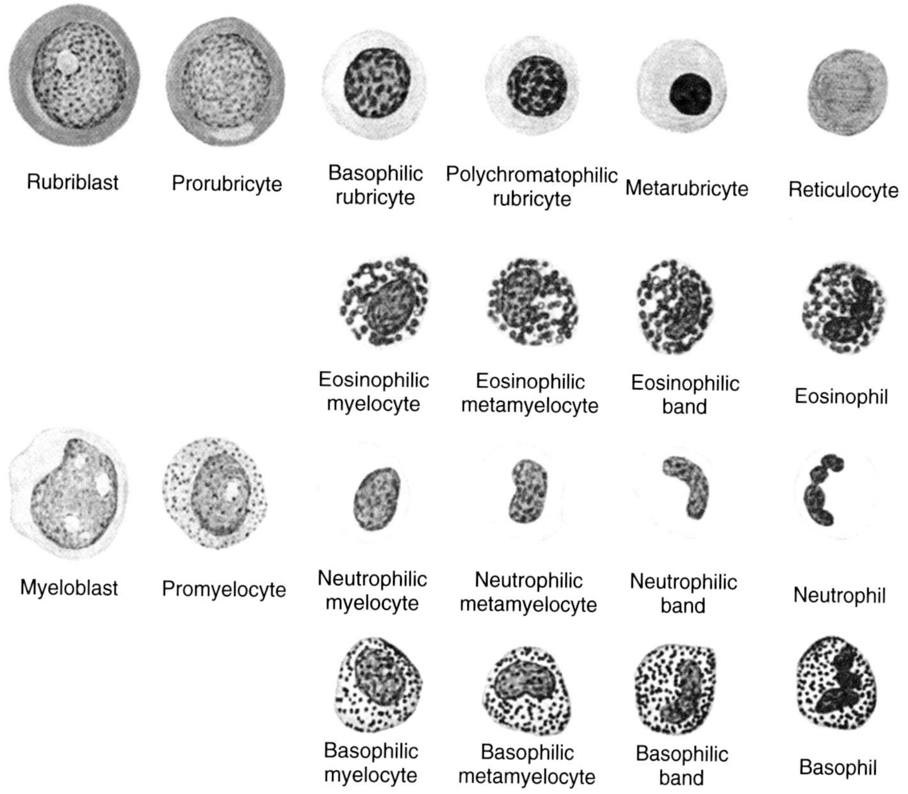

FIGURE 3-10

Maturation of canine erythroid and granulocytic cells as they appear in Wright-Giemsa-stained bone marrow aspirate smears.

Drawing by Perry Bain.

erythrocytes.[15] The loss of membrane protein and lipid components requires ATP and involves the formation of intracellular multivesicular endosomes that fuse with the plasma membrane, releasing vesicles (exosomes) extracellularly.[45,140] This is a highly selective process in which some proteins (e.g., transferrin receptor 1 and fibronectin receptor) are lost and cytoskeletal proteins (e.g., spectrin) and firmly bound transmembrane proteins (e.g., the anion transporter and glycophorin A) are retained and concentrated.[45,103]

The mitochondria undergo degenerative changes in a programmed death phenomenon (mitoptosis)[45] and are either digested or extruded following entrapment in structures resembling autophagic vacuoles (Fig. 3-12).[90,120] The polysomes separate into monosomes, decrease in number, and disappear as reticulocytes mature into erythrocytes. The degradation of ribosomes appears to be energy-dependent and presumably involves proteases and RNAases.[112]

Reticulocyte maturation begins in the bone marrow and is completed in the peripheral blood and spleen in dogs, cats, and pigs.[56] As reticulocytes mature, they lose the surface receptors needed to adhere to the fibronectin and thrombospondin components of the extracellular matrix, presumably facilitating their release from the bone marrow.[132] Reticulocytes become progressively more deformable as they mature, a characteristic that also facilitates their release from the marrow.[144] To exit the extravascular space of the marrow, reticulocytes press against the abluminal surfaces of endothelial cells making up the sinus wall. Cytoplasm thins and small pores develop in endothelial cells, which allow reticulocytes to be pushed through by a small pressure gradient across the sinus wall.[79,143] These pores apparently close after cell passage.

Relatively immature aggregate-type reticulocytes are released from canine bone marrow; consequently most of these cells appear polychromatophilic when they are viewed following routine blood-film staining procedures.[73] Reticulocytes are generally not released from bone marrow of nonanemic cats until they mature to punctate-type reticulocytes (Fig. 3-13); consequently few or no aggregate reticulocytes (less than 0.4%) but up to 10% punctate reticulocytes are found in blood from normal adult cats.[29] The high percentage of punctate reticulocytes results from a long maturation time with delayed degradation of RNA.[39] Reticulocytes are generally absent in the peripheral blood of healthy adult cattle and goats, but a small number of punctate types (0.5%) may occur in adult sheep.[56] Based on microscopic examination of blood films stained with new methylene blue, equine reticulocytes

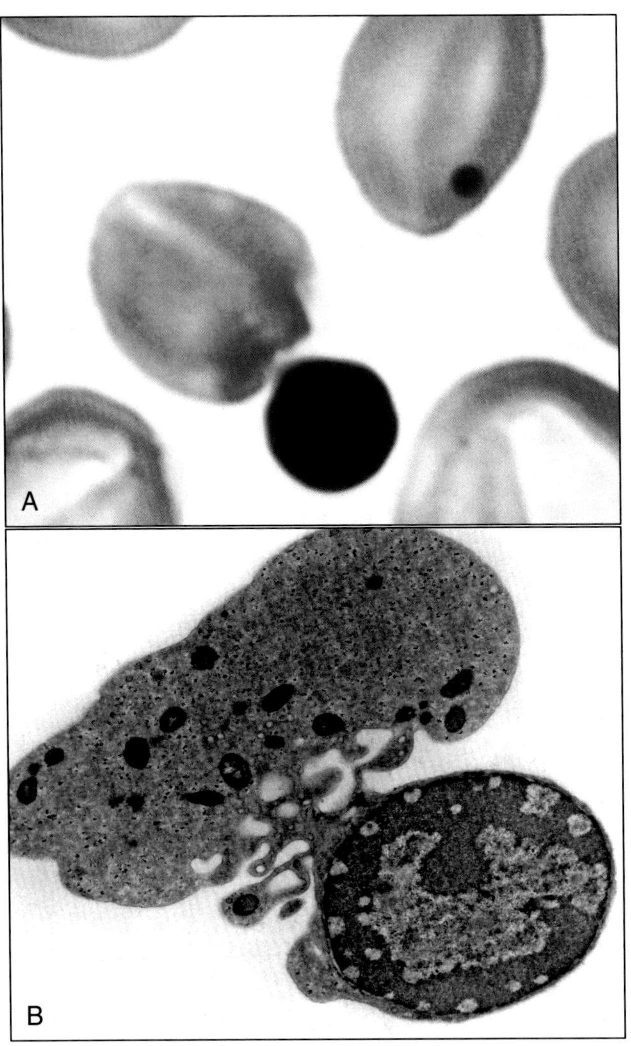

FIGURE 3-11

Nuclear extrusion of metarubricytes to form canine reticulocytes. **A,** Blood film from a dog with a hemolytic anemia secondary to hemangiosarcoma. Frictional forces during smear preparation may have contributed to the nuclear extrusion. **B,** Transmission electron microscopy of nuclear extrusion of a metarubricyte.

B, From Simpson CF, King JM. The mechanism of denucleation in circulating erythroblasts. J Cell Biol. *1967;35:237-245.*

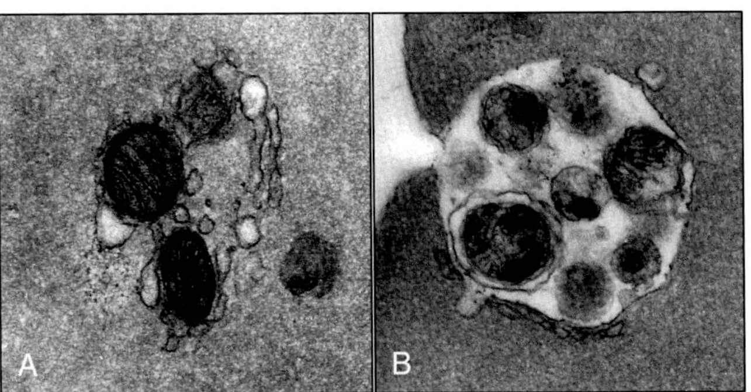

FIGURE 3-12

Transmission electron microscopy of mitochondrial extrusion from canine reticulocytes. **A,** A series of vesicles appear to be surrounding three mitochondria. **B,** Fusion of a vacuole containing mitochondria with the reticulocyte outer membrane, thereby promoting mitochondrial extrusion.

From Simpson CF, King JM. The mechanism of mitochondrial extrusion from phenylhydrazine-induced reticulocytes in the circulating blood. J Cell Biol. *1968;36:103-109.*

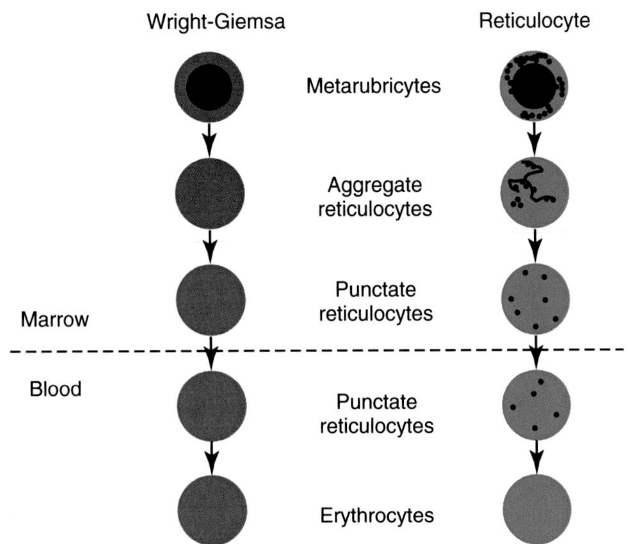

FIGURE 3-13

Cat erythroid cells demonstrating reticulocyte release into blood as it occurs in most normal cats. Note that punctate reticulocytes do not appear polychromatophilic when stained with Wright-Giemsa.

are normally absent from blood and are rarely released in response to anemia.

Control of Erythropoiesis

Early- and intermediate-acting growth factors—including SCF, IL-3, GM-CSF, and TPO—are utilized to produce EPs. EPO is the principal growth factor promoting the viability, proliferation, and differentiation of EPs (BFU-E and CFU-E) that express specific cell-surface EPO receptors. The main mechanism used to achieve these effects is inhibition of apoptosis.[124] Early BFU-E cells do not express EPO receptors, but more mature BFU-E cells do and are thus responsive to EPO. EPO receptor numbers on cell surfaces increase to maximum values in CFU-E cells, decline in rubriblasts, and continue to decrease in the later stages of erythroid development.[104,105] Because of their EPO receptor density, CFU-E cells readily respond to EPO, promoting their proliferation, differentiation, and transformation into rubriblasts, the first morphologically recognizable erythroid cell type. High concentrations of EPO may accelerate rubriblast entry into the first mitotic division, thus shortening the marrow transit time and resulting in the early release of stress reticulocytes.[105]

In the presence of EPO, other hormones—including androgens, glucocorticoid hormones, growth hormone, insulin, and insulin-like growth factors (IGFs)—can enhance the growth of erythroid progenitor cells in vitro.[76,88] The thyroid hormone 3,5,3′-triiodothyronine (T_3) promotes the differentiation and maturation of erythroid cells.[76] Thyroid hormones may also promote the synthesis of EPO in the kidney.[82] EPO production in adult mammals occurs primarily within peritubular interstitial cells located within the inner cortex and outer medulla of the kidney. The liver is an extrarenal source of EPO in adults and the major site of EPO production in the mammalian fetus.[59] Bone marrow macrophages and erythroid progenitor cells themselves can produce EPO, suggesting the possibility of short-range regulation of erythropoiesis.[126,141]

Hematopoietic cells die not only as a consequence of lack of HGFs but also in response to the presence of molecules that induce apoptosis. Inhibitors of erythropoiesis include TGF-β, TNF-α, IFN-γ, IL-6, and TNF-related apoptosis-inducing ligand (TRAIL).[26]

The ability to deliver oxygen to the tissues depends on cardiovascular integrity, oxygen content in arterial blood, and Hb oxygen affinity. Low oxygen content in the blood can result from a low partial pressure of oxygen (PO_2) in arterial blood, as occurs at high altitudes or with congenital heart defects in which some of the blood flow bypasses the pulmonary circulation. A low oxygen content in blood can also be present when arterial PO_2 is normal, as occurs with anemia and methemoglobinemia. An increased oxygen affinity of Hb within erythrocytes results in a decreased tendency to release oxygen to the tissues.[86] Regardless of the cause, EPO production is stimulated by tissue hypoxia (Fig. 3-14), which is mediated by hypoxia-inducible factors that control the transcription of the *EPO* gene in EPO-secreting cells.[50,59]

Other tissues also exhibit EPO receptors, and EPO stimulates nonhematopoietic actions, including promoting the proliferation and migration of endothelial cells, enhancing neovascularization, stimulating the production of modulators of vascular tone, and exerting cardioprotective and neuroprotective effects.[59]

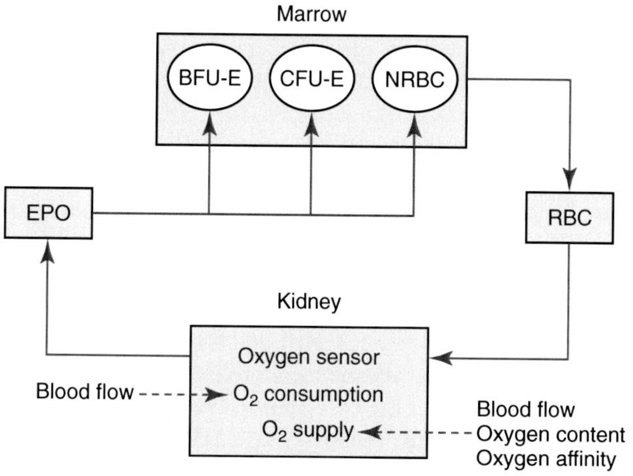

FIGURE 3-14
Central role of erythropoietin (EPO) in the control of erythropoiesis. BFU-E, burst-forming unit-erythroid; CFU-E, colony-forming unit-erythroid; NRBC, nucleated red blood cell.

LEUKOPOIESIS

Neutrophil Production

Neutrophilic cells within the bone marrow can be included in two pools (Fig. 3-15). The proliferation and maturation pool (mitotic pool) includes myeloblasts, promyelocytes, and myelocytes. Approximately four or five divisions occur over several days (Fig. 3-16). During this time primary (reddish purple) cytoplasmic granules are produced in late myeloblasts or early promyelocytes and secondary (specific) granules are synthesized within myelocytes (see Fig. 3-10). Once nuclear indentation and condensation become apparent, precursor

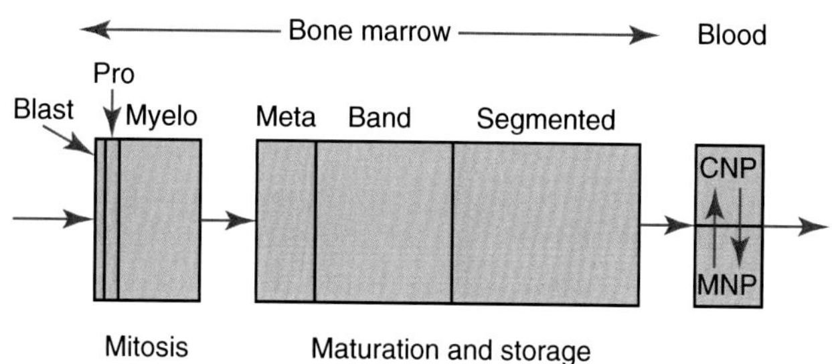

FIGURE 3-15
Approximate sizes of mitotic and postmitotic neutrophilic compartments within bone marrow.

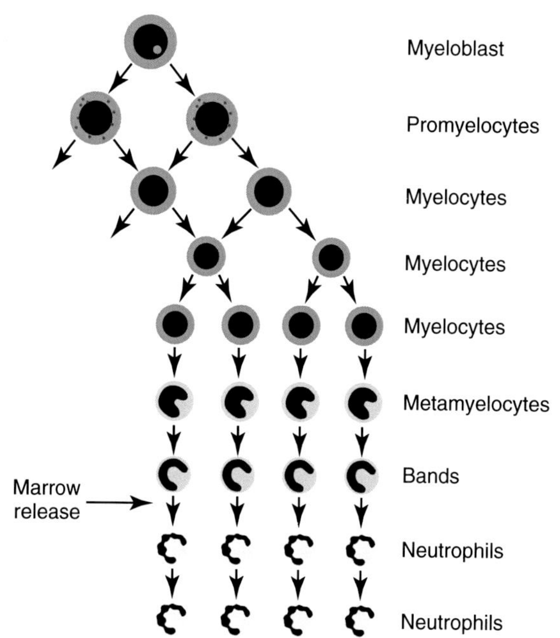

FIGURE 3-16
A diagram of granulopoiesis.

cells are no longer capable of division. The maturation and storage pool (postmitotic pool) includes metamyelocytes, bands, and segmented neutrophils. Cells within this pool normally undergo maturation and storage for several more days prior to the migration of mature neutrophils through the vascular endothelium and into the circulation.[123] The number of mature neutrophils stored in marrow is more than seven times the number present in the circulation of the dog.[32] The marrow transit time from myeloblast to release of mature neutrophils into the blood varies by species but is generally between 6 and 9 days. This time can be shortened considerably when inflammation is present.[108,123]

A variety of cytokines with overlapping specificities are important in neutrophil production (also called granulopoiesis). IL-3, GM-CSF, and G-CSF are of primary importance in the production of neutrophils. These cytokines act on various stages of development from CMPs to GMPs to GPs, depending on the array of growth factor receptors displayed on their surfaces. GPs are stimulated to proliferate and differentiate into myeloblasts by G-CSF. This cytokine appears to play a role in the basal regulation of granulopoiesis as well as to function as a primary regulator of the neutrophil response to inflammatory stimuli. G-CSF increases the number of cell divisions and reduces the time for granulocytic progenitors to develop into neutrophils. It also promotes the release of neutrophils from bone marrow into blood.[108,127]

As neutrophils mature, there is a progressive downregulation of certain surface receptors, including CXCR4 and the $\alpha_4\beta_1$ integrin, that adhere neutrophils to glycoproteins within the extravascular space. CXCR4 binds to CXCL12/SDF-1 produced by stromal cells, and the $\alpha_4\beta_1$ integrin binds to VCAM-1 on endothelial cells. Experimental neutralization of CXCR4 and VCAM-1 results in an increased release of neutrophils into blood. G-CSF promotes neutrophil release from bone marrow at least in part by decreasing CXCL12/SDF-1 production and decreasing CXCR4 expression on the surface of neutrophils.[127]

Activated helper T lymphocytes produce various growth factors including IL-3 and GM-CSF. Mononuclear phagocytes, fibroblasts, and endothelial cells can also produce GM-CSF and G-CSF when appropriately stimulated. Mononuclear phagocytes can not only synthesize HGFs when they contact bacterial products but can also stimulate other cells to produce them. The cytokines, IL-1 and TNF-α, produced by monocytes and macrophages stimulate the production of HGFs by other cell types. These monokines are important in the inflammatory response to foreign organisms and neoplastic cells, but their role in resting granulopoiesis is unclear.[66,123] IL-6 is a multifunctional cytokine that regulates inflammation (including the hepatic acute-phase response), the immune response, and hematopoiesis. In this latter role, it promotes granulopoiesis and thrombopoiesis during inflammation.[111]

Inhibition of neutrophil production is not well understood, but mature neutrophils may provide negative feedback inhibition on their own production in three ways. First, the addition of mature neutrophils to bone marrow culture inhibits neutrophilic colony formation. If this also happens in vivo, it might provide negative feedback for neutrophil production in the extravascular space of bone marrow.[71] One possible mechanism is the release of serine proteases, such as elastase, from neutrophils. Elastase appears to inhibit granulopoiesis by inactivating G-CSF.[35] Second, increased neutrophil numbers in blood are associated with the increased clearance of circulating G-CSF following binding to surface receptors on neutrophils, thereby decreasing the primary stimulus for their production.[65,75] Third, mature neutrophils indirectly inhibit granulopoiesis by the removal (through phagocytosis) of invading microorganisms that would otherwise stimulate the production of HGFs by tissue cells. Activated T lymphocytes may also inhibit neutrophil production by secreting the soluble molecule Fas-ligand and the cytokine IFN-γ.[99]

Eosinophil, Basophil, and Mast Cell Production

The eosinophil progenitor (EoP) or colony-forming unit eosinophil (CFU-Eo) is reported to develop from the CMP in humans but downstream from the GMP in mice.[89] Eosinophil production in the marrow parallels that of neutrophils. Eosinophil precursors become recognizable at the myelocyte stage, when their characteristic secondary granules appear (see Fig. 3-10). The marrow transit time is 1 week or less, with a significant storage pool of mature eosinophils.[142] As in the case of neutrophils, growth factors, including IL-3 and GM-CSF, are needed for the proliferation of early progenitors. In addition, activated T_H2 lymphocytes produce IL-5, which promotes the terminal maturation of eosinophils. IL-3, GM-CSF, and IL-5 also inhibit eosinophil apoptosis,[62] while inhibitors of eosinophil production include IL-12 and IFN-γ.[110]

The GMP reportedly produces the bipotential basophil-mast cell progenitor (BMaP), which gives rise to the basophil progenitor and the mast cell progenitor (MaP).[121] Like eosinophils, basophil precursors become recognizable at the myelocyte stage, when their characteristic secondary granules appear (see Fig. 3-10). A specific growth factor for the production of basophils has not been identified. IL-3 appears to be the major growth and differentiation factor for basophils, but other growth factors—including GM-CSF, IL-5, TGF-β, and nerve growth factor—also promote the production of basophils.[37]

In contrast to basophils, which mature in the bone marrow, maturation of mast cell progenitors into mast cells occurs in the tissues.[40] SCF appears to be the major growth and differentiation factor for mast cells. Additional cytokines—including IL-3, IL-4, IL-9, IL-10, and IL-13—also stimulate mast cell production.[54] Some local proliferation of mast cells can occur in tissues if they are appropriately stimulated.[41]

Production of Monocytes, Macrophages, Dendritic Cells, and Osteoclasts

Bone marrow MDPs give rise to monocytes and common dendritic cell progenitors (CDPs).[153] Monocytes are produced through the combined effects of IL-3, GM-CSF, M-CSF, and

IL-34 on the proliferation and differentiation of bone marrow progenitor cells.[44] Less time is required to produce monocytes than granulocytes, and there is little marrow reserve of these cells.

Monocytes have long been viewed primarily as precursors that develop into tissue macrophages and dendritic cells. However, it is now recognized that many macrophage and dendritic cells in tissues do not originate from monocytes under steady-state conditions because these cells are capable of self-replication. In addition, neither microglia (macrophages in the central nervous system) nor Langerhans cells (epidermal dendritic cells) depend on cells from the bone marrow for their renewal under steady-state conditions and possibly also during inflammation.[10] In fact, Langerhans cells appear to develop from embryonic progenitor cells that enter the epidermis before birth.[44]

Monocytes are important effector cells during inflammatory conditions. They exit the blood, respond to the tissue environment, and differentiate into subsets of macrophages and inflammatory dendritic cells. Exposure to M-CSF promotes the development of monocytes into macrophages. The addition of IFN-γ to M-CSF promotes the formation of M1-like macrophages, while the addition of IL-4 to M-CSF induces the differentiation of M2-like macrophages. The exposure of monocytes to GM-CSF, IL-4, and TNF-α promotes their development into inflammatory dendritic cells or TNF-α and inducible nitric oxide synthase (iNOS)-producing (TiP)-dendritic cells.[10,44,153]

CDPs can give rise to preclassic dendritic cells (Pre-cDC) and plasmacytoid dendritic cells (pDCs) in bone marrow.[96] Both cell types are released into blood and enter the tissues, where the Pre-cDCs develop into classic dendritic cells (cDC) in lymphoid organs and mucosal dendritic cells.[44,153] Cytokines—including Flt3L, GM-CSF, and lymphotoxin $\alpha_1\beta_2$—appear to be important for the development of cDCs and pDCs.[10,44]

Osteoclasts develop when monocyte progenitors are cultured with M-CSF and a soluble form of receptor activator of nuclear factor-κB ligand (RANKL).[9] IL-3 and GM-CSF inhibit osteoclast formation. The relative amounts of these growth factors and presumably others present in the microenvironment of a monocyte progenitor apparently determine whether macrophages, dendritic cells, or osteoclasts are formed.

Lymphocyte and NK Cell Production

The CLP is believed to give rise to B lymphocytes, T lymphocytes, and NK cells.[16] The development of B lymphocyte and T lymphocyte progenitors in bone marrow is antigen-independent. Both SCF and Flt3L appear to be involved in the production of early lymphoid progenitor cells in mice.[17]

B lymphocyte progenitors produce mature, naive B lymphocytes in the marrow in most mammals, in specialized ileal Peyer's patches in dogs, pigs, and ruminants, and in the bursa of Fabricius in birds.[83,135] Approximately 2 to 3 days are required for pre-B lymphocytes to develop into mature, naive B lymphocytes in the marrow and enter the circulation. Less than 20% of B lymphocytes produced in the marrow become part of the peripheral mature B lymphocyte pool, with most of the cells being culled in the bone marrow or after their entry into blood.[83] B lymphocytes also proliferate in peripheral lymphoid tissues in adults. As with other blood cells, the microenvironment of the marrow and lymphoid organs is important for lymphopoiesis. The production of antigen-sensitive, surface-immunoglobulin-positive B lymphocytes is marked by successive rearrangements of the immunoglobulin gene loci and selective expression of surface proteins. Although a number of cytokines—including SCF, Flt3L, SDF-1, and IGF—are involved in B lymphocyte production in marrow, IL-7 appears to be an especially important positive growth factor.[19,77] B lymphocyte lymphopoiesis is inhibited by several factors, including TGF-β, IFN-α, IFN-β, and IFN-γ.[77]

Recirculating B lymphocytes are activated by antigenic stimulation in the T lymphocyte region of secondary lymphoid organs, followed by migration to the cortex in lymph nodes and to follicles in jejunal Peyer's patches and the spleen in mammals.[135] B lymphocyte activation and differentiation into plasmablasts is induced by combinations of microbial products, cytokines, and molecules bound to the surfaces of T lymphocytes and dendritic cells. Plasmablasts can develop into plasma cells in the lymphoid organs where they are produced or can migrate through blood and develop into plasma cells in peripheral tissues or bone marrow. SDF-1 attracts circulating plasmablasts to the bone marrow, and factors including SDF-1 and IL-6 promote plasma cell development by preventing apoptosis.[91]

T lymphocyte progenitors leave the marrow and migrate to the thymus. Homing of these cells to the thymus depends on their interaction with various adhesion molecules on thymic endothelial cells and the production of specific chemotactic factors by thymic stromal cells. T lymphocyte progenitors develop into T lymphocytes under the influence of the thymic microenvironment and growth factors (including Flt3L and IL-7) produced in the thymus.[151] After maturation in the thymus, T lymphocytes accumulate within paracortical areas of lymph nodes, periarteriolar lymphoid sheaths of the spleen, and the interfollicular areas of jejunal Peyer's patches in mammals.[135]

Most NK cells are produced from progenitor cells in the bone marrow, where they undergo expansion and maturation for a week or more before their release into the blood.[155] Growth factors controlling their production need further characterization, but SCF, IL-2, IL-7, and IL-15 can stimulate NK cell development from progenitor cells in vitro.[3] Subsets of NK cells also develop in the thymus and possibly other organs, such as lymph nodes, liver, and spleen. These sites may depend on the trafficking of bone marrow–derived progenitor cells and/or immature NK cells into these organs from the blood, where they mature under the influence of microenvironmental factors.[49,55]

THROMBOPOIESIS

Blood platelets in mammals are produced from multinucleated giant cells in the bone marrow called megakaryocytes. The CMP gives rise to the MkEP, which can differentiate into megakaryocyte progenitors (MkPs) or erythroid progenitors (EPs). The earliest MkP is the burst-forming-unit megakaryocyte (BFU-Mk). When appropriately stimulated, this progenitor cell divides and differentiates into colony-forming-unit megakaryocyte (CFU-Mk) progenitor cells, which divide and differentiate into megakaryoblasts (Fig. 3-17).[68] Mitosis stops at this stage and endomitosis (nuclear reduplication without cell division) begins. Generally 2 to 5 nuclear reduplications occur resulting in 8 to 64 sets of chromosomes (8 N-64 N) in mature megakaryocytes, compared to two sets of chromosomes (2 N) in most cells in the body. Individual nuclei can be observed following the first two reduplications (promegakaryocytes), but a large polylobulated nucleus is seen when mature megakaryocytes are formed. The mean ploidy of human and mouse megakaryocytes (16 N) is lower than mean values (32 N to 64 N) reported for megakaryocytes in dogs, cats, and cattle.[18] The cytoplasm in promegakaryocytes is intensely basophilic. There is a progressive decrease in basophilia and increase in granularity as megakaryocytes mature. Cell volume increases with each reduplication; consequently, megakaryocytes are much larger than all other marrow cells except osteoclasts. In contrast to mature megakaryocytes, osteoclasts have multiple discrete nuclei.

Mature megakaryocytes develop just outside vascular sinuses. SDF-1 and fibroblast growth factor-4 promote the localization and binding of megakaryocyte progenitors in this vascular niche (via adhesion molecules VCAM-1 and the $\alpha_4\beta_1$ integrin), which promotes survival, maturation, and platelet production.[11] Protrusions of cytoplasm (proplatelets) from megakaryocytes form and extend into sinuses where they can be sheared off by the force of flowing blood (see Fig. 3-3). These beaded-appearing proplatelets eventually fragment into individual platelets within the sinuses and general circulation.[60] Megakaryocytes may rarely migrate through the vascular endothelium into the sinuses, enter the general venous circulation (see Fig. 2-34), and become lodged in pulmonary capillaries.[11] It is estimated that 1000 to 3000 platelets are produced from each megakaryocyte, depending on megakaryocyte size.[68] Megakaryocytes are not present in nonmammalian species. Like erythrocytes and leukocytes, the nucleated thrombocytes of nonmammalian species are produced by mitosis of precursor cells.

A number of cytokines can stimulate or enhance the proliferation and expansion of megakaryocyte progenitor cells. Factors that may be involved include SCF, Flt3L, IL-3, GM-CSF, IL-11, and EPO.[13,18,68] TPO is the key stimulator of platelet production by stimulating megakaryocyte proliferation, survival, and size (ploidy).[60,68] TPO also transiently enhances the aggregatory response of platelets to agonists.[4]

Although various cells in the body can produce TPO, including cells in the kidney and bone marrow stromal cells,[80,87] the major sites of TPO production appear to be the endothelial cells of the liver.[58,148] The amount of TPO produced in the body appears to be relatively constant. TPO receptors (c-Mpl receptors) on blood platelets and maturing megakaryocytes can bind, internalize, and degrade TPO, providing negative feedback on platelet production.[68] Consequently blood TPO concentration is remarkably high in the case of thrombocytopenia resulting from megakaryocytic hypoplasia. In contrast, blood TPO concentrations are much lower with ongoing immune-mediated thrombocytopenia, because megakaryocytes are generally increased in the marrow and rapid platelet turnover is occurring, resulting in increased binding and removal of TPO from blood.[52]

However, the number of maturing megakaryocytes and blood platelets present may not be the only determinants of blood TPO concentrations. IL-6 stimulates thrombopoiesis by increasing the production of TPO by the liver, which contributes to the thrombocytosis seen in some inflammatory conditions.[64] Conversely, platelet factor 4 (PF4), TGF-β, IL-4, and TNF-α appear to be inhibitors of megakaryocyte production.[13,137]

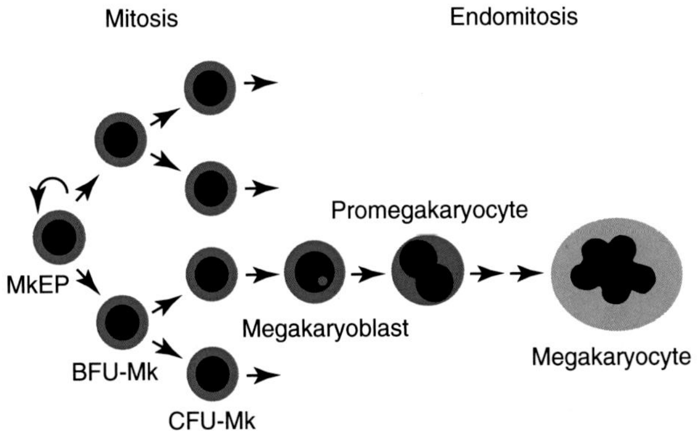

FIGURE 3-17
Stages of megakaryocyte development. MkEP, Megakaryocyte-erthroid progenitor; BFU-Mega, burst-forming unit megakaryocyte; CFU-Mega, colony-forming unit megakaryocyte.

REFERENCES

1. Abboud CN, Lichtman MA. Structure of the marrow and the hematopoietic microenvironment. In: Lichtman MA, Beutler E, Kipps TJ, et al, eds. *Williams Hematology.* 7th ed. New York: McGraw-Hill; 2006:35-72.
2. Abkowitz JL, Catlin SN, McCallie MT, et al. Evidence that the number of hematopoietic stem cells per animal is conserved in mammals. *Blood.* 2002;100:2665-2667.
3. Aiba Y, Hirayama F, Ogawa M. Clonal proliferation and cytokine requirement of murine progenitors for natural killer cells. *Blood.* 1997;89:4005-4012.
4. Akkerman JW. Thrombopoietin and platelet function. *Semin Thromb Hemost.* 2006;32:295-304.
5. Allender MC, Fry MM. Amphibian hematology. *Vet Clin North Am Exot Anim Pract.* 2008;11:463-480.
6. Alpen EL, Baum SJ. Modification of x-radiation lethality by autologous marrow infusion in dogs. *Blood.* 1958;13:1168-1175.
7. Alsaker RD. The formation, emergence, and maturation of the reticulocyte: a review. *Vet Clin Pathol.* 1977;6(3):7-12.

8. Arai F, Yoshihara H, Hosokawa K, et al. Niche regulation of hematopoietic stem cells in the endosteum. *Ann N Y Acad Sci.* 2009;1176:36-46.
9. Asagiri M, Takayanagi H. The molecular understanding of osteoclast differentiation. *Bone.* 2007;40:251-264.
10. Auffray C, Sieweke MH, Geissmann F. Blood monocytes: development, heterogeneity, and relationship with dendritic cells. *Annu Rev Immunol.* 2009;27:669-692.
11. Avecilla ST, Hattori K, Heissig B, et al. Chemokine-mediated interaction of hematopoietic progenitors with the bone marrow vascular niche is required for thrombopoiesis. *Nat Med.* 2004;10:64-71.
12. Barao I, Ascensao JL. Human natural killer cells. *Arch Immunol Ther Exp (Warsz).* 1998;46:213-229.
13. Battinelli EM, Hartwig JH, Italiano JE, Jr. Delivering new insight into the biology of megakaryopoiesis and thrombopoiesis. *Curr Opin Hematol.* 2007;14:419-426.
14. Bertrand JY, Jalil A, Klaine M, et al. Three pathways to mature macrophages in the early mouse yolk sac. *Blood.* 2005;106:3004-3011.
15. Bessis M. *Living Blood Cells and Their Ultrastructure.* New York: Springer-Verlag; 1973.
16. Blom B, Spits H. Development of human lymphoid cells. *Annu Rev Immunol.* 2006;24:287-320.
17. Borge OJ, Adolfsson J, Jacobsen AM. Lymphoid-restricted development from multipotent candidate murine stem cells: distinct and complimentary functions of the c-kit and flt3-ligands. *Blood.* 1999;94:3781-3790.
18. Boudreaux MK. Thrombopoiesis. In: Weiss DJ, Wardrop KJ, eds. *Schalm's Veterinary Hematology.* 6th ed. Ames, IA: Wiley-Blackwell; 2010:56-60.
19. Burkhard MJ. Lymphopoiesis. In: Weiss DJ, Wardrop KJ, eds. *Schalm's Veterinary Hematology.* 6th ed. Ames, IA: Wiley-Blackwell; 2010:61-64.
20. Campbell F. Fine structure of the bone marrow of the chicken and pigeon. *J Morphol.* 1967;123:405-439.
21. Carbonell F, Calvo W, Fliedner TM. Cellular composition of human fetal bone marrow. Histologic study in methacrylate sections. *Acta Anat (Basel).* 1982;113:371-375.
22. Carr BD. The hematopoietic system. In: Weiss DJ, Wardrop KJ, eds. *Schalm's Veterinary Hematology.* 6th ed. Ames, IA: Wiley-Blackwell; 2010:27-35.
23. Cecchini MG, Hofstetter W, Halasy J, et al. Role of CSF-1 in bone and bone marrow development. *Mol Reprod Dev.* 1997;46:75-83.
24. Chao H, Hirschi KK. Hemato-vascular origins of endothelial progenitor cells? *Microvasc Res.* 2010;79:169-173.
25. Chasis JA. Erythroblastic islands: specialized microenvironmental niches for erythropoiesis. *Curr Opin Hematol.* 2006;13:137-141.
26. Chasis JA, Mohandas N. Erythroblastic islands: niches for erythropoiesis. *Blood.* 2008;112:470-478.
27. Chute JP. Stem cell homing. *Curr Opin Hematol.* 2006;13:399-406.
28. Coombe DR. Biological implications of glycosaminoglycan interactions with haemopoietic cytokines. *Immunol Cell Biol.* 2008;86:598-607.
29. Cramer DV, Lewis RM. Reticulocyte response in the cat. *J Am Vet Med Assoc.* 1972;160:61-67.
30. Dabrowski Z, Sano MI, Tabarowski Z, et al. Haematopoiesis in snakes (Ophidia) in early postnatal development. *Cell Tissue Res.* 2007;328:291-299.
31. Dent AL, Kaplan MH. T cell regulation of hematopoiesis. *Front Biosci.* 2008;13: 6229-6236.
32. Deubelbeiss KA, Dancey JT, Harker LA, et al. Neutrophil kinetics in the dog. *J Clin Invest.* 1975;55:833-839.
33. Di Rosa F. T-lymphocyte interaction with stromal, bone and hematopoietic cells in the bone marrow. *Immunol Cell Biol.* 2009;87:20-29.
34. Durand C, Dzierzak E. Embryonic beginnings of adult hematopoietic stem cells. *Haematologica.* 2005;90:100-108.
35. El Ouriaghli F, Fujiwara H, Melenhorst JJ, et al. Neutrophil elastase enzymatically antagonizes the *in vitro* action of G-CSF: implications for the regulation of granulopoiesis. *Blood.* 2003;101:1752-1758.
36. Erslev AJ, Beutler E. Production and destruction of erythrocytes. In: Beutler E, Lichtman MA, Coller BS, et al, eds. *Williams Hematology.* 5th ed. New York: McGraw-Hill; 1995:425-441.
37. Falcone FH, Haas H, Gibbs BF. The human basophil: a new appreciation of its role in immune responses. *Blood.* 2000;96:4028-4038.
38. Faldyna M, Sinkora J, Knotigova P, et al. Flow cytometric analysis of bone marrow leukocytes in neonatal dogs. *Vet Immunol Immunopathol.* 2003;95:165-176.
39. Fan LC, Dorner JL, Hoffman WE. Reticulocyte response and maturation in experimental acute blood loss anemia in the cat. *J Am Anim Hosp Assoc.* 1978;14:219-224.
40. Födinger M, Fritsch G, Winkler K, et al. Origin of human mast cells: development from transplanted hematopoietic stem cells after allogeneic bone marrow transplantation. *Blood.* 1994;84:2954-2959.
41. Galli SJ, Metcalfe DD, Arber DA, et al. Basophils and mast cells and their disorders. In: Lichtman MA, Beutler E, Kipps TJ, et al, eds. *Williams Hematology.* 7th ed. New York: McGraw-Hill; 2006:879-897.
42. Galloway JL, Zon LI. Ontogeny of hematopoiesis: examining the emergence of hematopoietic cells in the vertebrate embryo. *Curr Top Dev Biol.* 2003;53: 139-158.
43. Gangenahalli GU, Singh VK, Verma YK, et al. Hematopoietic stem cell antigen CD34: role in adhesion or homing. *Stem Cells Dev.* 2006;15:305-313.
44. Geissmann F, Manz MG, Jung S, et al. Development of monocytes, macrophages, and dendritic cells. *Science.* 2010;327:656-661.
45. Geminard C, de Gassart A, Vidal M. Reticulocyte maturation: mitoptosis and exosome release. *Biocell.* 2002;26:205-215.
46. Gertz MA. Current status of stem cell mobilization. *Br J Haematol.* 2010;150: 647-662.
47. Gimble JM, Robinson CE, Wu X, et al. The function of adipocytes in the bone marrow stroma: an update. *Bone.* 1996;19:421-428.
48. Glomski CA, Tamburlin J, Chainani M. The phylogenetic odyssey of the erythrocyte. III. Fish, the lower vertebrate experience. *Histol Histopathol.* 1992;7:501-528.
49. Gregoire C, Chasson L, Luci C, et al. The trafficking of natural killer cells. *Immunol Rev.* 2007;220:169-182.
50. Gruber M, Hu CJ, Johnson RS, et al. Acute postnatal ablation of Hif-2α results in anemia. *Proc Natl Acad Sci U S A.* 2007;104:2301-2306.
51. Harvey JW. The erythrocyte: physiology, metabolism and biochemical disorders. In: Kaneko JJ, Harvey JW, Bruss ML, eds. *Clinical Biochemistry of Domestic Animals.* 6th ed. San Diego: Academic Press; 2008:173-240.
52. Hou M, Andersson PO, Stockelberg D, et al. Plasma thrombopoietin levels in thrombocytopenic states: implication for a regulatory role of bone marrow megakaryocytes. *Br J Haematol.* 1998;101:420-424.
53. Houwen B. Reticulocyte maturation. *Blood Cells.* 1992;18:167-186.
54. Hu ZQ, Zhao WH, Shimamura T. Regulation of mast cell development by inflammatory factors. *Curr Med Chem.* 2007;14:3044-3050.
55. Huntington ND, Vosshenrich CA, Di Santo JP. Developmental pathways that generate natural-killer-cell diversity in mice and humans. *Nat Rev Immunol.* 2007;7:703-714.
56. Jain NC. *Schalm's Veterinary Hematology.* 4th ed. Philadelphia: Lea & Febiger; 1986.
57. Jain NC. *Essentials of Veterinary Hematology.* Philadelphia: Lea & Febiger; 1993.
58. Jelkmann W. The role of the liver in the production of thrombopoietin compared with erythropoietin. *Eur J Gastroenterol Hepatol.* 2001;13:791-801.
59. Jelkmann W. Erythropoietin after a century of research: younger than ever. *Eur J Haematol.* 2007;78:183-205.
60. Junt T, Schulze H, Chen Z, et al. Dynamic visualization of thrombopoiesis within bone marrow. *Science.* 2007;317:1767-1770.
61. Kalinkovich A, Spiegel A, Shivtiel S, et al. Blood-forming stem cells are nervous: direct and indirect regulation of immature human CD34+ cells by the nervous system. *Brain Behav Immun.* 2009;23:1059-1065.
62. Kankaanranta H, Moilanen E, Zhang X. Pharmacological regulation of human eosinophil apoptosis. *Curr Drug Targets Inflamm Allergy.* 2005;4:433-445.
63. Kaplan RN, Psaila B, Lyden D. Niche-to-niche migration of bone-marrow-derived cells. *Trends Mol Med.* 2007;13:72-81.
64. Kaser A, Brandacher G, Steurer W, et al. Interleukin-6 stimulates thrombopoiesis through thrombopoietin: role in inflammatory thrombocytosis. *Blood.* 2001;98: 2720-2725.
65. Kastner M, Maurer HR. Pure bovine granulocytes as a source of granulopoiesis inhibitor (chalone). *Hoppe Seylers Z Physiol Chem.* 1980;361:197-200.
66. Kaushansky K. Hematopoietic stem cells, progenitors, and cytokines. In: Lichtman MA, Beutler E, Kipps TJ, et al, eds. *Williams Hematology.* 7th ed. New York: McGraw-Hill; 2006:201-220.
67. Kaushansky K. Lineage-specific hematopoietic growth factors. *N Engl J Med.* 2006;354:2034-2045.
68. Kaushansky K. Historical review: megakaryopoiesis and thrombopoiesis. *Blood.* 2008;111:981-986.
69. Kim DH, Yoo KH, Choi KS, et al. Gene expression profile of cytokine and growth factor during differentiation of bone marrow-derived mesenchymal stem cell. *Cytokine.* 2005;31:119-126.
70. Kingsley PD, Malik J, Fantauzzo KA, et al. Yolk sac-derived primitive erythroblasts enucleate during mammalian embryogenesis. *Blood.* 2004;104:19-25.
71. Kovacs P, Brunch C, Fliedner TM. Colony formation by canine hemopoietic cells *in vitro.* Inhibition by polymorphonuclear leukocytes. *Acta Haematol.* 1976;56:107-115.
72. Kucia M, Reca R, Jala VR, et al. Bone marrow as a home of heterogenous populations of nonhematopoietic stem cells. *Leukemia.* 2005;19:1118-1127.
73. Laber J, Perman V, Stevens JB. Polychromasia or reticulocytes—an assessment of the dog. *J Am Anim Hosp Assoc.* 1974;10:399-406.
74. Lancrin C, Sroczynska P, Serrano AG, et al. Blood cell generation from the hemangioblast. *J Mol Med.* 2010;88:167-172.
75. Layton JE, Hockman H, Sheridan WP, et al. Evidence for a novel control mechanism of granulopoiesis: mature cell related control of a regulatory growth factor. *Blood.* 1989;74:1303-1307.

76. Leberbauer C, Boulme F, Unfried G, et al. Different steroids co-regulate long-term expansion versus terminal differentiation in primary human erythroid progenitors. *Blood.* 2005;105:85-94.
77. Lebien TW. Lymphopoiesis. In: Lichtman MA, Beutler E, Kipps TJ, et al, eds. *Williams Hematology.* 7th ed. New York: McGraw-Hill; 2006:1039-1049.
78. Liang DC, Shih LY, Chai IJ, et al. The synergistic effect of thrombopoietin in erythropoiesis with erythropoietin and/or IL-3 and myelopoiesis with G-CSF or IL-3 from umbilical cord blood cells of premature neonates. *Pediatr Hematol Oncol.* 2002;19:399-405.
79. Lichtman MA, Santillo P. Red cell egress from the marrow. *Blood Cells.* 1986;12:11-23.
80. Linthorst GE, Folman CC, van Olden RW, et al. Plasma thrombopoietin levels in patients with chronic renal failure. *Hematol J.* 2002;3:38-42.
81. Liu ZJ, Zhuge Y, Velazquez OC. Trafficking and differentiation of mesenchymal stem cells. *J Cell Biochem.* 2009;106:984-991.
82. Ma Y, Freitag P, Zhou J, et al. Thyroid hormone induces erythropoietin gene expression through augmented accumulation of hypoxia-inducible factor-1. *Am J Physiol Regul Integr Comp Physiol.* 2004;287:R600-R607.
83. Macallan DC, Wallace DL, Zhang Y, et al. B-cell kinetics in humans: rapid turnover of peripheral blood memory cells. *Blood.* 2005;105:3633-3640.
84. Martin DR, Cox NR, Hathcock TL, et al. Isolation and characterization of multipotential mesenchymal stem cells from feline bone marrow. *Exp Hematol.* 2002;30: 879-886.
85. Mayani H, Guilbert LJ, Janowska-Wieczorek A. Biology of the hemopoietic microenvironment. *Eur J Haematol.* 1992;49:225-233.
86. McCully K, Chance B, Giger U. In vivo determination of altered hemoglobin saturation in dogs with M-type phosphofructokinase deficiency. *Muscle Nerve.* 1999;22: 621-627.
87. McIntosh B, Kaushansky K. Transcriptional regulation of bone marrow thrombopoietin by platelet proteins. *Exp Hematol.* 2008;36:799-806.
88. Miyagawa S, Kobayashi M, Konishi N, et al. Insulin and insulin-like growth factor I support the proliferation of erythroid progenitor cells in bone marrow through the sharing of receptors. *Br J Haematol.* 2000;109:555-562.
89. Mori Y, Iwasaki H, Kohno K, et al. Identification of the human eosinophil lineage-committed progenitor: revision of phenotypic definition of the human common myeloid progenitor. *J Exp Med.* 2009;206:183-193.
90. Mortensen M, Ferguson DJ, Simon AK. Mitochondrial clearance by autophagy in developing erythrocytes: Clearly important, but just how much so? *Cell Cycle.* 2010;15:1901-1906.
91. Moser K, Tokoyoda K, Radbruch A, et al. Stromal niches, plasma cell differentiation and survival. *Curr Opin Immunol.* 2006;18:265-270.
92. Nilsson SK, Simmons PJ. Transplantable stem cells: home to specific niches. *Curr Opin Hematol.* 2004;11:102-106.
93. Nobuhisa I, Takizawa M, Takaki S, et al. Regulation of hematopoietic development in the aorta-gonad-mesonephros region mediated by Lnk adaptor protein. *Mol Cell Biol.* 2003;23:8486-8494.
94. Oh IH, Kwon KR. Concise review: multiple niches for hematopoietic stem cell regulations. *Stem Cells.* 2010;28:1243-1249.
95. Ohishi M, Schipani E. Bone marrow mesenchymal stem cells. *J Cell Biochem.* 2010;109:277-282.
96. Onai N, Manz MG, Schmid MA. Isolation of common dendritic cell progenitors (CDP) from mouse bone marrow. *Methods Mol Biol.* 2010;595:195-203.
97. Palis J. Ontogeny of erythropoiesis. *Curr Opin Hematol.* 2008;15:155-161.
98. Palis J, Malik J, McGrath KE, et al. Primitive erythropoiesis in the mammalian embryo. *Int J Dev Biol.* 2010;54:1011-1018.
99. Papadaki HA, Stamatopoulos K, Damianaki A, et al. Activated T-lymphocytes with myelosuppressive properties in patients with chronic idiopathic neutropenia. *Br J Haematol.* 2005;128:863-876.
100. Penn PE, Jiang DZ, Fei RG, et al. Dissecting the hematopoietic microenvironment. IX. Further characterization of murine bone marrow stromal cells. *Blood.* 1993;81: 1205-1213.
101. Perkins PC, Grindem CB, Cullins LD. Flow cytometric analysis of punctate and aggregate reticulocyte responses in phlebotomized cats. *Am J Vet Res.* 1995; 56:1564-1569.
102. Pietila I, Vainio S. The embryonic aorta-gonad-mesonephros region as a generator of haematopoietic stem cells. *APMIS.* 2005;113:804-812.
103. Ponka P, Beaumont C, Richardson DR. Function and regulation of transferrin and ferritin. *Semin Hematol.* 1998;35:35-54.
104. Porter DL, Goldberg MA. Regulation of erythropoietin production. *Exp Hematol.* 1993;21:399-404.
105. Prchal JT. Production of erythrocytes. In: Lichtman MA, Beutler E, Kipps TJ, et al, eds. *Williams Hematology.* 7th ed. New York: McGraw-Hill; 2006:393-403.
106. Prosper F, Verfaillie CM. Regulation of hematopoiesis through adhesion receptors. *J Leukoc Biol.* 2001;69:307-316.
107. Qui LB, Dickson H, Hajibagheri N, et al. Extruded erythroblast nuclei are bound and phagocytosed by a novel macrophage receptor. *Blood.* 1995;85:1630-1639.
108. Radin MJ, Wellman ML. Granulopoiesis. In: Weiss DJ, Wardrop KJ, eds. *Schalm's Veterinary Hematology.* 6th ed. Ames, IA: Wiley-Blackwell; 2010:43-49.
109. Rafii S, Mohle R, Shapiro F, et al. Regulation of hematopoiesis by microvascular endothelium. *Leuk Lymphoma.* 1997;27:375-386.
110. Rais M, Wild JS, Choudhury BK, et al. Interleukin-12 inhibits eosinophil differentiation from bone marrow stem cells in an interferon-gamma-dependent manner in a mouse model of asthma. *Clin Exp Allergy.* 2002;32:627-632.
111. Raj DS. Role of interleukin-6 in the anemia of chronic disease. *Semin Arthritis Rheum.* 2009;38:382-388.
112. Rapoport SM. *The Reticulocyte.* Boca Raton, FL: CRC Press, Inc.; 1986.
113. Robinson SN, Seina SM, Gohr JC, et al. Hematopoietic progenitor cell mobilization by granulocyte colony-stimulating factor and erythropoietin in the absence of matrix metalloproteinase-9. *Stem Cells Dev.* 2005;14:317-328.
114. Sage PT, Carman CV. Settings and mechanisms for trans-cellular diapedesis. *Front Biosci.* 2009;14:5066-5083.
115. Satija NK, Singh VK, Verma YK, et al. Mesenchymal stem cell-based therapy: a new paradigm in regenerative medicine. *J Cell Mol Med.* 2009;13:4385-4402.
116. Sawada K, Krantz SB, Dai CH, et al. Purification of human blood burst-forming units-erythroid and demonstration of the evolution of erythropoietin receptors. *J Cell Physiol.* 1990;142:219-230.
117. Segel GB, Palis J. Hematology of the newborn. In: Lichtman MA, Beutler E, Kipps TJ, et al, eds. *Williams Hematology.* 7th ed. New York: McGraw-Hill; 2006:81-99.
118. Silva GV, Litovsky S, Assad JA, et al. Mesenchymal stem cells differentiate into an endothelial phenotype, enhance vascular density, and improve heart function in a canine chronic ischemia model. *Circulation.* 2005;111:150-156.
119. Simpson CF, Kling JM. The mechanism of denucleation in circulating erythroblasts. *J Cell Biol.* 1967;35:237-245.
120. Simpson CF, Kling JM. The mechanism of mitochondrial extrusion from phenylhydrazine-induced reticulocytes in the circulating blood. *J Cell Biol.* 1968;36:103-109.
121. Siracusa MC, Perrigoue JG, Comeau MR, et al. New paradigms in basophil development, regulation and function. *Immunol Cell Biol.* 2010;88:275-284.
122. Sitnicka E, Wang QR, Tsai S, et al. Support versus inhibition of hematopoiesis by two characterized stromal cell types. *Stem Cells.* 1995;13:655-665.
123. Smith CW. Production, distribution, and fate of neutrophils. In: Lichtman MA, Beutler E, Kipps TJ, et al, eds. *Williams Hematology.* 7th ed. New York: McGraw-Hill; 2006:855-861.
124. Socolovsky M. Molecular insights into stress erythropoiesis. *Curr Opin Hematol.* 2007;14:215-224.
125. Sorrell JM, Weiss L. Cell interactions between hematopoietic and stromal cells in the embryonic chick bone marrow. *Anat Rec.* 1980;197:1-19.
126. Stopka T, Zivny JH, Stopkova P, et al. Human hematopoietic progenitors express erythropoietin. *Blood.* 1998;91:3766-3772.
127. Summers C, Rankin SM, Condliffe AM, et al. Neutrophil kinetics in health and disease. *Trends Immunol.* 2010;31:318-324.
128. Suter SE, Gouthro TA, McSweeney PA, et al. Isolation and characterization of pediatric canine bone marrow CD34+ cells. *Vet Immunol Immunopathol.* 2004;101:31-47.
129. Tavassoli M. Embryonic and fetal hemopoiesis: an overview. *Blood Cells.* 1991;17:269-281.
130. Tavian M, Biasch K, Sinka L, et al. Embryonic origin of human hematopoiesis. *Int J Dev Biol.* 2010;54:1061-1065.
131. Tavian M, Peault B. The changing cellular environments of hematopoiesis in human development in utero. *Exp Hematol.* 2005;33:1062-1069.
132. Telen MJ. Red blood cell surface adhesion molecules: their possible roles in normal human physiology and disease. *Semin Hematol.* 2000;37:130-142.
133. Tiedemann K. On the yolk sac of the cat. II. Erythropoietic phases, ultrastructure of aging primitive erythroblasts, and blood vessels. *Cell Tissue Res.* 1977;183:71-89.
134. Tiedemann K, van Ooyen B. Prenatal hematopoiesis and blood characteristics of the cat. *Anat Embryol (Berl).* 1978;153:243-267.
135. Tizard IR. *Veterinary Immunology. An Introduction.* 8th ed. Philadelphia: Saunders Elsevier; 2009.
136. Tober J, Koniski A, McGrath KE, et al. The megakaryocyte lineage originates from hemangioblast precursors and is an integral component both of primitive and of definitive hematopoiesis. *Blood.* 2007;109:1433-1441.
137. Tornquist SJ, Crawford TB. Suppression of megakaryocyte colony growth by plasma from foals infected with equine infectious anemia virus. *Blood.* 1997;90:2357-2363.
138. Tsuji-Takayama K, Otani T, Inoue T, et al. Erythropoietin induces sustained phosphorylation of STAT5 in primitive but not definitive erythrocytes generated from mouse embryonic stem cells. *Exp Hematol.* 2006;34:1323-1332.
139. Ueno H, Weissman IL. The origin and fate of yolk sac hematopoiesis: application of chimera analyses to developmental studies. *Int J Dev Biol.* 2010;54:1019-1031.

140. Vidal M. Exosomes in erythropoiesis. *Transfus Clin Biol.* 2010;17:131-137.
141. Vogt C, Pentz S, Rich IN. The role for the macrophage in normal hematopoiesis: III. In: vitro and in vivo erythropoietin gene expression in macrophages detected by in situ hybridization. *Exp Hematol.* 1989;17:391-397.
142. Wardlaw A. Eosinophils and their disorders. In: Lichtman MA, Beutler E, Kipps TJ, et al, eds. *Williams Hematology.* 7th ed. New York: McGraw-Hill; 2006:863-878.
143. Waugh RE. Reticulocyte rigidity and passage through endothelial-like pores. *Blood.* 1991;78:3037-3042.
144. Waugh RE, Mantalaris A, Bauserman RG, et al. Membrane instability in late-stage erythropoiesis. *Blood.* 2001;97:1869-1875.
145. Weiss G, Goodnough LT. Anemia of chronic disease. *N Engl J Med.* 2005;352:1011-1023.
146. Weiss L. The hematopoietic microenvironment of the bone marrow: an ultrastructural study of the stroma in rats. *Anat Rec.* 1976;186:161-184.
147. Weiss L. *The Blood Cells and Hematopoietic Tissues.* New York: Elsevier; 1984.
148. Wolber EM, Jelkmann W. Thrombopoietin: the novel hepatic hormone. *News Physiol Sci.* 2002;17:6-10.
149. Wu H, Riha GM, Yang H, et al. Differentiation and proliferation of endothelial progenitor cells from canine peripheral blood mononuclear cells. *J Surg Res.* 2005;126:193-198.
150. Yao H, Liu B, Wang X, et al. Identification of high proliferative potential precursors with hemangioblastic activity in the mouse aorta-gonad-mesonephros region. *Stem Cells.* 2007;25:1423-1430.
151. Ye M, Graf T. Early decisions in lymphoid development. *Curr Opin Immunol.* 2007;19:123-128.
152. Yin T, Li L. The stem cell niches in bone. *J Clin Invest.* 2006;116:1195-1201.
153. Yona S, Jung S. Monocytes: subsets, origins, fates and functions. *Curr Opin Hematol.* 2010;17:53-59.
154. Zermati Y, Fichelson S, Valensi F, et al. Transforming growth factor inhibits erythropoiesis by blocking proliferation and accelerating differentiation of erythroid progenitors. *Exp Hematol.* 2000;28:885-894.
155. Zhang Y, Wallace DL, de Lara CM, et al. In vivo kinetics of human natural killer cells: the effects of ageing and acute and chronic viral infection. *Immunology.* 2007;121:258-265.

CHAPTER

4

EVALUATION OF ERYTHROCYTES

NORMAL ERYTHROCYTES

Erythrocyte Morphology

Erythrocytes from all mammals are anucleated, and most are in the shape of biconcave discs called discocytes (Figs. 4-1, 4-2).[205] The biconcave shape results in the central pallor of erythrocytes observed in stained blood films. Among common domestic animals, biconcavity and central pallor are most pronounced in dogs (Figs. 4-3, 4-4), which also have the largest erythrocytes. Other species do not consistently exhibit central pallor in erythrocytes on stained blood films. The apparent benefit of the biconcave shape is that it gives erythrocytes high surface area : volume ratios and allows for deformations that must take place as they circulate. Erythrocytes from goats generally have a flat surface with little surface depression; a variety of irregularly shaped erythrocytes (poikilocytes) may be present in clinically normal goats (Fig. 4-5). Erythrocytes from animals in the Camelidae family (camels, llamas, vicuñas, and alpacas) are anucleated, thin, elliptical cells termed elliptocytes or ovalocytes (Fig. 4-6). They are not biconcave in shape and are minimally deformable.[437] Erythrocytes from birds (Fig. 4-7), reptiles, and amphibians are also elliptical in shape, but they contain nuclei and are larger than mammalian erythrocytes. Blood cells in salamanders are the largest recognized (Fig. 4-8).

Erythrocyte Functions

Mammalian erythrocytes normally circulate for several months in blood despite limited synthetic capacities and repeated exposures to mechanical and metabolic insults. Erythrocytes have three functions: transport of oxygen (O_2) to tissue, transport of carbon dioxide (CO_2) to the lungs, and buffering of hydrogen ions (H^+). In nonanemic animals, the presence of hemoglobin within erythrocytes increases the O_2-carrying capacity of blood more than 50 times that of plasma without erythrocytes. The O_2 content of blood depends on the blood hemoglobin content, the partial pressure of dissolved oxygen (PO_2) in blood, and the affinity of hemoglobin for O_2.

Each hemoglobin tetramer is capable of binding four molecules of O_2 when fully oxygenated. The initial binding of a molecule of O_2 to a monomer of tetrameric deoxygenated hemoglobin facilitates further binding of O_2 to the hemoglobin molecule. The changing O_2 affinity of hemoglobin with oxygenation results in a sigmoid O_2 dissociation curve (Fig. 4-9), when the percent saturation of hemoglobin with O_2 is graphed against the PO_2. The steepness of the middle portion of the curve is of great physiologic significance because it covers the range of O_2 tensions present in tissues. Consequently a relatively small decrease in O_2 tension in tissues results in substantial O_2 release from hemoglobin. The overall affinity of hemoglobin for O_2 is decreased by increasing H^+, CO_2, temperature, and, in most mammals, 2,3-diphosphoglycerate (2,3DPG). There is a direct correlation between body weight and the O_2 affinity of hemoglobin in whole blood (lower body weight, lower O_2 affinity) when various species of mammals are compared.[205]

The O_2 affinity of fetal blood is greater than that of maternal blood except in the cat. Differences in fetal versus maternal O_2 affinity may potentiate O_2 transport from the mother to the fetus. However, the fetus is subjected to low arterial O_2 tensions, and the increased O_2 affinity of fetal blood is likely needed to more fully saturate hemoglobin with O_2.[205]

The ability of plasma to carry CO_2 is small, but the carbonic anhydrase reaction in erythrocytes increases the CO_2-carrying capacity of blood 17-fold by rapidly converting CO_2 to carbonic acid (H_2CO_3). The H_2CO_3 spontaneously ionizes to H^+ and bicarbonate (HCO_3^-). The HCO_3^- diffuses out of the cell down a concentration gradient and chloride (Cl^-) moves in (chloride shift) to maintain electrical neutrality. These processes are reversed at the lungs. Some CO_2 is also transported bound to hemoglobin as carbamino groups. Deoxyhemoglobin binds about twice the CO_2 that oxyhemoglobin does.[205]

Hemoglobin is the major protein buffer in blood. Deoxyhemoglobin is a weaker acid than oxyhemoglobin. Consequently, when oxyhemoglobin releases its O_2 in the tissues, the formation of deoxyhemoglobin results in increased binding

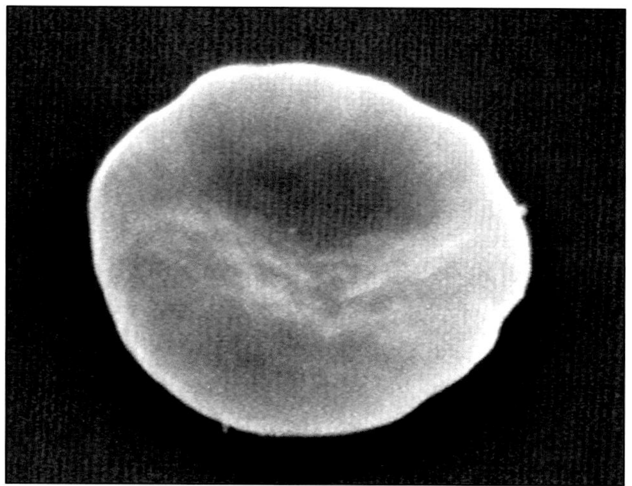

FIGURE 4-1
Scanning electron photomicrograph of a normal horse erythrocyte called a discocyte.

From Stockham SL, Harvey JW, Kinden DA. Equine glucose-6-phosphate dehydrogenase deficiency. Vet Pathol. *94;31:518-527.*

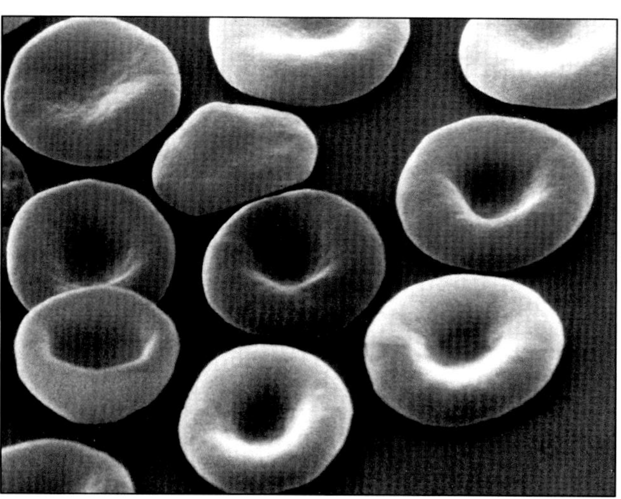

FIGURE 4-3
Scanning electron photomicrograph of dog erythrocytes (discocytes).

Courtesy of K. S. Keeton and N. C. Jain.

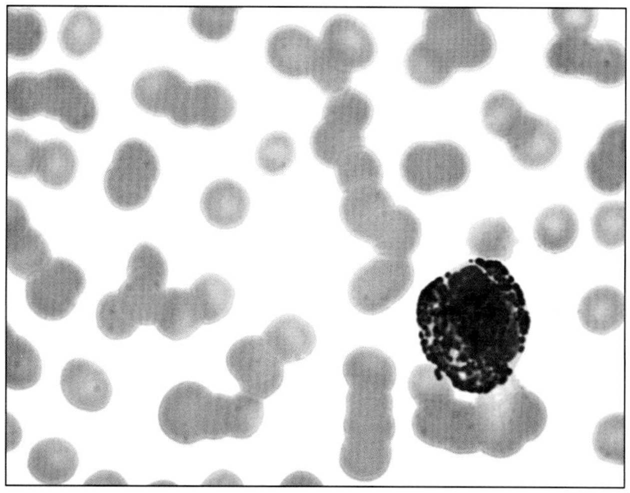

FIGURE 4-2
Blood film from a horse. Most erythrocytes are adhered together like stacks of coins (rouleaux), a normal finding in this species. Individual nonadherent erythrocytes exhibit central pallor as a result of their biconcave shape. A basophil with purple granules is present in the bottom right of the image. Wright-Giemsa stain.

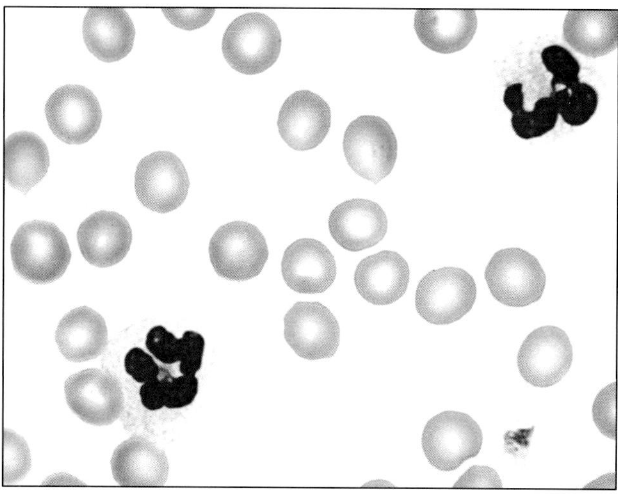

FIGURE 4-4
Blood from a dog with acute blood-loss anemia and normal erythrocyte morphology. Erythrocytes exhibit prominent central pallor. Two mature neutrophils and a platelet *(bottom right corner)* are also present. Wright-Giemsa stain.

of H^+. Hemoglobin buffers the effects of H_2CO_3 and allows for the isohydric transport of CO_2. Hemoglobin also buffers organic acids produced during metabolism.[205]

Erythrocyte Biochemistry

Membrane Structure and Function

The erythrocyte membrane contains a phospholipid bilayer with molecules of unesterified cholesterol intercalated between fatty acid chains. Phospholipids can move in various ways and contribute to membrane fluidity. Glycolipids are located on the outer layer of the membrane, with carbohydrate groups extending outward. Some blood group antigens are glycolipids, with their specificity residing in the carbohydrate moieties (see Chapter 6 for a discussion of clinically significant blood groups).[205]

Membrane proteins consist of integral membrane proteins that penetrate the lipid portion, often spanning the bilayer, and skeletal proteins that form or attach to the internal surface of the lipid bilayer. Glycoproteins associated with the membrane are integral membrane proteins with the carbohydrate residues extending from the outside surface of the cell

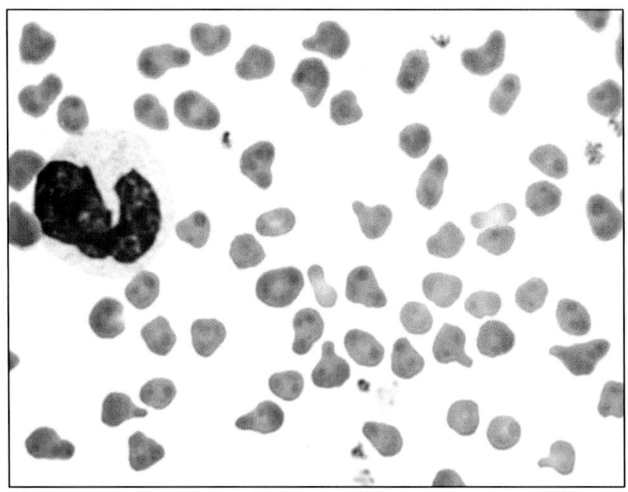

FIGURE 4-5
Poikilocytes in blood from a normal goat. Note the small size of the erythrocytes compared with the neutrophil in the left part of the image. Wright-Giemsa stain.

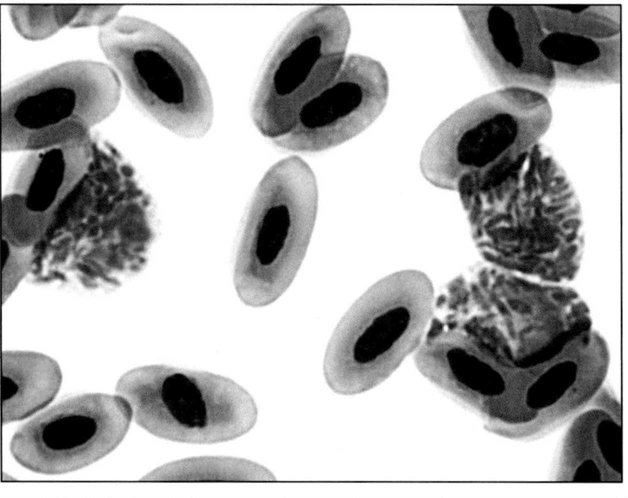

FIGURE 4-7
Blood film from a macaw. Nucleated erythrocytes and three heterophils are present.

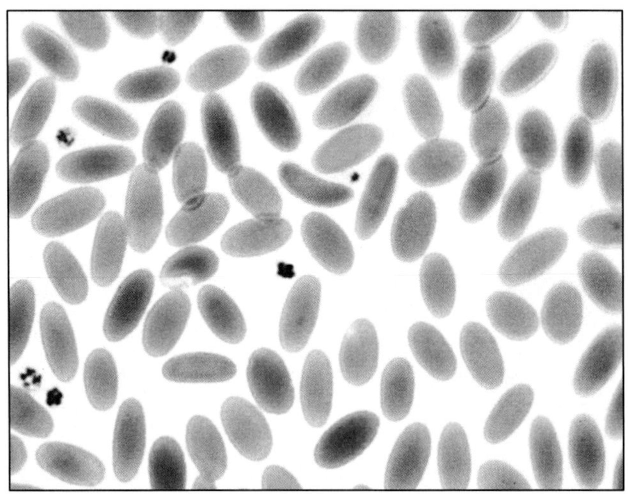

FIGURE 4-6
Elliptocytes in blood from a normal llama. Wright-Giemsa stain.

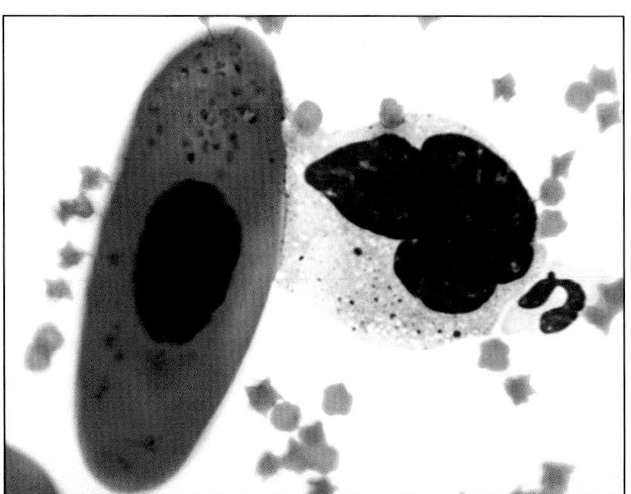

FIGURE 4-8
Blood film prepared by mixing equal parts of blood from a salamander *(Amphiuma means)* with that of a domestic cat to demonstrate the large size of the nucleated erythrocytes and a neutrophil in the salamander. Most of the cat erythrocytes are echinocytes, a shape artifact of sample handling in this instance. Wright-Giemsa stain.

Courtesy of H. L. Wamsley.

membrane. They carry erythrocyte antigens and function as receptors or transport proteins (e.g., band 3 is an anion transporter). The membrane skeleton is composed of various proteins located in a lattice-like arrangement on the inner surface of the erythrocyte membrane. This meshwork is attached to the membrane by binding to transmembrane proteins. The membrane skeleton is a major determining factor of membrane shape, deformability, and durability. It is in a condensed configuration in intact cells and can be stretched considerably without rupturing.[205]

Inherited membrane defects can result in abnormally shaped erythrocytes with shortened erythrocyte life spans and variable degrees of anemia. Band 3 deficiency in cattle results in marked spherocytosis with membrane instability and severe anemia.[232] Hereditary elliptocytosis has been reported in one dog with protein 4.1 deficiency and another with mutant β-spectrin.[122,205] Neither dog with elliptocytosis was anemic, but the protein 4.1-deficient dog had a reticulocytosis, indicating a shortened erythrocyte life span. Hereditary stomatocytosis occurs in multiple dog breeds, but the specific membrane defects have not been reported.[205]

ATP Generation

Mammalian erythrocytes lack nuclei; therefore they cannot synthesize DNA or RNA. They also lack ribosomes,

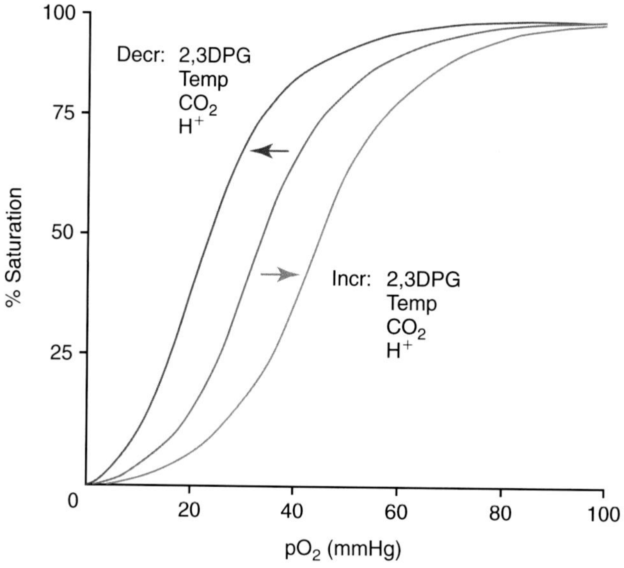

FIGURE 4-9

Hemoglobin-oxygen dissociation curve and factors influencing the position of the curve.

From Harvey JW. The erythrocyte: physiology, metabolism, and biochemical disorders. In: Kaneko JJ, Harvey JW, Bruss ML, eds. Clinical Biochemistry of Domestic Animals, *6th ed. San Diego, CA: Academic Press; 2008: 173-240.*

mitochondria, and endoplasmic reticula; consequently they have no Krebs cycle or electron transport system and are unable to synthesize proteins or lipids de novo. Glucose is the primary substrate for the energy needs of erythrocytes from all species except the pig, where inosine appears to be the major substrate. Mature erythrocytes depend on anaerobic glycolysis for energy (Fig. 4-10). The ATP generated by glycolysis is needed for the maintenance of erythrocyte ionic composition, shape, and deformability and for limited synthetic activities such as glutathione synthesis. Hypophosphatemia results in decreased erythrocyte glycolytic rates and decreased ATP generation. Hemolytic anemia resulting from hypophosphatemia has been reported in diabetic cats and in a diabetic dog following insulin therapy, in a cat with hepatic lipidosis, and in postparturient cattle and buffaloes.[109,205] Deficiencies of rate-controlling enzymes in glycolysis also result in insufficient ATP generation and shortened erythrocyte survival. Pyruvate kinase (PK)-deficient dogs and cats have mild to severe regenerative hemolytic anemia. Phosphofructokinase (PFK)-deficient dogs have compensated hemolytic anemia plus sporadic episodes of intravascular hemolysis and hemoglobinuria.[203]

2,3DPG Pathway

2,3DPG binds to hemoglobin and reduces the affinity of hemoglobin for oxygen in erythrocytes from most mammals. It is produced from a side pathway of the anaerobic glycolysis pathway. No net ATP is generated when molecules traverse this DPG pathway. The formation of 2,3DPG in erythrocytes is stimulated by increased blood inorganic phosphate (P_i) concentration and increased blood pH, both of which stimulate anaerobic glycolysis. 2,3DPG is the most abundant organic phosphate in the erythrocytes of most species but its concentration is low in erythrocytes of Felidae (including domestic cats), Bovidae (cattle, sheep, and goats), and Cervidae (deer).[415] Animals with high erythrocyte 2,3DPG concentrations, including dogs and horses, have the potential to alter their hemoglobin O_2 affinity to meet their metabolic needs. The significance (and, in some cases, the appropriateness) of alterations in 2,3DPG in disease states is not always clear. Erythrocyte 2,3DPG concentration increases in some anemic animals, and the resultant decrease in hemoglobin O_2 affinity would seem to be beneficial.[205] Increased 2,3DPG has also been reported in erythrocytes from horses with hypoxic conditions.[173] In the case of severe hypoxic hypoxemia, the response might be detrimental because hemoglobin cannot be fully saturated.[241] High-altitude camelids (including llamas, alpacas, guanacos, and vicuñas) have erythrocytes with high hemoglobin oxygen affinity, even though their erythrocytes have relatively high 2,3DPG concentrations, because their hemoglobin exhibits low reactivity toward 2,3DPG.[377] The P_{50} for greyhound erythrocytes in whole blood is lower than that for mongrel dogs, yet the groups have similar 2,3DPG concentrations.[458] The cause of this difference remains to be determined, but it could reflect a low reactivity to 2,3DPG. It is suggested that the higher hematocrit found in greyhound dogs may represent a compensatory response to a higher oxygen affinity of hemoglobin in this species.

PFK deficiency inhibits glycolysis above the DPG pathway, resulting in markedly decreased 2,3DPG concentrations, which makes dog erythrocytes alkaline-fragile. Episodes of intravascular hemolysis occur when PFK-deficient dogs develop alkalemia secondary to hyperventilation.[203]

Oxidant Injury

Animals are exposed to low levels of oxidants in their environments and from normal metabolic processes in the body. Reactive oxygen species and reactive nitrogen species are formed as products of normal cellular metabolism. When they are generated at higher concentrations in disease states, these free radicals (and the even more potent oxidative metabolites that they produce) can overwhelm protective systems within the body, producing cellular injury and/or destruction.[492]

Oxidative reactions can damage hemoglobin, enzymes (sulfhydryl groups especially), and the membrane lipids of erythrocytes. Methemoglobin forms when hemoglobin iron is oxidized from the +2 to the +3 state. Heinz bodies are inclusions that form within erythrocytes following the oxidative denaturation of the globin portion of hemoglobin. Membrane damage can result in intravascular hemolysis or erythrophagocytosis and shortened erythrocyte life spans.[205]

Protection against Oxidant Injury. NADPH generated in the pentose phosphate pathway (PPP) provides electrons for protection against oxidants. It is needed to maintain glutathione and thioredoxin in their reduced states, and it is

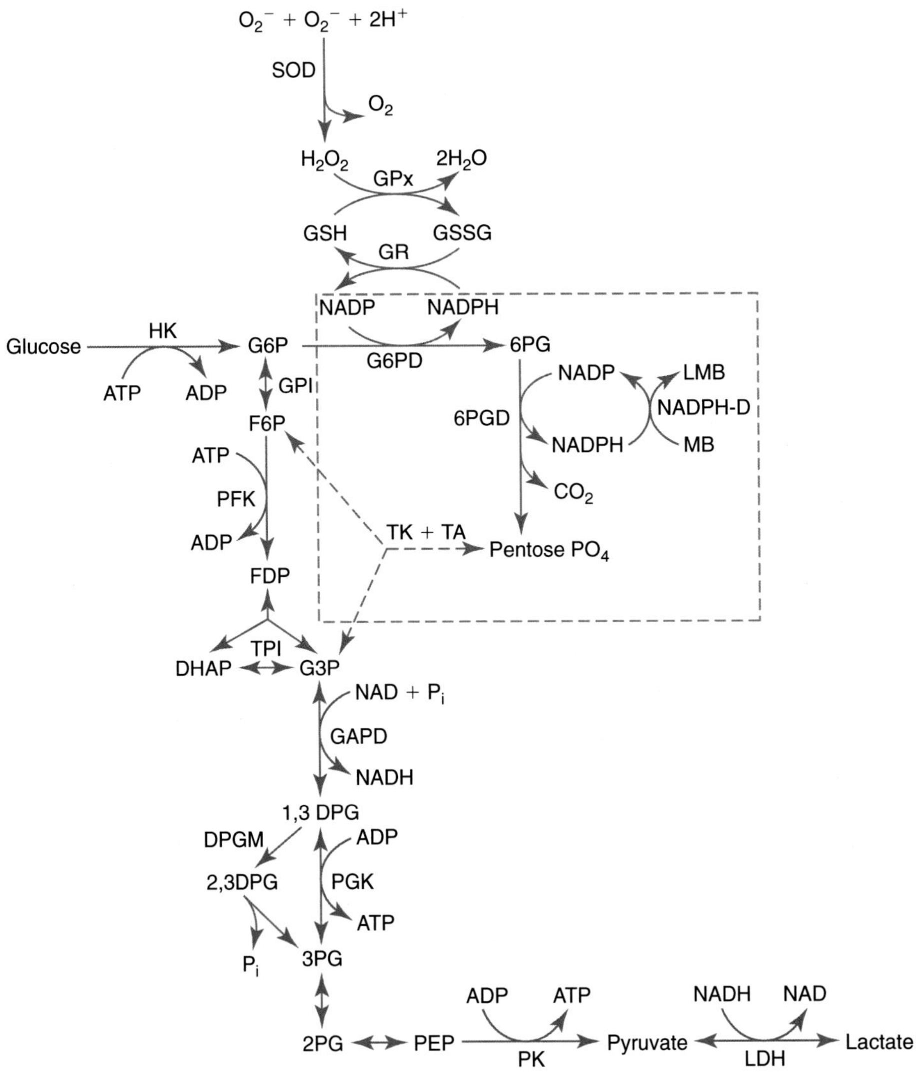

FIGURE 4-10

Metabolic pathways of the mature erythrocyte. HK, hexokinase; GPI, glucose phosphate isomerase; PFK, phosphofructokinase; TPI, triosephosphate isomerase; GAPD, glyceraldehyde-3-phosphate dehydrogenase; PGK, phosphoglycerate kinase; MPGM, monophosphoglycerate mutase; DPGM, diphosphoglycerate mutase; PK, pyruvate kinase; G6PD, glucose-6-phosphate dehydrogenase; 6PGD, 6-phosphogluconate dehydrogenase; LDH, lactate dehydrogenase; GR, glutathione reductase; GPx, glutathione peroxidase; TK, transketolase; TA, transaldolase; GSSG, oxidized glutathione; G6P, glucose 6-phosphate; F6P, fructose 6-phosphate; FDP, fructose 1,6-diphosphate; DHAP, dihydroxyacetone phosphate; GAP, glyceraldehyde 3-phosphate; 1,3DPG, 1,3-diphosphoglycerate; 2,3DPG, 2,3-diphosphoglycerate; 3PG, 3-phosphoglycerate; 2PG, 2-phosphoglycerate; PEP, phosphoenolpyruvate; ADP, adenosine diphosphate; ATP, adenosine triphosphate; NAD, nicotinamide adenine dinucleotide; NADH, reduced nicotinamide adenine dinucleotide; NADP, nicotinamide adenine dinucleotide phosphate; NADPH, reduced nicotinamide adenine dinucleotide phosphate; GSH, reduced glutathione; P_i, inorganic phosphate; SOD, superoxide dismutase.

From Harvey JW. The erythrocyte: physiology, metabolism, and biochemical disorders. In: Kaneko JJ, Harvey JW, Bruss ML, eds. Clinical Biochemistry of Domestic Animals, *6th ed. San Diego, CA: Academic Press; 2008:173-240.*

important in maintaining catalase in a functional form. Defects in the PPP can render erythrocytes susceptible to endogenous and exogenous oxidant injury. Glucose-6-phosphate dehydrogenase (G6PD) is the rate-controlling enzyme in the PPP. A persistent hemolytic anemia with eccentrocytosis has been described in an American saddlebred colt with less than 1% of normal G6PD activity.[452]

Reduced glutathione (GSH) is a tripeptide containing a highly reactive sulfhydryl group that may act nonenzymatically as a free radical acceptor to counteract oxidant damage.

GSH also functions as an electron donor in various reductive enzyme reactions including glutathione peroxidase (GPx), phospholipid hydroperoxide glutathione peroxidase, glutathione S-transferase, and glutaredoxin. Following oxidation, glutathione forms a disulfide (GSSG) that can be reduced back to GSH by the flavin adenine dinucleotide (FAD)-dependent glutathione reductase (GR) enzyme, using NADPH as the source of electrons (see Fig. 4-10). Horses with erythrocyte FAD deficiency have markedly reduced GR activity, decreased GSH concentration, and prominent eccentrocytosis.[203,212]

Selenium acts as an antioxidant when incorporated as selenocysteine at the active site of a wide range of selenoproteins, including GPx, phospholipid hydroperoxide glutathione peroxidase, and thioredoxin reductase in erythrocytes.[73] Heinz body hemolytic anemia has been reported in selenium-deficient cattle grazing on St. Augustine grass.[327] Catalase is an enzyme that can catalyze the conversion of H_2O_2 to water and O_2 without using energy.

Recent studies suggest that peroxiredoxins may be more important in protecting against H_2O_2 than GPx or catalase.[285] Oxidized peroxiredoxins are regenerated using reduced thioredoxin, and oxidized thioredoxin is reduced by NADPH using thioredoxin reductase.[277] Ascorbate functions as an antioxidant by donating one or two electrons to a variety of oxidants, including oxygen free radicals and peroxides. Vitamin E is lipid-soluble and acts as a free radical scavenger in the membrane.[205]

Methemoglobin Formation and Reduction

About 3% of hemoglobin (Fe^{+2}) is oxidized to methemoglobin (Fe^{+3}) each day. Methemoglobin is unable to bind O_2. To prevent hypoxemia, which would result from the accumulation of a high level of methemoglobin, the methemoglobin formed is reduced back to functional hemoglobin in a reaction that requires the cytochrome-b_5 reductase (Cb_5R) enzyme and NADH generated by anaerobic glycolysis.[205] An inherited deficiency in Cb_5R in dogs and cats results in persistent methemoglobinemia with minimal or no clinical signs.[203] Methemoglobinemia also occurs in horses that have decreased Cb_5R activity secondary to erythrocyte FAD deficiency.[212]

Iron Metabolism

Iron metabolism is presented in this chapter because more iron is needed for the production of erythrocytes than for all other cells in the body combined. Iron is absorbed from the diet in the small intestine and transferred to plasma, where it is bound to transferrin for transport to cells within the body. Once inside the body, iron cycles in a nearly closed system (Fig. 4-11) because little iron is lost in domestic animals unless hemorrhage occurs. About 75% of the iron present in plasma will be transported to the bone marrow for incorporation into hemoglobin in developing erythroid cells.[436] The remaining plasma iron is taken up by nonerythroid tissues, primarily the liver.[266] Erythrocytes containing hemoglobin normally circulate for several months before being phagocytized by macrophages when senescent. After phagocytosis, erythrocytes are lysed, hemoglobin is degraded, and iron is released. Most iron released from degraded hemoglobin is quickly released back into plasma, but a small amount may be stored as ferritin or hemosiderin within macrophages, which is released more slowly into plasma. The vast majority of iron entering plasma each day comes from macrophage release.[204]

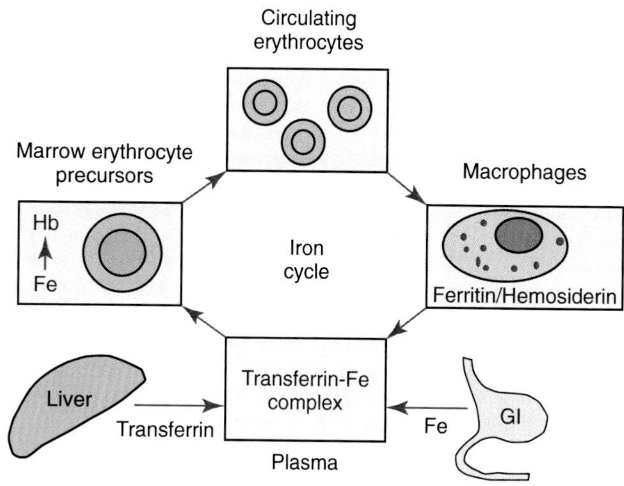

FIGURE 4-11

Iron cycle. Iron (Fe) is highly conserved in the body. Iron in plasma is bound to transferrin, a transport protein that is synthesized in the liver. Iron is transported to all tissues, but most iron is utilized to synthesize hemoglobin in developing erythroid cells. Aged blood erythrocytes are phagocytized by macrophages and hemoglobin is degraded. Released iron is either returned to plasma or stored in macrophages as ferritin and hemosiderin. Nearly all of the iron in plasma under normal conditions comes from the release of iron by macrophages that have phagocytized and degraded erythrocytes. Only about 3% of the iron in plasma results from gastrointestinal (GI) enterocyte absorption in normal individuals.

From Harvey JW. Iron metabolisms and its disorders. In: Kaneko JJ, Harvey JW, Bruss ML, eds. Clinical Biochemistry of Domestic Animals, *6th ed. San Diego, CA: Academic Press; 2008:259-285.*

About 60% to 70% of total body iron is present in hemoglobin (3.4 mg iron per gram of hemoglobin). About a third of total body iron is stored as ferritin and hemosiderin (primarily within macrophages), 3% to 7% is present in myoglobin (with the higher values occurring in dogs and horses), 1% is present in hemoprotein and flavoprotein enzymes, and only 0.1% is bound to transferrin in plasma.[204]

Iron Absorption. The absorption of iron from the diet depends upon age, species, iron stores, rate of erythropoiesis, inflammation, and pregnancy, as well as the amount and chemical form of iron ingested. A low percentage of dietary iron is absorbed in normal adult animals. Iron absorption occurs through enterocytes of the duodenum and proximal jejunum. Iron can be taken in by enterocytes as free ions or as heme by different pathways (Fig. 4-12). The relative importance of these pathways varies depending on species and diet.[204]

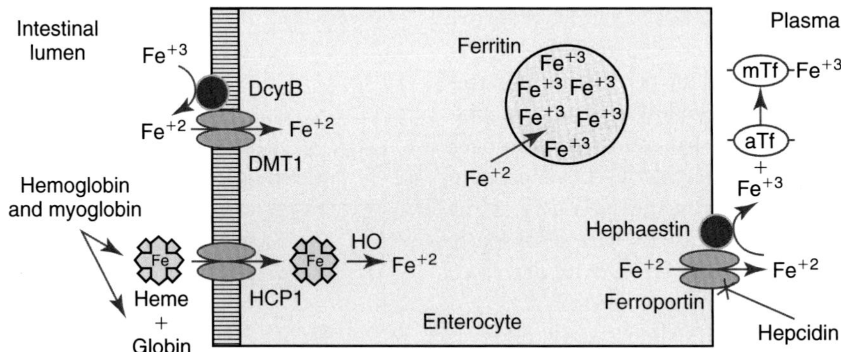

FIGURE 4-12

Mechanisms of iron absorption. Ferrous iron (Fe^{+2}) ions are transported into enterocytes in the duodenum by the divalent transporter-1 (DMT1) after reduction of ferric iron (Fe^{+3}) ions using a duodenal cytochrome b (DcytB). Heme is transported into enterocytes using heme carrier protein-1 (HCP1). Once inside, inorganic iron is released from heme by the action of the heme oxygenase (HO) reaction. Fe^{+2} ions are exported from enterocytes using ferroportin, oxidized to Fe^{+3} using hephaestin, and bound by apotransferrin (aTf) to form monoferric transferrin (mTf) and diferric transferrin (not shown). Hepcidin in plasma inhibits iron export to plasma by interacting directly with ferroportin, leading to ferroportin's internalization and lysosomal degradation. Fe^{+2} not transported to plasma is stored as ferritin following oxidation to Fe^{+3}. Iron stored as ferritin is returned to the lumen of the small intestine when enterocytes are sloughed at the tip of the villus.

From Harvey JW. Iron metabolism and its disorders. In: Kaneko JJ, Harvey JW, Bruss ML, eds. Clinical Biochemistry of Domestic Animals. *6th ed. San Diego, CA: Academic Press; 2008:259-285.*

Most inorganic iron in the diet is in the ferric (Fe^{+3}) state. Fe^{+3} iron is solubilized from food by hydrochloric acid in the stomach and binds to mucins and various small molecules in the stomach, which keep the iron soluble and available for absorption in the more alkaline environment of the small intestine. The most important pathway for nonheme iron uptake utilizes the divalent metal transporter-1 (DMT1). Fe^{+3} ions must be reduced to ferrous (Fe^{+2}) ions before they can be transported into the enterocyte via the DMT1. Although some Fe^{+3} ion reduction may occur by direct interaction with dietary ascorbic acid, most reduction appears to rely on duodenal cytochrome b (DcytB) and possibly other brush border ferrireductase enzymes. Although humans absorb Fe^{+2} salts more readily from the intestine than Fe^{+3} salts, dogs are reported to absorb both valence forms equally well.[204]

Heme is released from dietary myoglobin and hemoglobin by the action of digestive enzymes. Dietary heme iron is generally more bioavailable than is nonheme iron and is an important nutritional source of iron in carnivores and omnivores. Heme enters duodenal enterocytes as an intact metalloporphyrin, possibly using a brush border transporter named heme carrier protein 1 (HCP1). However, this protein transports folate more efficiently than heme; consequently, its physiologic role in intestinal heme uptake remains to be clearly defined. After heme absorption, iron is released from heme by the action of the heme oxygenase reaction.[20]

Once within the enterocyte, intracellular iron molecules are likely bound to one or more chaperone molecules. A potential chaperone named poly (rC)-binding protein 1 (PCBP1) has been described.[422] Iron taken up by enterocytes has one of two fates, export or storage, depending on the body's iron needs. If iron is required by the body, molecules will be transported from enterocytes to transferrin in plasma. This transportation is mediated by ferroportin, an iron transport protein located on the basolateral surface of mature enterocytes. In addition to ferroportin, the efflux of iron from enterocytes requires a copper-containing protein called hephaestin, which is also located on the basolateral membranes of mature enterocytes. Hephaestin is a membrane-bound ferroxidase that has significant homology to the plasma protein ceruloplasmin. Hephaestin's function may relate to its ability to oxidize Fe^{+2} ions to Fe^{+3} ions for binding to transferrin in plasma.[20]

If body iron requirements are low, enterocyte cytoplasmic iron accumulates. Free iron is toxic; consequently the mucosal cell protects itself by increasing apoferritin synthesis and incorporating the excess iron into ferritin. Each ferritin molecule is composed of a protein shell of 24 apoferritin subunits surrounding a central core of up to 4500 iron atoms as ferric oxyhydroxide. Ferritin is a storage protein that prevents free iron from catalyzing oxidative reactions, which would injure the cell. Ferritin within mucosal cells is returned to the small intestine lumen when enterocytes are sloughed at the tip of the villus after 1 to 2 days.[445]

Iron absorption is increased when total body iron content is low or erythropoiesis is increased. Iron absorption is decreased when total body iron content is high or inflammation is present.[204] Components of brush-border iron uptake, including DMT1 and DcytB, are strongly influenced by the iron concentration within enterocytes, with increased components expressed when intracellular iron content is low and decreased components expressed when iron content is high. These locally responsive changes in brush-border transport components help buffer the body against the absorption of excessive iron, but it is the control of the basolateral transport of iron from enterocytes to plasma that represents the primary site at which iron absorption is regulated.[445]

Systemic Control of Iron Metabolism. Hepcidin, a peptide secreted by hepatocytes into the circulation, is an important systemic regulator of iron metabolism.[153] Its production is modulated by body iron requirements, which are largely influenced by the magnitude of erythropoiesis present.[354] Hepcidin inhibits iron export from enterocytes, macrophages, and hepatocytes by interacting directly with ferroportin, leading to the internalization and lysosomal degradation of this iron export protein.[20] Hepcidin production is decreased in iron deficiency and disorders resulting in increased erythropoiesis, which increase the demand for iron.[152] As a result, ferroportin receptors are abundant on cell surfaces and dietary iron absorption is increased, as is the export of iron from macrophages and hepatocytes. Conversely, hepcidin production is increased and ferroportin transporter expression on cell surfaces is decreased when iron overload is present. Hepcidin production is also increased during inflammation by a pathway not dependent on body iron requirements.[445]

Plasma Iron. Nearly all of the iron in plasma is bound to the protein apotransferrin to form transferrin. The binding of iron to apotransferrin keeps iron molecules soluble and prevents iron-catalyzed oxidative reactions. Apotransferrin is a β-globulin with two binding sites for Fe^{+3}. Normally, 25% to 50% of the iron-binding sites are saturated with iron. Plasma iron turns over rapidly in 3 hours or less.[436] Nearly all of the iron in plasma under normal conditions comes from the release of iron by macrophages that have phagocytized and degraded erythrocytes. In contrast, in normal individuals, only about 3% of the iron in plasma results from enterocyte absorption.[372]

Iron Uptake by Erythroid Cells. The delivery of iron from plasma to developing erythroid cells and other cell types except macrophages is dependent on transferrin.[266] Transferrin (especially diferric transferrin) molecules bind to transferrin receptor 1 (TfR1) on the surface of cells, and these transferrin-TfR1 complexes invaginate to initiate endocytosis. After the transferrin-TfR1 complexes are internalized as endosomes, a proton pump decreases the pH in the endosome, resulting in conformational changes in the proteins and subsequent release of iron ions from transferrin. The released iron is exported from the endosome using DMT1.[349] The resultant apotransferrin-TfR1 complex is recycled to the cell membrane, where apotransferrin is released from the cell, and the TfR1 is again available for binding additional iron-containing transferrin molecules. Erythroid precursor cells in the bone marrow and reticulocytes that synthesize hemoglobin have TfR1 on their surfaces for iron uptake, but reticulocytes lose their TfR1 as they develop into mature erythrocytes.[372]

After its release from transferrin, iron is transported to the mitochondria, where it is incorporated into protoporphyrin to form heme. A direct interorganelle transfer of iron occurs between endosomes and mitochondria in developing erythroid cells.[419] Some iron is presumably released from endosomes into a cytoplasmic labile iron pool, with excess cytoplasmic iron stored as ferritin. TfR and apoferritin synthesis are regulated by the amount of intracellular iron present. High iron content stimulates apoferritin synthesis and inhibits TfR expression to minimize the potential of iron toxicity to the cell. Low iron content results in decreased apoferritin synthesis and increased TfR expression on cell surfaces to maximize iron uptake and use for heme synthesis. Free heme concentration within erythroid cells controls hemoglobin synthesis. An increase in free heme promotes the synthesis of globin chains and inhibits the uptake of iron from transferrin.[204]

Macrophage Iron Metabolism. Little iron enters macrophages, in contrast to other cell types in the body, via plasma transferrin. Rather, nearly all iron enters macrophages by the phagocytosis of aged or prematurely damaged erythrocytes (Fig. 4-13).[373] Following phagocytosis, erythrocytes are lysed and hemoglobin is degraded to heme and globin. The microsomal heme oxygenase reaction degrades heme and releases iron. Most of the iron released from degraded heme is quickly exported from the macrophage and bound to plasma transferrin for transport to other cells (especially erythrocyte

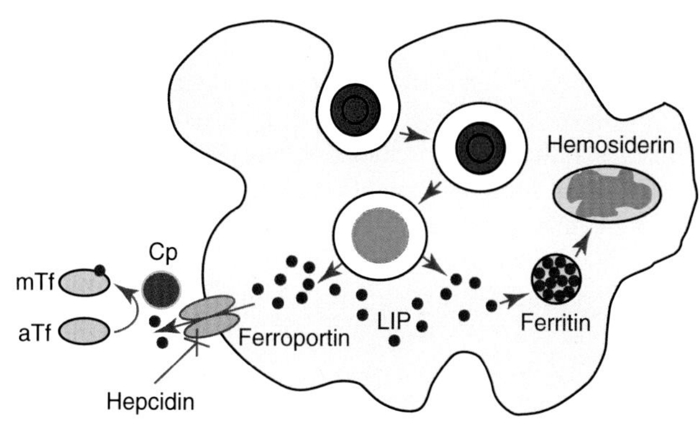

FIGURE 4-13

Iron metabolism in macrophages. Nearly all iron enters macrophages by the phagocytosis of aged or prematurely damaged erythrocytes. Following phagocytosis, erythrocytes are lysed, and hemoglobin is degraded to heme and globin. The microsomal heme oxygenase reaction within macrophages degrades heme and releases iron to the labile iron pool (LIP). Most of the released iron is exported from the macrophage by ferroportin as ferrous iron, oxidized to ferric iron by ceruloplasmin (Cp) in plasma, and bound to apotransferrin (aTf) to form monoferric transferrin (mTf) or diferric transferrin (not shown). Hepcidin in plasma inhibits iron export by interacting directly with ferroportin, leading to ferroportin's internalization and lysosomal degradation. Iron not rapidly released to plasma is stored within macrophages as ferritin, which may be degraded to hemosiderin within lysosomes.

From Harvey JW. Iron metabolism and its disorders. In: Kaneko JJ, Harvey JW, Bruss ML, eds. Clinical Biochemistry of Domestic Animals. *6th ed. San Diego, CA: Academic Press; 2008:259-285.*

precursors in the bone marrow).[204] The export of iron from macrophages is mediated by ferroportin and controlled by hepcidin, as has been discussed for enterocytes.[495] The copper-containing plasma protein ceruloplasmin oxidizes Fe^{+2} ions to Fe^{+3} ions for binding to transferrin in plasma.[341]

The mononuclear phagocyte system accounts for much of the total body iron stores. Iron not rapidly released to plasma is stored within macrophages as ferritin and hemosiderin. Free cytoplasmic ferritin molecules are visible by electron microscopy but not by light microscopy. Hemosiderin is composed of aggregates of protein and iron within lysosomes. It is insoluble in water and thought to result from the degradation of ferritin. Hemosiderin is visible by light microscopy when it is stained with an iron stain (Prussian blue stain). Iron in the storage pool turns over slowly unless there is an increased need for iron for hemoglobin synthesis.[45]

ERYTHROCYTE DESTRUCTION

Normal Removal of Aged Erythrocytes

Most erythrocytes circulate in blood for a finite time period (survival time or life span) ranging from 2 to 5 months in domestic animals, depending on the species. Erythrocyte life spans are related to body weight (and consequently metabolic rate), with the smallest animals (highest metabolic rate) having the shortest erythrocyte life spans. Greyhound dogs are often used as blood donors. The erythrocyte life span of 6 greyhound dogs (mean 93 days) was not significantly different from that of 3 nongreyhound dogs (103 days).[158] Aged erythrocytes are phagocytized by macrophages of the mononuclear phagocyte system. Oxidative injury, especially near the end of their life span, appears to be responsible for normal erythrocyte aging and removal.[205] Oxidative damage and other stressors can induce suicidal death of erythrocytes (eryptosis), with reactions similar to some of those that occur during apoptosis of nucleated cells. Eryptosis is characterized by Ca^{+2} entry, erythrocyte shrinkage, membrane blebbing (microvesicle formation), and cell membrane phospholipid scrambling, with phosphatidylserine exposure on the cell surface.[271]

Surface membrane alterations on aged or damaged cells that may be recognized by macrophages include exposure of phosphatidylserine on the external surface, modified external membrane carbohydrate residues (e.g., desialation of sialoglycoproteins), and/or modified membrane proteins (e.g., partially degraded band 3); these are possible signals for removal.[57,246,265] Phosphatidylserine is normally localized in the inner leaflet of the lipid bilayer, but with cell damage phosphatidylserine may be exposed on the outer leaflet of the lipid bilayer, where it can be bound by phosphatidylserine receptors such as CD36 on the surface of macrophages.[249] Other macrophage receptors can recognize altered carbohydrate moieties on the surface of erythrocytes.

The appearance of a senescent cell antigen may be an important signal in the removal of aged erythrocytes.[246] This senescent cell antigen is derived from the band 3 anion transporter. The specific alteration required for band 3 to become antigenic remains to be clarified, but oxidative mechanisms are probably involved. A natural antibody against the senescent cell antigen is present in human plasma. This antibody binds to senescent cell antigens on the surface of aged cells and, together with bound complement, promotes the phagocytosis of aged erythrocytes by macrophages that exhibit Fc and C3b surface receptors. Senescent dog erythrocytes accumulate surface-associated immunoglobulin, which is believed to promote their removal by macrophages.[395] The relative importance of the immune- and nonimmune-mediated phagocytosis of senescent erythrocytes remains to be clarified.

Erythrocytes lose volume by shedding microvesicles as they age. The composition of the resultant microvesicles varies, but they typically contain hemoglobin. Other components that may be present include glycophorin A, breakdown products of band 3 (senescent antigen), IgG, and exposed phosphatidylserine. They do not contain the skeletal proteins spectrin and ankyrin.[186,536] Microvesicles are rapidly cleared from the circulation by macrophages, using receptors discussed above for aged erythrocytes.[186] It may be that this process of microvesiculation removes patches of damaged membrane that would otherwise bind to macrophages and result in the early removal of otherwise healthy erythrocytes.[536]

Following phagocytosis by macrophages of the spleen, liver, and other organs, erythrocytes and erythrocyte microvesicles are lysed and hemoglobin is degraded to heme and globin (Fig. 4-14). Globin is catabolized to constituent amino acids, and the microsomal heme oxygenase reaction within macrophages degrades heme to iron, biliverdin, and carbon

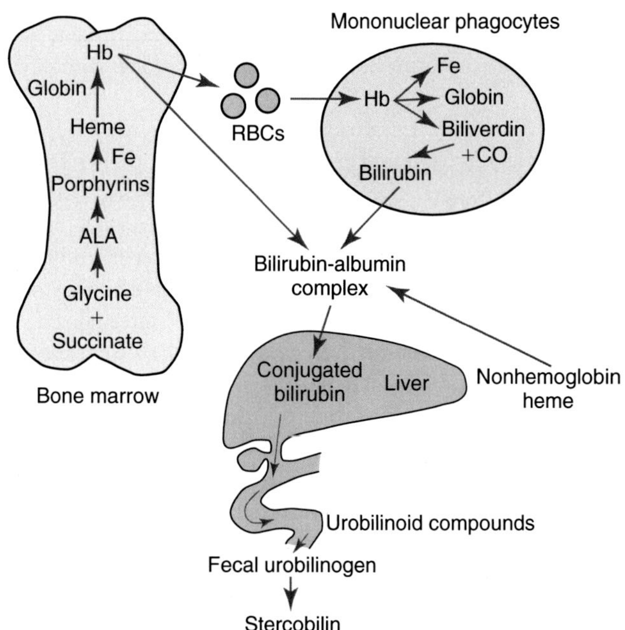

FIGURE 4-14
Overview of erythrocyte production, erythrocyte phagocytosis by mononuclear phagocytes, hemoglobin degradation, and bilirubin metabolism.

monoxide. Biliverdin is reduced to bilirubin via biliverdin reductase in nearly all mammals. Biliverdin reductase activity is low in rabbits and nutria and almost completely lacking in birds; consequently biliverdin is the predominant bile pigment in these species.[101,476] Considerable heterogeneity exists in reptiles, amphibians, and fish in the production of bilirubin versus biliverdin.[101] Bilirubin is released from macrophages and bound to albumin for transport to the liver for conjugation and excretion. Approximately 80% of the bilirubin produced in the body comes from the degradation of hemoglobin, with the remainder coming from the degradation of other heme-containing proteins.[476]

Pathologic Destruction of Erythrocytes

Increased membrane injury associated with various pathologic disorders can result in increased phagocytosis of erythrocytes by macrophages (see previous discussion concerning the removal of aged erythrocytes). Anemia develops if the rate of erythrocyte destruction exceeds the ability of the bone marrow to respond by producing new erythrocytes. Lysis of erythrocytes within macrophages after phagocytosis is sometimes referred to as extravascular hemolysis. Hyperbilirubinemia may be present within a few hours following substantial erythrocyte destruction.

Increased eryptosis (similar to the apoptosis of nucleated cells) may contribute to the development of anemia in some disorders. As discussed earlier, eryptosis is characterized by Ca^{+2} entry, erythrocyte shrinkage, and membrane blebbing with ectosome formation (Fig. 4-15).[271] Reported triggers of eryptosis include oxidative stress, energy depletion, osmotic shock, lipid-derived signaling molecules, certain bacterial exotoxins, various drugs, and metals including lead, copper, zinc, and mercury. Diseases associated with accelerated eryptosis in humans include sepsis, malaria, hemoglobinopathies, G6PD deficiency, phosphate depletion, iron deficiency, and hemolytic uremic syndrome.[270]

Almost no lysis of erythrocytes occurs within the circulation of normal individuals, but intravascular hemolysis can be present when severe membrane damage occurs in disease states (Fig. 4-16). Following lysis, hemoglobin in plasma (hemoglobinemia) reversibly dissociates into dimers that bind almost irreversibly to haptoglobin, an α_2-glycoprotein in plasma. The hemoglobin-haptoglobin complex is too large to be filtered through the kidney and is rapidly removed from the circulation following binding to the hemoglobin scavenger receptor CD163 on macrophages. Once inside the cell, hemoglobin-haptoglobin complexes are transported to lysosomes for degradation, and receptors are recycled to the cell surface.[229] The hemoglobin is degraded and iron is conserved, as discussed previously.

Once plasma haptoglobin is saturated (about 50 to 150 mg/dL of hemoglobin-binding capacity in dogs, cats, and horses), remaining free hemoglobin dimers are small enough to be readily filtered by the kidney.[196] Some hemoglobin is reabsorbed by the proximal tubules, but once that capacity is exceeded, hemoglobin appears in the urine (hemoglobinuria).[211] Plasma appears red when as little as 50 mg/dL of hemoglobin is present; consequently hemoglobinemia may be observed in the absence of hemoglobinuria. Hemoglobin absorbed by the proximal tubules is rapidly catabolized, and iron is stored as ferritin and hemosiderin.[203] Iron that is not reutilized is lost when tubular epithelial cells slough into the urine.

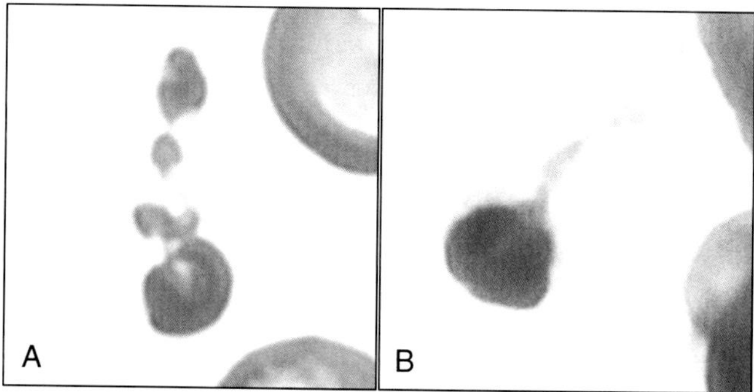

FIGURE 4-15
Presumptive eryptosis with erythrocyte shrinkage and vesicle formation in blood from dogs. **A,** Blood from a dog with regenerative anemia and hemangiosarcoma. Frequent acanthocytes and echinocytes and occasional schistocytes and keratocytes were also noted in the stained blood film. Wright-Giemsa stain. **B,** Blood from a febrile dog with mild nonregenerative anemia and lymphoma. Low numbers of eccentrocytes and pyknoctyes and rare hemoglobin crystals were also noted in the stained blood film. Wright-Giemsa stain.

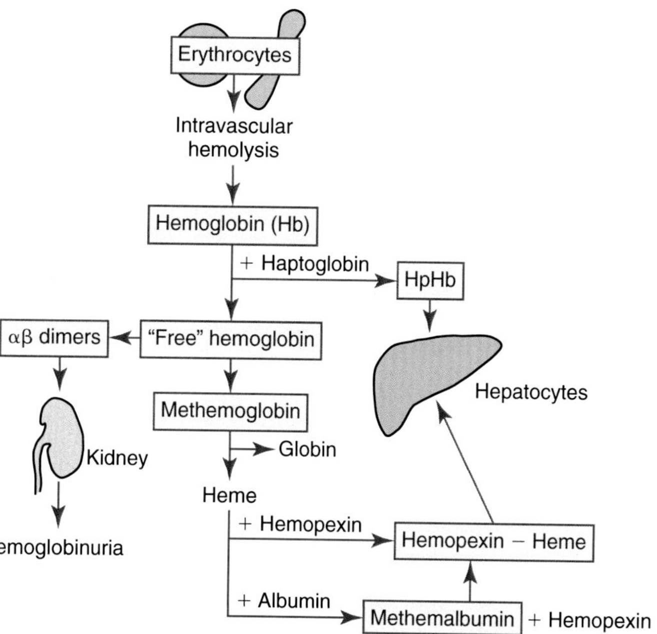

FIGURE 4-16
Pathophysiology of intravascular hemolysis. Methemalbumin forms in primates but not in common domestic animals. Hp, haptoglobin.

Free hemoglobin in plasma can spontaneously oxidize to form methemoglobin, which tends to dissociate into ferriheme (hemin) and globin. Free heme binds to a plasma protein called hemopexin. The heme-hemopexin complexes undergo endocytosis after binding to CD91 on the surface of macrophages and hepatocytes.[229] The binding to hemopexin protects cell membranes from toxic effects of free heme, and it also conserves iron. Albumin from primates can also bind heme to form methemalbumin, but albumin from common domestic animals does not bind heme.[163]

ABNORMAL ERYTHROCYTE MORPHOLOGY

Rouleaux

Erythrocytes on blood films from healthy horses, cats, and pigs often exhibit rouleaux (aggregations of erythrocytes grouped together like a stack of coins) formations (see Fig. 4-2). Rouleaux formation depends on both the nature of the erythrocytes and the composition of plasma.[37] Erythrocytes that are more deformable and have greater membrane fluidity with less negative charge on their surfaces (weaker electrostatic repulsive force) aggregate more readily than cells with the opposite characteristics.[37,443,460] Rouleaux formation also depends on the presence of high-molecular-weight proteins in plasma.[132] Increased concentrations of globulin proteins—including fibrinogen, haptoglobin, and immunoglobulins—potentiate rouleaux formation in association with inflammatory conditions.[11,532] Rouleaux formation can also occur in association with some lymphoproliferative disorders in which one or more immunoglobulins are secreted in high amounts (Fig. 4-17). Prominent rouleaux formation in species other than horses, cats, or pigs should be noted as an abnormal finding.

Prominent rouleaux formation results in rapid erythrocyte sedimentation in whole blood samples allowed to stand undisturbed. This characteristic formed the basis of an erythrocyte sedimentation rate test that was done with special sedimentation tubes. Increased sedimentation rates after 1 hour were suggestive of increased globulins in plasma, as typically seen with inflammation. Unfortunately the sedimentation rate increases as the hematocrit decreases, so correction factors were required for the HCT. The sedimentation rate has largely been replaced by making direct measurements of total globulins and fibrinogen and other acute-phase proteins.

Agglutination

Aggregation or clumping of erythrocytes in clusters (not in chains, as in rouleaux) is termed agglutination (Fig. 4-18). Agglutination is caused by the occurrence of immunoglobulins bound to erythrocyte surfaces. Because of their pentavalent nature, IgM immunoglobulins have the greatest propensity to produce agglutination.[129] EDTA-dependent IgM-mediated erythrocyte agglutination has been reported in a cat without evidence of hemolysis. Agglutination did not occur if blood was collected in heparin or citrate.[411] High-dose unfractionated heparin treatment in horses also causes erythrocyte agglutination by an undefined mechanism.[319,322]

Polychromasia

The presence of bluish-red erythrocytes in stained blood films is called polychromasia (Fig. 4-19). Polychromatophilic erythrocytes are reticulocytes that stain bluish-red owing to the combined presence of hemoglobin (red staining) and

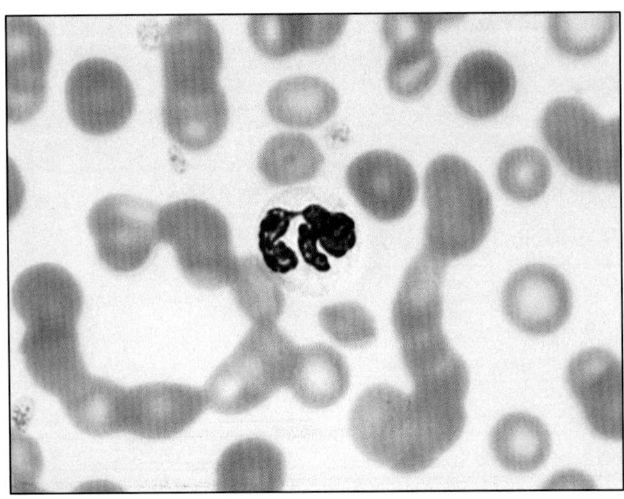

FIGURE 4-17

Rouleaux formation in blood from a dog with multiple myeloma and a monoclonal hyperglobulinemia. The cytoplasm of a neutrophil present is pale compared to the background that stains blue because of the increased protein present in the blood. Wright-Giemsa stain.

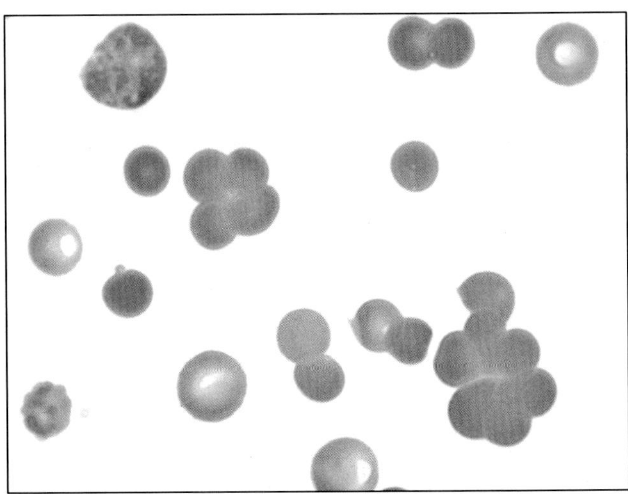

FIGURE 4-18

Erythrocyte agglutination and spherocyte formation in blood from a dog with von Willebrand's disease after transfusion. A large basophilic erythrocyte (macroreticulocyte or stress reticulocyte) is present in the upper left corner and an echinocyte is present in the lower left corner. Wright-Giemsa stain.

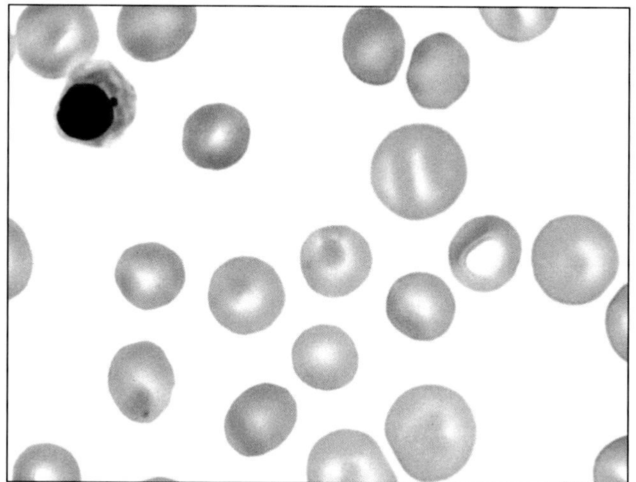

FIGURE 4-19
Increased polychromasia and anisocytosis in blood from a dog with a hemolytic anemia caused by *Mycoplasma haemocanis*, although no organisms are present in this field. Three large polychromatophilic erythrocytes (reticulocytes) are present in the central area. A nucleated erythrocyte (metarubricyte) is present in the upper left. Wright-Giemsa stain.

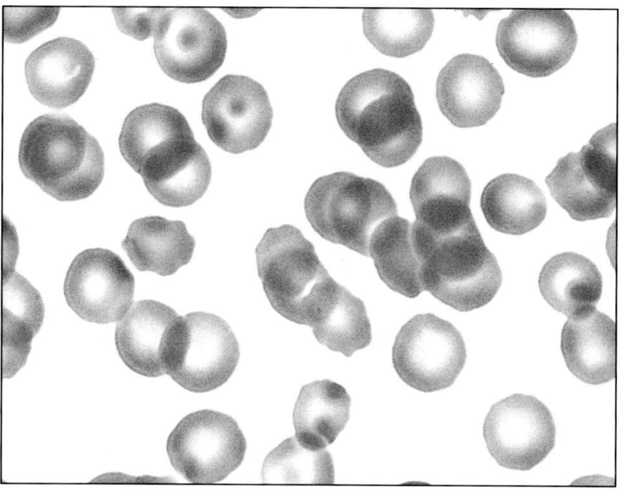

FIGURE 4-20
Blood from a dog with a nonregenerative aplastic anemia secondary to trimethoprim-sulfadiazine therapy. Erythrocyte morphology is normal except for several erythrocytes with scalloped borders (echinocytes). Wright-Giemsa stain.

individual ribosomes and polyribosomes (blue staining). Low numbers of polychromatophilic erythrocytes are usually seen in blood from normal dogs and pigs, because up to 1.5% reticulocytes may be present in dogs and up to 1% reticulocytes may be present in pigs even when the HCT is normal.[238] Slight polychromasia may be present in normal cats, but many normal cats exhibit no polychromasia in stained blood films. Polychromasia is absent in stained blood films from normal cattle, sheep, goats, and horses because reticulocytes with sufficient RNA to impart a bluish color are not normally present in the blood in these species.

The most useful approach in the classification of anemia is to determine whether or not evidence of a bone marrow response to the anemia is present in blood. For all species except the horse, this involves determining whether absolute reticulocyte numbers are increased in blood. Horses rarely release reticulocytes from the bone marrow even when an increased production of erythrocytes occurs. When an absolute reticulocytosis is present, the animal is said to have a regenerative anemia. The presence of a regenerative response suggests that the anemia results from either increased erythrocyte destruction or hemorrhage. A nonregenerative anemia generally indicates that the anemia is the result of decreased erythrocyte production (Fig. 4-20); however, about 3 to 5 days are required for increased reticulocyte production and release by the bone marrow in response to an acute anemia.[15,65,146,364] Consequently the anemia appears nonregenerative shortly after hemolysis or hemorrhage has occurred (see Fig. 4-4).

Increased polychromasia is usually present in regenerative anemias because many reticulocytes stain bluish-red with routine blood stains (see Fig. 4-19). When the degree of anemia is severe, basophilic macroreticulocytes or so-called stress reticulocytes or shift reticulocytes may be released into the blood (Fig. 4-21). High concentrations of erythropoietin shorten the marrow transit time for erythroid cells, resulting in the early release of immature reticulocytes that are twice the normal size.[379] There is a direct correlation between the percentage of polychromatophilic erythrocytes and the percentage of reticulocytes in dogs (and presumably in pigs) and between the percentage of polychromatophilic erythrocytes and percentage of aggregate reticulocytes in cats (Fig. 4-22).[15,269] Cats with mild anemia may not release aggregate reticulocytes from the marrow but will release punctate reticulocytes (Fig. 4-23, *A*).[15] Because punctate reticulocytes do not

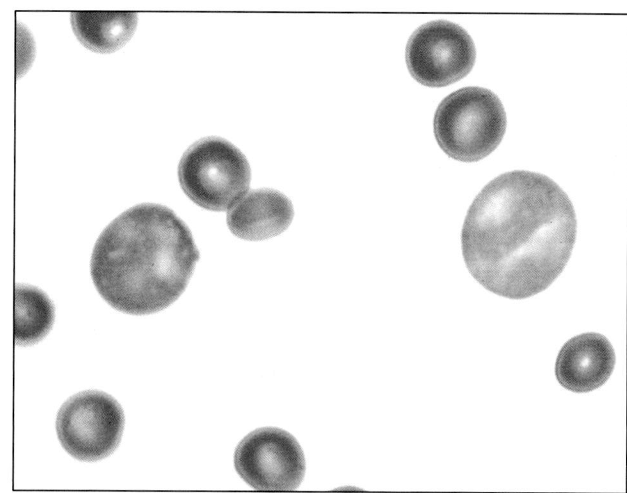

FIGURE 4-21
Two exceptionally large basophilic erythrocytes (macroreticulocytes or stress reticulocytes) are present in blood from a dog with immune-mediated hemolytic anemia. Wright-Giemsa stain.

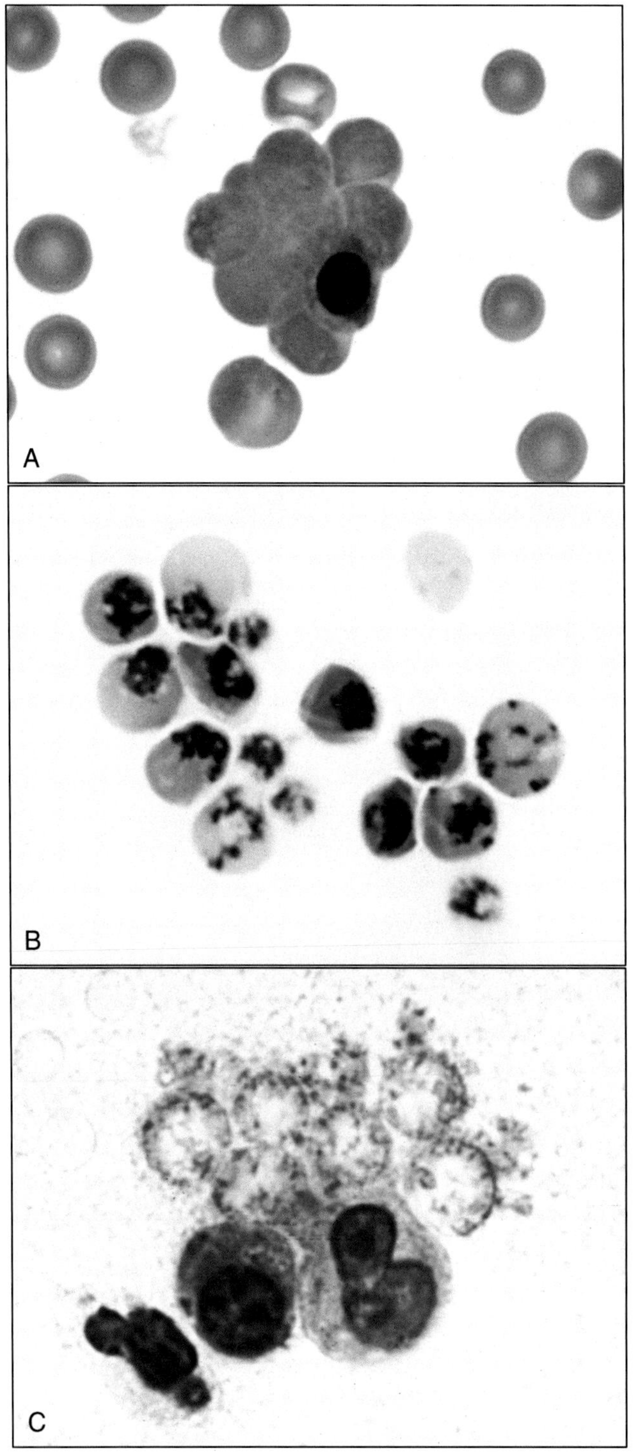

FIGURE 4-22
Agglutination of aggregate reticulocytes in blood from a cat with a Coombs'-positive hemolytic anemia. **A,** Agglutination of polychromatophilic erythrocytes and a metarubricyte. Wright-Giemsa stain. **B,** Agglutination of aggregate reticulocytes. New methylene blue reticulocyte stain. **C,** Agglutination of aggregate reticulocytes. New methylene blue wet mount preparation.

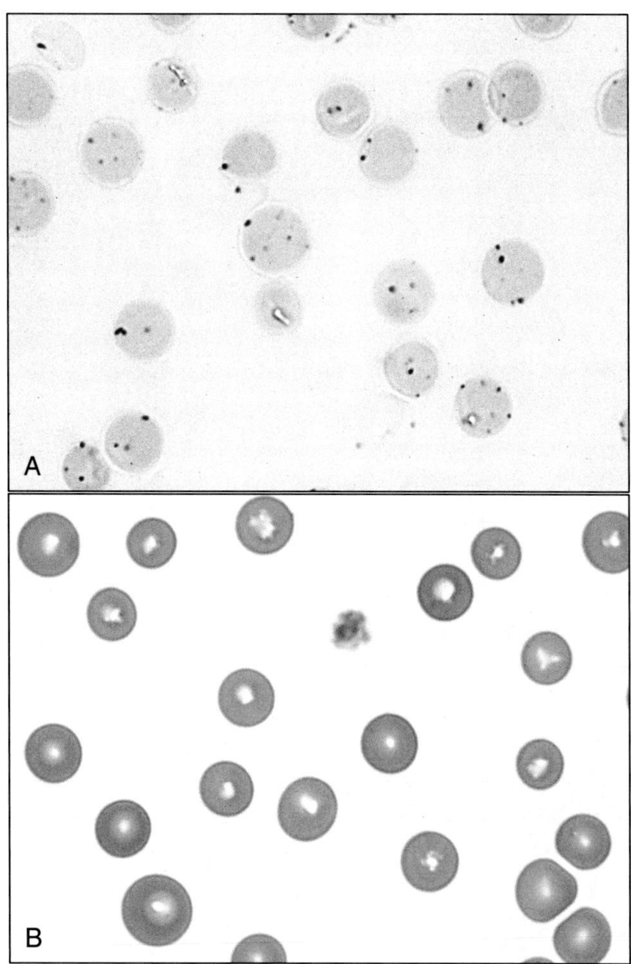

FIGURE 4-23
Blood from a FeLV-positive cat with a macrocytic normochromic anemia (HCT = 23%, MCV = 70 fL, MCHC = 33 g/dL). **A,** Low numbers of aggregate reticulocytes but markedly increased punctate reticulocytes (83% uncorrected) are present. Methylene blue reticulocyte stain. **B,** Increased anisocytosis is present but polychromasia is not apparent, even though most of the blood cells present are punctate reticulocytes, because there is insufficient RNA present to impart a blue color to the cytoplasm of these cells. Wright-Giemsa stain.

contain sufficient numbers of ribosomes to impart a bluish color to the cytoplasm, mild regenerative anemia in cats may lack polychromasia in stained blood films (Fig. 4-23, *B*).

Anisocytosis

Variation in erythrocyte diameters in stained blood films is called anisocytosis (see Fig. 4-23, *B*). It is greater in normal cattle than in other normal domestic animals.[238] Anisocytosis is increased when different populations of cells are present, as can occur following a transfusion (Fig. 4-24). Anisocytosis may occur when substantial numbers of smaller than normal cells are produced, as occurs with iron deficiency, or when substantial numbers of larger than normal cells are produced, as occurs when increased numbers of reticulocytes are

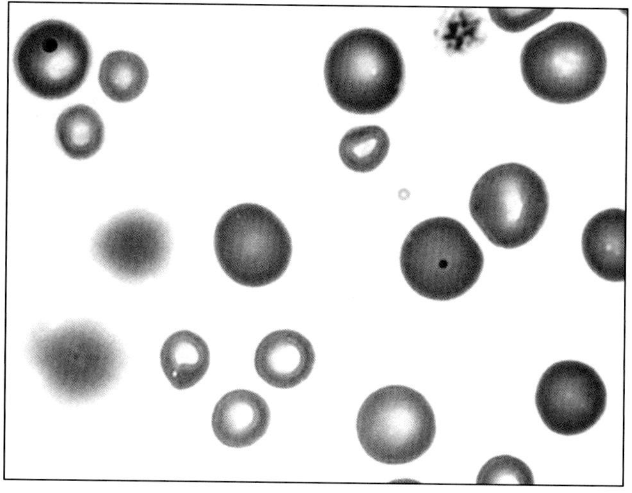

FIGURE 4-24
Marked anisocytosis in blood from a 6-week-old kitten after a blood transfusion. The RDW (43%) was also markedly increased. The kitten presented with marked lipemia and a severe iron-deficiency anemia. The small hypochromic erythrocytes are from the kitten and the larger erythrocytes from the blood donor cat. Two lysed erythrocytes (red smudges) are present *(left center)* because lipemia enhances erythrocyte lysis during blood film preparation. Wright-Giemsa stain.

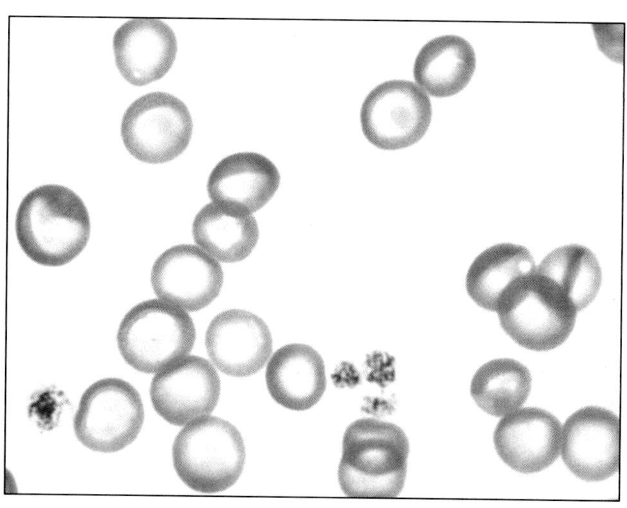

FIGURE 4-26
Hypochromic erythrocytes in blood from a dog with iron deficiency secondary to chronic blood loss resulting from a persistent flea infestation. Not only is the center of each cell paler than normal but the diameter of the area of central pallor is increased relative to the red-staining periphery of the cell. A polychromatophilic erythrocyte (reticulocyte) is present near the left edge of the image. Wright-Giemsa stain.

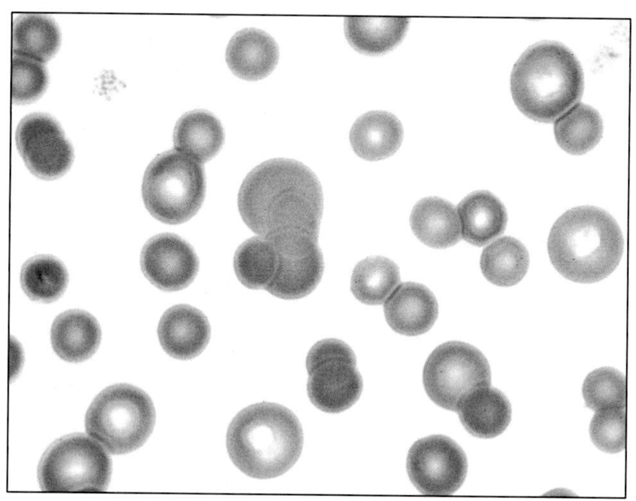

FIGURE 4-25
Increased anisocytosis in blood from a horse with a regenerative anemia resulting from internal hemorrhage. Horses almost never release reticulocytes in response to anemia; therefore no polychromasia is present. Wright-Giemsa stain.

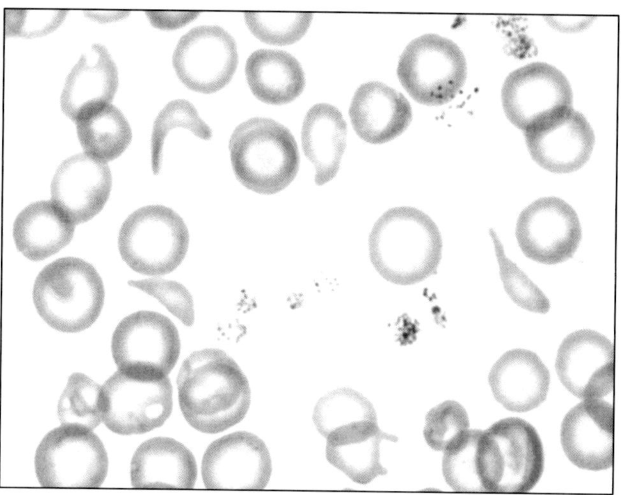

FIGURE 4-27
Hypochromic erythrocytes in blood from a dog with iron deficiency secondary to chronic gastrointestinal blood loss. A microcytic hypochromic anemia with poikilocytosis (including keratocytes, schistocytes, and dacryocytes) were present.

produced. Consequently increased anisocytosis is usually present in regenerative anemia (see Figs. 4-18, 4-19, 4-21), but it may be present in some cases of nonregenerative anemia resulting from dyserythropoiesis.[199] Anisocytosis without polychromasia may be seen in horses with intensely regenerative anemia (Fig. 4-25).

Hypochromasia

The presence of erythrocytes with decreased hemoglobin concentration and increased central pallor is called hypochromasia (Figs. 4-26 through 4-32). Not only is the center of the cell paler than normal but the diameter of the area of central pallor is increased relative to the red-staining periphery of the

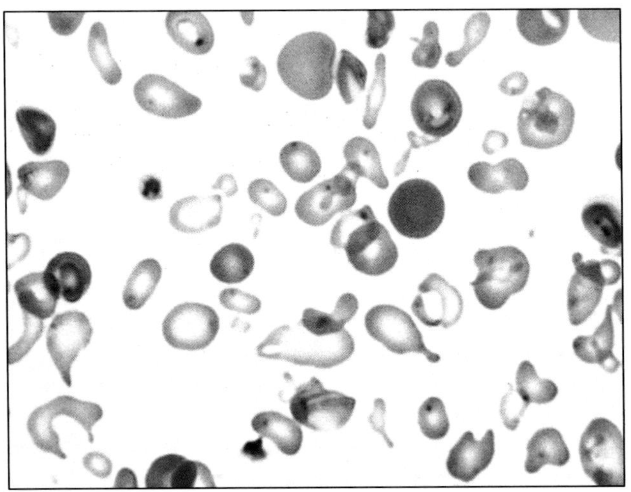

FIGURE 4-28
Marked poikilocytosis and hypochromasia in blood from a 6-week-old lamb with microcytic hypochromic iron-deficiency anemia. Wright-Giemsa stain.

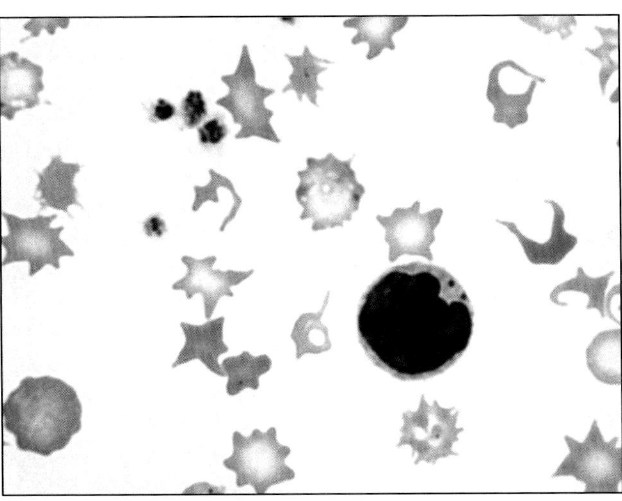

FIGURE 4-30
Marked poikilocytosis and hypochromasia in blood from a piglet with microcytic hypochromic iron-deficiency anemia resulting from a failure to provide iron injections that are part of the husbandry required in raising piglets on slated floors. Wright-Giemsa stain.

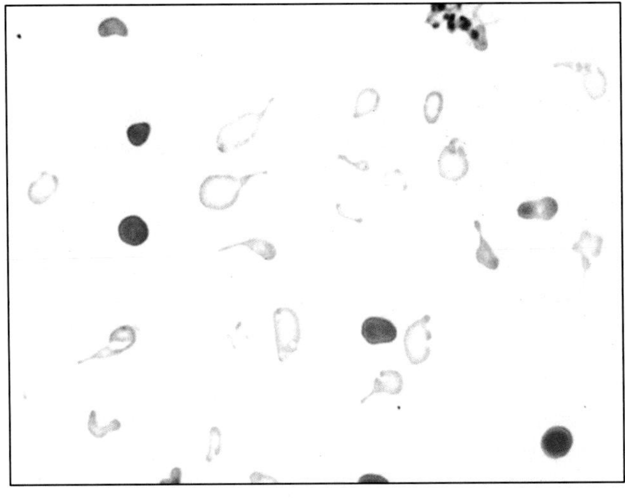

FIGURE 4-29
Marked poikilocytosis (primarily dacryocytes) and hypochromasia in blood from a goat with microcytic hypochromic iron-deficiency anemia secondary to chronic blood loss resulting from *Haemonchus* gastrointestinal parasites. Wright-Giemsa stain.

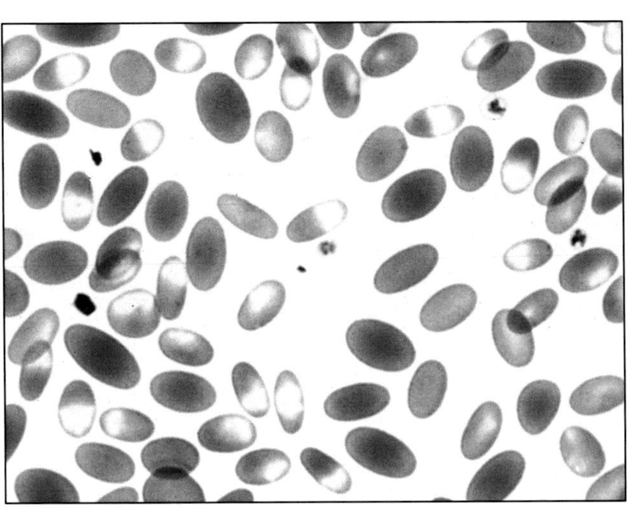

FIGURE 4-31
Microcytic erythrocytes in blood from an iron-deficient llama exhibiting irregular or eccentric areas of hypochromasia within the cells. Wright-Giemsa stain.

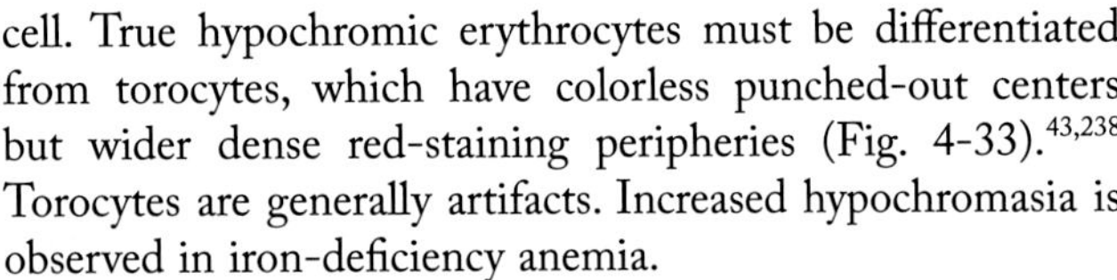

cell. True hypochromic erythrocytes must be differentiated from torocytes, which have colorless punched-out centers but wider dense red-staining peripheries (Fig. 4-33).[43,238] Torocytes are generally artifacts. Increased hypochromasia is observed in iron-deficiency anemia.

Erythrocytes from dogs, ruminants, and pigs with iron-deficiency anemia often appear hypochromic on stained blood smears. Hypochromasia is less prominent (see Fig. 4-24) and generally not recognized in iron-deficient cats and horses. Hypochromasia in iron deficiency results from both decreased hemoglobin concentration within cells and from the fact that the cells are thin leptocytes (Fig. 4-34, *A*). Because these microcytic leptocytes have increased diameter-to-volume ratios, they may not appear as small cells when viewed in stained blood films (Fig. 4-34, *B*).[210] Microcytic erythrocytes from iron-deficient llamas and alpacas exhibit irregular or eccentric areas of hypochromasia within the cells (see Figs. 4-31, 4-32).[326]

Poikilocytosis

Erythrocytes can assume a wide variety of shapes. *Poikilocytosis* is a general term used to describe the presence of abnormally shaped erythrocytes. Although specific terminology is used

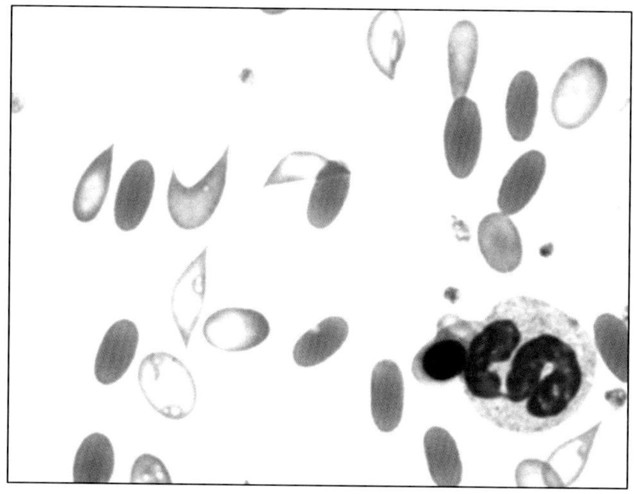

FIGURE 4-32
Blood from an iron-deficient alpaca with dacryocytes and spindle-shaped hypochromic erythrocytes. Wright-Giemsa stain.

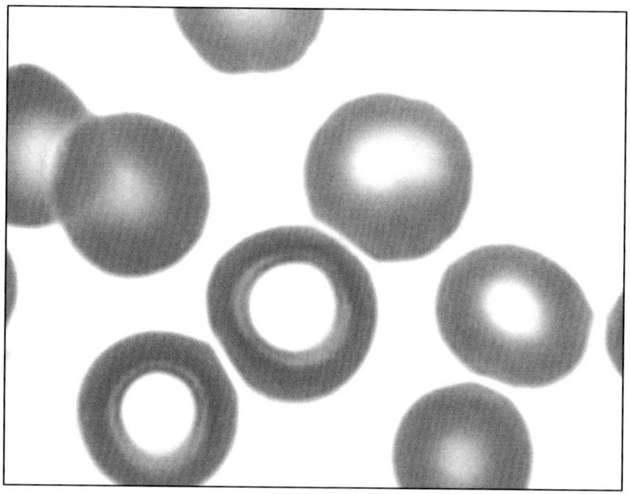

FIGURE 4-33
Two torocytes *(center and bottom left)* with colorless punched-out centers and wide dense red-staining peripheries in blood from a dog. Wright-Giemsa stain.

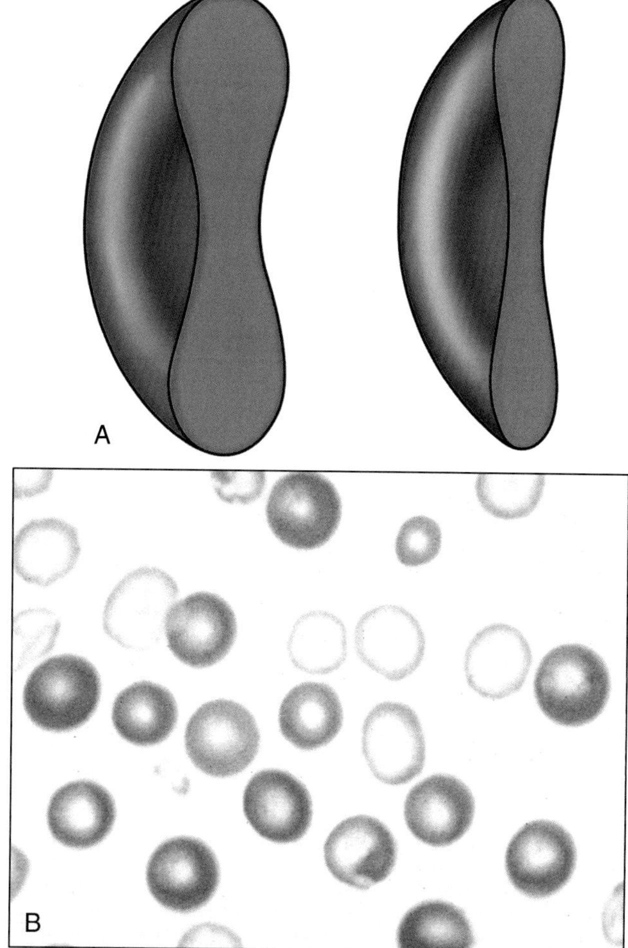

FIGURE 4-34
Comparison of discocytes to leptocytes. **A,** The profile of a normal discocyte is compared to a leptocyte with similar diameter but smaller volume. **B,** Blood from a dog with a microcytic hypochromic (MCV = 32 fL, MCHC = 23 g/dL) iron-deficiency anemia was mixed with an equal volume of blood from a normal dog (MCV = 70 fL, MCHC = 34 g/dL) prior to blood film preparation. Because the hypochromic cells are leptocytes, they have diameters similar to normal cells even though they are microcytic cells. Wright-Giemsa stain.

From Harvey JW, French TW, Meyer DJ. Chronic iron deficiency anemia in dogs. J Am Anim Hosp Assoc. *1982;18:946-960.*

for certain abnormal shapes, it is less important to quantify each type of shape change than it is to determine the cause of the shape change.[509] Poikilocytosis may be present in clinically normal goats and young cattle (Figs. 4-5, 4-35).[225,409] In some instances, these shapes appear to be related to the hemoglobin types present, but an abnormality in protein 4.2 in the membrane has been suggested as a causative factor in calves.[352] Increased numbers of poikilocytes are also present in human preterm and term neonates.[403]

Poikilocytosis forms in various disorders associated with erythrocyte fragmentation, including disseminated intravascular coagulation (DIC), liver disease, myeloid neoplasms, myelofibrosis, glomerulonephritis, and hemangiosarcoma (dogs).[392] For unknown reasons, severe iron-deficiency anemia in dogs, pigs, and ruminants may exhibit pronounced poikilocytosis (see Figs. 4-27 through 4-32).[201] Poikilocytes can form when oxidant injury results in Heinz body formation and/or membrane injury. One or more blunt erythrocyte surface projections may form as the membrane adheres to Heinz bodies bound to its internal surface.[392] Various abnormalities in erythrocyte shape were reported in horses with intravascular hemolysis resulting from severe cutaneous burn injuries. Membrane blebbing with fragmentation was prominent (Fig. 4-36).[347] A variety of abnormal erythrocyte shapes have been reported in dogs and cats with doxorubicin toxicity[32,348] and in dogs with dyserythropoiesis.[223]

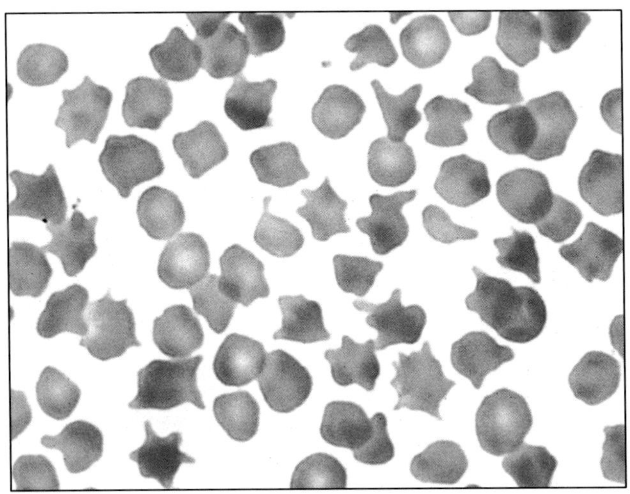

FIGURE 4-35
Poikilocytosis (acanthocytes and echinocytes) in blood from a nonanemic young calf. Wright-Giemsa stain.

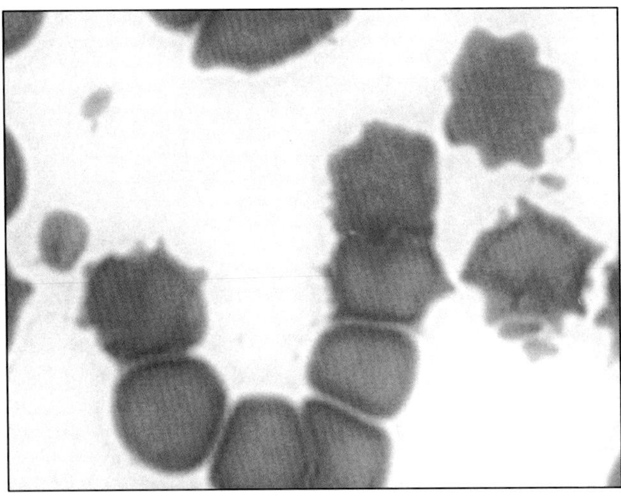

FIGURE 4-36
Echinocytes with membrane blebbing and fragmentation in blood from a horse with intravascular hemolysis resulting from severe cutaneous burn injuries. Wright stain.

Photograph of a stained blood film from a 2004 ASVCP slide review case submitted by E. Spangler, M. Johnson, A. Kessell, B. Weeks, T. Norman, and K. Chaffin.

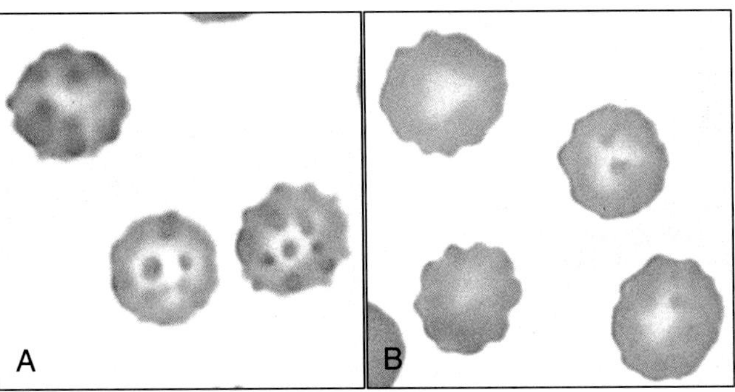

FIGURE 4-37
Echinocytes in blood from a dog with histiocytic sarcoma. **A,** Spicules of similar length are regularly spaced. **B,** Echinocytes, in a thinner area of the same blood film, appear as erythrocytes with scalloped borders. Wright-Giemsa stain.

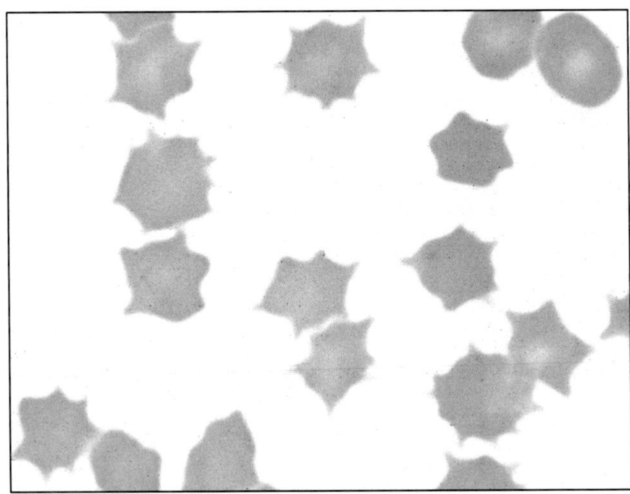

FIGURE 4-38
Echinocytes in blood from a normal pig appear as erythrocytes with scalloped borders; consequently the term *crenation,* from Latin meaning "notched," has previously been used for echinocytes. Wright-Giemsa stain.

Echinocytes (Crenated Erythrocytes)

Echinocytes are spiculated erythrocytes in which the spicules are relatively evenly spaced and of similar size.[523] Spicules may be sharp or blunt. When observed in stained blood films, echinocytosis is usually an artifact that results from excess EDTA, improper smear preparation, or prolonged sample storage before blood film preparation. The appearance of the echinocytes can vary depending on the thickness of the blood film (Fig. 4-37). They are common in normal pig blood smears (Fig. 4-38), forming in vitro.[238] The morphology of echinocytes varies from slightly spiculated echinodiscocytes to highly spiculated spheroechinocytes, which have been called burr cells (Fig. 4-39, *A*). The most advanced echinocytes are those that have lost most of their spicules and have nearly become spherocytes (Fig. 4-39, *B*). Echinocytes form when the surface area of the outer lipid monolayer increases relative to the inner monolayer.[438]

Echinocytic transformation occurs in the presence of fatty acids, lysophospholipids, and amphiphatic drugs that distribute preferentially in the outer half of the lipid bilayer.[205] Transient echinocytosis occurs in horses with *Clostridium perfringens* infection[526] and in dogs following rattlesnake (see Fig. 4-39, *A*),[70,191] coral snake (see Fig. 4-39, *B*),[301] water moccasin (Fig. 4-40), and asp viper (*Vipera aspis*) envenomation,[303]

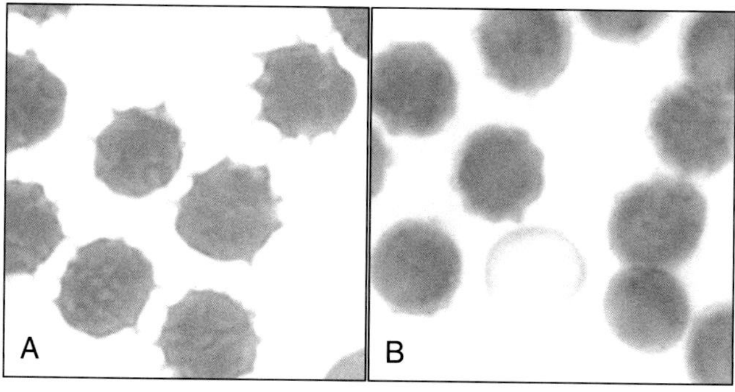

FIGURE 4-39
Echinocytes in the blood of dogs following snake bites. **A,** Highly spiculated echinocytes (burr cells) in blood from a dog following an Eastern diamondback rattlesnake bite. **B,** Spheroechinocytes and a lysed erythrocyte "ghost" *(bottom center)* in blood from a dog following a coral snake bite. Wright-Giemsa stain.

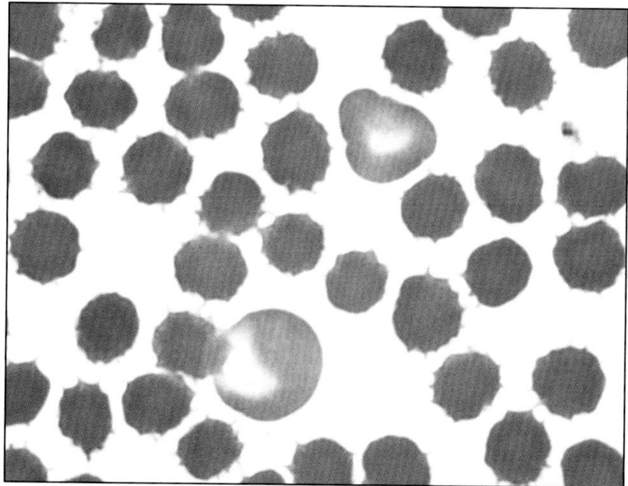

FIGURE 4-40
Highly spiculated echinocytes in blood from a dog following a water moccasin bite. Two large polychromatophilic erythrocytes (reticulocytes) are also present. Wright-Giemsa stain.

presumably secondary to the action of phospholipases present in venom.[498] Depending on the time course and dose of venom received, either echinocytosis or spherocytosis may be observed after these snakebites.

Echinocytes may occur in uremic animals and immediately after transfusion of stored blood.[392] They have been seen with increased frequency in dogs with glomerulonephritis and neoplasia (lymphoma, hemangiosarcoma, mast cell tumor, and carcinoma).[391,523] Echinocytes are the predominant erythrocyte shape abnormality in human burn patients, and this was one of the shape abnormalities recognized in horses with severe cutaneous burn injuries (see Fig. 4-36).[195,347]

Echinocytes also form when erythrocytes are dehydrated, pH is increased, ATP is depleted, and intracellular calcium is increased.[31,205] Echinocytosis occurs in horses when total body depletion of cations has occurred (endurance exercise, furosemide treatment, diarrhea, systemic disease).[162,205]

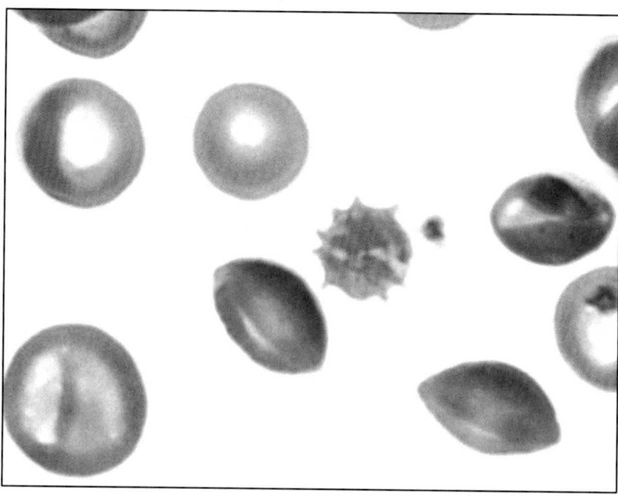

FIGURE 4-41
An echinocyte *(center)* and four polychromatophilic erythrocytes in blood from a pyruvate kinase-deficient beagle dog. Wright-Giemsa stain.

Although the mechanisms are not fully understood, ATP is required for the maintenance of normal shape and deformability of erythrocytes.[205] Phospholipids are asymmetrically arranged in the plasma membrane, with anionic amino-containing phospholipids (predominantly phosphatidylserine) located in the inner leaflet of the bilaminar membrane. These anionic phospholipids are shuttled (flipped) from the outer leaflet to the inner leaflet by an ATP-dependent aminophospholipid-specific translocase or flippase.[553] ATP also provides the energy needed to pump Ca^{+2} out of cells. Increased Ca^{+2} activates neutral proteases (calpains), which can degrade membrane skeletal proteins; phospholipase C, which cleaves phosphoinositides; and scramblase, which accelerates the bidirectional transbilayer movement of phospholipids.[205,540] The inhibition of the flippase and/or the activation of the scramblase can result in increased phosphatidylserine in the outer layer, which appears to promote echinocyte formation, as well as coagulation and erythrophagocytosis.[116,295,406]

Echinocytes and other shape abnormalities have been recognized in dogs with erythrocyte pyruvate kinase deficiency (Fig. 4-41), which results in a decreased ability to generate ATP.[86,328,412] Occasional echinocytes may also be seen in dogs with erythrocyte phosphofructokinase deficiency (Fig. 4-42). PFK-deficient erythrocytes have decreased ATP and increased Ca^{+2} concentrations.[404]

Acanthocytes

Erythrocytes with irregularly spaced, variably sized spicules are called acanthocytes or spur cells (Fig. 4-43).[43] Acanthocytes form when erythrocyte membranes contain excess cholesterol compared to phospholipids. If cholesterol and phospholipids are increased to a similar degree, codocyte formation is more likely than acanthocyte formation.[98] Alterations in erythrocyte membrane lipids can result from increased blood cholesterol content or due to the presence of

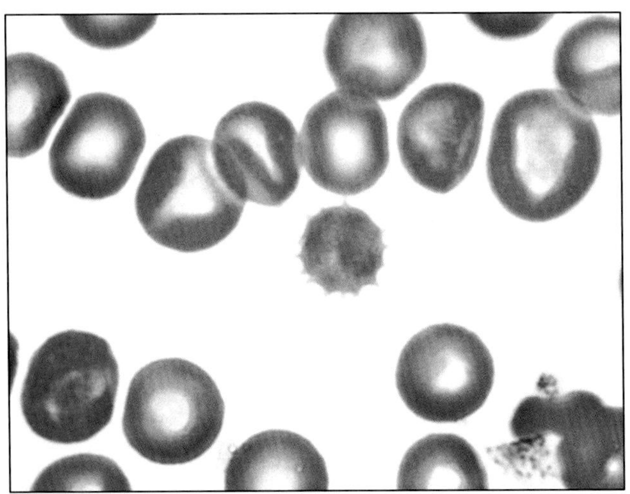

FIGURE 4-42
An echinocyte *(center)* and four polychromatophilic erythrocytes in blood from a phosphofructokinase-deficient English springer spaniel dog. Wright-Giemsa stain.

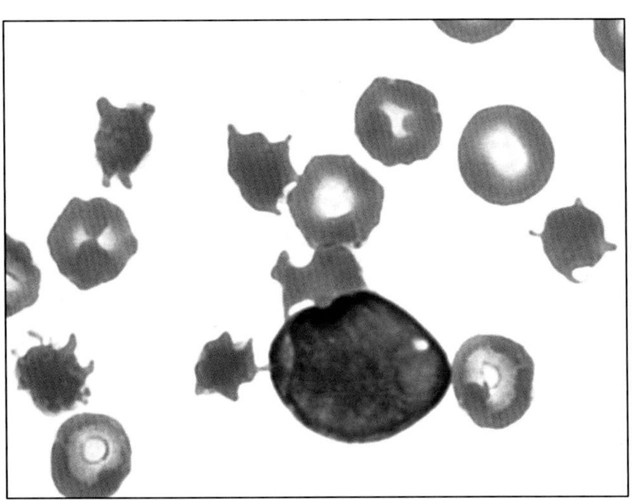

FIGURE 4-44
Acanthocytes in blood from a dog with neoplastic lymphoid infiltrates in the liver. A neoplastic lymphoblast is also present. Wright-Giemsa stain.

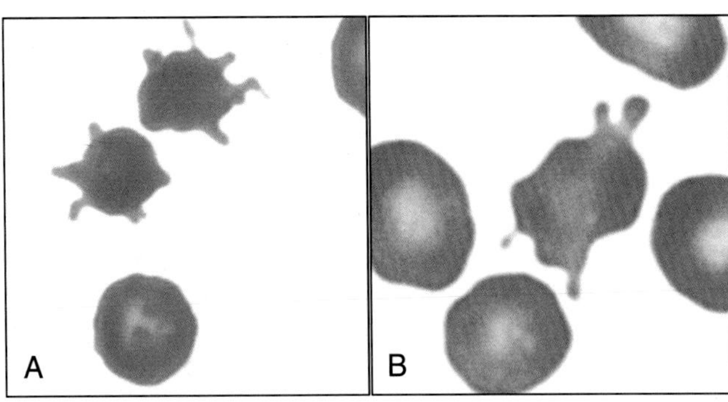

FIGURE 4-43
Acanthocytes in blood from a dog and cat. **A,** Two acanthocytes *(above)* with irregularly spaced, variably sized spicules in blood from a dog with neoplastic lymphoid infiltrates in the liver. **B,** An acanthocyte in blood of a cat with hepatic lipidosis. Wright-Giemsa stain.

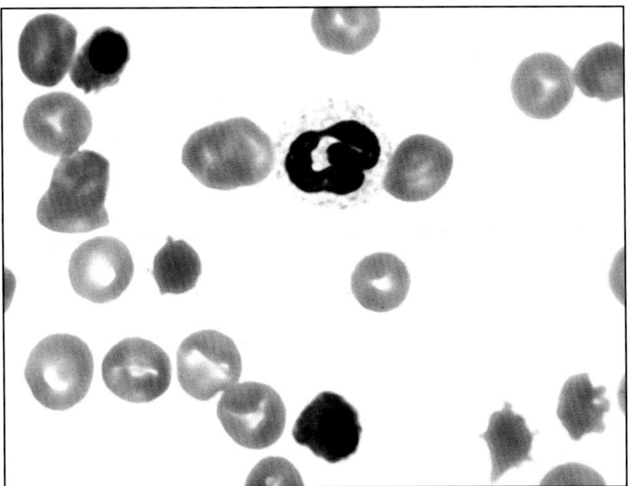

FIGURE 4-45
Three acanthocytes, four polychromatophilic erythrocytes, two metarubricytes, and a neutrophil in blood from a dog with hemangiosarcoma. Wright-Giemsa stain.

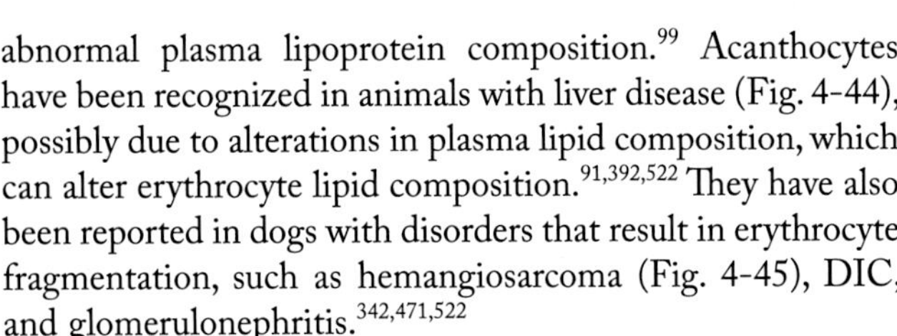

abnormal plasma lipoprotein composition.[99] Acanthocytes have been recognized in animals with liver disease (Fig. 4-44), possibly due to alterations in plasma lipid composition, which can alter erythrocyte lipid composition.[91,392,522] They have also been reported in dogs with disorders that result in erythrocyte fragmentation, such as hemangiosarcoma (Fig. 4-45), DIC, and glomerulonephritis.[342,471,522]

Marked acanthocytosis is reported to occur in young goats and some young cattle (see Fig. 4-35). Acanthocytosis of young goats occurs as a result of the presence of hemoglobin C at this early stage of development.[205]

Keratocytes

Erythrocytes containing one or more intact holes are called prekeratocytes, and erythrocytes with ruptured holes are called keratocytes (Figs. 4-46 and 4-47).[140] The rupture of the hole results in the formation of one or two projections. Keratocytes have been recognized in various disorders including iron-deficiency anemia,[201] liver disorders,[91] doxorubicin toxicity in cats,[348] myelodysplastic syndrome,[524] and in various disorders in dogs having concomitant echinocytosis or acanthocytosis.[342,522,523]

Stomatocytes

Cup-shaped erythrocytes that have oval or elongated areas of central pallor when viewed in stained blood films are called stomatocytes (Fig. 4-48, *A*). They most often occur as artifacts in thick blood film preparations. Stomatocytes form when pH

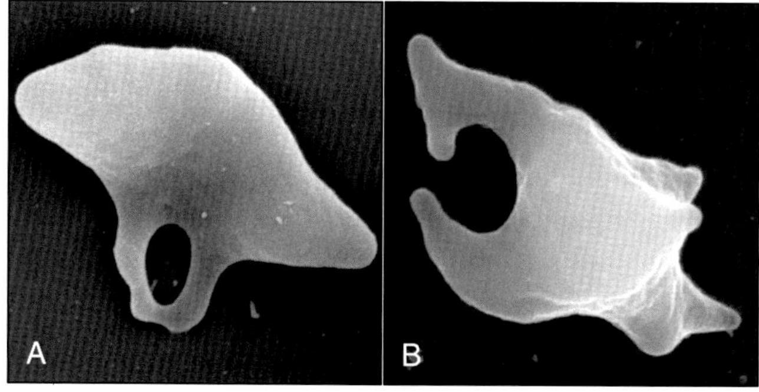

FIGURE 4-46
Scanning electron photomicrographs of cat keratocytes. **A,** A prekeratocyte contains a hole completely through the cell. **B,** A keratocyte forms when the hole in the prekeratocyte ruptures, resulting in the formation of one or two projections. This cell might be considered an echinokeratocyte because of its additional projections.

Photomicrographs were provided by C. L. Flint and M. A. Scott.

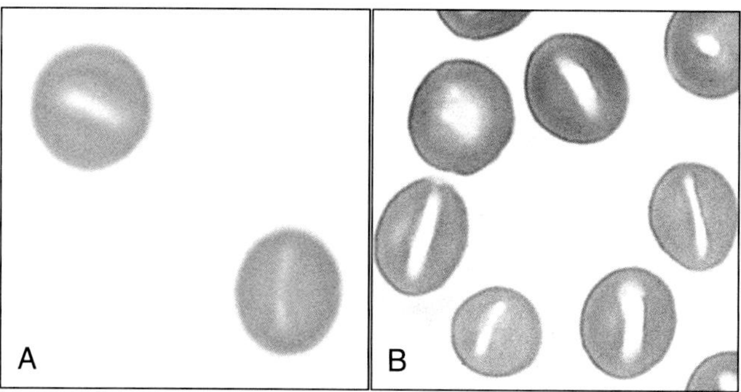

FIGURE 4-48
Stomatocytes with elongated areas of central pallor in blood. **A,** Blood from a cat with hemolytic anemia. The stomatocytes were not uniformly present in the blood film and were considered to be an artifact. Wright-Giemsa stain. **B,** Stomatocytes in blood from an asymptomatic Pomeranian dog with persistent stomatocytosis associated with macrocytic hypochromic erythrocytes. As in dogs reported to have hereditary stomatocytosis, these erythrocytes were osmotically fragile and had a low concentration of reduced glutathione. Wright-Giemsa stain.

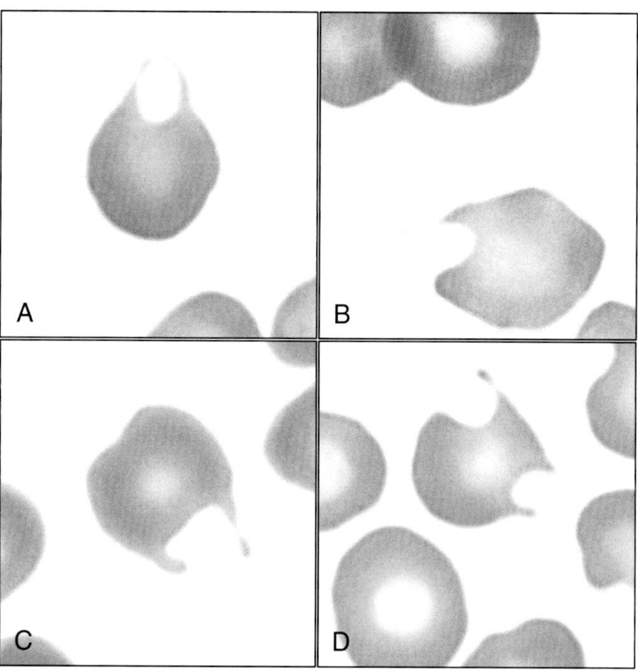

FIGURE 4-47
Keratocytes in blood from a cat with hepatic lipidosis. **A,** Prekeratocyte with a hole. **B,** Keratocyte where the hole has ruptured, producing a single horn. **C,** Keratocyte where hole has ruptured, producing two horns. **D,** Keratocyte where two holes have ruptured. Wright-Giemsa stain.

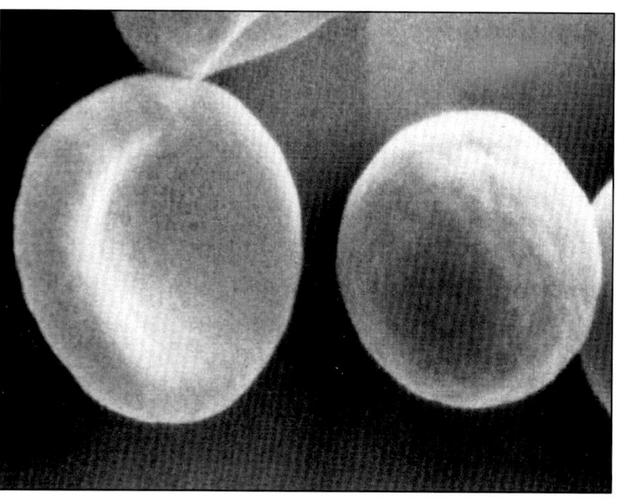

FIGURE 4-49
Scanning electron photomicrograph of a discocyte *(left)* and spherocyte *(right)* in blood from a dog.

Courtesy of K. S. Keeton and N. C. Jain.

is decreased[160] and amphiphatic drugs are present that distribute preferentially in the inner leaflet of the lipid bilayer.[205]

Stomatocytes also form when the water content of erythrocytes is increased, as occurs in at least three different inherited syndromes in dogs.[205] No clinical signs occur in miniature schnauzers,[71,170] standard schnauzers,[59,355] or Pomeranians (Fig. 4-48, *B*) with hereditary stomatocytosis. Chondrodysplasia (short-limbed dwarfism) occurs along with stomatocytosis in Alaskan malamutes.[139] Stomatocytosis in Drentse patrijshond dogs is associated with severe polysystemic disease and shortened life span.[433]

Spherocytes

Spherical erythrocytes that result from cell swelling and/or loss of cell membrane are referred to as spherocytes (Fig. 4-49). Spherocytes lack central pallor and have smaller diameters than normal on stained blood films (Fig. 4-50, *A*). Spherical erythrocytes with slight indentations on one side

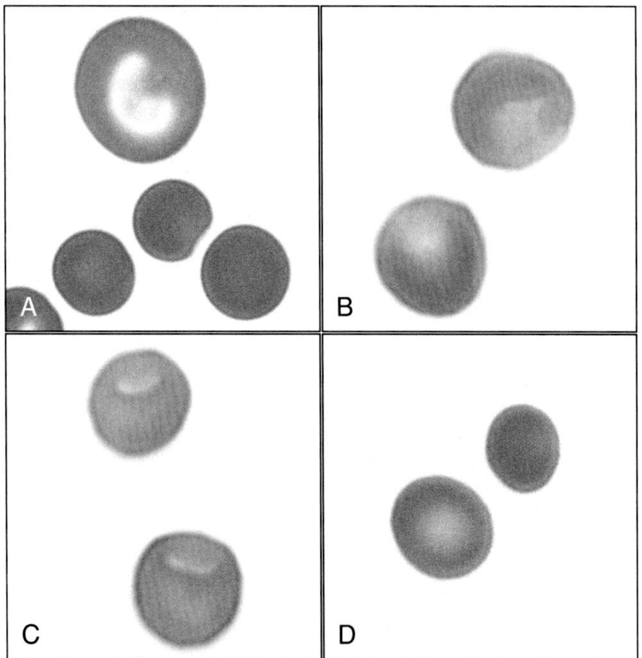

FIGURE 4-50
Spherocytes and stomatospherocytes in animal blood samples. **A,** Three spherocytes *(bottom)* and a large polychromatophilic erythrocyte or reticulocyte *(top)* in blood from a dog with immune-mediated hemolytic anemia. **B,** Two stomatospherocytes in blood from a dog with primary immune-mediated hemolytic anemia. The stomatospherocytes are not perfect spheres; rather, each has a slight indentation on one side. **C,** Two stomatospherocytes in blood from a cat with *Mycoplasma haemofelis* infection. **D,** A spherocyte *(top)* and a discocyte *(bottom)* in blood from a foal with immune-mediated neonatal isoerythrolysis. Wright-Giemsa stain.

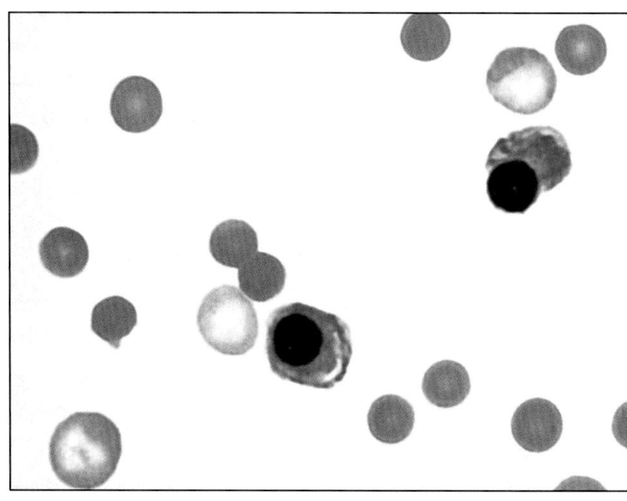

FIGURE 4-51
Spherocytes, polychromatophilic erythrocytes, and two rubricytes in blood from a dog with primary immune-mediated hemolytic anemia. Wright-Giemsa stain.

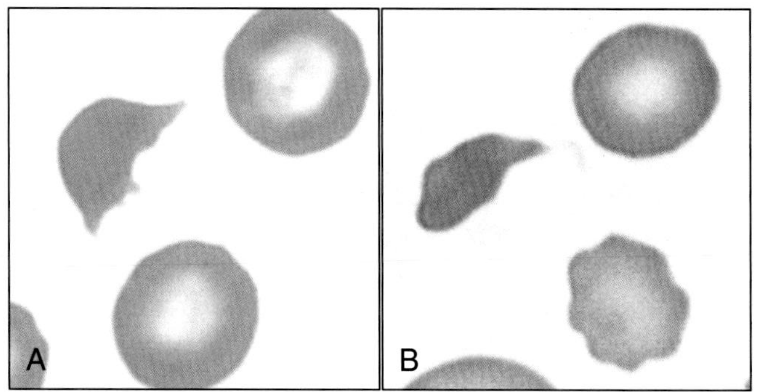

FIGURE 4-52
Schistocytes in dog blood. **A,** A fragmented erythrocyte (schistocyte) and two discocytes in blood from a dog with disseminated intravascular coagulation (DIC). **B,** A schistocyte *(left)*, discocyte *(top)*, and echinocyte *(bottom)* in blood from a dog with DIC. Wright-Giemsa stain.

may be called stomatospherocytes (Fig. 4-50, *B,C*). Since erythrocytes from other common domestic animals exhibit less central pallor than those of dogs, it is difficult to be certain when spherocytes are present in these noncanine species (Fig. 4-50, *D*).

Spherocytes and stomatospherocytes occur most frequently in association with immune-mediated hemolytic anemia in dogs (Fig. 4-51).[33,368] Other potential causes of spherocyte formation include snake envenomations,[301,303,498] bee stings,[344,543] zinc toxicity,[64] erythrocyte parasites,[3] transfusion of stored blood, and a familial dyserythropoiesis in dogs.[223] Spherocytes have been reported in cattle with anaplasmosis[463] and *Theileria buffeli* infection[453] and in horses with cutaneous burns.[347]

Defects in ankyrin, band 3, protein 4.2, and certain defects in α-spectrin and β-spectrin result in hereditary spherocytosis in mice and humans.[116] A complete absence of band 3 results in hereditary spherocytosis in Japanese black cattle.[34,232] Hereditary spherocytosis has been reported in golden retriever dogs with reductions in erythrocyte membrane spectrin[432]; however, spherocytes were not recognized in stained blood films.[434]

Schistocytes

Erythrocyte fragments with pointed extremities are called schistocytes or schizocytes (Fig. 4-52), and they are smaller than normal discocytes. Schistocytes may be seen in dogs with microangiopathic hemolytic anemia associated with DIC, where they can be formed by the impact of erythrocytes with fibrin strands in flowing blood (Fig. 4-53).[392] Schistocytes are less consistently seen in cats, horses, and cattle with DIC,[234,477] possibly because the erythrocytes of these species are smaller and less likely to be split by fibrin strands in the circulation.

Schistocytes have also been seen in severe iron-deficiency anemia (see Fig. 4-27),[201] myelofibrosis,[128,281,420] heart failure, glomerulonephritis, hemolytic uremic syndrome, hemophagocytic histiocytic disorders, hemangiosarcoma in dogs,

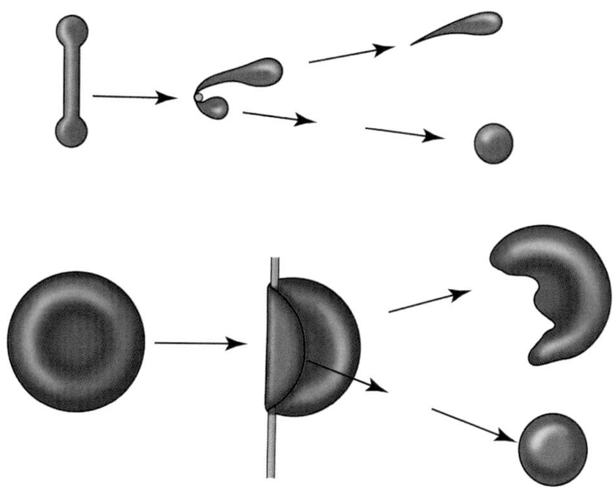

FIGURE 4-53
Drawing of schistocyte and microspherocyte formation when an erythrocyte impacts a fibrin strand under flow conditions.

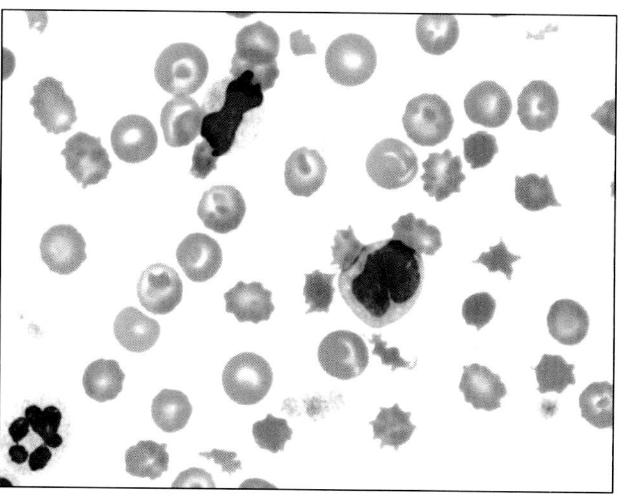

FIGURE 4-55
Echinocytes, acanthocytes, and echinoschistocytes in blood from a splenectomized pyruvate kinase-deficient Cairn terrier dog. Wright-Giemsa stain.

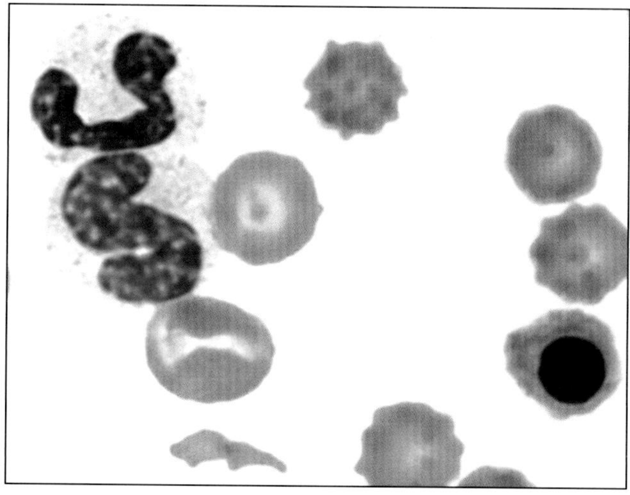

FIGURE 4-54
Echinocytes, a polychromatophilic erythrocyte, a metarubricyte and a schistocyte *(bottom)* in blood from a dog with intravascular hemolysis, resulting from dirofilariasis and caudal vena cava syndrome. A neutrophil and band neutrophil are also present. Wright-Giemsa stain.

caudal vena cava syndrome of dirofilariasis in dogs (Fig. 4-54), and congenital and acquired dyserythropoiesis in dogs.* Marked poikilocytosis with schistocytes and acanthocytes has been recognized in pyruvate kinase-deficient dogs after splenectomy (Fig. 4-55).[378,412] It is assumed that the spleen had previously removed these fragmented erythrocytes. Schistocytes have been described in cats with liver disease, in cats and dogs with doxorubicin toxicity,[91,348] and in horses with severe cutaneous burns.[347]

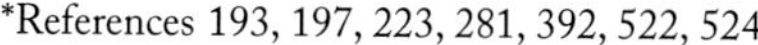

*References 193, 197, 223, 281, 392, 522, 524.

Leptocytes

These cells are thin, often hypochromic-appearing erythrocytes with increased membrane-to-volume ratios. Some leptocytes appear folded (Fig. 4-56, *A*), some appear as triconcave knizocytes (Fig. 4-57) that give the impression that the erythrocyte has a central bar of hemoglobin (Fig. 4-56, *B*, *C*), and others appear as codocytes (Fig. 4-58). Codocytes (target cells) are bell-shaped cells that exhibit a central density or "bull's-eye" in stained blood films. Small numbers of codocytes are often seen in normal dog blood, and both codocytes and knizocytes are increased in regenerative anemia in dogs. Codocytes are especially increased in dogs with a congenital dyserythropoiesis.[223] Leptocytes may be seen in iron-deficiency anemia (Fig. 4-58, *B*)[201] and rarely in hepatic insufficiency (Fig. 4-58, *C*), resulting in a balanced accumulation of membrane phospholipids and cholesterol.[98] Polychromatophilic erythrocytes can sometimes appear as leptocytes.

Eccentrocytes

An erythrocyte in which the hemoglobin is localized to part of the cell, leaving a hemoglobin-poor area visible in the remaining part of the cell, is termed an eccentrocyte (Figs. 4-59, 4-60). Other terms used to refer to eccentrocytes include *hemighosts, irregularly contracted cells, double-colored cells*, and *cross-bonded erythrocytes*.[24] Oxidant damage to erythrocyte membranes results in the adhesion of opposing areas of the cytoplasmic face of the erythrocyte membrane.[24,137] It has been suggested that eccentrocytes form in vivo when adhesive, damaged membranes are brought together by osmotic shrinkage in the kidney and/or from squeezing through the microcirculation.[138]

Eccentrocytes have been recognized in dogs secondary to increased endogenous oxidants associated with ketoacidotic diabetes, inflammation (Fig. 4-61), neoplasia (especially

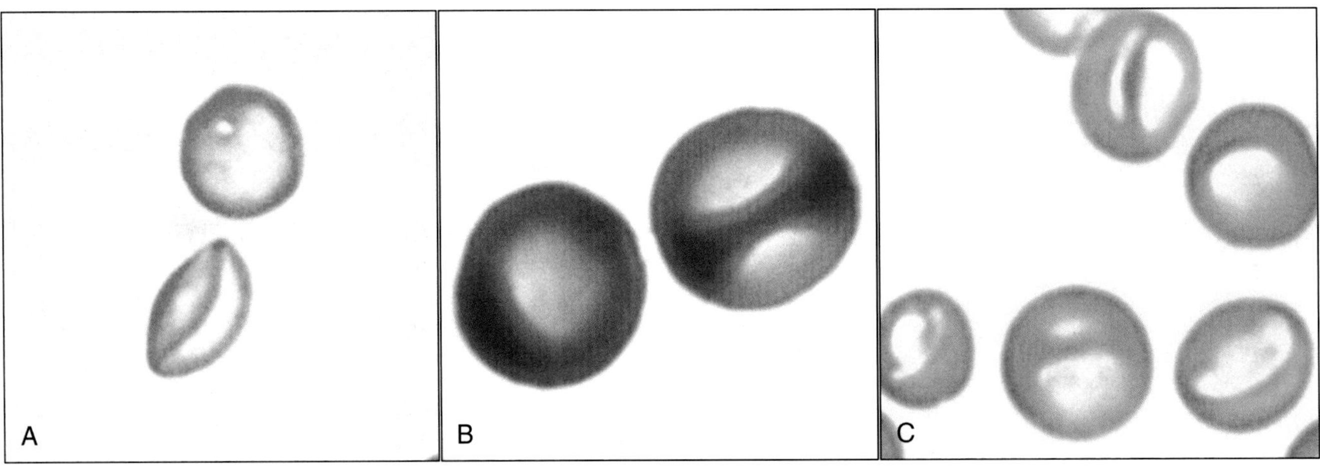

FIGURE 4-56

Leptocytes in blood from dogs. **A,** Two thin, flat, hypochromic-appearing erythrocytes (leptocytes) with increased membrane-to-volume ratios are present in blood from a dog with severe iron-deficiency anemia. The bottom leptocyte is folded. **B,** A discocyte and triconcave knizocyte in blood from a dog with a mild nonregenerative anemia associated with a hepatocellular carcinoma. **C,** Leptocytes, including two knizocytes *(top and bottom center),* are present in blood of a dog with iron-deficiency anemia. Wright-Giemsa stain.

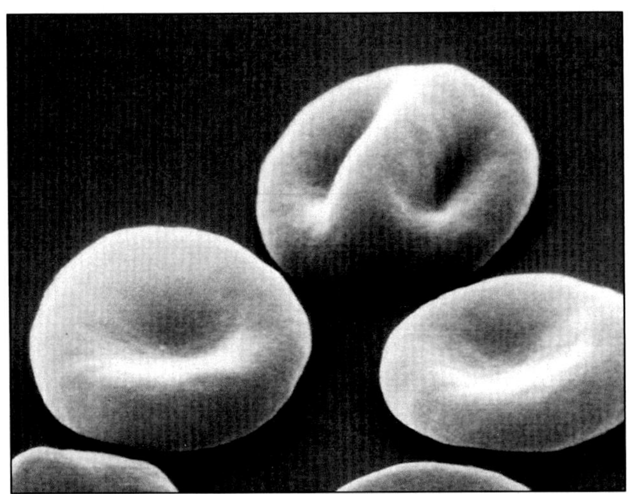

FIGURE 4-57

Scanning electron photomicrograph of two discocytes and a knizocyte *(top)* in blood from a dog.

Courtesy of K. S. Keeton and N. C. Jain.

lymphoma), and *Babesia canis canis* infection.[77,82] Eccentrocytes have been seen in dogs ingesting or receiving oxidants including onions and garlic, acetaminophen (see Fig. 4-59, *C*) and nonsteroidal anti-inflammatory drugs, vitamin K and vitamin K antagonist rodenticides, naphthalene, and prolonged propofol anesthesia (Fig. 4-62).[77,120,200,276] Eccentrocyte formation also occurs in cats following oxidant damage (Fig. 4-63).

Eccentrocytosis was recognized in a cow treated with intravenous hydrogen peroxide as a "home remedy."[291] Eccentrocytes have been reported in horses ingesting red maple leaves and in those with severe cutaneous burns.[347,389] Finally, eccentrocytes have been seen in horses with inherited G6PD deficiency (see Fig. 4-59, *B*) and glutathione reductase deficiency secondary to erythrocyte FAD deficiency (Fig. 4-64).[212,452] Both of these hereditary disorders result in the decreased ability of erythrocytes to protect against endogenous oxidants.

Pyknocytes

Irregularly spherical erythrocytes with small cytoplasmic projections are called pyknocytes (see Figs. 4-59, *D*, 4-60, D). Like eccentrocytes, pyknocytes appear to be a product of oxidant injury.[131,452] They may develop from eccentrocytes following the loss of much of the fused membrane.[212] Pyknocytes are appreciably smaller in diameter and stain more densely (especially with new methylene blue) than discocytes (Fig. 4-64).[203] These contracted erythrocytes have higher hemoglobin concentrations than normal[131] and presumably represent erythrocytes undergoing eryptosis.

Elliptocytes (Ovalocytes)

Erythrocytes from nonmammals and animals in the Camelidae family are elliptical or oval in shape (see Fig. 4-6). They are generally flat rather than biconcave. Abnormal elliptocytes have been recognized in cats with bone marrow abnormalities (myeloid neoplasms and acute lymphoblastic leukemia),[281] hepatic lipidosis,[91] portosystemic shunts,[410] and doxorubicin toxicity[348] and in dogs with myelofibrosis,[222,420] myelodysplastic syndrome,[524] and glomerulonephritis, in which the

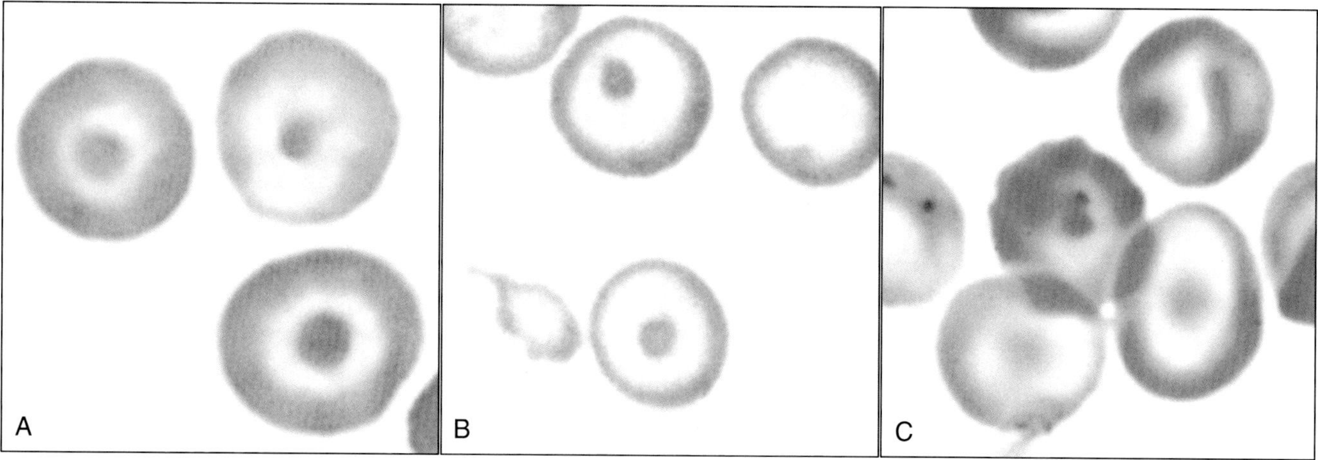

FIGURE 4-58

Codocytes in blood from dogs. These erythrocytes exhibit a central density or "bull's-eye" and are often referred to as target cells. **A,** Three codocytes in blood from a Cairn terrier dog with a regenerative anemia and hepatic hemochromatosis secondary to pyruvate kinase deficiency. **B,** Two codocytes *(top and bottom center)* and a schistocyte *(bottom left)* in blood from a dog with severe iron-deficiency anemia. **C,** Codocytes in blood from a dog with liver disease. Wright-Giemsa stain.

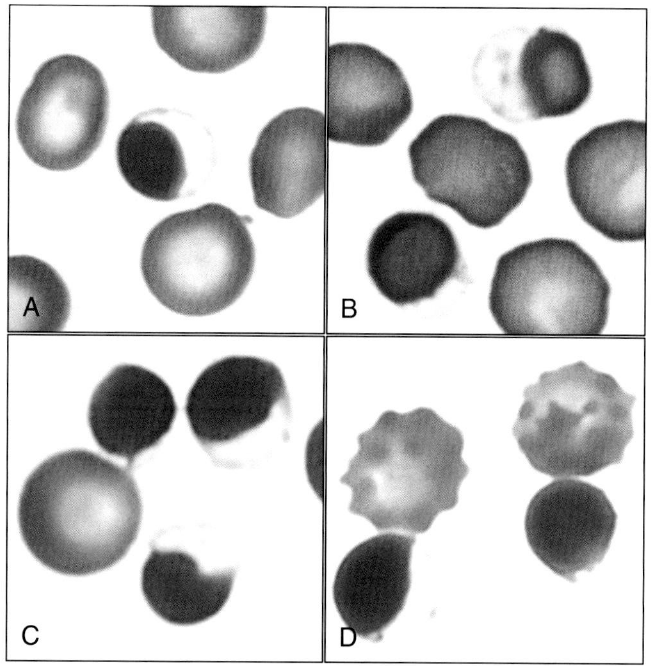

FIGURE 4-59

Eccentrocytes in blood from dogs and a horse. **A,** An eccentrocyte *(center)* in blood from a dog with prolonged propofol anesthesia. **B,** Two eccentrocytes in blood from a horse with inherited erythrocyte glucose-6-phosphate dehydrogenase (G6PD) deficiency. **C,** Two eccentrocytes and a discocyte *(left)* in blood from a dog with oxidant injury induced by the administration of acetaminophen. The cell at top center appears spherical with a small tag of cytoplasm and is classified as a pyknocyte. **D,** Two echinocytes *(top)*, an eccentrocyte *(bottom left)* and a pyknocyte *(bottom right)* in blood from a dog with diabetes mellitus and septic hepatitis. Wright-Giemsa stain.

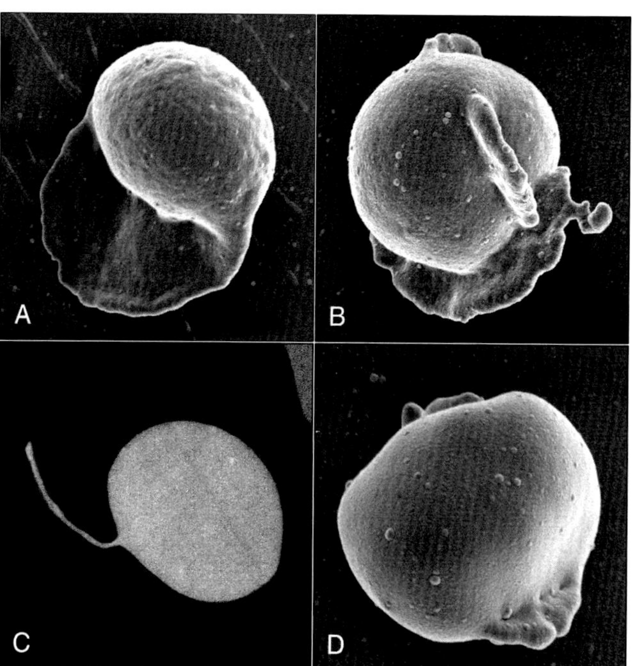

FIGURE 4-60

Scanning and transmission electron photomicrographs of eccentrocytes and a pyknocyte in blood from a horse with erythrocyte flavin adenine dinucleotide (FAD) deficiency. **A,** Scanning electron photomicrograph of an eccentrocyte showing a fused membrane leaf in the left portion and a spheroid region containing hemoglobin in the right portion of an erythrocyte. **B,** Scanning electron photomicrograph of an eccentrocyte showing fused membranes in different planes. **C,** Transmission electron photomicrograph of an eccentrocyte showing a fused membrane leaf in the left portion and a spheroid region containing hemoglobin in the right portion of an erythrocyte. **D,** Scanning electron photomicrograph of a spheroid pyknocyte with only tags of cytoplasm remaining.

From Harvey JW, Stockham SL, Scott MA, et al. Methemoglobinemia and eccentrocytosis in equine erythrocyte flavin adenine dinucleotide deficiency. Vet Pathol. *2003;40:632-642.*

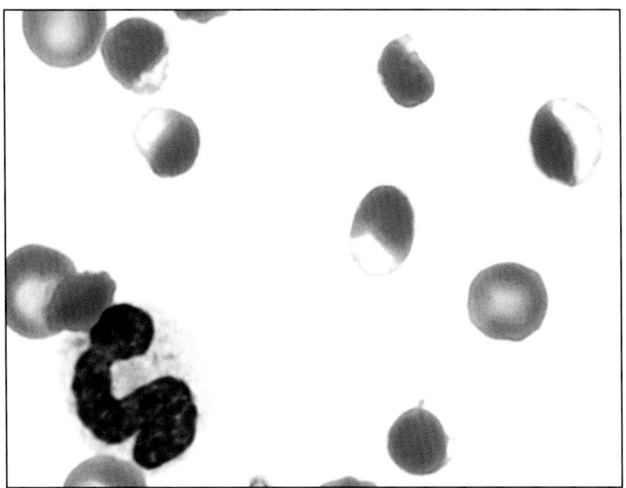

FIGURE 4-61
Blood from a dog with diabetes mellitus and septic hepatitis. Four eccentrocytes, two pyknocytes, and a toxic band neutrophil are present. Wright-Giemsa stain.

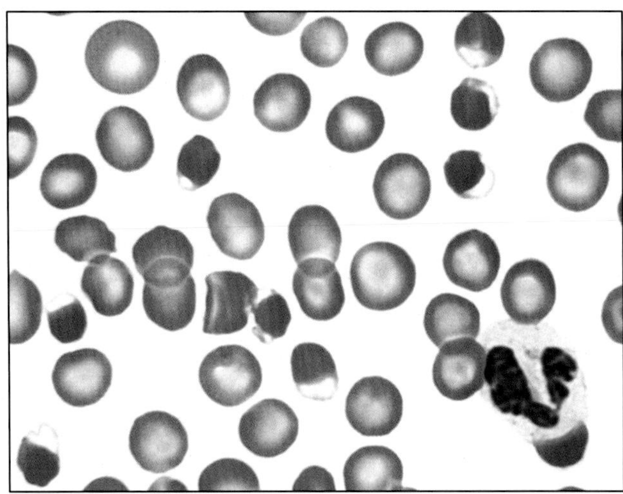

FIGURE 4-62
Eight eccentrocytes in blood from a dog subjected to prolonged propofol anesthesia. A neutrophil is present at bottom right. Wright-Giemsa stain.

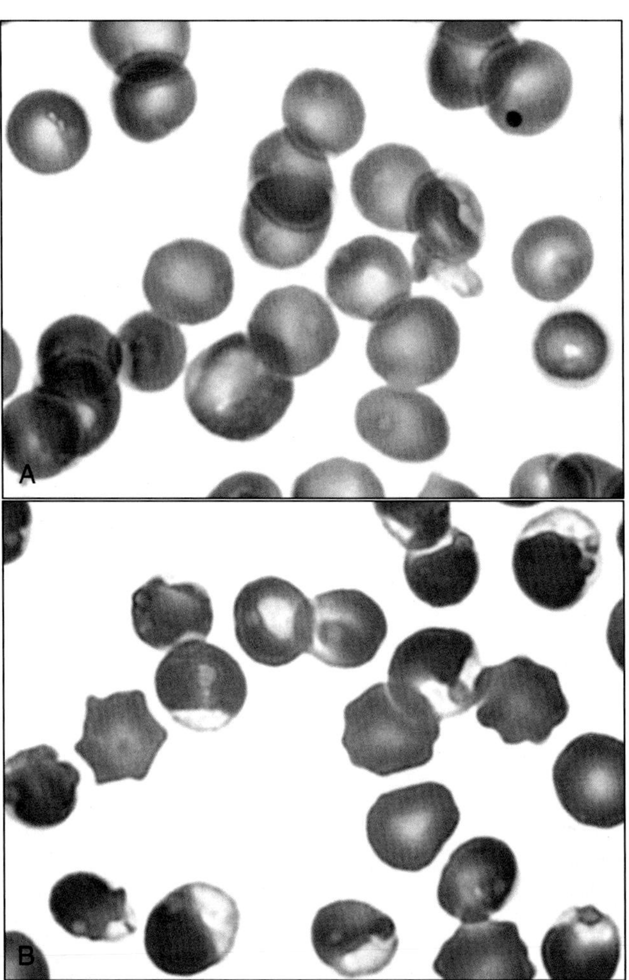

FIGURE 4-63
Heinz body and eccentrocyte formation in blood from a cat with acetaminophen toxicity. **A,** Heinz bodies are barely discernible as pale spots in erythrocytes. A polychromatophilic erythrocyte *(left lower quadrant)* and an erythrocyte containing a Howell-Jolly body *(top right)* are also present. **B,** Eccentrocytes and pale-staining Heinz bodies are visible in blood collected 2 days after the sample shown in **(A).**

elliptocytes may be spiculated (Fig. 4-65).[391] Hereditary elliptocytosis has been reported in a dog with a membrane protein 4.1 deficiency and in another with a mutant β-spectrin (Fig. 4-66).[122,439]

Dacryocytes

These erythrocytes are teardrop-shaped with single elongated or pointed extremities (Fig. 4-67, *A,B*). Dacryocytosis is a common feature of myelofibrosis in humans, but dacryocytes are not as commonly recognized in dogs with myelofibrosis.[281,388,420] Dacryocytes have also been seen in the blood of dogs and cats with myeloid neoplasms,[238] dogs with glomerulonephritis, and a dog with hypersplenism.[267] Dacryocytes are common erythrocyte shape abnormalities in iron-deficient ruminants, including llamas and alpacas (Fig. 4-67, *C,D*).[326,483]

Drepanocytes (Sickle Cells)

These fusiform or spindle-shaped erythrocytes were first recognized in deer blood in 1840 and in a human with sickle cell anemia in 1910.[44] Drepanocytes are often observed in blood from normal deer (Figs. 4-68, *A,* 4-69).[474] They develop secondary to hemoglobin polymerization, and drepanocyte shape in deer depends on the hemoglobin types present. This is an in vitro phenomenon that occurs when oxygen tension is high and pH is above 7.4. Members of the Cervidae family whose erythrocytes do not sickle in vitro include reindeer, caribou, and muntjac deer.[479]

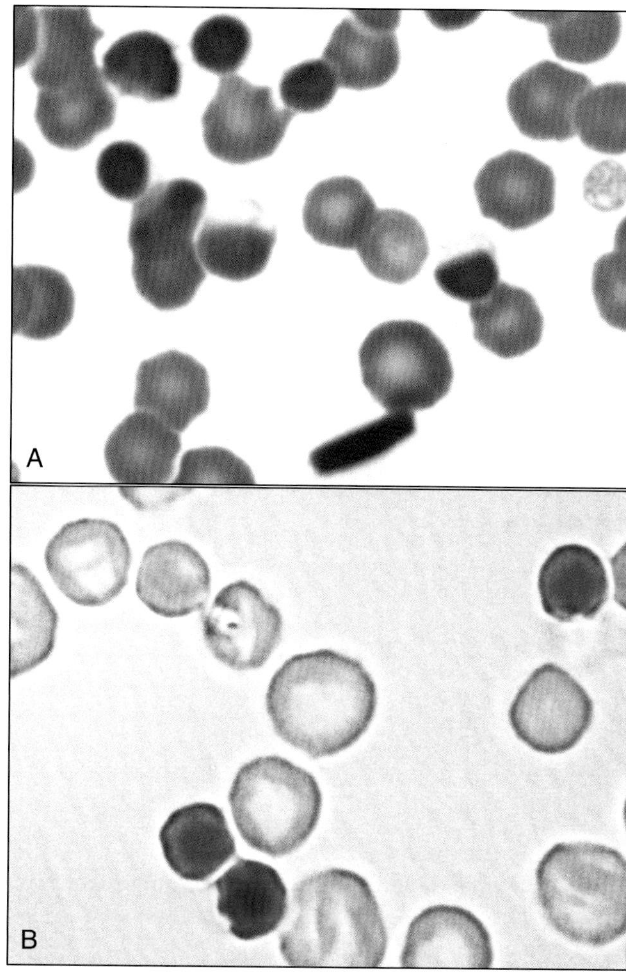

FIGURE 4-64

Pyknocytes and eccentrocytes in blood from horses with erythrocyte flavin adenine dinucleotide (FAD) deficiency. **A,** Two eccentrocytes *(center),* three pyknocytes *(upper left quadrant),* and an erythrocyte containing an eccentrically located hemoglobin crystal *(bottom)* in a stained-blood film from a mustang mare with FAD deficiency. Wright-Giemsa. **B,** Dark blue-staining eccentrocytes and pyknocytes in a blood film from a Kentucky mountain saddle horse gelding with FAD deficiency. New methylene blue reticulocyte stain.

From Harvey JW. Pathogenesis, laboratory diagnosis, and clinical implications of erythrocyte enzyme deficiencies in dogs, cats, and horses. Vet Clin Pathol. *2006;35:144-156.*

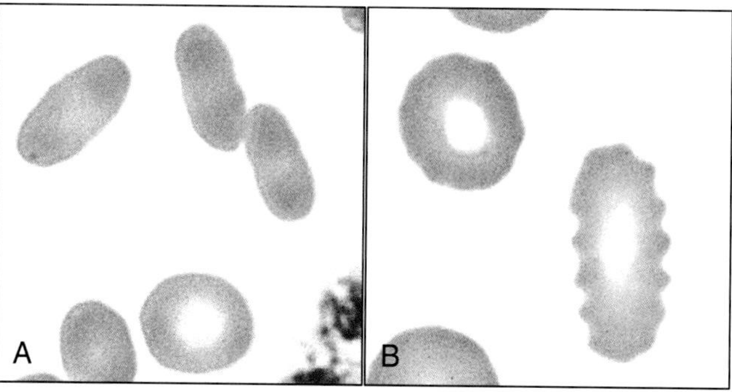

FIGURE 4-65

Elliptocytes in blood from a cat and a dog. **A,** Three elliptocytes *(top)* and a discocyte in blood from a diabetic cat with mild anemia. Radiographs revealed diffuse interstitial lung disease of unknown etiology. **B,** A discocyte *(left)* and an echinoelliptocyte *(right)* in blood from a dog with glomerulonephritis. Wright-Giemsa stain.

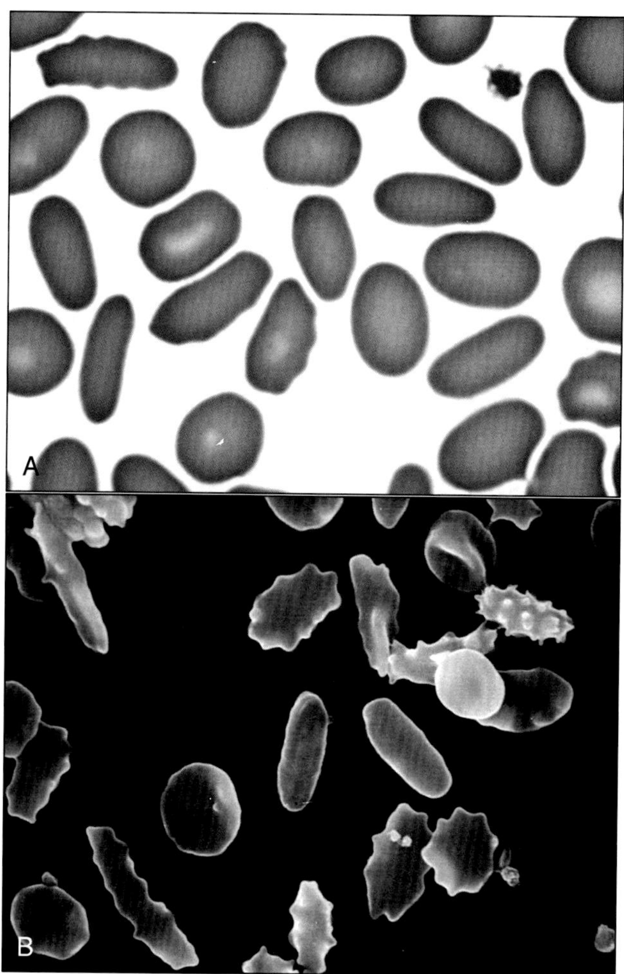

FIGURE 4-66

Elliptocytosis in blood from a dog with a mutant β-spectrin. **A,** Elliptocytes and echinoelliptocytes in blood from a dog. Wright-Giemsa stain. **B,** Scanning electron photomicrograph of elliptocytes and echinoelliptocytes in blood from a dog.

From Di Terlizzi R, Gallagher PG, Mohandas N, et al. Canine elliptocytosis due to a mutant beta-spectrin. Vet Clin Pathol. *2009;38:52-58.*

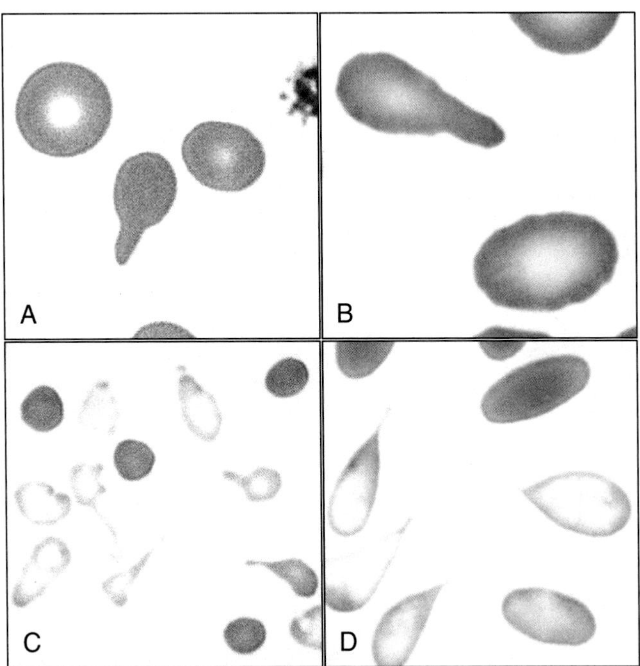

FIGURE 4-67

Dacryocytes in the blood of animals. **A,** A dacryocyte *(bottom)* and two discocytes in blood from a cat. Wright-Giemsa stain. **B,** A dacryocyte *(top)* and elliptocyte *(bottom)* in blood from a dog with glomerulonephritis. **C,** Hypochromic dacryocytes in blood from a goat with severe iron-deficiency anemia. **D,** Hypochromic dacryocytes in blood from a llama with severe iron-deficiency anemia. The presence of the normal llama elliptocyte *(above right)* is the result of a blood transfusion. Wright-Giemsa stain.

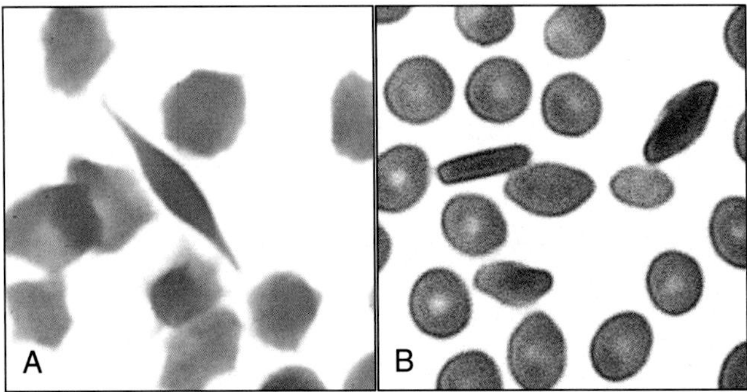

FIGURE 4-68

Drepanocytes and fusiform erythrocytes in a deer and goat. **A,** Elongated drepanocyte (sickle cell) in blood from a white-tailed deer. **B,** Erythrocytes containing hemoglobin inclusions in blood from a mixed-breed goat. Some erythrocytes appeared as rectangles but most appeared more fusiform and may represent polymerization of hemoglobin in tubular filaments, as occurs in drepanocytes. Wright-Giemsa stain.

Polymerization of hemoglobin in tubular filaments occurs in some normal adult Angora goats[239,240] and some breeds of British sheep.[130] The resultant fusiform or spindle-shaped erythrocytes resemble drepanocytes in deer; they have been called acuminocytes by some authors (Fig. 4-68, *B*).[238] The proportion of fusiform cells in Angora goats varies

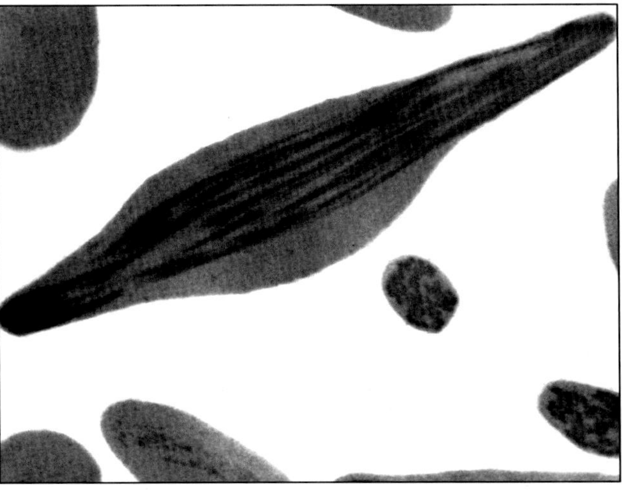

FIGURE 4-69

Transmission electron photomicrograph of a matchstick-shaped drepanocyte in blood from a deer showing filamentous aggregates of hemoglobin.

From Taylor WJ, Simpson CF. Ultrastructure of sickled deer erythrocytes. II. The matchstick cell. Blood. *1974;43:907-914.*

depending on the individual goat and on in vitro alterations in temperature, pH, and oxygenation. The number of these cells decreases during anemia, probably because of the synthesis of hemoglobin C.[239]

Crystallized Hemoglobin

The presence of large hemoglobin crystals within erythrocytes is occasionally recognized in blood films from cats (Figs. 4-70, *A*, 4-71, *A*)[16,17,428] and dogs (Fig. 4-70, *B*)[287] and frequently in the blood of llamas and alpacas (Fig. 4-70, *C*).[483] No hemoglobin abnormalities have been recognized by hemoglobin electrophoresis in animals with hemoglobin crystals.

In addition to eccentrocytes and pyknocytes, intraerythrocytic crystals have been recognized in low number in horses with erythrocyte G6PD and FAD deficiencies (Figs. 4-70, *D*, 4-71, *B*).[212] Large hemoglobin crystals were reported in horses with experimental *Babesia equi* infections treated with imidocarb dipropionate (Fig. 4-71, *C*).[429] Low numbers of intraerythrocytic hemoglobin crystals have been reported in two dogs with multiple erythroid abnormalities including prominent siderotic inclusions in their erythrocytes (Fig. 4-71, *D*).[81,209] Hemoglobin crystals may also develop as sample storage artifacts.[38]

The mechanism or mechanisms of hemoglobin crystal formation are unknown, but based on studies of humans with hemoglobin C disease, crystal formation may be influenced by factors such as pH, degree of oxygen saturation, and cellular dehydration/increased intracellular hemoglobin concentration.[76] Their potential relationships to oxidant injury, eccentrocytes, and eryptosis need further study.[212]

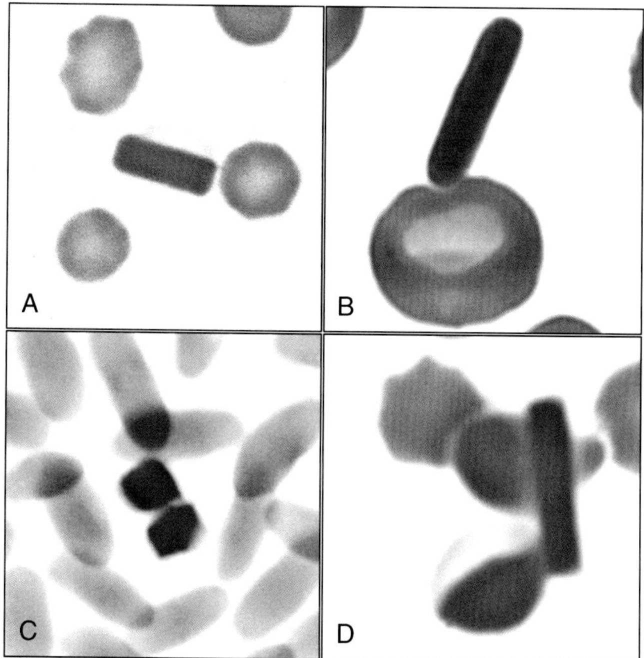

FIGURE 4-70

Hemoglobin crystals in stained blood films. **A,** Crystallized hemoglobin in an erythrocyte from a cat. **B,** Discocyte and erythrocyte with crystallized hemoglobin in the blood from a dog with a mild nonregenerative anemia associated with a hepatocellular carcinoma. **C,** Crystallized hemoglobin in two erythrocytes from a llama. **D,** An eccentrocyte *(bottom)* and hemoglobin crystal in blood from mustang mare with FAD deficiency. Wright-Giemsa stain.

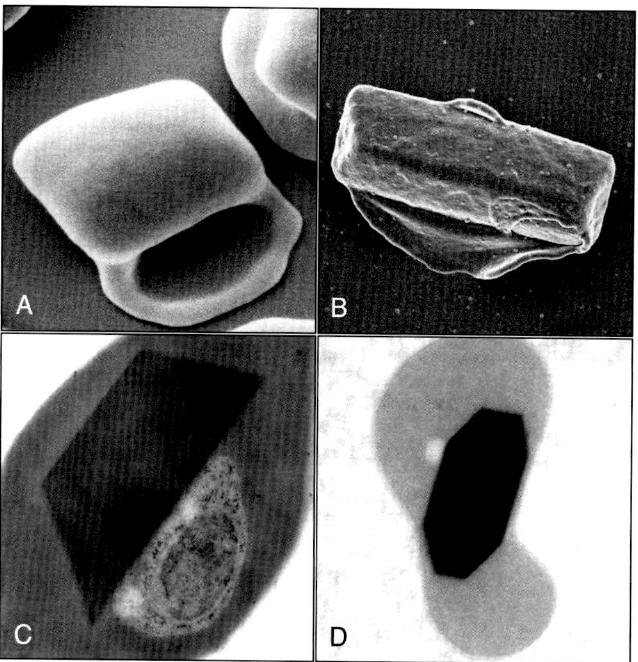

FIGURE 4-71

Scanning and transmission electron photomicrographs of hemoglobin crystals. **A,** Scanning electron photomicrograph of a cat erythrocyte containing crystallized hemoglobin. **B,** Scanning electron photomicrograph of an erythrocyte containing a hemoglobin crystal in blood from a mustang mare with FAD deficiency. **C,** Transmission electron photomicrograph of a horse erythrocyte containing both a hemoglobin crystal and a *Babesia equi* organism. The horse had been treated with imidocarb. **D,** Transmission electron photomicrograph of a dog erythrocyte containing a hemoglobin crystal. The dog had microcytic hypochromic erythrocytes that also contained siderotic inclusions and Heinz bodies.

***A,** From Jain NC.* Schalm's Veterinary Hematology. *4th ed. Philadelphia, Lea & Febiger, 1986.* ***B,** From Harvey JW, Stockham SL, Scott MA, et al. Methemoglobinemia and eccentrocytosis in equine erythrocyte flavin adenine dinucleotide deficiency.* Vet Pathol. *2003;40:632-642.* ***C,** From Simpson CF, Taylor WJ, Kitchen H. Crystalline inclusions in erythrocytes parasitized with* Babesia equi *following treatment of ponies with imidocarb.* Am J Vet Res. *1980;41:1336-1340.* ***D,** Courtesy of W. L. Clapp.*

Lysed Erythrocytes

The presence of erythrocyte "ghosts" in peripheral blood films indicates that the cells lysed prior to blood film preparation (Fig. 4-72, *A*). Erythrocyte membranes are rapidly cleared from the circulation following intravascular hemolysis; consequently the presence of erythrocyte ghosts indicates either recent intravascular hemolysis or in vitro hemolysis in the blood tube after collection. If the hemolysis is caused by an oxidant, Heinz bodies may be visible within erythrocyte ghosts (Fig. 4-72, *B*). When erythrocytes lyse during blood film preparation, they appear as red smudges (see Figs. 4-24, 4-72, *C*). These smudged erythrocytes are commonly seen in lipemic samples.

Erythroid Loops

In addition to echinocytes, spherocytes, and erythrocyte ghosts, moderate numbers of unusual erythrocyte membrane-like structures (termed erythroid loops) have been found in the blood of dogs bitten by the asp viper (Fig. 4-73).[303] Although generally round, these loops were sometimes disrupted and appeared as thin, pale reddish-blue bands. They are believed to be a consequence of erythrocyte hemolysis, but the mechanism of their formation is unknown.

Erythrocyte Vesicles

Erythrocyte injury can result in the formation of variably sized erythrocyte vesicles (Fig. 4-74, *A–C*). They are classified as microvesicles when their diameter is less than 1 μm. The small size of microvesicles makes them difficult to identify in stained blood films and difficult to count using flow cytometers.

Erythrocytes, leukocytes, platelets, and endothelial cells all release membrane-bound microvesicles (also called microparticles) into the circulation, even in healthy individuals. Depending on the cell type and stimulus, these microvesicles may be either exosomes or ectosomes. Exosomes are microvesicles that form following inward budding of membranes to form multivesicular bodies, and multivesicular bodies subsequently fuse with the external cell membrane, releasing

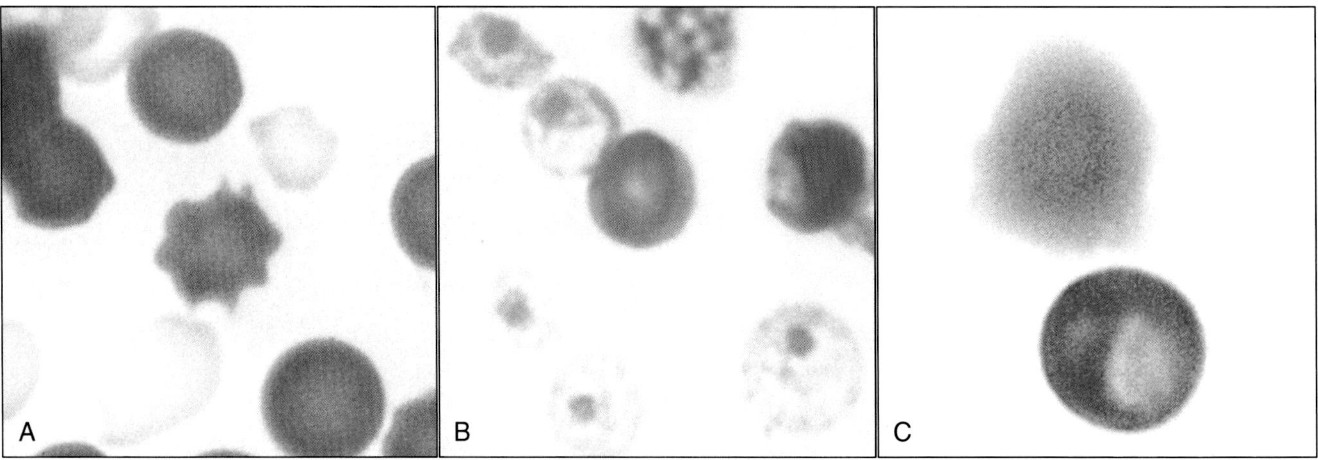

FIGURE 4-72
Lysed erythrocytes in blood films. **A,** Red-staining intact erythrocytes (echinocyte in the center) and pale-staining erythrocyte ghosts in blood from a horse in which intravascular hemolysis was produced by the intravenous and intraperitoneal administration of hypotonic fluid believed isotonic at the time of administration. **B,** Erythrocyte ghosts, each containing a single red-staining Heinz body, in erythrocytes from a cat with intravascular hemolysis caused by acetaminophen administration. **C,** A lysed erythrocyte *(red smudge at top)* and discocyte in blood from a dog with lipemia. The lysis occurred during smear preparation. Wright-Giemsa stain.

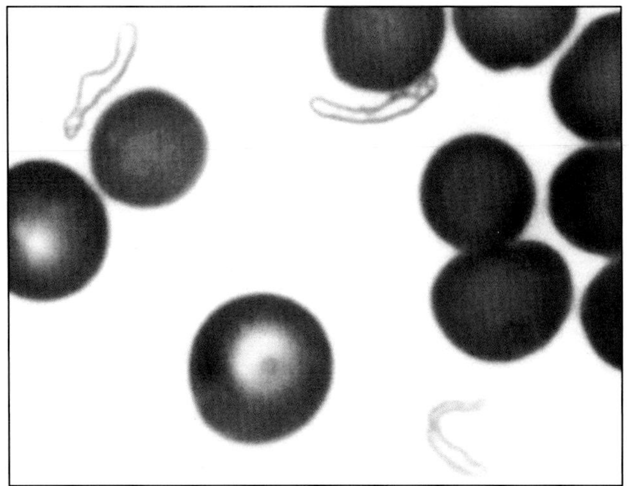

FIGURE 4-73
Three erythroid loops in blood from a dog bitten by a snake *(Vipera aspis).*

From Masserdotti C. Unusual "erythroid loops" in canine blood smears after viper-bite envenomation. Vet Clin Pathol. *2009;38:321-325.*

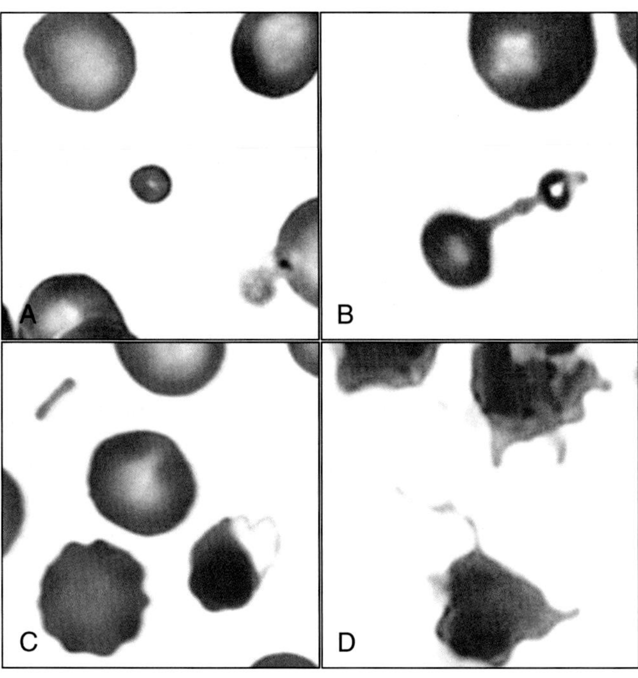

FIGURE 4-74
Erythrocyte vesicles in blood films. **A,** Erythrocyte vesicle *(center)* in blood from a febrile dog with mild nonregenerative anemia and lymphoma. Low numbers of eccentrocytes and pyknoctyes and rare hemoglobin crystals were also noted in the stained blood film. **B,** Erythrocyte vesicle formation in blood from a cat with eccentrocytes and erythrocytes containing Heinz bodies. The cat was a ketoacidotic diabetic with hepatic lipidosis. **C,** Elongated erythrocyte vesicle *(top left)* and eccentrocyte *(bottom right)* in blood from a dog subjected to prolonged propofol anesthesia. **D,** Microvesiculation from an acanthocyte in blood from a dog with neoplastic lymphoid infiltrates in the liver.

preformed exosomes.[405] As presented in Chapter 3, as reticulocytes mature into erythrocytes, this process is used by reticulocytes to eliminate unneeded proteins, such as transferrin receptors and Na^+, K^+ ATPase transporters (in dogs) from their surfaces.[263]

Ectosomes are shed by many cells, including erythrocytes, following the budding of microvesicles directly from the cell membrane (Fig. 4-74, *D*). The mean numbers of erythrocyte microvesicles in healthy humans are reported to vary from about 30 to 300/μL of plasma, depending on the methods used to measure them.[40,335,536] Erythrocytic ectosomes have both procoagulant and anti-inflammatory/immunosuppressive activities.[405] They are released in increased numbers during conditions that result in eryptosis (see Fig. 4-15), as discussed earlier in this chapter.[270] Increased total microvesicles, including erythrocyte microvesicles, are present in the blood of humans with metabolic syndrome and oxidative stress.[216] Large numbers of microvesicles can form in blood stored for transfusion when ATP depletion results in echinocyte formation and blebbing of ectosomes from the tips of echinocytic spicules.[186]

Erythrocyte microvesicles are rapidly cleared by macrophages in the liver.[537] The spleen also appears to be important in this regard because erythrocyte microvesicles are higher in splenectomized compared with nonsplenectomized humans with immune-mediated thrombocytopenia.[143]

Nucleated Erythrocytes

Rubricytes and metarubricytes (Fig. 4-75, *A,B*) are seldom present in the blood of normal adult mammals, although low numbers may occur in some normal dogs and cats.[490] Metarubricytosis (generally called normoblastemia in human hematology) is often seen in blood in association with a regenerative anemia; however, their presence does not necessarily indicate that a regenerative response is present.[296]

FIGURE 4-75 **Nucleated erythroid cells and nuclear fragmentation**

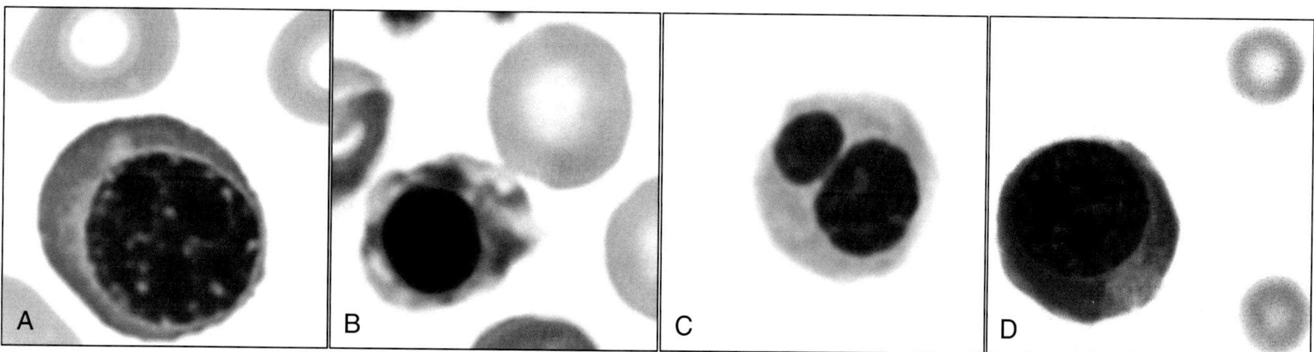

A, Polychromatophilic rubricyte in blood from a dog with regenerative anemia. **B,** Metarubricyte in blood from a beagle with erythrocyte pyruvate kinase deficiency. **C,** Nuclear lobulation in a polychromatophilic rubricyte in blood from a cat with acute myelogenous leukemia (AML-M6) and a nonregenerative anemia. **D,** Exceptionally large basophilic rubricyte in blood from a cat with myelodysplastic syndrome and a nonregenerative anemia.

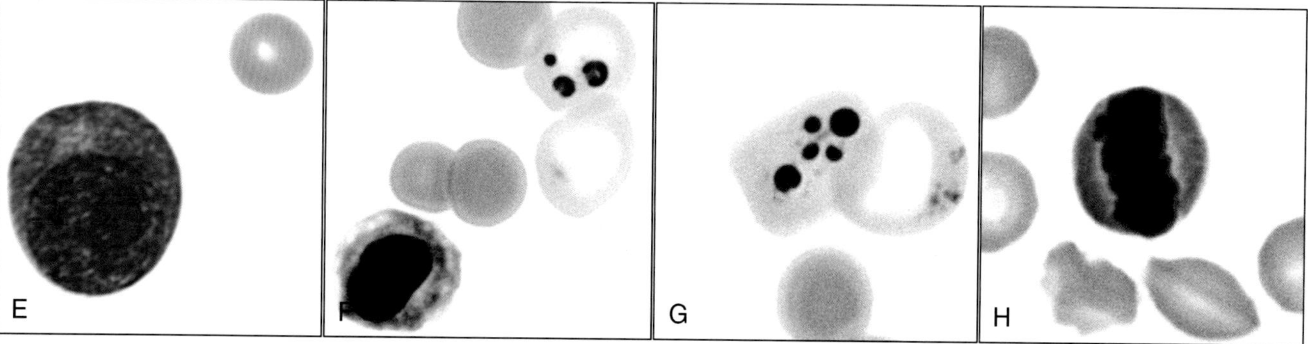

E, Rubriblast in blood from a cat with acute myelogenous leukemia (AML-M6) and a nonregenerative anemia. **F,** Polychromatophilic metarubricyte with elongated nucleus and erythrocyte containing nuclear fragments in blood from a dog with immune-mediated hemolytic anemia and thrombocytopenia 5 days after treatment with vincristine. **G,** Erythrocyte containing nuclear fragments in blood from a dog with immune-mediated hemolytic anemia and thrombocytopenia 5 days after treatment with vincristine. **H,** Mitotic rubricyte in blood from a dog with hemangiosarcoma and a regenerative anemia. Wright-Giemsa stain.

Nucleated erythrocytes are rarely seen in horses with regenerative anemia.

Nucleated erythrocytes may be seen in animals with lead poisoning, in which there is minimal or no anemia,[164,325] and in nonanemic conditions in which the bone marrow is damaged, such as septicemia, endotoxic shock, and drug administrations.[117,490,534] Nucleated erythrocytes are present in the blood of most dogs presented with heat stroke.[25] Low numbers of nucleated erythrocytes are seen in a wide variety of conditions in dogs, including cardiovascular disease, trauma, hyperadrenocorticism, and various inflammatory conditions.[296]

When frequent nucleated erythrocyte precursors are present in the blood of an animal with nonregenerative anemia (Fig. 4-75, *C-E*), conditions including myelodysplasia, hematopoietic neoplasia,[238,296] infiltrative marrow disease,[217,490] impaired splenic function,[490] and inherited dyserythropoietic disorders[223,446] should be considered. The presence of rubriblasts in blood from an animal with nonregenerative anemia strongly suggests that a myeloid neoplasm is present (Fig. 4-75, *E*). Nucleated erythrocytes may be excessively large (Fig. 4-75, *D*) and erythrocyte nuclei may be lobulated or fragmented in animals with myeloid neoplasms (Fig. 4-75, *C*)[105,125,416] or following vincristine therapy (Fig. 4-75, *F, G*). Nucleated erythroid precursors are capable of division earlier than metarubricytes; consequently, mitotic nucleated erythrocytes may be seen in blood (Fig. 4-75, *H*).

INCLUSIONS OF ERYTHROCYTES

Howell-Jolly Bodies (Micronuclei)

These small spherical nuclear remnants (Fig. 4-76) form in the bone marrow following nuclear fragmentation or rupture of the nuclear membrane, with nuclear material left behind when the nucleus is expelled (Fig. 4-77).[43,76] They have generally been called Howell-Jolly bodies by hematologists and micronuclei by toxicologists.[194,552] The latter term is advantageous because it describes their composition. Howell-Jolly bodies are removed or "pitted" by the spleen as reticulocytes and erythrocytes squeeze through interendothelial slits of the splenic sinus.[76,528] They may be present in low numbers in erythrocytes of normal horses and cats (Fig. 4-76, *A*). They are often present in association with regenerative anemia or following splenectomy in other species.[76,384,494] Howell-Jolly bodies may be increased in animals receiving glucocorticoid therapy (Fig. 4-76, *B*),[238] in benign poodle macrocytosis (Fig. 4-76, *C*),[238] and in animals being treated with chemotherapeutic agents that induce nuclear fragmentation, such as vincristine, colchicine, cytosine arabinoside, and cyclophosphamide (see Fig. 4-75, *F, G*).[194,552]

Heinz Bodies

These inclusions are large aggregates of oxidized, precipitated hemoglobin attached to the internal surfaces of erythrocyte membranes. In contrast to Howell-Jolly bodies, which stain dark blue, Heinz bodies stain red to pale pink with Romanowsky-type stains (Fig. 4-78, *A, C*). Heinz bodies stain lighter blue than Howell-Jolly bodies when stained with reticulocyte stains (Fig. 4-78, *B, D*). They can also be visualized as dark refractile inclusions in new methylene blue wet mount preparations (Fig. 4-78, *E*). Heinz bodies may also be visible within eccentrocytes (Fig. 4-78, *F*). If they bind extensively to the inner surface of erythrocyte membranes, they may be recognized as small surface projections when the membrane binds around much of an inclusion (Figs. 4-78, *F, G*, 4-79, 4-80). When intravascular hemolysis occurs, they may be visible as red inclusions within erythrocyte ghosts (Figs. 4-72, *B*, 4-78, *G*, 4-79, *C*).

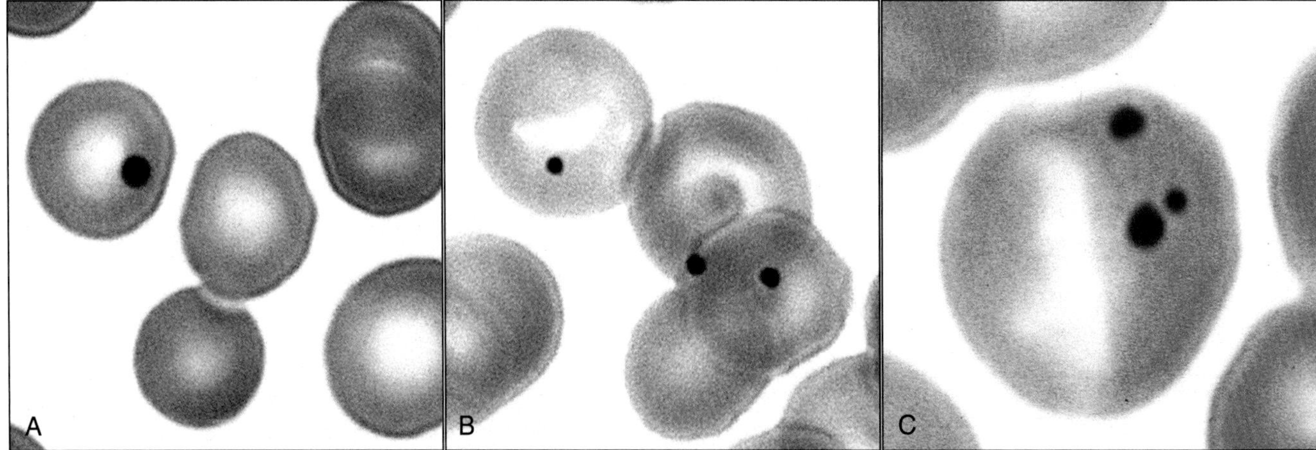

FIGURE 4-76

Howell-Jolly bodies (spherical nuclear remnants) in erythrocytes. **A,** Erythrocyte *(left)* containing a Howell-Jolly body in blood from a cat. **B,** Three Howell-Jolly bodies in erythrocytes in blood from a dog being treated with glucocorticoid steroids. **C,** Three Howell-Jolly bodies in a single erythrocyte from a poodle with benign macrocytosis.

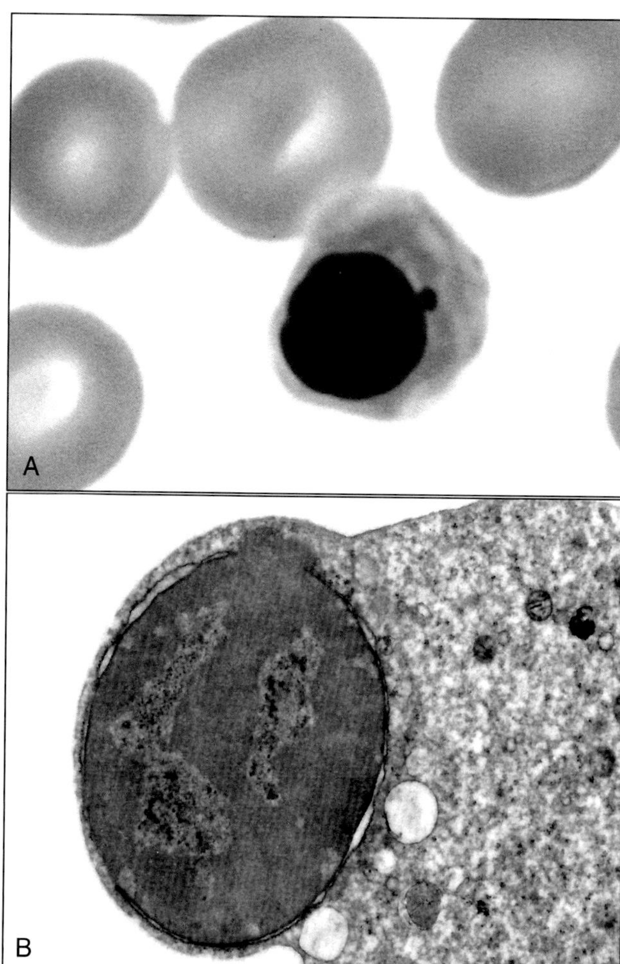

FIGURE 4-77

Formation of Howell-Jolly bodies. **A,** Apparent rupture of the nuclear membrane of a metarubricyte, allowing nuclear material to enter the cytoplasm and potentially form a Howell-Jolly body. **B,** Transmission electron photomicrograph of a nucleated erythroid cell with expanded nuclear pore or rupture of the nuclear membrane, allowing nuclear material to enter the cytoplasm and potentially form a Howell-Jolly body.

From Simpson CF, Kling JM. The mechanism of denucleation in circulating erythroblasts. J Cell Biol. *1967;35:237-245.*

In contrast to other domestic animal species, normal cats may have up to 5% Heinz bodies within their erythrocytes.[90] Small Heinz bodies may be seen in other species following splenectomy.[238] Not only is cat hemoglobin more susceptible to denaturation by endogenous oxidants,[205] but the cat spleen is less efficient in the removal (pitting) of Heinz bodies from erythrocytes than are spleens of other species.[55] Increased numbers of Heinz bodies may occur in cats with spontaneous diseases such as diabetes mellitus (especially when ketoacidosis is present), hyperthyroidism, and lymphoma.[89,90] Increased numbers of Heinz bodies have been seen in kittens fed fish-based diets[218] and in cats fed commercial soft-moist diets containing propylene glycol.[92,218] Increased Heinz body formation can also occur in cats with repeated propofol anesthesia.[21,304] Although erythrocyte survival tends to be shortened, anemia is either absent or mild in the above conditions. Causes of Heinz body hemolytic anemia are presented under "Hemolytic Anemias," below.

Basophilic Stippling

Reticulocytes usually stain as polychromatophilic erythrocytes with Romanowsky-type blood stains owing to the presence of dispersed ribosomes and polyribosomes; however, sometimes the ribosomes and polyribosomes aggregate together, forming blue-staining punctate inclusions referred to as basophilic stippling (Fig. 4-81).[43] These aggregates are similar to those produced using reticulocyte stains, but they form during the process of cell drying prior to staining with Romanowsky-type blood stains. Diffuse basophilic stippling commonly occurs in regenerative anemia in ruminants (Fig. 4-81, *A,B*) and occasionally in regenerative anemia in other species (Fig. 4-81, *C*).[238] It may be prominent in any species in the presence of lead poisoning (Fig. 4-81, *D*).[164,325] Diffuse basophilic stippling was reported in a dog with dyserythropoiesis and Cabot rings within erythrocytes.[286]

Siderotic Inclusions

Anucleated erythrocytes containing siderotic (iron-positive) inclusions are called siderocytes. Nucleated siderocytes have been called sideroblasts in human hematology. In contrast to diffuse basophilic stippling, which is distributed throughout the erythrocyte, siderotic inclusions generally appear as focal basophilic inclusions located near the periphery of erythrocytes (Fig. 4-81, *E,F*). A Prussian blue staining procedure is used to verify the presence of iron-positive material (Fig. 4-81, *G*). Siderotic inclusions in erythroid cells may consist of cytoplasmic ferritin aggregates or iron-loaded mitochondria. Ferritin aggregates can occur normally in nucleated erythroid cells of humans, dogs, and pigs, but the presence of iron-loaded mitochondria (Fig. 4-82) is a pathologic finding.[205] Iron-loaded degenerative mitochondria may be contained within autophagic vacuoles (lysosomes).[43] These inclusions have been called Pappenheimer bodies in human hematology.[60] Electron microscopy is used to identify the nature of siderotic inclusions; however, the location of iron-positive inclusions in a ring around the nucleus of a nucleated siderocyte (termed ringed sideroblast in human hematology) strongly suggests the presence of iron-loaded mitochondria.[60]

Except for iron deficiency, disorders of mitochondrial iron metabolism have the potential to cause excess iron accumulation in mitochondria. Erythrocytes may be microcytic and/or hypochromic secondary to defective heme synthesis.[233] Experimental pyridoxine deficiency and experimental chronic copper deficiency have both resulted in mitochondrial iron overload in nucleated erythroid cells in the bone marrow of deficient pigs.[205] Drugs or chemicals reported to cause siderocytes and/or nucleated siderocytes in dogs include chloramphenicol (see Fig. 4-81, *E*), lead, hydroxyzine (Fig. 4-83), zinc, and an oxazolidinone antibiotic.[213,288,370]

FIGURE 4-78 **Staining characteristics and appearance of Heinz bodies**

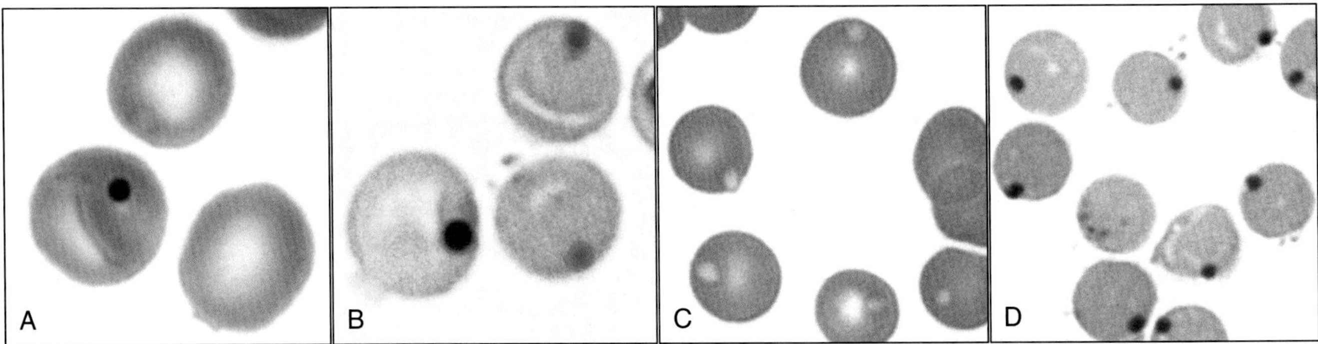

A, The erythrocyte at the top contains a pale-pink staining Heinz body at the margin at the 7 o'clock position. This cat had a Heinz body hemolytic anemia resulting from acetaminophen toxicity. In contrast, the erythrocyte at the bottom contains a Howell-Jolly body that stains dark blue. Wright-Giemsa stain. **B,** For comparison, erythrocytes from the same cat presented in **(A)** were stained with a new methylene blue reticulocyte stain. The erythrocyte on the left contains a dark blue-staining Howell-Jolly body and the other two cells each contain a light blue-staining Heinz body. **C,** Heinz bodies in blood from a cat appearing as pale "spots" within erythrocytes. Wright-Giemsa stain. **D,** Heinz bodies in blood from a cat. New methylene blue reticulocyte stain.

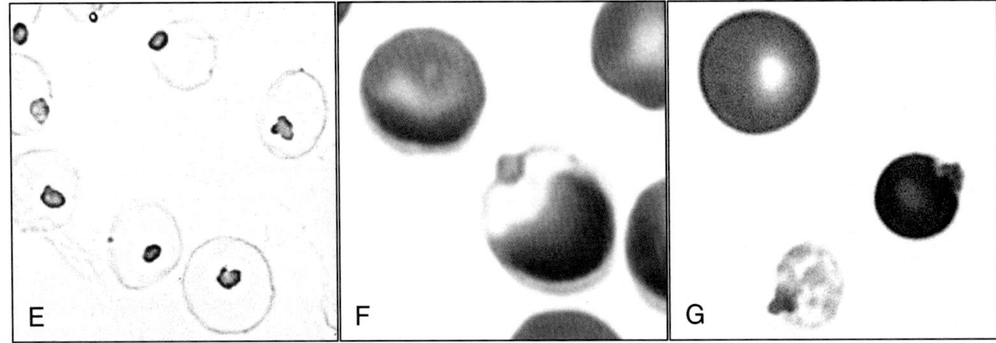

E, Heinz bodies in blood from a cat. New methylene blue wet mount preparation. **F,** Eccentrocyte with a visible Heinz body in blood of a cat with acetaminophen toxicity. **G,** A large polychromatophilic erythrocyte *(top),* erythrocyte "ghost" containing a Heinz body *(bottom),* and an intact erythrocyte containing a Heinz body projecting from its surface *(right)* in blood from a dog with a hemolytic anemia resulting from the ingestion of several pennies containing zinc. Wright-Giemsa stain.

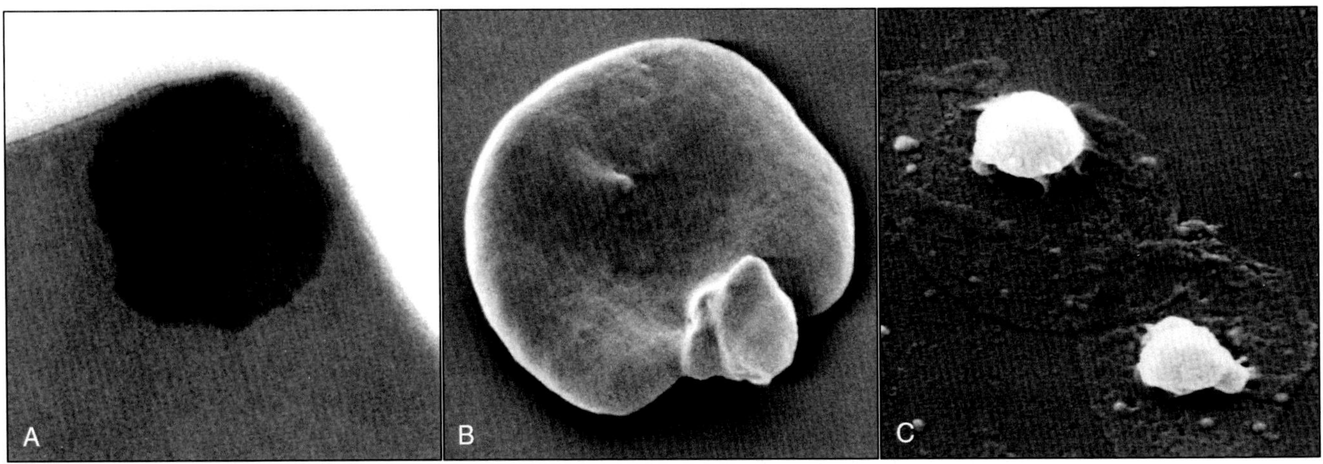

FIGURE 4-79

Transmission and scanning electron photomicrographs of Heinz bodies. **A,** Transmission electron photomicrograph of a Heinz body bound to the inner membrane of a horse erythrocyte. **B,** Scanning electron photomicrograph of a Heinz body protruding from a cat erythrocyte. **C,** Scanning electron photomicrograph of two erythrocyte ghosts, each containing a Heinz body.

A, From Simpson CF. The ultrastructure of Heinz bodies in horse, dog, and turkey erythrocytes. Cornell Vet. *1971;61:228-238. **B,** From Jain NC.* Schalm's Veterinary Hematology. *4th ed. Philadelphia: Lea & Febiger, 1986. C, From Jain NC.* Schalm's Veterinary Hematology. *4th ed. Philadelphia: Lea & Febiger; 1986.*

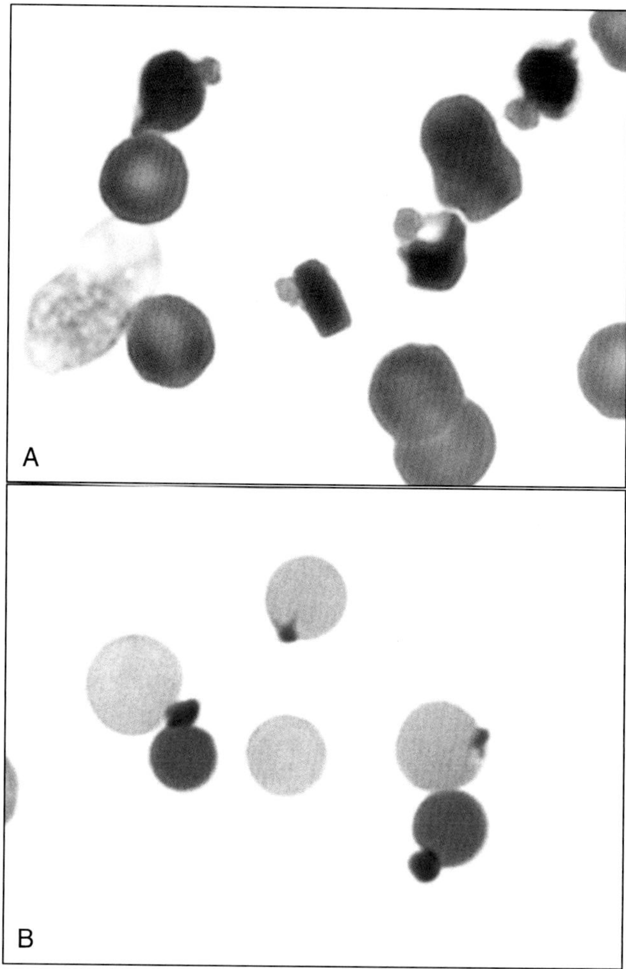

FIGURE 4-80

Idiopathic Heinz body hemolytic anemia in a horse. **A,** Heinz bodies protruding from erythrocytes, including two erythrocytes that also contain hemoglobin crystals. A large platelet is located on the left side. Wright-Giemsa stain. **B,** Heinz bodies protruding from erythrocytes. Apparently shrunken erythrocytes with larger Heinz bodies stain more basophilic. New methylene blue reticulocyte stain.

Siderotic inclusions in erythroid cells have been recognized in some dogs and cats with myeloid neoplasms.[56,524] Acquired dyserythropoiesis with siderocytes has been reported in dogs in which specific etiologies could not be determined, although some of these animals had inflammatory disorders.[81,513] Congenital anemias with ringed nucleated siderocytes have been reported in humans.[60,233] Persistent siderotic inclusions have been recognized in microcytic hypochromic erythrocytes from an English bulldog; they were composed of degenerate iron-loaded mitochondria (see Fig. 4-82). Echinocytes and acanthocytes were present and erythrocytes contained Heinz bodies and low numbers of hemoglobin crystals (see Fig. 4-83).[209] A congenital defect resulting in mitochondrial iron overload and secondary oxidant injury was suspected but not identified.

Cabot Rings

Cabot rings are reddish purple-staining threadlike loops or figure-eight structures that are primarily found in reticulocytes in humans.[189] Diffuse basophilic stippling is usually also present. Spectral analysis indicates that Cabot rings contain arginine-rich histones but not DNA.[401] They may be remnants of mitotic spindle microtubules. Cabot rings have been reported in erythrocytes from humans with cobalamin and folate deficiency, dyserythropoiesis, and myelodysplastic syndrome.[189]

Cabot rings have been observed in normal camel and llama erythrocytes stained with reticulocyte stains (Fig. 4-84, *A,B*) and less frequently in llama erythrocytes prepared with May-Grunwald-Giemsa stain.[30,321,483] Studies of lysed camelid erythrocytes demonstrate thin elliptical and figure-eight-shaped structures in reticulocytes that presumably represent Cabot rings. When examined by transmission electron microscopy, these structures were described as marginal bands that are composed of microtubules and associated proteins. These marginal bands disappear as the cell matures.[94]

Cabot rings have been reported in a May-Grunwald-Giemsa-stained blood film from a dog with dyserythropoiesis (Fig. 4-84, *C,D*).[286] As in humans, most Cabot rings occurred in polychromatophilic erythrocytes.

INFECTIOUS AGENTS OF ERYTHROCYTES

A number of infectious agents are recognized to occur in or on erythrocytes. These include intracellular protozoal parasites (*Babesia* species, *Theileria* species, and *Cytauxzoon felis*), intracellular rickettsial organisms (*Anaplasma* species), and epicellular *Mycoplasma* species. The erythrocyte protozoal organisms (piroplasms) of the order Piroplasmida each have a nucleus within their cytoplasm. In contrast to *Plasmodium* and *Haemoproteus* genera, these organisms do not form pigment in infected erythrocytes even though they also consume hemoglobin.[491] The rickettsia and mycoplasma organisms are bacteria and therefore lack nuclei. These infectious agents generally cause mild to severe hemolytic anemia depending on the pathogenicity of the organism and the susceptibility of the host. Distemper virus inclusions may also be seen in dog erythrocytes.

Babesia Species

More than 100 species of *Babesia* are recognized to infect domestic animals, wild animals, and humans worldwide.[228,491] When stained with Romanowsky-type blood stains, a babesial organism (piroplasm) generally has colorless to light-blue cytoplasm with a red to purple nucleus (Fig. 4-85). Babesial parasites vary considerably in size from large (2.5-5.0 μm), easily visualized *Babesia canis* parasites (Fig. 4-85, *A*) to small (1.0-2.5 μm in diameter), difficult-to-see *Babesia gibsoni* (Fig. 4-85, *B*) and *Babesia felis* (Fig. 4-85, *C*) parasites. Large

FIGURE 4-81 **Diffuse and focal basophilic stippling**

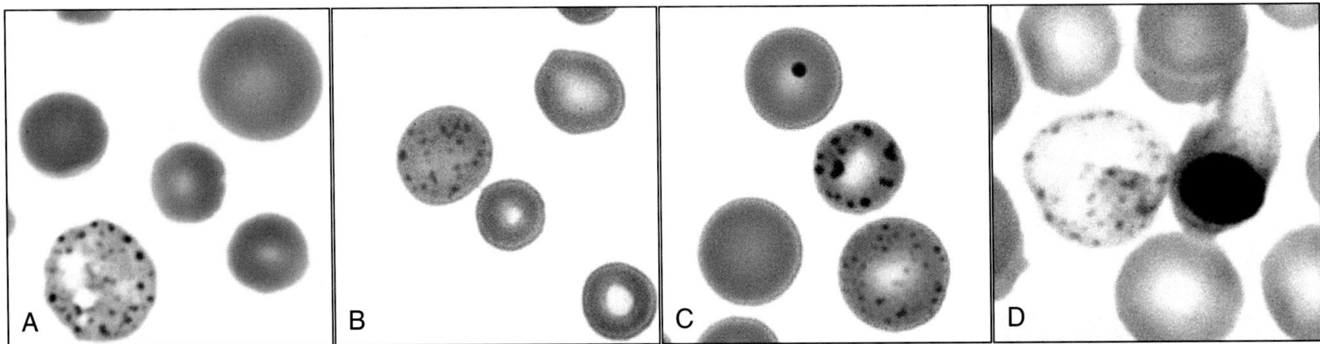

A, Diffuse basophilic stippling *(bottom left)* in a macrocytic polychromatophilic erythrocyte, a macrocytic erythrocyte *(top right),* and three normal-sized erythrocytes in blood from a cow with anaplasmosis (no organisms present) and a subsequent regenerative anemia. Wright-Giemsa stain. **B,** Diffuse basophilic stippling in a large erythrocyte *(left)* in blood from a sheep with a regenerative anemia. Wright-Giemsa stain. **C,** Erythrocytes containing a Howell-Jolly body *(top),* diffuse coarse basophilic stippling *(middle),* and diffuse fine basophilic stippling *(bottom)* in blood from a cat with *Mycoplasma haemofelis* infection (no organisms present) and a regenerative anemia. Wright-Giemsa stain. **D,** A polychromatophilic erythrocyte with basophilic stippling *(left)* and a polychromatophilic metarubricyte *(right)* in blood from a dog with lead toxicity. Wright-Giemsa stain.

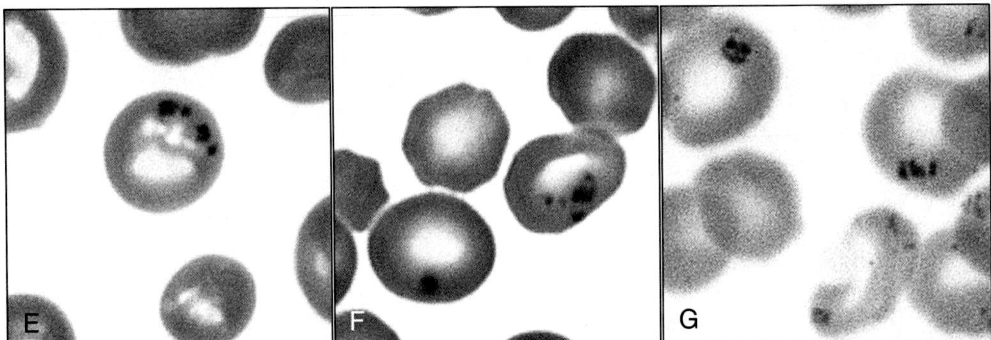

E, Focal basophilic stippling in an erythrocyte in blood from a dog treated with chloramphenicol. The inclusions were shown to contain iron using the Prussian blue staining procedure and can therefore be called siderocytes. Wright-Giemsa stain. **F,** Focal basophilic stippling in two erythrocytes (siderocytes) in blood from a male Sheltie dog that had many siderocytes in his blood when examined several times over 4 years. Erythrocytes were microcytic but the dog was not anemic. The dog was treated with hydroxyzine. Abnormalities in copper, zinc, and pyridoxine metabolism were ruled out, as was lead toxicity. Wright-Giemsa stain. **G,** Iron-positive inclusions in erythrocytes (siderocytes) in blood from the same dog as shown in **(F),** Prussian blue stain.

F-G, Blood samples and case information provided by M. Plier.

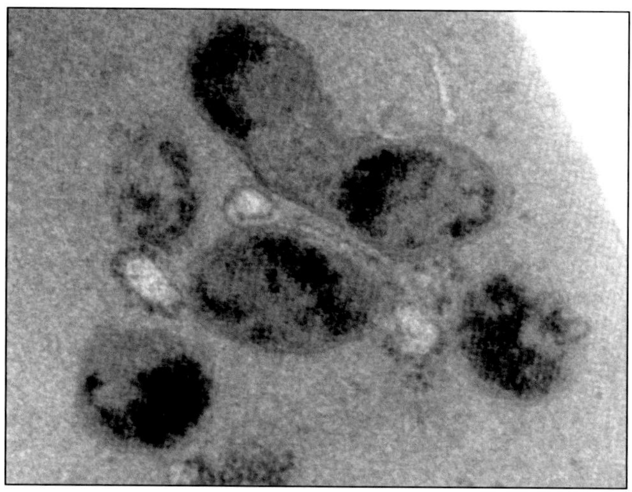

FIGURE 4-82

Transmission electron photomicrograph of a cluster of iron-loaded *(dark material)* degenerating mitochondria in a circulating erythrocyte from an English bulldog, which produced focal basophilic stippling seen in erythrocytes by light microscopy in this animal (see Fig. 4-83).

Courtesy of W. L. Clapp.

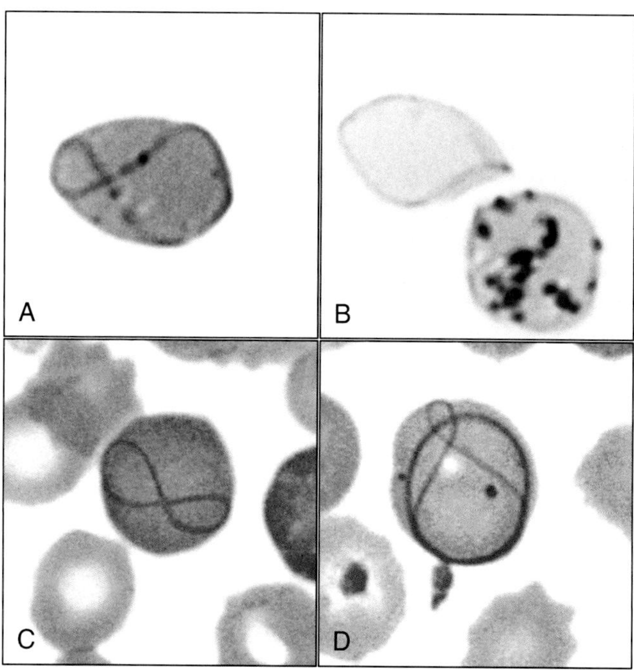

FIGURE 4-84

Cabot rings in erythrocytes. **A,** Cabot ring with a figure-eight shape in an erythrocyte from an adult alpaca with a moderately regenerative hypochromic iron-deficient anemia secondary to gastric ulceration and hemorrhage. New methylene blue reticulocyte stain. **B,** Erythrocyte with a Cabot ring at the periphery and a reticulocyte *(bottom right)* in blood from an adult alpaca with a moderately regenerative hypochromic iron-deficient anemia secondary to gastric ulceration and hemorrhage. New methylene blue reticulocyte stain. **C,** Cabot ring with a figure-eight shape in an erythrocyte from a dog with dyserythropoiesis. **D,** Cabot rings in an erythrocyte from a dog with dyserythropoiesis. May-Grunwald-Giemsa stain.

A, *From a stained blood film from a 2009 ASVCP slide review case submitted by B. Fierro and M. Scott.* **B,** *From a stained blood film from a 2009 ASVCP slide review case submitted by B. Fierro and M. Scott.* **C and D,** *From Lukaszewska J, Lewandowski K. Cabot rings as a result of severe dyserythropoiesis in a dog.* Vet Clin Pathol. *2008;37:180-183.*

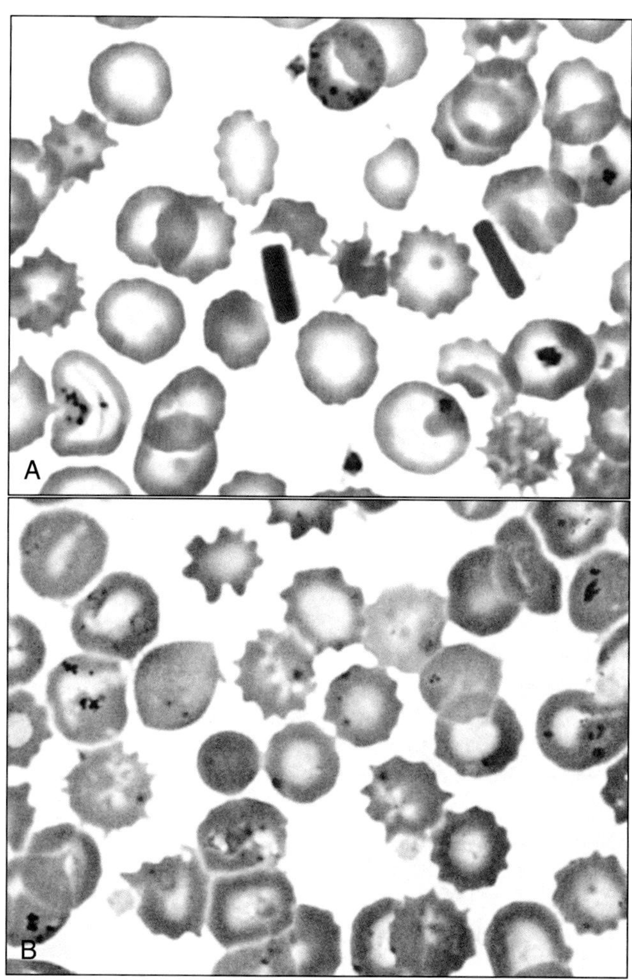

FIGURE 4-83

Siderotic inclusions in microcytic hypochromic erythrocytes in a blood film from an English bulldog with a presumptive defect in mitochondrial iron metabolism. **A,** Basophilic stippling is diffuse in one erythrocyte *(top center)* but focal in other erythrocytes. Echinocytes and acanthocytes are present, and two erythrocytes contain hemoglobin crystals. Wright-Giemsa stain. **B,** Focal (iron-positive) basophilic inclusions are present in a blood film from the same dog presented in **(A).** These siderotic inclusions were composed of degenerate, iron-loaded mitochondria (see Fig. 4-82). Prussian blue stain.

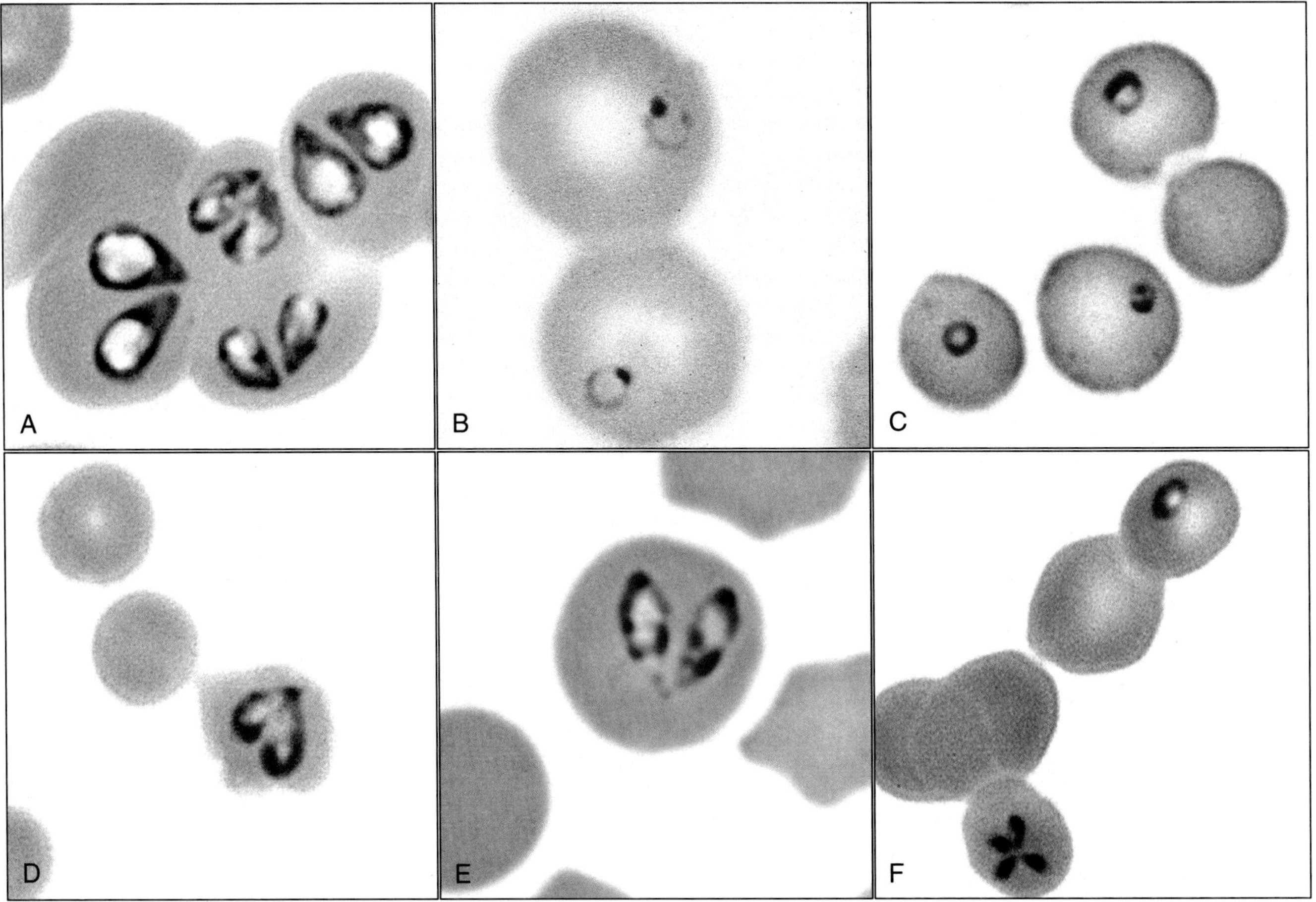

FIGURE 4-85 ***Babesia* organisms in erythrocytes**

A, Two pear-shaped *Babesia canis* organisms in each of four erythrocytes in blood from a puppy with hemolytic anemia. Infected erythrocytes often were seen to be adhering to one another. Wright-Giemsa stain. **B,** Single small *Babesia gibsoni* organisms in two erythrocytes from a dog. **C,** Single *Babesia felis* organisms in three erythrocytes in blood from a domestic cat from South Africa. Wright stain. **D,** Two *Babesia bigemina* organisms in an erythrocyte from a cow. Wright-Giemsa stain. **E,** Two pear-shaped *Babesia caballi* organisms in a horse erythrocyte. Wright-Giemsa stain. **F,** A single *Babesia equi* organism in one erythrocyte *(top)* and a Maltese cross of four organisms in another erythrocyte *(bottom)* in blood from a horse. Wright-Giemsa stain.

babesial organisms generally appear pear-shaped and commonly occur in pairs. Small babesial organisms are more often round in shape. Aside from size, the morphology of protozoal organisms infecting erythrocytes is similar; therefore polymerase chain reaction (PCR) and 18S rRNA gene sequencing is required to specifically identify these organisms.[228] New organisms will continue to be identified using genetic analysis.

Three genetically distinct large *B. canis* subspecies (*B. canis canis, B. canis vogeli,* and *B. canis rossi*) have been identified as causing disease in dogs.[467] In reality, these organisms appear to be different species; consequently they may be renamed *B. canis, B. vogeli* (Fig. 4-85, *A*), and *B. rossi*, respectively.[491] In addition, a large *Babesia* species was originally described in dogs in North Carolina; it has yet to be named.[51,226,427] At least three small protozoal species, *B. gibsoni* (Fig. 4-85, *B*), *Babesia conradae,* and a *Babesia microti*-like organism cause disease in dogs. *B. microti* organisms exhibit characteristics of *Theileria* species, and a *B. microcoti*-like organism in dogs has been called *Theileria annae*, but a new genus may be required for this group of organisms.[491]

B. felis (Fig. 4-85, *C*) causes hemolytic anemia in cats in South Africa.[362] Additional piroplasms have been identified by PCR in domestic cats, but their clinical significance remains to be determined.[491] The two most important *Babesia* species infecting cattle appear to be *Babesia bigemina* (Fig. 4-85, *D*) and *Babesia bovis*. The two most important piroplasms infecting horses are the large *Babesia caballi* parasite (Fig. 4-85, *F*) and the smaller, more pleomorphic *Babesia. equi* parasite (Figs. 4-85, *E*, 4-86). Some investigators have recommended that *B. equi* be renamed *Theileria equi* based on genetic studies as well as finding schizonts transiently in lymphocytes.[318] Other investigators believe *B. equi* belongs in a new genus that is distinct from both *Babesia* and *Theileria*.[14,491]

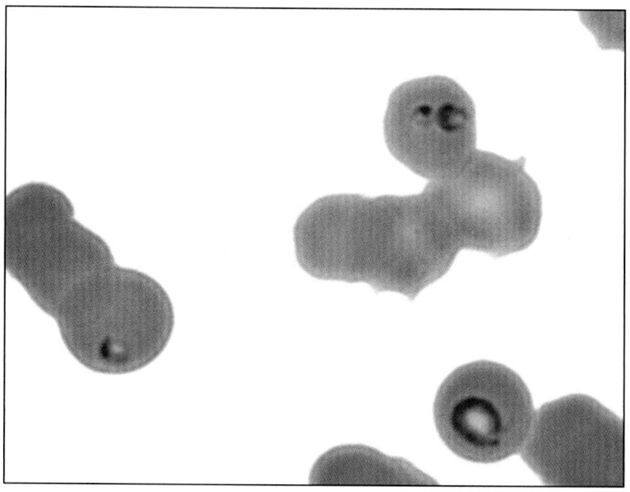

FIGURE 4-86

Babesia equi organisms in erythrocytes from a horse with clinical disease. Although pleomorphism (including variation in organism size) was prominent, PCR and gene sequencing of the *18S rDNA* gene identified a single infective agent. Wright-Giemsa stain.

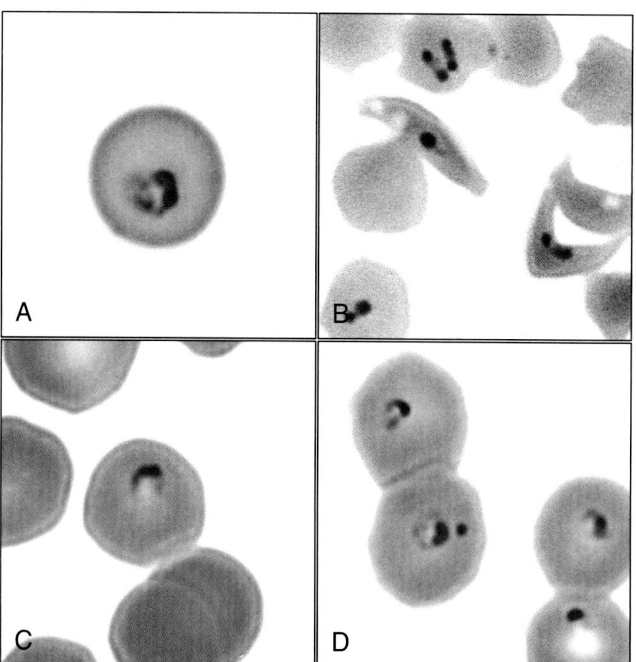

FIGURE 4-87

Theileria and *Cytauxzoon* organisms in erythrocytes. **A,** *Theileria buffeli* organism in an erythrocyte in blood from a cow. Wright stain. *(Photograph from a 2001 ASVCP slide review case submitted by A. Boisvert and R. Pillars.)* **B,** *Theileria cervi* organisms in erythrocytes in blood from a white-tailed deer. Several drepanocytes (sickle erythrocytes) are present. Wright-Giemsa stain. **C,** A *Cytauxzoon felis* organism in a domestic cat erythrocyte. Wright-Giemsa stain. **D,** Single *Cytauxzoon felis* organisms in several domestic cat erythrocytes. Wright-Giemsa stain.

Theileria Species

Theilerial organisms appear similar to babesial organisms when observed on stained blood films (Fig. 4-87, *A*). The genus *Theileria* differs from the genus *Babesia* in that the former species has a tissue phase as well as an erythrocyte stage of development. Schizonts develop in lymphoid cells and, when mature, release merozoites, which enter erythrocytes. *Babesia* organisms proliferate only in erythrocytes.

Theilerial species (*Theileria parva* and *Theileria annulata*) cause important diseases in ruminants in Africa, Asia, and the Middle East[274]; however, the theilerial organisms present in ruminants in the United States are usually nonpathogenic.[245,453] Piroplasms are commonly observed in deer blood in the United States (Fig.4-87, *B*). They are generally considered of low pathogenicity but may cause hemolytic anemia under some circumstances.[544]

Cytauxzoon felis

Cytauxzoon felis (Fig. 4-87, *C,D*), as its name implies, infects feline erythrocytes.[185] It is similar in morphology to *B. felis* in erythrocytes (see Fig. 4-85, *C*). Like *Theileria*, the genus *Cytauxzoon* has both a tissue phase and an erythrocyte phase. In contrast to *Theileria*, the schizonts of *Cytauxzoon* develop in macrophages rather than in lymphocytes.

Anaplasma Species

Anaplasma organisms appear as round to oval basophilic inclusions in ruminant erythrocytes (Fig. 4-88), which must be differentiated from Howell-Jolly bodies.[500] Although morulae are not appreciated by light microscopy, the inclusions consist of one to several subunits within a membrane-lined vesicle (Fig. 4-89). The size of an inclusion seen by light microscopy is directly related to the number of subunits present. Unlike Howell-Jolly bodies, *Anaplasma* organisms are generally not perfect spheres, and most are smaller than Howell-Jolly bodies. *Anaplasma marginale* is an important pathogen of cattle. Organisms are often located at the margin in erythrocytes when viewed on stained blood films (see Fig. 4-88). *Anaplasma centrale* is less pathogenic and organisms are more often located more centrally in erythrocytes when viewed on stained blood films.[159] *Anaplasma ovis* (see Fig. 4-88, *C*) is pathogenic for sheep, goats, and some wild ruminants.[112]

Distemper Inclusions

Viral inclusions may be seen in the blood cells of some dogs during the viremic stage of canine distemper virus infection.[181,504] These inclusions can be difficult to visualize when routine Wright or Giemsa stains are used. In erythrocytes, they appear as variably sized round, oval, or irregular blue-gray inclusions that most often occur in polychromatophilic cells (Fig. 4-90, *A*). For an unknown reason, distemper inclusions typically stain red and are easier to see in erythrocytes stained with the aqueous Diff-Quik stain (Fig. 4-90, *B*), which is a rapid modified Wright stain.[13,198]

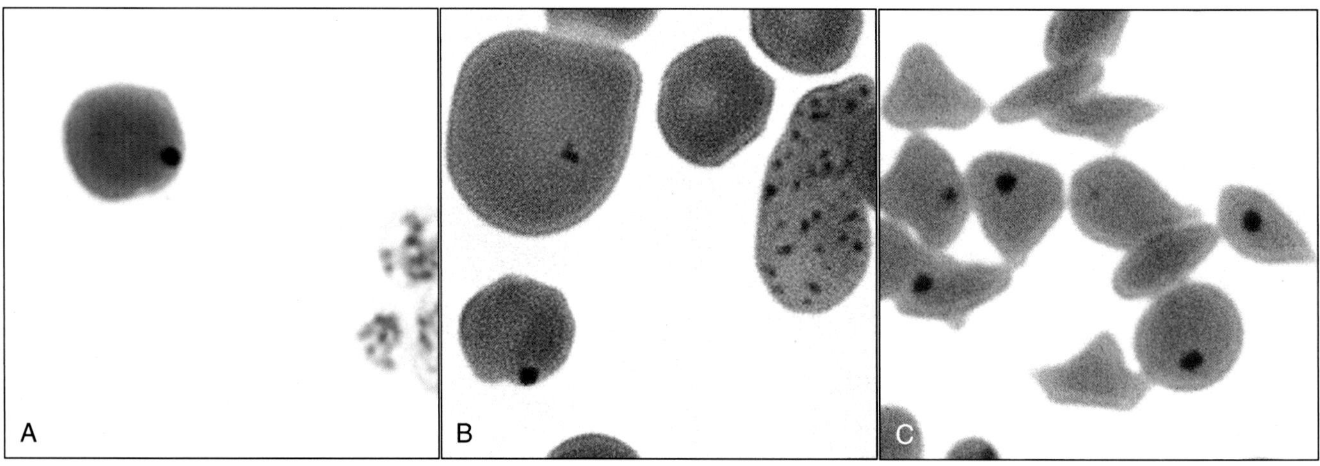

FIGURE 4-88

Anaplasma organisms in erythrocytes. **A,** *Anaplasma marginale* organism located within an erythrocyte in blood from a Holstein cow. Three platelets are also visible *(right)*. Wright-Giemsa stain. **B,** An erythrocyte containing an *Anaplasma marginale* organism *(bottom left)*, a macrocytic erythrocyte *(top left)*, and an abnormally shaped erythrocyte with basophilic stippling *(right)* in blood from a Holstein cow. Wright-Giemsa stain. **C,** *Anaplasma ovis* organisms in blood from a 6-month-old goat with esophageal perforation and intestinal *Trichostrongylus* infestation. Wright-Giemsa stain.

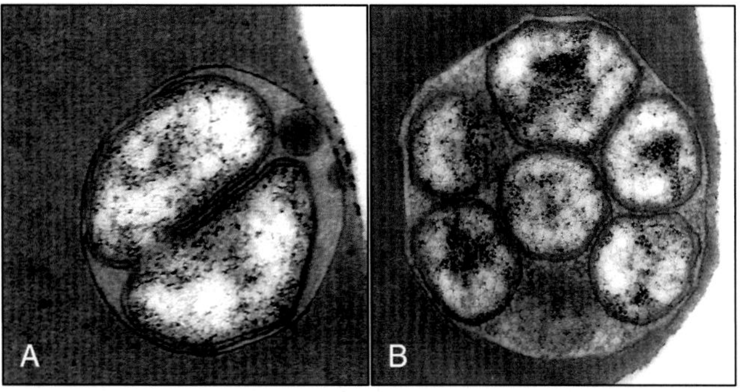

FIGURE 4-89

Transmission electron photomicrograph of *Anaplasma marginale* organisms in bovine erythrocytes. **A,** Binary fission of an *Anaplasma* organism within an erythrocytic vacuole. **B,** Six *Anaplasma* organisms within an erythrocytic vacuole.

From Simpson CF, Kling JM, Love JN. Morphologic and histochemical nature of Anaplasma marginale. Am J Vet Res. *1967;28:1055-1065.*

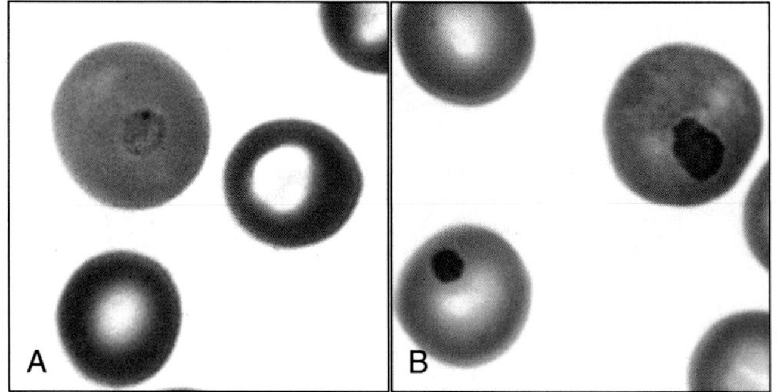

FIGURE 4-90

Distemper inclusions in dog erythrocytes. **A,** Round blue-gray distemper inclusion in a polychromatophilic erythrocyte *(top left)*. Wright-Giemsa stain. **B,** Two round reddish distemper inclusions in erythrocytes in blood from the same dog as shown in **(A).** The inclusion at top right is in a large polychromatophilic erythrocyte. Diff-Quik stain.

Distemper inclusions are composed of aggregates of viral nucleocapsids.[310] The presence of viral inclusions in anucleated cells is explained by the fact that they form within nucleated erythroid precursors in the bone marrow and persist following expulsion of the nucleus.[181]

Hemotropic Mycoplasmas (Hemoplasmas)

Hemotropic mycoplasmas are gram-negative non-acid-fast bacteria that attach to the external surfaces of erythrocytes (Figs. 4-91, 4-92, 4-93), although evidence that *Mycoplasma suis* can enter erythrocytes has recently been published.[187] *Hemoplasmas* has been proposed as a trivial name for these hemotropic mycoplasmas.[340]

Hemoplasmas appear as small (generally 0.5 to 1 μm) blue-staining cocci, rods, or rings on erythrocytes in blood films stained with Wright-type blood stains (Fig. 4-94, *A,B*). Reticulocyte stains cannot be used to search for mycoplasmas because the basophilic ribosomal material in reticulocytes can appear similar to the organisms. These organisms were classified as rickettsia in the genus *Haemobartonella* or the genus *Eperythrozoon* for many years.[202] Organisms that were tightly bound to erythrocyte surfaces, with prominent cocci and rod

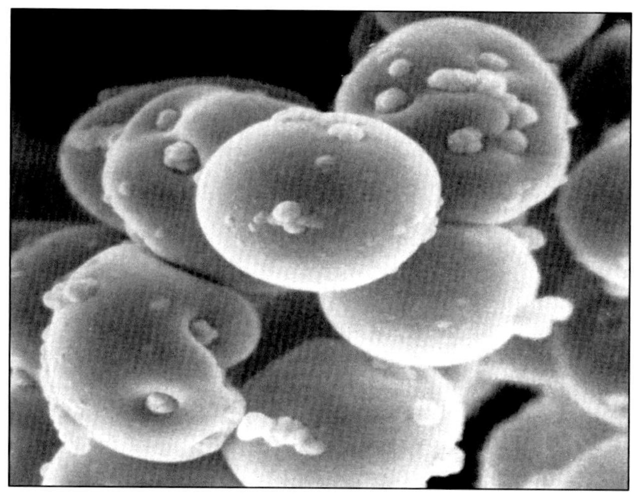

FIGURE 4-91
Scanning electron photomicrograph of erythrocytes from a cat infected with *Mycoplasma haemofelis.*

From Harvey JW. Hemotrophic mycoplasmosis (hemobartonellosis). In: Greene CE, ed. Infectious Diseases of the Dog and Cat. *3rd ed. Philadelphia: Saunders Elsevier; 2006:252-260.*

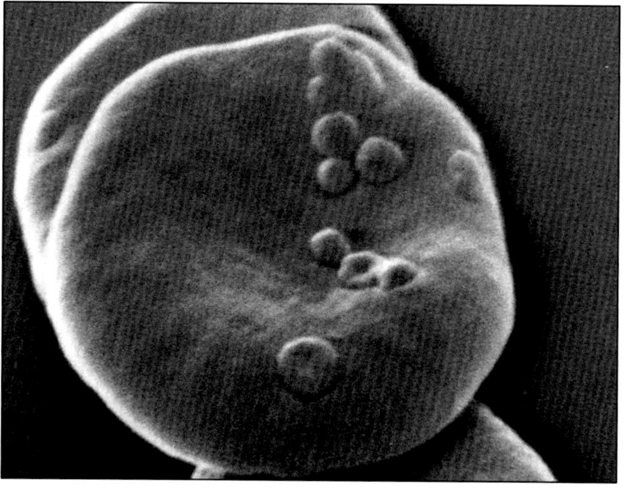

FIGURE 4-93
Scanning electron photomicrograph of a bovine erythrocyte parasitized with *M. wenyoni.*

From Keeton KS, Jain NC. Eperythrozoon wenyoni: a scanning electron microscopy study. J Parasitol. *1973;59:867-873.*

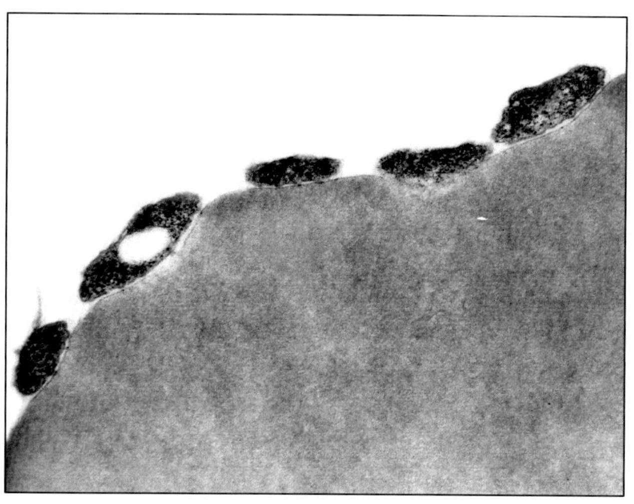

FIGURE 4-92
Transmission photomicrograph of *Mycoplasma haemofelis* organisms attached to the external surface of a cat erythrocyte.

From Simpson CF, Gaskin JM, Harvey JW. Ultrastructure of erythrocytes parasitized by Haemobartonella felis. J Parasitol. *1978;64:504-511.*

forms, were classified in the *Haemobartonella* genus. Organisms that were often found between erythrocytes, as well as adhered to erythrocytes, with prominent ring forms, were classified in the *Eperythrozoon* genus. These criteria seemed inadequate for the establishment of two genera, especially since the frequency of ring forms and the number of free organisms can be influenced to some degree simply by the manner in which a blood film is prepared. In addition, organisms detach from erythrocytes over time in blood samples collected using EDTA as an anticoagulant (Fig. 4-94, *C*).[12]

Results from sequencing of the *16S rRNA* gene indicate that all of these epicelluar erythrocyte parasites are mycoplasmas.[202,539] Consequently the *Haemobartonella* and *Eperythrozoon* genera have been discarded and organisms in these genera were moved to the genus *Mycoplasma.* Species names often include the prefix haemo (e.g., *Mycoplasma haemofelis*) to identify these unique mycoplasmas that attach to erythrocytes.

Three different hemoplasmas have been identified in cats based on *16S rRNA* gene sequences, *Mycoplasma haemofelis* (formerly called the large form of *Haemobartonella felis*), Candidatus *Mycoplasma haemominutum* (formerly called the small form of *Haemobartonella felis*), and Candidatus *Mycoplasma turicensis.*[473,539] *M. haemofelis* is more pathogenic than either of the other organisms.[473]

M. haemofelis organisms appear as small blue-staining cocci, rods, or rings on feline erythrocytes (see Fig. 4-94, *A*). Chains of organisms may be present on the surface of heavily parasitized erythrocytes (Fig. 4-95). Ring- and rod-shaped organisms are seen more readily in thin blood films. Organisms are pleomorphic and vary in size, but most are between 0.5 and 1.5 μm in diameter or length. They appear to be partially buried in indented foci on the surface of the erythrocytes (Fig. 4-96). Parasitized erythrocytes may lose their normal biconcave shape and become spherocytes or stomatospherocytes (see Fig. 4-91). Organisms occur in cyclic parasitemias; consequently they are not always identifiable in blood even during acute infections.[202]

FIGURE 4-94 **Hemotrophic mycoplasmas (hemoplasmas)**

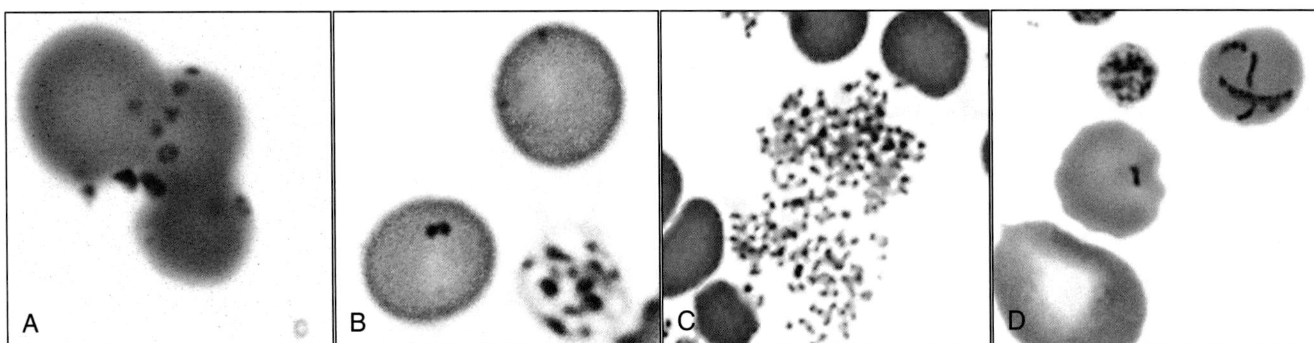

A, *Mycoplasma haemofelis* organisms located on the surface of erythrocytes in blood from a cat. Some organisms appear as rings, including the unattached one at the bottom right. Wright-Giemsa stain. **B,** *Mycoplasma haemominutum* organisms on the outside of an erythrocyte. **C,** An aggregate of free *Mycoplasma haemofelis* organisms that have detached from erythrocytes following 3 days in transit to the laboratory of infected blood collected with EDTA as the anticoagulant. Wright stain. **D,** *Mycoplasma haemocanis* organisms located on the outside of erythrocytes in blood from a dog. One erythrocyte *(center)* has a rod-shaped structure on its surface that may be composed of two closely associated organisms, while another erythrocyte *(top right)* has many organisms forming filamentous chains in deep grooves on its surface. A platelet and large polychromatophilic erythrocyte are also present. Wright-Giemsa stain.

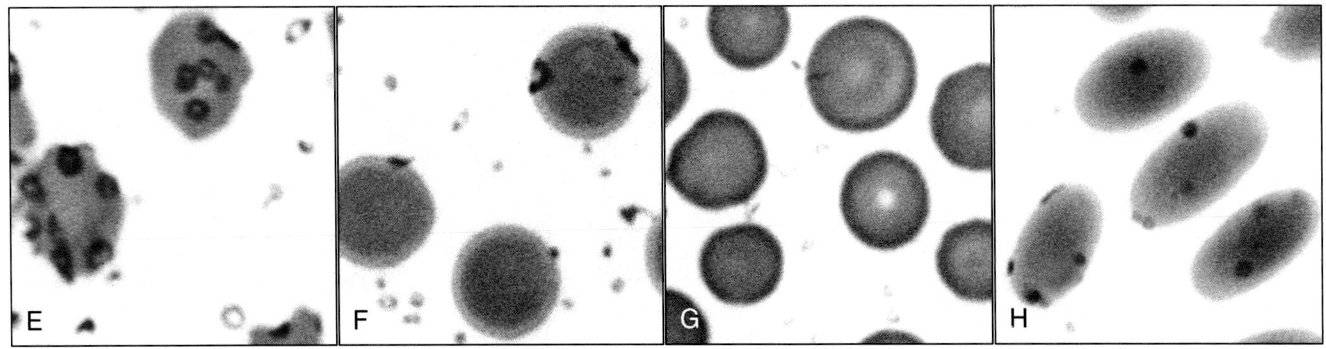

E, *Mycoplasma suis* organisms on the surface of erythrocytes and between erythrocytes in blood from a splenectomized pig. Erythrocytes appear as echinocytes, a normal finding in pig blood. Wright stain. **F,** *Mycoplasma ovis* organisms between erythrocytes in blood from a sheep. Wright-Giemsa stain. **G,** *Mycoplasma wenyoni* organisms between erythrocytes in blood from a Charolais bull. Wright stain. **H,** *Mycoplasma haemolamae* organisms on the surface of erythrocytes and between erythrocytes in blood from a llama. Wright-Giemsa stain.

***B,** Courtesy of J. B. Messick.* ***C,** From Allison RW, Fielder SE, Meinkoth JH. What is your diagnosis? Blood film from an icteric cat.* Vet Clin Pathol. *2010;39:125-126.* ***E,** Photograph of a stained blood film from a 1980 ASVCP slide review case submitted by G. Searcy.* ***F,** Photograph of a stained blood film from a 1993 ASVCP slide review case submitted by E. G. Welles, J. W. Tyler, and D. F. Wolfe.*

Candidatus *M. haemominutum* organisms (see Fig. 4-94, *B*) are rarely recognized in stained blood films. When seen, they appear as small rods or coccoid organisms and infrequently as ring forms, which stain less densely and measure about half the size (approximately 0.3 μm) of *M. haemofelis.*[142,165] However, this reported size difference has been challenged by the finding of a Candidatus *M. haemominutum* isolate in Great Britain that is about 0.6 μm in diameter.[472] Consequently morphologic appearance is not reliable in distinguishing these isolates; genetic analysis is needed for specific identification. Candidatus *M. turicensis* has been documented in blood from many cats using PCR-based assays, but it has not yet been identified in stained blood films from infected cats, presumably because of the low numbers of organisms present.[539]

Three hemoplasmas have been reported in dogs based on *16S rRNA* gene sequences. Organisms are generally observed only in splenectomized or immunosuppressed dogs.[202] Single *Mycoplasma haemocanis* (formerly *Haemobartonella canis*) organisms dimple the surface of host erythrocytes in a manner

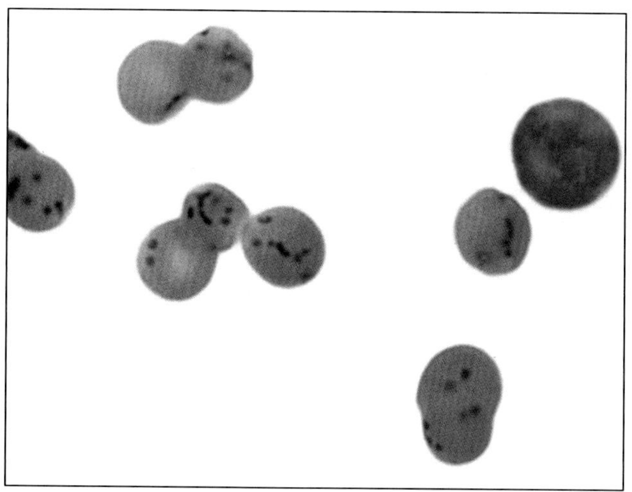

FIGURE 4-95
Large numbers of *Mycoplasma haemofelis* organisms (including ones forming chains) located on the outside of erythrocytes in blood from a cat. A large polychromatophilic erythrocyte (aggregate reticulocyte) is also present *(upper right)*. Wright-Giemsa stain.

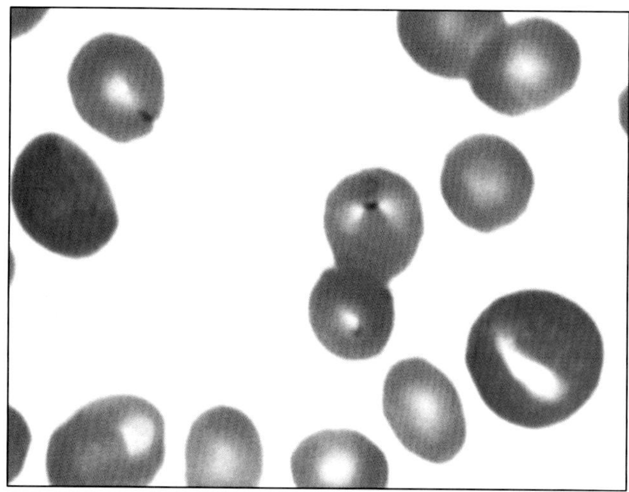

FIGURE 4-96
Blood film from a cat with *Mycoplasma haemofelis* infection demonstrating features that help distinguish this parasite from stain precipitation. An organism indents the membrane of the erythrocyte in the upper left. A second organism *(center right)* binds two areas of an erythrocyte membrane together. Two polychromatophilic erythrocytes (aggregate reticulocytes) are also present.

similar to *M. haemofelis* and chains of organisms are frequently found in grooves or deep folds, which can markedly distort the erythrocyte shape and appear as filamentous structures on the surface of erythrocytes (see Fig. 4-94, *D*). *M. haemocanis* has long been considered to be a distinctly different organism from *M. haemofelis,* but the sequence of the *16S rRNA* gene of a *M. haemocanis* isolate from one dog was remarkably similar (99% homology) to that of *M. haemofelis.*[67] More recent studies evaluating RNase P gene sequences demonstrated a lower degree of sequence homology between the two organisms (about 95%), suggesting that the organisms may represent different species.[48]

A hemoplasma with 99% *16S rRNA* gene homology to Candidatus *M. haemominutum* has been identified in a dog in China.[551] Another hemoplasma with somewhat less *16S rRNA* gene homology has been identified in multiple countries and classified as Candidatus *Mycoplasma haematoparvum.*[35,465,539] Candidatus *Mycoplasma haematoparvum* appeared as small (0.3 μm), basophilic coccoid bodies on the surface of erythrocytes in a stained blood film from a dog.[464]

Hemoplasmas, previously classified as *Eperythrozoon* organisms, infect pigs (*Mycoplasma suis,* Fig. 4-94, *E*),[221] sheep and goats (*Mycoplasma ovis,* Fig. 4-94,*G*),[339] cattle (*Mycoplasma wenyoni* [Figs. 4-93, 4-94, *F*], and Candidatus *Mycoplasma haemobos* or the synonymous Candidatus *Mycoplasma haemobovis*),[343,457,493] and llamas and alpacas (Candidatus *Mycoplasma haemolamae,* Fig. 4-94, *H*).[315,390]

Hemoplasma infections have been recognized for many years in animals but, using PCR assays, have only recently been documented in humans. These human organisms were related to *M. suis, M. wenyoni,* and *M. ovis.*[95,466] Based on the widespread use of PCR assays, new hemoplasmas will undoubtably be identified in animals and humans.

Bartonella Species

Members of the *Bartonella* species are small gram-negative bacteria. Cats and dogs are infected with multiple *Bartonella* species.[88] *Bartonella henselae* appears to be the primary cause of cat-scratch disease in humans. This organism causes mild illness and anemia in cats during the initial infection; subsequently, however, cats generally become carriers without evidence of disease.[63] This small rod-shaped bacterium occurs within erythrocytes[264] but is rarely appreciated in blood films of bacteremic cats (Fig. 4-97, *A*), even though the organism can be cultured from the blood of many healthy cats.[63]

Artifacts Resembling Infectious Agents

Erythrocyte parasites (especially hemoplasmas) must be differentiated from precipitated stain, refractile drying or fixation artifacts (Fig. 4-97, *B*), poorly staining Howell-Jolly bodies, and basophilic stippling. Platelets overlying erythrocytes (Fig. 4-97, *C*) may also be confused with erythrocyte parasites, especially *Babesia* species.

ERYTHROCYTE ASSAYS

Erythrocyte Counts, Hematocrit, and Hemoglobin Content

Erythrocytes in blood are quantified by cell counting (number of cells per microliter), by determining blood hemoglobin content (grams per deciliter), and by determining the hematocrit (HCT) as a percentage of blood volume. Because essentially all hemoglobin is present within erythrocytes, the erythrocyte count or red blood cell (RBC) count, HCT, and

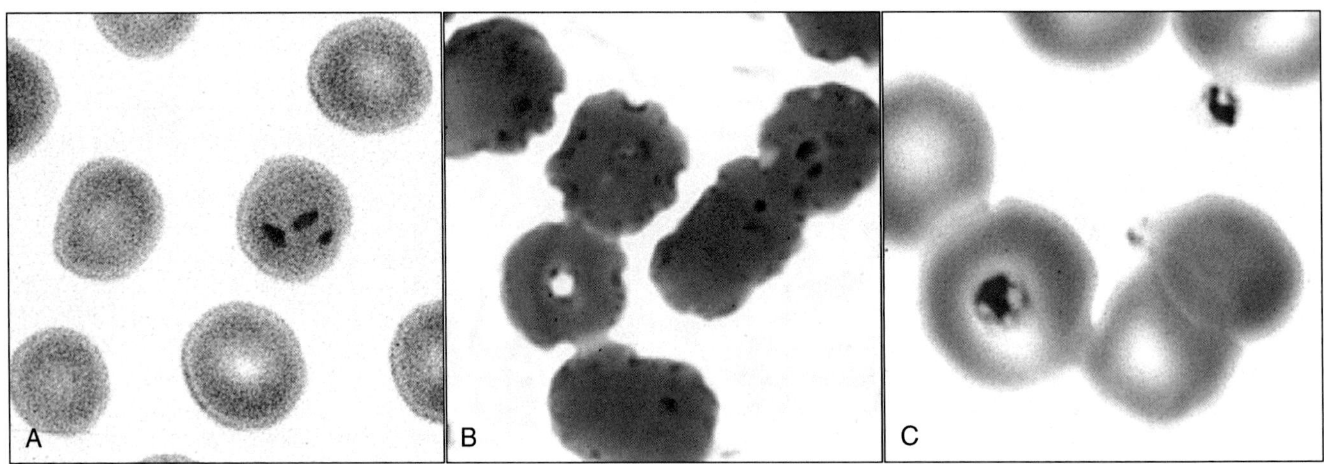

FIGURE 4-97

Bartonella organisms and artifacts that might be confused with erythrocyte parasites. **A,** *Bartonella henselae* organisms in an erythrocyte *(center right)* from a confirmed bacteremic cat. In addition to blood culture, organisms were identified in fixed erythrocytes using a fluorescent-labeled antibody. Wright-Giemsa stain. **B,** Drying artifact and precipitated stain present in this blood film from a cat may be confused with blood parasites. Wright-Giemsa stain. **C,** A platelet overlying an erythrocyte *(bottom left)* may be confused with a blood parasite in this blood film from a dog. Wright-Giemsa stain.

A, Courtesy of R. E. Raskin.

hemoglobin content parallel each other when a change occurs. The *term packed cell volume* (PCV) is often used when the HCT is measured by centrifugation of blood in a microhematocrit centrifuge. The PCV is the easiest and most reproducible test available for quantifying erythrocytes in clinical practice. The RBC count and hemoglobin content need to be measured only when erythrocyte indices are to be calculated.

The RBC count and mean cell volume (MCV) are accurate if they are measured using an electronic cell counter that has been designed or adjusted to measure the variably sized erythrocytes of animals. Hemoglobin concentration is measured spectrophotometrically. Modern electronic cell counters calculate the HCT using the measured RBC count and MCV. This efficiency negates the need to centrifuge a microhematocrit tube of blood. Unfortunately, useful information concerning the appearance of plasma is missed when the HCT is determined electronically unless a serum sample is also prepared for clinical chemistry tests.

Cats, dogs, hot-blooded horses, and some marine diving mammals (e.g., seals) have large (as much as one-third of the total blood volume in horses) contractile spleens.[449] This provides a blood reservoir that can be released into the general circulation in response to sympathetic stimulation induced by exercise, hypoxia, hemorrhage, or excitement. The capacity of the spleen to expand and contract results in substantial changes in the peripheral blood HCT in these species because the HCT in the spleen (about 80%-90%) is much higher than that in peripheral blood.[110,449] Maximal splenic contraction increases the HCT 1.3- to 1.5-fold above resting levels in these species.[66,110,309] The HCT is slightly higher in spleen-intact versus splenectomized dogs, presumably because basal sympathetic tone keeps the spleen slightly contracted during the awake resting state.[110] A slight postprandial increase in HCT has been reported after feeding dogs and sheep; this persists for several hours, and most of this change in dogs and about half of this change in sheep is attributable to splenic contraction.[123,268] HCT increases associated with splenic contraction in ruminants and pigs are smaller than increases in cats, dogs, and horses.[376,448] Conversely, anesthesia (especially with barbiturates) can produce splenic enlargement, causing the HCT to drop below reference intervals.[66]

Maximum information can be gained by interpretating the HCT and plasma protein concentrations simultaneously. Various combinations of low, normal, or high HCT values may occur with low, normal, or high plasma protein concentrations. The various combinations and examples of how they can be interpreted are given in Box 4-1.

Reticulocyte Counts

Manual methods used in performing reticulocyte staining and counting are given in Chapter 2. Reticulocytes in cats are classified as aggregate (if coarse clumping is observed) or punctate (if small individual inclusions are present). In healthy cats as well as cats with regenerative anemia, the number of punctate reticulocytes is much greater than that seen in other species.[15] In contrast to those of the cat, most reticulocytes in other species are of the aggregate type; consequently no attempt is made to differentiate stages of reticulocytes except in cats. The higher number of punctate reticulocytes occurs in cats because the maturation (loss of ribosomes) of reticulocytes in cats is slower than that in other species. Aggregate reticulocytes in the circulation mature to punctate

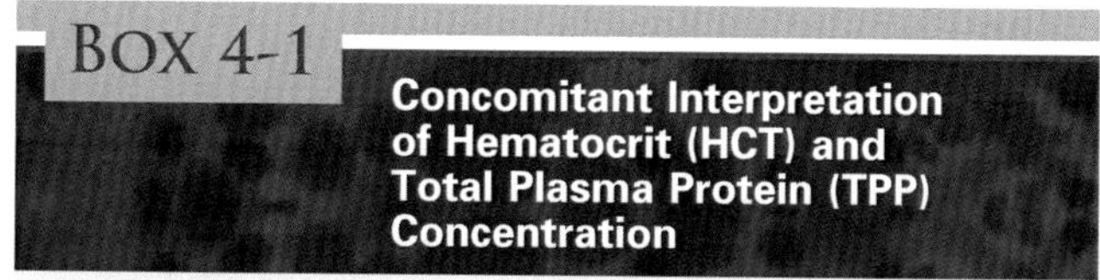

Concomitant Interpretation of Hematocrit (HCT) and Total Plasma Protein (TPP) Concentration

Normal HCT with
- **Low TPP:** Gastrointestinal protein loss, proteinuria, severe liver disease, vasculitis
- **Normal TPP:** Normal
- **High TPP**–Increased globulin synthesis, dehydration-masked anemia

High HCT with
- **Low TPP:** A combination of splenic contraction and a source of protein loss
- **Normal TPP:** Splenic contraction, primary or secondary erythrocytosis, dehydration-masked hypoproteinemia
- **High TPP:** Dehydration

Low HCT with
- **Low TPP:** Substantial ongoing or recent blood loss, overhydration
- **Normal TPP:** Increased erythrocyte destruction, decreased erythrocyte production, chronic blood loss
- **High TPP:** Anemia of inflammatory disease, multiple myeloma, lymphoproliferative diseases, hepatocellular carcinoma (one report in a dog)[97]

reticulocytes in a day or less, but a week or more is required for maturation (total disappearance of ribosomes) of punctate reticulocytes in cat blood.[133] Percentages of both types should be reported separately in cats. Manual reticulocyte counts were done in blood from 41 healthy cats. Aggregate reticulocyte counts were between 0% and 0.9% and punctate reticulocyte counts were between 0% and 7.4%.

Raw (uncorrected) manual reticulocyte counts can be misleading when moderate to severe anemia is present because reticulocytes are quantified as a percentage of the total number of erythrocytes (reticulocytes plus mature erythrocytes) counted. The raw reticulocyte count (percent) would be higher in an anemic animal (with a lower number of mature erythrocytes) than it would be in a normal animal (with a higher number of mature erythrocytes), even if the actual number of reticulocytes per microliter in the circulation was the same in each animal. Consequently reticulocyte counts should either be corrected for the degree of anemia using the HCT or an absolute reticulocyte count should be calculated using the total RBC count. The reticulocyte count is corrected by dividing the patient's HCT by the mean normal HCT for the species and then multiplying this value by the raw reticulocyte count to obtain a corrected reticulocyte count.

Corrected reticulocyte count
= (patient's HCT/mean normal HCT for species)
× raw reticulocyte count in percent

For example, if the raw reticulocyte count was determined to be 6% in a dog with an HCT of 9%, the corrected reticulocyte count would be 9 divided by 45 (mean normal HCT for dogs) times 6% = 1.2%. The corrected reticulocyte count is used to determine whether reticulocytes are truly increased in blood. Although the raw reticulocyte count (6%) suggests that the reticulocyte numbers were increased substantially in blood, the corrected reticulocyte count demonstrates that little increase in reticulocyte numbers was present in blood. Normal dogs generally have no more than about 1% reticulocytes when this value is determined by manual methods.

If the total RBC count is known, an absolute reticulocyte count (reticulocytes per microliter) can be determined. This is done by multiplying the percentage of reticulocytes counted (expressed as a fraction) by the total RBC count.

Absolute reticulocyte count (per microliter)
= RBC count (per microliter)
× raw reticulocyte count (fraction)

It should be noted that the calculations of absolute reticulocyte counts and corrected reticulocyte counts are independent calculations, with each one using the original raw reticulocyte count.

Absolute reticulocyte counts in normal dog are generally less than $80 \times 10^3/\mu L$ when manual counts are done. Determined manually, absolute aggregate reticulocyte counts in 41 normal cats were between 0 and $95 \times 10^3/\mu L$ and absolute punctate reticulocyte counts were between 0 and $650 \times 10^3/\mu L$.

Absolute reticulocyte counts can also be determined directly by flow cytometry with some automated hematology analyzers. These instruments provide more rapid results with better precision than the manual method. Their use is also much less labor-intensive. However, it is essential that these automated counts be validated by comparing automated counts against manual counts for accuracy. Automated reference intervals can vary considerably depending on the instrument used. In cats, it is especially important to determine whether some punctate reticulocytes are counted by the machine, along with the aggregate reticulocytes, before the reticulocyte counts can be interpreted appropriately. The Advia 120 (Siemens Healthcare Diagnostics, Inc., Tarrytown, NY) hematology analyzer appears to count primarily aggregate reticulocytes in cats; reticulocyte counts from the same 41 normal cats listed above were between $8 \times 10^3/\mu L$ and $57 \times 10^3/\mu L$, when measured by the Advia 120. This was similar to the absolute reticulocyte counts in 58 normal dogs, which were between $8 \times 10^3/\mu L$ and $65 \times 10^3/\mu L$ when measured using the Advia 120.

The corrected reticulocyte response to blood loss anemia in the cat is shown in Figure 4-98.[15] As in other species, about 4 days are required to obtain a maximal aggregate reticulocyte response to anemia because of the time needed for the production of aggregate reticulocytes from progenitor cells. The maximal punctate response occurs considerably later, primarily because of the long time required for punctate reticulocytes to mature to erythrocytes. As can be seen in Figure 4-98,

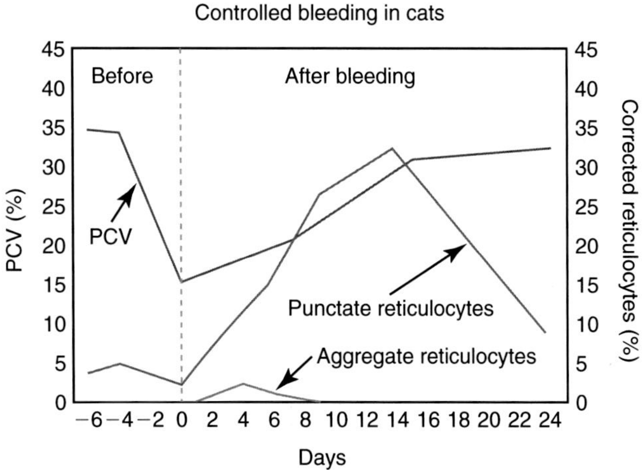

FIGURE 4-98
Reticulocyte response following controlled bleeding in cats. Reticulocyte counts have been corrected using packed cell volume (PCV) values.

Data from Alsaker RD, Laber J, Stevens JB, et al. A comparison of polychromasia and reticulocyte counts in assessing erythrocyte regenerative response in the cat. J Am Vet Med Assoc. *1977;170:39.*

punctate reticulocyte continue to be released from bone marrow after the HCT begins to increase and aggregate reticulocyte release has ceased. Consequently cats with mild regenerative anemia may have increased punctate reticulocyte counts and normal aggregate reticulocyte counts (see Fig. 4-23, *A*).

Lower HCTs typically result in higher plasma erythropoietin concentrations,[351] which lead to higher absolute blood reticulocyte counts (except in horses) if the marrow is able to respond appropriately. High erythropoietin concentrations also lead to the early release of reticulocytes from the bone marrow into the blood.[7] Instead of continuing to mature in the bone marrow, these more immature reticulocytes mature in the circulation. This reticulocyte maturation time or residence time increases from about 0.5 day to 1 day in sheep following a phlebotomy removing more than half of the circulating erythrocyte mass.[146] Absolute reticulocyte counts are generally higher in response to hemolytic anemia than they are in response to hemorrhage, presumably because plasma iron concentration is high in animals with hemolytic anemia and normal or low in animals following hemorrhage. Consequently the presence of a marked reticulocytosis indicates the likelihood that increased erythrocyte destruction is the cause of the anemia. When the degree of anemia is severe, basophilic macroreticulocytes or so-called stress reticulocytes may be released into the blood (see Fig. 4-21). It is proposed that one less mitotic division occurs during production and that large immature reticulocytes are released. Although a portion of these macroreticulocytes may be rapidly removed from the circulation, it appears from studies in cats that some can mature into large (macrocytic) erythrocytes with relatively normal life spans.[506]

Erythrocyte Indices

Determination of erythrocyte indices can assist in the differential diagnosis of anemia. Of the erythrocyte parameters routinely determined or calculated, the MCV is the most useful.

Mean Cell Volume

The MCV represents the average volume of a single erythrocyte in femtoliters (10^{-15} L) in a population of erythrocytes (typically whole blood). Erythrocytes lose volume and hemoglobin through vesiculation as they age. The MCV measured in an aged human erythrocyte population was decreased by 30%, while the mean cell hemoglobin concentration (MCHC) was increased by 15%.[535] The MCV is determined most accurately by direct measurement with electronic cell counters. It can be determined indirectly by dividing the HCT (as a percentage) by the RBC count (in millions of cells per microliter) and multiplying by 10, but this calculated value is less accurate because two separate measurements are required. The MCV varies greatly depending on species. Mammals have smaller erythrocytes than birds, reptiles, or amphibians.[215] Erythrocytes (and other blood cell types) are especially large in amphibians with MCVs in excess of 10,000 fL in the *Amphiuma* salamander (see Fig. 4-8).[175] Species with larger erythrocytes have lower RBC counts, resulting in similar HCTs and hemoglobin concentrations in mammals and birds.[215] MCVs can vary with age, with higher MCVs reported in older horses and cattle.[84,238] Slight increases in MCVs are reported with exercise in horses.[302,329]

When identified, high MCV values (macrocytosis) are usually associated with regenerative anemias because the volumes of individual reticulocytes (especially stress reticulocytes) are larger than the volumes of mature erythrocytes. However, it is important to remember that many macrocytic cells must be present to increase the MCV above the normal reference interval; consequently the MCV is usually within reference intervals in animals with regenerative anemia.[119] Some dogs with nonregenerative immune-mediated anemia and/or myelofibrosis also have a macrocytosis.[454] High MCVs may occur in animals with myeloid neoplasms and nonregenerative anemia.[125,257,527] Macrocytosis is often seen in feline leukemia virus (FeLV)-positive cats with nonregenerative anemias.[507] Folate deficiency has been reported as a cause of macrocytic nonregenerative anemia in a cat.[332] Macrocytosis (without anemia or reticulocytosis) occurs in some apparently healthy miniature and toy poodle dogs that have variable megaloblastic abnormalities in the bone marrow and normal serum folate and cobalamin values.[80] Dogs with hereditary stomatocytosis may have high MCVs, with normal or only slightly increased reticulocyte counts.[59,231] Some cats with hyperthyroidism have slightly increased MCVs with normal or increased HCTs.[365] Macrocytic anemia has been reported in Hereford calves with congenital dyserythropoiesis. In these calves, many nucleated erythrocytes are present in blood but reticulocyte counts are only slightly increased.[447]

High MCVs may occur as an artifact secondary to agglutination of erythrocytes, as can occur in immune-mediated disorders or following heparin administration to horses.[322,374,489,550] MCVs may also be spuriously increased in cats and dogs with persistent hypernatremia because the cells can swell in vitro when diluted with counting fluid prior to sizing in an electronic cell counter.[58] Finally, MCVs increase with prolonged storage of blood samples; however, the increase may not be sufficient to elevate the value beyond the reference interval.[156,311]

Macrocytosis is more likely to occur in response to hemolytic anemia than to hemorrhage, at least in part because serum iron concentration is increased in animals with hemolytic anemia. While iron does not stimulate erythropoiesis, decreased iron availability may limit the erythropoietic response following hemorrhage. Reticulocytes, especially those produced in response to severe anemia (stress reticulocytes), are larger than mature erythrocytes. A week or more is required before macrocytosis occurs in response to hemolytic anemia. Although the bone marrow normally contains some reticulocytes undergoing maturation, most reticulocytes released from the bone marrow in response to anemia must be formed de novo. A minimum of 4 days is required for a peak reticulocyte response to occur,[15,136,364] and then the newly produced, larger cells must comprise a high enough percentage of the total erythrocytes present to increase the MCV above the reference interval. Although there is a reduction in size as reticulocytes mature into erythrocytes, larger-than-normal reticulocytes produce larger-than-normal erythrocytes.[506]

The erythrocytes produced in the fetus are larger than those produced in the adult.[10,62,334] There is a gradual decrease in MCV during fetal development. The MCV is within adult reference intervals in horses and cattle at birth.[207,238] The MCV is above adult reference intervals in dogs and cats at birth, and it declines as the larger erythrocytes formed in the fetus are replaced by smaller erythrocytes produced after birth.[126,508]

Microcytic (low-MCV) anemias usually indicate the presence of chronic iron deficiency.[204] Microcytic iron-deficiency anemia in adult animals is almost always due to chronic hemorrhage. Depending on the initial MCV and the magnitude of ongoing blood loss, one or more months are required before the MCV decreases below the reference interval. Body iron stores must be depleted and then the microcytes formed must comprise a high enough percentage of the total erythrocytes present to decrease the MCV below the reference interval. Microcytic anemia rarely occurs as a result of dietary iron deficiency in adult animals. However, iron deficiency without blood loss is common in nursing animals, because milk is low in iron and these rapidly growing animals have an increased demand for iron.[204] Although microcytes are often formed in nursing animals, the MCV may not be reduced in iron-deficient neonatal dogs and cats because of the persistence of macrocytes formed before birth.[508] Even if body iron stores have not been depleted, erythrocytes may become microcytic in dogs given long-term recombinant canine erythropoietin (rcEPO) therapy.[387] Microcytosis apparently occurs because iron delivery to the developing erythroid cells is not sufficient to fully support the accelerated erythropoiesis accompanying rcEPO administration.

Copper is needed for optimal iron absorption and release from body iron stores. Consequently prolonged copper deficiency results in microcytic anemia in some species. Pyridoxine is required for the first step in heme synthesis. Although natural cases of pyridoxine deficiency have not been documented in domestic animals, microcytic anemias with high serum iron values have been produced experimentally in dogs, cats, and pigs with dietary pyridoxine deficiency.[205]

The MCV may be slightly decreased in association with the anemia of inflammatory disease, but the MCV is at the low end of the reference interval in most cases. Microcytosis is common in dogs with portosystemic shunts.[243] In these cases, the MCV is seldom more than 7 fL below the reference interval and the HCT is within the reference interval or only slightly decreased.[201] This modest decrease in MCV may be masked if blood is stored for 24 hours before being assayed.[178] Some cats with portosystemic shunts and hepatic lipidosis exhibit slight microcytosis.[85,280] Drugs or chemicals that interfere with heme synthesis, such as chloramphenicol, lead, and probably hydroxyzine (dogs) have the potential for causing the formation of microcytic erythrocytes with siderotic inclusions.[205] Microcytic anemia may also occur in myeloid neoplasms exhibiting iron accumulation in erythroid cells.[524] Persistent siderotic inclusions have been recognized in microcytic hypochromic erythrocytes from an English bulldog (see Fig. 4-83, *A,B*). These erythrocytes also contained Heinz bodies and rare hemoglobin crystals.[209] A congenital defect resulting in mitochondrial iron overload and secondary oxidant injury was suspected but not identified. A nonregenerative microcytic anemia with many circulating nucleated erythrocytes has been reported in related English springer spaniels with dyserythropoiesis, polymyopathy, and heart disease.[223] Microcytosis has been described in a crossbred dog with persistent elliptocytosis resulting from a lack of erythrocyte membrane protein band 4.1. Although the animal was not anemic, the reticulocyte count was about twice normal in response to a shortened erythrocyte life span.[205] Some Japanese breeds (Akita and Shiba) normally have MCV values below the reference intervals established for other breeds of dogs, but they are not anemic.[115,179]

Spurious microcytosis may occur when platelets are included with erythrocytes in MCV calculations in severely anemic animals or animals with marked thrombocytosis.[550] MCVs may also be spuriously decreased in dogs with persistent hyponatremia because the erythrocytes shrink when they are diluted in vitro with counting fluid prior to sizing in an electronic cell counter.[58]

Mean Cell Hemoglobin Concentration

The MCHC represents the average hemoglobin concentration within erythrocytes. It is calculated by dividing the whole blood hemoglobin value (in grams per deciliter) by the

HCT (as a percentage) and multiplying by 100. The MCHC is expressed as grams per deciliter of erythrocytes. (Note: Hemoglobin values in blood are expressed as grams per deciliter of whole blood.) Electronic cell counters calculate the MCHC using three measured parameters (RBC count, MCV, and hemoglobin concentration); consequently the MCHC can provide a form of quality control for these measured parameters.

High MCHC values are artifacts. They may result from in vivo or in vitro hemolysis, lipemia, the presence of Heinz bodies within erythrocytes, cryoproteins that precipitate when the sample is cooled, or paraprotein precipitation in the analyzer diluent.[100,297,550] In the case of hemolysis, some hemoglobin is free in plasma; but the formula used to calculate the MCHC assumes that all measured hemoglobin is contained within erythrocytes. Lipemia, protein precipitation, and Heinz bodies cause turbidity in the spectrophotometric assay for hemoglobin, thereby giving erroneously elevated hemoglobin values. A high MCHC may also occur if there is agglutination of erythrocytes when the specimen is assayed in an electronic cell counter, as can happen with cold-acting autoantibodies or following heparin therapy in some horses.[322,489,550] Large erythrocyte aggregates are too large to be considered erythrocytes; consequently cell counters are programmed to exclude them from erythrocyte measurements. This results in erroneously low HCT values and consequently erroneously high MCHC values. Agglutination should not interfere with HCT values determined by centrifugation as long as the blood samples are well mixed before the microhematocrit tubes are filled. In addition to the standard MCHC calculation, the Advia 120 (Siemens Healthcare Diagnostics, Inc., Tarrytown, NY) determines the hemoglobin concentration within individual erythrocytes based on deflection of light that occurs when a laser beam strikes individual cells. The mean of hemoglobin concentrations within erythrocytes determined in this manner is calculated and referred to as the cell hemoglobin concentration mean (CHCM). The CHCM provides an accurate measure of mean hemoglobin concentration within erythrocytes even when hemoglobinemia and lipemia are present.[297] For example, a kitten with marked lipemia and a microcytic anemia (HCT 12%, MCV 33 fL) had a calculated MCHC of 122 g/dL but a CHCM of 26 g/dL.

MCHC values may be decreased in animals with regenerative anemia, especially those with high percentages of stress reticulocytes. Hemoglobin synthesis is not complete until late in reticulocyte maturation. Consequently hemoglobin synthesis is less complete in stress reticulocytes because these cells are released from the bone marrow earlier than would occur normally.[205]

Low MCHC values may also occur in animals with chronic iron-deficiency anemia. When it is determined using an electronic cell counter, the MCHC may be normal in animals with slight microcytosis, but it is usually low when the MCV is markedly reduced.[201] The MCHC is low in iron deficiency because there is inadequate iron to support the synthesis of normal amounts of hemoglobin. Low MCHC values occur in dogs with hereditary stomatocytosis because the increased intracellular water, which occurs in this condition, dilutes the hemoglobin concentration within the cells.[59,231] MCHCs may be spuriously decreased in cats and dogs with persistent hypernatremia because the cells can swell when they are diluted with counting fluid prior to analysis in an electronic cell counter.[58]

Mean Cell Hemoglobin

The mean cell hemoglobin (MCH) is calculated by dividing the hemoglobin value (in grams per deciliter) by the RBC count (in millions of cells per microliter) and multiplying by 10. The MCH provides no added value because it depends on the MCV and MCHC. It usually correlates directly with the MCV except in animals with macrocytic hypochromic erythrocytes.

Red Cell Distribution Width

The red cell distribution width (RDW) is an electronic measure of anisocytosis or erythrocyte volume heterogeneity. A histogram of the volume of individual erythrocytes reveals a plot approximating a Gaussian distribution. Consequently one can calculate the degree of size variation by determining the standard deviation (SD) of erythrocyte volumes. However, the SD depends on the size of the cells as well as the degree of size variation around the MCV. To provide a measure of size variation that does not depend on how large the cells are, the coefficient of variation of erythrocyte volume is calculated by dividing the SD by the MCV and then multiplying by 100. In short, the RDW is the SD of erythrocyte volumes expressed as a percentage of the mean erythrocyte volume.

Reference values vary depending on the instrument used to measure the RDW. Cattle and horses normally have somewhat higher RDW values than cats and dogs.[505] One need only refer to the upper limit of a reference interval in examining data from a patient, because there is no pathologic state in which erythrocytes have greater volume homogeneity (lower RDW) than in the normal state.

Examination of the RDW has not been extensively utilized in veterinary medicine. It is expected to be increased in cases where the degree of anisocytosis (as estimated on the stained blood film) is increased. It is often increased in regenerative anemias because reticulocytes and young erythrocytes are larger than mature erythrocytes.[127,338,382] Like the MCV, the number of large erythrocytes in blood must reach a certain level before the RDW of a given patient exceeds the reference interval. As an animal responds to anemia and young erythrocytes become the predominant population, the RDW will begin to decline and may return to the reference interval even though the MCV is still high.

The RDW is also expected to increase in iron-deficiency anemia, where smaller than normal erythrocytes are produced. As in regenerative anemia, the increase is most likely to be seen during the phase of disease when a significant number of normally and abnormally sized erythrocytes are present simultaneously.[201] In severe chronic iron-deficiency anemia, the RDW might decrease toward normal once the whole population of erythrocytes is small. The RDW may increase again following iron therapy, as normally sized erythrocytes are produced.

Other potential causes of increased RDW include conditions in which substantial fragmentation of erythrocytes is occurring and following transfusion of blood from a donor animal in which the MCV is substantially different from that of the recipient. The RDW is also increased in dogs with hereditary stomatocytosis.[59] Animals with nonregenerative anemias will have normal RDW values unless significant dyserythropoiesis is present. Spuriously increased RDW values may occur when agglutination is present or platelets are included with erythrocytes in calculations of cell volume distribution in severely anemic animals.[183]

Erythrocyte Volume Histograms and Erythrocyte Cytograms

Although quite useful when abnormal, MCV and MCHC values are relatively insensitive in identifying the presence of erythrocytes with abnormal volumes or hemoglobin concentrations. Many microcytic or macrocytic erythrocytes are required to move the MCV below or above the reference interval, and many hypochromic erythrocytes are needed to move the MCHC below the reference interval. In addition to counting cells, electronic cell counters can determine and plot the volume of individual erythrocytes, and examination of these erythrocyte volume histograms can reveal the presence of increased numbers of microcytes or macrocytes even when the MCV is within the reference interval (Fig. 4-99, *A*). Some electronic cell counters, such as the Advia 120, can also determine the hemoglobin concentration of individual erythrocytes from the deflection of light that occurs when a laser beam strikes individual cells. This allows for the generation of hemoglobin concentration histograms (Fig. 4-99, *B*). Inspection of hemoglobin concentration histograms can reveal the presence of increased numbers of hypochromic erythrocytes even when MCHC has not decreased below the reference interval. Individual erythrocytes can be further characterized by creating a cytogram in which the erythrocyte volumes of individual cells are plotted against their respective hemoglobin concentrations (Fig. 4-100).

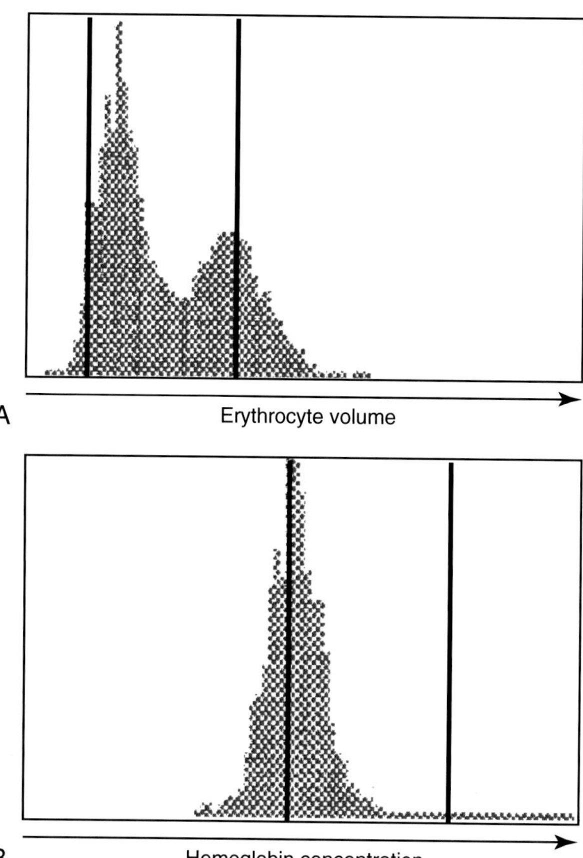

FIGURE 4-99

Erythrocyte histograms from a 6-week-old kitten after a blood transfusion. The kitten presented with marked lipemia and a severe iron deficiency anemia. The animal was obtained from a shelter and was no longer nursing. An image from the stained blood film prepared from this cat is shown in Figure 4-24. Most erythrocytes from normal animals are expected to be between the vertical lines. **A,** Erythrocyte volume histogram demonstrates a population of small erythrocytes from the patient and a population of large erythrocytes from the blood donor. The MCV was 47 fL and the RDW was 43%. **B,** Erythrocyte hemoglobin concentration histogram revealed hypochromic cells but did not demonstrate two distinct cell populations. Histograms were generated using an Advia 120 hematology analyzer.

Direct Antiglobulin Test

A direct antiglobulin (Coombs') test is done when autoagglutination is absent but immune-mediated hemolytic anemia is still suspected. Species-specific antisera against IgG, IgM, and the third component of complement (C_3) are used to detect the presence of one or more of these factors on the surface of erythrocytes.[502] This test is discussed in greater detail in Chapter 6.

Methemoglobin Determination

Methemoglobin differs from hemoglobin only in that the iron moiety of heme groups has been oxidized to the ferric (+3) state. The term *methemoglobinemia* refers to methemoglobin content in blood above 1.5% of total hemoglobin. Clinical signs associated with methemoglobinemia are the result of tissue hypoxia, because methemoglobin cannot bind O_2. Both low blood O_2 tension and methemoglobinemia can result in cyanotic-appearing mucous membranes and dark-colored blood samples. Hypoxemia is documented by measuring a low Po_2 in arterial blood (Pao_2). Methemoglobinemia is suspected when arterial blood with normal or increased Pao_2 is dark-colored. Methemoglobin is quantified spectrophotometrically, but a spot test can be used to determine whether clinically significant levels of methemoglobin are present (see Fig. 2-4).

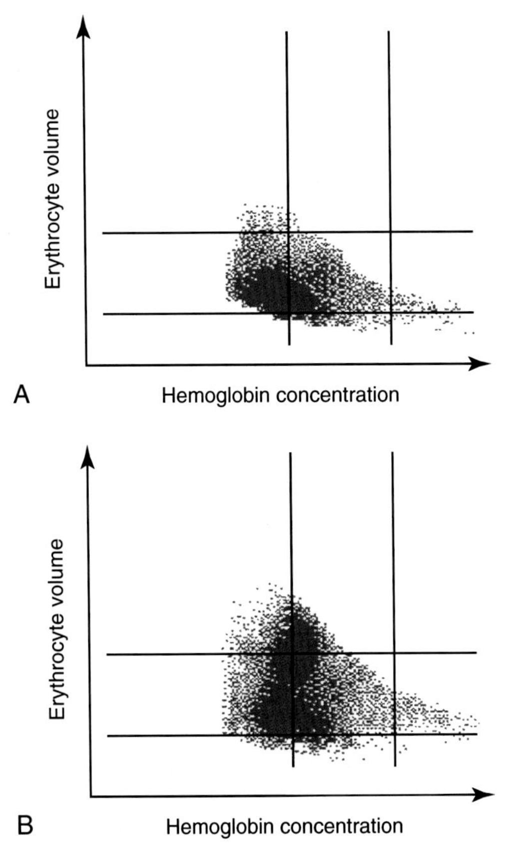

FIGURE 4-100

Erythrocyte volume versus hemoglobin concentration (V/HC) cytograms. Most erythrocytes from normal animals are expected to be within the square formed by the double vertical and horizontal lines. **A,** Erythrocyte V/HC cytogram from a 6-week-old kitten with marked lipemia and a severe iron-deficiency anemia that was a littermate of the cat presented in Figures 4-24 and 4-99. A population of microcytic hypochromic cells is clearly visible. The HCT was 12%, MCV was 33 fL, RDW was 30%, MCHC was 122 g/dL, and CHCM was 26 g/dL. The MCHC was spuriously increased because of the lipemia. **B,** Erythrocyte V/HC cytogram from a 6-week-old kitten with lipemia and severe iron deficiency that is also presented in Figures 4-24 and 4-99. The kitten was given a whole-blood transfusion prior to sample analysis. The HCT was 23%, MCV was 47 fL, RDW was 43%, MCHC was 40 g/dL, and CHCM was 27 g/dL. Two populations of erythrocytes are visible. The kitten's cells are concentrated in the bottom left area of the cytogram. Erythrocyte V/HC cytograms were generated using an Advia 120 hematology analyzer.

Toxic Methemoglobinemia

Methemoglobinemia results from either increased production of methemoglobin by oxidants or decreased reduction of methemoglobin associated with a deficiency in the erythrocyte Cb_5R (also called methemoglobin reductase) enzyme.[203] Experimental studies indicate that many drugs can produce methemoglobinemia in animals. Significant methemoglobinemia has been associated with clinical cases of benzocaine toxicity in several species, acetaminophen and phenazopyridine toxicities in cats, skunk musk in dogs, chlorate toxicity in cattle, copper toxicity in sheep and goats, and red maple toxicity in horses.[53,205] These oxidants can also produce Heinz body hemolytic anemia. Methemoglobinemia without Heinz bodies or eccentrocytes has been reported in a dog with hydroxycarbamide (hydroxyurea) toxicity.[542] Nitrite produces methemoglobinemia without Heinz body formation or development of anemia. Methemoglobinemia occurs in ruminants eating nitrate-accumulating plants, especially when those plants have been fertilized with nitrogenous compounds. Nitrate is relatively nontoxic, but it is reduced to nitrite by ruminal microorganisms.[205] Nitrite toxicity has been reported in dogs and cats fed a commercial pet food that had sodium nitrite added as a preservative.[541]

Cytochrome-b_5 Reductase Deficiency

Persistent methemoglobinemia resulting from erythrocyte Cb_5R deficiency has been recognized in many breeds of dogs and in domestic shorthaired cats.[203] Methemoglobin content is generally higher in cats (44% to 52%) than in dogs (13% to 51%) with this deficiency because of lower enzyme activity in deficient cats compared with deficient dogs. Flavin adenine dinucleotide (FAD) is a cofactor for the Cb_5R enzyme, and persistent methemoglobinemia (26% to 48%) has also been recognized in horses with Cb_5R deficiency secondary to erythrocyte FAD deficiency.[203] Animals with Cb_5R deficiency, in contrast to those with methemoglobinemia produced by oxidant drugs and compounds, usually exhibit few or no clinical signs of illness. The diagnosis of this deficiency is made by measuring enzyme activity within erythrocytes.

SERUM IRON ASSAYS

Serum Iron

Serum iron concentration is generally increased in animals with hemolytic anemia, dyserythropoiesis, hypoplastic or aplastic anemia, iron overload, acute iron toxicity, chronic hepatopathy (dogs), experimental pyridoxine deficiency (pigs), and following the administration of glucocorticoid steroids to dogs and horses.[192,205] Serum iron values may be spuriously increased if laboratory tubes or pipettes that are used to handle blood or serum are contaminated with iron.

Serum iron concentration is generally low in iron deficiency and with inflammation.[108,204,236] It is also low in about half of the dogs with portosystemic shunts.[204] Serum iron may be decreased when demands for erythropoiesis exceed the iron flow from the diet and storage pools, such as might occur with erythropoietin administration or following acute hemorrhage.[204,356] Serum iron concentration is decreased following glucocorticoid administration to cattle and goats.[204]

True iron deficiency may be differentiated from other causes of hypoferremia by examination of bone marrow for stainable iron, which is minimal or absent in iron deficiency and normal or high in other disorders (see Chapter 8). However, stainable iron is not present in the bone marrow of normal cats; consequently a lack of stainable iron does not suggest iron deficiency in this species.[204]

Total Iron-Binding Capacity

The total iron-binding capacity (TIBC) of serum is a measure of serum transferrin concentration because insignificant amounts of circulating iron are bound to other proteins. TIBC is calculated by measuring serum iron and serum unsaturated iron-binding capacity and summing these values. Serum TIBC is low normal or decreased in association with inflammatory disorders and increased in iron-deficient humans, rabbits, pigs, horses, and cattle.[204] A slight increase in serum TIBC was reported in an experimental study of diet-induced iron-deficiency anemia in young growing dogs,[151] but serum TIBC is generally normal in dogs with naturally occurring iron-deficiency anemia.[204] About half of the dogs with portosystemic shunts exhibited hypoferremia with normal or slightly decreased serum TIBC.[204] TIBC may be increased in some animals with iron overload and in dogs with chronic hepatopathy.[204,441]

Serum Ferritin

Ferritin is secreted by cells into the blood rather than leaking from the cytoplasm of damaged cells. Serum ferritin typically has a much lower iron content than does intracellular ferritin. The macrophage appears to be the primary cell involved in secreting ferritin into the blood, at least under steady-state conditions, but other cells, including kidney proximal tubular cells and hepatocytes, may also secrete ferritin into the blood.[93,486]

Serum ferritin concentration correlates with tissue iron stores in domestic animals, including cats. Consequently serum ferritin concentration can help differentiate true iron deficiency (serum ferritin is low) from the anemia of inflammatory disease (serum ferritin is normal or high).[204] Increased serum ferritin occurs in animals with increased storage iron, as may occur with hemolytic anemia, hemophagocytic histiocytic sarcoma (in dogs), and repeated blood transfusions. An increase has also been reported in dogs with inflammation, liver disease, and lymphoma.[148] It is transiently increased in horses after moderate to severe exercise and in foals following consumption of colostrum. Serum ferritin is an acute-phase protein; consequently increased values are expected in inflammatory conditions in addition to conditions with increased iron stores.[204] It should be remembered that true iron deficiency can be missed if concomitant inflammation is present, resulting in increased ferritin secretion into blood. Commercial assay kits are not available for serum ferritin assays in animals, but ferritin assays may be performed for several species at the Kansas State University College of Veterinary Medicine.

ERYTHROPOIETIN ASSAY

Erythropoietin (EPO) is a glycoprotein hormone that stimulates erythropoiesis in a number of ways. Radioimmunoassays or enzyme-linked immunosorbent assays (ELISAs) may be used to measure EPO, but commercial tests developed for human assays may not always cross-react sufficiently for use in other species. Consequently individual tests require validation for each species to be assayed before they can be used clinically. Serum EPO is increased in response to various anemias except the anemia of chronic renal disease, in which EPO production is decreased.[96,350,361] Serum EPO concentration appears to be regulated not only by the rate of renal production but also by the rate of utilization by erythroid cells. At any given blood hemoglobin concentration, the serum EPO concentration is likely to be highest in disorders with low marrow erythroid activity (e.g., erythroid aplasia).[83] The EPO assay has received limited use in veterinary medicine. EPO has been assayed in serum to assist in differentiating primary erythrocytosis (where EPO values should be normal or low) from secondary erythrocytosis (where EPO values should be high).[182,214,248,408] Unfortunately there is considerable overlap among patients with primary and secondary erythrocytosis, thus limiting the diagnostic value of the EPO assay.[96]

DIFFERENTIAL DIAGNOSIS OF ANEMIA

True or absolute anemia is defined as a decrease in erythrocyte mass within the body. HCT, hemoglobin, and RBC count values are usually below their reference intervals; however, the anemia can sometimes be masked by concomitant dehydration. Low erythrocyte parameters may also be present in blood when the total-body erythrocyte mass is normal (relative anemia). This can result from overhydration resulting in erythrocyte dilution and from splenic sequestration of erythrocytes as occurs with splenic relaxation during anesthesia, heparin-induced erythrocyte agglutination in horses, and various causes of splenomegaly.[66,319]

Anemia is a condition, not a diagnosis. Anemia is classified in various ways to assist in determining its specific cause so that effective therapy can be given. In addition to past history, presenting complaints, and laboratory findings, results of other test procedures (e.g., diagnostic imaging) are important in reaching a final diagnosis.

Anemia may occur following blood loss, increased erythrocyte destruction, or decreased erythrocyte production. Factors that can be useful in categorizing anemia into these broad causes (and often into more specific causes) include reticulocyte counts, erythrocyte indices, erythrocyte morphology on stained blood films, the appearance of the plasma, plasma protein concentration, serum iron measurements, serum bilirubin determination, direct antiglobulin test, and bone marrow evaluation.

Anemia may also develop as a result of the expansion of the vascular space faster than the expansion of the total-body erythrocyte mass. This hemodilution contributes to the anemia of the neonate (to be discussed later) and to the mild anemia that develops during pregnancy in most domestic animals, the horse being an exception.[8,41,208,531]

REGENERATIVE VERSUS NONREGENERATIVE ANEMIA

The most useful approach in the classification of anemia is to determine whether evidence of a bone marrow response to the anemia is present in blood. For all common domestic animals except the horse, this involves determining whether absolute reticulocyte numbers are increased in blood. Horses rarely release reticulocytes from the bone marrow even when an increased production of erythrocytes occurs. MCV and/or RDW values are increased in some horses responding to anemia, but others recover from anemia without having these parameters exceed reference intervals.[127,382] Consequently bone marrow evaluation is often needed to determine whether an appropriate response to anemia is present in a horse. Myeloid to erythroid (M:E) ratios below 0.5 and bone marrow reticulocyte counts above 5% suggest a regenerative response to anemia.[238]

Increased polychromasia is usually present in regenerative anemias because many reticulocytes stain bluish red with routine blood stains (see Figs. 4-18, 4-19, 4-21, 4-22). Cats with mild anemias may not release aggregate reticulocytes from the marrow but will release punctate reticulocytes. Because punctate reticulocytes do not contain sufficient numbers of ribosomes within them to impart a bluish color to the cytoplasm, mild regenerative anemias in cats may lack polychromasia in stained blood films (see Fig. 4-23, *A,B*). Increased anisocytosis is often present in regenerative anemias because of the presence of large immature erythrocytes (see Figs. 4-18, 4-19, 4-21), although anisocytosis may be marked in some nonregenerative anemias as well.

Except in horses, some nucleated erythrocytes (rubricytes and metarubricytes) are often seen on blood films in association with regenerative anemia; however, nucleated erythrocytes may also be present in anemic and nonanemic disorders with minimal or no reticulocytosis (see Fig. 4-75, *C-E*). Therefore the presence of nucleated erythrocytes in blood is a much less reliable indicator of a regenerative response to anemia than is an increased reticulocyte count.

Howell-Jolly bodies are often present within erythrocytes in regenerative anemias, but they also occur in normal cats (see Fig. 4-76, *A*) and horses and in splenectomized animals of other species. Basophilic stippling occurs in regenerative anemias in ruminants (see Fig. 4-81, *A,B*) but rarely in other species (see Fig. 4-81, *C*). Basophilic stippling can also occur in erythrocytes of any species with lead toxicity whether or not anemia is present (see Fig. 4-81, *D*).

The presence of compensatory reticulocytosis indicates that the anemia has resulted from either blood loss or increased erythrocyte destruction. Several factors should be kept in mind in interpreting the magnitude of a reticulocyte response. In regenerative anemias, animals with lower HCTs should have higher absolute reticulocyte counts. Severe anemia evokes a greater stimulus for increased erythrocyte production than does mild anemia.[351] Also, in response to severe anemia, reticulocytes can be released from the marrow earlier in their development than normally occurs. These large "stress" reticulocytes (see Fig. 4-21) apparently remain in the circulation longer than other reticulocytes before maturation is complete.[146] Factors have been utilized in an attempt to correct for this longer reticulocyte circulation time in humans, and some veterinary authors have empirically applied these same factors to anemic dogs to calculate what has been called the reticulocyte index. This approach has not been validated in dogs.

Hemolytic anemia usually elicits a more dramatic regenerative response than hemorrhagic anemia at least in part due to the greater availability of iron. There are also species differences in the ability to increase erythrocyte production. The HCT increases about 1 percentage point per day following experimental phlebotomy in dogs and cats, with a slightly lower response in cattle and horses.[15,65,364]

Anemias with no or minimal increase in blood reticulocyte counts are classified as nonregenerative and poorly regenerative respectively. The lack of a reticulocyte response in nonequine species generally indicates that the anemia results from insufficient erythrocyte production in the marrow. A minimal reticulocyte response may be present if the anemia develops acutely following hemorrhage or hemolysis because about 4 days are required for a substantial reticulocyte response to occur. Mild anemias may have minimally increased reticulocyte counts.

Classification of Anemia Using Erythrocyte Indices

An anemia can also be classified using the MCV and MCHC values to assist in determining its cause. The terms used to indicate size are *macrocytic* (increased MCV), *normocytic* (normal MCV), and *microcytic* (decreased MCV). The terms used to describe MCHC values are *normochromic* (normal MCHC) and *hypochromic* (decreased MCHC). Anemias are not classified as hyperchromic because high MCHC values are artifacts. A comparison of erythrocyte indices and causes of anemia is given in Box 4-2.

HEMOLYTIC ANEMIAS

Hemolytic anemias occur as a result of increased erythrocyte destruction within the body. Causes of hemolytic anemia in animals are given in Box 4-3. Erythrocytes may be lysed within the circulation (intravascular hemolysis), but more frequently they are lysed following phagocytosis by cells of the mononuclear phagocyte system (extravascular hemolysis).

Hemolytic anemias are generally regenerative if sufficient time has elapsed for a bone marrow response to the anemia. They are initially normocytic normochromic but may be macrocytic hypochromic or macrocytic normochromic if sufficient time has elapsed for the release of a significant number of large reticulocytes from the bone marrow. Macrocytic hypochromic erythrocytes may also occur in hereditary stomatocytosis in dogs as a result of membrane abnormalities and erythrocyte swelling.[205] An example of a hemolytic anemia that is usually nonregenerative and normocytic normochromic

BOX 4-2 Comparison of Classification of Anemias by Erythrocyte Indices and Etiology

Normocytic Normochromic

1. Hemolytic anemia if reticulocyte response is mild or if sufficient time has not elapsed for a prominent reticulocyte response to occur.
2. Hemorrhage if reticulocyte response is mild or if sufficient time has not elapsed for a prominent reticulocyte response to occur.
3. Early iron-deficiency anemia before microcytes predominate
4. Chronic inflammation and neoplasia (sometimes slightly microcytic)
5. Chronic renal disease
6. Endocrine deficiencies
7. Selective erythroid aplasia
8. Aplastic and hypoplastic bone marrows
9. Lead toxicity (may not be anemic)
10. Cobalamin deficiency

Macrocytic Hypochromic

1. Regenerative anemias with marked reticulocytosis
2. Hereditary stomatocytosis in dogs (often slight reticulocytosis)
3. Abyssinian and Somali cats with increased erythrocyte osmotic fragility (a reticulocytosis is usually present)
4. Spurious with prolonged storage of blood sample

Macrocytic Normochromic

1. Regenerative anemias (decreased MCHC is not always present)
2. FeLV infections with no reticulocytosis (common)
3. Erythroleukemia (AML-M6) and myelodysplastic syndromes
4. Nonregenerative immune-mediated anemia and/or myelofibrosis in dogs
5. Poodle macrocytosis (healthy miniature poodles with no anemia)
6. Hyperthyroid cats (slight macrocytosis without anemia)
7. Folate deficiency (rare)
8. Congenital dyserythropoiesis of Hereford calves
9. Spurious with erythrocyte agglutination
10. Spurious in cats and dogs with persistent hypernatremia (may be hypochromic)

Microcytic Normochromic/Hypochromic[a]

1. Chronic iron deficiency (months in adults, weeks in nursing animals)
2. Portosystemic shunts in dogs and cats (often not anemic)
3. Anemia of inflammatory disease (usually normocytic)
4. Hepatic lipidosis in cats (usually normocytic)
5. Normal Akita and Shiba dogs (not anemic)
6. Prolonged recombinant erythropoietin treatment (mild)
7. Copper deficiency (rare)
8. Drugs or compounds that inhibit heme synthesis
9. Myeloid neoplasms with abnormal iron metabolism (rare)
10. Pyridoxine deficiency (experimental)
11. Familial dyserythropoiesis of English springer spaniel dogs (rare)
12. Hereditary elliptocytosis in dogs (rare)
13. Spurious when platelets are included in erythrocyte histograms
14. Spurious in dogs with persistent hyponatremia (not typically anemic)

[a]The presence of low MCHC along with low MCV strongly suggests iron-deficiency anemia.

is cytauxzoonosis in cats. Most cats die before there is time for a regenerative response to the anemia to occur.[185] Increased erythrocyte phagocytosis occurs in animals with hemophagocytic syndrome (macrophage activation syndrome), but the anemia may not be regenerative because the associated release of inflammatory mediators interferes with normal erythropoiesis.[499,516]

An increase in the plasma bilirubin concentration imparts a yellow color to the plasma (see Fig. 2-9, *B*). Mucous membranes and skin may also appear yellow (icteric) in extreme cases of hyperbilirubinemia (Fig. 4-101). Hyperbilirubinemia associated with a substantial decrease in the HCT suggests increased phagocytosis of erythrocytes.

If substantial intravascular hemolysis occurs rapidly, hemoglobinemia (see Fig. 2-9, *C*, *D*) and subsequently hemoglobinuria may be observed. Disorders where significant intravascular hemolysis sometimes occurs include immune-mediated hemolytic anemia, oxidant chemical and plant toxicities, severe hypophosphatemia, leptospiral and clostridial infections, coral snake and rattlesnake envenomation, zinc toxicity, copper toxicity, severe babesiosis, hypo-osmolality,

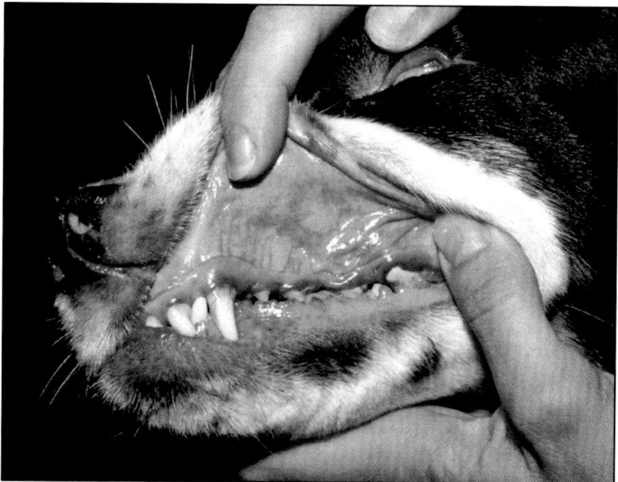

FIGURE 4-101
Icteric mucous membranes in an English springer spaniel dog with a hemolytic crises associated with PFK deficiency.

BOX 4-3 Causes of Hemolytic Anemias in Domestic Animals

1. **Immune-mediated erythrocyte destruction:** Primary or autoimmune hemolytic anemia (common in dogs); neonatal isoerythrolysis (primarily horses and cats); lupus erythematosus (primarily dogs); incompatible blood transfusions; drugs, including penicillin (horses), cephalosporins (dogs), levamisole (dogs), sulfonamides (horses and dogs), pirimicarb (insecticide in dogs), and propylthiouracil (cats)
2. **Erythrocyte parasites (may have an immune-mediated component):** *Anaplasma* spp. (ruminants), erythrocytic *Mycoplasma* spp. (except horses), *Babesia* spp., *Cytauxzoon felis*, *Theileria* spp. (ruminants)
3. **Other infectious agents (may have an immune-mediated component):** *Leptospira* and *Clostridium* spp. (primarily ruminants and horses), FeLV (seldom hemolytic), equine infectious anemia virus (multifactorial, also with decreased production), *Sarcocystis* spp. (cattle and sheep), *Trypanosoma* spp. (primarily outside the United States)
4. **Chemicals and plants (most are oxidants):** Onions, red maple (horses), *Brassica* spp. (ruminants), lush winter rye (cattle), copper (sheep and goats), phenothiazine (horses), acetaminophen (cats and dogs), methylene blue (cats and dogs), benzocaine (cats and dogs), phenazopyridine (cats), methionine (cats), vitamin K (dogs), propylene glycol (cats), naphthalene (dogs?), zinc (dogs and ruminants), indole (experimental in cattle and horses), tryptophan (experimental in horses), crude oil (marine birds), venoms (snakes, bees, wasps, and spiders)
5. **Fragmentation:** Disseminated intravascular coagulation (primarily dogs), dirofilariasis (especially posterior vena cava syndrome) in dogs, hemangiosarcoma (dogs), vasculitis, hemolytic uremia syndrome
6. **Hypo-osmolality:** Hypotonic fluid administration, water intoxication (primarily in cattle)
7. **Hypophosphatemia:** Postparturient hemoglobinuria (cattle), ketoacidotic diabetic animals following insulin therapy (cats and dogs), hepatic lipidosis (cats)
8. **Hereditary erythrocyte defects:** Pyruvate kinase deficiency (dogs and cats), phosphofructokinase deficiency (dogs), glucose-6-phosphate dehydrogenase deficiency (horses), hereditary stomatocytosis (mild anemia in dogs), erythropoietic porphyria (cattle and cats), hereditary nonspherocytic hemolytic anemias of unknown etiology (poodle and beagle dogs), idiopathic increased erythrocyte osmotic fragility (cats), erythrocyte flavin adenine dinucleotide deficiency in horses (methemoglobinemia and sometimes mild anemia), hereditary spherocytosis in cattle
9. **Miscellaneous:** Liver failure (horses), hypersplenism, hemophagocytic histiocytic sarcoma, splenic torsion (dogs), selenium deficiency in cattle grazing on St. Augustine grass, postparturient hemoglobinuria in cattle not associated with hypophosphatemia

caudal vena cava syndrome of dirofilariasis in dogs, hepatic failure in horses, phosphofructokinase deficiency in dogs, inherited idiopathic increased erythrocyte osmotic fragility in Abyssinian and Somali cats, postparturient cattle without hypophosphatemia, and splenic torsion in dogs. In most of these disorders, however, erythrocyte destruction occurs primarily by increased phagocytosis.

Immune-Mediated Hemolytic Anemia

The binding of antibodies and/or complement to erythrocyte surfaces can result in phagocytosis by macrophages and, in some cases, intravascular hemolysis. Immune-mediated hemolytic anemia (IMHA) may be primary or it may occur secondarily to rickettsial, bacterial, protozoal, viral, or hemotropic mycoplasmal infections; neoplasia (especially lymphomas); and toxin or drug exposure. Additional information concerning IMHA is given in Chapter 6.

Primary IMHA

A diagnosis of primary IMHA, also called autoimmune hemolytic anemia, is reached by ruling out other disorders known to have concomitant IMHA. Primary IMHA is common in dogs,[33] less common in cats,[261] and rare in other domestic animal species. About two-thirds of the dogs with IMHA appear to have primary IMHA.[394] In contrast, IMHA in noncanine species is usually a secondary rather than a primary, disorder. Primary IMHA may be associated with immune-mediated thrombocytopenia; it may also be part of systemic lupus erythematosus, a multisystemic autoimmune disease.[167,480]

Neonatal Isoerythrolysis

Neonatal isoerythrolysis is an IMHA that develops in neonatal animals following ingestion of colostrum containing antibodies against antigens on their erythrocytes.[480] It occurs primarily in horses, mules, and cats. In horses, dams become sensitized to foreign erythrocyte antigens from leakage of fetal erythrocytes through the placenta during pregnancy or from exposure to fetal erythrocytes of the same blood type during a previous parturition. Antibodies are produced against these antigens and secreted in colostrum.[61,371] Neonatal isoerythrolysis can occur in kittens with blood type A born to queens with blood type B who have had no prior exposure to blood type A antigens, because all adult cats with type B blood naturally have high anti-A antibody titers.[171]

Transfusion Reactions

Hemolytic transfusion reactions may occur when plasma of the recipient contains antibodies against one or more antigens on the surface of donor erythrocytes. Erythrocyte destruction may also occur when plasma of the donor contains antibodies against one or more antigens on the surface of recipient erythrocytes, but the amount of antibody present to react with erythrocytes is considerably less. With the exception of cats, naturally occurring antierythrocyte antibodies of clinical significance seldom occur in animals. Rather, antibody formation results from prior exposure to different erythrocyte antigens via transfusion, pregnancy, or vaccination with products containing blood group antigens. Consequently severe hemolytic transfusion reactions generally do not occur at the time of the first blood transfusion. Cats with blood type B have naturally occurring anti-A antibodies with high hemolytic titers. Therefore the transfusion of type A blood into a type B cat can result in a life-threatening intravascular hemolytic reaction the first time such a transfusion is given.

Erythrocyte Parasites

Erythrocyte parasites include intracellular protozoal parasites (*Babesia* species, *Theileria* species, and *Cytauxzoon felis*), intracellular rickettsial organisms (*Anaplasma* species), and epicellular *Mycoplasma* species. The morphology of these organisms is presented earlier in this chapter. These infectious agents generally cause mild to severe hemolytic anemia, depending on the pathogenicity of the organism and the susceptibility of the host. Some damage to erythrocytes is caused directly by a parasite, but secondary immune-mediated injury may be more important in the pathogenesis of anemia in some cases.[314] Antierythrocyte antibodies are often present and spherocytes may be seen in stained blood films; therefore it is important to differentiate these infectious diseases from primary IMHA.[82,176] Macrophage activation with increased erythrophagocytosis may also contribute to the development of anemia.[330]

Except in horses, reticulocytosis is generally present if sufficient time (about 4 days) has elapsed for a bone marrow response to occur. The anemia may be nonregenerative if a concomitant inflammatory response inhibits erythropoiesis (see "Anemia of Inflammatory Disease," below), and/or if the infection results in decreased hematopoietic precursors, as reported with *Theileria parva* infection in cattle.[305] Thrombocytopenia is usually present with protozoal infections of erythrocytes. Platelet consumption may occur in association with DIC in severe disorders,[185,467] but thrombocytopenia is probably more often associated with increased phagocytosis of platelets in response to antibodies on their surfaces and/or because of macrophage activation by inflammatory cytokines such as M-CSF and IFN-γ.[2,159,331] Thrombocytopenia is not generally present with erythrocytic *Anaplasma* and hemoplasma infections.

Babesia *Species*

Three genetically distinct large *B. canis* subspecies (*B. canis canis*, *B. canis vogeli*, and *B. canis rossi*) have been identified. *B. canis vogeli* in the United States generally causes mild or inapparent disease in adults (unless they are immunosuppressed) but severe hemolytic anemia in pups. *B. canis rossi* in South Africa can cause severe disease and death in adult dogs. *B. canis canis* occurs primarily in Europe and Asia and is of intermediate pathogenicity.[467] In addition, an unnamed large *Babesia* species has been described in the United States in immunosuppressed dogs.[51,226,427]

B. gibsoni is a small *Babesia* species infecting dogs; it is endemic in Africa, the Middle East, and Asia. There has been a rapid increase in the number of cases reported in various parts of the United States, predominantly in American pit bull terriers.[547] Although ticks are considered the primary vector in much of the world, it appears that transmission of infected blood through dog bites is a major mechanism of transmission of this organism in the United States.[49] A second small *Babesia* species called *Babesia conradae* has been recognized in California. Like *B. gibsoni,* it causes severe clinical disease in adult dogs.[252] It is closely related to piroplasms isolated from wildlife and humans in the western United States. A third small piroplasm has been identified causing hemolytic anemia in dogs; it is closely related to *Babesia microti,* a previously recognized parasite of rodents and humans. A provisional name of *Theileria annae* has been assigned to this organism based on its *18S rRNA* gene sequence.[79]

B. felis causes hemolytic anemia in cats in South Africa.[362] Additional piroplasms have been identified by PCR in domestic cats, but their clinical significance remains to be determined.[491]

The two most important *Babesia* species infecting cattle are *B. bigemina* and *B. bovis.* Both are capable of causing life-threatening hemolytic anemia.[176] The two most important piroplasms infecting horses are the large *B. caballi* parasite, and the smaller, more pleomorphic *B. equi* parasite.[491] The anemia is generally more severe in *B. equi*-infected than in *B. caballi*-infected horses.[78]

Theileria *Species*

Theileria parva and *Theileria annulata* cause important diseases in ruminants in Africa, Asia, and the Middle East.[274] The associated anemia may be regenerative or nonregenerative.[353,430] Theilerial organisms present in domestic ruminants in the United States are usually nonpathogenic.[245,453] Likewise, *Theileria* in deer are generally considered of low pathogenicity, but may cause hemolytic anemia under some circumstances.[544] Some investigators have proposed that *B. equi* and *B. microti* be moved to the genus *Theileria*, but others believe that they belong in a new genus that is distinct from both *Babesia* and *Theileria.*[14,491]

Cytauxzoon felis

Like *Theileria*, the genus *Cytauxzoon* has both a tissue phase and an erythrocyte phase. In contrast to *Theileria*, the schizonts of *Cytauxzoon* develop exclusively in macrophages rather than in lymphocytes.[459] Most domestic cats with acute cytauxzoonosis die.[185] Cats generally have icteric plasma in the terminal stage of the disease. The HCT may be in the low thirties but is usually in the twenties. Reticulocyte counts are not increased in response to the anemia. Cats become thrombocytopenic during the late stage of disease.

Coagulation tests may be prolonged or remain normal, tests for fibrin degradation products (FDPs) may be positive, and the total serum protein concentration is variably decreased. White blood cell counts are variable, but leukopenia generally develops terminally. Parasitemia occurs late in the disease. Since domestic cats with acute cytauxzoonosis generally die in a matter of days, they are believed to be dead-end hosts. Bobcats, however, usually do not die when infected with *C. felis* and serve as a reservoir of infection for transmission to domestic cats by ticks. A low percentage of cats have been reported to survive.[190] This may, in large part, be because of infection with a less virulent strain of the organism; however, studies are needed to determine if these cats can serve as a reservoir for *C. felis* transmission that would result in disease in other domestic cats.[72]

Anaplasma *Species*

Anaplasma marginale is an important pathogen causing mild to severe hemolytic anemia and sometimes death in naive adult cattle.[255] Infected calves generally do not become ill but become carriers of the organism. *Anaplasma centrale* is much less pathogenic in cattle and has been used as a vaccine against *A. marginale.*[159,313] *Anaplasma ovis* is pathogenic for sheep, goats, and some wild ruminants.[112]

Hemotropic Mycoplasmas (Hemoplasmas)

Hemotropic mycoplasmas are bacteria that attach to the external surfaces of erythrocytes. In contrast to erythrocyte protozoal parasites, thrombocytopenia is not a feature of hemoplasma infections. Three different hemoplasmas have been identified in cats based on *16S rRNA* gene sequences.[473,539] *Mycoplasma haemofelis* generally produces anemia and clinical signs of disease, while Candidatus *Mycoplasma haemominutum* generally results in unapparent infection and minimal change in HCT unless the infection is complicated by other disorders such as FeLV infection, feline immunodeficiency virus (FIV) infection, and neoplasia.[113,141,165,242,533] Candidatus *Mycoplasma turicensis* can be pathogenic in cats, causing a moderate to severe hemolytic anemia. Early reports suggest that the clinical signs of infection are worsened in cats having concurrent FIV infections or following the administration of corticosteroids.[538]

Three hemoplasmas have been reported in dogs based on *16S rRNA* gene sequences. *Mycoplasma haemocanis* is closely related to *M. haemofelis.*[48,67] A hemoplasma closely related to Candidatus *M. haemominutum* has been identified in a dog in China.[551] Another hemoplasma has been identified in multiple countries and classified as Candidatus *Mycoplasma haematoparvum.*[35,465,539] Splenectomy, splenic pathology, or immunosuppression is generally required before hemoplasmas are recognized in stained blood films, and hemolytic anemia develops in dogs.[202]

Mycoplasma suis causes hemolytic anemia with icterus in young piglets. Hemolytic anemia may also occur in pigs at weaning, in feeder pigs under stress, and in pregnant sows immediately prepartum.[314] However, *M. suis* has more often been associated with growth retardation and mild anemia in feeder pigs and unthriftiness with poor reproductive performance in sows.[221,397]

M. ovis generally causes hemolytic anemia in young sheep and goats, with mild or unapparent disease in adults.[314,339] However, severe hemolytic anemia and death have been described in an outbreak in adult sheep that were also infected with *A. ovis.*[227]

Systemic illness with edema has been reported in cattle infected with *M. wenyoni*[435,530]; however, this syndrome could not be reproduced experimentally.[529] *M. wenyoni* is not reported to produce significant anemia in cattle unless they have been splenectomized.

Variable anemia has been reported in llamas and alpacas infected with Candidatus *M. haemolamae*, but most infections appear to be subclinical. Camelids that are immune-compromised or have other concurrent disorders are more likely to be ill and anemic.[483] The anemia may not be regenerative if it is complicated by inflammatory disease.[390]

Other Infectious Agents

In addition to erythrocyte parasites, infections with other agents may result in hemolytic anemia. As in the case of erythrocyte parasites, the enhanced erythrocyte destruction may have an immune-mediated component. *Leptospira* species have been reported to cause hemolytic anemia in cattle, sheep, and pigs.[47,114,451] *Clostridium* species have been reported to cause hemolytic anemia in cattle,[469] sheep,[307,385] and horses.[393,526]

Hemolytic anemia has been described in experimental acute *Sarcocystis* infections in cattle,[147,293] goats,[124] and pigs.[36] Several *Trypanosoma* species cause hemolytic anemia in cattle, sheep, and goats in tropical and subtropical regions, except in the United States, even though the parasite is not directly associated with erythrocytes.[23,52,230] Nonpathogenic trypanosomes, including *T. theileri,* occur worldwide in cattle.[134,413]

The anemia associated with equine infectious anemia (EIA) virus infection is multifactorial. It includes both an immune-mediated destruction of erythrocytes and bone marrow suppression.[308,417,461] Macrophages within the marrow are important components of the erythropoietic microenvironment, where they can produce erythropoietic stimulatory and inhibitory factors (see Chapter 3). The EIA virus replicates in macrophages, including those in the bone marrow,[462] and macrophages produce proinflammatory cytokines in response to EIA infection that may inhibit both erythrocyte and platelet production.[283,461,484]

A transient regenerative anemia was reported in some kittens experimentally infected with FeLV,[290] and immune-mediated hemolytic anemia has infrequently been reported in naturally infected cats,[261] although some of these animals might have had concomitant hemoplasma infections.[165,174] However, the anemia seen in FeLV-infected cats is typically nonregenerative because it is secondary to bone marrow proliferative abnormalities, discussed later in this chapter and in Chapter 9.[174,421]

Chemicals and Plants

Oxidants

Most chemicals and plants that cause hemolytic anemia are oxidants. Consequently Heinz bodies, eccentrocytes, and/or methemoglobinemia may be present. Dietary causes of Heinz body hemolytic anemia (with or without eccentrocytosis and/or methemoglobinemia) include consumption of onions and garlic in small and large animals, consumption of kale and other *Brassica* species by ruminants, consumption of lush winter rye by cattle, and consumption of red maple leaves by horses and alpacas.* Heinz bodies have been recognized in erythrocytes from selenium-deficient Florida cattle grazing on St. Augustine grass pastures and in postparturient New Zealand cattle grazing primarily on perennial ryegrass.[205] Copper toxicity results in Heinz body formation in sheep and goats.[39] Heinz body formation has been reported in dogs ingesting zinc-containing objects (e.g., U.S. pennies minted after 1982).[46,205] Naphthalene ingestion may have caused Heinz body formation in a dog.[120]

Heinz body hemolytic anemia has occurred following the administration of a variety of drugs including acetaminophen and methylene blue in cats and dogs, methionine and phenazopyridine in cats, menadione (vitamin K_3) in dogs, and phenothiazine in horses. The application of benzocaine to inflamed dog skin can result in Heinz body formation, but methemoglobinemia is more prominent.[205]

Heinz body hemolytic anemia has been reported in a dog that had been sprayed with skunk musk.[549] The ingestion of crude oil by marine birds results in Heinz body hemolytic anemia.[278,488]

Heinz bodies were consistently present in erythrocytes from a male English bulldog with multiple erythroid abnormalities including prominent siderotic inclusions in his erythrocytes.[209] A prominent Heinz body hemolytic anemia (see Fig. 4-80, *A,B*), with an HCT of 14% to 24% and a mild methemoglobinemia (about 13%), persisted in a rescued quarter horse colt during 3 months of study. A source of dietary oxidants was not identified, and hemoglobin electrophoresis appeared normal. Erythrocyte reduced glutathione concentration was below the reference interval. An erythrocyte metabolic defect was suspected, but erythrocyte enzyme assays failed to identify a cause. (J. W. Harvey, unpublished).

Venoms

Venoms from snakes, bees, wasps, and brown recluse spiders are complex mixtures of proteins, peptides, enzymes, and chemicals that have multiple pathologic effects, including hemolytic anemia and other forms of tissue injury.[301,303,344,431] Phospholipase enzymes (especially phospholipase A_2) in venoms appear to be important in causing erythrocyte injury.[396,407,431,498]

*References 18, 27, 121, 205, 470, 545.

Drugs Causing Immune-Mediated Anemia

A number of drugs are reported to produce secondary IMHA in animals. These drugs include penicillin (horses),[306,398] cephalosporins (dogs),[54] levamisole (dogs),[28] sulfonamides (horses and dogs),[478,487] pirimicarb (insecticide in dogs),[235] and propylthiouracil (cats).[29]

Fragmentation

Microangiopathic hemolytic anemia may occur when erythrocytes are forced to flow through altered vascular channels or exposed to turbulent blood flow. Erythrocyte fragments with pointed extremities are called schistocytes. Erythrocyte fragmentation may be seen in animals (especially dogs) with DIC. Mechanical fragmentation occurs as the cells pass through the fibrin meshwork of a microthrombus (see Fig. 4-53). Fragmentation anemia is especially common in dogs with hemangiosarcoma and in dogs with caudal vena cava syndrome, resulting from a rapid blockage of the posterior vena cava with large numbers of adult heartworms.[197,392,456]

Erythrocyte fragmentation is a component of the hemolytic-uremic syndrome. This rare syndrome is characterized by hemolytic anemia, thrombocytopenia, and acute renal failure.[345] In humans (and probably animals), the syndrome is usually initiated by certain toxins produced by *Escherichia coli* (and less often other bacteria) infecting the gastrointestinal tract; however, atypical cases have also been associated with nongastrointestinal infections, cancer, parturition, immunosuppressive drug therapy, organ transplants, and autoimmune diseases.[26,118,224,345] Absorbed bacterial toxins can result in endothelial injury, activation of hemostasis, the formation of microthrombi, erythrocyte fragmentation, and reduced blood flow with injury to the kidney and other affected organs.[345] Atypical cases have been attributed to the overactivation of the alternative complement pathway. The glomerular capillary bed of the kidney may be at increased risk because of its fenestrated endothelium, which continually exposes the subendothelial matrix to a variety of circulating proteins and peptides.[346] Additional disorders where erythrocyte fragmentation may be observed are described under "Schistocytes," above.

Hypo-osmolality

Intravascular hemolysis can occur in calves that drink excessive amounts of water following a period of water deprivation.[172] Water intoxication decreases plasma osmolality, and water moves into erythrocytes causing them to swell and lyse. Hemolysis has been reported in juvenile pygmy goats fed water using a nipple bottle for human infants,[316] and hemolysis may occur when hypotonic fluid is administered intravenously (see Fig. 4-72, *A*).

Hypophosphatemia

Hemolytic anemia can occur secondary to hypophosphatemia because hypophosphatemia decreases the erythrocyte glycolytic rate, which results in a decreased ATP concentration. Hemolytic anemia resulting from hypophosphatemia has been reported in diabetic cats and in a diabetic dog following insulin therapy, in a cat with hepatic lipidosis, and in postparturient cattle and buffaloes.[109,205] In addition to having low ATP concentrations, dog erythrocytes might hemolyze as a result of decreased erythrocyte 2,3DPG concentration, because dog erythrocytes with low 2,3DPG are more alkaline-fragile than those of normal dogs and may hemolyze at physiologic pH values.[205]

Hereditary Erythrocyte Defects

Pyruvate Kinase Deficiency in Dogs and Cats

Pyruvate kinase (PK) deficiency is transmitted as an autosomal recessive trait in many breeds of dogs, with highest prevalence reported in basenji and beagle dogs. Homozygously affected animals have decreased exercise tolerance, pale mucous membranes, tachycardia, and splenomegaly. Affected animals have a macrocytic hypochromic anemia (HCT 16% to 28%) with marked reticulocytosis (15% to 50% uncorrected reticulocyte count) when young. Myelofibrosis and osteosclerosis develop in the bone marrow, and hemochromatosis and cirrhosis develop in the liver as the dogs age. HCT and reticulocyte counts decrease as myelofibrosis and osteosclerosis become severe. Affected dogs generally die between 1 and 5 years of age because of bone marrow failure and/or liver failure.[169,203]

PK deficiency has been reported in Abyssinian, Somali, and domestic shorthaired cats. Affected cats are often asymptomatic, but lethargy, pale mucous membranes, and inappetence may be recognized. The HCT is generally normal or mildly decreased, but severe anemia may occur during intermittent hemolytic crises. The MCV is usually mildly increased. The MCHC is sometimes decreased. An aggregate reticulocytosis is present in 90% of cases.[259] Splenectomy may reduce the severity of the anemia in cats. In contrast to dogs, bone marrow and liver failure have not been reported in cats; consequently the life expectancy in cats with PK deficiency is generally longer than that in dogs with this defect.[169]

PK deficiency can be diagnosed by measuring erythrocyte enzyme activity in affected cats, but it can be difficult to diagnose by measuring enzyme activities in affected dogs because their erythrocytes contain an unstable M_2 isozyme that is usually lost as erythroid precursors develop into erythrocytes.[206] All PK-deficient cats identified thus far have had the same mutation; therefore a single DNA-based diagnostic test may be used to identify deficient cats.[259] Unfortunately several different genetic mutations have been identified in dogs with PK deficiency. Consequently different DNA-based diagnostic assays must be developed and/or validated for each affected dog breed.[169]

Phosphofructokinase Deficiency in Dogs

Autosomal recessive inherited erythrocyte PFK deficiency occurs in English springer spaniel, American cocker spaniel, mixed-breed, wachtelhund, and whippet dogs.[166,205] Homozygously affected dogs have persistent compensated hemolytic anemias and sporadic episodes of intravascular hemolysis with hemoglobinuria. HCTs are generally between 30% and 40%, except during hemolytic crises, when the HCT may decrease to 15% or less. MCVs are usually between 80 and 90 fL and reticulocyte counts are generally between 10% and 30% even when the HCT is within the reference range. Lethargy, weakness, pale or icteric mucous membranes, mild hepatosplenomegaly, muscle wasting, and fever as high as 41°C may occur during hemolytic crises, which occur secondary to hyperventilation-induced alkalemia.

Affected dogs appear to tire more easily than normal, and a myopathy with cramping is infrequently observed. Progressive cardiac disease was reported in two whippets. In contrast to PK deficiency, myelofibrosis and liver failure have not been recognized in dogs with PFK deficiency.

Homozygous affected animals more than 3 months of age can easily be identified by measuring erythrocyte PFK activity. A DNA test using PCR technology has been developed that can clearly differentiate normal, carrier, and affected dogs of all breeds except wachtelhunds, which have a different genetic mutation.[205]

Increased Erythrocyte Osmotic Fragility in Cats

A hemolytic anemia with markedly increased osmotic fragility occurs in Abyssinian and Somali cats.[260] Splenomegaly and polyclonal hyperglobulinemia are common. The HCT is generally between 15% and 25%, but values as low as 5% have been recognized. A macrocytosis with mild to moderate reticulocytosis is present in most cats. Most samples exhibit extreme hemolysis after 1 day of refrigeration; however, in vivo intravascular hemolysis also occurs, as evidenced by hemoglobinuria in some cats. An erythrocyte membrane defect is suspected.

Hereditary Spherocytosis in Cattle

Severe hemolytic anemia with icterus and splenomegaly is present shortly after birth in Japanese black cattle that lack band 3 in their erythrocyte membranes. The mortality rate is high in affected animals, especially during the first week of life. Those that survive exhibit a persistent mild hemolytic anemia (HCT 25% to 35%), with marked spherocytosis and anisocytosis but no reticulocytosis. This defect is inherited as an autosomal dominant trait, and osmotic fragility is increased in both heterozygous and homozygous cattle.[231]

Glucose-6-Phosphate Dehydrogenase Deficiency in a Horse

Persistent hemolytic anemia and hyperbilirubinemia have been described in an American standard-bred colt with severe G6PD activity. Morphologic abnormalities of erythrocytes included eccentrocytosis, pyknocytosis, increased anisocytosis, increased Howell-Jolly bodies, and rare hemoglobin crystals. Heinz bodies were not observed in erythrocytes stained with new methylene blue.[452]

Erythrocyte Flavin Adenine Dinucleotide Deficiency in Horses

Eccentrocytosis, pyknocytosis, and variable numbers of hemoglobin crystals have also been seen in FAD-deficient horses, but HCTs were normal or only slightly decreased. Affected horses have undetectable glutathione reductase and reduced Cb_5R enzyme activities because FAD is a cofactor for these enzymes. A persistent methemoglobinemia (25% to 46%) is present because of the Cb_5R deficiency.[203]

Hereditary Stomatocytosis in Dogs

Stomatocytosis is recognized in association with three different inherited syndromes in dogs that result in one or more membrane defects causing erythrocytes to swell. Hemoglobin values and erythrocyte counts are low-normal or slightly reduced, but HCTs are normal in Malamutes, schnauzers, and Pomeranians. The MCV is increased and MCHC decreased even though reticulocyte counts are normal or only slightly increased. Affected Drentse patrijshond dogs have lower HCTs and higher reticulocyte counts than those found in the other breeds. Erythrocytes from all breeds have increased osmotic fragility and shortened erythrocyte survival.[205]

Additional Hereditary Defects

Familial nonspherocytic hemolytic anemia has been reported in poodles. Despite extensive studies, the defect in this disorder could not be determined, but PK deficiency cannot be ruled out. A mild hemolytic anemia with reticulocytosis, slightly increased erythrocyte osmotic fragility, shortened erythrocyte life span, and normal erythrocyte morphology has been reported in beagle dogs. A membrane defect was suspected. Persistent elliptocytosis and microcytosis have been described in a crossbred dog that lacked erythrocyte membrane protein 4.1. Although the animal was not anemic, the reticulocyte count was about twice normal in compensation for a shortened erythrocyte life span.[205]

Miscellaneous Causes of Hemolytic Anemia

Splenic Disorders

Disorders that cause splenomegaly may result in a syndrome called hypersplenism, where phagocytosis of blood cells is increased.[442] Increased erythrophagocytosis and anemia occur in various hemophagocytic disorders,[516] most notably in hemophagocytic histiocytic sarcoma, which typically involve the spleen.[149,324] Erythrocyte destruction can occur secondary to splenic torsion, where stagnation and breakdown of blood results in hemoglobinuria.[336]

Liver Failure in Horses

Marked intravascular hemolysis has been reported in horses with liver failure. The mechanism of this hemolysis is unknown, but bile acids or their salts have been considered possible hemolytic factors in horses.[383]

Postparturient Hemoglobinuria in Dairy Cattle

Postparturient hemoglobinuria in dairy cattle has been associated with hypophosphatemia.[450] The anemia appears to develop because affected animals have decreased erythrocyte ATP concentrations.[205] An apparently different syndrome of postparturient hemoglobinuria has been reported in cattle in New Zealand grazing primarily on perennial ryegrass *(Lolium perenne)*. The presence of Heinz bodies in these animals indicates an oxidant etiology. Postparturient cattle may be more susceptible to the development of anemia because increased food consumption associated with lactation could increase exposure to an unidentified dietary oxidant. Copper deficiency may contribute to the severity of the anemia in these cattle by rendering their erythrocytes more susceptible to oxidants.[292]

BLOOD-LOSS ANEMIAS

Causes of blood-loss anemia are given in Box 4-4.* In some cases the diagnosis of blood-loss anemia and its cause is apparent from the history and/or physical findings. In other

*References 6, 107, 145, 161, 168, 284, 298, 312, 380, 414, 444.

BOX 4-4 Causes of Blood-Loss Anemias in Domestic Animals

1. **Trauma:** Accidents, fights, gastrointestinal foreign bodies, surgery
2. **Parasites:** Hookworms, fleas, blood-sucking lice, *Haemonchus* spp. (small ruminants), liver flukes, *Coccidia* spp.
3. **Coagulation disorders:** Vitamin K deficiency, sweet clover (dicoumarol) toxicity (cattle), rodenticide toxicity, bracken fern toxicity (cattle and sheep), disseminated intravascular coagulation, inherited coagulation factor deficiencies (see Chapter 7)
4. **Platelet disorders:** Thrombocytopenia and inherited platelet function defects (see Chapter 7)
5. **Neoplasia:** Gastric tumors including carcinomas, leiomyosarcoma, and lymphoma; transitional cell carcinoma and transitional cell papilloma of urogenital system; and ruptured hemangioma, hemangiosarcoma, and adrenal gland tumors with bleeding into body cavities and tissues
6. **Gastrointestinal ulcers:** Glucocorticoids, nonsteroidal anti-inflammatory drugs, mast cell tumors, gastrinoma, stress, metabolic diseases (uremia, liver failure, hypoadrenocorticism)
7. **Vascular abnormalities:** Arteriovenous fistula and vascular ectasia in the gastrointestinal or urogenital tracts
8. **Phenylephrine-induced hemorrhage:** Presumably associated with hypertension in aged horses treated for nephrosplenic entrapment of the large colon

cases hemorrhage is apparent but its cause must be determined. Finally, blood-loss anemia and its cause may not be recognized until laboratory tests and other diagnostic tests are done. The gastrointestinal and urogenital tracts are common sites of occult hemorrhage. Tests that may assist in the diagnosis of gastrointestinal hemorrhage include the occult blood test in feces, fecal examination for parasite ova, and diagnostic imaging to identify tumors or ulcers. Urinalysis and diagnostic imaging of the urinary system may assist in the diagnosis of renal or bladder hemorrhage.

Although total blood volume is decreased, HCT and plasma protein concentration are normal immediately after substantial acute blood loss has occurred because there is a balanced loss of erythrocytes and plasma. The HCT may even be increased shortly after acute blood loss in horses and dogs because splenic contraction occurs, which releases blood with a higher HCT into the general circulation.[237] After several hours, the HCT and plasma protein concentration decrease as fluid moves from the digestive tract and extravascular spaces into the circulation to return the blood volume toward normal. If no further hemorrhage occurs, the plasma protein concentration will return to normal within a few days. Consequently the occurrence of a low plasma protein concentration in association with anemia suggests the presence of recent or ongoing hemorrhage. Considerably more time is required for the HCT to return to normal than is required for the plasma protein concentration to return to normal. The HCT increases about 1 percentage point per day following experimental phlebotomy in dogs and cats, with a slightly lower response in cattle and horses.[15,65,364]

The anemia appears nonregenerative shortly after blood loss because approximately 4 days are required for production of reticulocytes by the marrow. The MCV may not be increased following blood loss in animals because the reticulocyte response may not be of sufficient magnitude to result in a high MCV. Few reticulocytes are released from the marrow in response to blood-loss anemia in cattle and no reticulocytes are released following hemorrhage in horses.

Chronic external blood loss can result in iron deficiency. Iron-deficiency anemia is common in adult dogs and ruminants but seldom occurs in adult cats and horses because parasitism causing significant blood loss is uncommon in these species. If iron deficiency persists for several weeks, the anemia can become microcytic and hypochromic. Reticulocyte counts may be slightly to moderately increased in early iron-deficiency anemia in dogs; however, as iron deficiency becomes more severe, the regenerative response will be attenuated (see discussion of iron deficiency under "Abnormalities in Heme Synthesis," later in this chapter).[204] Internal hemorrhage can share some characteristics of hemolytic anemias. Iron is conserved so that hypoferremia does not occur. Slight hyperbilirubinemia may occur due to phagocytosis and degradation of erythrocytes at the sites of widespread hemorrhage. Some plasma proteins may be reabsorbed when hemorrhage occurs in body cavities, thus shortening the return of plasma protein concentrations to normal.

ANEMIAS RESULTING FROM DECREASED ERYTHROCYTE PRODUCTION

Anemia resulting from decreased erythrocyte production lacks evidence of bone marrow response to the anemia (e.g., the absolute reticulocyte count in blood is not increased or only minimally raised for the degree of anemia). Nonregenerative anemias result from reduced or defective erythropoiesis (Box 4-5). They are usually normocytic. Exceptions include microcytic anemia associated with chronic iron-deficiency anemia, copper deficiency, pyridoxine deficiency, and dyserythropoiesis in English springer spaniel dogs and macrocytic anemia associated with folate deficiency, FeLV infection in cats, erythroleukemia, some myelodysplastic disorders, and dyserythropoiesis in polled Hereford calves.[201,257] Bone marrow biopsies are often required to delineate the nature of nonregenerative anemias.

BOX 4-5 Anemias Resulting from Decreased Erythrocyte Production in Domestic Animals

Reduced Erythropoiesis

1. **Chronic renal disease:** Primarily lack of erythropoietin
2. **Endocrine deficiencies:** Hypothyroidism, hypoadrenocorticism, hypopituitarism, hypoandrogenism
3. **Inflammatory disease:** Inflammation and neoplasia
4. **Cytotoxic damage to the marrow:** Bracken fern poisoning (cattle), cytotoxic anticancer drugs, estrogen toxicity (dogs and ferrets), chloramphenicol (cats, usually not anemic), phenylbutazone (dogs), trimethoprim-sulfadiazine (dogs), radiation, albendazole (dogs, cats, alpacas), griseofulvin (cats), trichloroethylene (cattle)
5. **Infectious agents:** *Ehrlichia* spp. (dogs, horses, and cats), FeLV, nonbloodsucking trichostrongyloid parasites (ruminants), parvovirus (pups)
6. **Immune-mediated:** Nonregenerative anemia, selective erythroid aplasia, continued treatment with recombinant human erythropoietin, idiopathic aplastic anemia (?)
7. **Congenital/inherited:** Foals and dogs?
8. **Myelophthisis:** Myeloid leukemias, lymphoid leukemias, myelodysplastic syndromes, multiple myeloma, myelofibrosis, osteosclerosis, metastatic lymphomas, metastatic mast cell tumors

Defective Erythropoiesis

1. **Disorders of heme synthesis:** Iron, copper, and pyridoxine deficiencies; lead toxicity; drugs
2. **Disorders of nucleic acid synthesis:** Folate and cobalamin deficiencies
3. **Abnormal maturation:** Erythroleukemia or AML-M6 (primarily cats), myelodysplastic syndromes with erythroid predominance (MDS-Er), inherited dyserythropoiesis of Hereford calves, inherited dyserythropoiesis of English springer spaniels

Nonregenerative Anemias without Leukopenia or Thrombocytopenia

A nonregenerative anemia without an accompanying leukopenia or thrombocytopenia in blood suggests a bone marrow abnormality affecting only erythroid cells. Mild to moderate anemia of this type may occur in association with chronic renal disease, endocrine deficiencies, and the anemia of inflammatory disease. Erythroid production is reduced in these disorders, but often not enough to result in an M:E ratio in the marrow that is increased above the reference interval.

Hormone Deficiencies

Because the kidney is the major site of EPO production in the body, chronic renal disease can result in a mild to moderate nonregenerative anemia secondary to reduced EPO production.[250,360] Disorders such as hypopituitarism, hypoadrenocorticism, and hypothyroidism may result in mild nonregenerative anemia because these hormones enhance the growth of erythroid progenitor cells in the presence of EPO.[205,282,357] Glucocorticoids appear to be important in stress erythropoiesis (e.g., following hemorrhage or increased erythrocyte destruction, when a substantial increase in erythropoiesis is required). Thyroid hormones may also promote the synthesis of EPO in the kidney.[205]

Anemia of Inflammatory Disease (Anemia of Chronic Disease)

A mild to moderate nonregenerative anemia often accompanies chronic inflammatory and neoplastic disorders. The cause of the anemia is multifactorial and only partially understood. Abnormalities that can contribute to the anemia include low serum iron, the production of inflammatory mediators that can inhibit erythropoiesis, and shortened erythrocyte life spans, presumably secondary to membrane damage caused by endogenous oxidants generated during inflammation.[204]

Disorders of Nucleic Acid Synthesis

Anemia resulting from folate deficiency is rarely reported in animals. Macrocytic anemia has been produced experimentally in pigs and a clinical case of folate deficiency has been recognized in a cat.[205] Cobalamin (vitamin B_{12}) deficiency in humans, who require cobalamin for normal folate metabolism, causes hematologic abnormalities similar to folate deficiency. In contrast, cobalamin deficiency does not cause macrocytic anemia in any animal species. Anemia has been reported in some experimental animal studies, but erythrocytes were of normal size. Cobalamin deficiency occurs secondarily to an inherited malabsorption of cobalamin in dogs. Affected animals have normocytic, nonregenerative anemia with increased anisocytosis. Additional findings include neutropenia with hypersegmented neutrophils and giant platelets. A normocytic nonregenerative anemia was also present in a cobalamin-deficient cat that probably had an inherited defect in cobalamin absorption.[205]

Abnormalities in Heme Synthesis

Iron deficiency in adult domestic animals usually results from blood loss. The absolute reticulocyte count may be increased early in response to hemorrhage, but as iron deficiency becomes more severe, a minimal regenerative response is present. Microcytic erythrocytes form when iron becomes limiting because erythroid cells apparently undergo additional divisions, resulting in smaller-than-normal cells. If sufficient time has elapsed for these small cells to account for a substantial portion of the total erythrocyte population, the MCV will decrease below the normal reference interval. When the MCV is only slightly decreased, the MCHC is usually normal. When the MCV is substantially below normal, the MCHC will also be decreased.[204] Erythrocytes in these microcytic hypochromic anemias will appear hypochromic (pale cells with prominent areas of central pallor) on stained blood films. A low MCHC is seldom present and hypochromasia is usually not apparent in stained blood films from iron-deficient horses and adult cats. Hematologic aspects of iron deficiency are compared to the anemia of inflammatory disease in Table 4-1.

Milk contains little iron; consequently nursing animals can deplete body iron stores as they grow. Microcytic erythrocytes are produced in response to iron deficiency, but a low MCV may not develop postnatally in species such as dogs and cats in which the MCV is above adult values at birth. The potential for development of severe iron deficiency in young animals appears to be less in species that begin to eat food at an early age. Piglets are especially susceptible to the development of iron deficiency when they are not raised on dirt; thus the practice of iron injections of piglets.[204]

Prolonged copper deficiency usually results in anemia in mammals. Because copper is required for normal iron

TABLE 4-1

Laboratory Findings in Chronic Iron-Deficiency Anemia versus the Anemia of Inflammatory Disease

Parameter	Chronic Iron Deficiency	Anemia of Inflammatory Disease
HCT	Slight to marked decrease	Slight to moderate decrease
MCV	Slight to marked decrease	Normal to slight decrease
Serum iron	Slight to marked decrease	Slight to moderate decrease
Serum TIBC	Normal to increased	Normal to decreased
Serum ferritin	Decreased	Normal to increased
Marrow hemosiderin	Decreased or absent	Normal to increased

HCT, Hematocrit; MCV, mean cell volume; TIBC, total iron-binding capacity.

metabolism, the anemia that develops is generally microcytic, but it may be normocytic. Pyridoxine (vitamin B_6) is required for the first step in heme synthesis. While natural cases of pyridoxine deficiency have not been documented in domestic animals, microcytic anemias with high serum iron values have been produced experimentally in dogs, cats, and pigs with dietary pyridoxine deficiency.[205]

Nonregenerative Immune-Mediated Anemia

Erythroid cellularity in the marrow varies from hypocellular to hypercellular in dogs and cats with nonregenerative immune-mediated anemia. Erythroid maturation may be complete to the polychromatophilic erythrocyte stage or a maturation arrest may occur at an earlier stage of erythrocyte development.[244,261,454,517] A nonregenerative immune-mediated anemia with maturation arrest has also been reported in a ferret.[294] An antibody or cell-mediated response may be directed against one or more maturation antigens present on nucleated erythrocyte precursors and/or reticulocytes. Erythroid hypoplasia occurs when the immune response is directed at earlier stages of erythroid development.[517]

Selective Erythroid Aplasia

Pure red cell aplasia or selective erythroid aplasia can result in severe anemia in dogs and cats. Most cases appear to be acquired, but congenital erythroid aplasia may occur in dogs.[320] Some cases in adult dogs and cats appear to be immune-mediated.[511,517] Selective erythroid aplasia occurs in cats infected with FeLV subgroup C, but not in cats infected only with subgroups A or B.[155] Colony-forming-unit-erythrocyte (CFU-E) numbers are markedly decreased but burst-forming-unit-erythrocyte (BFU-E) numbers are normal in infected cats.[1] FeLV-C binds to a heme exporter on bone marrow CFU-E cells, and it is hypothesized that this binding inhibits heme export from these cells, resulting in their destruction because free heme is toxic to cells.[381] High doses of chloramphenicol cause reversible erythroid hypoplasia in some dogs and erythroid aplasia in cats.[205] Marked erythroid hypoplasia has been reported in dogs, cats, and horses given recombinant human EPO.[106,369] Antibodies made against this human recombinant glycoprotein apparently cross-react with the animals' endogenous EPO.[369] A recombinant cat EPO produced in a hamster cell line has also caused erythroid aplasia in cats.[386]

Dyserythropoiesis

The term *dyserythropoiesis* refers to various disorders in which abnormal erythrocyte maturation and/or morphology is associated with ineffective erythropoiesis (see dyserythropoiesis section in Chapter 9). Dyserythropoiesis is a prominent component of some congenital (presumably inherited) disorders in Hereford calves and English springer spaniel dogs.[223,447] Dyserythropoiesis has been reported in association with immune-mediated disorders, drug toxicities, and myelofibrosis.[9,518] Dyserythropoiesis with Cabot rings has been reported in a dog with a metastatic carcinoma.[286] Dyserythropoiesis may be a prominent feature of some hematopoietic neoplasms, especially erythroleukemia, and some myelodysplastic syndromes.[56,125,518] However, leukopenia and/or thrombocytopenia are usually present along with nonregenerative anemia in these latter disorders, which in cats are usually associated with FeLV infections.[56]

Nonregenerative Anemias with Leukopenia and/or Thrombocytopenia

The pattern of a pancytopenia with a nonregenerative anemia suggests a defect in the production of blood cells in bone marrow. The bone marrow may be hypocellular, with low numbers of cells (including hematopoietic precursors) present, or high numbers of abnormal cells may have replaced the normal hematopoietic precursors in marrow (myelophthisis).[520] However, pancytopenia with nonregenerative anemia may sometimes be present in disorders other than marrow hypoplasia/aplasia and myelophthisis. These disorders generally have increased numbers of macrophages (histiocytes) in bone marrow and/or peripheral tissues, and the destruction of blood cells is a component of the pathogenesis of the cytopenias in these histiocytic disorders. Histiocytic inflammatory conditions that may have accompanying pancytopenia include the terminal stage of cytauxzoonosis in cats,[50] histoplasmosis,[157] leishmaniasis,[300] and mycobacteriosis.[363] Bicytopenia or pancytopenia has been reported in dogs classified as having the hemophagocytic syndrome (activated macrophage syndrome) with greater than 2% hemophagocytic macrophages in bone marrow.[516] This syndrome develops secondary to some infectious, neoplastic, and immune-mediated conditions, but an underlying disease may not always be identified.[499,516] Cytopenias may also occur with hypersplenism, associated with splenomegaly and increased phagocytosis of blood cells by the spleen.[87,420,442,520] Hemophagocytic histiocytic sarcoma may also result in multiple cytopenias.[149,514,520] The anemia is generally nonregenerative in most of these histiocytic disorders because of accompanying inflammation (see "Anemia of Inflammatory Disease," above), but the anemia may be regenerative in response to erythrocyte phagocytosis in some histiocytic disorders.

Hypocellular/Aplastic Bone Marrow

A marrow is classified as hypoplastic when 5% to 25% of the hematopoietic space consists of bone marrow cells. Generalized necrosis may result in hypocellular marrow,[247,420,426,525] but generally fat replaces lost hematopoietic cells in hypocellular marrow. When all hematopoietic cell types—erythrocytic, granulocytic, and megakaryocytic—are absent or markedly reduced (less than 5% of the hematopoietic space consists of hemic cells), the marrow is said to be aplastic. Anemic animals with generalized marrow aplasia in which nearly all of the marrow space is occupied by fat are reported to have aplastic anemia. When only one cell line is reduced or absent, more restrictive terms, such as *granulocytic hypoplasia* or *erythroid aplasia,* are used to describe the abnormalities present. Hypocellular or aplastic bone marrow may result from insufficient numbers of stem cells, abnormalities in the hematopoietic microenvironment or abnormal humoral or cellular control of hematopoiesis. These factors are interrelated, and the specific defect in a given disorder is usually unknown.

Drug-induced causes of aplastic anemia or generalized marrow hypoplasia in animals include estrogen toxicity in dogs,[440] phenylbutazone toxicity in dogs (and possibly horses),[521] trimethoprim-sulfadiazine administration in dogs,[144] bracken fern poisoning in cattle and sheep,[496] trichloroethylene-extracted soybean meal in cattle,[180] albendazole toxicity in dogs, cats, and alpacas,[188,455] griseofulvin toxicity in cats,[402] methimazole toxicity in cats,[515] various cancer chemotherapeutic agents, immunosuppressive drugs, such as azathioprine, and radiation.[150,180,359,366,510] Thiacetarsamide, meclofenamic acid, and quinidine have also been incriminated as potential causes of aplastic anemia in dogs.[521]

In addition to exogenous estrogen injections, aplastic anemia can occur in dogs because of high levels of endogenous estrogens produced by Sertoli cell, interstitial cell, and granulosa cell tumors.[440] Functional cystic ovaries also have the potential of inducing myelotoxicity in dogs.[69] Ferrets have induced ovulations and may remain in estrus for long periods of time when they are not bred. This prolonged exposure to a high endogenous estrogen concentration can result in aplastic anemia.[258]

Acute parvovirus infections may cause transient marrow hypoplasia, but not true aplastic anemia. Parvovirus infections can cause erythroid hypoplasia, as well as myeloid hypoplasia in canine pups,[375,399] but generally only myeloid hypoplasia in adult dogs and cats.[68,272,273] Either affected animals die acutely or the bone marrow returns to normal within a week. If present, anemia is usually mild, unless GI hemorrhage is severe, because of the long erythrocyte life span. Thrombocytopenia, if present, is generally mild unless DIC occurs as part of the disease process.[184,520]

Although some degree of marrow hypoplasia and/or dysplasia often occurs in cats with FeLV infections,[103] true aplastic anemia is not a well-documented sequela,[400] but it may rarely occur.[515] Hypocellular bone marrow has been reported in experimental cats coinfected with FeLV and feline parvovirus.[289]

Dogs with acute *Ehrlichia canis* infections may spontaneously recover or develop chronic disease that generally exhibits some degree of marrow hypoplasia. Although rare, aplastic anemia may develop in association with severe chronic ehrlichiosis in dogs.[75,333,337] Natural cases of East Coast fever (*Theileria parva* infection) have been described in cattle with generalized marrow hypoplasia and pancytopenia.[305]

Aplastic anemia has been reported in five cats with chronic renal failure. These cats also exhibited prolonged anorexia and/or emaciation, and it was suggested that starvation played a role in the development of marrow aplasia in these cases.[515]

Idiopathic aplastic anemia has been reported in dogs,[497,520] cats,[515] and horses.[275,317] One case of erythroid and myeloid aplasia with normal megakaryocyte numbers has been reported in a horse; the etiology was unknown.[501] In humans, most cases of aplastic anemia are immune-mediated, and activated type-1 cytotoxic T cells have been implicated.[548] Consequently most cases of idiopathic aplastic anemia in animals may be immune-mediated, if the pathophysiology is similar to that in humans.

Congenital aplastic anemia, renal abnormalities, and skin lesions have been reported in newborn foals whose mothers were treated for equine protozoal myeloencephalitis with sulfonamides and/or pyrimethamine during pregnancy.[482] Aplastic anemia has been described in 11- and 14-day-old Holstein calves that may have also developed in utero.[19,424] An in utero toxic insult was suspected in a 9-week-old Clydesdale foal with aplastic anemia.[317] Generalized bone marrow hypoplasia has been reported in eight young standard-bred horses sired by the same stallion, suggesting an inherited etiology.[262]

Myelophthisic Disorders

Myelophthisic disorders are characterized by the replacement of normal hematopoietic cells with abnormal ones. Examples include myelogenous leukemias, lymphoid leukemias, multiple myeloma, myelodysplastic syndromes, and myelofibrosis (often associated with anemia but less often with pancytopenia). Nonregenerative anemia with leukopenia and/or thrombocytopenia are often recognized in cats infected with FeLV and less often with cats infected with FIV.[154,174] Examination of bone marrow generally reveals the presence of a myelodysplastic syndrome or less often leukemia.[154,512] Multiple cytopenias may sometimes be present secondary to the extensive metastasis of lymphomas, carcinomas, and mast cell tumors.* Myelophthisic disorders do not simply "crowd out" normal cells, but also alter the marrow microenvironment so that normal hematopoiesis is compromised. In the case of myelodysplastic syndromes, increased apoptosis probably accounts for the ineffective hematopoiesis that is present.[425]

Physiologic Anemia of Neonatal Animals

HCT and hemoglobin values increase during fetal development, reaching values near those of adult animals upon birth (Fig. 4-102). Following birth, there is a rapid decrease in these parameters during the first few weeks of life, followed by a gradual increase to adult values by 4 months of age in most species (Fig. 4-103). Factors involved in the development of the anemia of the neonate include absorption of colostral proteins during the first day of life (increases plasma volume through an osmotic effect), decreased erythrocyte production during the early neonatal period, shortened life span of erythrocytes formed in utero, and rapid growth with hemodilution resulting from total plasma volume expansion, which occurs more rapidly than the increase in total erythrocyte mass.[205]

In some species, production of erythrocytes is decreased because of low EPO concentrations at birth. The decreased stimulus for EPO production at birth may occur as a result of a placental blood transfusion that increases erythrocyte mass

*References 4, 22, 135, 154, 220, 279, 299, 420, 514, 519, 520.

immediately after birth, a rapid increase in PaO_2 associated with breathing air, and a decrease in hemoglobin O_2 affinity due to an increase in erythrocyte 2,3DPG content after birth. Although not involved in the early, rapid decrease in HCT, iron availability may limit the response to anemia in some rapidly growing animals.[204]

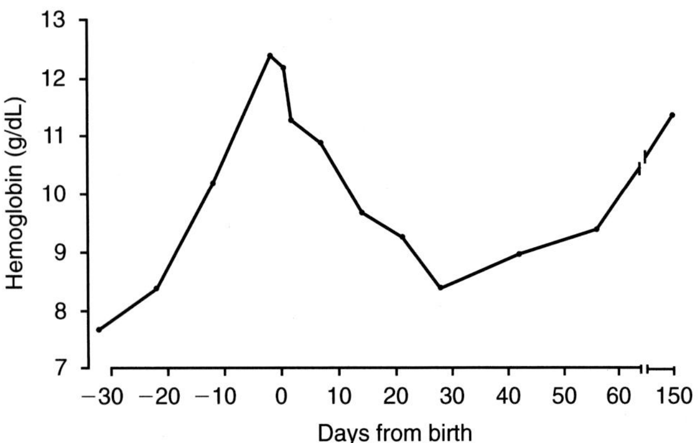

FIGURE 4-102
Blood hemoglobin values in prenatal and postnatal cats.

Data from Windle WF, Sweet M, Whitehead WH. Some aspects of prenatal and postnatal development of the blood of cats. Anat Rec. *1940;78:321.*

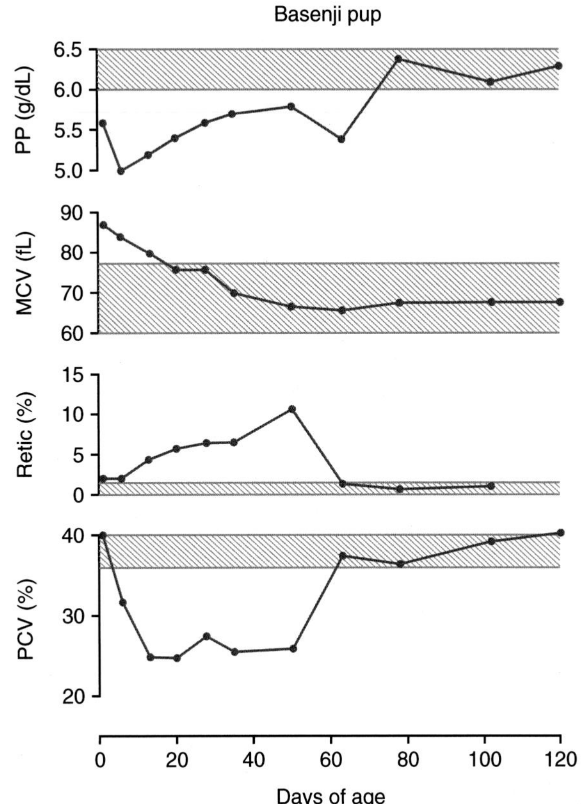

FIGURE 4-103
Age-related changes in total plasma protein (PP) concentration, mean cell volume (MCV), reticulocyte (Retic) count, and packed cell volume (PCV) in blood from a basenji dog.

ERYTHROCYTOSIS (POLYCYTHEMIA)

Erythrocytosis refers to an increase in HCT, hemoglobin, and RBC count above the normal reference interval. The reference interval can sometimes vary by breed as well as by species. The HCTs of hot-blooded horses (e.g., thoroughbreds, quarter horses, and Arabians) are usually higher than those of draft horses because of the larger spleens, relative to body weight, in the hot-blooded group.[254] Some sighthound breeds (greyhounds, whippets, Afghan hounds, and salukis) have higher HCTs than other breeds.[238,481] The reference interval for the HCT in adult greyhound dogs is reported to be 48% to 64%.[423] A reference interval of 50% to 69% was reported using blood from healthy adult whippets, Afghan hounds, and salukis.[219] In addition, slightly increased HCTs are sometimes measured in individuals from some non-sighthound breeds (i.e., poodle, German shepherd, boxer, beagle, dachshund, and Chihuahua).[238] These somewhat higher values may result from splenic contraction in animals with a high normal erythrocyte mass.

Relative Erythrocytosis

Erythrocytosis is either relative (spurious) or absolute (Box 4-6). A relative erythrocytosis is one in which the HCT is high but the total erythrocyte mass in the body is normal. It is caused by splenic contraction or dehydration. Splenic contraction results from sympathetic stimulation as occurs with excitement, fear, pain, or exercise. The HCT measured in blood from peripheral veins increases because the HCT in the spleen is considerably higher than that in the general circulation.[110,449] Splenic contraction results in higher (30% to 50%)

BOX 4-6 Erythrocytosis in Domestic Animals

Relative Erythrocytosis

1. Splenic contraction: Excitement, exercise, pain (primarily in horses, dogs, and cats)
2. Dehydration: Water loss, water deprivation, shock with fluid shift into tissues

Absolute Erythrocytosis

1. Primary erythrocytosis: A myeloproliferative neoplasm in adult dogs and cats
2. Familial erythrocytosis in young Jersey cattle: Etiology unknown
3. Hypoxemia with compensatory increased erythropoietin production: Chronic lung disease, heart disease with right-to-left shunting of blood, chronic methemoglobinemia (rare in dogs and cats)
4. Inappropriate erythropoietin production: Renal lesions (primarily tumors), nonrenal erythropoietin secreting tumors (rare)

increases in HCT in dogs, cats, and hot-blooded horses than in ruminants, pigs, or draft horses because the former group have large, contractile spleens.[449,485]

Dehydration results from increased water loss (diarrhea, vomiting, excessive diuresis, or sweating) or from water deprivation. The plasma protein concentration is also usually increased. The HCT may also be high when increased vascular permeability results in water loss from the circulation into the tissues, as occurs in endotoxic shock.[5,111,251]

Absolute Erythrocytosis

An absolute erythrocytosis is one in which the HCT is high because the total erythrocyte mass in the body is increased. Absolute erythrocytosis may occur secondary to increased EPO production (secondary erythrocytosis) or in disorders where increased erythrocyte proliferation occurs in the presence of normal or low blood EPO values (primary erythrocytosis). Causes of secondary erythrocytosis include chronic hypoxemia (heart defects with right-to-left shunting of blood,[102,323,418] diffuse lung disease,[42,367] persistent methemoglobinemia[203]), renal disorders causing local tissue hypoxia (renal tumors[74,253] and localized inflammation[248]), and tumors that secrete EPO, EPO-like proteins, or other hormones such as androgens that might enhance the effects of EPO.[104,177,256,408,546]

Primary erythrocytosis (polycythemia vera) is considered to be a myeloproliferative neoplasm that results from an autonomous (erythropoietin-independent) proliferation of erythroid precursor cells, resulting in high numbers of mature erythrocytes in blood.[358,503] In contrast to humans with polycythemia vera, blood granulocyte and platelet numbers are generally not increased in animals; consequently, in veterinary medicine, the term *primary erythrocytosis* is more appropriate than *polycythemia vera*. A diagnosis of primary erythrocytosis is ultimately made by ruling out causes of the secondary erythrocytosis.

Familial erythrocytosis (HCTs of 60% to 80%) has been described in calves from a highly inbred Jersey herd.[475] The cause of this defect was not determined. Affected calves had normal hemoglobin types and arterial blood gas values and lacked measurable EPO in plasma. The majority of the affected calves died by 6 months of age. HCTs of surviving animals returned slowly to normal by maturity. Erythrocytosis of unknown etiology has also been diagnosed in an 8-month-old Japanese black heifer.[468] A variety of familial and congenital erythrocytosis syndromes have been described in humans. They include altered hypoxia sensing, mutations in the EPO receptor gene, high-affinity hemoglobins, and 2,3DPG deficiency.[205]

Differential Diagnosis of Erythrocytosis

Splenic contraction is considered a likely cause of erythrocytosis when the HCT is slightly to moderately increased in the absence of evidence of dehydration. A slight to moderate increase in HCT with increased plasma protein concentration suggests that dehydration is present. This interpretation is confirmed by finding evidence of dehydration on physical examination.

The persistence of a moderate or marked increase in HCT suggests that an absolute erythrocytosis is present. Tests that may help determine the cause of the absolute erythrocytosis include arterial blood gas measurements, diagnostic imaging, a methemoglobin screening test, and a validated EPO test. The cytologic examination of bone marrow is not useful. When present, methemoglobinemia is easily recognized using a simple spot test (see "Methemoglobin Determination," above). The presence of low PaO_2 suggests that either a heart defect (with right-to-left shunting of blood) or chronic lung disease is present. Diagnostic imaging procedures are used to differentiate heart and lung disease and search for renal lesions and tumors. Plasma EPO values should be increased when hypoxemia, renal lesions, or EPO-secreting tumors cause the erythrocytosis, but are low when primary erythrocytosis is present. Unfortunately, there is considerable overlap among patients with primary and secondary erythrocytosis, limiting the diagnostic value of the EPO assay.[96] A diagnosis of primary erythrocytosis is reached after ruling out other potential causes of persistent erythrocytosis.

REFERENCES

1. Abkowitz JL. Retrovirus-induced feline pure red blood cell aplasia: pathogenesis and response to suramin. *Blood.* 1991;77:1442-1451.
2. Abrams K, Yunusov MY, Slichter S, et al. Recombinant human macrophage colony-stimulating factor-induced thrombocytopenia in dogs. *Br J Haematol.* 2003;121:614-622.
3. Adachi K, Makimura S. Changes in anti-erythrocyte membrane antibody level of dogs experimentally infected with *Babesia gibsoni. J Vet Med Sci.* 1992;54:1221-1223.
4. Adam F, Villiers E, Watson S, et al. Clinical pathological and epidemiological assessment of morphologically and immunologically confirmed canine leukaemia. *Vet Comp Oncol.* 2009;7:181-195.
5. Adams T Jr, Traber DL. The effects of a prostaglandin synthetase inhibitor, ibuprofen, on the cardiopulmonary response to endotoxin in sheep. *Circ Shock.* 1982;9:481-489.
6. Aird B. Acute blood loss. In: Feldman BF, Zinkl JG, Jain NC, eds. *Schalm's Veterinary Hematology,* 5th ed. Philadelphia: Lippincott Williams & Wilkins; 2000:151-153.
7. Al-Huniti NH, Widness JA, Schmidt RL, et al. Pharmacodynamic analysis of changes in reticulocyte subtype distribution in phlebotomy-induced stress erythropoiesis. *J Pharmacokinet Pharmacodyn.* 2005;32:359-376.
8. Allard RL, Carlos AD, Faltin EC. Canine hematologic changes during gestation and lactation. *Compan Anim Pract.* 1989;19:3-6.
9. Alleman AR, Harvey JW. The morphologic effects of vincristine sulfate on canine bone marrow cells. *Vet Clin Pathol.* 1993;22:36-41.
10. Allen AL, Meyers SL, Searcy GP, et al. Hematology of equine fetuses with comparisons to their dams. *Vet Clin Pathol.* 1998;27:93-100.
11. Allen BV. Relationships between the erythrocyte sedimentation rate, plasma proteins and viscosity, and leucocyte counts in thoroughbred racehorses. *Vet Rec.* 1988;122:329-332.
12. Allison RW, Fielder SE, Meinkoth JH. What is your diagnosis? Blood film from an icteric cat. *Vet Clin Pathol.* 2010;39:125-126.
13. Allison RW, Velguth KE. Appearance of granulated cells in blood films stained by automated aqueous versus methanolic Romanowsky methods. *Vet Clin Pathol.* 2010;39:99-104.
14. Allsopp MT, Cavalier-Smith T, De Waal DT, et al. Phylogeny and evolution of the piroplasms. *Parasitology.* 1994;108(Pt 2):147-152.
15. Alsaker RD, Laber J, Stevens JB, et al. A comparison of polychromasia and reticulocyte counts in assessing erythrocyte regenerative response in the cat. *J Am Vet Med Assoc.* 1977;170:39-41.
16. Altman NH. Intraerythrocytic crystalloid bodies in cats and their comparison with hemoglobinopathies of man. *Ann N Y Acad Sci.* 1974;241:589-593.

17. Altman NH, Melby EC, Squire RA. Intraerythrocytic crystalloid bodies in cats. *Blood.* 1972;39:801-803.
18. Alward A, Corriher CA, Barton MH, et al. Red maple (Acer rubrum) leaf toxicosis in horses: a retrospective study of 32 cases. *J Vet Intern Med.* 2006;20:1197-1201.
19. Ammann VJ, Fecteau G, Helie P, et al. Pancytopenia associated with bone marrow aplasia in a Holstein heifer. *Can Vet J.* 1996;37:493-495.
20. Anderson GJ, Frazer DM, McLaren GD. Iron absorption and metabolism. *Curr Opin Gastroenterol.* 2009;25:129-135.
21. Andress JL, Day TK, Day D. The effects of consecutive day propofol anesthesia on feline red blood cells. *Vet Surg.* 1995;24:277-282.
22. Angel KL, Spano JS, Schumacher J, et al. Myelophthisic pancytopenia in a pony mare. *J Am Vet Med Assoc.* 1991;198:1039-1042.
23. Anosa VO, Logan-Henfrey LL, Wells CW. The haematology of *Trypanosoma congolense* infection in cattle I. Sequential cytomorphological changes in the blood and bone marrow of Boran cattle. *Comp Haematol Int.* 1997;7:14-22.
24. Arese P, De Flora A. Denaturation of normal and abnormal erythrocytes II. Pathophysiology of hemolysis in glucose-6-phosphate dehydrogenase deficiency. *Semin Hematol.* 1990;27:1-40.
25. Aroch I, Segev G, Loeb E, et al. Peripheral nucleated red blood cells as a prognostic indicator in heatstroke in dogs. *J Vet Intern Med.* 2009;23:544-551.
26. Aronson LR, Gregory C. Possible hemolytic uremic syndrome in three cats after renal transplantation and cyclosporine therapy. *Vet Surg.* 1999;28:135-140.
27. Aslani MR, Mohri M, Movassaghi AR. Heinz body anaemia associated with onion (*Allium cepa*) toxicosis in a flock of sheep. *Comp Clin Path.* 2005;14:118-120.
28. Atwell RB, Johnstone I, Read R, et al. Haemolytic anaemia in two dogs suspected to have been induced by levamisole. *Aust Vet J.* 1979;55:292-294.
29. Aucoin DP, Peterson ME, Hurvitz AI, et al. Propylthiouracil-induced immune-mediated disease in the cat. *J Pharmacol Exp Ther.* 1985;234:13-18.
30. Azwai SM, Abdouslam OE, Al-Bassam LS, et al. Morphologic characteristics of blood cells in clinically normal adult llamas (*Lama glama*). *Veterinarski Arhiv.* 2007;77:69-79.
31. Backman L, Jonasson JB, Horstedt P. Phosphoinositide metabolism and shape control in sheep red blood cells. *Mol Membr Biol.* 1998;15:27-32.
32. Badylak SF, Van Vleet JF, Herman EH, et al. Poikilocytosis in dogs with chronic doxorubicin toxicosis. *Am J Vet Res.* 1985;46:505-508.
33. Balch A, Mackin A. Canine immune-mediated hemolytic anemia: pathophysiology, clinical signs, and diagnosis. *Compend Contin Educ Vet.* 2007;29:217-225.
34. Ban A, Ogata Y, Kato T, et al. Erythrocyte morphology and the frequency of spherocytes in hereditary erythrocyte membrane protein disorder in Japanese Black cattle. *Bull Nippon Vet Anim Sci Univ.* 1995;44:21-27.
35. Barker EN, Tasker S, Day MJ, et al. Development and use of real-time PCR to detect and quantify *Mycoplasma haemocanis* and "*Candidatus* Mycoplasma haematoparvum" in dogs. *Vet Microbiol.* 2010;140:167-170.
36. Barrows PL, Prestwood AK, Green CE. Experimental *Sarcocystis suicanis* infections: disease in growing pigs. *Am J Vet Res.* 1982;43:1409-1412.
37. Baskurt OK, Farley RA, Meiselman HJ. Erythrocyte aggregation tendency and cellular properties in horse, human, and rat: a comparative study. *Am J Physiol.* 1997;273:H2604-H2612.
38. Beaudoin S, Lanevschi A, Dunn M, et al. Peripheral blood smear from a dog [hemoglobin crystals]. *Vet Clin Pathol.* 2002;31:33-35.
39. Belford CJ, Raven CR, Black H. Chronic copper poisoning in Angora kids. *New Zealand Veterinary Journal.* 1989;37:152-154.
40. Berckmans RJ, Neiuwland R, Boing AN, et al. Cell-derived microparticles circulate in healthy humans and support low grade thrombin generation. *Thromb Haemost.* 2001;85:639-646.
41. Berman E. Hemograms of the cat during pregnancy and lactation and after lactation. *Am J Vet Res.* 1974;35:457-460.
42. Bertazzolo W, Zuliani D, Pogliani E, et al. Diffuse bronchiolo-alveolar carcinoma in a dog. *J Small Anim Pract.* 2002;43:265-268.
43. Bessis M. *Living Blood Cells and Their Ultrastructure.* New York: Springer-Verlag; 1973.
44. Bessis M, Delpech G. Sickle cell shape and structure: images and concepts (1840-1980). *Blood Cells.* 1982;8:359-435.
45. Beutler E. Disorders of iron metabolism. In: Lichtman MA, Beutler E, Kipps TJ, et al, eds. *Williams Hematology.* 7th ed. New York: McGraw-Hill; 2006:511-553.
46. Bexfield N, Archer J, Herrtage M. Heinz body haemolytic anaemia in a dog secondary to ingestion of a zinc toy: A case report. *Vet J.* 2007;174:414-417.
47. Bhasin JL, Freeman MJ, Morter RL. Properties of a cold hemagglutin associated with leptospiral hemolytic anemia of sheep. *Infect Immun.* 1971;3:398-404.
48. Birkenheuer AJ, Breitschwerdt EB, Alleman AR, et al. Differentiation of *Haemobartonella canis* and *Mycoplasma haemofelis* on the basis of comparative analysis of gene sequences. *Am J Vet Res.* 2002;63:1385-1388.
49. Birkenheuer AJ, Correa MT, Levy MG, et al. Geographic distribution of babesiosis among dogs in the United States and association with dog bites: 150 cases (2000-2003). *J Am Vet Med Assoc.* 2005;227:942-947.
50. Birkenheuer AJ, Le JA, Valenzisi AM, et al. *Cytauxzoon felis* infection in cats in the mid-Atlantic states: 34 cases (1998-2004). *J Am Vet Med Assoc.* 2006;228:568-571.
51. Birkenheuer AJ, Neel J, Ruslander D, et al. Detection and molecular characterization of a novel large *Babesia* species in a dog. *Vet Parasitol.* 2004;124:151-160.
52. Biryomumaisho S, Katunguka-Rwakishaya E. The pathogenesis of anaemia in goats experimentally infected with *Trypanosoma congolense* or *Trypanosoma brucei*: use of the myeloid:erythroid ratio. *Vet Parasitol.* 2007;143:354-357.
53. Blakley BR, Fraser LM, Waldner C. Chlorate poisoning in beef cattle. *Can Vet J.* 2007;48:1071-1073.
54. Bloom JC, Thiem PA, Sellers TS, et al. Cephalosporin-induced immune cytopenia in the dog: demonstration of erythrocyte-, neutrophil-, and platelet-associated IgG following treatment with cefazedone. *Am J Hematol.* 1988;28:71-78.
55. Blue J, Weiss L. Vascular pathways in nonsinusal red pulp—an electron microscope study of the cat spleen. *Am J Anat.* 1981;161:135-168.
56. Blue JT, French TW, Kranz JS. Non-lymphoid hematopoietic neoplasia in cats: a retrospective study of 60 cases. *Cornell Vet.* 1988;78:21-42.
57. Boas FE, Forman L, Beutler E. Phosphatidylserine exposure and red cell viability in red cell aging and in hemolytic anemia. *Proc Natl Acad Sci U S A.* 1998;95:3077-3081.
58. Boisvert AM, Tvedten HW, Scott MA. Artifactual effects of hypernatremia and hyponatremia on red cell analytes measured by the Bayer H*1 Analyzer. *Vet Clin Pathol.* 1999;28:91-96.
59. Bonfanti U, Comazzi S, Paltrinieri S, et al. Stomatocytosis in 7 related Standard Schnauzers. *Vet Clin Pathol.* 2004;33:234-239.
60. Bottomley SS. Sideroblastic anemias. In: Greer JP, Foerster J, Lukens JN, et al, eds. *Wintrobe's Clinical Hematology.* 11th ed. Philadelphia: Lippincott Williams & Williams; 2004:1011-1033.
61. Boyle AG, Magdesian KG, Ruby RE. Neonatal isoerythrolysis in horse foals and a mule foal: 18 cases (1988-2003). *J Am Vet Med Assoc.* 2005;227:1276-1283.
62. Brace RA, Langendorfer C, Song TB, et al. Red blood cell life span in the ovine fetus. *Am J Physiol Regul Integr Comp Physiol.* 2000;279:R1196-R1204.
63. Breitschwerdt EB. Feline bartonellosis and cat scratch disease. *Vet Immunol Immunopathol.* 2008;123:167-171.
64. Breitschwerdt EB, Armstrong PJ, Robinette CL, et al. Three cases of acute zinc toxicosis in dogs. *Vet Hum Toxicol.* 1986;28:109-117.
65. Bremner KC. The reticulocyte response in calves made anaemic by phlebotomy. *Aust J Exp Biol Med Sci.* 1966;44:251-258.
66. Breznock EM, Strack D. Effects of the spleen, epinephrine, and splenectomy on determination of blood volume in cats. *Am J Vet Res.* 1982;43:2062-2066.
67. Brinson JJ, Messick JB. Use of polymerase chain reaction assay for detection of *Haemobartonella canis* in a dog. *J Am Vet Med Assoc.* 2001;218:1943-1945.
68. Brock KV, Jones JB, Shull RM, et al. Effect of canine parvovirus on erythroid progenitors in phenylhydrazine-induced regenerative hemolytic anemia in dogs. *Am J Vet Res.* 1989;50:965-969.
69. Brockus CW. Endogenous estrogen myelotoxicity associated with functional cystic ovaries in a dog. *Vet Clin Pathol.* 1998;27:55-56.
70. Brown DE, Meyer DJ, Wingfield WE, et al. Echinocytosis associated with rattlesnake envenomation in dogs. *Vet Pathol.* 1994;31:654-657.
71. Brown DE, Weiser MG, Thrall MA, et al. Erythrocyte indices and volume distribution in a dog with stomatocytosis. *Vet Pathol.* 1994;31:247-250.
72. Brown HM, Berghaus RD, Latimer KS, et al. Genetic variability of *Cytauxzoon felis* from 88 infected domestic cats in Arkansas and Georgia. *J Vet Diagn Invest.* 2009;21:59-63.
73. Brown KM, Arthur JR. Selenium, selenoproteins and human health: a review. *Public Health Nutr.* 2001;4:593-599.
74. Bryan JN, Henry CJ, Turnquist SE, et al. Primary renal neoplasia of dogs. *J Vet Intern Med.* 2006;20:1155-1160.
75. Buhles WC Jr, Huxsoll DL, Hildebrandt PK. Tropical canine pancytopenia: role of aplastic anaemia in the pathogenesis of severe disease. *J Comp Pathol.* 1975;85:511-521.
76. Bull BS. Morphology of the erythron. In: Lichtman MA, Beutler E, Kipps TJ, et al, eds. *Williams Hematology.* 7th ed. New York: McGraw-Hill; 2006:369-385.
77. Caldin M, Carli E, Furlanello T, et al. A retrospective study of 60 cases of eccentrocytosis in the dog. *Vet Clin Pathol.* 2005;34:224-231.
78. Camacho AT, Guitian FJ, Pallas E, et al. *Theileria* (*Babesia*) *equi* and *Babesia caballi* infections in horses in Galicia, Spain. *Trop Anim Health Prod.* 2005;37:293-302.
79. Camacho AT, Pallas E, Gestal JJ, et al. Infection of dogs in north-west Spain with a *Babesia microti*-like agent. *Vet Rec.* 2001;149:552-555.
80. Canfield PJ, Watson ADJ. Investigations of bone marrow dyscrasia in a poodle with macrocytosis. *J Comp Pathol.* 1989;101:269-278.
81. Canfield PJ, Watson ADJ, Ratcliffe RCC. Dyserythropoiesis, sideroblasts/siderocytes and hemoglobin crystallization in a dog. *Vet Clin Pathol.* 1987;16(1):21-28.

82. Carli E, Tasca S, Trotta M, et al. Detection of erythrocyte binding IgM and IgG by flow cytometry in sick dogs with *Babesia canis canis* or *Babesia canis vogeli* infection. *Vet Parasitol.* 2009;162:51-57.
83. Cazzola M, Guarnone R, Cerani P, et al. Red blood cell precursor mass as an independent determinant of serum erythropoietin level. *Blood.* 1998;91:2139-2145.
84. Cebulj-Kadunc N, Bozic M, Kosec M, et al. The influence of age and gender on haematological parameters in Lipizzan horses. *J Vet Med A Physiol Pathol Clin Med.* 2002;49:217-221.
85. Center SA, Crawford MA, Guida L, et al. A retrospective study of 77 cats with severe hepatic lipidosis: 1975-1990. *J Vet Intern Med.* 1993;7:349-359.
86. Chandler FW, Prasse KW, Callaway CS. Surface ultrastructure of pyruvate kinase-deficient erythrocytes in the basenji dog. *Am J Vet Res.* 1975;36:1477-1480.
87. Chen Y, Zhang Q, Liao Y, et al. A modified canine model of portal hypertension with hypersplenism. *Scand J Gastroenterol.* 2009;44:478-485.
88. Chomel BB, Boulouis HJ, Maruyama S, et al. *Bartonella* spp. in pets and effect on human health. *Emerg Infect Dis.* 2006;12:389-394.
89. Christopher MM. Relation of endogenous Heinz bodies to disease and anemia in cats: 120 cases (1978-1987). *J Am Vet Med Assoc.* 1989;194:1089-1095.
90. Christopher MM, Broussard JD, Peterson ME. Heinz body formation associated with ketoacidosis in diabetic cats. *J Vet Intern Med.* 1995;9:24-31.
91. Christopher MM, Lee SE. Red cell morphologic alterations in cats with hepatic disease. *Vet Clin Pathol.* 1994;23:7-12.
92. Christopher MM, Perman V, Eaton JW. Contribution of propylene glycol-induced Heinz body formation to anemia in cats. *J Am Vet Med Assoc.* 1989;194:1045-1056.
93. Cohen LA, Gutierrez L, Weiss A, et al. Serum ferritin is derived primarily from macrophages through a nonclassical secretory pathway. *Blood.* 2010;116:1574-1584.
94. Cohen WD, Terwilliger NB. Marginal bands in camel erythrocytes. *J Cell Sci.* 1979;36:97-107.
95. Congbin Y, Aibin L, Congli Y, et al. Overexpression of complement receptor type I (CR1, CD35) on erythrocytes in patients with hemoplasma infection. *Microbiol Immunol.* 2010;54:460-465.
96. Cook SM, Lothrop CD Jr. Serum erythropoietin concentrations measured by radioimmunoassay in normal, polycythemic, and anemic dogs and cats. *J Vet Intern Med.* 1994;8:18-25.
97. Cooper ES, Wellman ML, Carsillo ME. Hyperalbuminemia associated with hepatocellular carcinoma in a dog. *Vet Clin Pathol.* 2009;38:516-520.
98. Cooper RA, Diloy-Puray M, Lando P, et al. An analysis of lipoproteins, bile acids, and red cell membranes associated with target cells and spur cells in patients with liver disease. *J Clin Invest.* 1972;51:3182-3192.
99. Cooper RA, Leslie MH, Knight D, et al. Red cell cholesterol enrichment and spur cell anemia in dogs fed a cholesterol-enriched atherogenic diet. *J Lipid Res.* 1980;21:1082-1089.
100. Corn SC, Wellman ML, Burkhard MJ, et al. IgM paraprotein interference with hemoglobin measurement using the CELL-DYN 3500. *Vet Clin Pathol.* 2008;37:61-65.
101. Cornelius CE. Bile pigments in fishes: a review. *Vet Clin Pathol.* 1991;20:106-115.
102. Cote E, Ettinger SJ. Long-term clinical management of right-to-left ("reversed") patent ductus arteriosus in 3 dogs. *J Vet Intern Med.* 2001;15:39-42.
103. Cotter SM. Anemia associated with feline leukemia virus infection. *J Am Vet Med Assoc.* 1979;175:1191-1194.
104. Couto CG, Boudrieau RJ, Zanjani ED. Tumor-associated erythrocytosis in a dog with nasal fibrosarcoma. *J Vet Intern Med.* 1989;3:183-185.
105. Couto CG, Kallet AJ. Preleukemic syndrome in a dog. *J Am Vet Med Assoc.* 1984;184:1389-1392.
106. Cowgill LD, James KM, Levy JK, et al. Use of recombinant human erythropoietin for management of anemia in dogs and cats with renal failure. *J Am Vet Med Assoc.* 1998;212:521-528.
107. Crystal MA, Cotter SM. Acute hemorrhage: A hematologic emergency in dogs. *Comp Cont Ed Pract Vet.* 1992;14:60-67.
108. Da Silva AS, Hoehne L, Tonin AA, et al. *Trypanosoma evansi*: levels of copper, iron and zinc in the bloodstream of infected cats. *Exp Parasitol.* 2009;123:35-38.
109. Dalir-Naghadeh B, Seifi HA, Asri RS, et al. Post-parturient haemoglobinuria in Iranian river buffaloes: a preliminary study. *Comp Clin Path.* 2006;14:225.
110. Dane DM, Hsia CC, Wu EY, et al. Splenectomy impairs diffusive oxygen transport in the lung of dogs. *J Appl Physiol.* 2006;101:289-297.
111. de Carvalho H, Matos JA, Bouskela E, et al. Vascular permeability increase and plasma volume loss induced by endotoxin was attenuated by hypertonic saline with or without dextran. *Shock.* 1999;12:75-80.
112. de la Fuente J, Atkinson MW, Naranjo V, et al. Sequence analysis of the msp4 gene of *Anaplasma ovis* strains. *Vet Microbiol.* 2007;119:375-381.
113. De Lorimier LP, Messick JB. Anemia associated with "*Candidatus* Mycoplasma haemominutum" in a feline leukemia virus-negative cat with lymphoma. *J Am Anim Hosp Assoc.* 2004;40:423-427.
114. Decker MJ, Freeman MJ, Morter RL. Evaluation of mechanisms of leptospiral hemolytic anemia. *Am J Vet Res.* 1970;31:873-878.
115. Degen M. Pseudohyperkalemia in Akitas. *J Am Vet Med Assoc.* 1987;190:541-543.
116. Delaunay J. The molecular basis of hereditary red cell membrane disorders. *Blood Rev.* 2007;21:1-20.
117. Deldar A, Lewis H, Bloom J, et al. Cephalosporin-induced changes in the ultrastructure of canine bone marrow. *Vet Pathol.* 1988;25:211-218.
118. Dell'Orco M, Bertazzolo W, Pagliaro L, et al. Hemolytic-uremic syndrome in a dog. *Vet Clin Pathol.* 2005;34:264-269.
119. DeNicola DB, Matthews JA, Fernandes PJ, et al. Comparison of reticulocyte counts with mean corpuscular volume and mean corpuscular hemoglobin concentration in anemic cats (abstract). *Vet Pathol.* 2008;45:732.
120. Desnoyers M, Hebert P. Heinz body anemia in a dog following possible naphthalene ingestion. *Vet Clin Pathol.* 1995;24:124-125.
121. Dewitt SF, Bedenice D, Mazan MR. Hemolysis and Heinz body formation associated with ingestion of red maple leaves in two alpacas. *J Am Vet Med Assoc.* 2004;225:578-583.
122. Di Terlizzi R, Gallagher PG, Mohandas N, et al. Canine elliptocytosis due to a mutant beta-spectrin. *Vet Clin Pathol.* 2009;38:52-58.
123. Dooley PC, Williams VJ. Changes in plasma volume and haematocrit in intact and splenectomized sheep during feeding. *Aust J Biol Sci.* 1976;29:533-544.
124. Dubey JP, Weisbrode SE, Speer CA, et al. Sarcocystosis in goats: clinical signs and pathologic and hematologic findings. *J Am Vet Med Assoc.* 1981;178:683-699.
125. Durando MM, Alleman AR, Harvey JW. Myelodysplastic syndrome in a quarter horse gelding. *Equine Vet J.* 1994;26:83-85.
126. Earl FL, Melveger BE, Wilson RL. The hemogram and bone marrow profile of normal neonatal and weanling beagle dogs. *Lab Anim Sci.* 1973;23:690-695.
127. Easley JR. Erythrogram and red cell distribution width of equidae with experimentally induced anemia. *Am J Vet Res.* 1985;46:2378-2384.
128. English RV, Breitschwerdt EB, Grindem CB, et al. Zollinger-Ellison syndrome and myelofibrosis in a dog. *J Am Vet Med Assoc.* 1988;192:1430-1434.
129. Ernst M, Meier D, Sonneborn HH. From IgG monoclonals to IgM-like molecules. *Hum Antibodies.* 1999;9:165-170.
130. Evans ETR. Sickling phenomenon in sheep. *Nature.* 1968;217:74-75.
131. Eyssette-Guerreau S, Bader-Meunier B, Garcon L, et al. Infantile pyknocytosis: a cause of haemolytic anaemia of the newborn. *Br J Haematol.* 2006;133:439-442.
132. Fabry TL. Mechanism of erythrocyte aggregation and sedimentation. *Blood.* 1987;70:1572-1576.
133. Fan LC, Dorner JL, Hoffman WE. Reticulocyte response and maturation in experimental acute blood loss anemia in the cat. *J Am Anim Hosp Assoc.* 1978;14:219-224.
134. Farrar RG, Klei TR. Prevalence of *Trypanosoma theileri* in Louisiana cattle. *J Parasitol.* 1990;76:734-736.
135. Feldman BF, Soares CJ, Kitchell BE, et al. Hemorrhage in a cat caused by inhibition of factor XI (plasma thromboplastin antecedent). *J Am Vet Med Assoc.* 1983;182:589-591.
136. Fernandez FR, Grindem CB. Reticulocyte response. In: Feldman BF, Zinkl JG, Jain NC, eds. *Schalm's Veterinary Hematology.* 5th ed. Philadelphia: Lippincott Williams & Wilkins; 2000:110-116.
137. Fischer TM. Role of spectrin in cross bonding of the red cell membrane. *Blood Cells.* 1988;13:377-394.
138. Fischer TM, Meloni T, Pescarmona GP, et al. Membrane cross bonding in red cells in favic crises: a missing link in the mechanism of extravascular haemolysis. *Br J Haematol.* 1985;59:159-169.
139. Fletch SM, Pinkerton PH, Brueckner PJ. The Alaskan Malamute chondrodysplasia (dwarfism—anemia) syndrome—in review. *J Am Anim Hosp Assoc.* 1975;11:353-361.
140. Flint CL, Scott MA. Do keratocytes form in EDTA-anticoagulated feline blood (abstract)? *Vet Clin Pathol.* 2009;38:E6.
141. Foley JE, Harrus S, Poland A, et al. Molecular, clinical, and pathologic comparison of two distinct strains of *Haemobartonella felis* in domestic cats. *Am J Vet Res.* 1998;59:1581-1588.
142. Foley JE, Pedersen NC. "*Candidatus* Mycoplasma haemominutum", a low-virulence epierythrocytic parasite of cats. *Int J Syst Evol Microbiol.* 2001;51:815-817.
143. Fontana V, Jy W, Ahn ER, et al. Increased procoagulant cell-derived microparticles (C-MP) in splenectomized patients with ITP. *Thromb Res.* 2008;122:599-603.
144. Fox LE, Ford S, Alleman AR, et al. Aplastic anemia associated with prolonged high-dose trimethoprim-sulfadiazine administration in two dogs. *Vet Clin Pathol.* 1993;22:89-92.
145. Frederick J, Giguère S, Butterworth K, et al. Severe phenylephrine-associated hemorrhage in five aged horses. *J Am Vet Med Assoc.* 2010;237:830-834.
146. Freise KJ, Widness JA, Schmidt RL, et al. Pharmacodynamic analysis of time-variant cellular disposition: reticulocyte disposition changes in phlebotomized sheep. *J Pharmacokinet Pharmacodyn.* 2007;34:519-547.

147. Frelier PF, Lewis RM. Hematologic and coagulation abnormalities in acute bovine sarcocystosis. *Am J Vet Res.* 1984;45:40-48.
148. Friedrichs KR, Thomas C, Plier M, et al. Evaluation of serum ferritin as a tumor marker for canine histiocytic sarcoma. *J Vet Intern Med.* 2010;24:904-911.
149. Friedrichs KR, Young KM. Histiocytic sarcoma of macrophage origin in a cat: case report with a literature review of feline histiocytic malignancies and comparison with canine hemophagocytic histiocytic sarcoma. *Vet Clin Pathol.* 2008;37:121-128.
150. Fry MM, Forman MA. 5-fluorouracil toxicity with severe bone marrow suppression in a dog. *Vet Hum Toxicol.* 2004;46:178-180.
151. Fry MM, Kirk CA. Reticulocyte indices in a canine model of nutritional iron deficiency. *Vet Clin Pathol.* 2006;35:172-181.
152. Fry MM, Kirk CA, Liggett JL, et al. Changes in hepatic gene expression in dogs with experimentally induced nutritional iron deficiency. *Vet Clin Pathol.* 2009;38:13-19.
153. Fry MM, Liggett JL, Baek SJ. Molecular cloning and expression of canine hepcidin. *Vet Clin Pathol.* 2004;33:223-227.
154. Fujino Y, Horiuchi H, Mizukoshi F, et al. Prevalence of hematological abnormalities and detection of infected bone marrow cells in asymptomatic cats with feline immunodeficiency virus infection. *Vet Microbiol.* 2009;136:217-225.
155. Fujino Y, Ohno K, Tsujimoto H. Molecular pathogenesis of feline leukemia virus-induced malignancies: insertional mutagenesis. *Vet Immunol Immunopathol.* 2008;123:138-143.
156. Furlanello T, Tasca S, Caldin M, et al. Artifactual changes in canine blood following storage, detected using the ADVIA 120 hematology analyzer. *Vet Clin Pathol.* 2006;35:42-46.
157. Gabbert NH, Campbell TW, Beiermann RL. Pancytopenia associated with disseminated histoplasmosis in a cat. *J Am Anim Hosp Assoc.* 1984;20:119-122.
158. Garon CL, Cohn LA, Scott MA. Erythrocyte survival time in Greyhounds as assessed by use of in vivo biotinylation. *Am J Vet Res.* 2010;71:1033-1038.
159. Gaunt SD. Hemolytic anemias caused by blood rickettsial agents and protozoa. In: Feldman BF, Zinkl JG, Jain NC, eds. *Schalm's Veterinary Hematology.* 5th ed. Philadelphia: Lippincott Williams & Wilkins; 2000:154-162.
160. Gedde MM, Davis DK, Huestis WH. Cytoplasmic pH and human erythrocyte shape. *Biophys J.* 1997;72:1234-1246.
161. Gelens HC, Moreau RE, Stalis IH, et al. Arteriovenous fistula of the jejunum associated with gastrointestinal hemorrhage in a dog. *J Am Vet Med Assoc.* 1993;202:1867-1868.
162. Geor RJ, Lund EM, Weiss DJ. Echinocytosis in horses: 54 cases (1990). *J Am Vet Med Assoc.* 1993;202:976-980.
163. George JW. Methemalbumin: reality and myth. *Vet Clin Pathol.* 1988;17:43-46.
164. George JW, Duncan JR. The hematology of lead poisoning in man and animals. *Vet Clin Pathol.* 1979;8:23-30.
165. George JW, Rideout BA, Griffey SM, et al. Effect of preexisting FeLV infection or FeLV and feline immunodeficiency virus coinfection on pathogenicity of the small variant of *Haemobartonella felis* in cats. *Am J Vet Res.* 2002;63:1172-1178.
166. Gerber K, Harvey JW, D'Agorne S, et al. Hemolysis, myopathy, and cardiac disease associated with hereditary phosphofructokinase deficiency in two Whippets. *Vet Clin Pathol.* 2009;38:46-51.
167. Gershwin LJ. Antinuclear antibodies in domestic animals. *Ann N Y Acad Sci.* 2005;1050:364-370.
168. Gerspach C, Hull BL, Rings DM, et al. Hematuria and transitional cell papilloma of the renal pelvis treated via unilateral nephrectomy in an alpaca. *J Am Vet Med Assoc.* 2008;232:1206-1209.
169. Giger U. Erythrocyte phosphofructokinase and pyruvate kinase deficiencies. In: Feldman BF, Zinkl JG, Jain NC, eds. *Schalm's Veterinary Hematology.* 5th ed. Philadelphia: Lippincott Williams & Wilkins; 2000:1020-1025.
170. Giger U, Amador A, Meyers-Wallen V, et al. Stomatocytosis in miniature schnauzers. *Proc ACVIM Forum.* 1988;754.
171. Giger U, Casal ML. Feline colostrum–friend or foe: maternal antibodies in queens and kittens. *J Reprod Fertil Suppl.* 1997;51:313-316.
172. Gilchrist F. Water intoxication in weaned beef calves. *Can Vet J.* 1996;37:490-491.
173. Giordano A, Salvadori M, Pieralisi C, et al. Increases in 2,3-diphosphoglycerate concentration in blood from horses with poor performance due to respiratory disorders. *Comp Clin Path.* 2005;14:24.
174. Gleich S, Hartmann K. Hematology and serum biochemistry of feline immunodeficiency virus-infected and feline leukemia virus-infected cats. *J Vet Intern Med.* 2009;23:552-558.
175. Glomski CA, Tamburlin J, Hard R, et al. The phylogenetic odyssey of the erythrocyte. IV. The amphibians. *Histol Histopathol.* 1997;12:147-170.
176. Goes TS, Goes VS, Ribeiro MF, et al. Bovine babesiosis: anti-erythrocyte antibodies purification from the sera of naturally infected cattle. *Vet Immunol Immunopathol.* 2007;116:215-218.
177. Gold JR, Warren AL, French TW, et al. What is your diagnosis? Biopsy impression smear of a hepatic mass in a yearling Thoroughbred filly. *Vet Clin Pathol.* 2008;37:339-343.
178. Goodfellow M, Papasouliotis K, Cue S, et al. Effect of storage on microcytosis observed in dogs with portosystemic vascular anomalies. *Res Vet Sci.* 2008;84:490-493.
179. Gookin JL, Bunch SE, Rush LJ, et al. Evaluation of microcytosis in 18 Shibas. *J Am Vet Med Assoc.* 1998;212:1258-1259.
180. Gossett KA. Anemias associated with drugs and chemicals. In: Feldman BF, Zinkl JG, Jain NC, eds. *Schalm's Veterinary Hematology.* 5th ed. Philadelphia: Lippincott Williams & Wilkins; 2000:185-189.
181. Gossett KA, MacWilliams PS, Fulton RW. Viral inclusions in hematopoietic precursors in a dog with distemper. *J Am Vet Med Assoc.* 1982;181:387-388.
182. Gray HE, Weigand CM, Cottrill NB, et al. Polycythemia vera in a dog presenting with uveitis. *J Am Anim Hosp Assoc.* 2003;39:355-360.
183. Green RA. Spurious platelet effects on erythrocyte indices using the Cell-Dyne 3500 Automated Hematology System. *Vet Clin Pathol.* 1999;28:47-49.
184. Greene CE, Addie DD. Feline parvovirus infections. In: Greene CE, ed. *Infectious Diseases of the Dog and Cat.* 3rd ed. Philadelphia: Saunders Elsevier; 2006:78-88.
185. Greene CE, Meinkoth J, Kocan AA. Cytauxzoonosis. In: Greene CE, ed. *Infectious Diseases of the Dog and Cat.* 3rd ed. St. Louis: Saunders Elsevier; 2006:716-722.
186. Greenwalt TJ. The how and why of exocytic vesicles. *Transfusion.* 2006;46:143-152.
187. Groebel K, Hoelzle K, Wittenbrink MM, et al. *Mycoplasma suis* invades porcine erythrocytes. *Infect Immun.* 2009;77:576-584.
188. Gruntman A, Nolen-Walston R, Parry N, et al. Presumptive albendazole toxicosis in 12 alpacas. *J Vet Intern Med.* 2009;23:945-949.
189. Gulati G, Caro J. *Blood Cells: An Atlas of Morphology With Clinical Relevance.* Singapore: American Society for Clinical Pathology Press; 2007.
190. Haber MD, Tucker MD, Marr HS, et al. The detection of *Cytauxzoon felis* in apparently healthy free-roaming cats in the USA. *Vet Parasitol.* 2007;146:316-320.
191. Hackett TB, Wingfield WE, Mazzaferro EM, et al. Clinical findings associated with prairie rattlesnake bites in dogs: 100 cases (1989-1998). *J Am Vet Med Assoc.* 2002;220:1675-1680.
192. Haldane SL, Davis RM. Acute toxicity in five dogs after ingestion of a commercial snail and slug bait containing iron EDTA. *Aust Vet J.* 2009;87:284-286.
193. Hammer AS, Couto CG, Swardson C, et al. Hemostatic abnormalities in dogs with hemangiosarcoma. *J Vet Intern Med.* 1991;5:11-14.
194. Harper SB, Dertinger SD, Bishop ME, et al. Flow cytometric analysis of micronuclei in peripheral blood reticulocytes. III. An efficient method of monitoring chromosomal damage in the beagle dog. *Toxicol Sci.* 2007;100:406-414.
195. Harris RL, Cottam GL, Johnston JM, et al. The pathogenesis of abnormal erythrocyte morphology in burns. *J Trauma.* 1981;21:13-21.
196. Harvey JW. Quantitative determinations of normal horse, cat, and dog haptoglobins. *Theriogenology.* 1976;6:133-138.
197. Harvey JW. Canine hemolytic anemias. *J Am Vet Med Assoc.* 1980;176:970-974.
198. Harvey JW. Hematology tip—stains for distemper inclusions. *Vet Clin Pathol.* 1982;11:12.
199. Harvey JW. Canine bone marrow: normal hematopoiesis, biopsy techniques, and cell identification and evaluation. *Comp Cont Ed Pract Vet.* 1984;6:909-926.
200. Harvey JW. Methemoglobinemia and Heinz body hemolytic anemia. In: Bonagura JD, ed. *Kirk's Current Veterinary Therapy XII. Small Animal Practice.* Philadelphia: W.B. Saunders Co.; 1995:443-446.
201. Harvey JW. Microcytic anemias. In: Feldman BF, Zinkl JG, Jain NC, eds. *Schalm's Veterinary Hematology.* 5th ed. Philadelphia: Lippincott Williams & Wilkins; 2000:200-204.
202. Harvey JW. Hemotrophic mycoplasmosis (hemobartonellosis). In: Greene CE, ed. *Infectious Diseases of the Dog and Cat.* 3rd ed. Philadelphia: Saunders Elsevier; 2006:252-260.
203. Harvey JW. Pathogenesis, laboratory diagnosis, and clinical implications of erythrocyte enzyme deficiencies in dogs, cats, and horses. *Vet Clin Pathol.* 2006;35:144-156.
204. Harvey JW. Iron metabolism and its disorders. In: Kaneko JJ, Harvey JW, Bruss ML, eds. *Clinical Biochemistry of Domestic Animals.* 6th ed. San Diego: Academic Press; 2008:259-285.
205. Harvey JW. The erythrocyte: physiology, metabolism and biochemical disorders. In: Kaneko JJ, Harvey JW, Bruss ML, eds. *Clinical Biochemistry of Domestic Animals.* 6th ed. San Diego: Academic Press; 2008:173-240.
206. Harvey JW. Red blood cell enzyme activity. In: Vaden SL, Knoll JS, Smith FWK, et al, eds. *Blackwell's Five-Minute Veterinary Consult: Laboratory Tests and Diagnostic Procedures.* Ames, Iowa: Wiley-Blackwell; 2009:520-521.
207. Harvey JW, Asquith RL, McNulty PK, et al. Haematology of foals up to one year old. *Equine Vet J.* 1984;16:347-353.

208. Harvey JW, Asquith RL, Pate MG, et al. Haematological findings in pregnant, post-parturient and nursing mares. *Comp Haematol Int.* 1994;4:25-29.
209. Harvey JW, Clapp WL, Yao Y, et al. Microcytic hypochromic erythrocytes containing siderotic inclusions, Heinz bodies, and hemoglobin crystals in a dog (abstract). *Vet Clin Pathol.* 2007;36:313-314.
210. Harvey JW, French TW, Meyer DJ. Chronic iron deficiency anemia in dogs. *J Am Anim Hosp Assoc.* 1982;18:946-960.
211. Harvey JW, Gaskin JM. Feline haptoglobin. *Am J Vet Res.* 1978;39:549-553.
212. Harvey JW, Stockham SL, Scott MA, et al. Methemoglobinemia and eccentrocytosis in equine erythrocyte flavin adenine dinucleotide deficiency. *Vet Pathol.* 2003; 40:632-642.
213. Harvey JW, Wolfsheimer KJ, Simpson CF, et al. Pathologic sideroblasts and siderocytes associated with chloramphenicol therapy in a dog. *Vet Clin Pathol.* 1985; 14(1):36-42.
214. Hasler AH, Giger U. Serum erythropoietin values in polycythemic cats. *J Am Anim Hosp Assoc.* 1996;32:294-301.
215. Hawkey CM, Bennett PM, Gascoyne SC, et al. Erythrocyte size, number and haemoglobin content in vertebrates. *Br J Haematol.* 1991;77:392-397.
216. Helal O, Defoort C, Robert S, et al. Increased levels of microparticles originating from endothelial cells, platelets and erythrocytes in subjects with metabolic syndrome: relationship with oxidative stress. *Nutr Metab Cardiovasc Dis.* 2010; (Epub 2010 Apr 14).
217. Henson KL, Alleman AR, Fox LE, et al. Diagnosis of disseminated adenocarcinoma by bone marrow aspiration in a dog with leukoerythroblastosis and fever of unknown origin. *Vet Clin Pathol.* 1998;27:80-84.
218. Hickman MA, Rogers QR, Morris JG. Effect of diet on Heinz body formation in kittens. *Am J Vet Res.* 1990;51:475-478.
219. Hilppo M. Some haematological and clinical-chemical parameters of sight hounds (Afghan hound, saluki and whippet). *Nord Vet Med.* 1986;38:148-155.
220. Hisasue M, Nagashima N, Nishigaki K, et al. Myelodysplastic syndromes and acute myeloid leukemia in cats infected with feline leukemia virus clone33 containing a unique long terminal repeat. *Int J Cancer.* 2009;124:1133-1141.
221. Hoelzle LE. Haemotrophic mycoplasmas: recent advances in *Mycoplasma suis. Vet Microbiol.* 2008;130:215-226.
222. Hoff B, Lumsden JH, Valli VE. An appraisal of bone marrow biopsy in assessment of sick dogs. *Can J Comp Med.* 1985;49:34-42.
223. Holland CT, Canfield PJ, Watson ADJ, et al. Dyserythropoiesis, polymyopathy, and cardiac disease in three related English springer spaniels. *J Vet Intern Med.* 1991; 5:151-159.
224. Holloway S, Senior D, Roth L, et al. Hemolytic uremic syndrome in dogs. *J Vet Intern Med.* 1993;7:220-227.
225. Holman HH, Drew SM. The blood picture of the goat. II. Changes in erythrocyte shape, size and number associated with age. *Res Vet Sci.* 1964;5:274-285.
226. Holman PJ, Backlund BB, Wilcox AL, et al. Detection of a large unnamed *Babesia* piroplasm originally identified in dogs in North Carolina in a dog with no history of travel to that state. *J Am Vet Med Assoc.* 2009;235:851-854.
227. Hornok S, Meli ML, Erdos A, et al. Molecular characterization of two different strains of haemotropic mycoplasmas from a sheep flock with fatal haemolytic anaemia and concomitant *Anaplasma ovis* infection. *Vet Microbiol.* 2009;136:372-377.
228. Hunfeld KP, Hildebrandt A, Gray JS. Babesiosis: Recent insights into an ancient disease. *Int J Parasitol.* 2008;38:1219-1237.
229. Hvidberg V, Maniecki MB, Jacobsen C, et al. Identification of the receptor scavenging hemopexin-heme complexes. *Blood.* 2005;106:2572-2579.
230. Igbokwe IO, Anosa VO. Response to anaemia in experimental *Trypanosoma vivax* infection of sheep. *J Comp Pathol.* 1989;100:111-118.
231. Inaba M. Red blood cell membrane defects. In: Feldman BF, Zinkl JG, Jain NC, eds. *Schalm's Veterinary Hematology.* 5th ed. Philadelphia: Lippincott Williams & Wilkins; 2000:1012-1019.
232. Inaba M, Yawata A, Koshino I, et al. Defective anion transport and marked spherocytosis with membrane instability caused by hereditary total deficiency of red cell band 3 in cattle due to a nonsense mutation. *J Clin Invest.* 1996;97:1804-1817.
233. Iolascon A, De Falco L, Beaumont C. Molecular basis of inherited microcytic anemia due to defects in iron acquisition or heme synthesis. *Haematologica.* 2009;94: 395-408.
234. Irmak K, Sen I, Col R, et al. The evaluation of coagulation profiles in calves with suspected septic shock. *Vet Res Commun.* 2006;30:497-503.
235. Jackson JA, Chart IS, Sanderson JH, et al. Pirimicarb induced immune haemolytic anaemia in dogs. *Scand J Haematol.* 1977;19:360-366.
236. Jacobsen S, Nielsen JV, Kjelgaard-Hansen M, et al. Acute phase response to surgery of varying intensity in horses: a preliminary study. *Vet Surg.* 2009;38:762-769.
237. Jain NC. *Schalm's Veterinary Hematology.* 4th ed. Philadelphia: Lea & Febiger; 1986.
238. Jain NC. *Essentials of Veterinary Hematology*, Philadelphia: Lea & Febiger; 1993.
239. Jain NC, Kono CS. Fusiform erythrocytes in angora goats resembling sickle cells: influence of temperature, pH, and oxygenation on cell shape. *Am J Vet Res.* 1977; 38:983-990.
240. Jain NC, Kono CS, Myers A, et al. Fusiform erythrocytes resembling sickle cells in angora goats: observations on osmotic and mechanical fragilities and reversal of shape during anaemia. *Res Vet Sci.* 1980;28:25-35.
241. Jensen FB. Red blood cell pH, the Bohr effect, and other oxygenation-linked phenomena in blood O_2 and CO_2 transport. *Acta Physiol Scand.* 2004;182:215-227.
242. Jensen WA, Lappin MR, Kamkar S, et al. Use of a polymerase chain reaction assay to detect and differentiate two strains of *Haemobartonella felis* in naturally infected cats. *Am J Vet Res.* 2001;62:604-608.
243. Johnson CA, Armstrong PJ, Hauptman JG. Congenital portosystemic shunts in dogs: 46 cases (1979-1986). *J Am Vet Med Assoc.* 1987;191:1478-1483.
244. Jonas LD, Thrall MA, Weiser MG. Nonregenerative form of immune-mediated hemolytic anemia in dogs. *J Am Anim Hosp Assoc.* 1987;23:201-204.
245. Kawazu S, Kamio T, Sekizaki T, et al. *Theileria sergenti* and *T. buffeli*: polymerase chain reaction-based marker system for differentiating the parasite species from infected cattle blood and infected tick salivary gland. *Exp Parasitol.* 1995;81:430-435.
246. Kay M. Immunoregulation of cellular life span. *Ann N Y Acad Sci.* 2005;1057: 85-111.
247. Kelton DR, Holbrook TC, Gilliam LL, et al. Bone marrow necrosis and myelophthisis: manifestations of T-cell lymphoma in a horse. *Vet Clin Pathol.* 2008;37:403-408.
248. Kessler M. Secondary polycythaemia associated with high plasma erythropoietin concentrations in a dog with a necrotising pyelonephritis. *J Small Anim Pract.* 2008;49:363-366.
249. Kiefer CR, Snyder LM. Oxidation and erythrocyte senescence. *Curr Opin Hematol.* 2000;7:113-116.
250. King LG, Giger U, Diserens D, et al. Anemia of chronic renal failure in dogs. *J Vet Intern Med.* 1992;6:264-270.
251. Kirkebo A, Tyssebotn I. Renal blood flow distribution during E. coli endotoxin shock in dog. *Acta Physiol Scand.* 1980;108:367-372.
252. Kjemtrup AM, Wainwright K, Miller M, et al. *Babesia conradae*, sp. Nov., a small canine *Babesia* identified in California. *Vet Parasitol.* 2006;138:103-111.
253. Klainbart S, Segev G, Loeb E, et al. Resolution of renal adenocarcinoma-induced secondary inappropriate polycythaemia after nephrectomy in two cats. *J Feline Med Surg.* 2008;10:264-268.
254. Kline H, Foreman JH. Heart and spleen weights as a function of breed and somatotype. *Equine Exercise Physiology.* 1991;3:17-21.
255. Kocan KM, de la Fuente J, Blouin EF, et al. The natural history of *Anaplasma marginale. Vet Parasitol.* 2010;167:95-107.
256. Koch TG, Wen X, Bienzle D. Lymphoma, erythrocytosis, and tumor erythropoietin gene expression in a horse. *J Vet Intern Med.* 2006;20:1251-1255.
257. Kociba GJ. Macrocytosis. In: Feldman BF, Zinkl JG, Jain NC, eds. *Schalm's Veterinary Hematology.* 5th ed. Philadelphia: Lippincott Williams & Wilkins; 2000:196-199.
258. Kociba GJ, Caputo CA. Aplastic anemia associated with estrus in pet ferrets. *J Am Vet Med Assoc.* 1981;178:1293-1294.
259. Kohn B, Fumi C. Clinical course of pyruvate kinase deficiency in Abyssinian and Somali cats. *J Feline Med Surg.* 2008;10:145-153.
260. Kohn B, Goldschmidt MH, Hohenhaus AE, et al. Anemia, splenomegaly, and increased osmotic fragility of erythrocytes in Abyssinian and Somali cats. *J Am Vet Med Assoc.* 2000;217:1483-1491.
261. Kohn B, Weingart C, Eckmann V, et al. Primary immune-mediated hemolytic anemia in 19 cats: diagnosis, therapy, and outcome (1998-2004). *J Vet Intern Med.* 2006;20:159-166.
262. Kohn CW, Swardson C, Provost P, et al. Myeloid and megakaryocytic hypoplasia in related standardbreds. *J Vet Intern Med.* 1995;9:315-323.
263. Komatsu T, Arashiki N, Otsuka Y, et al. Extrusion of Na,K-ATPase and transferrin receptor with lipid raft-associated proteins in different populations of exosomes during reticulocyte maturation in dogs. *Jpn J Vet Res.* 2010;58:17-27.
264. Kordick DL, Breitschwerdt EB. Intraerythrocytic presence of *Bartonella henselae. J Clin Microbiol.* 1995;33:1655-1656.
265. Kosower NS. Altered properties of erythrocytes in the aged. *Am J Hematol.* 1993;42:241-247.
266. Koury MJ, Ponka P. New insights into erythropoiesis: the roles of folate, vitamin B_{12}, and iron. *Annu Rev Nutr.* 2004;24:105-131.
267. Kuehn NF, Gaunt SD. Hypocellular marrow and extramedullary hematopoiesis in a dog: hematologic recovery after splenectomy. *J Am Vet Med Assoc.* 1986;188: 1313-1315.
268. Kurata M, Nakamura H, Baba A, et al. Postprandial change in canine blood viscosity. *Comp Biochem Physiol Comp Physiol.* 1993;105:587-592.
269. Laber J, Perman V, Stevens JB. Polychromasia or reticulocytes—an assessment of the dog. *J Am Anim Hosp Assoc.* 1974;10:399-406.
270. Lang F, Gulbins E, Lerche H, et al. Eryptosis, a window to systemic disease. *Cell Physiol Biochem.* 2008;22:373-380.
271. Lang F, Lang KS, Lang PA, et al. Mechanisms and significance of eryptosis. *Antioxid Redox Signal.* 2006;8:1183-1192.

272. Langheinrich KA, Nielsen SW. Histopathology of feline panleukopenia: a report of 65 cases. *J Am Vet Med Assoc.* 1971;158:863-872.
273. Larsen S, Flagstad A, Aalbaek B. Experimental panleukopenia in the conventional cat. *Vet Pathol.* 1976;13:216-240.
274. Lau AO. An overview of the *Babesia, Plasmodium* and *Theileria* genomes: a comparative perspective. *Mol Biochem Parasitol.* 2009;164:1-8.
275. Lavoie JP, Morris DD, Zinkl JG, et al. Pancytopenia caused by marrow aplasia in a horse. *J Am Vet Med Assoc.* 1987;191:1462-1464.
276. Lee KW, Yamato O, Tajima M, et al. Hematologic changes associated with the appearance of eccentrocytes after intragastric administration of garlic extract to dogs. *Am J Vet Res.* 2000;61:1446-1450.
277. Lee TH, Kim SU, Yu SL, et al. Peroxiredoxin II is essential for sustaining life span of erythrocytes in mice. *Blood.* 2003;101:5033-5038.
278. Leighton FA, Peakall DB, Butler RG. Heinz body hemolytic anemia from the ingestion of crude oil: a primary toxic effect in marine birds. *Science.* 1983;220:871-873.
279. Lester GD, Alleman AR, Raskin RE, et al. Pancytopenia secondary to lymphoid leukemia in three horses. *J Vet Intern Med.* 1993;7:360-363.
280. Levy JK, Bunch SE, Komtebedde J. Feline portosystemic vascular shunts. In: Bondagura JD, ed. *Kirk's Current Veterinary Therapy XII. Small Animal Practice.* Philadelphia: W.B. Saunders; 1995:743-749.
281. Lewis HB, Rebar AH. *Bone Marrow Evaluation in Veterinary Practice.* St. Louis: Ralston Purina Co.; 1979.
282. Lifton SJ, King LG, Zerbe CA. Glucocorticoid deficient hypoadrenocorticism in dogs: 18 cases (1986-1995). *J Am Vet Med Assoc.* 1996;209:2076-2081.
283. Lim WS, Payne SL, Edwards JF, et al. Differential effects of virulent and avirulent equine infectious anemia virus on macrophage cytokine expression. *Virology.* 2005;332:295-306.
284. Littman MP, Niebauer GW, Hendrick MJ. Macrohematuria and life-threatening anemia attributable to subepithelial vascular ectasia of the urinary bladder in a dog. *J Am Vet Med Assoc.* 1990;196:1487-1489.
285. Low FM, Hampton MB, Peskin AV, et al. Peroxiredoxin 2 functions as a noncatalytic scavenger of low-level hydrogen peroxide in the erythrocyte. *Blood.* 2007;109: 2611-2617.
286. Lukaszewska J, Lewandowski K. Cabot rings as a result of severe dyserythropoiesis in a dog. *Vet Clin Pathol.* 2008;37:180-183.
287. Lund JE. Hemoglobin crystals in canine blood. *Am J Vet Res.* 1974;35:575-577.
288. Lund JE, Brown PK. Hypersegmented megakaryocytes and megakaryocytes with multiple separate nuclei in dogs treated with PNU-100592, an oxazolidinone antibiotic. *Toxicol Pathol.* 1997;25:339-343.
289. Lutz H, Castelli I, Ehrensperger F, et al. Panleukopenia-like syndrome of FeLV caused by co-infection with FeLV and feline panleukopenia virus. *Vet Immunol Immunopathol.* 1995;46:21-33.
290. Mackey L, Jarrett W, Jarrett O, et al. Anemia associated with feline leukemia virus infection in cats. *J Natl Cancer Inst.* 1975;54:209-217.
291. MacWilliams P, Meadows R. Unpublished case submitted to the 1993 ASVCP microscopic slide review. 1993, personal communication.
292. MacWilliams PS, Searcy GP, Bellamy JEC: Bovine postparturient hemoglobinuria: a review of the literature. *Can Vet J.* 1982;23:309-312.
293. Mahaffey EA, George JW, Duncan JR, et al. Hematologic values in calves infected with *Sarcocystis cruzi. Vet Parasitol.* 1986;19:275-280.
294. Malka S, Hawkins MG, Zabolotzky SM, et al. Immune-mediated pure red cell aplasia in a domestic ferret. *J Am Vet Med Assoc.* 2010;237:695-700.
295. Mandal D, Mazumder A, Das P, et al. Fas-, caspase 8-, and caspase 3-dependent signaling regulates the activity of the aminophospholipid translocase and phosphatidylserine externalization in human erythrocytes. *J Biol Chem.* 2005;280: 39460-39467.
296. Mandell CP, Jain NC, Farver TB. The significance of normoblastemia and leukoerythroblastic reaction in the dog. *J Am Anim Hosp Assoc.* 1989;25:665-672.
297. March H, Barger A, McCullough S, et al. Use of the ADVIA 120 for differentiating extracellular and intracellular hemoglobin. *Vet Clin Pathol.* 2005;34:106-109.
298. Marchetti V, Benetti C, Citi S, et al. Paraneoplastic hypereosinophilia in a dog with intestinal T-cell lymphoma. *Vet Clin Pathol.* 2005;34:259-263.
299. Marconato L, Bettini G, Giacoboni C, et al. Clinicopathological features and outcome for dogs with mast cell tumors and bone marrow involvement. *J Vet Intern Med.* 2008;22:1001-1007.
300. Marcos R, Santos M, Malhao F, et al. Pancytopenia in a cat with visceral leishmaniasis. *Vet Clin Pathol.* 2009;38:201-205.
301. Marks SL, Mannella C, Schaer M. Coral snake envenomation in the dog: Report of four cases and review of the literature. *J Am Anim Hosp Assoc.* 1990;26:629-634.
302. Masini AP, Baragli P, Tedeschi D, et al. Behavior of mean erythrocyte volume during submaximal treadmill exercise in the horse. *Comp Haematol Int.* 2000;10:38-42.
303. Masserdotti C. Unusual "erythroid loops" in canine blood smears after viper-bite envenomation. *Vet Clin Pathol.* 2009;38:321-325.
304. Matthews NS, Brown RM, Barling KS, et al. Repetitive propofol administration in dogs and cats. *J Am Anim Hosp Assoc.* 2004;40:255-260.
305. Mbassa GK, Balemba O, Maselle RM, et al. Severe anaemia due to haematopoietic precursor cell destruction in field cases of East Coast Fever in Tanzania. *Vet Parasitol.* 1994;52:243-256.
306. McConnico RS, Roberts MC, Tompkins M. Penicillin-induced immune-mediated hemolytic anemia in a horse. *J Am Vet Med Assoc.* 1992;201:1402-1403.
307. McDonnell AM, Holmes LA. Haemoglobinuria due to *Clostridium perfringens* type A mastitis in a ewe. *Br Vet J.* 1990;146:380-381.
308. McGuire TC, Henson JB, Quist SE. Impaired bone marrow response in equine infectious anemia. *Am J Vet Res.* 1969;30:2099-2104.
309. McKeever KH, Hinchcliff KW, Reed SM, et al. Role of decreased plasma volume in hematocrit alterations during incremental treadmill exercise in horses. *Am J Physiol.* 1993;265:R404-R408.
310. McLaughlin BG, Adams PS, Cornell WD, et al. Canine distemper viral inclusions in blood cells of four vaccinated dogs. *Can Vet J.* 1985;26:368-372.
311. Medaille C, Briend-Marchal A, Braun JP. Stability of selected hematology variables in canine blood kept at room temperature in EDTA for 24 and 48 hours. *Vet Clin Pathol.* 2006;35:18-23.
312. Medinger TL, Williams DA, Bruyette DS. Severe gastrointestinal tract hemorrhage in three dogs with hypoadrenocorticism. *J Am Vet Med Assoc.* 1993;202: 1869-1872.
313. Melendez RD, Toro BM, Niccita G, et al. Humoral immune response and hematologic evaluation of pregnant Jersey cows after vaccination with *Anaplasma centrale. Vet Microbiol.* 2003;94:335-339.
314. Messick JB. Hemotrophic mycoplasmas (hemoplasmas): a review and new insights into pathogenic potential. *Vet Clin Pathol.* 2004;33:2-13.
315. Messick JB, Walker PG, Raphael W, et al. "*Candidatus* Mycoplasma haemodidelphidis" sp. nov., "*Candidatus* Mycoplasma haemolamae" sp. nov. and *Mycoplasma haemocanis* comb. nov., haemotrophic parasites from a naturally infected opossum (*Didelphis virginiana*), alpaca (*Lama pacos*) and dog (*Canis familiaris*): phylogenetic and secondary structural relatedness of their 16S rRNA genes to other mycoplasmas. *Int J Syst Evol Microbiol.* 2002;52:693-698.
316. Middleton JR, Katz L, Angelos JA, et al. Hemolysis associated with water administration using a nipple bottle for human infants in juvenile pygmy goats. *J Vet Intern Med.* 1997;11:382-384.
317. Milne EM, Pyrah ITG, Smith KC, et al. Aplastic anemia in a Clydesdale foal: a case report. *J Equine Vet Sci.* 1995;15:129-131.
318. Moltmann UG, Mehlhorn H, Schein E, et al. Fine structure of *Babesia equi* Laveran, 1901 within lymphocytes and erythrocytes of horses: an in vivo and in vitro study. *J Parasitol.* 1983;69:111-120.
319. Monreal L, Villatoro AJ, Monreal M, et al. Comparison of the effects of low-molecular-weight and unfractioned heparin in horses. *Am J Vet Res.* 1995;56:1281-1285.
320. Moore AH, Day MJ, Graham MW. Congenital pure red blood cell aplasia (Diamond-Blackfan anaemia) in a dog. *Vet Rec.* 1993;132:414-415.
321. Moore DM. Hematology of camelid species: llamas and camels. In: Feldman BF, Zinkl JG, Jain NC, eds. *Schalm's Veterinary Hematology.* 5th ed. Philadelphia: Lippincott Williams & Wilkins; 2000:1184-1190.
322. Moore JN, Mahaffey EA, Zboran M. Heparin-induced agglutination of erythrocytes in horses. *Am J Vet Res.* 1987;48:68-71.
323. Moore KW, Stepien RL. Hydroxyurea for treatment of polycythemia secondary to right-to-left shunting patent ductus arteriosus in 4 dogs. *J Vet Intern Med.* 2001;15:418-421.
324. Moore PF, Affolter VK, Vernau W. Canine hemophagocytic histiocytic sarcoma: a proliferative disorder of CD11d+ macrophages. *Vet Pathol.* 2006;43:632-645.
325. Morgan RV, Moore FM, Pearce LK, et al. Clinical and laboratory findings in small companion animals with lead poisoning: 347 cases (1977-1986). *J Am Vet Med Assoc.* 1991;199:93-97.
326. Morin DE, Garry FB, Weiser MG. Hematologic responses in llamas with experimentally-induced iron deficiency anemia. *Vet Clin Pathol.* 1993;22:81-85.
327. Morris JG, Cripe WS, Chapman HL, et al. Selenium deficiency in cattle associated with Heinz bodies and anemia. *Science.* 1984;223:491-493.
328. Muller-Soyano A, Platt O, Glader BE. Pyruvate kinase deficiency in dog and human erythrocytes: effects of energy depletion on cation composition and cellular hydration. *Am J Hematol.* 1986;23:217-221.
329. Munoz A, Riber C, Santisteban R, et al. Cardiovascular and metabolic adaptations in horses competing in cross-country events. *J Vet Med Sci.* 1999;61:13-20.
330. Murase T, Maede Y. Increased erythrophagocytic activity of macrophages in dogs with *Babesia gibsoni* infection. *Nippon Juigaku Zasshi.* 1990;52:321-327.
331. Musaji A, Cormont F, Thirion G, et al. Exacerbation of autoantibody-mediated thrombocytopenic purpura by infection with mouse viruses. *Blood.* 2004;104:2102-2106.
332. Myers S, Wiks K, Giger U. Macrocytic anemia caused by naturally occurring folate-deficiency in the cat (abstract). *Vet Clin Pathol.* 1996;25:30.
333. Mylonakis ME, Day MJ, Siarkou V, et al. Absence of myelofibrosis in dogs with myelosuppression induced by *Ehrlichia canis* infection. *J Comp Pathol.* 2010;142:328-331.

334. Nakage AP, Santana AE, de Capua ML, et al. Characterization and quantification of blood cells from the umbilical cord of dogs. *Vet Clin Pathol.* 2005;34:394-396.
335. Nantakomol D, Imwong M, Soontarawirat I, et al. The absolute counting of red cell-derived microparticles with red cell bead by flow rate based assay. *Cytometry B Clin Cytom.* 2009;76:191-198.
336. Neath PJ, Brockman DJ, Saunders HM. Retrospective analysis of 19 cases of isolated torsion of the splenic pedicle in dogs. *J Small Anim Pract.* 1997;38: 387-392.
337. Neer TM, Harrus S. Canine monocytotropic ehrlichiosis and neorickettsiosis (*E. canis, E. chaffeensis, E. ruminatium, N. sennetsu,* and *N. risticii* infections). In: Greene CE, ed. *Infectious Diseases of the Dog and Cat.* 3rd ed. St. Louis: Saunders Elsevier; 2006:203-219.
338. Neiger R, Hadley J, Pfeiffer DU. Differentiation of dogs with regenerative and non-regenerative anaemia on the basis of their red cell distribution width and mean corpuscular volume. *Vet Rec.* 2002;150:431-434.
339. Neimark H, Hoff B, Ganter M. *Mycoplasma ovis* comb. nov. (formerly *Eperythrozoon ovis*), an epierythrocytic agent of haemolytic anaemia in sheep and goats. *Int J Syst Evol Microbiol.* 2004;54:365-371.
340. Neimark H, Johansson KE, Rikihisa Y, et al. Proposal to transfer some members of the genera *Haemobartonella* and *Eperythrozoon* to the genus *Mycoplasma* with descriptions of "*Candidatus* Mycoplasma haemofelis", "*Candidatus* Mycoplasma haemomuris", "*Candidatus* Mycoplasma haemosuis" and "*Candidatus* Mycoplasma wenyonii". *Int J Syst Evol Microbiol.* 2001;51:891-899.
341. Nemeth E, Tuttle MS, Powelson J, et al. Hepcidin regulates cellular iron efflux by binding to ferroportin and inducing its internalization. *Science.* 2004;306: 2090-2093.
342. Ng CY, Mills JN. Clinical and haematological features of haemangiosarcoma in dogs. *Aust Vet J.* 1985;62:1-4.
343. Nishizawa I, Sato M, Fujihara M, et al. Differential detection of hemotropic *Mycoplasma* species in cattle by melting curve analysis of PCR products. *J Vet Med Sci.* 2010;72:77-79.
344. Noble SJ, Armstrong PJ. Bee sting envenomation resulting in secondary immune-mediated hemolytic anemia in two dogs. *J Am Vet Med Assoc.* 1999;214: 1021-1026.
345. Noris M, Remuzzi G. Hemolytic uremic syndrome. *J Am Soc Nephrol.* 2005;16: 1035-1050.
346. Noris M, Remuzzi G. Atypical hemolytic-uremic syndrome. *N Engl J Med.* 2009;361: 1676-1687.
347. Norman TE, Chaffin MK, Johnson MC, et al. Intravascular hemolysis associated with severe cutaneous burn injuries in five horses. *J Am Vet Med Assoc.* 2005;226: 2039-2043.
348. O'Keefe DA, Schaeffer DJ. Hematologic toxicosis associated with doxorubicin administration in cats. *J Vet Intern Med.* 1992;6:276-283.
349. Ohgami RS, Campagna DR, Greer EL, et al. Identification of a ferrireductase required for efficient transferrin-dependent iron uptake in erythroid cells. *Nat Genet.* 2005;37:1264-1269.
350. Oishi A, Sakamoto H, Shimizu R. Canine plasma erythropoietin levels in 124 cases of anemia. *J Vet Med Sci.* 1995;57:747-749.
351. Oishi A, Sakamoto H, Shimizu R, et al. Evaluation of phlebotomy-induced erythropoietin production in the dog. *J Vet Med Sci.* 1993;55:51-58.
352. Okabe J, Tajima S, Yamato O, et al. Hemoglobin types, erythrocyte membrane skeleton and plasma iron concentration in calves with poikilocytosis. *J Vet Med Sci.* 1996;58:629-634.
353. Omer OH, El Malik KH, Mahmoud OM, et al. Haematological profiles in pure bred cattle naturally infected with *Theileria annulata* in Saudi Arabia. *Vet Parasitol.* 2002;107:161-168.
354. Pak M, Lopez MA, Gabayan V, et al. Suppression of hepcidin during anemia requires erythropoietic activity. *Blood.* 2006;108:3730-3735.
355. Paltrinieri S, Comazzi S, Ceciliani F, et al. Stomatocytosis of Standard Schnauzers is not associated with stomatin deficiency. *Vet J.* 2007;173:202-205.
356. Paltrinieri S, Preatoni M, Rossi S. Microcytosis does not predict serum iron concentrations in anaemic dogs. *Vet J.* 2010;185:341-343.
357. Panciera DL. Conditions associated with canine hypothyroidism. *Vet Clin North Am Small Anim Pract.* 2001;31:935-950.
358. Patnaik MM, Tefferi A. The complete evaluation of erythrocytosis: congenital and acquired. *Leukemia.* 2009;23:834-844.
359. Paul AL, Shaw SP, Bandt C. Aplastic anemia in two kittens following a prescription error. *J Am Anim Hosp Assoc.* 2008;44:25-31.
360. Pechereau D, Martel P, Braun JP. Plasma erythropoietin concentrations in dogs and cats: reference values and changes with anaemia and/or chronic renal failure. *Res Vet Sci.* 1997;62:185-188.
361. Pechereau D, Martel P, Braun JP. Plasma erythropoietin concentrations in dogs and cats: reference values and changes with anaemia and/or chronic renal failure. *Res Vet Sci.* 1997;62:185-188.
362. Penzhorn BL, Schoeman T, Jacobson LS. Feline babesiosis in South Africa: a review. *Ann N Y Acad Sci.* 2004;1026:183-186.
363. Perkins PC, Grindem CB, Levy JK. What is your diagnosis? Mycobacteriosis. *Vet Clin Pathol.* 1995;24:77.
364. Perman V, Schall WD. Diseases of the red cells. In: Ettinger SJ, ed. *Textbook of Veterinary Internal Medicine: Diseases of the Dog and Cat.* 2nd ed. Philadelphia: W.B. Saunders Co; 1983:1938-2000.
365. Peterson ME, Kintzer PP, Cavanaugh PG, et al. Feline hyperthyroidism : pretreatment clinical and laboratory evaluation of 131 cases. *J Am Vet Med Assoc.* 1983;183: 103-110.
366. Phillips B. Severe, prolonged bone marrow hypoplasia secondary to the use of carboplatin in an azotemic dog. *J Am Vet Med Assoc.* 1999;215:1250-1252.
367. Phillips S, Barr S, Dykes N, et al. Bronchiolitis obliterans with organizing pneumonia in a dog. *J Vet Intern Med.* 2000;14:204-207.
368. Piek CJ, Junius G, Dekker A, et al. Idiopathic immune-mediated hemolytic anemia: treatment outcome and prognostic factors in 149 dogs. *J Vet Intern Med.* 2008;22:366-373.
369. Piercy RJ, Swardson CJ, Hinchcliff KW. Erythroid hypoplasia and anemia following administration of recombinant human erythropoietin to two horses. *J Am Vet Med Assoc.* 1998;212:244-247.
370. Plier M. Unpublished studies. 2000, personal communication.
371. Polkes AC, Giguère S, Lester GD, et al. Factors associated with outcome in foals with neonatal isoerythrolysis (72 cases, 1988-2003). *J Vet Intern Med.* 2008;22: 1216-1222.
372. Ponka P, Beaumont C, Richardson DR. Function and regulation of transferrin and ferritin. *Semin Hematol.* 1998;35:35-54.
373. Ponka P, Richardson DR. Can ferritin provide iron for hemoglobin synthesis? *Blood.* 1997;89:2611-2612.
374. Porter RE, Weiser MG. Effect of immune-mediated erythrocyte agglutination on analysis of canine blood using a multichannel blood cell counting system. *Vet Clin Pathol.* 1990;19:45-50.
375. Potgieter LN, Jones JB, Patton CS, et al. Experimental parvovirus infection in dogs. *Can J Comp Med.* 1981;45:212-216.
376. Potocnik SJ, Wintour EM. Development of the spleen as a red blood cell reservoir in lambs. *Reprod Fertil Dev.* 1996;8:311-315.
377. Poyart C, Wajcman H, Kister J. Molecular adaptation of hemoglobin function in mammals. *Respir Physiol.* 1992;90:3-17.
378. Prasse KW, Crouser D, Beutler E, et al. Pyruvate kinase deficiency anemia with terminal myelofibrosis and osteosclerosis in a beagle. *J Am Vet Med Assoc.* 1975;166:1170-1175.
379. Prchal JT. Production of erythrocytes. In: Lichtman MA, Beutler E, Kipps TJ, et al, eds. *Williams Hematology.* 7th ed. New York: McGraw-Hill; 2006:393-403.
380. Pusterla N, Fecteau ME, Madigan JE, et al. Acute hemoperitoneum in horses: a review of 19 cases (1992-2003). *J Vet Intern Med.* 2005;19:344-347.
381. Quigley JG, Yang Z, Worthington MT, et al. Identification of a human heme exporter that is essential for erythropoiesis. *Cell.* 2004;118:757-766.
382. Radin MJ, Eubank MC, Weiser MG. Electronic measurement of erythrocyte volume and volume heterogeneity in horses during erythrocyte regeneration associated with experimental anemias. *Vet Pathol.* 1986;23:656-660.
383. Ramaiah SK, Harvey JW, Giguère S, et al. Intravascular hemolysis associated with liver disease in a horse with marked neutrophil hypersegmentation. *J Vet Intern Med.* 2003;17:360-363.
384. Ramirez-Munoz MP, Zuniga G, Torres-Bugarin O, et al. Evaluation of the micronucleus test in peripheral blood erythrocytes by use of the splenectomized model. *Lab Anim Sci.* 1999;49:418-420.
385. Randhawa SS, Sharma DK, Randhawa CS, et al. An outbreak of bacillary haemoglobinuria in sheep in India. *Trop Anim Health Prod.* 1995;27:31-36.
386. Randolph JE, Scarlett JM, Stokol T, et al. Expression, bioactivity, and clinical assessment of recombinant feline erythropoietin. *Am J Vet Res.* 2004;65: 1355-1366.
387. Randolph JF, Stokol T, Scarlett JM, et al. Comparison of biological activity and safety of recombinant canine erythropoietin with that of recombinant human erythropoietin in clinically normal dogs. *Am J Vet Res.* 1999;60:636-642.
388. Reagan WJ. A review of myelofibrosis in dogs. *Toxicol Pathol.* 1993;21:164-169.
389. Reagan WJ, Carter C, Turek J. Eccentrocytosis in equine red maple leaf toxicosis. *Vet Clin Pathol.* 1994;23:123-127.
390. Reagan WJ, Garry F, Thrall MA, et al. The clinicopathologic, light, and scanning electron microscopic features of eperythrozoonosis in four naturally infected llamas. *Vet Pathol.* 1990;27:426-431.
391. Rebar AH. *Hemogram Interpretation for Dogs and Cats.* St. Louis: Ralston Purina Co.; 1998.
392. Rebar AH, Lewis HB, DeNicola DB, et al. Red cell fragmentation in the dog: an editorial review. *Vet Pathol.* 1981;18:415-426.
393. Reef VB. *Clostridium perfringens* cellulitis and immune-mediated hemolytic anemia in a horse. *J Am Vet Med Assoc.* 1983;182:251-254.

394. Reimer ME, Troy GC, Warnick LD. Immune-mediated hemolytic anemia: 70 cases (1988-1996). *J Am Anim Hosp Assoc.* 1999;35:384-391.
395. Rettig MP, Low PS, Gimm JA, et al. Evaluation of biochemical changes during in vivo erythrocyte senescence in the dog. *Blood.* 1999;93:376-384.
396. Ribeiro RO, Chaim OM, da Silveira RB, et al. Biological and structural comparison of recombinant phospholipase D toxins from *Loxosceles intermedia* (brown spider) venom. *Toxicon.* 2007;50:1162-1174.
397. Ritzmann M, Grimm J, Heinritzi K, et al. Prevalence of *Mycoplasma suis* in slaughter pigs, with correlation of PCR results to hematological findings. *Vet Microbiol.* 2009;133:84-91.
398. Robbins RL, Wallace SS, Brunner CJ, et al. Immune-mediated haemolytic disease after penicillin therapy in a horse. *Equine Vet J.* 1993;25:462-465.
399. Robinson WF, Wilcox GE, Fowler RLP: Canine parvoviral disease: experimental reproduction of the enteric form with a parvovirus isolated from a case of myocarditis. *Vet Pathol.* 1980;17:589-599.
400. Rojko JL, Olsen RG. The immunobiology of the feline leukemia virus. *Vet Immunol Immunopathol.* 1984;6:107-165.
401. Rothmann C, Malik Z, Cohen AM. Spectrally resolved imaging of Cabot rings and Howell-Jolly bodies. *Photochem Photobiol.* 1998;68:584-587.
402. Rottman JB, English RV, Breitschwerdt EB, et al. Bone marrow hypoplasia in a cat treated with griseofulvin. *J Am Vet Med Assoc.* 1991;198:429-431.
403. Ruef P, Linderkamp O. Deformability and geometry of neonatal erythrocytes with irregular shapes. *Pediatr Res.* 1999;45:114-119.
404. Sabina RL, Woodliff JE, Giger U. Disturbed erythrocyte calcium homeostasis and adenine nucleotide dysregulation in canine phosphofructokinase deficiency. *Comp Clin Path.* 2008;17:117-123.
405. Sadallah S, Eken C, Schifferli JA. Ectosomes as modulators of inflammation and immunity. *Clin Exp Immunol* 2011;163:26-32.
406. Sakthivel R, Farooq SM, Kalaiselvi P, et al. Investigation on the early events of apoptosis in senescent erythrocytes with special emphasis on intracellular free calcium and loss of phospholipid asymmetry in chronic renal failure. *Clin Chim Acta.* 2007;382:1-7.
407. Santos LD, Santos KS, de Souza BM, et al. Purification, sequencing and structural characterization of the phospholipase A1 from the venom of the social wasp *Polybia paulista* (Hymenoptera, Vespidae). *Toxicon.* 2007;50:923-937.
408. Sato K, Hikasa Y, Morita T, et al. Secondary erythrocytosis associated with high plasma erythropoietin concentrations in a dog with cecal leiomyosarcoma. *J Am Vet Med Assoc.* 2002;220:486-490, 464.
409. Sato T, Mizuno M. Poikilocytosis of newborn calves. *Nippon Juigaku Zasshi.* 1982;44:801-805.
410. Scavelli TD, Hornbuckle WE, Roth L, et al. Portosystemic shunts in cats: seven cases (1976-1984). *J Am Vet Med Assoc.* 1986;189:317-325.
411. Schaefer DM, Priest H, Stokol T, et al. Anticoagulant-dependent in vitro hemagglutination in a cat. *Vet Clin Pathol.* 2009;38:194-200.
412. Schaer M, Harvey JW, Calderwood Mays MB, et al. Pyruvate kinase deficiency causing hemolytic anemia with secondary hemochromatosis in a Cairn terrier dog. *J Am Anim Hosp Assoc.* 1992;28:233-239.
413. Schlafer DH. *Trypanosoma theileri*: a literature review and report of incidence in New York cattle. *Cornell Vet.* 1979;69:411-425.
414. Schoofs SH. Lingual hemangioma in a puppy: a case report and literature review. *J Am Anim Hosp Assoc.* 1997;33:161-165.
415. Scott AF, Bunn HF, Brush AH. The phylogenetic distribution of red cell 2,3 diphosphoglycerate and its interaction with mammalian hemoglobins. *J Exp Zool.* 1977;201:269-288.
416. Searcy GP, Orr JP. Chronic granulocytic leukemia in a horse. *Can Vet J.* 1981;22: 148-151.
417. Sentsui H, Kono Y. Complement-mediated hemolysis of horse erythrocytes treated with equine infectious anemia virus. *Arch Virol.* 1987;95:53-66.
418. Serres F, Chetboul V, Sampedrano CC, et al. Ante-mortem diagnosis of persistent truncus arteriosus in an 8-year-old asymptomatic dog. *J Vet Cardiol.* 2009;11: 59-65.
419. Sheftel AD, Zhang AS, Brown C, et al. Direct interorganellar transfer of iron from endosome to mitochondrion. *Blood.* 2007;110:125-132.
420. Shelly SM. Causes of canine pancytopenia. *Comp Cont Ed Pract Vet.* 1988;10:9-16.
421. Shelton GH, Linenberger ML. Hematologic abnormalities associated with retroviral infections in the cat. *Semin Vet Med Surg (Small Anim).* 1995;10:220-233.
422. Shi H, Bencze KZ, Stemmler TL, et al. A cytosolic iron chaperone that delivers iron to ferritin. *Science.* 2008;320:1207-1210.
423. Shiel RE, Brennan SF, O'Rourke LG, et al. Hematologic values in young pretraining healthy Greyhounds. *Vet Clin Pathol.* 2007;36:274-277.
424. Shimada A, Onozato T, Hoshi E, et al. Pancytopenia with bleeding tendency associated with bone marrow aplasia in a Holstein calf. *J Vet Med Sci.* 2007;69: 1317-1319.
425. Shimazaki K, Ohshima K, Suzumiya J, et al. Apoptosis and prognostic factors in myelodysplastic syndromes. *Leuk Lymphoma.* 2002;43:257-260.
426. Shimoda T, Shiranaga N, Mashita T, et al. Bone marrow necrosis in a cat infected with feline leukemia virus. *J Vet Med Sci.* 2000;62:113-115.
427. Sikorski LE, Birkenheuer AJ, Holowaychuk MK, et al. Babesiosis caused by a large *Babesia* species in 7 immunocompromised dogs. *J Vet Intern Med.* 2010;24: 127-131.
428. Simpson CF, Gaskin JM, Harvey JW. Ultrastructure of erythrocytes parasitized by *Haemobartonella felis. J Parasitol.* 1978;64:504-511.
429. Simpson CF, Taylor WJ, Kitchen H. Crystalline inclusions in erythrocytes parasitized with *Babesia equi* following treatment of ponies with imidocarb. *Am J Vet Res.* 1980;41:1336-1340.
430. Singh A, Singh J, Grewal AS, et al. Studies on some blood parameters of crossbred calves with experimental *Theileria annulata* infections. *Vet Res Commun.* 2001;25:289-300.
431. Sitprija V. Animal toxins and the kidney. *Nat Clin Pract Nephrol.* 2008;4:616-627.
432. Slappendel RJ. Hereditary spherocytosis associated with spectrin deficiency in golden retrievers (abstract). *Eur Soc Vet Intern Med.* 1998;131.
433. Slappendel RJ, Van der Gaag I, Van Nes JJ, et al. Familial stomatocytosis–Hypertrophic gastritis (FSHG), a newly recognized disease in the dog (Drentse patrijshond). *Vet Q.* 1991;13:30-40.
434. Slappendel RJ, van Zwieten R, Van Leeuwen M, et al. Hereditary spectrin deficiency in Golden Retriever dogs. *J Vet Intern Med.* 2005;19:187-192.
435. Smith JA, Thrall MA, Smith JL, et al. *Eperythrozoon wenyonii* infection in dairy cattle. *J Am Vet Med Assoc.* 1990;196:1244-1250.
436. Smith JE. Iron metabolism and its disorders. In: Kaneko JJ, Harvey JW, Bruss ML, eds. *Clinical Biochemistry of Domestic Animals.* 5th ed. San Diego: Academic Press; 1997:223-238.
437. Smith JE, Mohandas N, Shohet SB. Variability in erythrocyte deformability among various mammals. *Am J Physiol.* 1979;236:H725-H730.
438. Smith JE, Mohandas N, Shohet SB. Interaction of amphipathic drugs with erythrocytes from various species. *Am J Vet Res.* 1982;43:1041-1048.
439. Smith JE, Moore K, Arens M, et al. Hereditary elliptocytosis with protein band 4.1 deficiency in the dog. *Blood.* 1983;61:373-377.
440. Sontas HB, Dokuzeylu B, Turna O, et al. Estrogen-induced myelotoxicity in dogs: A review. *Can Vet J.* 2009;50:1054-1058.
441. Soubasis N, Rallis TS, Vlemmas J, et al. Serum and liver iron concentration in dogs with experimentally induced hepatopathy. *J Gastroenterol Hepatol.* 2006;21: 599-604.
442. Spangler WL, Kass PH. Splenic myeloid metaplasia, histiocytosis, and hypersplenism in the dog (65 cases). *Vet Pathol.* 1999;36:583-593.
443. Spengler MI, Bertoluzzo SM, Catalani G, et al. Study on membrane fluidity and erythrocyte aggregation in equine, bovine and human species. *Clin Hemorheol Microcirc.* 2008;38:171-176.
444. Stanton ME, Bright RM. Gastroduodenal ulceration in dogs. Retrospective study of 43 cases and literature review. *J Vet Intern Med.* 1989;3:238-244.
445. Steele TM, Frazer DM, Anderson GJ. Systemic regulation of intestinal iron absorption. *IUBMB Life.* 2005;57:499-503.
446. Steffen DJ, Elliott GS, Leipold HW, et al. Congenital dyserythropoiesis and progressive alopecia in Polled Hereford calves: hematologic, biochemical, bone marrow cytologic, electrophoretic, and flow cytometric findings. *J Vet Diagn Invest.* 1992; 4:31-37.
447. Steffen DJ, Leipold HW, Gibb J, et al. Congenital anemia, dyskeratosis, and progressive alopecia in polled Hereford calves. *Vet Pathol.* 1991;28:234-240.
448. Steinhardt M, Petzold K, Lyhs L. Blood storage function of the spleen in the domestic pig. I. Effect of adrenaline and bodily exercise on the haematocrit value and the haemoglobin content. *Arch Exp Vet Med.* 1970;24:817-824.
449. Stewart IB, McKenzie DC. The human spleen during physiological stress. *Sports Med.* 2002;32:361-369.
450. Stockdale CR, Moyes TE, Dyson R. Acute post-parturient haemoglobinuria in dairy cows and phosphorus status. *Aust Vet J.* 2005;83:362-366.
451. Stockham SL. Anemia associated wit bacterial and viral infections. In: Feldman BF, Zinkl JG, Jain NC, eds. *Schalm's Veterinary Hematology.* 5th ed. Philadelphia: Lippincott Williams & Wilkins; 2000:163-168.
452. Stockham SL, Harvey JW, Kinden DA. Equine glucose-6-phosphate dehydrogenase deficiency. *Vet Pathol.* 1994;31:518-527.
453. Stockham SL, Kjemtrup AM, Conrad PA, et al. Theilerosis in a Missouri beef herd caused by *Theileria buffeli*: case report, herd investigation, ultrastructure, phylogenetic analysis, and experimental transmission. *Vet Pathol.* 2000;37:11-21.
454. Stokol T, Blue JT, French TW. Idiopathic pure red cell aplasia and nonregenerative immune-mediated anemia in dogs: 43 cases (1988-1999). *J Am Vet Med Assoc.* 2000;216:1429-1436.
455. Stokol T, Randolph JF, Nachbar S, et al. Development of bone marrow toxicosis after albendazole administration in a dog and cat. *J Am Vet Med Assoc.* 1997;210: 1753-1756.
456. Strickland KN. Canine and feline caval syndrome. *Clin Tech Small Anim Pract.* 1998;13:88-95.

457. Su QL, Song HQ, Lin RQ, et al. The detection of "*Candidatus* Mycoplasma haemobos" in cattle and buffalo in China. *Trop Anim Health Prod.* 2010;42:1805-1808.
458. Sullivan PS, Evans HL, McDonald TP. Platelet concentration and hemoglobin function in Greyhounds. *J Am Vet Med Assoc.* 1994;205:838-841.
459. Susta L, Torres-Velez F, Zhang J, et al. An in situ hybridization and immunohistochemical study of cytauxzoonosis in domestic cats. *Vet Pathol.* 2009;46:1197-1204.
460. Suzuki Y, Tateishi N, Cicha I, et al. Aggregation and sedimentation of mixtures of erythrocytes with different properties. *Clin Hemorheol Microcirc.* 2001;25:105-117.
461. Swardson CJ, Kociba GJ, Perryman LE. Effects of equine infectious anemia virus on hematopoietic progenitors in vitro. *Am J Vet Res.* 1992;53:1176-1179.
462. Swardson CJ, Lichtenstein DL, Wang S, et al. Infection of bone marrow macrophages by equine infectious anemia virus. *Am J Vet Res.* 1997;58:1402-1407.
463. Swenson C, Jacobs R. Spherocytosis associated with anaplasmosis in two cows. *J Am Vet Med Assoc.* 1986;188:1061-1063.
464. Sykes JE, Bailiff NL, Ball LM, et al. Identification of a novel hemotropic *Mycoplasma* in a splenectomized dog with hemic neoplasia. *J Am Vet Med Assoc.* 2004;224: 1946-1951.
465. Sykes JE, Ball LM, Bailiff NL, et al. "*Candidatus* Mycoplasma haematoparvum", a novel small haemotropic *Mycoplasma* from a dog. *Int J Syst Evol Microbiol.* 2005;55: 27-30.
466. Sykes JE, Lindsay LL, Maggi RG, et al. Human coinfection with *Bartonella henselae* and two hemotropic *Mycoplasma* variants resembling *Mycoplasma ovis*. *J Clin Microbiol.* 2010;48:3782-3785.
467. Taboada J, Lobetti R. Babesiosis. In: Greene CE, ed. *Infectious Diseases of the Dog and Cat.* 3rd ed. St. Louis: Saunders Elsevier; 2006:722-736.
468. Takagi M, Takagaki K, Kamimura S, et al. Primary erythrocytosis in a Japanese black calf: a case report. *J Vet Med A Physiol Pathol Clin Med.* 2006;53:296-299.
469. Takagi M, Yamato O, Sasaki Y, et al. Successful treatment of bacillary hemoglobinuria in Japanese Black cows. *J Vet Med Sci.* 2009;71:1105-1108.
470. Tang X, Xia Z, Yu J. An experimental study of hemolysis induced by onion (Allium cepa) poisoning in dogs. *J Vet Pharmacol Ther.* 2008;31:143-149.
471. Tant MS, Lumsden JH, Jacobs RM, et al. Evaluation of acanthocyte count as a diagnostic test for canine hemangiosarcoma. *Comp Clin Path.* 2004;12:174-181.
472. Tasker S, Helps CR, Belford CJ, et al. 16S rDNA comparison demonstrates near identity between a United Kingdom *Haemobartonella felis* strain and the American California strain. *Vet Microbiol.* 2001;81:73-78.
473. Tasker S, Peters IR, Papasouliotis K, et al. Description of outcomes of experimental infection with feline haemoplasmas: copy numbers, haematology, Coombs' testing and blood glucose concentrations. *Vet Microbiol.* 2009;139:323-332.
474. Taylor WJ. Sickled red cells in the Cervidae. *Adv Vet Sci Comp Med.* 1983;27:77-98.
475. Tennant B, Harrold D, Reina-Guerra M, et al. Arterial pH, PO_2, and PCO_2 of calves with familial bovine polycythemia. *Cornell Vet.* 1969;59:594-604.
476. Tennant BC, Center SA. Hepatic function. In: Kaneko JJ, Harvey JW, Bruss ML, eds. *Clinical Biochemistry of Domestic Animals.* 6th ed. San Diego: Academic Press; 2008:379-412.
477. Tholen I, Weingart C, Kohn B. Concentration of D-dimers in healthy cats and sick cats with and without disseminated intravascular coagulation (DIC). *J Feline Med Surg.* 2009;11:842-846.
478. Thomas HL, Livesey MA. Immune-mediated hemolytic anemia associated with trimethoprim-sulphamethoxazole administration in a horse. *Can Vet J.* 1998;39: 171-173.
479. Thorn CE. Normal hematology of the deer. In: Feldman BF, Zinkl JG, Jain NC, eds. *Schalm's Veterinary Hematology.* 5th ed. Philadelphia: Lippincott Williams & Wilkins; 2000:1179-1183.
480. Tizard IR. *Veterinary Immunology. An Introduction.* 8th ed. Philadelphia: Saunders Elsevier; 2009.
481. Toll PW, Gaehtgens P, Neuhaus D, et al. Fluid, electrolyte, and packed cell volume shifts in racing greyhounds. *Am J Vet Res.* 1995;56:227-232.
482. Toribio RE, Bain FT, Mrad DR, et al. Congenital defects in newborn foals of mares treated for equine protozoal myeloencephalitis during pregnancy. *J Am Vet Med Assoc.* 1998;212:697-701.
483. Tornquist SJ. Clinical pathology of llamas and alpacas. *Vet Clin North Am Food Anim Pract.* 2009;25:311-322.
484. Tornquist SJ, Crawford TB. Suppression of megakaryocyte colony growth by plasma from foals infected with equine infectious anemia virus. *Blood.* 1997;90:2357-2363.
485. Torten M, Schalm OW. Influence of equine spleen on rapid changes in the concentration of erythrocytes in peripheral blood. *Am J Vet Res.* 1964;25:500-504.
486. Tran TN, Eubanks SK, Schaffer KJ, et al. Secretion of ferritin by rat hepatoma cells and its regulation by inflammatory cytokines and iron. *Blood.* 1997;90:4979-4986.
487. Trepanier LA, Danhof R, Toll J, et al. Clinical findings in 40 dogs with hypersensitivity associated with administration of potentiated sulfonamides. *J Vet Intern Med.* 2003;17:647-652.
488. Troisi G, Borjesson L, Bexton S, et al. Biomarkers of polycyclic aromatic hydrocarbon (PAH)-associated hemolytic anemia in oiled wildlife. *Environ Res.* 2007;105: 324-329.
489. Tvedten HW, Tetens J. What is your diagnosis? [Heparin induced erythrocyte agglutination in a horse]. *Vet Clin Pathol.* 1996;25(5):27-28.
490. Tyler RD, Cowell RL. Normoblastemia. In: August JR, ed. *Consultations in Feline Internal Medicine 3.* Philadelphia: W.B. Saunders; 1997:483-487.
491. Uilenberg G. *Babesia*—a historical overview. *Vet Parasitol.* 2006;138:3-10.
492. Valko M, Leibfritz D, Moncol J, et al. Free radicals and antioxidants in normal physiological functions and human disease. *Int J Biochem Cell Biol.* 2007;39:44-84.
493. Vandervoort JM, Bourne C, Carson RL, et al. Use of a polymerase chain reaction assay to detect infection with *Eperythrozoon wenyoni* in cattle. *J Am Vet Med Assoc.* 2001;219:1432-1434.
494. Velcek FT, Kugaczewski JT, Jongco B, et al. Function of the replanted spleen in dogs. *J Trauma.* 1982;22:502-506.
495. Verga Falzacappa MV, Muckenthaler MU. Hepcidin: iron-hormone and anti-microbial peptide. *Gene.* 2005;364:37-44.
496. Vetter J. A biological hazard of our age: bracken fern [*Pteridium aquilinum* (L.) Kuhn]—a review. *Acta Vet Hung.* 2009;57:183-196.
497. Walker D, Cowell RL, Clinkenbeard KD, et al. Bone marrow mast cell hyperplasia in dogs with aplastic anemia. *Vet Clin Pathol.* 1997;26:106-111.
498. Walton RM, Brown DE, Hamar DW, et al. Mechanisms of echinocytosis induced by *Crotalus atrox* venom. *Vet Pathol.* 1997;34:442-449.
499. Walton RM, Modiano JF, Thrall MA, et al. Bone marrow cytological findings in 4 dogs and a cat with hemophagocytic syndrome. *J Vet Intern Med.* 1996;10:7-14.
500. Wanduragala L, Ristic M. Anaplasmosis. In: Woldehiwet Z, Ristic M, eds. *Rickettsial and Chlamydial Diseases of Domestic Animals.* New York: Pergamon Press; 1993:65-87.
501. Ward MV, Mountan PC, Dodds WJ. Severe idiopathic refractory anemia and leukopenia in a horse. *Calif Vet.* 1980;12:19-22.
502. Wardrop KJ. The Coombs' test in veterinary medicine: past, present, future. *Vet Clin Pathol.* 2005;34:325-334.
503. Watson ADJ: Erythrocytosis and polycythemia. In: Feldman BF, Zinkl JG, Jain NC, eds. *Schalm's Veterinary Hematology.* 5th ed. Philadelphia: Lippincott Williams & Wilkins; 2000:217-221.
504. Watson ADJ, Wright RG. The ultrastructure of inclusions in blood cells of dogs with distemper. *J Comp Pathol.* 1974;84:417-427.
505. Weiser MG. Erythrocyte volume distribution analysis in healthy dogs, cats, horses and dairy cows. *Am J Vet Res.* 1982;43:163-166.
506. Weiser MG, Kociba GJ. Persistent macrocytosis assessed by erythrocyte subpopulation analysis following erythrocyte regeneration in cats. *Blood.* 1982; 60:295-303.
507. Weiser MG, Kociba GJ. Erythrocyte macrocytosis in feline leukemia virus associated anemia. *Vet Pathol.* 1983;20:687-697.
508. Weiser MG, Kociba GJ. Sequential changes in erythrocyte volume distribution and microcytosis associated with iron deficiency in kittens. *Vet Pathol.* 1983;20: 1-12.
509. Weiss DJ. Uniform evaluation and semiquantitative reporting of hematologic data in veterinary laboratories. *Vet Clin Pathol.* 1984;13:27-31.
510. Weiss DJ. Aplastic anemia. In: Feldman BF, Zinkl JG, Jain NC, eds. *Schalm's Veterinary Hematology.* 5th ed. Philadelphia: Lippincott Williams & Wilkins; 2000: 212-215.
511. Weiss DJ. Primary pure red cell aplasia in dogs: 13 cases (1996-2000). *J Am Vet Med Assoc.* 2002;221:93-95.
512. Weiss DJ. New insights into the physiology and treatment of acquired myelodysplastic syndromes and aplastic pancytopenia. *Vet Clin North Am Small Anim Pract.* 2003;33:1317-1334.
513. Weiss DJ. Sideroblastic anemia in 7 dogs (1996-2002). *J Vet Intern Med.* 2005;19:325-328.
514. Weiss DJ. A retrospective study of the incidence and the classification of bone marrow disorders in the dog at a veterinary teaching hospital (1996-2004). *J Vet Intern Med.* 2006;20:955-961.
515. Weiss DJ. Aplastic anemia in cats—clinicopathological features and associated disease conditions 1996-2004. *J Feline Med Surg.* 2006;8:203-206.
516. Weiss DJ. Hemophagocytic syndrome in dogs: 24 cases (1996-2005). *J Am Vet Med Assoc.* 2007;230:697-701.
517. Weiss DJ. Bone marrow pathology in dogs and cats with non-regenerative immune-mediated haemolytic anaemia and pure red cell aplasia. *J Comp Pathol.* 2008;138: 46-53.
518. Weiss DJ, Aird B. Cytologic evaluation of primary and secondary myelodysplastic syndromes in the dog. *Vet Clin Pathol.* 2001;30:67-75.
519. Weiss DJ, Evanson OA. A retrospective study of feline pancytopenia. *Comp Haematol Int.* 2000;10:50-55.
520. Weiss DJ, Evanson OA, Sykes J. A retrospective study of canine pancytopenia. *Vet Clin Pathol.* 1999;28:83-88.

521. Weiss DJ, Klausner JS. Drug-associated aplastic anemia in dogs: eight cases (1984-1988). *J Am Vet Med Assoc.* 1990;196:472-475.
522. Weiss DJ, Kristensen A, Papenfuss N. Quantitative evaluation of irregularly spiculated red blood cells in the dog. *Vet Clin Pathol.* 1993;22:117-121.
523. Weiss DJ, Kristensen A, Papenfuss N, et al. Quantitative evaluation of echinocytes in the dog. *Vet Clin Pathol.* 1990;19:114-118.
524. Weiss DJ, Lulich J. Myelodysplastic syndrome with sideroblastic differentiation in a dog. *Vet Clin Pathol.* 1999;28:59-63.
525. Weiss DJ, Miller DC. Bone marrow necrosis associated with pancytopenia in a cow. *Vet Pathol.* 1985;22:90-92.
526. Weiss DJ, Moritz A. Equine immune-mediated hemolytic anemia associated with *Clostridium perfringens* infection. *Vet Clin Pathol.* 2003;32:22-26.
527. Weiss DJ, Raskin RE, Zerbe C. Myelodysplastic syndrome in two dogs. *J Am Vet Med Assoc.* 1985;187:1038-1040.
528. Weiss L. *The Blood Cells and Hematopoietic Tissues.* New York: Elsevier, 1984.
529. Welles EG, Tyler JW, Wolfe DF. Hematologic and semen quality changes in bulls with experimental eperythrozoon infection. *Theriogenology.* 1995;43:427-437.
530. Welles EG, Tyler JW, Wolfe DF, et al. Eperythrozoon infection in young bulls with scrotal and hindlimb edema, a herd outbreak. *Theriogenology.* 1995;43: 557-567.
531. Wells MY, Decobecq CP, Decouvelaere DM, et al. Changes in clinical pathology parameters during gestation in the New Zealand white rabbit. *Toxicol Pathol.* 1999;27:370-379.
532. Weng XD, Cloutier G, Beaulieu R, et al. Influence of acute-phase proteins on erythrocyte aggregation. *Am J Physiol Heart Circ Physiol.* 1996;271:H2346-H2352.
533. Westfall DS, Jensen WA, Reagan WJ, et al. Inoculation of two genotypes of *Hemobartonella felis* (California and Ohio variants) to induce infection in cats and the response to treatment with azithromycin. *Am J Vet Res.* 2001;62:687-691.
534. Wilcox A, Russell KE. Hematologic changes associated with Adderall toxicity in a dog. *Vet Clin Pathol.* 2008;37:184-189.
535. Willekens FL, Roerdinkholder-Stoelwinder B, Groenen-Dopp YA, et al. Hemoglobin loss from erythrocytes: in vivo results from spleen-facilitated vesiculation. *Blood.* 2003;101:747-751.
536. Willekens FL, Werre JM, Groenen-Dopp YA, et al. Erythrocyte vesiculation: a self-protective mechanism? *Br J Haematol.* 2008;141:549-556.
537. Willekens FL, Werre JM, Kruijt JK, et al. Liver Kupffer cells rapidly remove red blood cell-derived vesicles from the circulation by scavenger receptors. *Blood.* 2005;105: 2141-2145.
538. Willi B, Boretti FS, Cattori V, et al. Identification, molecular characterization, and experimental transmission of a new hemoplasma isolate from a cat with hemolytic anemia in Switzerland. *J Clin Microbiol.* 2005;43:2581-2585.
539. Willi B, Boretti FS, Tasker S, et al. From Haemobartonella to hemoplasma: molecular methods provide new insights. *Vet Microbiol.* 2007;125:197-209.
540. Wolfs JL, Comfurius P, Bevers EM, et al. Influence of erythrocyte shape on the rate of Ca^{2+}-induced scrambling of phosphatidylserine. *Mol Membr Biol.* 2003;20:83-91.
541. Worth AJ, Ainsworth SJ, Brocklehurst PJ, et al. Nitrite poisoning in cats and dogs fed a commercial pet food. *N Z Vet J.* 1997;45:193-195.
542. Wray JD. Methaemoglobinaemia caused by hydroxycarbamide (hydroxyurea) ingestion in a dog. *J Small Anim Pract.* 2008;49:211-215.
543. Wysoke JM, Berg BB, Marshall C. Bee sting-induced haemolysis, spherocytosis and neural dysfunction in three dogs. *J S Afr Vet Assoc.* 1990;61:29-32.
544. Yabsley MJ, Quick TC, Little SE. Theileriosis in a white-tailed deer (*Odocoileus virginianus*) fawn. *J Wildl Dis.* 2005;41:806-809.
545. Yamato O, Kasai E, Katsura T, et al. Heinz body hemolytic anemia with eccentrocytosis from ingestion of Chinese chive (*Allium tuberosum*) and garlic (*Allium sativum*) in a dog. *J Am Anim Hosp Assoc.* 2005;41:68-73.
546. Yamauchi A, Ohta T, Okada T, et al. Secondary erythrocytosis associated with schwannoma in a dog. *J Vet Med Sci.* 2004;66:1605-1608.
547. Yeagley TJ, Reichard MV, Hempstead JE, et al. Detection of *Babesia gibsoni* and the canine small *Babesia* "Spanish isolate" in blood samples obtained from dogs confiscated from dogfighting operations. *J Am Vet Med Assoc.* 2009;235:535-539.
548. Young NS, Calado RT, Scheinberg P. Current concepts in the pathophysiology and treatment of aplastic anemia. *Blood.* 2006;108:2509-2519.
549. Zaks KL, Tan EO, Thrall MA. Heinz body anemia in a dog that had been sprayed with skunk musk. *J Am Vet Med Assoc.* 2005;226:1516-1518.
550. Zandecki M, Genevieve F, Gerard J, et al. Spurious counts and spurious results on haematology analysers: a review. Part II. white blood cells, red blood cells, haemoglobin, red cell indices and reticulocytes. *Int J Lab Hematol.* 2007;29:21-41.
551. Zhuang QJ, Zhang HJ, Lin RQ, et al. The occurrence of the feline "*Candidatus* Mycoplasma haemominutum" in dog in China confirmed by sequence-based analysis of ribosomal DNA. *Trop Anim Health Prod.* 2009;41:689-692.
552. Zuniga Gonzalez G, Ramirez Munoz MP, Torres Bugarin O, et al. Induction of micronuclei in the domestic cat (*Felis domesticus*) peripheral blood by colchicine and cytosine-arabinoside. *Mutat Res.* 1998;413:187-189.
553. Zwaal RF, Comfurius P, Bevers EM. Mechanism and function of changes in membrane-phospholipid asymmetry in platelets and erythrocytes. *Biochem Soc Trans.* 1993;21:248-253.

CHAPTER

5

EVALUATION OF LEUKOCYTIC DISORDERS

LEUKOCYTE TYPES AND NUMBERS IN BLOOD

Mammalian leukocytes or white blood cells have been classified as either polymorphonuclear leukocytes (PMNs) or mononuclear leukocytes. The PMNs have condensed, segmented nuclei. They are commonly referred to as granulocytes because they contain large numbers of cytoplasmic granules (Fig. 5-1). The term *granulocyte* is preferred in veterinary medicine because nuclear segmentation does not occur in the granulocytes of most reptiles and it is not as prominent in birds as it is in mammals. The granules in these cells are lysosomes containing hydrolytic enzymes, antibacterial agents, and other compounds. Primary granules are synthesized in the cytoplasm of late myeloblasts or early promyelocytes. They appear reddish purple when stained with routine blood stains such as Wright-Giemsa (see Chapter 8). Secondary (specific) granules appear at the myelocyte stage of development in the bone marrow. Three types of granulocytes (neutrophils, eosinophils, basophils) are identified by the staining characteristics of their secondary granules (Fig. 5-2).

Mononuclear leukocytes in blood are classified as either lymphocytes or monocytes (Fig. 5-3). These cells are not devoid of granules but rather have lower numbers of cytoplasmic granules than do granulocytes. Lymphocytes have high nuclear-to-cytoplasmic (N:C) ratios. Their nuclei have coarsely clumped chromatin and are usually round, but they may be oval or slightly indented. A low percentage of lymphocytes in blood have focal accumulations of red- or purple-staining granules within the cytoplasm (Fig. 5-4). These granular lymphocytes may be cytotoxic T lymphocytes or natural killer (NK) cells. Monocytes are usually larger than lymphocytes, have nuclei with finer chromatin clumping that are more variable in shape (round-, kidney-, or band-shaped), and have N:C ratios of 1 or less. They often exhibit cytoplasmic vacuoles in films prepared from blood collected with an anticoagulant.

The total number of leukocytes varies considerably by species. Among common domestic animals, the mean total leukocyte count is highest in pigs (16,000/μL) and lowest in cattle and sheep (8000/μL).[226] Neutrophils and lymphocytes are the most numerous leukocyte types present in the blood of healthy domestic mammals. Dogs, cats, and horses usually have more neutrophils in blood than lymphocytes. In contrast, lymphocytes are usually more numerous in pigs, cattle, sheep, goats, and rodents.[226] Numbers of neutrophils and lymphocytes change with age after birth. The neutrophil-to-lymphocyte ratio tends to be higher at birth than in later life, in part because of the increased blood cortisol concentration at birth.[84,249,312,331,460] Cortisol causes circulating neutrophil numbers to increase and circulating lymphocyte numbers to decrease. Calves have neutrophil-to-lymphocyte ratios well above 1.0 at birth owing to neutrophil numbers above and lymphocyte numbers below those of adults. Within a week, neutrophil numbers decrease and lymphocyte numbers increase to counts that are approximately equal, with lymphocyte counts above neutrophil counts by 3 weeks of age.[249,331] Low numbers of monocytes, eosinophils, and basophils are present in normal mammals. Basophil numbers are especially low in dogs and cats, with none being seen in blood from many healthy animals.

LEUKOCYTE KINETICS

In contrast to erythrocytes, leukocytes do not exhibit a life span in blood but rather leave blood at random times in response to chemoattractant stimuli. Except for lymphocytes that recirculate, it was thought that leukocytes did not reenter the circulation after migration into the tissues. However, there is evidence that some tissue eosinophils return to the circulation via lymphatics[478] and that, in the absence of inflammation, some monocytes may shuttle back to the bone marrow.[506]

Neutrophils

Following release from the bone marrow, neutrophils are normally present in blood for a short time (half-life about 5 to 10 hours) before they egress into the tissues.[75,116,383,433] Neutrophils appear to survive no more than a few days in tissues.[433] Neutrophils that remain in blood spontaneously undergo apoptosis and are removed by macrophages in the spleen,

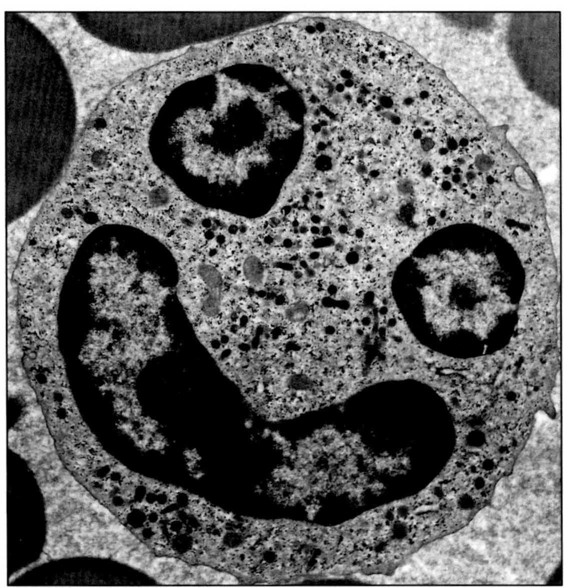

FIGURE 5-1
Transmission electron photomicrograph of a cat neutrophil containing many characteristically small cytoplasmic granules. The thin sectioning of the sample creates the appearance of the nucleus as being in three parts.

Courtesy of C. F. Simpson.

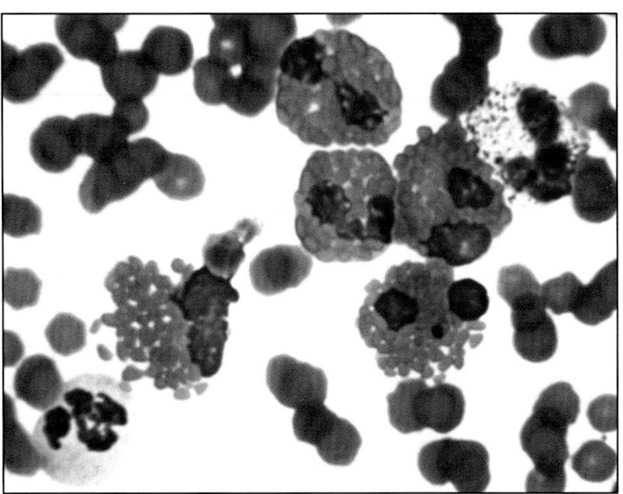

FIGURE 5-2
Blood film from a horse demonstrating the types of granulocytes normally present in blood. Granulocytes present include a neutrophil *(bottom left),* five eosinophils *(middle),* and a basophil *(top right).* Granules in the basophil stained poorly, which is a characteristic of the aqueous stain used. Diff-Quik stain.

liver, and bone marrow via a phagocytic process (termed efferocytosis) that does not generate an inflammatory reaction.[162,328,422]

Neutrophils occur in circulating and marginating pools in blood, with 50% or less of the total blood neutrophil pool being present in the circulating pool (Fig. 5-5).[226,433] The

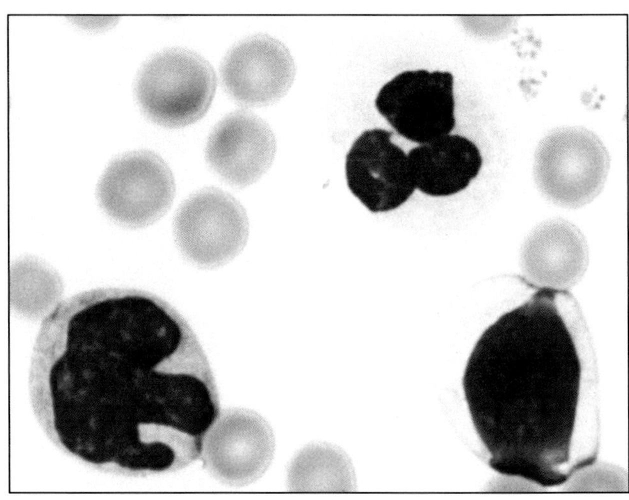

FIGURE 5-3
Blood film from a cow demonstrating the types of mononuclear leukocytes normally present in blood. Nucleated cells present include a monocyte *(lower left),* a large lymphocyte *(lower right),* and a neutrophil *(top).* Wright-Giemsa stain.

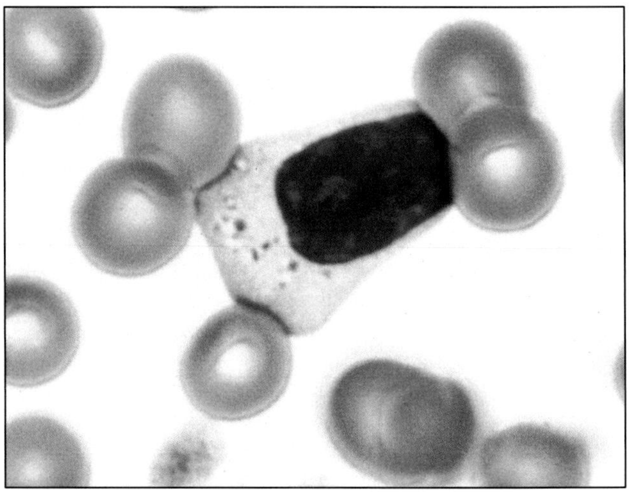

FIGURE 5-4
Granular lymphocyte in blood from a dog. Wright-Giemsa stain.

circulating neutrophil pool (CNP) is assessed by routine blood sample collection. The marginating neutrophil pool (MNP) consists of neutrophils that are transiently retained in capillaries and veins. The lung has long been considered the predominant organ contributing to the MNP[121,309]; however, recent studies suggest that the liver, spleen, and bone marrow may contribute substantially to the MNP.[445] The retention of neutrophils in the vasculature does not appear to involve neutrophil adhesion to endothelial cells.[260] The size of the MNP in an organ is related to its blood flow and the neutrophil intravascular transit time through the organ.[445] Neutrophil margination is increased in lungs when blood flow is reduced and decreased when blood flow is increased.[455] The absolute neutrophil count measured in blood samples can be affected

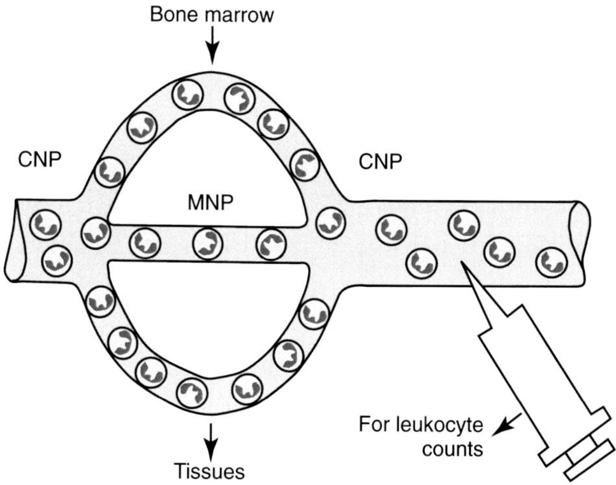

FIGURE 5-5
Neutrophil distribution in blood. Neutrophils occur in the circulating neutrophil pool (CNP) and marginating neutrophil pool (MNP), with 50% or less of the total blood neutrophil pool being present in the CNP.

by cell movements between the MNP and CNP. A net movement of neutrophils from the MNP to the CNP increases the circulating blood neutrophil count. A net movement in the opposite direction results in a decreased circulating blood neutrophil count.[435]

Eosinophils and Basophils

The half-life reported for human eosinophils ranges from 8 to 18 hours.[368] Little information is available concerning blood basophil kinetics, but a half-life of 2 to 3 days has been reported for humans.[440] Basophils appear to survive no more than a few days in tissues.[164] In contrast, eosinophils may remain in tissues for weeks to months unless they migrate into airways or the gastrointestinal tract.[478]

Monocytes

The half-life for monocytes in blood is reported to vary from 0.5 to 3 days in rabbits, mice, and humans.[185,506] Monocytes also have a marginating pool within pulmonary capillaries.[121] Monocytes develop into macrophages and dendritic cells in the tissues, where they survive for variable time periods.[506] Macrophages may survive up to 3 months in tissues.[165] Dendritic cells in lymphoid organs are reported to survive 10 to 14 days.[284] In contrast, dendritic cells in skin (Langerhans cells) are reported to survive more than a year.[322]

Lymphocytes

Most lymphocytes reside within lymphoid organs (lymph nodes, thymus, spleen, and bone marrow). Only about 2% to 5% of lymphocytes circulate in blood.[50,458] Like neutrophils and monocytes, lymphocytes have a MNP within pulmonary capillaries.[121,455] Depending on the species and individual variability, about 50% to 75% of blood lymphocytes are T lymphocytes and about 10% to 40% are B lymphocytes. NK cells account for 5% to 10% of blood lymphocytes.[458] Some NK cells appear as granular lymphocytes, but not all. A subset of $CD8^+$ T lymphocytes also appear as granular lymphocytes.[33]

A majority of blood lymphocytes are naive T and B lymphocytes, and most of the remaining blood lymphocytes are antigen-primed memory T and B lymphocytes.[140] The fraction of memory lymphocytes increases and the fraction of naive lymphocytes decreases in the blood of humans as they age.[293] Most lymphocytes in blood have come from peripheral lymphoid organs (primarily lymph nodes). Lymphocytes circulate for a short time in blood (half-life about 30 minutes), exit, migrate through lymphoid tissues (and to some degree extralymphoid tissues), and return to blood via lymphatics.[50] B and T lymphocytes migrate through lymph nodes with average velocities of around 6 and 12 μm/min, respectively. It is estimated that it takes about 1 day for a recirculating lymphocyte to migrate through a lymph node.[40,507] Recirculation allows lymphocytes, with their complete repertoire of unique antigen receptors, to be available for immune reactions throughout the body.

Naive lymphocytes have a propensity to recirculate through lymph nodes. They migrate into lymph nodes through high endothelial venules (HEVs) because these venules have adhesion molecules and chemokines on their surfaces that recognize complementary adhesion and chemokine receptors expressed on naive lymphocyte surfaces.[399] Recirculating lymphocytes generally exit the lymph nodes via the efferent lymphatics; however, they appear to emigrate from lymph nodes via paracortical postcapillary venules in pigs.[51] Efferent lymphatics join together to form large lymphatic vessels, the largest of which is the thoracic duct, and drain into the blood at the level of the heart (Fig. 5-6).

Dendritic cells are exposed to antigens in tissues and migrate to draining lymph nodes. When naive T and B lymphocytes are exposed to their cognate antigens presented by dendritic cells in lymph nodes, they proliferate and form effector lymphocytes and long-lived memory lymphocytes. Dendritic cells present not only antigens but also environmental signals (including vitamin A and D_3 metabolites) that program migration pathways.[428] Memory lymphocytes develop an array of adhesion molecules and chemokine receptors that target their subsequent migration to specific tissues including skin, intestinal mucosa, and lungs.[50,399] Tissue lymphocytes are picked up by afferent lymphatics and are carried to lymph nodes, where they exit by efferent lymphatics, traverse large lymphatic vessels, and reenter the blood (see Fig. 5-6). Most plasma cells and proliferating lymphocytes, such as those present in germinal centers, do not express the adhesion molecules necessary for migration.[458]

Lymphocytes generally survive much longer than granulocytes. Naive T lymphocytes are reported to have a half-life of about 40 days in mice. $CD8^+$ memory T lymphocytes and some $CD4^+$ memory T lymphocytes are long-lived in mice (many months), but other $CD4^+$ memory T lymphocytes survive only about 2 months. Memory T lymphocytes are reported to survive for many years in humans.[309] Long-term survival may require cell proliferation; therefore it may be a matter of semantics whether long-term survival refers to an individual lymphocyte or a population of lymphocytes.

The $t_{1/2}$ disappearance rate for B lymphocytes from the recirculating pool is reported to be 2 to 3 weeks in humans. Long-term-memory B lymphocytes appear to be maintained as proliferating clones of cells rather than as individual cells that survive for a long time.[293] Plasma cells survive for variable periods of time. Those that develop in sites of inflammation disappear when the inflammation is resolved. However, some plasma cells may survive for years in humans, especially within stromal niches in bone marrow.[339]

An NK cell's half-life in the circulation is about 7 to 10 days in mice and 12 days in humans under normal conditions. NK cells leave the circulation by entering tissues during steady-state conditions or through cell death. NK cell survival is promoted by the cytokine, interleukin-15 (IL-15).[513] NK cells are located in many organs including spleen, lung, bone marrow, lymph nodes, liver, intestine, skin, and thymus (low numbers). Some NK cells recirculate through blood and lymph.[117,187] The spleen and bone marrow appear to provide NK cell reserves that can rapidly enter the blood and subsequently migrate into tissues in response to inflammation. NK cell migration from blood to inflammatory sites occurs by mechanisms similar to those described for granulocytes. These include initial adhesion to endothelial cells via selectins, followed by tighter adhesion to endothelial cells via integrins and chemoattractant-directed migration. Chemoattractants include certain chemokines as well as bacterial products, leukotrienes, and C5a. Marked infiltrates of NK cells are also present in the uterus during pregnancy.[187]

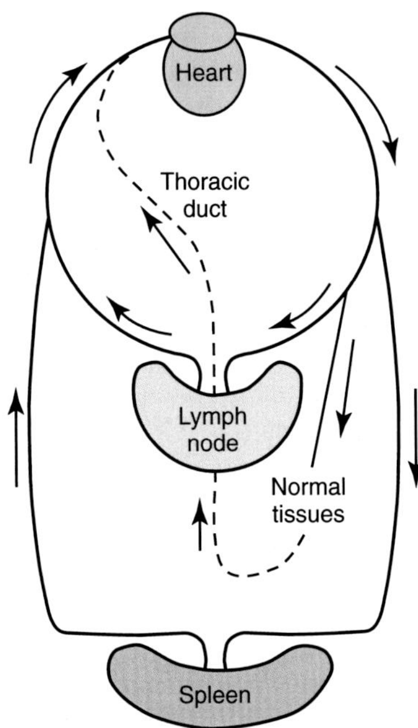

FIGURE 5-6
Circulation routes for lymphocytes. Solid lines represent blood vessels and dashed lines represent lymphatic vessels. Naive lymphocytes circulate primarily through lymph nodes and memory lymphocytes circulate through tissues.

LEUKOCYTE FUNCTIONS

Neutrophil Functions

Neutrophils are essential in the defense against invading microorganisms, primarily bacteria. To be effective, they must recognize inflammatory signals, leave the blood, migrate through tissue to a site where bacteria are present, and then neutralize the bacteria. Neutrophils display glycoprotein adhesion molecules on their surfaces that are needed for various adhesion-dependent functions, including adhesion to endothelium and subendothelial structures, spreading, haptotaxis, and phagocytosis.[106] Unless they are activated, neutrophils and endothelial cells exhibit little tendency to adhere to each other. Following the stimulation of endothelial cells by mediators—such as thrombin, histamine, and oxygen radicals—P-selectin is rapidly mobilized from storage granules and expressed on the surfaces of endothelial cells. Inflammatory mediators, including interleukin-1 (IL-1) and tumor necrosis factor (TNF), promote the expression of E-selectin adhesion molecules on the surface of activated endothelial cells within 1 to 2 hours.[58] These oligosaccharide-binding selectin molecules, acting in concert with the L-selectin adhesion molecule expressed on the surface neutrophils, bind to their counterligands, most notably P-selectin glycoprotein ligand-1 (PSGL-1), which results in the initial adhesion of unstimulated neutrophils to activated endothelial cells (Fig. 5-7).[511] As a result of selectin binding between neutrophils and activated endothelial cells, the velocity of neutrophils in the circulation is markedly decreased and they are seen to roll along the endothelium.[510]

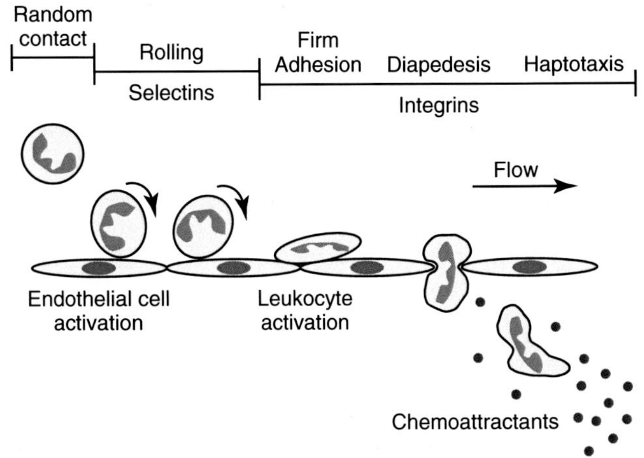

FIGURE 5-7
Endothelial cell activation, neutrophil rolling along vessel walls, tight adhesion between neutrophils and endothelial cells, diapedesis, and haptotaxis.

Activated endothelial cells produce factors including interleukin-8 (IL-8) and platelet activating factor (PAF, a biologically active phospholipid) that result in neutrophil activation. Other mediators that can activate neutrophils include opsonized particles, immune complexes, N-formylated bacterial peptides, granulocyte-macrophage colony-stimulating factor (GM-CSF), granulocyte colony-stimulating factor (G-CSF), and chemoattractants produced during inflammation.[58] Neutrophil activation results in increased expression and enhanced binding affinity of β_2 integrin adhesion molecules and shedding of L-selectin molecules. β_2 integrins (CD11a,b,c/CD18) are heterodimers that bind with variable affinity to intercellular adhesion molecules (ICAMs). β_2 integrin binding further slows rolling and ultimately results in the firm adhesion of neutrophils to endothelial cells. Adherent (activated) neutrophils then spread and exhibit pseudopod formation. Neutrophil activation also promotes degranulation, superoxide generation, and the production of arachidonate metabolites, to be discussed later.[58]

In addition to increased β_2 integrin affinity, activated neutrophils have increased numbers of surface receptors and/or enhanced receptor affinity for chemoattractants.[432] These receptors are also found in granules, suggesting that they are mobilized to the cell surface during neutrophil activation. When they are exposed to chemoattractants, neutrophils penetrate the wall of postcapillary venules, primarily by moving between endothelial cells.[58] Less than 5 minutes is required for neutrophils to pass between endothelial cells, but 15 minutes or more may be required for them to pass through the vascular basement membrane.[277] Once outside the vessel, the active directional migration of neutrophils in tissues occurs largely by haptotaxis, which means migration up a gradient of immobilized chemoattractants rather than soluble chemoattractants (chemotaxis). A wide variety of substances can function as a chemoattractant, including IL-8 and other chemokines, C5a (complement fragment), leukotriene B_4 (a product of arachidonic acid metabolism via the lipoxygenase pathway), PAF (1-0-alkyl-2-acetyl *sn*-glyceryl phosphorylcholine) and bacterial products (e.g., N-formyl-methionyl oligopeptides) recognized by Toll-like receptors.[58,106]

During their movement toward increasing concentrations of chemoattractants, neutrophils become elongated, with a frontal pseudopod extending in the direction of movement and a distal uropod that consists of fine trailing appendages. Membrane sheets (lamellipodia) on the leading edge of the pseudopod are in continual motion, orienting in the direction of chemoattractants.[441] Neutrophils crawl (10-12 μm/min) toward the source of the chemoattractant by the binding of integrin surface molecules to their respective ligands within the extracellular matrix at the frontal pseudopod and detaching from these ligands at the distal uropod. Although present in only small amounts on the surfaces of circulating blood neutrophils, activated neutrophils express increased surface β_1 integrins, which appear to be the most important class of integrins for migration. Members of the β_1 integrin family have high affinity for proteins in the extracellular matrix, including collagen, laminin, fibronectin, and vitronectin.[280] Movement depends on actomyosin-mediated contractions at the leading edge for pseudopod advancement and in the trailing end to break adhesive contacts.[441]

For phagocytosis to occur, neutrophils must be able to first bind invading bacteria to their surfaces (Fig. 5-8). This adherence is greatly potentiated if bacteria have been opsonized (have antibodies and complement components bound to their surfaces) because neutrophils have immunoglobulin Fc and C3b receptors on their surfaces. Following binding, bacteria are engulfed by the neutrophils' cytoplasmic processes, which extend around the organisms. The membranes of the neutrophils' cytoplasmic processes fuse to form phagocytic vacuoles surrounding the engulfed bacteria.[58,106]

Bacterial killing involves a multitude of mechanisms that are set into motion by two cellular events, initiation of the respiratory burst and degranulation. The respiratory burst is initiated by the activation of an NADPH oxidase enzyme (Fig. 5-9). This enzyme is normally "inactive" in resting or unstimulated phagocytes. Enzyme activation depends on the assembly of multiple components, some of which are already membrane-bound and others that must be translocated from the cytoplasm to the membrane. Activated NADPH oxidase is located in the plasma membrane and becomes incorporated into the phagocytic vacuole. It catalyzes the one-step reduction of O_2 to form superoxide (O_2^-).[106] The NADPH needed to generate superoxide is formed in the pentose phosphate pathway. The superoxide thus formed undergoes dismutation to form hydrogen peroxide, as shown below:

$$2O_2 + NADPH \rightarrow 2O_2^- + NADP^+ + H^+ \text{ (oxidation)}$$

$$2O_2^- + 2H^+ \rightarrow O_2 + H_2O_2 \text{ (dismutation)}$$

Hydrogen peroxide and superoxide can diffuse from the phagocytic vacuole into the cytoplasm of the cell. Activated

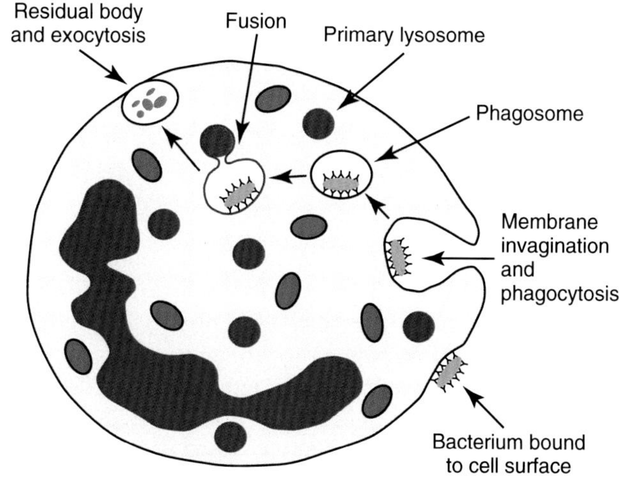

FIGURE 5-8
Basic events involved in the phagocytosis, killing, and the discharge of killed bacteria and degraded bacterial products.

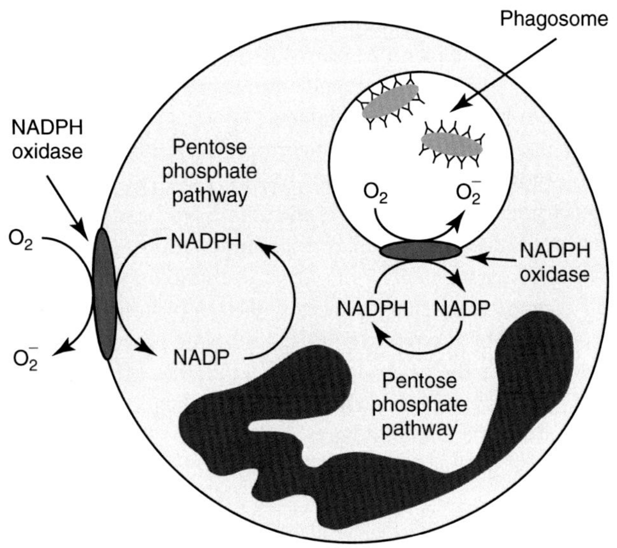

FIGURE 5-9

Generation of superoxide free radicals by the membrane-associated NADPH oxidase enzyme.

neutrophils utilize the superoxide dismutase and glutathione peroxidase reactions to protect themselves from these oxidants. The latter reaction requires that additional NADPH be generated to maintain glutathione in the reduced form. Activation of the respiratory burst requires neither phagocytosis nor degranulation to occur. In addition to opsonized particles, chemoattractants, such as C5a, can activate the respiratory burst.[106]

Superoxide, other free radicals (e.g., hydroxyl radical), and H_2O_2 may be involved directly in the killing of bacteria, but killing is potentiated by degranulation, which results in the fusion and release of the contents of lysosomal granules into the phagocytic vacuole (see Fig. 5-8). Myeloperoxidase is an iron-containing enzyme located in the primary granules of neutrophils. The myeloperoxidase reaction greatly enhances the bactericidal potency of H_2O_2. This reaction catalyzes the oxidation of chloride to hypochlorous acid, resulting in halogenation of bacterial cell walls (see below) and loss of integrity.[106]

$$Cl^- + H_2O_2 + H^+ \rightarrow HOCl + H_2O$$

$$R\text{-}NH_2 + HOCl \rightarrow R\text{-}NHCl + H_2O$$

Other enzymes are also present in primary and secondary granules of neutrophils.[432] These include collagenase, acid and neutral hydrolases, and lysozyme, which hydrolyzes glycosidic linkages in the cell walls of certain bacteria. These enzymes are probably more important in digestion than in killing. Nonenzymatic agents are also involved in neutrophil defense. A number of cationic proteins and peptides in neutrophil granules have antimicrobial properties.[432] Of these molecules, defensins appear to be the most common. With the lowest molecular weight, defensins are small (4 kD) antimicrobial peptides within primary granules that act against bacteria and other microorganisms by altering their membrane permeability. They are inserted into the lipid bilayer, disrupting interaction between lipid molecules. In addition, lactoferrin occurs within secondary granules and chelates iron required for microbial growth.[432]

The growth factors G-CSF and GM-CSF are important, not only in the production of neutrophils but also in promoting neutrophil survival and function. G-CSF and GM-CSF are produced by macrophages, neutrophils, and other cell types at inflammatory sites.[137] They prime neutrophils in ways that enhance their functions and inhibit apoptosis of neutrophils at sites of inflammation.[106,360] Neutrophils become more adhesive and responsive to other stimuli, including chemoattractants, and their respiratory burst is enhanced after they bind these growth factors.[106,137,304,499]

Following the killing and digestion of bacteria, the phagocytic vacuole fuses with the plasma membrane and discharges the killed bacteria, products of degraded bacteria, and contents of granules to the outside of the cell in a process called exocytosis (see Fig. 5-8). Discharge of granules can also occur following activation of neutrophils in the absence of phagocytosis. Considerable tissue injury occurs in areas where neutrophils are activated because of the oxidants they produce and the granule contents they release.

Neutrophils can trap and kill bacteria and fungi without phagocytosis by releasing neutrophil extracellular traps (NETs). These NETs consist of fibers (composed of DNA, histones, and proteins from granules) that can kill microbes.[158] Initial reports indicated that these NETs were generated by neutrophils undergoing cell death[158]; however, more recent reports indicate that NET formation can occur without neutrophil death.[365,509] NET production is an active process, not the result of leakage during cellular disintegration. The NETs formed by living neutrophils contain mitochondrial DNA but no nuclear DNA.[509] In addition to mammalian neutrophils,[192,477] neutrophils from fish and heterophils from birds produce NETs when they are appropriately stimulated.[85,365]

Several pathogens have co-opted phagocytic and killing processes to survive within phagocytes. These include *Listeria*, *Yersinia*, and *Mycobacterium* species.[106]

Eosinophil Functions

Most tissue eosinophils reside in the gastrointestinal mucosa.[335] Eosinophils have less phagocytic ability than neutrophils and provide poor host defense against bacterial or viral agents.[207] However, eosinophils are an important component of the type 2 cytokine-induced inflammatory response that is critical in the host defense against helminth infections and is responsible for the pathogenesis of type 1 hypersensitivity allergic reactions. $CD4^+$, type 2 helper T (T_H2) lymphocytes secrete a group of cytokines that result in the recruitment and/or activation of effector cells including B lymphocytes producing IgE, mast cells, basophils, and eosinophils.[346]

Rather than simply responding to an otherwise innocuous environmental antigen by producing IgG or IgA antibodies, some animals respond to environmental antigens with an exaggerated T_H2 response that produces excessive amounts of IgE. IL-4 and IL-13 from T_H2 lymphocytes and the presence of activated mast cells, basophils, and eosinophils stimulate B lymphocytes to switch to IgE production.[381,431] This excess IgE binds to receptors (FcεRI) on mast cells in the tissues and primes the mast cells to bind the environmental antigen (allergen) that stimulated the IgE response. When the primed mast cell encounters the allergen and it cross-links two of the bound IgE molecules, the mast cell will degranulate and release a mixture of inflammatory mediators and potent chemoattractants for eosinophils into the surrounding tissues.[458] These chemoattractants include histamine and small C-C chemokine proteins, including eotaxins (CCL11, CCL24, and CCL26) and CCL5, which appear to be particularly important in the selective recruitment of eosinophils. Other factors such as PAF and leukotriene B_4 also function as chemoattractants, but these factors are not specific for eosinophils. T_H2 lymphocytes and activated mast cells produce factors (IL-5, IL-3, and GM-CSF) that not only stimulate the production and release of eosinophils but also activate eosinophils and promote their survival.[458]

Helminths stimulate both humoral and cellular immunity, but they are resistant to killing by conventional immune mechanisms. B lymphocytes produce IgG antibodies that may bind to the parasites, but their extracellular cuticles cannot be penetrated by the complement membrane attack complex or T lymphocyte perforins. As previously discussed for allergens, specific IgE antibodies against parasite antigens are also produced, and these IgE molecules bind to mast cells. The binding of parasite antigens to these IgE antibodies results in mast cell activation and degranulation and release of inflammatory mediators and potent chemoattractants for eosinophils.[458]

Like molecules associated with neutrophil adhesive processes, selectins and β_2 integrins are involved in eosinophil adhesion to activated endothelial cells. In addition, endothelial cells activated by IL-4 and IL-13 express vascular cell adhesion molecule-1 (VCAM-1), which binds to very late antigen-4 (VLA-4) on the surfaces of eosinophils. This integrin is not expressed on neutrophils and presumably helps to provide specificity for eosinophil localization.[478]

Eosinophils migrate into the tissues in response to chemoattractants generated in response to helminths. Initially, migration is stimulated primarily by mast cell- and/or parasite-derived attractants, including chitin (N-acetyl-beta-D-glucosamine), a widespread polymer that provides structural rigidity to helminths, insects, crustaceans, and fungi.[393] A second wave of migration is supported by IL-5 and other cytokines produced by T_H2 lymphocytes.[458]

Eosinophils bind to the opsonized parasites via their surface receptors to IgG and complement. The parasites are much too large for eosinophils to ingest, but when activated, eosinophils exhibit dramatic NADPH oxidase activity, which generates extracellular oxidants. They also exocytose their granules in the area of the invading parasite. Eosinophil peroxidase released from granules interacts with hydrogen peroxide generated from the respiratory burst and halide ions. This complex—along with other oxygen metabolites, major basic protein, eosinophil cationic protein, and eosinophil neurotoxin released from secondary granules—is primarily involved in the killing of helminths.[458,478]

The eosinophil has been perceived as a terminal effector cell in the T_H2 inflammatory response. However, recent work indicates that eosinophils have the ability to modulate T lymphocyte responses. Eosinophils can present antigens to T lymphocytes and produce cytokines (primarily IL-4 and IL-13) that induce T_H2-cell development and recruit additional T_H2 cells to sites of inflammation.[438]

Basophil Functions

Basophils generally occur in low numbers in the circulation. They contain most of the histamine measured in blood. Histamine in granules is bound to proteoglycans (such as chondroitin sulfate and heparin), which are responsible for the metachromatic staining (purple color with blue dyes) of the granules. Basophils have biochemical characteristics similar to those of mast cells and share a common progenitor cell with mast cells in bone marrow, but they are clearly different cell types.[164] Basophils have segmented nuclei and mast cells have round nuclei. Mast cells usually have more cytoplasmic granules than basophils. In cats, both primary and secondary granules in basophils are morphologically different from mast cell granules.

Basophils have functions similar to those of mast cells, including being important in the protective immunity against helminths.[361] In contrast to mast cells, which develop and reside in tissues, basophils are recruited from blood into sites of inflammation after exposure to allergens, helminths, and ectoparasites.[476] Among chemoattractants, chemokines that bind to C-C chemokine receptor type 3 (CCR3) are the most potent basophil chemoattractants. These chemokines include the eotaxins (CCL11, CCL24, and CCL26) and CCL5, CCL7, and CCL13.[470] IL-33 has recently been identified as an interleukin that targets basophils. It enhances histamine release by IgE-dependent stimuli as well as the secretion of IL-4, IL-8, and IL-13 by blood basophils. IL-33 may also help regulate basophil binding to endothelium and migration into the tissues.[470]

Following the binding of an antigen to a specific, surface-bound IgE antibody, basophils are activated and release histamine and other mediators that contribute to the inflammation present in immediate hypersensitivity reactions. In addition to IgE-mediated antigenic activation, other substances including C5a, various bacterial peptides, and chemokines can also activate basophils.[470] Recent studies reveal that basophils perform essential nonredundant functions in T_H2 cytokine-dependent immunity. In particular, basophils migrate to lymph nodes and function as antigen-presenting cells, which appears to be critical for the induction of T_H2-cell differentiation.[411,431] In concert with IL-3, stem cell factor (SCF) prolongs basophil survival by delaying apoptosis.[208]

Monocyte/Macrophage/Dendritic-Cell Functions

Monocyte Functions

Monocytes are present in mammals, birds, amphibians, and fish.[27] Several subsets of monocytes are reported to occur in mice and humans.[27] One subset of monocytes appears to crawl along the luminal endothelium of blood vessels during the steady state, patrolling the endothelium independent of the direction of blood flow.[27] Monocytes and their progeny have at least three major functions in mammals: phagocytosis, antigen presentation to T lymphocytes, and immunomodulation associated with the production of an array of cytokines involved in the regulation of inflammation and hematopoiesis. Monocytes may circulate in blood and return to the bone marrow under steady-state conditions or they may migrate into tissues, where they can differentiate into macrophages and dendritic cells. They are rapidly mobilized from the bone marrow in response to inflammatory conditions.[506] Chemokines, including CCL2 and CCL7, promote this egress from bone marrow.[27] Monocytes migrate in tissues in response to a similar array of chemoattractants to which neutrophils respond, including various chemokines, C5a, leukotriene B_4, PAF, and bacterial products.[106,160]

Macrophage Functions

Macrophage colony-stimulating factor (M-CSF) stimulates not only monocyte production but also the transformation of monocytes into macrophages.[122] M1 macrophages are activated by lipopolysaccharides (LPS) and interferon-γ (IFN-γ). They have potent antimicrobial properties, promote inflammation, and secrete IL-12, which stimulates T-helper 1 (T_H1) responses. M2 macrophages appear to be more important in wound repair, tissue remodeling, and immunomodulation by stimulating T_H2 responses.[27,170]

The development of monocytes into macrophages is associated with a marked increase in size, an increase in granules (lysosomes), an increase in the size and number of mitochondria, and an increase in phagocytic capacity. Macrophage function is augmented by various cytokines, the most potent of which is reported to be IFN-γ. M-CSF and GM-CSF also enhance macrophage function. The mononuclear phagocyte system consists of various macrophage subsets, including Kupffer cells in the liver, littoral cells in spleen, nurse cells in marrow, peritoneal and pleural macrophages, alveolar macrophages, and multinucleated giant cells that may form during chronic inflammatory conditions from a fusion of mononuclear phagocytes.[160]

Macrophages move more slowly and are generally less potent in killing bacteria, but they are notably more active against viral, fungal, protozoal, and helminth infections than are neutrophils. Macrophages can synthesize new membrane material and replace expended lysosomes. Therefore they have more staying power in combating infections than do neutrophils, which have limited synthetic abilities.[106,160]

Macrophages play important roles in linking the innate and adaptive immune responses. As part of the innate immune response, they express an array of microbial pattern-recognition receptors, including Toll-like receptors, which allow them to recognize a variety of bacterial molecules such as LPS from Gram-negative bacilli. Macrophages also have Fc receptors for antibodies and complement receptors, which promote their phagocytosis of opsonized microorganisms.[160]

The antimicrobial properties of macrophages are less well understood than those of neutrophils. NADPH oxidase and myeloperoxidase activities are present, although the activity of myeloperoxidase is considerably less than it is in neutrophils. Lysozyme is present, but few organisms are sensitive to it in their native states. Nitric oxide, a free radical generated from L-arginine, generally appears to be important in microbial killing by macrophages, especially after nitric oxide interacts with superoxide to generate toxic derivatives, including peroxynitrite.[108,160,341]

Macrophage scavenger receptors recognize not only microorganisms but also lipids and dying or dead cells.[27] Macrophages demonstrate necrotaxis and necrophagocytosis (phagocytosis of devitalized tissue). Opsonization of necrotic tissue is not required for necrophagocytosis to occur. Consequently macrophages serve an important function in cleaning up necrotic tissue and other debris within the body.[160]

Macrophages have important functions in the modulation of immunity, including antigen processing; killing of tumor cells after sensitization by T lymphocytes; and synthesis of CSFs, interleukins, complement components, IFN, and TNF-α. Macrophages also remove aged or damaged erythrocytes. Most of the iron released from these phagocytized erythrocytes is rapidly returned back into the circulation, but some of it is stored in macrophages in the form of ferritin and hemosiderin. Macrophages are also necessary for normal wound healing.[160] Macrophages in the liver and spleen are most important in clearing blood-borne pathogens of dogs, rodents, rabbits, monkeys, and humans, but intravenous pulmonary macrophages are most important in defending against blood-borne pathogens in cats, ruminants, pigs, and horses.[62,430]

Dendritic-Cell Functions

Classic dendritic cells are antigen-presenting cells that are present in nearly all tissues. They are essential in the initiation and control of acquired immunity as well as in maintaining immunologic tolerance. They continually present antigenic peptides, processed from self and foreign proteins within the body, to a spectrum of T lymphocytes. This communication with T lymphocytes requires that antigenic peptides be presented in the context of major histocompatibility complex class I (MHC-I) and major histocompatibility complex class II (MHC-II) molecules on the surfaces of dendritic cells.

Dendritic cells develop from immature dendritic cells that leave the bone marrow, enter blood, and migrate into the tissues. Immature dendritic cells are estimated to account for about 5% of the monocyte-like cells in the blood of humans.[27,506] Immature dendritic cells are capable of recognizing invading pathogens because they have pattern-recognition receptors (PRRs), including Toll-like receptors and nucleotide-binding oligomerization domain (NOD) receptors, on their surfaces, which bind to pathogen-associated molecular patterns (PAMPs), such as lipopolysaccharides and microbial nucleic acids. Once immature dendritic cells bind and phagocytize an exogenous antigen, they rapidly mature and develop enhanced antigen-processing abilities. Engulfed antigens are partially digested when phagosomes containing antigens fuse with lysosomes. Resultant endosomes containing peptide fragments fuse with other endosomes containing newly formed MHC-II molecules. The MHC-II molecules combine with peptide antigens to form MHC-peptide complexes, which are presented on the cell surface for binding to CD4$^+$ T lymphocytes with complementary T cell receptors (TCRs).

A subset of dendritic cells can process endogenous antigen and express both MHC-I and MHC-II on their surfaces. The antigen bound to MHC-I may be acquired if the dendritic cells are infected with a pathogen, or they may acquire the antigen from dying cells. Dendritic cells with foreign antigen bound to MHC-I and MHC-II molecules on their surfaces migrate to lymph nodes and present antigen to naive CD8$^+$ and CD4$^+$ lymphocytes, respectively.[458]

Plasmacytoid dendritic cells are produced in the bone marrow and migrate to the tissues. Although they can also process antigens and control T lymphocyte responses, they are specialized cells that respond to viral infections with a massive production of IFN-α.[170]

Monocytes can develop into inflammatory dendritic cells or TNF-α- and iNOS-producing (TiP) dendritic cells under inflammatory conditions. The main function of monocyte-derived inflammatory dendritic cells may be to kill organisms rather than to process antigens and regulate T lymphocyte function.[27]

Lymphocyte and NK Cell Functions

Lymphocytes are divided into T lymphocytes, B lymphocytes, and NK cells. A thorough discussion of the functions of these cells is beyond the scope of this text; the reader is therefore referred to immunology textbooks such as the one by Tizard[458] for more detailed information.

T lymphocytes are largely responsible for cellular immunity. They are involved in immune regulation, cytotoxicity, delayed-type hypersensitivity, and graft-versus-host reactions. T lymphocytes are also actively involved in the control of hematopoiesis. To produce these effects, different subpopulations produce a large number of cytokines with diverse biological activities. Most T lymphocytes express TCRs composed of α and β chains. These TCRs recognize peptide antigens bound to MHC-I or MHC-II molecules. Peptides bound to MHC-I molecules are synthesized intracellularly by most cell types in the body, while peptides bound to MHC-II molecules are formed from extracellular antigens that have been endocytosed and processed by professional antigen-presenting cells, with dendritic cells being most important. Surface proteins CD8 and CD4 are coreceptors that bind to MHC-I and MHC-II, respectively.[458]

CD4$^+$ T Lymphocyte Functions

Naive CD4$^+$ T lymphocytes develop into subsets of T-helper (T_H1, T_H2, and T_H17) lymphocytes through maturational processes induced by binding of processed antigens (bound to MHC-II on the surface of antigen-presenting cells) to complementary TCRs on the surface of the lymphocytes. Different sets of cytokines promote lineage differentiation.[514] The binding of an antigen to its complementary TCR sends a signal through CD3 proteins that triggers a clonal proliferation of cells and the production of short-lived effector cells and long-lived memory cells. When these antigen-specific memory cells recognize the same antigen at a later date, they undergo a secondary heightened proliferative response. Dendritic cells are particularly important as antigen-presenting cells and appear to be required to activate naive T lymphocytes. Macrophages and B lymphocytes can also function as antigen-presenting cells with MHC-II on their surfaces.[458]

T_H lymphocytes exert their control in defending against pathogens and neoplasia by recruiting and activating other immune cells, including B lymphocytes, CD8$^+$ T lymphocytes, macrophages, mast cells, neutrophils, eosinophils, and basophils.[514] T_H1 lymphocytes produce IFN-γ, TNF-β, IL-2, and IL-3; support cellular immunity; and are particularly important in the defense against intracellular pathogens. T_H2 lymphocytes produce IL-4, IL-5, IL-6, IL-10, IL-13, and IL-25; they also support humoral immunity and are essential in the defense against helminths and other extracellular pathogens. T_H17 lymphocytes secrete IL-17, IL-21, and IL-22; generate strong proinflammatory effects; and are involved in fighting gram-negative bacteria, fungi, and some protozoa.[144] Considerable heterogeneity and variable plasticity exist between T_H lymphocytes.[514]

CD4$^+$ T lymphocytes can also differentiate into regulatory T (Treg) lymphocytes. These Treg lymphocytes synthesize IL-10 and appear to suppress potentially deleterious effects of T_H cytokine production. CD8$^+$ Treg lymphocytes have also been identified but are less well studied. Altered T lymphocyte function may result in the development of autoimmune and allergic inflammation; Treg lymphocytes may help prevent the development of these disorders.[96,172,231]

CD8$^+$ T Lymphocyte Functions

CD8$^+$ cytotoxic T lymphocytes are antigen-dependent cells that can destroy target cells (e.g., virus-infected cells and neoplastic cells) by a contact-dependent MHC-I-dependent nonphagocytic process. With the exception of erythrocytes, neurons, gametes, and trophoblasts, MHC-I molecules are generally expressed in all tissue cells. When tissue cells synthesize proteins, samples are processed to form small peptides that are transported to the surface bound to MHC-I molecules. Abnormal cells, such as neoplastic cells or virus-infected cells, express abnormal antigens as well as normal self antigens bound to MHC-I on their surfaces. Self antigens are not recognized by TCRs on CD8$^+$ lymphocytes; however, the recognition and binding of abnormal antigens by TCRs triggers lymphocytes to respond.

Dendritic cells with foreign antigen bound to MHC-I migrate to lymph nodes and present the antigen to naive $CD8^+$ lymphocytes. The activation of naive $CD8^+$ lymphocytes also requires IL-12 from activated dendritic cells and IL-2 and IFN-γ from T_H1 lymphocytes that recognize the same antigen. Stimulated naive and memory $CD8^+$ lymphocytes proliferate and develop into short-lived cytotoxic T lymphocytes and long-lived memory cells. When these antigen-specific memory cells recognize the same antigen at a later date, they undergo a secondary heightened proliferative response.[458]

Immunologic synapses form when TCR-CD8 complexes on the surface of cytotoxic T lymphocytes bind to target cells expressing complementary peptide antigens bound to MHC-I molecules on the surfaces of target cells. Following adhesion, cytotoxic proteins (including perforin, granzymes, and granulysin) within secretory lysosomes of cytotoxic T lymphocytes are exocytosed. Released perforin creates transmembrane channels that facilitate the entry of granzymes and granulysin into the cytoplasm of target cells, and these molecules induce apoptosis. Cytotoxic T lymphocytes also mediate apoptosis of target cells by binding between CD95L (Fas-ligand) expressed on their surfaces to CD95 (Fas) on the surface of target cells. This death receptor pathway is important as a mechanism for removing excess or self-reactive T lymphocytes.[458]

B Lymphocyte Functions

B lymphocytes are primarily responsible for humoral immunity; however, immunoglobulin production also requires the participation of T lymphocytes, dendritic cells, and macrophages. Soluble antigens can enter lymph nodes and spleen by afferent lymph and blood, respectively. Immature dendritic cells beneath the skin and mucosal epithelium also carry antigens to regional lymph nodes.

Naive B lymphocytes are exposed to antigens in lymph nodes and spleen. These recirculating cells enter lymph nodes through HEVs in the paracortex, a region that contains resident dendritic cells, recently migrated dendritic cells that have collected antigen from peripheral tissues, and $CD4^+$ T_H lymphocytes needed for the maximal activation of B lymphocytes to produce antibody and to undergo class switching and affinity maturation. A separate T_H lineage termed follicular helper T lymphocytes (TF_H) has been reported to promote B lymphocyte activation,[282] but some authors have suggested that TF_H cells may be a different state of one or more of the other T_H lineages.[514] These activated B lymphocytes may develop into extrafollicular plasma cells which mount early antibody responses to antigen, or they may migrate to follicles and promote the formation of germinal centers, which generate plasma cells that can secrete high-affinity antibody and memory B lymphocytes, which provide long-lasting protection against a repeated challenge with the same antigen.[40]

Most B lymphocytes in lymph nodes are located in follicles; consequently antigens in afferent lymph that enters the subcapsular sinus must gain access to follicular B lymphocytes. For small antigens, such as low-molecular-weight toxins, this may occur by diffusion; but dendritic cells, macrophages, or B lymphocytes appear to be required to carry large antigens (particulates, immune complexes, viruses, and bacteria) to the follicles. Resident follicular dendritic cells mediate the retention of antigens and function as potent accessory cells during B lymphocyte activation.[40]

Although B lymphocytes can interact with antigens in various forms, it appears that membrane-bound antigens are the predominant forms that initiate B lymphocyte activation. In contrast to the need to process protein antigens to small peptides for binding to TCRs on T lymphocytes, intact antigens are recognized and bound by B cell receptors (BCRs) on B lymphocytes. It is unclear whether antigens are internalized into nondegradative intracellular compartments and then recycled to the surfaces of macrophages, dendritic cells, and B lymphocytes or simply retained as antigen on the surface of these antigen-presenting cells. Macrophages and dendritic cells may bind antigens to a variety of surface receptors, including Fc receptors, complement receptors, pattern-recognition receptors, and/or lectin receptors that could present unprocessed antigen to B lymphocytes, and B lymphocytes are reported to bind antigen to complement receptors, thereby transporting antigen independently of their BCRs.[40]

B lymphocyte activation is initiated following the binding of antigens to their cognate BCRs. Not only does antigen binding initiate their activation, but B lymphocytes can process the bound antigen and present it along with MHC-II to specific $CD4^+$ T_H lymphocytes, which secrete cytokines that stimulate B lymphocyte proliferation and differentiation. IL-21, produced by T_H lymphocytes (especially TF_H lymphocytes), is a potent cytokine for the activation and proliferation of human B lymphocytes, for differentiation of these cells into plasma cells, and for stimulating antibody production by plasma cells. This interaction between B and T lymphocytes results in the simultaneous stimulation of humoral and cellular immunity.[40,282,410] B cell activating factor (BAFF) also induces B lymphocyte proliferation and differentiation into plasma cells. This glycoprotein member of the TNF family is secreted by activated innate immune cells and appears to be an important factor in B lymphocyte homeostasis.[102]

Following activation, B lymphocytes are transformed into immunoglobulin-producing immunoblasts and subsequently plasma cells. IgM is initially produced by these cells, but with continued antigenic stimulation, IgG becomes the predominant antibody type produced. Clonal amplification of these cells results in the production of greater amounts of antibody against the foreign antigen. In addition to immunoglobulins, B lymphocytes produce cytokines that may influence the proliferation and/or function of other blood cell types.[40,458]

B lymphocytes provide a link between innate and adaptive immunity because B lymphocytes express Toll-like receptors in addition to antigen-specific BCRs. Antigen binding to Toll-like receptors on memory B lymphocytes may result in their activation and differentiation into immunoglobulin-secreting plasma cells independent of T lymphocytes.[102]

NK Cell Functions

NK cells appear as granular lymphocytes in most species. They do not have antigen receptors on their surfaces, like T and B lymphocytes. NK cells have receptors for MCH-I molecules that are present on the surfaces of normal cells, and they have a NKG2D receptor that recognizes several proteins, including MHC-I chain-related A and B (MICA and MICB), which are expressed on stressed cells but not on normal cells. Target cell destruction by NK cells is triggered if target cells express MICA or MICB, but destruction is inhibited if target cells express appropriate MHC-I molecules. Tumor cells and virus-infected cells are destroyed by NK cells because these cells have upregulated proteins like MICA and MICB and decreased amounts of normal MCH-I molecules on their surfaces. NK cells also have Fc receptors and can bind to and kill cells with antibodies on their surfaces through a process called antibody-dependent cellular cytotoxicity.[458,461]

After activation, $CD8^+$ lymphocytes typically proliferate and exhibit clonal expansion before acquiring cytotoxic potential. In contrast, NK cells become cytotoxic rapidly following activation by IFN-γ and a number of cytokines without going through a phase of proliferation and expansion.[513] Activated NK cells bind to target cells and induce apoptosis using mechanisms like those described previously for cytotoxic T lymphocytes.[461] Activated NK cells also secrete an array of cytokines (including TNF and IFN-γ) and chemokines that recruit and activate other hematopoietic cells into sites of inflammation.[117]

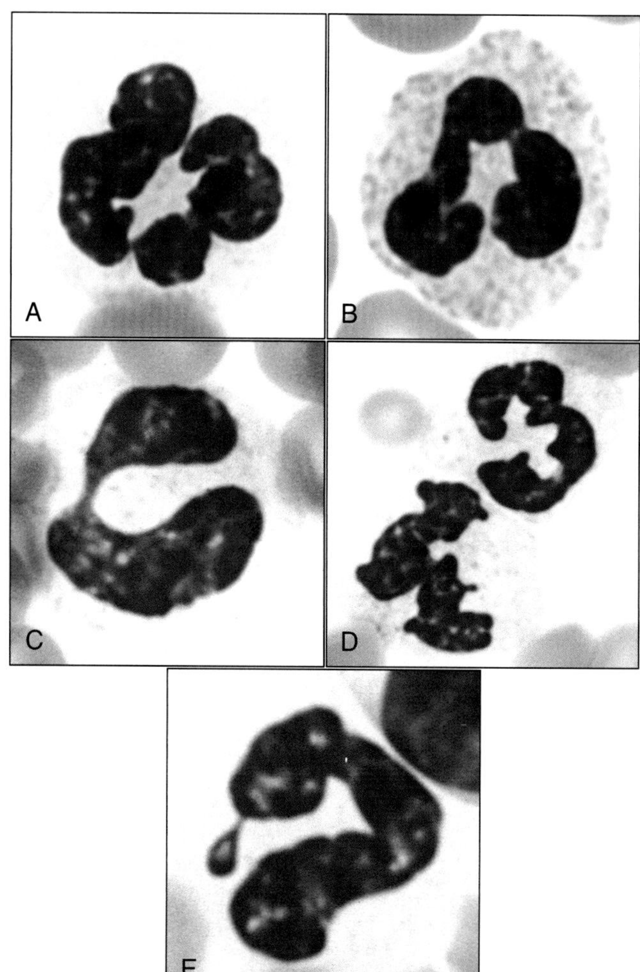

FIGURE 5-10

Normal neutrophil morphology. **A,** Neutrophil in blood from a dog with nearly colorless granules. Wright-Giemsa stain. **B,** Neutrophil in blood from a dog with pink-staining granules. Wright stain. **C,** Bilobed neutrophil in blood from a cow. Wright-Giemsa stain. **D,** Two neutrophils in blood from a horse. Wright-Giemsa stain. **E,** Neutrophil in blood from a female dog exhibiting a sex chromatin lobe or Barr body. Wright-Giemsa stain.

NEUTROPHILS

Normal Neutrophil Morphology

Normal neutrophil morphology is similar in common domestic mammalian species. The chromatin of the nucleus is condensed (dark-staining clumped areas separated by lighter-staining areas) and segmented (lobulated) and stains purple to blue (Fig. 5-10, *A,B*). Nuclear lobes may be joined by fine filaments, but generally there is simply a narrowing of the nucleus between lobes without true filament formation. When an area of the nucleus has a diameter less than two-thirds the diameter of any other area of the nucleus, the neutrophil is classified as mature, even if only two lobes are present (Fig. 5-10, *C*). The nuclear outline is more scalloped (jagged) in horses than in other species (Fig. 5-10, *D*).

Most invertebrates and most reptiles, including turtles and snakes, have oval or round nuclei in mature granulocytes.[49] Neutrophils in amphibians are lobulated and exceptionally large, like their erythrocytes (see Fig. 4-8). Some species of lizards, including the green iguana, have lobed nuclei.[74] Avian granulocytes generally have less nuclear segmentation than mammalian neutrophils. Granulocytes have lobulated nuclei in some species of fish, but many have round or oval nuclei.[74] Some neutrophil nuclei are ring-shaped in mice.[49]

A Barr body (sex chromatin lobe or drumstick) is present in a low percentage of neutrophils from female mammals (Fig. 5-10, *E*).[226] This round basophilic body is attached to a terminal lobe of the nucleus by a thin chromatin strand. It contains the inactivated X chromosome.[239] The background cytoplasm of neutrophils generally appears colorless but may appear pale pink or faintly basophilic. In most mammalian species, neutrophil granules either do not stain or appear light pink with routine blood stains (see Fig. 5-10, *B*).

In birds, reptiles, fish, and some mammalian species (e.g., rabbits, guinea pigs, and manatees), the granules of these cells stain red and the cells are called heterophils (Fig. 5-11, *A*). They must be differentiated from eosinophils, which also have red-staining granules. The granular shape can often help to differentiate these cells. Heterophils usually have rod-shaped or oval granules and eosinophils usually have round granules (Fig. 5-11, B). In addition, the cytoplasm tends to be more basophilic in eosinophils than in heterophils.[203]

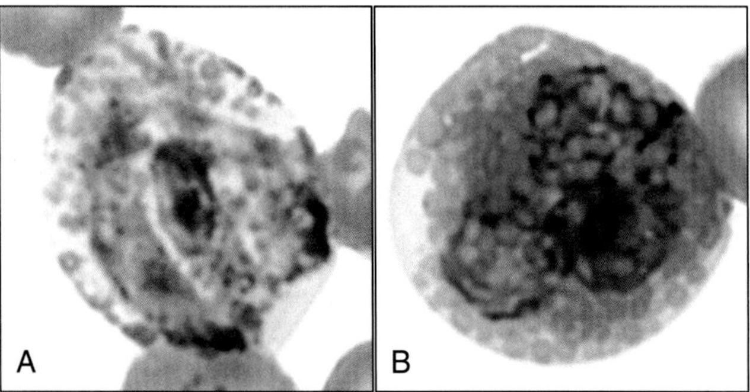

FIGURE 5-11
Morphology of a rabbit heterophil **(A)** compared with a rabbit eosinophil **(B)**. Wright-Giemsa stain.

Morphology of Left Shifts

Mature segmented neutrophils and sometimes low numbers of band neutrophils are released from bone marrow into blood in normal animals. When increased numbers of nonsegmented neutrophilic cells are present in blood, their presence is referred to as a left shift.

Band neutrophils are commonly seen in blood, with metamyelocytes and myelocytes present less often and promyelocytes and myeloblasts rarely encountered. Morphologic changes that occur as cells of the granulocytic series undergo maturation from myeloblasts to mature granulocytes in the bone marrow include a slight diminution in size, a decrease in nucleus : cytoplasm (N : C) ratio, progressive nuclear condensation, changes in nuclear shape, and the appearance of cytoplasmic granules. In the absence of toxicity, the background (i.e., nongranular) cytoplasm color changes from gray-blue in myeloblasts to nearly colorless in mature neutrophils. However, cytoplasmic toxicity is often present in animals with pronounced left shifts in their blood.

Myeloblasts

The morphology of myeloblasts is described under "Blast Cells or Poorly Differentiated Cells," below. Their presence indicates the likelihood of a myeloid neoplasm (Fig. 5-12, *A*).

Promyelocytes

Promyelocytes or progranulocytes have round to oval nuclei with lacy to coarse chromatin. Their most identifiable characteristic is the presence of many magenta-staining primary granules within light-blue cytoplasm (Fig. 5-12, *B*).

Myelocytes

Myelocytes have round nuclei (Fig. 5-12, *C*), but they are generally smaller with more nuclear condensation and lighter-blue cytoplasm than promyelocytes. The primary magenta-staining granules characteristic of promyelocytes are no longer visible in myelocytes. Secondary granules that characterize neutrophils are present but are difficult to visualize because of their neutral-staining characteristics.

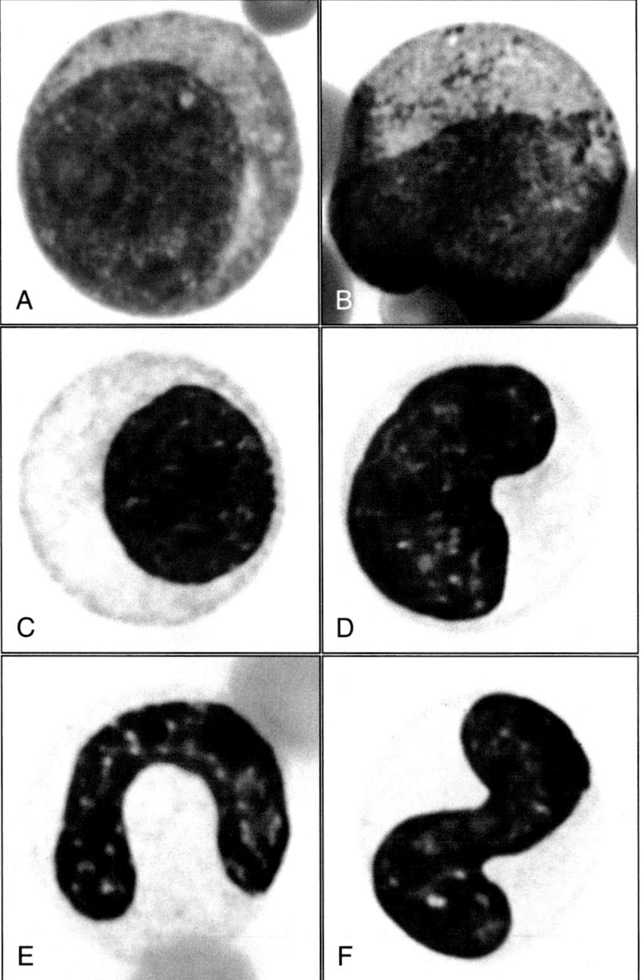

FIGURE 5-12
Neutrophil precursor cells. **A,** Myeloblast in blood from a cat with acute myeloid leukemia (AML). **B,** Promyelocyte with purple cytoplasmic granules in blood from a dog with acute myelomonocytic leukemia (AML-M4). **C,** Neutrophilic myelocyte in blood from a dog with chronic myeloid leukemia. **D,** Neutrophilic metamyelocyte in blood from a dog with chronic myeloid leukemia. **E,** Band neutrophil in blood from a dog with immune-mediated hemolytic anemia. **F,** S-shaped band neutrophil in blood from a dog with immune-mediated hemolytic anemia. Wright-Giemsa stain.

Metamyelocytes

Nuclei with slight indentations are still classified as myelocytes, but once the nuclear indentation extends more than 25% into the nucleus, the cell is called a metamyelocyte (Fig. 5-12, *D*). Nuclear condensation becomes readily apparent at this stage of maturation.

Band Neutrophils

Various criteria have been used to differentiate bands from mature neutrophils in humans. The National Committee for Clinical Laboratory Standards and the College of American Pathologists differentiate a band from a segmented neutrophil by requiring a segmented neutrophil to have a complete separation of the lobes, with a clearly visible strand that appears as a solid thread-like dark line, containing no visible chromatin between the margins.[95] This criterion is not appropriate for most animal species, because neutrophils do not have the degree of segmentation seen in humans. Generally speaking, band neutrophils have rod-shaped nuclei with parallel sides (Fig. 5-12, *E*). Because few cells will have perfectly parallel sides, it is recommended that no area of the nucleus should have a diameter less than two-thirds the diameter of any other area of the nucleus; otherwise the cell is classified as a mature neutrophil. Band neutrophil nuclei twist to conform to the space within the cytoplasm, and U-shaped or S-shaped nuclei (Fig. 5-12, *F*) are common. Chromatin condensation is prominent, and the cytoplasm's appearance is essentially the same as that seen in mature neutrophils. Once nuclear segments form, the cell is called a mature neutrophil even if only two lobes are present (see Fig. 5-10, *C*).

Disorders with Left Shifts

Left shifts are usually associated with inflammatory conditions.[99,412,452,493] These conditions are often infectious but they may be noninfectious, as in immune-mediated disorders and infiltrative marrow disease.[213,317] Left shifts are also present in animals with chronic myeloid leukemia and Pelger-Huët anomaly.[270,471]

Inflammation

The presence of a significant left shift in animals with an inflammatory disorder indicates that the stimulus for release of neutrophils from bone marrow is greater than can be accommodated by release from mature neutrophil stores alone. The magnitude of a left shift in response to inflammation can vary from slightly increased numbers of bands to severe left shifts with metamyelocytes, myelocytes, and, rarely, even promyelocytes present in blood. The total neutrophil count may be low, normal, or high depending on the number of these cells released from the bone marrow versus the number utilized in the inflammatory process. Toxic cytoplasm is often present in animals with left shifts in response to inflammatory disorders (Fig. 5-13). Other abnormalities that may be present include donut-shaped nuclei and giant neutrophils (Figs. 5-14, 5-15).

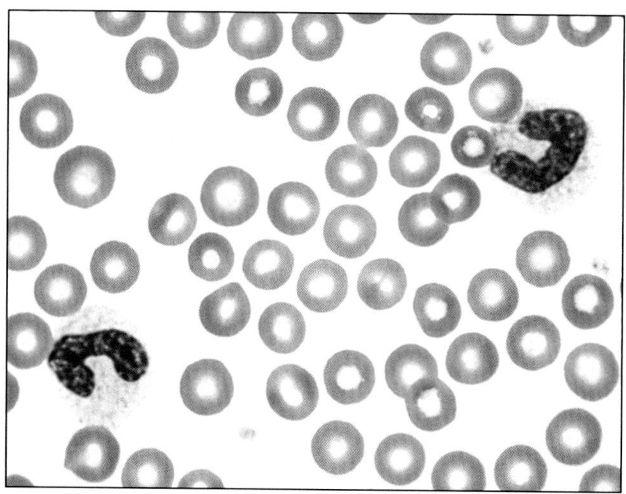

FIGURE 5-13
Toxic left shift in blood from a dog with a septic peritonitis. Two band neutrophils with toxic cytoplasm are present.

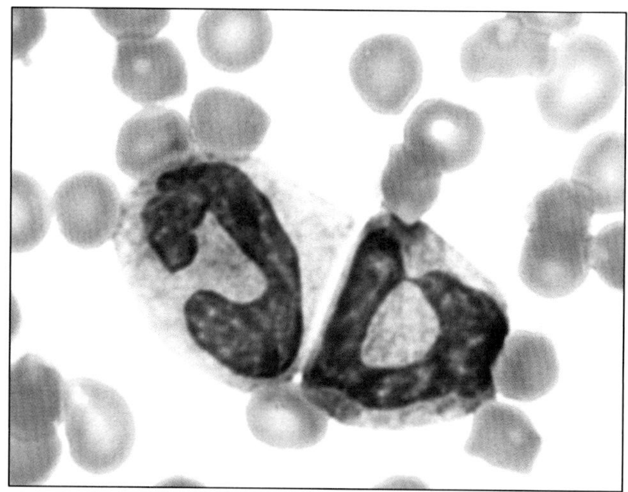

FIGURE 5-14
Toxic left shift in the blood of a cat with diabetes mellitus and fungal pneumonia. A band neutrophil and a neutrophilic cell with a donut-shaped nucleus are present. Pale inclusions in erythrocytes are Heinz bodies. Wright-Giemsa stain.

Chronic Myeloid Leukemia

Chronic myeloid leukemia (CML) presents with a high total leukocyte count (usually greater than 50,000/µL) with a marked neutrophilic left shift in blood (Fig. 5-16).[195,273,450] In domestic animals, CML is primarily seen in dogs. Increased numbers of monocytes, eosinophils, and/or basophils may also be present. Myeloblasts are either absent or present in low numbers in blood. CML is suspected when no inflammatory disorder can be found to explain the extreme left shift. The left shift present in CML is usually less orderly than that seen in leukemoid reactions. The presence of dysplastic abnormalities in other blood cell types also supports a diagnosis of CML. On the other hand, the presence of moderate to marked cytoplasmic toxicity, increased inflammatory plasma proteins, and physical evidence of inflammation suggests that a leukemoid reaction is present rather than CML.

Pelger-Huët Anomaly (Hyposegmentation)

The term *hyposegmentation* refers to a left shift with condensed nuclear chromatin and few or no nuclear constrictions (Figs. 5-17, 5-18, 5-19). Nuclei may be round, oval, kidney-shaped, band-shaped, peanut-shaped, or bilobed. Hyposegmentation occurs as an inherited Pelger-Huët anomaly in dogs, cats, horses, rabbits, and humans.[175,196,268] Eosinophils and basophils may also be affected. This abnormality in humans is

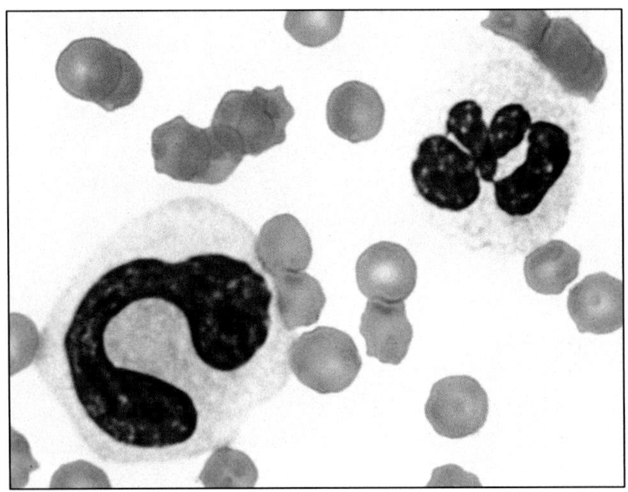

FIGURE 5-15
Giant neutrophil *(bottom)* in the blood of a cat with a leukemoid reaction secondary to a bacterial infection that resulted in the formation of multiple draining abscesses. Wright-Giemsa stain.

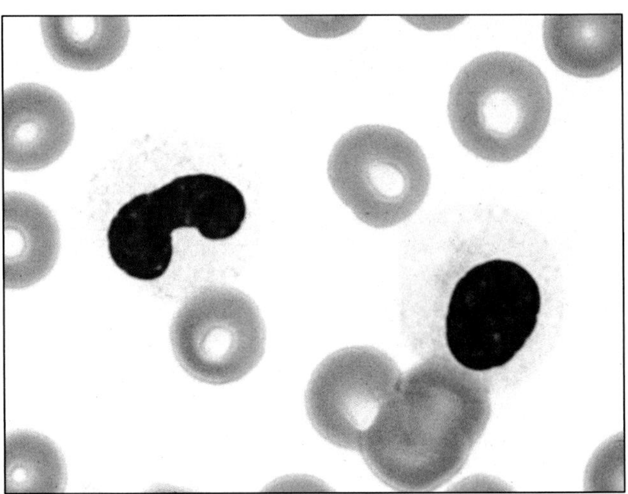

FIGURE 5-17
Band neutrophil *(left)* and neutrophilic myelocyte *(right)* in the blood of a dog with Pelger-Huët anomaly. Wright-Giemsa stain.

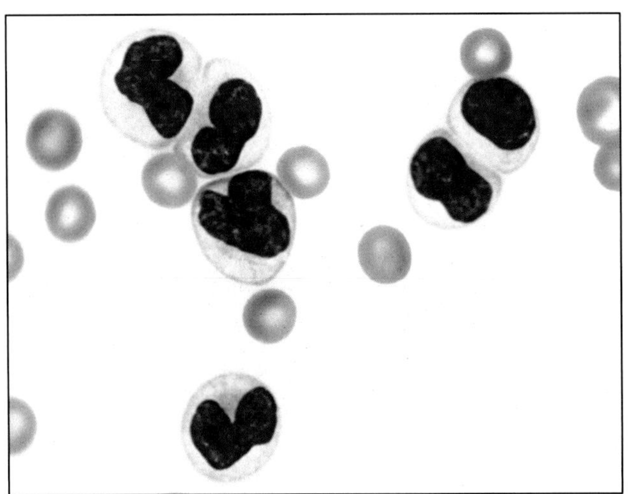

FIGURE 5-16
Left shift in the blood of a dog with chronic myeloid leukemia. Band neutrophils, neutrophilic metamyelocytes, and a neutrophilic myelocyte are present. Wright-Giemsa stain.

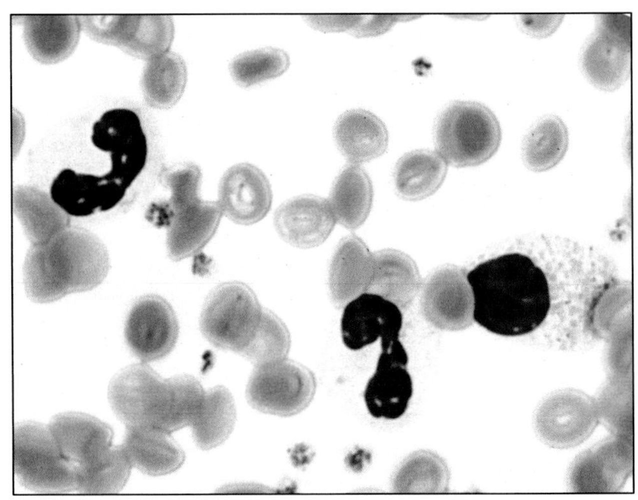

FIGURE 5-18
Band neutrophil *(left),* bilobed neutrophil *(center),* and eosinophilic myelocyte *(right)* in the blood of a cat with Pelger-Huët anomaly. Wright-Giemsa stain.

caused by a defect in the lamin B receptor (LBR) gene. LBR is an integral membrane protein in the nuclear envelope.[218]

No clinical signs are associated with animals that are heterozygous for this disorder. Homozygous affected animals exhibit skeletal deformities and die in utero or shortly after birth.[218] The Pelger-Huët anomaly is common in Australian shepherd dogs, where it appears to be transmitted as an autosomal dominant trait with incomplete or decreased penetrance.[270] A pseudo-Pelger-Huët anomaly may occur in myeloid neoplasms, transiently with infections, or rarely with the administration of certain drugs. In contrast to hereditary Pelger-Huët anomaly, a minority of neutrophils are generally hyposegmented in disorders exhibiting pseudo-Pelger-Huët cells.[105,414,427]

Hypersegmentation

Hypersegmentation (right shift) has generally been defined as the presence of five or more distinct nuclear lobes within neutrophils of domestic animals (Fig. 5-20). However, nuclei of horse neutrophils have large clumps of dense chromatin projecting from their surfaces, making them appear more segmented than the neutrophils of other common domestic animals. Normal horse neutrophils average about five lobes, where a lobe is defined as a rounded part of the nucleus that

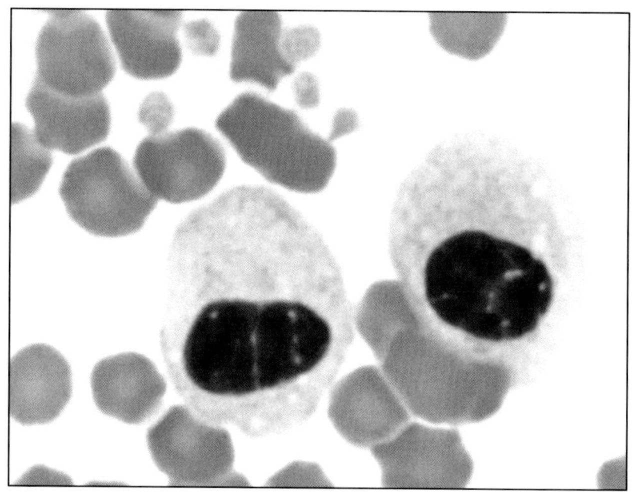

FIGURE 5-19

Neutrophilic myelocytes in the blood of a horse with Pelger-Huët anomaly.

From Grondin TM, Dewitt SF, Keeton KS. Pelger-Huët anomaly in an Arabian horse. Vet Clin Pathol. *2007;36:306-310.*

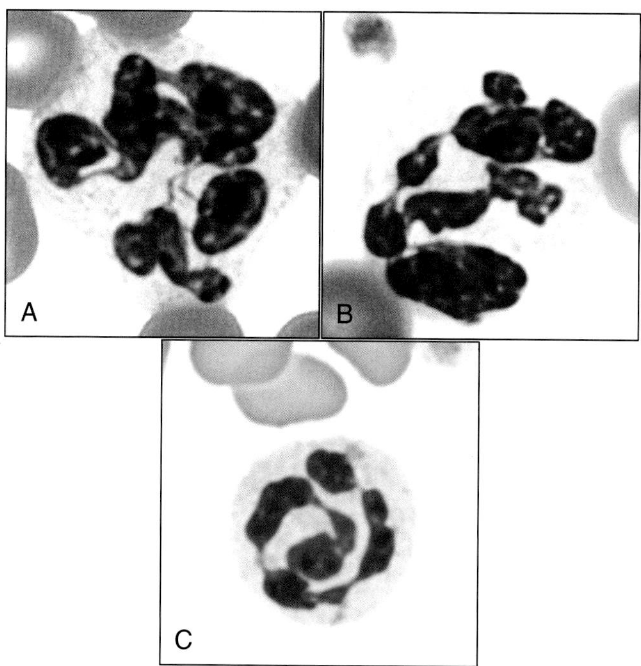

FIGURE 5-20

Hypersegmented neutrophils. **A,** Hypersegmented neutrophil in blood from a dog with systemic mastocytosis treated with vincristine and prednisone. **B,** Hypersegmented neutrophil in blood from a dog with AML-M4. **C,** Hypersegmented neutrophil in blood from a cat with folate deficiency. Wright-Giemsa stain.

C, Courtesy of S. Myers.

is focal and distinct. Consequently it has been suggested that seven or more lobes are required before a horse neutrophil is considered to be hypersegmented.[465] Hypersegmentation in rats has been defined as six or more lobes.[44]

Hypersegmentation occurs as a normal aging process and may reflect prolonged transit time in blood, as can occur with resolving chronic inflammation, glucocorticoid administration, or hyperadrenocorticism.[131] Hypersegmentation may also be present in myeloid neoplasms.[387,492] Idiopathic (presumably inherited) hypersegmentation has been reported in quarter horses (Fig. 5-21).[382,386,465] The presence of hypersegmentation in these horses does not appear to be associated with clinical disease. Neutrophilic hypersegmentation has been described in dogs with an inherited defect in cobalamin absorption and in a cat with folate deficiency (see Fig. 5-20, *C*).[163,344] Finally, neutrophilic hypersegmentation has been described in association with oxazolidinone and amphetamine toxicity[291,496] and with long-term phenytoin administration in dogs.[70]

Toxic Cytoplasm

When the cytoplasm of a neutrophilic cell has increased basophilia, foamy vacuolation, and/or contains Döhle bodies, it is said to be toxic. Criteria for classifying the degree of toxicity are given in Table 2-1. These morphologic abnormalities develop in neutrophilic cells within the bone marrow prior to their release into the circulation.[182,183] Toxic cytoplasm is primarily seen in association with strong inflammatory conditions. Nuclear abnormalities—including karyolysis,

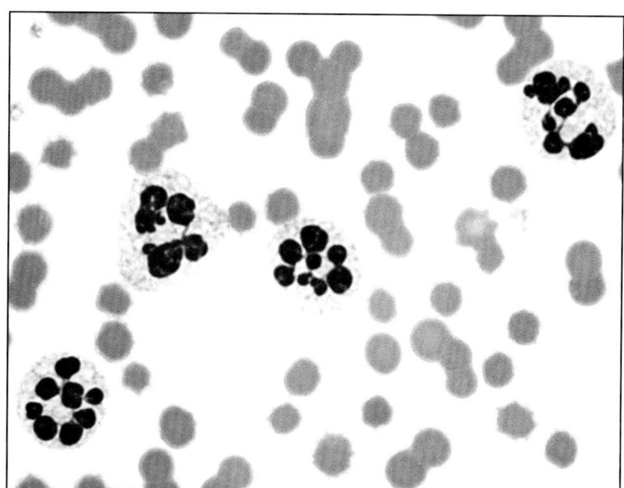

FIGURE 5-21

Persistent (presumably inherited) hypersegmentation in blood from a quarter horse. Echinocytosis with intravascular hemolysis was also present; it was attributed to transient liver disease.

From Ramaiah SK, Harvey JW, Giguère S, et al. Intravascular hemolysis associated with liver disease in a horse with marked neutrophil hypersegmentation. J Vet Intern Med. *2003;17:360-363.*

karyorrhexis, hyposegmentation, ring formation and binucleation—may also be present in neutrophils with toxic cytoplasm. Giant neutrophils with nuclear abnormalities are most often seen in cats.[226] Animals with toxic neutrophils generally exhibit severe signs of illness, require longer hospitalizations, and have higher mortality (at least among dogs) than animals without toxic neutrophils.[22,415] Although toxic neutrophils are most often associated with bacterial infections (e.g., pneumonia, peritonitis, septicemia, pyometra),[22,285,338,415] they may also be observed in viral infections (e.g., parvovirus in dogs and cats, upper respiratory viruses in cats),[415] immune-mediated hemolytic anemia in dogs,[317] and some severe metabolic disorders (e.g., acute renal failure, ketoacidotic diabetes, hepatic lipidosis in cats).[22,415]

Foamy Basophilia

Foamy basophilia often occurs with severe bacterial infections but can occur with other causes of toxemia (Fig. 5-22, *A-H*). When viewed by electron microscopy, foamy vacuolation appears as irregular, electron-lucent areas that are not membrane bound. Cytoplasmic basophilia results from the persistence of large amounts of rough endoplasmic reticulum and polyribosomes.[182]

Döhle Bodies

Döhle bodies are bluish angular cytoplasmic inclusions of neutrophils and their precursors (Fig. 5-22, *D-I*). They are composed of retained aggregates of rough endoplasmic reticula.[47] By themselves, these inclusions represent evidence of mild toxicity and are sometimes seen in neutrophils of cats that do not exhibit signs of illness (Fig. 5-22, *I*). Döhle bodies must be differentiated from iron-positive granules, distemper inclusions in dogs, and granules present in neutrophils from cats with inherited Chédiak-Higashi syndrome.

Toxic Granulation

Toxic granulation refers to the presence of magenta-staining cytoplasmic granules (Fig. 5-22, *J-L*).[47] These granules are primary granules that have retained the staining intensity normally observed in promyelocytes in the bone marrow. The presence of toxic granulation and cytoplasmic basophilia suggests severe toxemia. Toxic granulation is most often seen in horses and rarely in dogs and cats.[226] It should not be confused with the pink staining of secondary granules, which is not a sign of toxicity. Toxic granulation must be differentiated from the granules present in some Birman cats, granules in animals with certain lysosomal storage disorders, and miscellaneous granules and inclusions to be discussed subsequently.

Granules and Inclusions

Normal Foals

Purple granules are often seen in neutrophils from foals without other evidence of cytoplasmic toxicity (Fig. 5-23, *A*). The percentage of neutrophils with purple granules varied from 0% to 70% (mean 13%) in 38 healthy newborn thoroughbred foals, and the percentage of neutrophils with granules tended to be maintained in each foal through 30 days of age (J. W. Harvey, unpublished data). It is assumed that like toxic granules, these are primary granules that have retained the staining intensity normally observed in promyelocytes in the bone marrow.

Lipemia in a Horse

Purple granules were present in neutrophils from a Paso Fino mare with hyperlipidemia and hepatic lipidosis (Fig. 5-23, *B*). As in the normal foals described above, no other cytoplasmic evidence of toxicity was present. Consequently caution must be exercised in using the term *toxic granulation* with regard to horses.

Lysosomal Storage Diseases

The lysosomal system is the principal site of intracellular degradation. Lysosomes are membrane-bound organelles that contain more than 40 acid hydrolases capable of degrading most biologically important macromolecules. An inherited deficiency in one of these enzymes can result in the accumulation of undegraded substances (e.g., glycosaminoglycans, complex oligosaccharides, cerebrosides, etc.) within lysosomes; hence the name *lysosomal storage disease.*[204] Blue- to magenta-staining granulation occurs in the cytoplasm of neutrophils from animals with certain lysosomal storage disorders, including mucopolysaccharidosis type VI (Fig. 5-23, *C,D*),[11,98,349] mucopolysaccharidosis type VII (Fig. 5-23, *E,F*),[177,205,429] and GM_2-gangliosidosis (Fig. 5-23, *G*).[230,256]

Birman Cats

Small reddish granules have been reported as an inherited anomaly in Birman cats without evidence of illness.[217] These granules were of normal size when examined by transmission electron microscopy. They did not stain with alcian blue or toluidine blue, indicating that the animals did not have an inherited mucopolysaccharidosis.

Reddish Granulation in Cats

We have observed persistent reddish granulation in neutrophils of five cats (Fig. 5-23, *H*) that appeared similar to that reported in Birman cats. Affected animals have included several Siamese and Himalayan cats. The granules were negative when they were stained with toluidine blue. No clinical signs could be associated with the presence of the granules, which were found even when animals were healthy.

Chédiak-Higashi Syndrome

The Chédiak-Higashi syndrome is an inherited disorder characterized by partial oculocutaneous albinism, increased susceptibility to infections, hemorrhagic tendencies, and the presence of enlarged membrane-bound granules in many cell types including blood leukocytes. It has been described in Persian cats, several species of cattle, Aleutian mink, foxes, beige rats, and a killer whale.[325] Neutrophils from affected cattle[30,358] and Persian cats[272] contain large pink-to-purple granules (Fig. 5-23, *I,J*). The giant granules may arise from

FIGURE 5-22 **Toxic cytoplasm in neutrophils**

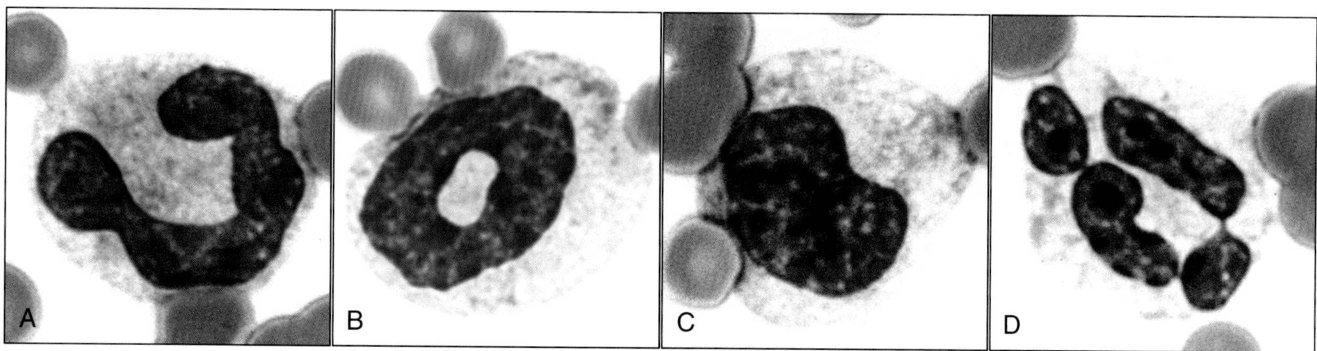

A, Neutrophil with foamy basophilia (toxicity) of the cytoplasm in blood from a cat with septic peritonitis. **B,** Neutrophil with donut-shaped nucleus and foamy basophilia (toxicity) of the cytoplasm in blood from a horse with a *Babesia equi* infection. **C,** Toxic metamyelocyte with foamy basophilia of the cytoplasm in blood from a cat with septic peritonitis. **D,** Toxic neutrophil with foamy basophilia and Döhle bodies (angular blue inclusions) in the cytoplasm in blood from a cat with septic peritonitis.

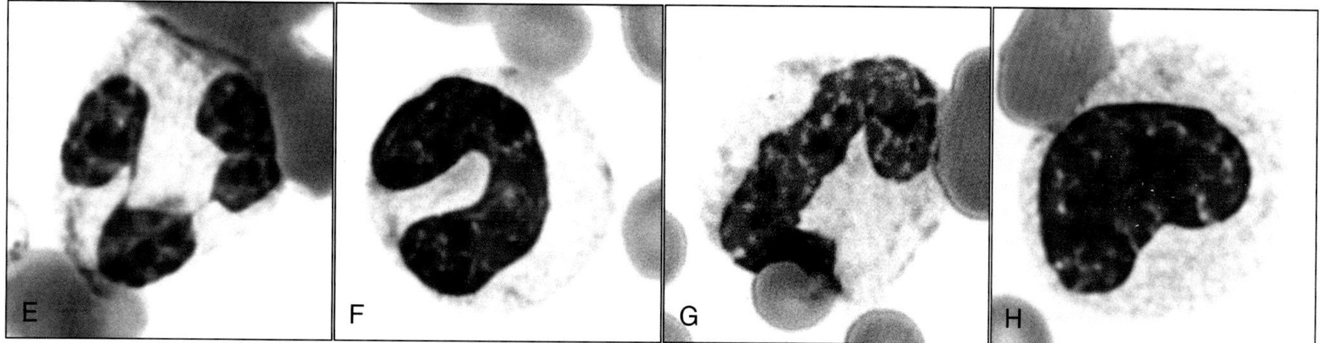

E, Toxic neutrophil with foamy basophilia and Döhle bodies in the cytoplasm in blood from a cat with a marked left shift (leukemoid reaction) secondary to a bacterial infection that resulted in the formation of multiple draining abscesses. **F,** Band neutrophil with lightly basophilic cytoplasm containing Döhle bodies in blood from a horse. **G,** Toxic band neutrophil with foamy basophilia and Döhle bodies in the cytoplasm in blood from a cat with septic peritonitis. **H,** Toxic neutrophilic metamyelocyte with foamy basophilia and faintly staining Döhle bodies in the cytoplasm in blood from a cat with a leukemoid reaction secondary to a bacterial infection that resulted in the formation of multiple draining abscesses.

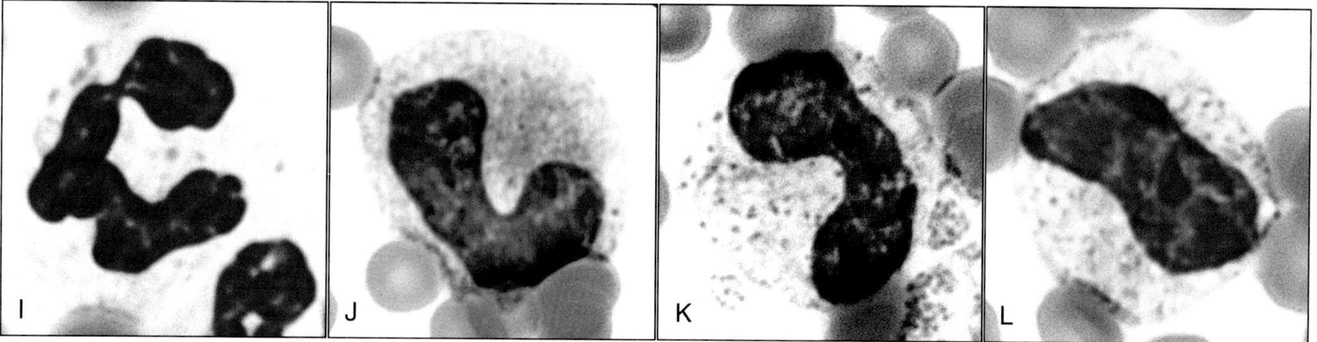

I, Döhle bodies in the cytoplasm of a neutrophil in blood from a cat without other cytoplasmic evidence of toxicity. **J,** Band neutrophil with toxic granulation in blood from a horse with acute salmonellosis. **K,** Band neutrophil with basophilic cytoplasm and toxic granulation in blood from a Holstein cow with a bacterial infection. **L,** Neutrophilic metamyelocyte with toxic granulation in blood from a Holstein cow with a bacterial infection. Wright-Giemsa stain.

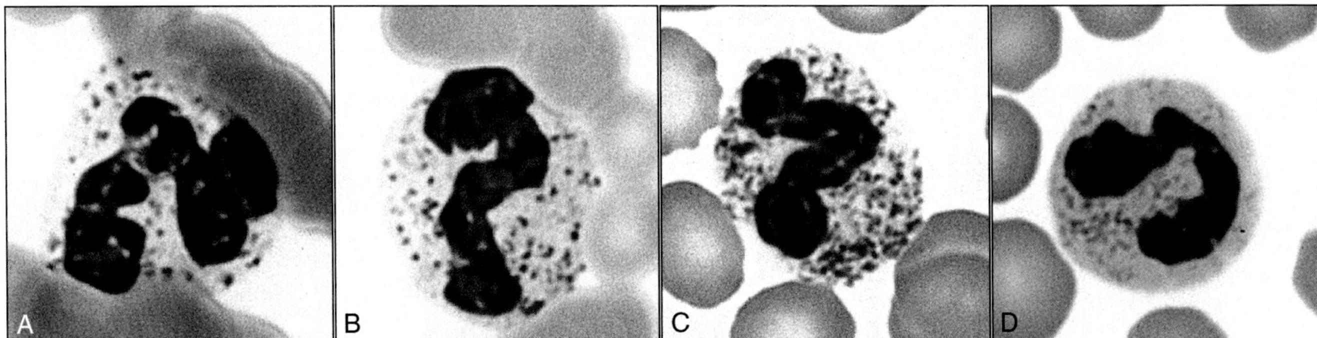

A, Neutrophil with basophilic cytoplasmic granules in the blood of a normal foal. Wright-Giemsa stain. **B,** Neutrophil with cytoplasmic granules in the blood of a hyperlipemic 7-year-old Paso Fino mare with hepatic lipidosis. Wright stain. **C,** Neutrophil with cytoplasmic granules in the blood of a 7-month-old miniature schnauzer dog with mucopolysaccharidosis type VI. Wright-Giemsa stain. **D,** Neutrophil with cytoplasmic granules in the blood of a 1-year-old domestic shorthair cat with inherited mucopolysaccharidosis type VI. Wright stain.

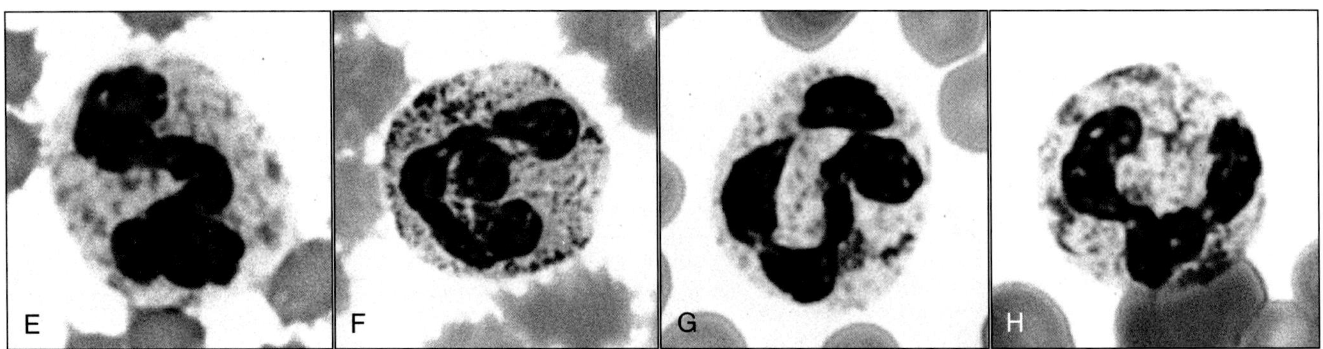

E, Neutrophil with cytoplasmic granules in the blood of an 8-month-old domestic shorthair cat with inherited mucopolysaccharidosis type VII. Wright stain. **F,** Neutrophil with cytoplasmic granules in the blood of a 3-month-old German shepherd dog with inherited mucopolysaccharidosis type VII. Wright stain. **G,** Neutrophil with cytoplasmic granules in the blood of a korat cat with inherited GM_2-gangliosidosis. Wright-Giemsa stain. **H,** Neutrophil with reddish cytoplasmic granulation in blood from a Siamese cat without clinical signs attributable to a lysosomal storage disease. Wright-Giemsa stain.

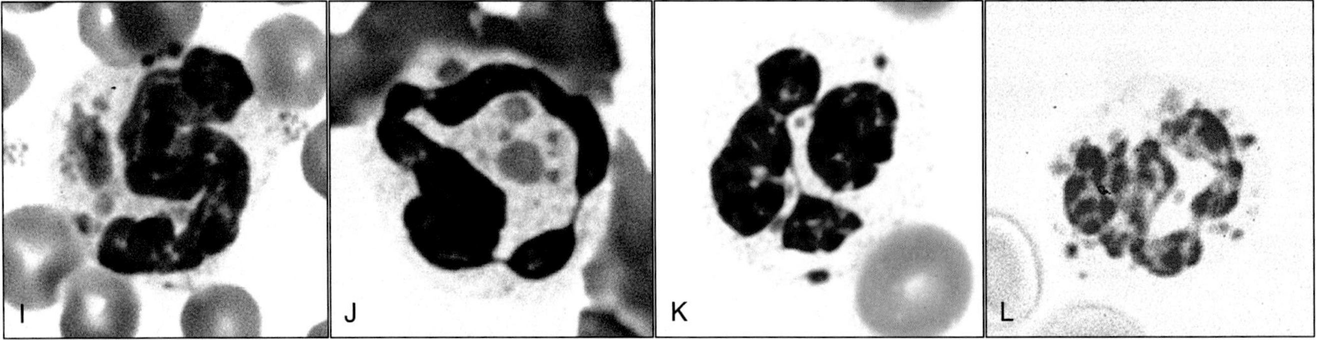

I, Neutrophil with large cytoplasmic granules in blood from a 15-month-old Hereford female with Chédiak-Higashi syndrome. Wright stain. **J,** Neutrophil with large cytoplasmic granules in blood from a Persian cat with Chédiak-Higashi syndrome. Wright stain. **K,** Neutrophil with siderotic cytoplasmic inclusions in blood from a horse with equine infectious anemia. Wright-Giemsa stain. **L,** Neutrophil with siderotic cytoplasmic inclusions in blood from a horse with equine infectious anemia (same blood sample as shown in **K**). **K,** Blue-staining inclusions indicate the presence of iron. Prussian blue stain.

__B,__ Photograph of a stained blood film from a 1983 ASVCP slide review case submitted by J. R. Duncan and E. A. Mahaffey. __C,__ Photograph of a stained blood film from a 1995 ASVCP slide review case submitted by P. R. Avery, D. E. Brown, M. A. Thrall, and D. A. Wenger. __D,__ Photograph of a stained blood film from a 1995 ASVCP slide review case submitted by D. A. Andrews, D. B. DeNicola, S. Jakovljevic, J. Turek, and U. Giger. __E,__ Photograph of a stained blood film from a 1996 ASVCP slide review case submitted by M. A. Thrall, L. Vap, S. Gardner, and D. Wenger. __F,__ Photograph of a stained blood film from a 1997 ASVCP slide review case submitted by D. I. Bounous, D. C. Silverstein, K. S. Latimer, and K. P. Carmichael. __I,__ Photograph of a stained blood film from a 1987 ASVCP slide review case submitted by M. Menard and K. J. Wardrop. __J,__ Photograph taken from a stained slide provided by J. W. Kramer.

unregulated fusion of primary lysosomes during cell development.

May-Hegglin Anomaly

The May-Hegglin anomaly is characterized by a triad of leukocyte inclusions, thrombocytopenia, and macroplatelets (macrothrombocytes). It results from a mutation in the *MYH9* gene that encodes for the heavy chain of nonmuscle myosin IIA. It is an inherited autosomal dominant disorder in humans, where only heterozygous mutations have been identified. This genetic defect has recently been reported in a pug dog.[146] Neutrophils typically had one to four large blue fusiform inclusions in their cytoplasm (Fig. 5-24). The inclusions resembled Döhle bodies but were larger (up to 2 × 4 µm) and more distinct than Döhle bodies. When they were examined by transmission electron microscopy, the inclusions appeared as non-membrane-bound areas devoid of granules containing thin filaments oriented parallel to the longitudinal axis of the inclusions. Neutrophil function appeared to be normal, and there was no evidence of an increased bleeding tendency in this dog.

Siderotic Inclusions

Iron-positive inclusions (hemosiderin) may be seen in neutrophils and monocytes from animals with hemolytic anemia.[169] Prior to the development of definitive serologic tests, the presence of these inclusions in equine leukocytes (sideroleukocytes) was used to support a diagnosis of equine infectious anemia (Fig. 5-23, *K,L*).[212,403] These inclusions can be differentiated from Döhle bodies using the Prussian blue staining procedure because Döhle bodies do not stain positively for iron.

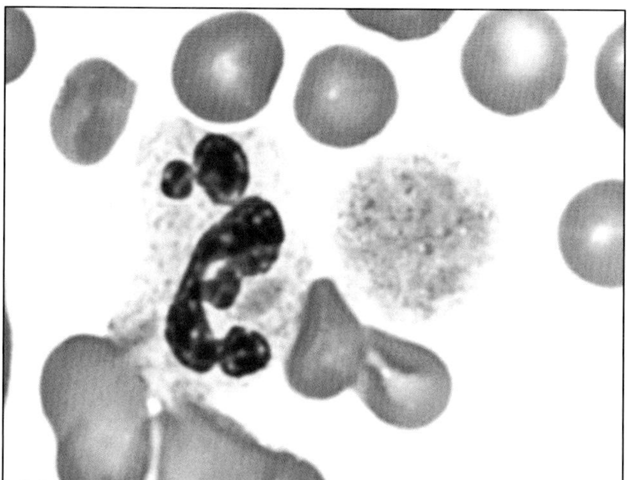

FIGURE 5-24

May-Hegglin anomaly in a dog. A neutrophil with two large blue fusiform cytoplasmic inclusions *(left)* and a macroplatelet (macrothrombocyte) are present. Wright stain.

Photograph of a stained blood film from a 2010 ASVCP slide review case submitted by B. Flatland, M. M. Fry, S. J. Baek, J. H. Bahn, C. J. LeBlanc, J. R. Dunlap, D. J. Kosiba, D. J. Millsaps, and S. E. Schleis.

Infectious Agents

Distemper Inclusions

Distemper viral inclusions are formed in bone marrow precursor cells and may be present in blood cells during the acute viremic stage of the disease.[81,184,314,480] These viral inclusions can be difficult to visualize in the cytoplasm of neutrophils in Wright- or Giemsa-stained blood films but can easily be seen as homogeneous round, oval, or irregularly shaped 1- to 4-µm red inclusions when they are stained with Diff-Quik (Fig. 5-25, *A*).[200]

Rickettsial Species

Rickettsial species infecting granulocytes include *Ehrlichia ewingii* and *Anaplasma phagocytophilum*. Morulae of *Ehrlichia* and *Anaplasma* species appear as tightly packed basophilic clusters of organisms within phagosomes in the cytoplasm (Fig. 5-25, *B-F*; Figs. 5-26, 5-27). Morulae are regularly found in neutrophils and infrequently in eosinophils during the acute stage of infection.[188,189]

In 2001, based on genetic findings obtained using PCR and sequencing of the 16S rRNA gene, *Ehrlichia equi*, *Ehrlichia phagocytophila*, and the human granulocytic *Ehrlichia* (HGE) organism were reorganized into a single species named *Anaplasma phagocytophilum*.[124] However, different variants or strains of *A. phagocytophilum* vary in their pathogenicity and host specificity. For example, a variant of *A. phagocytophilum* in Europe causes severe disease in cattle, but a California variant of *A. phagocytophilum* failed to induce such disease.[148] Similarly, the variant of *A. phagocytophilum* previously classified as HGE causes disease in dogs, but the variant previously classified as *Ehrlichia equi* does not.[130,276]

E. ewingii (see Fig. 5-25, *B*) and the HGE variant of *A. phagocytophilum* (see Fig. 5-25, *C*) cause similar, nonspecific signs of illness in dogs, including fever, lethargy, depression, and sometimes reluctance to move associated with inflammatory arthritis. In addition to blood neutrophils, morulae may be found in a low percentage of neutrophils within the joint fluid of *E. ewingii*-infected and *A. phagocytophilum*-infected dogs with polyarthritis.[5,79,173,189] Thrombocytopenia is the most common hematologic finding, followed by mild to moderate nonregenerative anemia. Lymphopenia is also reported to be a common finding in *A. phagocytophilum*-infected dogs.[5,188,189]

Infection with the equine variant (formerly *E. equi*) and the HGE variant of *A. phagocytophilum* cause high fever, depression, inappetence, ataxia, petechial hemorrhages, and edema, resulting from an associated vasculitis,[274] of the distal limbs in horses.[66,153,303] Hematologic findings include a transient leukopenia (neutropenia and lymphopenia), thrombocytopenia, and mild anemia. Morulae are present in neutrophils (see Fig. 5-25, *D,E*; Fig. 5-26) for about a week after clinical signs are apparent.[153] The disease is usually self-limiting and rarely fatal.[154]

A variant of *A. phagocytophilum* (formerly *E. phagocytophila*) causes tick-borne fever in sheep, goats, and cattle in Europe

FIGURE 5-25 **Infectious agents in neutrophils**

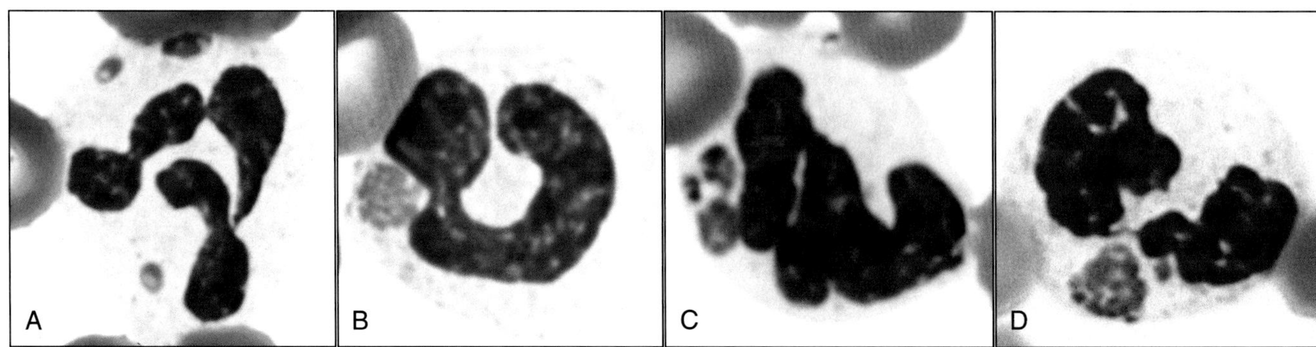

A, Three reddish distemper inclusions in the cytoplasm of a neutrophil in blood from a dog with canine distemper. Diff-Quik stain. **B,** *Ehrlichia ewingii* morula in the cytoplasm of a neutrophil in blood from a dog. Wright-Giemsa stain. **C,** *Anaplasma phagocytophilum* (formerly human granulocytic *Ehrlichia)* morulae in the cytoplasm of a neutrophil in blood from a dog from Minnesota. Wright-Giemsa stain. **D,** *Anaplasma phagocytophilum* (formerly *Ehrlichia equi*) morula in the cytoplasm of a neutrophil in blood from a horse. Wright-Giemsa stain.

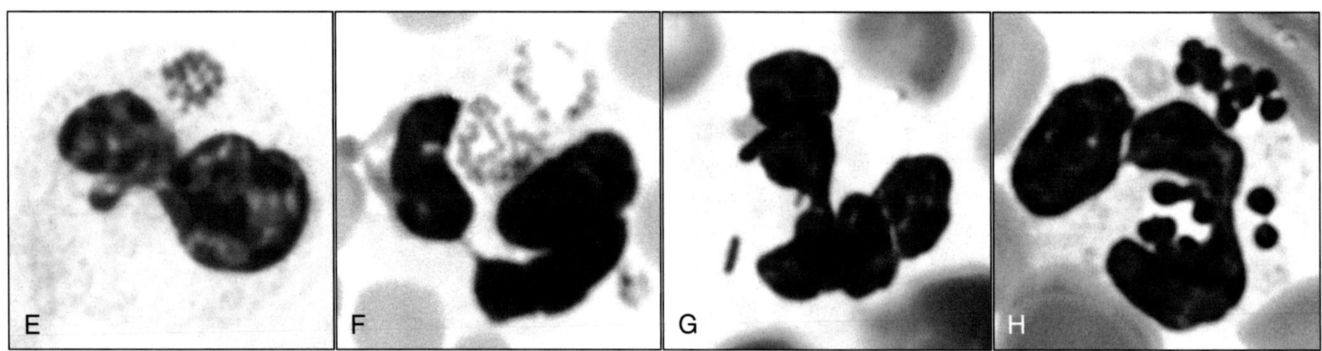

E, *Anaplasma phagocytophilum* (formerly *Ehrlichia equi*) morula in the cytoplasm of a neutrophil in blood from a horse stained using the new methylene blue wet mount procedure. **F,** Two *Anaplasma phagocytophilum* (formerly *Ehrlichia phagocytophila*) morulae in the cytoplasm of a neutrophil in blood from a goat. Wright-Giemsa stain. **G,** Bacterial rods phagocytized by a neutrophil in a buffy coat smear prepared from blood from a cat with a leukopenia and septicemia. Wright-Giemsa stain. **H,** Bacterial cocci phagocytized by a neutrophil in blood from a dog with urolithiasis, pyelonephritis, and septicemia. *Staphylococcus intermedius* was cultured from blood and urine. Wright-Giemsa stain.

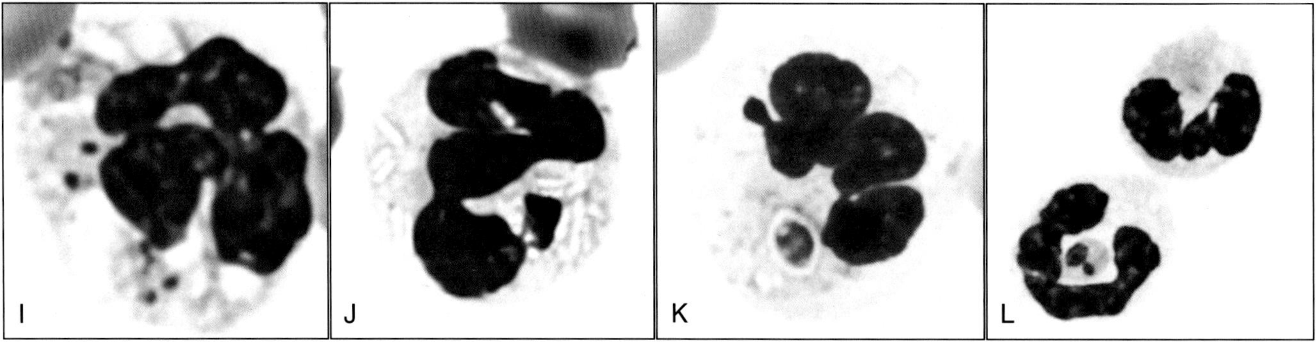

I, Toxic and degenerative neutrophil with multiple intracellular *Francisella philomiragia* organisms in a dog with septicemia and disseminated intravascular coagulation (DIC). Wright-Giemsa stain. **J,** *Mycobacterium* organisms in the cytoplasm of a neutrophil in blood from a dog. These organisms do not stain; they appear as linear clear areas. Wright-Giemsa stain. **K,** *Histoplasma capsulatum* organisms in the cytoplasm of a dog neutrophil. Modified Wright stain. **L,** Neutrophil containing a *Leishmania infantum* amastigote within its cytoplasm. Diff-Quik stain.

C, Image provided by H. L. Wamsley. I, Photograph of a stained blood film from a 2009 ASVCP slide review case submitted by M. Cora, J. Neel, and J. Tarigo. K, From Gingerich K, Gumptill L. Canine and feline histoplasmosis: a review of a widespread fungus. Vet Med. *2008;103:248-264. Image provided by C. A. Thompson. L, Image provided by M. Santos.*

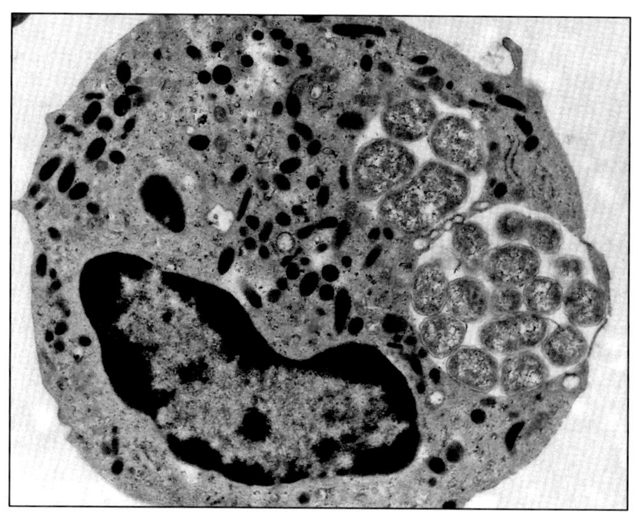

FIGURE 5-26
Transmission electron photomicrograph of a horse neutrophil containing two *Anaplasma phagocytophilum* (formerly *Ehrlichia equi*) morulae. Each morula consists of a membrane-lined vesicle containing multiple organisms.

From Brewer BD, Harvey JW, Mayhew IG, et al. Ehrlichiosis in a Florida horse. J Am Vet Med Assoc. *1984;184:446-447.*

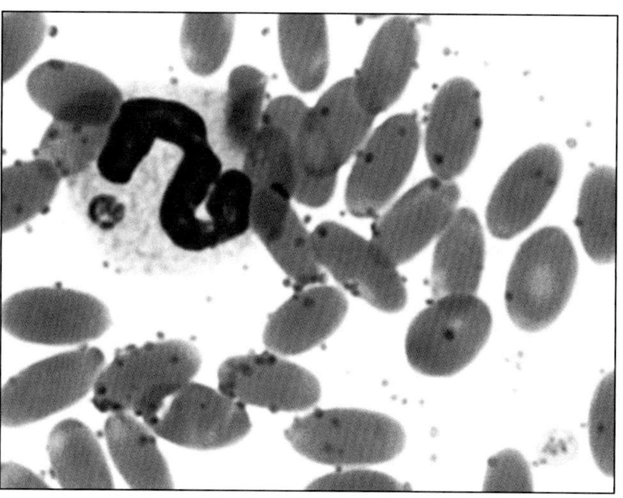

FIGURE 5-27
An *Anaplasma phagocytophilum* morula within a neutrophil and many small *Mycoplasma haemolamae* organisms between and attached to erythrocytes in blood from an alpaca. Wright stain.

From Lascola K, Vandis M, Bain P, et al. Concurrent infection with Anaplasma phagocytophilum and Mycoplasma haemolamae in a young alpaca. J Vet Intern Med. *2009;23:379-382.*

(see Fig. 5-25, *F*).[501] The disease is severe in sheep, causing abortion in adults, and high fever, lameness, and sometimes death in lambs. In addition to fever and respiratory signs, a drop in milk production is reported in infected dairy cattle. Hematologic findings in sheep include a prominent leukopenia (neutropenia and lymphopenia), thrombocytopenia, and generalized immunosuppression resulting in secondary bacterial infections. During the peak bacteremia, as many as 90% of granulocytes (neutrophils and eosinophils) may contain morulae.[501] *A. phagocytophilum* infection has also been reported in a llama and an alpaca (see Fig. 5-27).[36,267]

Hepatozoon *Species*

Hepatozoon is a protozoal parasite in the Apicomplexa phylum. Approximately 50 *Hepatozoon* species are recognized to infect mammals, but only two species (*H. canis* and *H. americanum*) are currently documented to infect dogs.[283,380] *H. canis* infections generally cause mild or inapparent disease in dogs in temperate and tropical regions of the world, but severe illness may occur.[405] Gamonts of *H. canis* are often seen in the cytoplasm of circulating neutrophils. This organism was not reported to occur within the United States before 2008.[6]

In contrast, *H. americanum* has been documented to occur only in the United States, with most infections reported in dogs living in southeastern and south central states.[283,380] It causes a severe, debilitating illness in dogs that is characterized by fever, lethargy, musculoskeletal pain, lameness, and mucopurulent ocular discharge. Periosteal proliferation of the long bones may be observed on diagnostic imaging. Cysts, meronts, and pyogranulomatous inflammation occur in skeletal and cardiac muscle. A marked neutrophilic leukocytosis is often present. However, *H. americanum* gamonts are rarely seen in the cytoplasm of circulating neutrophils (Fig. 5-28) and monocytes. On routine blood staining, the gamonts appear as large oblong structures with a poorly staining nucleus.

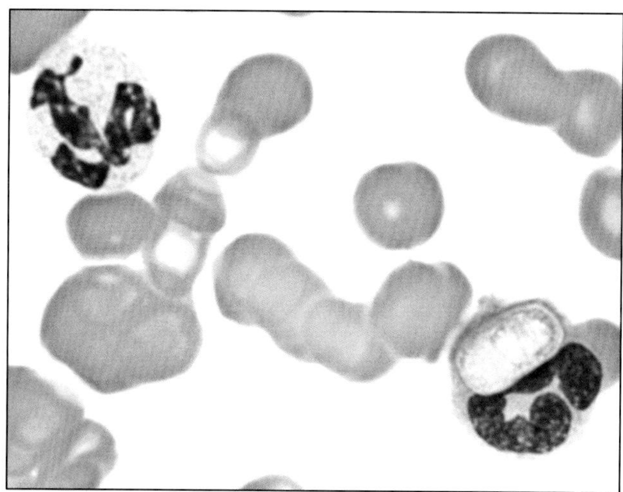

FIGURE 5-28
Hepatozoon americanum gamont in the cytoplasm of a neutrophil *(bottom right)* in blood from a dog. Modified Wright stain.

Photograph of a stained blood film from a 2002 ASVCP slide review case submitted by C. J. LeBlanc, K. A. Ryan, and S. D. Gaunt.

FIGURE 5-29 **Miscellaneous neutrophil abnormalities**

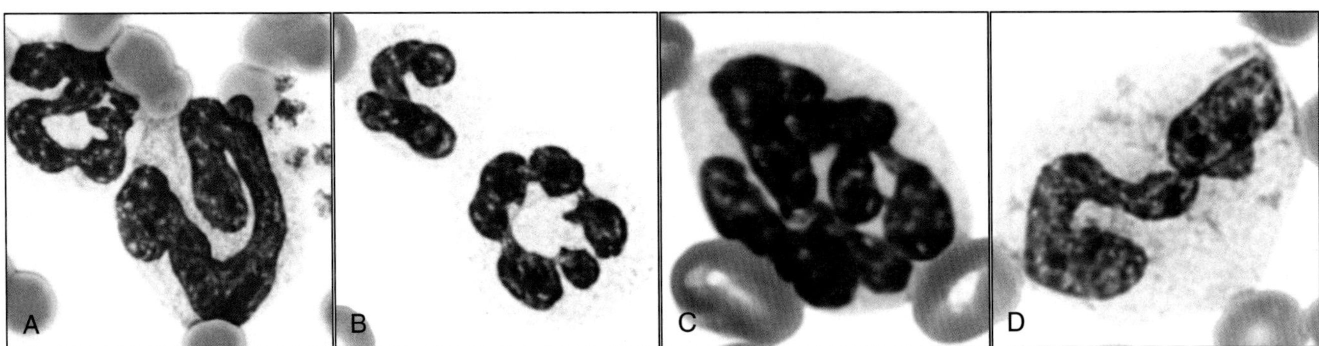

A, Giant neutrophil in blood from a cat with septic peritonitis. **B,** Giant hypersegmented neutrophil in blood from a dog with lymphoma. **C,** Giant hypersegmented neutrophil in blood from a dog with lymphoma that is being treated with chemotherapy. **D,** Giant toxic neutrophil in blood from a cat with diabetes mellitus and fungal pneumonia.

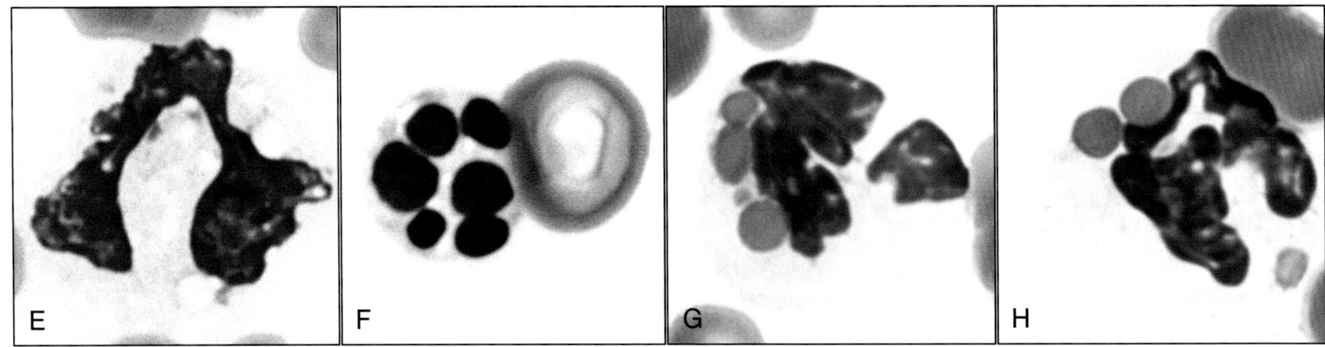

E, Toxic degenerate neutrophil exhibiting karyolysis (nuclear lysis) in blood from an FIV-positive leukopenic cat. **F,** Pyknosis and karyorrhexis in a neutrophil in blood from a dog with acute lymphoblastic leukemia (ALL). **G,H,** Phagocytized eosinophil granules in horse neutrophils. Wright-Giemsa stain.

H. canis has been identified in cats using PCR and sequencing of the *18S rRNA* gene,[103] but additional *Hepatozoon* species may also infect cats.[104] A wide variety of clinical signs have been reported in domestic cats with *Hepatozoon* infections, some of which may be the result of concomitant diseases.[34,35]

Miscellaneous Bacteria, Fungi, and Protozoa

Although bacteremia is common in animals, microorganisms are seldom numerous enough to be found in stained blood films. Because blood stains are easily contaminated with bacteria (especially when they are also used to stain exfoliative cytology), it is important that the bacteria be found phagocytized within cells before a diagnosis of a bacteremia is made (see Fig. 5-25, *G-I*). *Mycobacterium* organisms appear as unstained rods within the cytoplasm (see Fig. 5-25, *J*).[232,271] In addition to mononuclear phagocytes, neutrophils may also rarely contain phagocytized organisms in animals with systemic histoplasmosis (see Fig. 5-25, *K*)[53,90,176] and dogs and cats with leishmaniasis (see Fig. 5-25, *L*).[308,407]

Miscellaneous Neutrophil Morphologic Abnormalities

Giant Neutrophils

Large neutrophils may occur in animals (especially cats) with inflammatory diseases and/or dysgranulopoiesis.[226] They may exhibit normal nuclear morphology (Fig. 5-29, *A*) or appear hypersegmented (Fig. 5-29, *B-C*). Cytoplasmic toxicity may be prominent in inflammatory conditions (Fig. 5-29, *D*). Dysgranulopoiesis is seen in acute myeloid leukemias (AMLs), myelodysplastic syndromes, feline leukemia virus (FeLV) infections, and feline immunodeficiency virus (FIV) infections.[425,490] Giant neutrophils have also been reported in blood secondary to other disorders including lymphoma, immune-mediated thrombocytopenia (IMT), immune-mediated hemolytic anemia (IMHA), and pyometra in dogs.[490] Giant neutrophils have been reported in humans following administration of recombinant G-CSF.[73] They may occur transiently in animals recovering from granulocytic hypoplasia, such as panleukopenia in cats.

Karyolysis

The dissolution of the nucleus resulting in nuclear swelling and loss of affinity for basic dyes is referred to as karyolysis (Fig. 5-29, *E*). This degenerative change occurs outside the bone marrow. It is frequently observed in neutrophils present in septic exudates and may sometimes be observed in the mammalian blood.

Pyknosis and Karyorrhexis

Neutrophils that undergo programmed cell death (apoptosis) exhibit pyknosis and karyorrhexis.[359] Pyknosis involves the shrinkage or condensation of a cell with increased nuclear compactness or density; *karyorrhexis* refers to subsequent nuclear fragmentation (Fig. 5-29, *F*). Pyknosis and karyorrhexis are degenerative changes that are often observed in nonseptic exudates. They may be seen in blood neutrophils that have had prolonged time in the circulation. Pyknotic neutrophils are reported in increased numbers in inflammatory and neoplastic disorders in humans.[423] Neutrophil hypersegmentation and pyknosis were reported in a dog with amphetamine toxicity attributed to high body temperature and accelerated apoptosis.[496]

Cytoplasmic Vacuoles

Foamy vacuolation occurs in toxic neutrophils, but clear, discrete vacuoles in the absence of cytoplasmic basophilia usually represent an in vitro artifact. In addition to discrete vacuolation, uneven distribution of granules, irregular cell membranes, and pyknosis may occur in neutrophils in blood samples that have been collected in EDTA and kept at room temperature for several hours.[181] These artifacts are avoided by preparing blood films quickly after blood collection.

Phagocytized Eosinophil Granules

Intact granules can be extruded from eosinophils.[351] They may be phagocytized by neutrophils, as is shown in Figure 5-29, *G,H*. The significance of this finding is unclear.

Stain Precipitation

An inexperienced observer may confuse neutrophils with precipitated stain with basophils (Fig. 5-30, *A*). When this artifact is unevenly distributed, other areas of the blood film can be found that stain normally (Fig. 5-30, *B*).

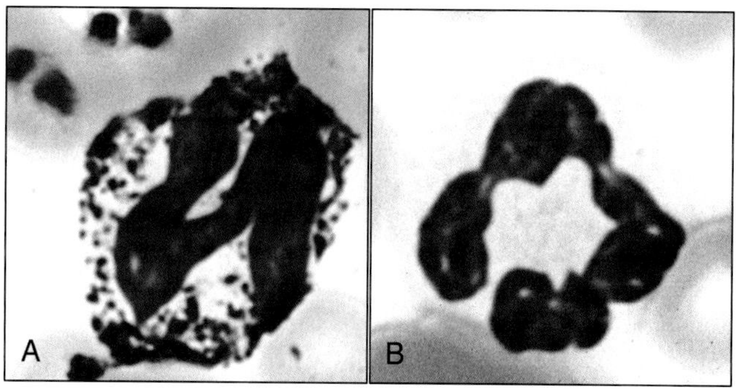

FIGURE 5-30
Stain precipitation artifact. **A,** Stain precipitation associated with a neutrophil in blood from a dog. **B,** Normal-appearing neutrophil, in blood from a dog, three oil immersion fields away from the neutrophil as shown in **(A)**. Wright-Giemsa stain.

TABLE 5-1

Expected Findings in Different Types of Neutrophilia

Type	Lymphocyte Count	Left Shift
Physiologic (epinephrine)	Normal or increased	None
Stress (glucocorticoids)	Usually decreased	None or slight
Inflammation	Often decreased	Often present

Neutrophilia

Neutrophilia may develop as a result of increased neutrophil production and/or release from the bone marrow, decreased movement of neutrophils from blood into the tissues, or net movement of neutrophils from the MNP to the CNP, as shown in Figure 5-31. Neutrophilia develops rapidly in blood following catecholamine (norepinephrine and epinephrine) release, as occurs in early exercise, fear, or excitement. This results from a shift of neutrophils from the MNP to the CNP.[43] The cell count usually does not increase above twice normal and no left shift occurs (Table 5-1). Sustained exercise, especially in a hot environment, also results in cortisol release, which can enhance the neutrophilia, as discussed subsequently.[65] Some animals may exhibit an accompanying lymphocytosis. Leukogram effects should return to normal within 30 minutes of removal of the stimulus.[226]

The increased endogenous release or exogenous administration of glucocorticoid steroids has profound effects on circulating blood cell numbers within a few hours after release or administration. Potential causes of increased endogenous release of glucocorticoids include pain, trauma, prolonged emotional stress, intense sustained exercise, high body temperature, and hyperadrenocorticism.[65,111] The duration of effects depends on the nature of the exogenous glucocorticoid administered (long- or short-acting). Neutrophilia occurs because glucocorticoids cause increased release of mature neutrophils from bone marrow stores and decreased egress of neutrophils from blood into tissues.[77,111,226] The glucocorticoid-induced release of neutrophils from bone marrow is reduced in elderly humans.[83] A higher proportion of neutrophils is also present in the CNP compared with the MNP, but the size of the MNP may not actually be decreased because the total blood neutrophil pool is increased. The absolute number of neutrophils seldom increases above twice normal and little or no left shift is present. Glucocorticoids also cause lymphopenia and eosinopenia in all domestic animals (see Table 5-1). Monocytosis is commonly observed in dogs and occasionally in cats.[226] The magnitude of the neutrophilia decreases with

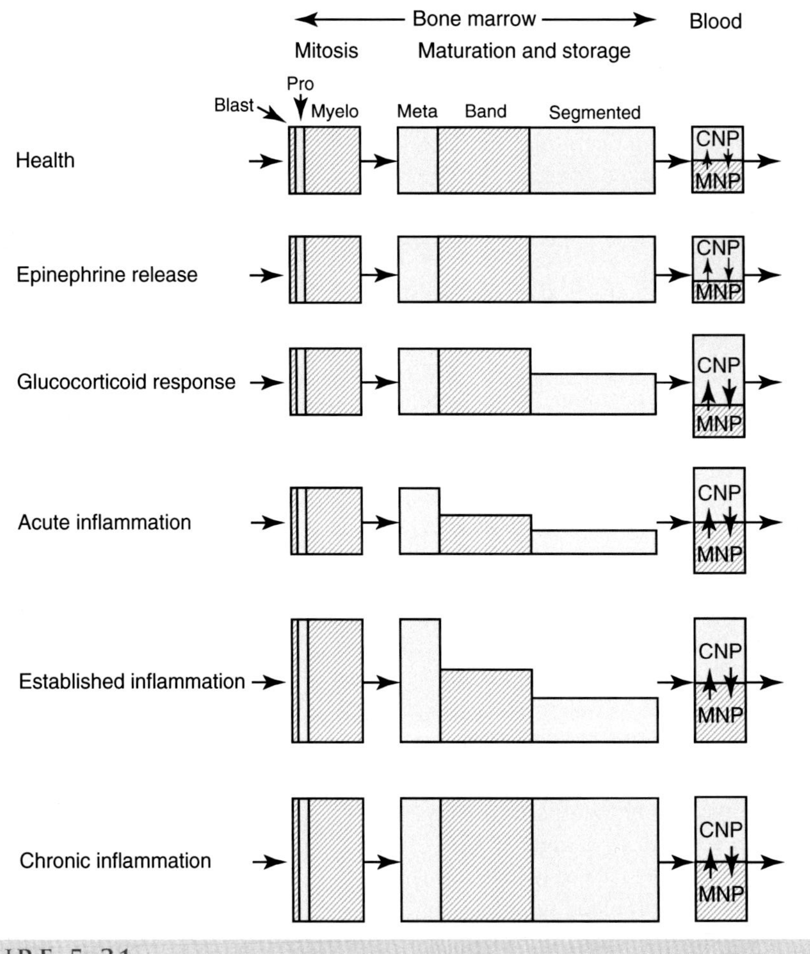

FIGURE 5-31
Mechanisms responsible for the production of a neutrophilia.

time, but the lymphopenia and eosinopenia persist as long as plasma glucocorticoid concentrations are increased. For example, most dogs with pituitary gland-dependent hyperadrenocorticism have lymphopenia and eosinopenia with normal neutrophil counts.[281,334]

Neutrophilia without a significant left shift may also be present in association with hemorrhage, hemolysis, necrosis, chemical and drug toxicities, malignancy, mild inflammation, and some chronic inflammatory conditions. The mechanism causing neutrophilia in these disorders is not always clear. Various conditions, including hyperthermia, can result in increased concentrations of hematopoietic growth factors (especially G-CSF) in the circulation that result in increased neutrophil production and release.[132,340,468] The inflammatory cytokines IL-1 and TNF-α induce neutrophilia by stimulating the production of growth factors such as G-CSF and GM-CSF.[421] In mild inflammatory conditions and some chronic inflammatory conditions, the increased peripheral demand for neutrophils is met by increased production and release of mature neutrophils from the marrow.

The neutrophil response to inflammatory stimuli is more muted in ruminants than in other domestic animals. Neutrophilia is less common and neutropenia is more common in response to acute bacterial infections in ruminants compared with other species. Total leukocyte counts of 20 to 30 $\times 10^3/\mu L$ are considered to be markedly elevated in ruminants. Detection of increased concentrations of acute-phase proteins, such as haptoglobin and fibrinogen, can provide evidence of chronic inflammation that may not be seen in the leukogram.[452]

Prominent left shifts are often associated with inflammatory conditions. These may be infectious (especially bacterial)[251,311] or noninfectious (tissue injury, immune-mediated) disorders.[17,215,247,317] The presence of a significant left shift indicates that the stimulus for release of neutrophils from bone marrow is greater than can be accommodated by release from mature neutrophil stores alone. Regenerative left shifts are generally viewed as an adequate marrow response at that moment. However, the presence of significant cytoplasmic toxicity requires a guarded prognosis. A marked leukocytosis (total leukocyte count of greater than 50,000/μL) with a neutrophilia and marked left shift back to at least myelocytes associated with an inflammatory condition is called a "leukemoid reaction" because it resembles the blood pattern seen in CML. Left shifts associated with leukemoid reactions are usually orderly, with mature segmented neutrophils being the most numerous neutrophilic cells present, bands being the next most numerous, metamyelocytes being less numerous, and myelocytes being present in the lowest numbers. A localized purulent inflammatory condition, such as pyometra, is suspected when a leukemoid response is present.[226]

Disorders that may stimulate extreme neutrophilic leukocytosis in dogs and cats (leukocyte counts above 50,000/μL with neutrophils greater than 25,000/μL) include infections (such as pyothorax, pyelonephritis, septic peritonitis, pyometra, abscess, pneumonia, and hepatitis), immune-mediated disorders (such as immune-mediated hemolytic anemia, glomerulonephritis, polyarthritis, and vasculitis), neoplasia (such as lymphoma, acute and chronic myeloid leukemia, and mast cell tumors), and tissue necrosis (caused by diseases such as trauma, pancreatitis, thrombosis, and bile peritonitis).[289,290] A neutrophilic leukocytosis as high as 200,000/μL has been reported in dogs with *H. americanum* infection, which causes pyogranulomatous myositis.[296] Extreme leukocytosis also occurs during the first 3 weeks after the injection of a toxic dose of estrogen in dogs. This neutrophilic hyperplastic phase in the marrow is followed by generalized hypoplasia or aplasia and death or slow recovery.[485] Neutrophilia in animals with a wide variety of tumors may result from inflammation or necrosis within the tumor; but neutrophilia may also occur as a paraneoplastic phenomenon secondary to the production of growth factors, such as G-CSF and GM-CSF, by the tumor.[301,418,456]

Animals with CML have persistent marked neutrophilia with a pronounced left shift that may extend to myeloblasts. This diagnosis is usually reached by ruling out inflammatory causes and documenting the concomitant occurrence of additional proliferative abnormalities in blood and bone marrow.[273,450]

Neutrophilia with or without a modest left shift is present in some animals with inherited neutrophil dysfunctions. Profound neutrophilia occurs in dogs and cattle with β_2 integrin adhesion molecule deficiency.[174,394] Both increased production of neutrophils and decreased egress of neutrophils from blood into the tissues contribute to the high number of neutrophils in blood of animals with this inherited defect.[18] A prominent neutrophilia with no or minimal left shift also occurred in a German shepherd dog with Kindlin-3 deficiency that failed to activate β_2 integrin normally, resulting in leukocyte and platelet function defects.[60] Inherited neutrophil dysfunctions should be included in the differential diagnosis when unexplained recurrent bacterial infections occur in a young animal.

Neutropenia

Neutropenia can develop from decreased release of neutrophils from bone marrow, increased egress of neutrophils from blood, destruction of neutrophils within the blood, or a shift of neutrophils from the CNP to the MNP (Fig. 5-32). Healthy Belgian Tervuren dogs living in North America are reported to frequently have physiologic leukopenia, with total leukocyte counts, absolute neutrophil counts, and absolute lymphocyte counts below reference intervals established for dogs.[186] However, leukopenia appears to be rare in this breed in Belgium, possibly due to genetic differences.[179]

Decreased release of neutrophils from bone marrow can result from decreased progenitor cells or from abnormal

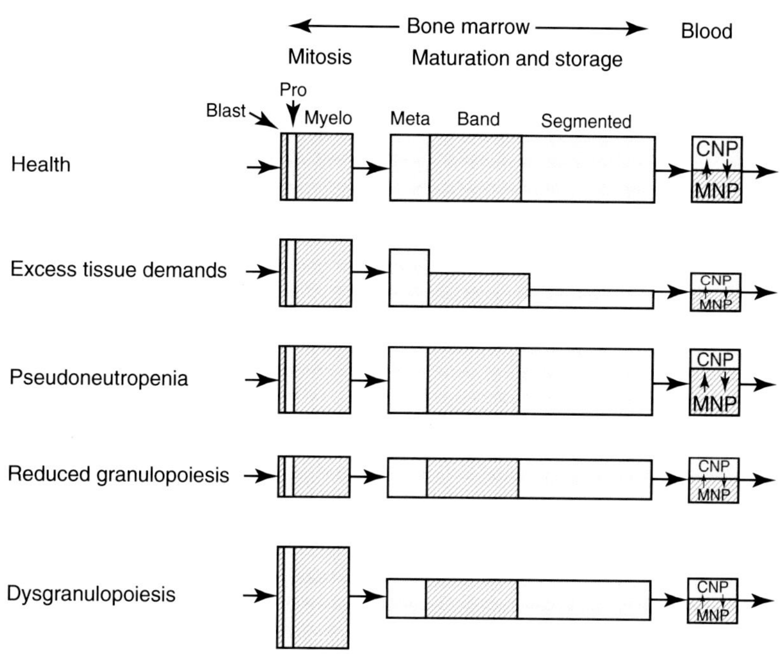

FIGURE 5-32
Mechanisms responsible for the production of a neutropenia.

precursor cell maturation called "dysgranulopoiesis." Conditions in which neutrophil precursors are present in normal or increased numbers in bone marrow but the release of mature neutrophils into blood is decreased include some AMLs, some myelodysplastic syndromes, secondary myelodysplasia, FeLV infections, and FIV infections.[55,159,420,488,489] Leukopenia has been reported in young dogs with inherited cobalamin deficiency and dysgranulopoiesis in the marrow.[163]

Decreased numbers of neutrophil precursors can occur in bone marrow when generalized marrow hypoplasia or selective neutrophil hypoplasia is present.[318] Hypoplastic conditions associated with decreased numbers of neutrophil precursor cells in the marrow include idiosyncratic drug reactions (e.g., phenylbutazone, trimethoprim/sulfadiazine, griseofulvin, cephalosporins, fenbendazole),[151,167,210,479,485] estrogen toxicity (exogenous or endogenous) in dogs and ferrets,[45,437] cytotoxic chemotherapy drugs,* viral diseases (e.g., parvovirus in dogs and cats and equine herpesvirus-1 in foals),[67,265,266,372] rickettsial diseases (*Ehrlichia canis* infection in dogs and *E. risticii* infection in horses),[345,515] and inherited disorders (cyclic hematopoiesis in gray collie dogs and some cats with Chédiak-Higashi syndrome).[18,220,384]

Phenobarbital toxicity is reported to cause neutropenia and thrombocytopenia in dogs, but its effects on the bone marrow need further study.[69,223,244] Marrow necrosis has been suggested in dogs, but bone marrow in neutropenic humans has appeared normal.[355,487] Lithium carbonate stimulates neutrophil production in dogs and humans, but it causes a bone marrow neutrophilic maturational arrest and neutropenia in cats.[119,402]

Familial neutropenia and thrombocytopenia have been reported in eight horses with severe neutrophilic hypoplasia/aplasia and megakaryocytic hypoplasia in bone marrow.[255] Chronic (possibly congenital) neutropenia has been described in a young Rottweiler dog with G-CSF deficiency. Bone marrow aspiration biopsy revealed a maturational arrest at the promyelocyte-myelocyte stage.[264] A hereditary defect has been suggested as a cause of chronic neutropenia with recurrent bacterial infections in border collie dogs, but myeloid hyperplasia is also reported in this disorder.[3]

Decreased numbers of neutrophil precursors can also occur in bone marrow when myelophthisis is present. Myelophthisic disorders are characterized by the replacement of normal hematopoietic cells with abnormal ones. Examples of myelophthisic disorders—where decreased numbers of neutrophil precursors may occur in marrow—include lymphoid leukemias, multiple myeloma, some myeloid leukemias, some myelodysplastic syndromes, myelofibrosis (often associated with anemia but less often with leukopenia or thrombocytopenia), and possibly metastases of lymphomas, carcinomas, and mast cell tumors.[2,69,369,390,451] Myelophthisic disorders do not simply "crowd out" normal cells but also alter the marrow microenvironment so that normal hematopoiesis is compromised.

*References 41, 157, 180, 370, 377, 486.

Primary immune-mediated neutropenia is difficult to diagnose in the absence of readily available and reliable diagnostic tests.[481] Neutrophilic precursors may be decreased or increased in the bone marrow, depending on the neutrophilic stage involved in the destruction.[297,318,373,473,491] Animals may be asymptomatic or may be ill because of secondary bacterial infections. The pathogenesis of some drug-induced neutropenias and some neutropenias associated with infectious agents probably also have an immune-mediated component. The neutropenia sometimes associated with *Anaplasma phagocytophilum* infections appears to be associated with increased neutrophil destruction following the appearance of organisms within neutrophils.[500]

The long-term use of a recombinant G-CSF from one species in a second species can result in a persistent neutropenia in the second species when antibodies made against the recombinant G-CSF also neutralize the endogenous G-CSF of the species receiving treatment.[199,391]

Neutropenia can develop in acute inflammatory conditions when the demand for neutrophils depletes the bone marrow storage pool and insufficient time has elapsed for increased granulopoiesis to occur. Neutropenia is common in overwhelming septic conditions (e.g., septicemia) and secondary to endotoxemia.* Degenerative left shifts are often present in these disorders. A common example of this type of presentation is acute salmonellosis in horses and calves.[343,408] Finally, neutropenia can occur following the net movement of neutrophils from the CNP to the MNP, as occurs during shock.[155,248,455]

Inherited Neutrophil Defects

Chédiak-Higashi Syndrome

The Chédiak-Higashi syndrome has been reported in cattle, Persian cats, Aleutian mink, the beige mouse, blue and silver foxes, and a killer whale, as well as in humans.[325] This disorder is characterized by partial oculocutaneous albinism, increased susceptibility to infections, hemorrhagic tendencies, and the presence of enlarged membrane-bound granules in many cell types, including melanocytes and blood leukocytes. The giant granules may arise from abnormal fusion or fission of lysosomes or lysosome-related organelles during cell development.[222] Neutrophils from affected animals exhibit reduced mobility and defective phagocytic and/or bactericidal responses, explaining these animals' increased susceptibility to bacterial infections.[325] A defect in the *Chédiak-Higashi syndrome 1 (CHS1)* gene (*beige* gene in deficient mice) has been identified in humans and mice. The protein produced by this gene appears to be involved in regulating vesicular size and trafficking.[237] Neutropenia has been reported in some humans with Chédiak-Higashi syndrome,[56] and neutropenia is a common finding in cats with this disorder.[384] An increased bleeding tendency is also present because platelets lack normal dense granules, resulting in a platelet storage pool deficiency.[101,406]

*References 22, 128, 306, 385, 415, 464.

β_2 *Integrin Adhesion Molecule Deficiencies*

An autosomal recessive deficiency in leukocyte surface adhesion glycoproteins (β_2 integrins), resulting from a defect in the CD18 β subunit, has been recognized in Irish setter dogs and Holstein cattle.[174,245] This leukocyte adhesion deficiency-I (LAD-I) defect results in decreased neutrophil adhesion, impaired chemotaxis and aggregation, and minimal bactericidal activity.[18] Similar defects also occur in monocytes. As a result, animals have recurrent bacterial and fungal infections without pus formation. Clinical signs include gingivitis, oral ulcers, periodontitis, chronic pneumonia, poor wound healing, and stunted growth. Marked neutrophilia with or without a modest left shift is usually present. Increased numbers of other blood leukocyte types may also occur at times. Mild to moderate nonregenerative anemia and a polyclonal hyperglobulinemia may be present.[174,463]

Kindlin-3 Deficiency

A mutation in the *Kindlin-3* gene in a German shepherd dog resulted in leukocyte adhesion deficiency III (LAD-III), a phenotype characterized by increased susceptibility to infection and increased risk of bleeding.[60] β-integrin proteins are important adhesion molecules on the surfaces of leukocytes and platelets. These integrin molecules bind poorly to their ligands when blood cells are quiescent, but they become adhesive following activation by inside-out signaling through other membrane receptors. The Kindlin-3 protein is critical in the pathway of β-integrin activation. Consequently a deficiency in the Kindlin-3 protein abolishes the activation of β integrins and prevents normal leukocyte and platelet adhesion. In the case of neutrophils, the lack of Kindlin-3 abolishes β_2-integrin activation, preventing the firm adhesion of neutrophils to activated endothelial cells.[60]

Unknown Neutrophil Function Defects

A less well-defined defect in neutrophils has been reported in Doberman pinscher dogs.[64] Neutrophil chemotaxis and phagocytosis are normal, but these cells have reduced bactericidal ability. The bactericidal defect appears to be the result of inadequate generation of superoxide radicals following stimulation. An inadequate oxidant burst may also occur in young Weimaraner dogs that present with recurrent infections.[97]

Cyclic Hematopoiesis

Cyclic hematopoiesis (previously termed cyclic neutropenia) is transmitted as an autosomal recessive trait in gray collie dogs. The "gray collie syndrome" is associated with several distinct abnormalities (abnormal hair pigmentation, bilateral scleral ectasia, enteropathy, and gonadal hypoplasia) in addition to cyclic hematopoiesis. Blood neutrophil counts exhibit 12- to 14-day cyclic fluctuations. Neutrophils may be completely absent from the blood during neutropenic episodes, which last for 2 to 4 days. Blood neutrophil counts return to normal or even increase above normal following neutropenic periods. Monocyte, platelet, and reticulocyte counts cycle in blood with the same periodicity, but they cycle out of phase with neutrophils and from normal to above-normal values in blood. Affected pups are susceptible to bacterial and fungal infections, especially during the neutropenic episodes. A defect in neutrophil bactericidal function also contributes to the recurrent infections that occur in these animals.[86] Affected pups usually die by 6 months of age. Animals that reach adulthood often die of systemic amyloidosis, which is believed to be the result of the repeated activation of the acute-phase response by inflammatory cytokines during periods of monocytosis.[354]

This defect in dogs results from a mutation in the *AP3B1* gene, which produces a subunit of the adaptor-related protein complex 3 (AP3) and is involved in trafficking of vesicular cargo proteins, including neutrophil elastase (NE), from the Golgi to lysosomes. Affected dogs have reduced amounts of mature NE (i.e., NE activity) in their primary granules but increased amounts of the inactive NE precursor protein bound to membranes, most likely in the trans-Golgi network.[321] It is noteworthy that some defects in *ELA2,* the gene that encodes NE, result in cyclic neutropenia in humans. NE appears to provide feedback inhibition in normal neutropoiesis, and it is postulated that a disruption in this feedback loop results in the cycling phenomenon.[220]

EOSINOPHILS

Eosinophil Morphology

Eosinophils are so named because their granules have an affinity for eosin, the red dye in routine blood stains. The size, shape, and number of eosinophil granules vary considerably. In most animal species, eosinophils have round granules, but those from domestic cats have rod-shaped ones (Fig. 5-33, *A,B*). Eosinophils from dogs often exhibit a few cytoplasmic vacuoles (Fig. 5-33, *C*), and the granules can sometimes be exceptionally large (Fig. 5-33, *D*). Eosinophils from greyhound dogs and occasionally from individual animals in other breeds appear highly vacuolated (Fig. 5-33, *E*) and may be mistaken for vacuolated neutrophils by inexperienced observers. Horse eosinophils have especially large granules (Fig. 5-33, *F*). Granules in ruminant and pig eosinophils are small (Fig. 5-33, *G*). The cytoplasm between the granules is usually faintly blue in color. Iguanas and psittacine birds have "eosinophils" with gray-blue-staining granules (Fig. 5-34).

Intact granules can be extruded from eosinophils (see Fig. 5-29, *G,H*). These extracellular granules express cytokine receptors on their membranes and function as independent secretory organelles that release granule constituents in response to appropriate cytokines.[351]

The nucleus of eosinophils is similar to that of neutrophils but tends to be less lobulated (often divided into only two lobes) and may be partially obscured by granules in some species, most notably the horse. Pyknosis and karyorrhexis may occur in eosinophils (see Fig. 5-33, *H*), as discussed previously for neutrophils.

FIGURE 5-33 **Morphology of eosinophils**

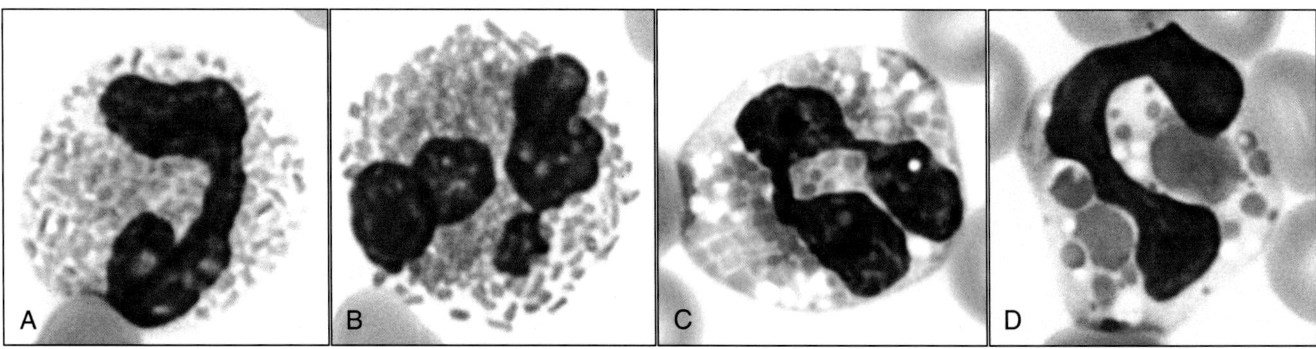

A, Eosinophil with rod-shaped granules in blood from a cat. **B,** Eosinophil with rod-shaped granules in blood from a cat. **C,** Eosinophil with round granules and a small cytoplasmic vacuole in blood from a dog. **D,** Eosinophil with two exceptionally large granules in blood from a dog.

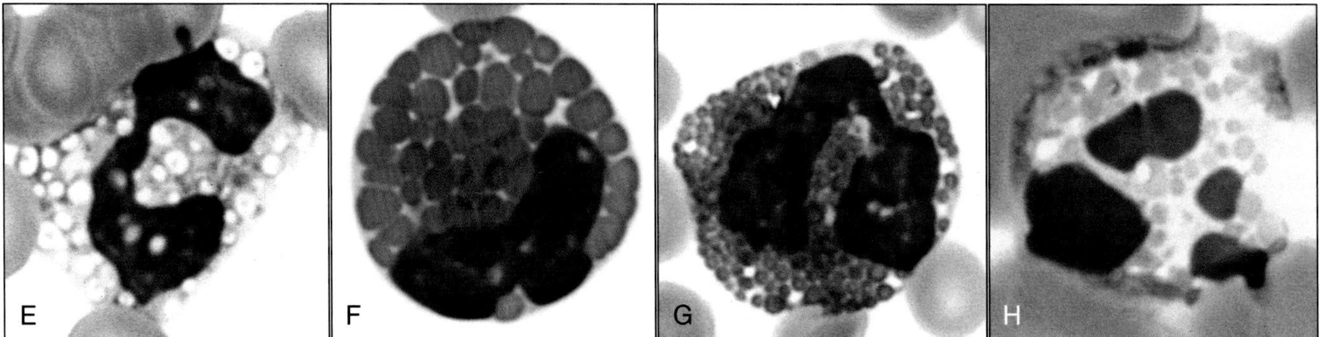

E, Heavily vacuolated eosinophil in blood from a greyhound dog. **F,** Eosinophil in blood from a horse, exhibiting numerous large granules typical of this species. **G,** Eosinophil in blood from a cow exhibiting numerous small round granules typical of this species. **H,** Eosinophil in 2-day-old blood from a dog exhibiting pyknosis and karyorrhexis.

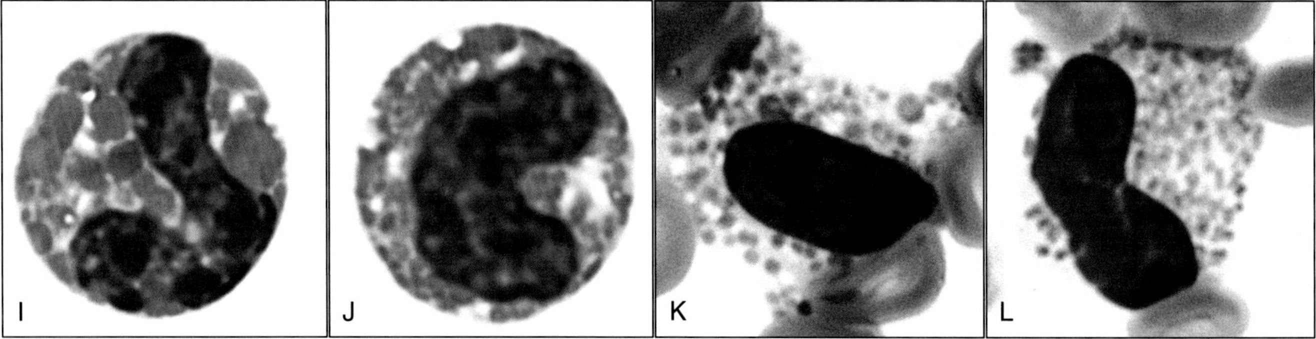

I, Band eosinophil from a dog with immune-mediated hemolytic anemia. **J,** Eosinophilic metamyelocyte from a dog with immune-mediated hemolytic anemia. **K,** Eosinophilic metamyelocyte in blood from a dog with Pelger-Huët anomaly. **L,** Eosinophilic metamyelocyte in blood from a cat with Pelger-Huët anomaly. Wright-Giemsa stain.

Band eosinophils are common in some animals (see Fig. 5-33, *I*) and eosinophilic metamyelocytes may sometimes be seen (see Fig. 5-33, *J*). They are not usually separated from segmented eosinophils during differential counts because they are generally of little clinical significance and may be difficult to identify with certainty when granules obscure the nucleus. Eosinophil maturational stages may be differentiated when extreme eosinophilia is present in an attempt to help separate hyperplastic from neoplastic disorders.[337,348,462] As in neutrophils, a pronounced left shift is present in eosinophils

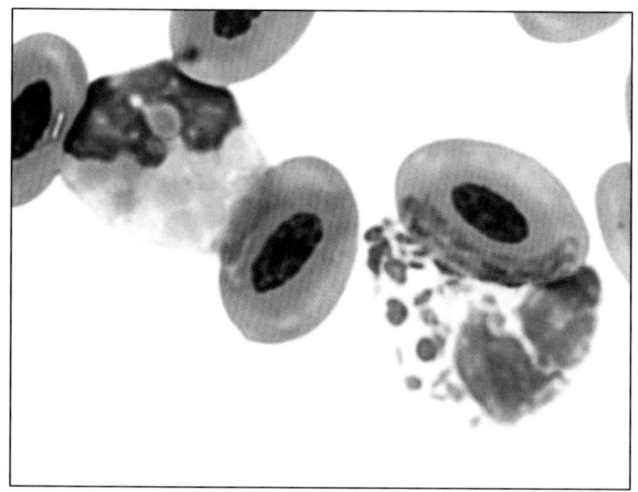

FIGURE 5-34
An "eosinophil" with gray-blue staining round granules *(left)* and a heterophil with red, primarily elongated, granules *(right)* in blood from an African gray parrot. Wright-Giemsa stain.

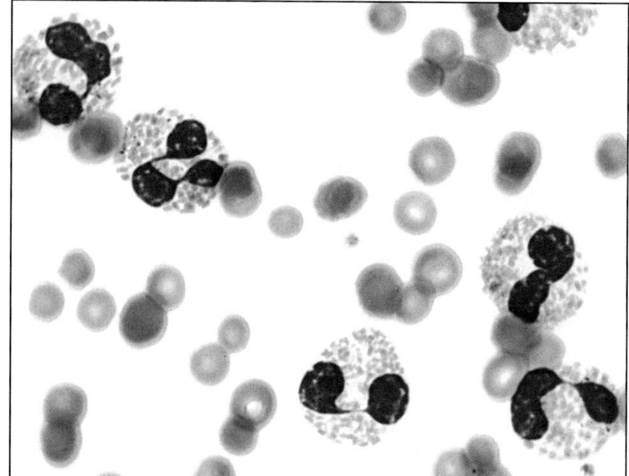

FIGURE 5-35
Eosinophilia in blood from a cat with dirofilariasis. Wright-Giemsa stain.

in the blood of animals with Pelger-Huët anomaly (see Fig. 5-33, *K,L*).[196] Increased numbers of hyposegmented (pseudo-Pelger-Huët) band eosinophils have been reported in a family of Samoyed dogs with accompanying ocular and skeletal abnormalities.[23]

Ehrlichia and *Anaplasma* organisms have rarely been reported in eosinophils,[302,443] and *Histoplasma* organisms have been identified in blood eosinophils from a dog.[89]

Eosinophilia

Eosinophilia occurs in disorders that result in increased IL-5 production.[257] The injection of recombinant IL-2 resulted in eosinophilia in dogs, which was likely mediated by IL-5 production.[209,294] Eosinophilia may accompany parasitic diseases, especially those caused by nematodes and flukes (Fig. 5-35).* Eosinophilia is not typically seen in animals with protozoal infections, but marked eosinophilia was reported in a puppy with hepatic sarcocystosis.[7] Eosinophilia is more likely present when intestinal nematodes are migrating within the body than when they are located only within the intestine.

Eosinophilia may occur in association with eosinophilic inflammatory conditions of organs that normally contain numerous mast cells, such as skin, lung, and intestine.† It may be present in animals with IgE-mediated allergic hypersensitivity reactions such as flea bite allergies and asthma.[94,279,310,392] Eosinophilia has also been reported with sarcoptic mange and nasal mite infestations.[278] Eosinophilia occurs in some animals with *Pythium* infections[46,127] and in some with idiopathic eosinophilic granulomas.[269,279] Eosinophilia has been reported in some hyperthyroid cats treated with methimazole or its prodrug carbimazole.[156,376]

*References 25, 61, 78, 82, 197, 259, 389, 453, 498.
†References 42, 87, 278, 279, 292, 508.

Although not usually present, eosinophilia may occur in animals with mast cell tumors (Fig. 5-36) and T lymphocyte lymphomas.* Eosinophilia rarely occurs in animals with lymphomatoid granulomatosis (T lymphocyte-rich large B lymphocyte lymphoma) and other tumor types.[32,143,287,416]

Marked eosinophilia with extensive eosinophilic organ infiltrates in animals (primarily cats) and humans has been classified as either chronic eosinophilic leukemia or hypereosinophilic syndrome.[24,221,261,449] However, criteria for separating this collection of heterogeneous disorders into two distinct entities have been difficult to define. Using new molecular and genetic diagnostic techniques, it appears that most human patients diagnosed with hypereosinophilic syndrome have neoplastic rather than reactive disorders.[31,367,419] This same phenomenon will likely occur in veterinary medicine as additional molecular and genetic techniques become available.[171,417] Eosinophilia may also be present in CML, where neutrophilia predominates, and in thrombocythemia.[145,329]

Marked eosinophilia with eosinophilic infiltration of multiple organs including liver, spleen, lungs, and lymph nodes has been described in Rottweiler dogs.[228,348,447] Three dogs were classified as having idiopathic hypereosinophilic syndrome because mean serum immunoglobulin E concentrations were markedly high and no karyotype abnormalities were identified on cytogenetic analysis.[447] One dog underwent a spontaneous remission.[228]

Eosinopenia

The absolute eosinophil count may be zero in some normal animals, making eosinopenia of limited significance. Endogenous and exogenous glucocorticoids rapidly induce eosinopenia in animals.[226,288] The presence of increased numbers of

*References 20, 38, 59, 100, 123, 262, 307, 396, 448.

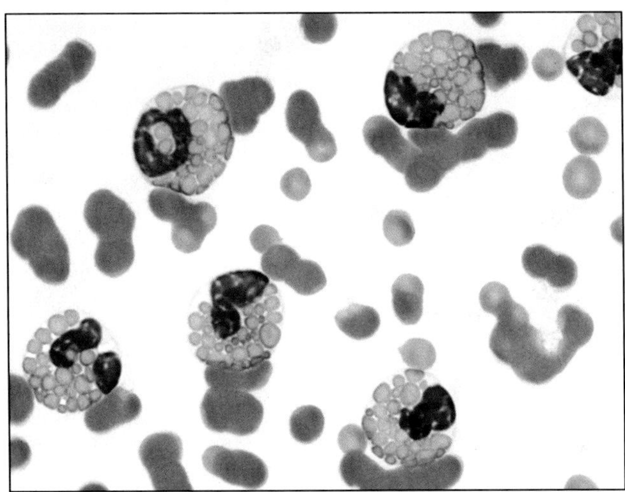

FIGURE 5-36
Eosinophilia in blood from a horse with an abdominal mast cell tumor. Wright-Giemsa stain.

eosinophilic cells in bone marrow together with eosinopenia in blood and reduced numbers of tissue eosinophils suggests decreased marrow release of eosinophils,[133] and glucorticoids are reported to inhibit eosinophil release from the bone marrow.[76] This might be the result of upregulation of α4 integrin adhesion molecules on the surfaces of immature eosinophils by glucocorticoids.[168] Glucorticoids also potentiate apoptosis of eosinophils.[236,478] Long-term glucocorticoid therapy may decrease eosinophil production by decreasing the production of growth factors from T lymphocytes. Eosinopenia is often present in acute inflammatory conditions, and endogenous glucorticoid production contributes to this decrease in eosinophil numbers.[508]

BASOPHILS

Basophil Morphology

The cytoplasm of basophils is generally pale blue in color, and basophil nuclei are often less segmented than neutrophil nuclei. Basophil granules are acidic and consequently have an affinity for the basic (blue) dyes in routine blood stains. The number, size, and staining characteristics of the granules vary considerably by species. Granules in dog basophils generally appear purple and are not numerous enough to fill the cytoplasm (Fig. 5-37, *A-C*). Degranulated basophils may have purple-staining cytoplasm in the absence of granules (Fig. 5-37, *D*).

The basophils of domestic cats are distinctive. Most of their granules are round or oval and stain light lavender or mauve in color (Fig. 5-37, *E,F*). Some basophils have large purple granules in addition to the light lavender ones (Fig. 5-37, *G*), as is seen in basophil precursors in the bone marrow. The granules typically fill the cytoplasm, giving the cat basophil nucleus a moth-eaten appearance. All of the granules stained dark purple in a cat with mucopolysaccharidosis type VI[98] and in two cats with reddish granulation of neutrophils of unknown etiology (Fig. 5-37, *H*).

Granules are often so numerous in ruminant and pig basophils that the nuclear shape is obscured (Fig. 5-37, *I*). In some instances, discrete granules are not seen but the cytoplasm stains purple (Fig. 5-37, *J*). Variable numbers of purple granules are present in horse basophils (Fig. 5-37, *K*). Basophils can be difficult to recognize in blood films stained with aqueous stains, such as Diff-Quik (Dade Behring Inc., Newark, DE), Hema 3 (Fisher Scientific, Pittsburgh, PA), and the Wright-type stain used in the automated stainer Aerospray 7120 (Westcore, Inc., Logan, UT), because granules do not stain as well with these stains (see Fig. 2-16, *B*).[10] Rickettsial morulae have been recognized in basophils from a dog (Fig. 5-37, *L*).

Band basophils are not usually separated from segmented basophils during differential counts because they are generally of little clinical significance and, except in dogs, may be difficult to identify with certainty when granules obscure the nucleus. Basophilic cell stages may be differentiated when extreme basophilia is present in an attempt to help separate hyperplastic from neoplastic disorders. A more pronounced left shift is expected in an animal with chronic basophilic leukemia than in one with an inflammatory basophilia.[295,305,320]

Basophilia

Basophilia is generally associated with IgE-mediated disorders. When it is present, basophilia usually accompanies eosinophilia.* Basophilia may occur in some animals with mast cell tumors, primarily noncutaneous types (Fig. 5-38),[4,59,110,134,356] and in dogs diagnosed with thrombocythemia.[125,141,219,329] It has been reported in dogs with pulmonary lymphomatoid granulomatosis.[32,378] Basophilia has rarely been reported in association with basophilic leukemia in animals.[295,305,320] Basophilic leukemia must be differentiated from mast cell neoplasia with mastocytemia (sometimes called mast cell leukemia). Mast cells have round nuclei and basophils have segmented nuclei.[20,110,216,448]

MAST CELLS

Mast cells are not normally found in blood.[57,166] They develop in tissues from precursor cells produced in the bone marrow. Mast cells have biochemical characteristics similar to those of basophils and share a common progenitor cell with basophils in bone marrow, but they are clearly different cell types.[164]

Mast Cell Morphology

Basophils have segmented nuclei and mast cells have round nuclei (Fig. 5-39, *A,B*). Mast cells usually have more

*References 26, 72, 120, 259, 389, 469.

FIGURE 5-37 **Morphology of basophils**

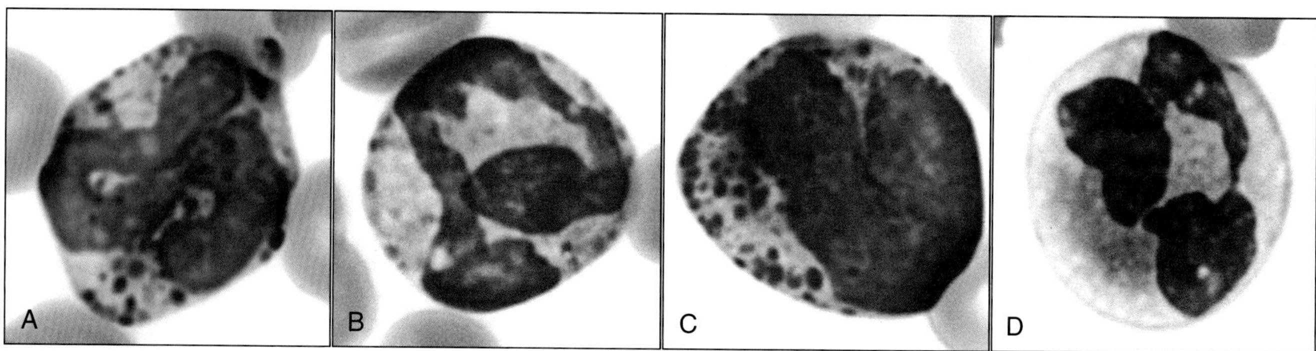

A, Basophil in blood from a dog. **B,** Basophil in blood from a dog. The nucleus is ribbonlike in shape and few granules are present. **C,** Band basophil in the blood of a dog with a basophilia. **D,** Degranulated basophil in blood from a dog with a basophilia. Wright-Giemsa stain.

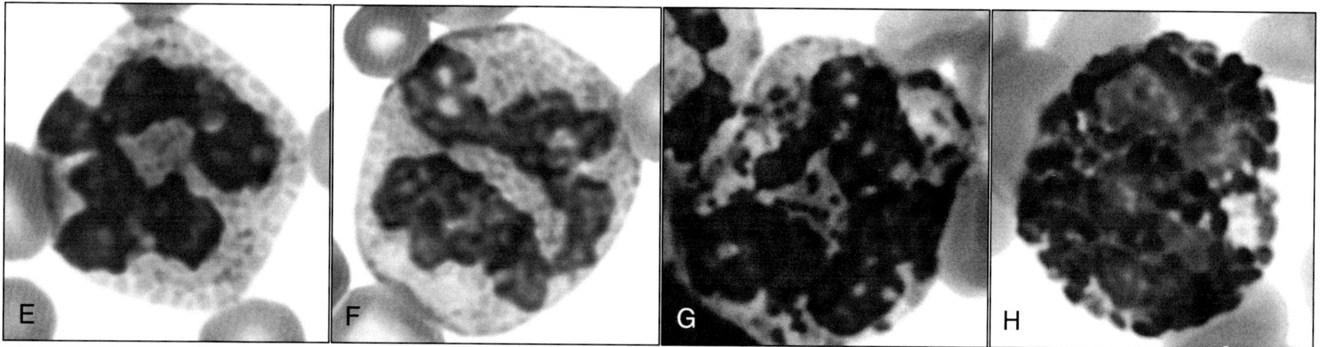

E, Basophil in blood from a cat with light-lavender granules filling the cytoplasm and giving the nucleus a moth-eaten appearance. **F,** Basophil in blood from a cat with light-lavender granules filling the cytoplasm and giving the nucleus a moth-eaten appearance. **G,** Basophil in blood from a cat with a mixture of light-lavender and purple granules filling the cytoplasm. **H,** Basophil with reddish purple granules filling the cytoplasm in blood from the same Siamese cat as described in Figure 5-23, *H.*

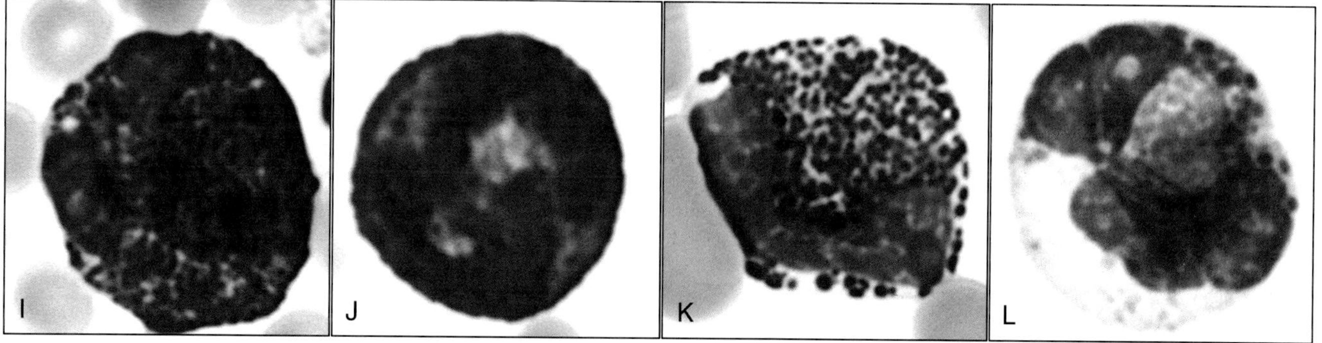

I, Basophil in blood from a cow. The granules are so numerous that they prevent evaluation of nuclear shape. **J,** Basophil in the blood of a goat. Few granules are visible, but the cytoplasm stains purple. **K,** Band basophil in the blood of a horse. **L,** Basophil with a rickettsial morula of unknown species in blood from a dog. The dog had a basophilia and organisms were found in several basophils. Wright-Giemsa stain.

cytoplasmic granules than do basophils. In cats, both primary and secondary granules in basophils are morphologically different from mast cell granules. Like basophils, granules in mast cells stain poorly if at all with Diff-Quik and other aqueous blood stains.[10]

Mastocytemia

Mastocytemia occurs in association with noncutaneous and metastatic cutaneous mast cell tumors.[20,110,448] Rarely, mast cells have been seen to phagocytize erythrocytes (Fig. 5-39, *C*).[20,298,300] Low numbers of mast cells may also

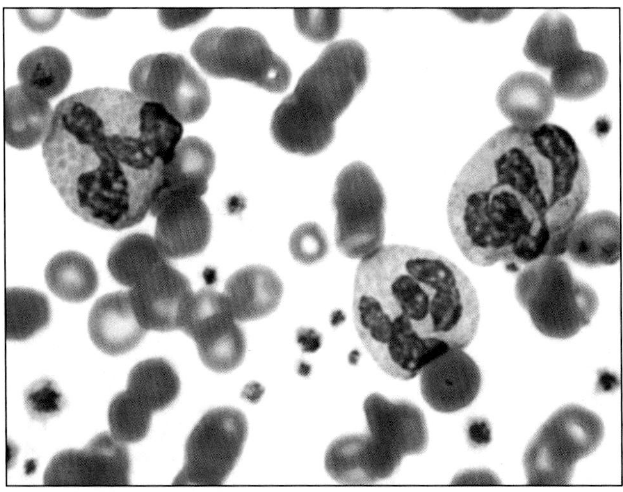

FIGURE 5-38
Marked basophilia (13 × 10^3/µL in a cat with splenic mastocytosis. Wright-Giemsa stain.

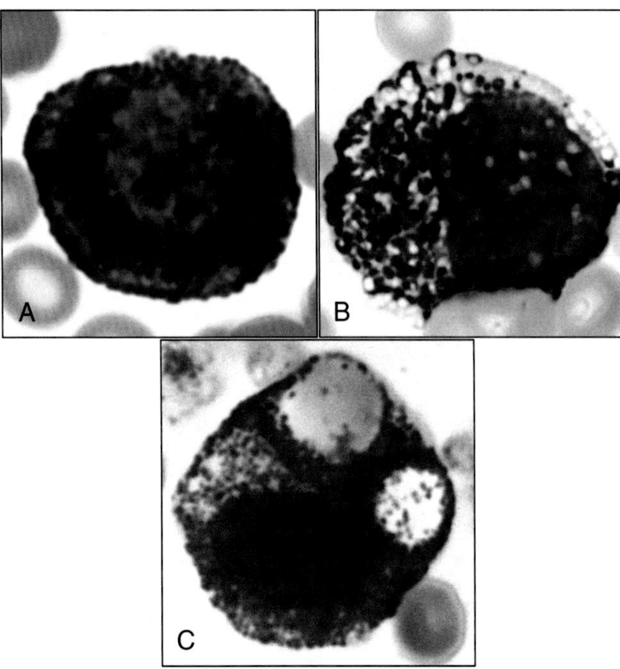

FIGURE 5-39
Morphology of mast cells. **A,** Mast cell in blood from a cat with splenic mastocytosis. **B,** Large mast cell with cytoplasmic vacuoles in addition to granules in blood from a dog with a noncutaneous mast cell neoplasm. **C,** Large mast cell exhibiting erythrophagocytosis in blood from a cat with a noncutaneous mast cell neoplasm. Wright-Giemsa stain.

be present in the blood of dogs with inflammatory diseases, necrosis, tissue injury, and severe regenerative anemia.[80,315,442] In contrast to findings in dogs, mast cells are rarely seen in the blood of cats in the absence of mast cell neoplasms.[166]

MONOCYTES

Monocyte Morphology

Mononuclear leukocytes in blood are classified as either lymphocytes or monocytes. These cells are not devoid of granules but rather have lower numbers of cytoplasmic granules than do granulocytes. Monocytes are usually larger than lymphocytes and have nuclei that are more variable in shape and have N:C ratios of 1.0 or less.

The monocyte nucleus may be round, kidney-shaped, band-shaped, or convoluted (ameboid) with chromatin that is diffuse or mildly clumped (Fig. 5-40, *A-H*). The cytoplasm is typically blue-gray and often contains variably sized vacuoles. Less often, dust-like pinkish or reddish purple granules may be visible in the cytoplasm (Fig. 5-40, *G,H*). Monocytes develop into macrophages after they leave the blood and enter tissue. In some disorders, mononuclear phagocytes in blood become activated and enlarged, resembling macrophages (Fig. 5-40, *I,J*).

Monocytes in dogs often have band-shaped nuclei (Fig. 5-40, *B,C*); consequently they may be confused with band neutrophils (Fig. 5-41). The cytoplasmic staining of the mature neutrophils should be examined. If no toxicity is present, the cells with band-shaped nuclei and blue-gray cytoplasm are identified as monocytes. Other potentially helpful criteria include the following: the ends of the band-like nucleus of the monocyte are often enlarged and knob-like and the nuclear chromatin of the monocyte is not clumped in the dark-light pattern to the degree commonly seen in band neutrophils. If marked toxicity is present in the cytoplasm of neutrophilic cells, differentiation becomes much more difficult.

Differentiation of monocytes with round nuclei from large lymphocytes can be difficult, especially in ruminants (Fig. 5-42). The N:C ratio is typically greater than 1.0 for large lymphocytes. Monocytes must also be differentiated from large reactive lymphocytes with convoluted nuclei. The cytoplasm of reactive lymphocytes is more basophilic (navy blue in color) than the cytoplasm of monocytes (Fig. 5-43). Finally, monocytes may sometimes be confused with basophils (Fig. 5-44).

Erythrophagocytosis may be present in monocytes in primary or secondary immune-mediated hemolytic anemia (Fig. 5-45, *A*)[202] and in neoplastic cells in dogs with hemophagocytic histiocytic sarcoma.[48] Like neutrophils, monocytes may phagocytize extruded eosinophil granules (Fig. 5-45, *B*). Monocytes may also contain hemosiderin, which stains gray-to-black with routine blood stains (Fig. 5-45, *C*) and blue with the Prussian blue stain (Fig. 5-45, *D*). Iron-positive inclusions may be seen in association with hemolytic anemia and/or marked inflammatory responses.[169] Mononuclear phagocytes containing melanin granules (melanophages) may rarely occur with malignant melanoma (Fig. 5-45, *E*).

Rickettsial organisms that infect mononuclear phagocytes include *Ehrlichia canis, E. chaffeensis,* and *Neorickettsia risticii.* In contrast to granulocytic rickettsial species, morulae of

FIGURE 5-40 **Morphology of monocytes**

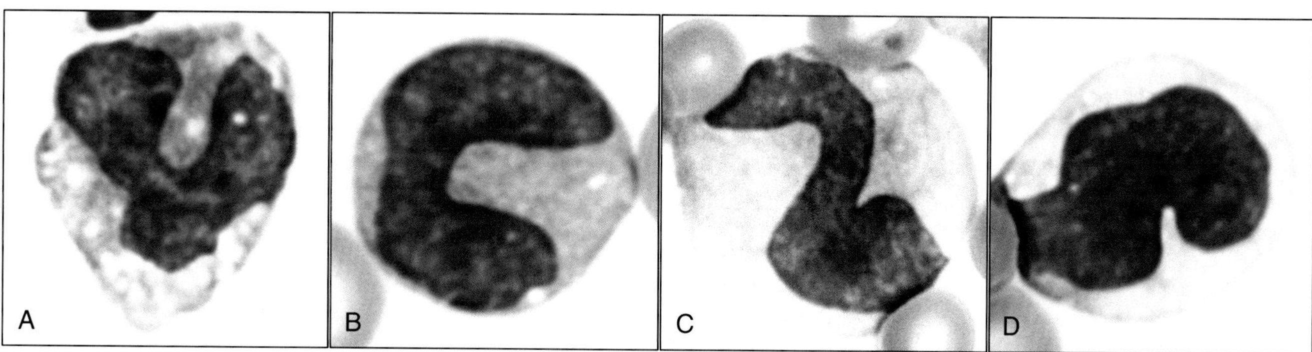

A, Monocyte in blood from a dog with band-shaped nucleus and prominent cytoplasmic vacuolation. **B,** Monocyte in blood from a dog with a band-shaped nucleus, basophilic cytoplasm and two vacuoles. **C,** Monocyte in blood from a dog with a band-shaped nucleus and basophilic cytoplasm **D,** Monocyte in blood of a dog with kidney-shaped nucleus.

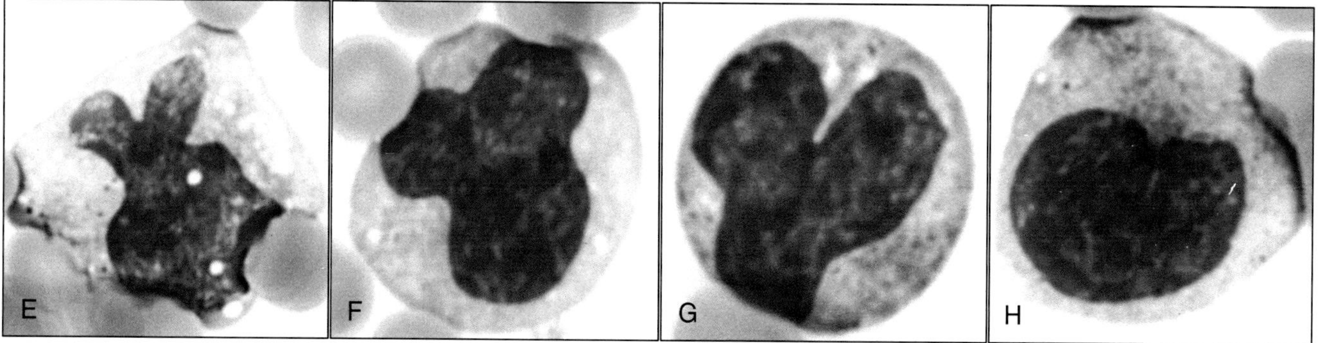

E, Monocyte in blood from a horse with a pleomorphic nucleus and basophilic cytoplasm containing vacuoles. **F,** Monocyte in blood from a cow with a pleomorphic nucleus and basophilic cytoplasm. **G,** Monocyte in blood from a dog with band-shaped nucleus and basophilic cytoplasm containing magenta-staining granules. **H,** Monocyte in blood from a horse with a kidney-shaped nucleus and basophilic cytoplasm containing magenta-staining granules.

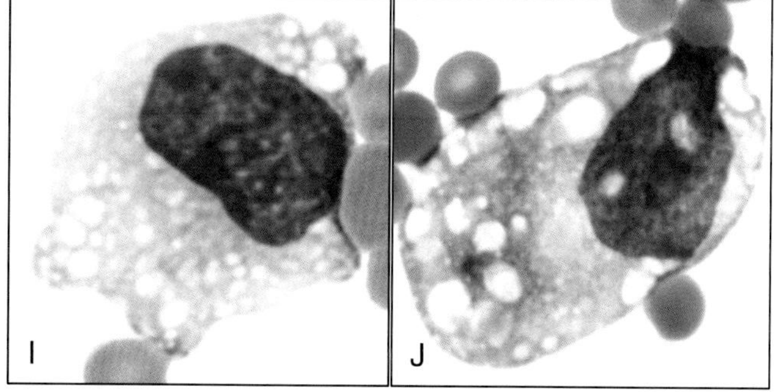

I, Large activated monocyte or macrophage with prominent vacuolation in blood from a horse with *Babesia equi* infection. **J,** Macrophage in blood from a cat with *Mycoplasma haemofelis* infection. Lower magnification than other images in this figure. Wright-Giemsa stain.

monocytic rickettsial species are rarely found in blood leukocytes. When present, these morulae appear as tightly packed basophilic clusters of organisms within the cytoplasm (Fig. 5-45, *F,G*; Fig. 5-46).

E. canis causes mild-to-severe disease in dogs. Clinical signs include fever, anorexia, weight loss, hemorrhagic diathesis (especially epistaxis), lymphadenopathy, and neurologic signs. Laboratory findings generally include marked thrombocytopenia, mild nonregenerative anemia, variably mild leukopenia, and hyperglobulinemia. Marked pancytopenia secondary to bone marrow aplasia is rarely seen in the United States.

E. chaffeensis (human monocytic ehrlichiosis) infects dogs. Clinical signs have not been reported following experimental

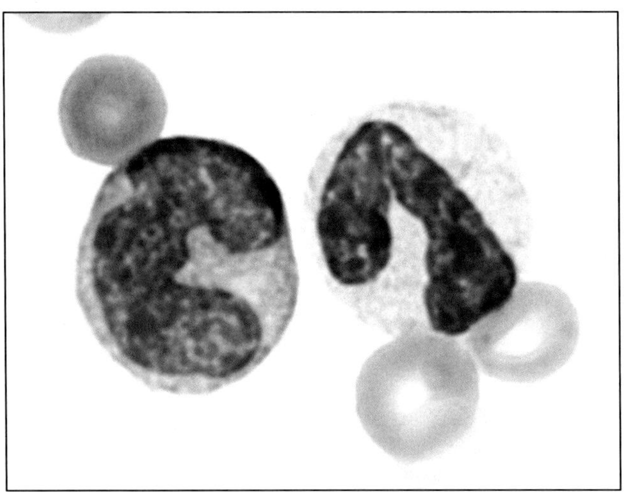

FIGURE 5-41
Monocyte *(left)* and band neutrophil *(right)* in blood from a dog with immune-mediated hemolytic anemia. Wright-Giemsa stain.

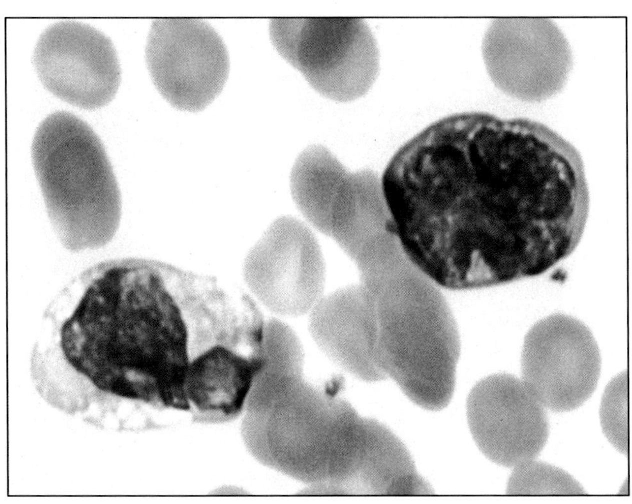

FIGURE 5-43
Monocyte *(left)* and a reactive lymphocyte with intensely basophilic cytoplasm *(right)* in blood from a dog after vaccination. Wright-Giemsa stain.

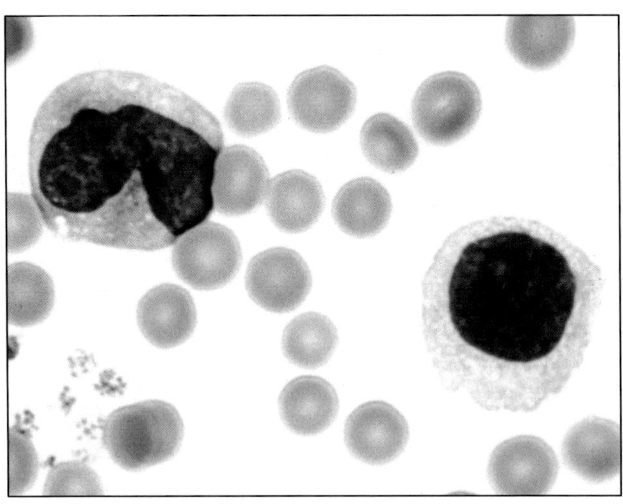

FIGURE 5-42
Monocyte *(left)* and large lymphocyte *(right)* in blood from a cow. Wright-Giemsa stain.

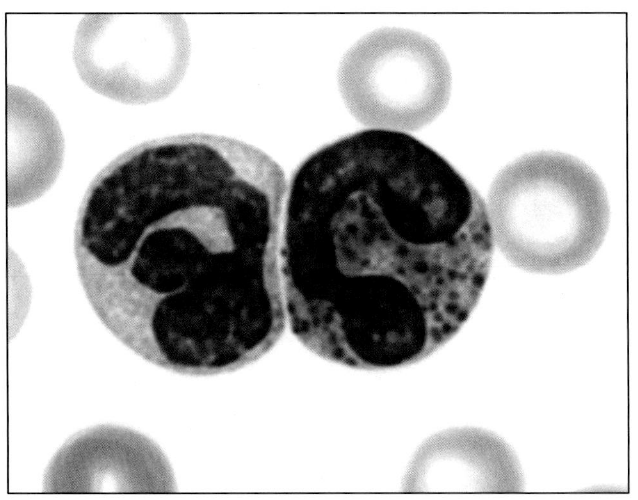

FIGURE 5-44
Monocyte *(left)* and basophil *(right)* in blood from a dog with a severe flea infestation. Wright-Giemsa stain.

infections,[113,512] but anterior uveitis, vomiting, epistaxis, and lymphadenopathy have been reported in clinical cases.[189] Thrombocytopenia has been reported in animals without evidence of illness.[189]

N. risticii is primarily pathogenic to horses (Potomac horse fever), where it causes fever, depression, anorexia, diarrhea, and variable leukopenia and thrombocytopenia.[126,515] *N. risticii* also infects other mammals including dogs and cats.[112,398,504] Clinical signs in dogs have varied from none to fever, lethargy, bleeding diathesis, and polyarthritis. Thrombocytopenia is often present even in asymptomatic dogs.[233,398]

Other infectious agents that may rarely be seen in blood mononuclear phagocytes include *Histoplasma capsulatum* (Fig. 5-45, *H*),[88,89] *Mycobacterium* species,[271] *Leishmania infantum*,[404] and remarkably large schizonts of *Cytauxzoon felis* (Fig. 5-47).[9,484]

Monocytosis

Monocytosis may occur in conditions that also cause neutrophilia (discussed earlier in this chapter). It may be present in both acute and chronic inflammation.* The injection of recombinant growth factors—including IL-3, GM-CSF, G-CSF, and M-CSF—results in a monocytosis.[347,357,421,466,482] Endogenous and exogenous glucocorticoid steroids can induce monocytosis in animals, especially in dogs.[16,226,241,363]

*References 139, 190, 229, 246, 247, 364, 469.

FIGURE 5-45 **Monocyte inclusions and infectious agents**

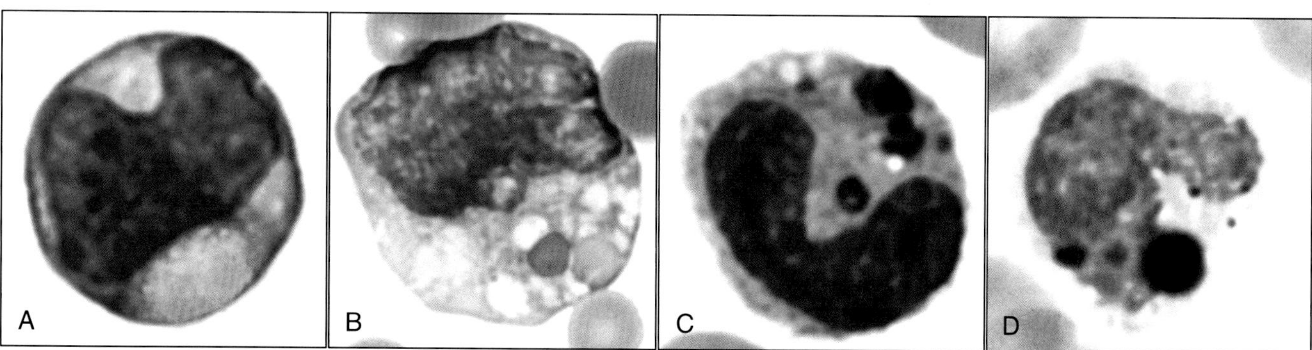

A, Monocyte with erythrophagocytosis in blood from a dog with immune-mediated hemolytic anemia. Wright-Giemsa stain. **B,** Monocyte that has phagocytized eosinophil granules in blood from a horse. Wright-Giemsa stain. **C,** Monocyte containing hemosiderin (dark inclusions in the cytoplasm) in blood from a dog with a hemolytic anemia. Wright-Giemsa stain. **D,** Monocyte containing hemosiderin (dark blue inclusions in the cytoplasm) in blood from a dog with a hemolytic anemia. Prussian blue stain.

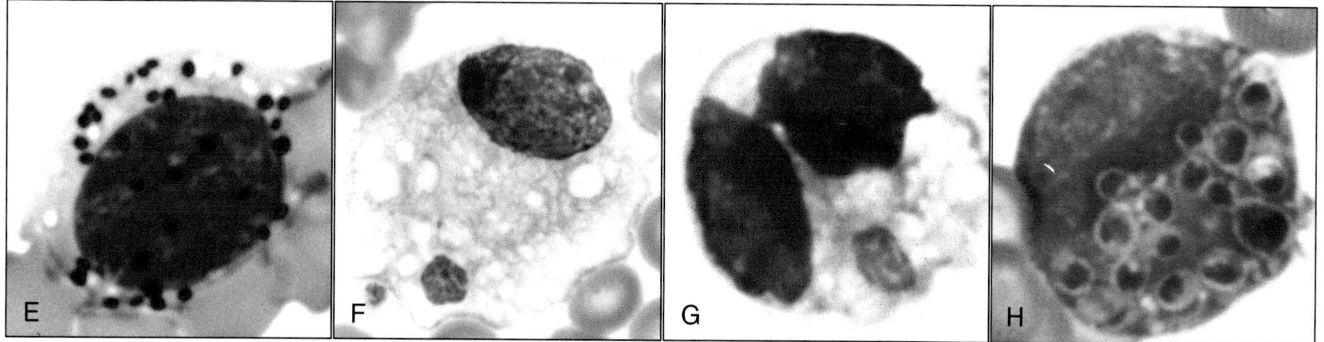

E, Mononuclear cell containing melanin granules (presumably a melanophage) in blood from an aged gray Arabian gelding with disseminated malignant melanoma. Wright stain. **F,** Macrophage with an *Ehrlichia canis* morula in the cytoplasm in a buffy coat smear from a dog. Wright-Giemsa stain. **G,** *Ehrlichia canis* morula in the cytoplasm of a dog monocyte. Wright-Giemsa stain. **H,** *Histoplasma capsulatum* in the cytoplasm of a monocyte in blood from a dog. Modified Wright stain.

E, Photograph of a stained blood film from a 1999 ASVCP slide review case submitted by J. Tarrant, T. Stokol, J. Bartol, and J. Wakshlag. H, Image provided by C. A. Thompson.

Monocytosis occurs in animals with acute monocytic or acute myelomonocytic leukemias.[194,323,401,426] Monocytosis sometimes accompanies histiocytic sarcoma in dogs.[252] Normal domestic animals may have few or no monocytes in blood; consequently the term *monocytopenia* is not usually used.

LYMPHOCYTES

Most lymphocytes reside within lymphoid organs (lymph nodes, thymus, spleen, and bone marrow), with only a small percentage circulating in blood. Depending on the species and individual variability, about 50% to 75% of blood lymphocytes are T lymphocytes and about 10% to 40% are B lymphocytes. NK cells account for 5% to 10% of blood lymphocytes. T lymphocytes and B lymphocytes cannot be differentiated from one another based on morphology in stained blood films.[458]

Lymphocyte Morphology

Normal Lymphocyte Morphology

Most lymphocytes have microvilli on their surfaces (Fig. 5-48, *A*).[47] They have high N:C ratios and vary considerably in size, with the highest N:C ratios in the smaller cells (Fig. 5-49, *A-F*). The cytoplasm of resting (unstimulated) blood lymphocytes is usually pale blue in color. Unstimulated lymphocytes have a few mitochondria and numerous ribosomes but little or no rough endoplasmic reticulum. Granules are generally absent or low in number unless the cell is a granular lymphocyte. Their nuclei are usually round but may be oval or slightly indented (Fig. 5-48, *B*).[224] Nuclear chromatin varies from condensed and densely staining to a pattern of light and dark

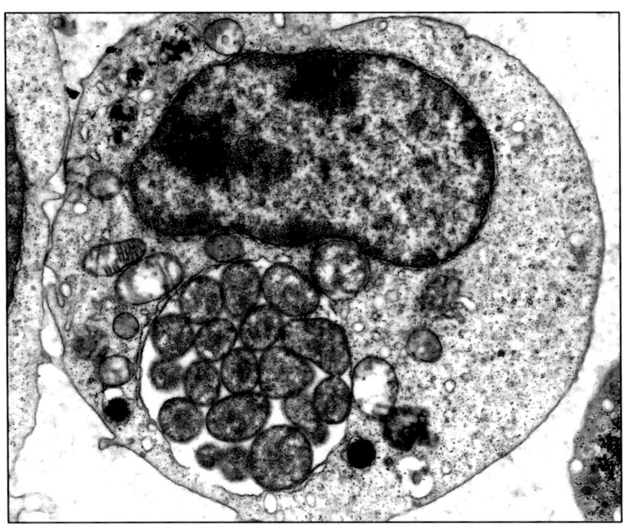

FIGURE 5-46

Transmission electron photomicrograph of an *Ehrlichia canis* morula in a monocyte from a dog. The morula consists of a membrane-lined vesicle containing multiple organisms.

Courtesy of C. F. Simpson.

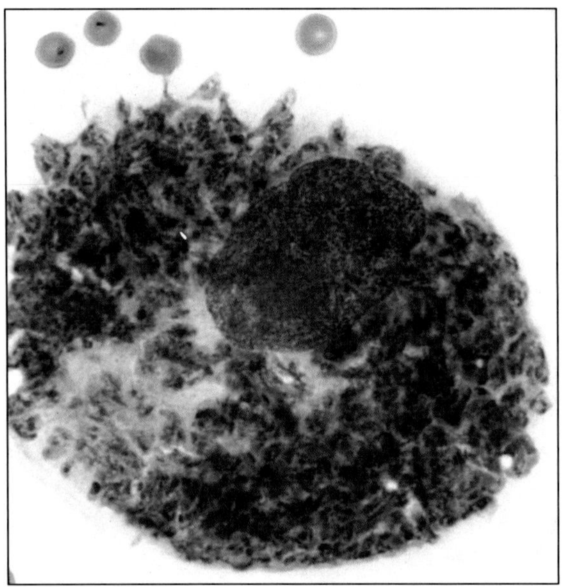

FIGURE 5-47

Cytauxzoon felis schizont development in a large macrophage in blood from a cat. Note the small size of the erythrocytes compared to the macrophage in this low-magnification image. Wright-Giemsa stain.

staining areas and to lighter-staining nuclei with a smooth chromatin pattern. Lymphocytes in healthy ruminants may have ring-like clumped chromatin patterns in their nuclei that may be confused with nucleoli (Fig. 5-49, *F*). Consequently caution should be taken in making a diagnosis of lymphoid neoplasia in cattle based on a finding of what appear to be

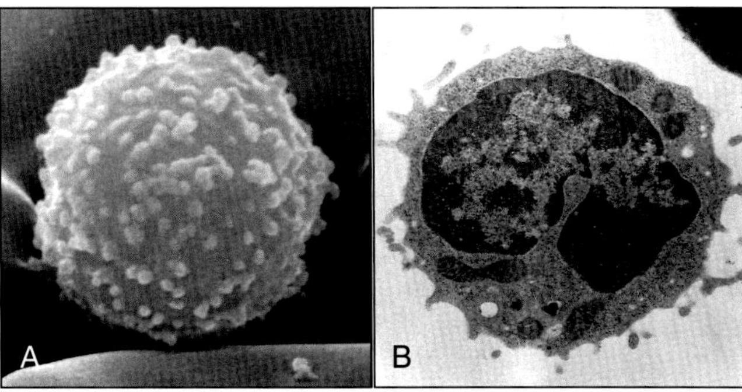

FIGURE 5-48

Electron microscopy of lymphocytes. **A,** Scanning electron photomicrograph of a small lymphocyte with numerous short microvilli on its surface in blood from a dog with chronic lymphocytic leukemia (CLL). **B,** Transmission electron photomicrograph of a small lymphocyte in blood from a dog with CLL. Abundant heterochromatin and single deep cleft are present in the nucleus. Many ribosomes, a few mitochondria, and one osmiophilic dense inclusion are present in the cytoplasm.

From Harvey JW, Terrell TG, Hyde DM, et al. Well-differentiated lymphocytic leukemia in a dog: long-term survival without therapy. Vet Pathol. *1981;18:37-47.*

low numbers of lymphoblasts in blood. Most lymphocytes in the blood of domestic animals are small to medium in size, but some large lymphocytes may be present. Lymphocytes in ruminants are often larger, with more cytoplasm than is seen in other species, sometimes making these cells difficult to differentiate from monocytes (see Fig. 5-42).[198] If it is unclear whether a cell is a lymphocyte or a monocyte, it is classified as a lymphocyte because cells of this type are usually much more numerous in blood than are monocytes.

A low percentage of lymphocytes in blood have red- or purple-staining (generally focal) granules within their cytoplasm (see Figs. 5-4, 5-49, *G,H*). These cells are generally medium to large in size and usually have more cytoplasm and lower N:C ratios than small lymphocytes. Granular lymphocytes appear to be either NK cells or a subset of cytotoxic T lymphocytes.[33] The granules in granular lymphocytes do not stain as well with aqueous blood stains (such as Diff-Quik) as they do with methanolic blood stains.[10]

Reactive Lymphocytes

Lymphocytes proliferate in response to antigenic stimulation. They increase in size and exhibit increased cytoplasmic basophilia (Fig. 5-50, *A-C*). Most of these antigenically stimulated cells remain in peripheral lymphoid tissues but some may enter the circulation, although usually in low numbers. Various terms including *reactive lymphocytes, transformed lymphocytes,* and *immunocytes* have been used to describe them. Some reactive lymphocytes are large, with convoluted nuclei (see Figs. 5-43, 5-50, *B,C*). They resemble monocytes except that their cytoplasm is more basophilic (navy blue in color) than cytoplasm seen in monocytes (see Fig. 5-43). These cells can also be difficult to differentiate from some neoplastic lymphocytes.

FIGURE 5-49 **Normal lymphocyte morphology**

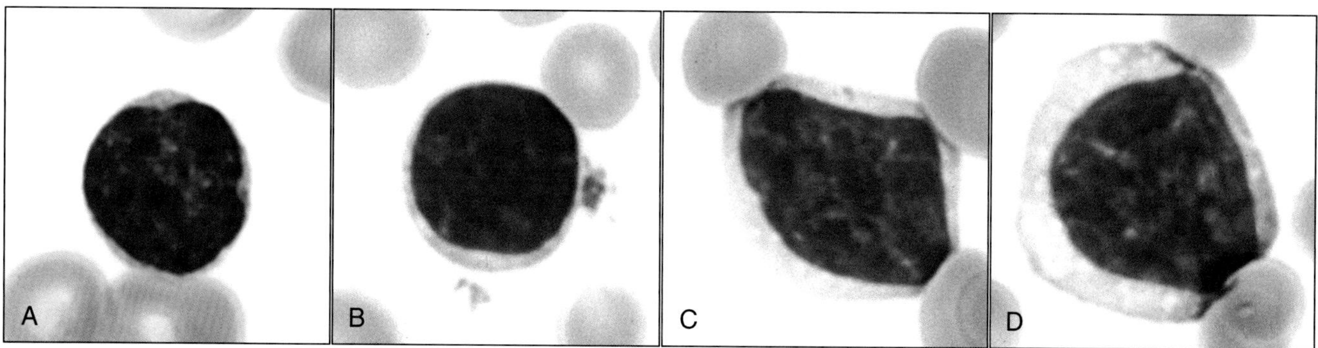

A, Small lymphocyte in blood from a dog. **B,** Small lymphocyte in blood from a cow. **C,** Medium-sized lymphocyte in blood from a horse. **D,** Medium to large lymphocyte in blood from a cow.

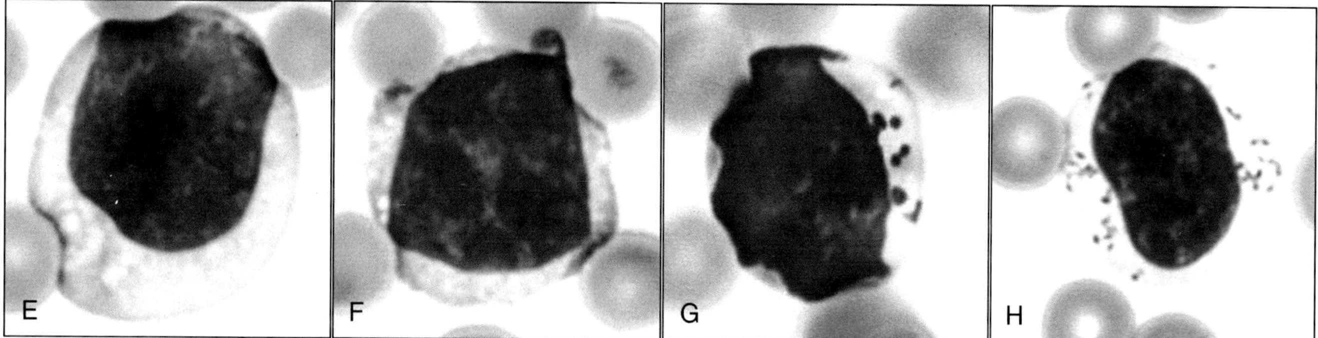

E, Large lymphocyte in blood from a cow. **F,** Medium to large lymphocyte in blood from a cow. The ringlike clumped chromatin patterns in the nucleus may be confused with nucleoli. **G,** Granular lymphocyte in blood from a cow. **H,** Granular lymphocyte in blood from a cat. Wright-Giemsa stain.

When it is not possible to decide whether a basophilic lymphocyte is reactive or neoplastic, the term *atypical lymphocyte* is sometimes used. Basophilic erythroid precursors may be confused with reactive lymphocytes. Some reactive lymphocytes are plasmacytoid (plasma-cell-like) in appearance (Fig. 5-50, *D,E*) and may rarely contain pinkish or bluish globules (Russell bodies) within their cytoplasm (Fig. 5-50, *F*). These inclusions are composed of dilated endoplasmic reticula containing immunoglobulins.[47] Lymphoid cells containing Russell bodies have been called Mott cells. Plasma cells are present in lymphoid organs except the thymus, but they are rarely observed in blood even when plasma cell neoplasia (e.g., multiple myeloma) is present.

Cytoplasmic Granules, Vacuoles, and Inclusions

A low percentage of lymphocytes in blood from normal animals contains cytoplasmic granules (see previous discussion of granular lymphocytes). Basophilic granules may be seen in the lymphocytes from animals with certain lysosomal storage diseases (Figs. 5-51, *A*; 5-52), including mucopolysaccharidosis type VI[11,349] and type VII[205,206] in dogs and cats and GM_2-gangliosidosis in pigs.[256]

Cytoplasmic vacuoles may be seen in lymphocytes from a variety of neoplastic and nonneoplastic disorders (Fig. 5-51, *B*). Discrete vacuoles may occur in the cytoplasm of lymphocytes from animals with inherited lysosomal storage diseases (Fig. 5-51, *C-E*), including mucopolysaccharidosis type VII in cats,[177] GM_2-gangliosidosis in cats,[230,350] GM_1-gangliosidosis in cats and dogs,[12,118,342] α-mannosidosis in cats,[11] β-mannosidosis in goats,[371] Niemann-Pick type C in cats,[68] and α-L-fucosidase in dogs.[243] Basophilic granules and vacuoles may not become apparent in some lysosomal disorders until the affected animal reaches adulthood.

Lymphocytes may also contain distemper inclusions as in other blood cell types.[314] Finally, *Sarcocystis neurona* organisms have been recognized in blood monocytes and lymphocytes (Fig. 5-51, *F*) from an immunosuppressed dog (R. Di Terlizzi, personal communication).

Neoplastic Large Granular Lymphocytes, Plasma Cells, and Mott Cells

Neoplasms involving lymphoid cells with large cytoplasmic magenta granules in cats have been called large granular lymphomas, globule leukocyte tumors, and granulated round cell tumors.[107,152,238,494] Most of these large granular lymphomas appear to originate as intestinal tumors composed of cytotoxic T lymphocytes. As with other lymphomas, neoplastic cells may sometimes be present in blood (Figs. 5-53, *A*; 5-54) and

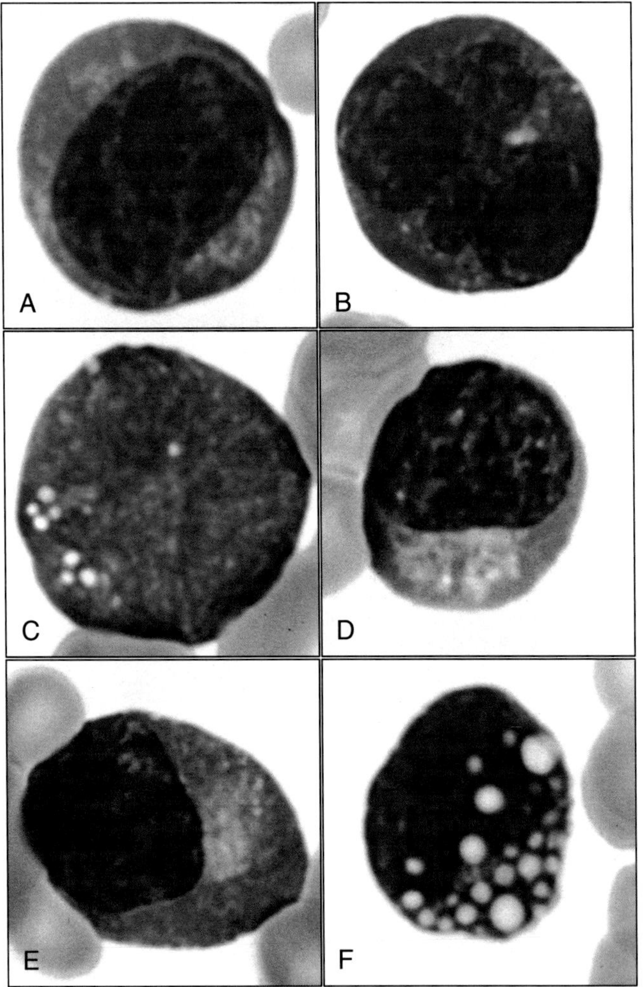

FIGURE 5-50

Morphology of reactive lymphocytes. **A,** Reactive lymphocyte with intensely basophilic cytoplasm in blood from a cow infected with bovine leukemia virus. **B,** Reactive lymphocyte with a convoluted nucleus and intensely basophilic cytoplasm in blood from a cat with a bacterial infection. **C,** Reactive lymphocyte with a convoluted nucleus and intensely basophilic cytoplasm in blood from a dog with a mild cough. **D,** Plasmacytoid lymphocyte with intensely basophilic cytoplasm in blood from a dog with babesiosis. **E,** Plasmacytoid lymphocyte with intensely basophilic cytoplasm in blood from a horse with *Anaplasma phagocytophilum* infection. **F,** Lymphocyte containing Russell bodies in the cytoplasm in blood from a horse. Wright-Giemsa stain.

bone marrow.[107,152] Similarly large granules have been described in blood lymphocytes from a horse with large granular lymphocyte leukemia.[258]

Plasma cells are present in lymphoid organs (except the thymus but they are rarely observed in blood even when plasma cell neoplasia (e.g., multiple myeloma) is present (Fig. 5-53, *B*).[129,369] Plasma cells have lower N:C ratios and greater cytoplasmic basophilia than resting lymphocytes. The presence of prominent Golgi may create a pale perinuclear area in the cytoplasm. Plasma cells typically have eccentrically located nuclei with coarse chromatin clumping in a mosaic pattern. In addition to reactive Mott cells, neoplastic Mott cells may

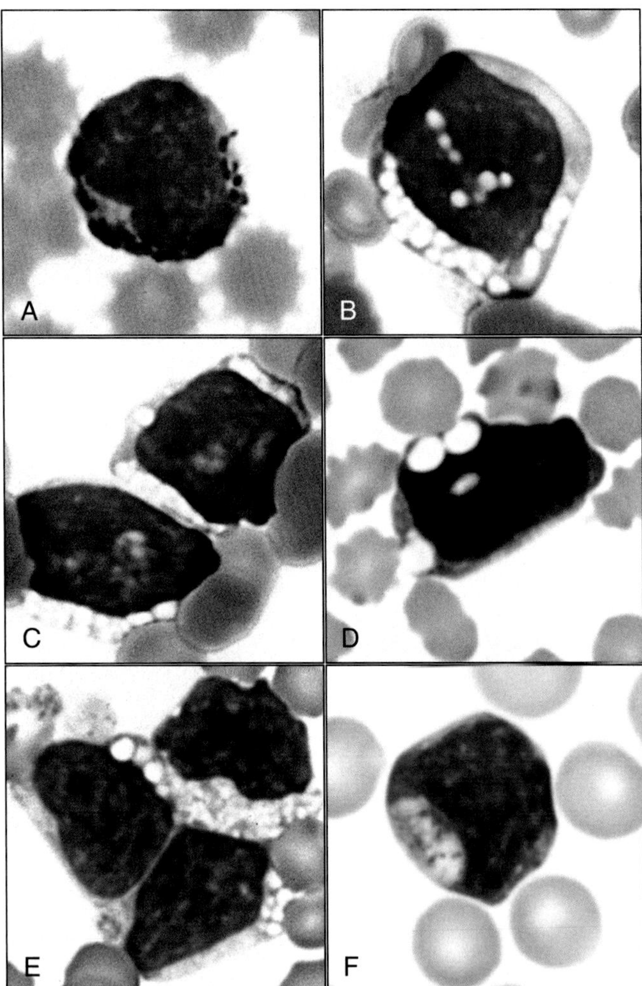

FIGURE 5-51

Cytoplasmic granules, vacuoles, and inclusions in lymphocytes. **A,** Lymphocyte containing basophilic granules in the blood of a 3-month-old German shepherd dog with inherited mucopolysaccharidosis type VII. Wright stain. **B,** One of many lymphocytes containing cytoplasmic vacuoles in blood from an 8-week-old foal with *Corynebacterium equi* pneumonia. Lymphocytes appeared normal after treatment and recovery. Wright-Giemsa stain. **C,** Lymphocytes with cytoplasmic vacuoles in the blood of a Korat cat with inherited GM_2-gangliosidosis. **D,** Lymphocytes with cytoplasmic vacuoles in the blood of a goat with presumptive diagnosis of inherited β-mannosidosis. Wright stain. **E,** Lymphocytes with cytoplasmic vacuoles in the blood of a domestic shorthair cat with inherited Niemann-Pick disease type C. Wright-Giemsa stain. **F,** Lymphocyte containing a *Sarcocystic neurona* organism in a lymphocyte. Wright stain.

A, *Photograph of a stained blood film from a 1997 ASVCP slide review case submitted by D. I. Bounous, D. C. Silverstein, K. S. Latimer, and K. P. Carmichael.* ***D,*** *Photograph of a stained blood film from a 1990 ASVCP slide review case submitted by W. Vernau.* ***E,*** *Photograph of a stained blood film from a 1993 ASVCP slide review case submitted by D. E. Brown and M. A. Thrall.* ***F,*** *Photograph from a 2007 ASVCP review case submitted by R. Di Terlizzi, H. Bender, K. Gibson-Corley, A. Ginman, J. Haynes, M. Lappin.*

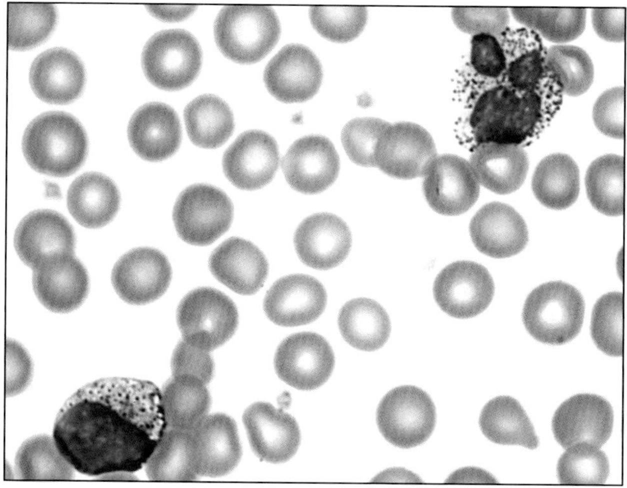

FIGURE 5-52
Blood from a bulldog with an inherited mucopolysaccharidosis with purple granules in a lymphocyte and a neutrophil. The general disorder was diagnosed using screening tests, but the specific type was not determined. Wright-Giemsa stain.

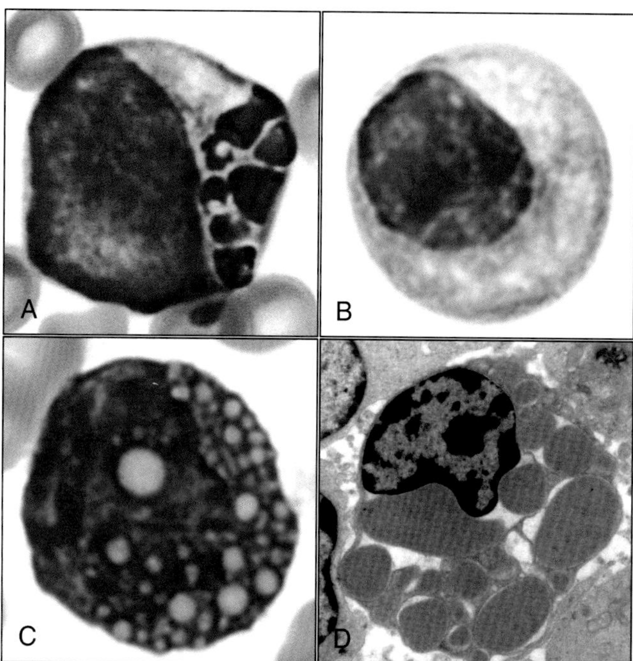

FIGURE 5-53
Neoplastic large granular lymphocytes, plasma cells, and Mott cells. **A,** Neoplastic large granular lymphocyte in blood from a cat with large granular lymphoma. Note the large size of the granules compared to the normal granular lymphocyte as shown in Figure 5-49, *H.* Wright-Giemsa stain. **B,** Plasma cell with eccentric nucleus in blood from a dog with multiple myeloma. Wright-Giemsa stain. **C,** Mott cell in the blood of a dog with lymphoma and Mott cell differentiation. Wright-Giemsa stain. **D,** Transmission electron photomicrograph of a Mott cell from a dog with lymphoma and Mott cell differentiation. Disorganized and dilated endoplasmic reticula containing immunoglobulin.

C,D, From Stacy NI, Nabity MB, Hackendahl N, et al. B-cell lymphoma with Mott cell differentiation in two young adult dogs. Vet Clin Pathol. *2009;38:113-120.*

be seen in low numbers in blood from dogs with B lymphocyte lymphoma with Mott cell differentiation (Fig. 5-53, *C,D*). In these neoplasms, Mott cells appeared to develop from lymphoblasts without first becoming plasma cells.[250,439]

Lymphocytosis

Lymphocyte numbers in blood vary with age. Absolute lymphocyte counts are lower in young animals than in adults of some species (e.g., horses) and higher in young animals than in adults of other species (e.g., cats).[201,326] Lymphocytosis is much less common than neutrophilia. Transient lymphocytosis sometimes occurs with excitement or exercise in animals (especially horses and cats).[400,436] Marginating lymphocyte pools are reported to occur in lungs and spleen, and lymphocytosis may occur secondary to increased blood flow and splenic contraction, respectively.[43,121,353] The increased lymphocytosis in humans associated with exercise, acute psychological stress, or the activation of β-adrenergic receptors (by infused isoproterenol) results from increased numbers of circulating NK cells and, to a lesser degree, increased numbers of γδ T lymphocytes and $CD8^+$ T lymphocytes.[15] Lymphocytosis has been reported in rats and humans after splenectomy.[242,495]

Although increased proliferation of lymphocytes is common in lymph nodes during response to foreign antigens, evidence of this reaction is often not present in blood. In some cases, reactive lymphocytes account for a substantial proportion of the total lymphocytes present in blood, but an absolute lymphocytosis is uncommon.

Lymphocytosis is sometimes present in animals with low-grade or chronic inflammatory conditions. In contrast, lymphopenia is more often present in acute and/or severe inflammatory conditions. The injection of recombinant growth factors—including IL-2, SCF, GM-CSF, and G-CSF—has resulted in lymphocytosis in animals.[19,161,209,347]

Parasitic diseases that may result in a lymphocytosis in a small percentage of cases include trypanosomiasis in several species,[37,138,240] *Spirocerca lupi* infection in dogs,[29] *Coenurus cerebralis* infection in sheep,[364] *Leishmania* infection in dogs,[29] experimental *Toxoplasma gondii* infection in cats, and *Babesia* infection in dogs.[397,516]

Bacterial diseases that may sometimes have an associated lymphocytosis include bartonellosis in cats and subclinical ehrlichiosis in dogs.[63,92,444] Lymphocytosis in dogs with subclinical *E. canis* infection results from an increase in $CD8^+$ lymphocytes, which may appear as granular lymphocytes in stained blood films.[214,286,483]

Viral diseases that may sometimes have an associated lymphocytosis include FeLV infection in cats,[178] caprine arthritis-encephalitis virus infections in goats,[319] and bovine leukemia virus (BLV) infection in cattle and sheep.[114] Although acute

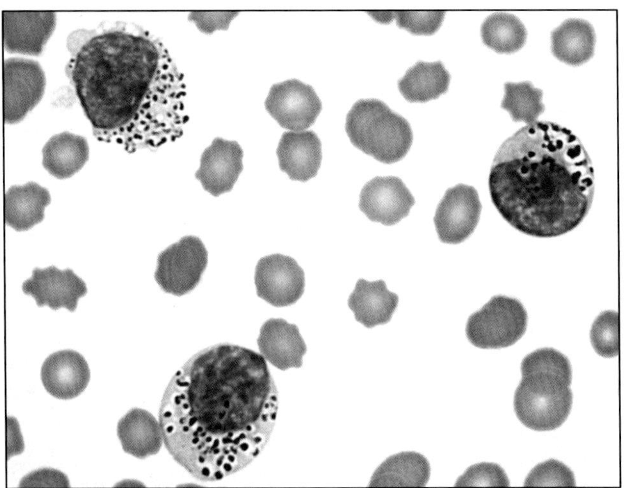

FIGURE 5-54
Three large granular lymphocytes in blood from a cat with an abdominal large granular lymphoma. Wright-Giemsa stain.

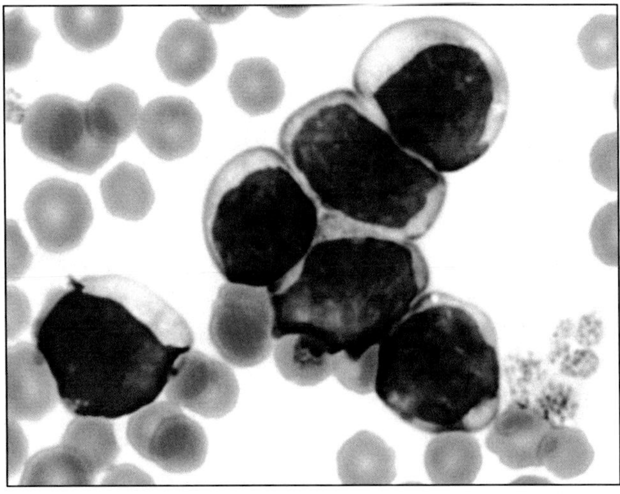

FIGURE 5-55
Nonneoplastic lymphocytosis in blood from a cow infected with bovine leukemia virus. Lymphocytes are medium to large in size with increased cytoplasmic basophilia. Wright-Giemsa stain.

parvovirus infection in dogs causes lymphopenia, lymphocytosis may occur during recovery from the infection.[379]

BLV is a B-lymphotrophic retrovirus that can produce a persistent lymphocytosis in cattle and sheep. Some reactive lymphocytes, as well as normal-appearing lymphocytes, may be seen in cattle with persistent lymphocytosis (Fig. 5-55).[142]

This persistent lymphocytosis is due to an increase in circulating B lymphocytes.[413] The lymphocytosis appears to develop because lymphocytes, in which the virus is transcriptionally silenced, survive and accumulate.[147] BLV infection can also produce lymphomas in cattle and sheep, which can have secondary lymphocytosis comprised of neoplastic lymphocytes.[142,362] A vaccine reaction has been considered a cause of

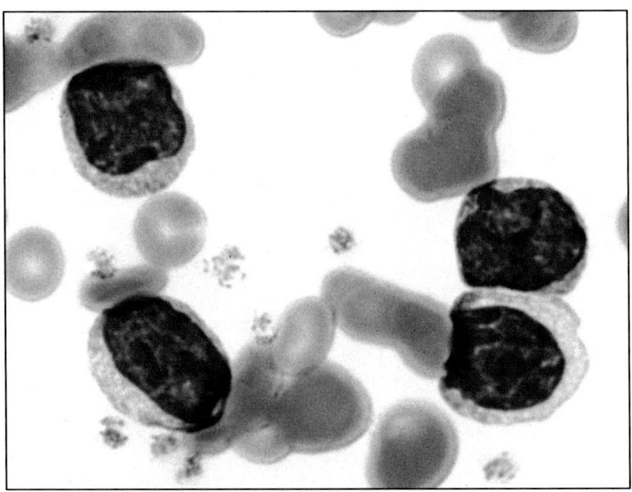

FIGURE 5-56
Chronic lymphocytic leukemia (CLL) in blood from a cat with normal-appearing lymphocytes. Wright-Giemsa stain.

reactive lymphocytosis in animals, but evidence for this phenomenon has not been substantiated in published studies.[29]

Persistent lymphocytosis has been described in association with an indolent lymphoproliferative disease in ferrets. This disorder appears to be caused by a virus other than FeLV or Aleutian disease virus.[135,136]

Lymphocytosis is reported in about 40% of cats with primary immune-mediated hemolytic anemia, but lymphocytosis is rarely recognized in dogs with autoimmune disease.[29,254] Lymphocytosis is common in Abyssinian and Somali cats with a disorder characterized by increased osmotic fragility of erythrocytes.[253]

Lymphocytosis has been reported to occur in a low percentage of dogs and cats with hypoadrenocorticism.[29] Lymphocytosis has also been reported in a low percentage of cats with hyperthyroidism in one study.[454] However, treatment of hyperthyroid cats with methimazole has also been reported to cause a lymphocytosis in some, raising the concern whether untreated hyperthyroidism causes lymphocytosis.[375,376]

Lymphocytosis has been reported in a low percentage of dogs, cats, and humans with thymoma.[29] Lymphocytosis in humans has been associated with invasive, lymphocyte-rich thymomas.[39,434] The lymphocytosis is attributable to nonneoplastic T lymphocytes whose proliferation is probably increased secondary to factors produced by neoplastic thymic epithelial cells. B lymphopenia is much more common than T lymphocytosis in humans with thymoma.[332]

Marked lymphocytosis, involving normal-appearing small to medium-sized lymphocytes, is present in the blood of animals with chronic lymphocytic leukemia (CLL) (Figs. 5-56, 5-57).[2,109,503] Although normal in appearance, these cells have abnormal function. CLL is uncommon and is reported most often in older dogs.[474,503] About three-fourths of dogs with CLL exhibit T lymphocytosis, and about three-fourths of these cases of T lymphocyte CLL appear as $CD8^+$ granular

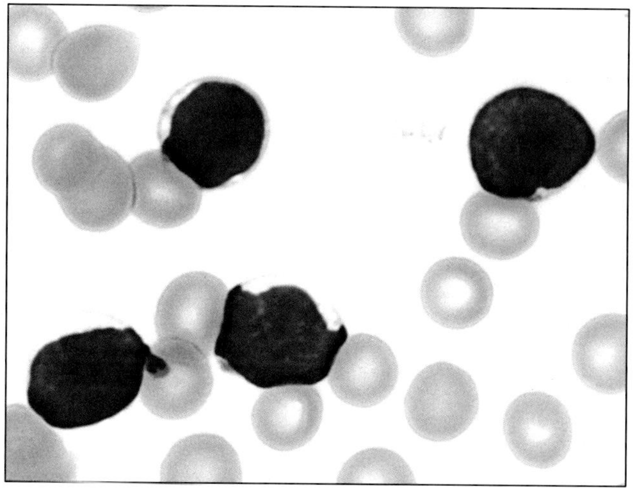

FIGURE 5-57
Chronic lymphocytic leukemia (CLL) involving normal-appearing small lymphocytes with scant cytoplasm in blood from a dog. Wright-Giemsa stain.

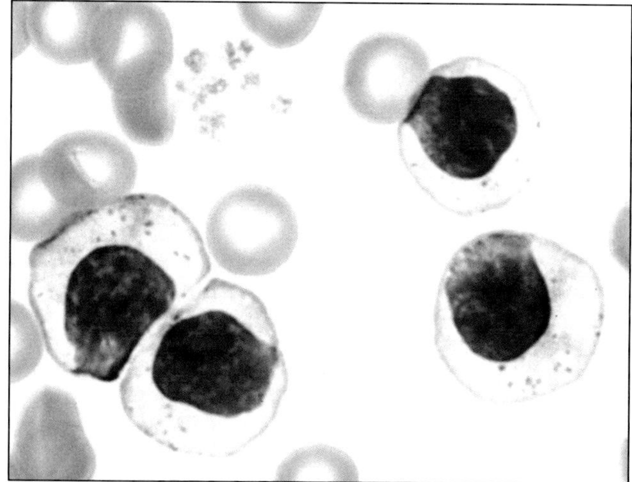

FIGURE 5-58
Chronic lymphocytic leukemia (CLL) involving granular lymphocytes with abundant cytoplasm in blood from a dog. Wright-Giemsa stain.

lymphocytes (Fig. 5-58).[474] CLL is much less common in cats than in dogs. Like dogs, most cats with CLL exhibit T lymphocytosis, but in contrast to dogs, the $CD4^+$ helper cells are the predominant type involved.[503]

Most cases of granular lymphocyte leukemia in dogs consist of mature-appearing lymphocytes and behave as a form of CLL, being indolent and slowly progressive. However, lymphocytes in some cases appear less well differentiated, with fine nuclear chromatin, and the disorder behaves more like acute lymphoblastic leukemia (ALL), being fulminant and rapidly fatal (Fig. 5-59).[474,494] A granular lymphocyte leukemia has also been reported in a horse.[258]

A lymphocytosis often occurs in animals with ALL. Most cases have increased numbers of circulating lymphoblasts of a

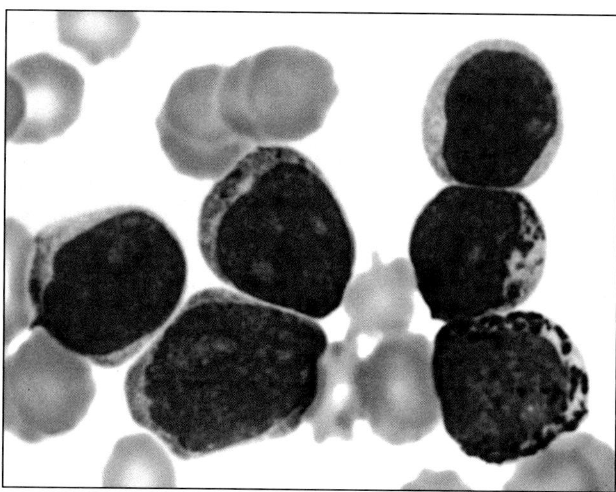

FIGURE 5-59
Acute lymphoblastic leukemia (ALL) involving granular lymphocytes in blood from a dog. Lymphoblasts with fine nuclear chromatin and nucleoli are present. Some of these cells contain cytoplasmic granules. Wright stain.

Photograph of a stained blood film from a 1989 ASVCP slide review case submitted by M. Wellman and G. Kociba.

single phenotype along with peripheral cytopenias. A lymphocytosis is occasionally present in animals with lymphomas. The morphology of the neoplastic lymphocytes in blood is generally reflective of the morphology of the lymphocytes in the solid tumors.[29]

Lymphopenia

Lymphopenia occurs in response to endogenous or exogenous glucocorticoids in animals.[1,93,235,424,505] This appears to result in part from the sequestration of lymphocytes in lymphoid organs, including bone marrow.[54,459] Glucocorticoids also potentiate apoptosis of sensitive lymphocytes.[14] The release of endogenous glucocorticoids in response to severe systemic disorders may play a major role in the production of the lymphopenia that often accompanies these disorders.[191] Lymphopenia occurs following the experimental injection of IL-1 and TNF and often accompanies severe systemic bacterial infections.[421,467,472] Lymphopenia also accompanies many viral infections in animals.[21,52,115,263,366] It appears to be induced primarily by type 1 IFNs (especially IFN-α) produced in response to viral infections and immune stimulation.[28,211,352,395] Transient lymphopenia that develops in response to type 1 IFNs may result from lymphocyte activation and binding to endothelium[234]; however, high concentrations of type 1 IFNs can result in lymphocyte apoptosis and lymphoid depletion.[395] Lymphopenia also occurs following the use of immunosuppressive drugs and irradiation, which result in lymphocyte destruction.[458]

Lymphocytes are present in afferent lymph from gastrointestinal and bronchial lymphoid tissues and efferent lymph from lymph nodes. The loss of lymphocyte-rich afferent lymph (e.g., lymphangiectasia) or efferent lymph (e.g., thoracic duct rupture) results in lymphopenia because most blood lymphocytes recirculate through lymphoid tissues. Lymphopenia can also occur when lymph node architecture is disrupted (e.g., multicentric lymphoma or generalized granulomatous inflammation), preventing the normal recirculation of lymphocytes.[226]

Lymphopenia occurs with inherited severe combined immunodeficiency (SCID) in horses and dogs.[374] Details concerning these disorders are given in Chapter 6.

BLAST CELLS OR POORLY DIFFERENTIATED CELLS

Blast cells in blood generally have single round nuclei with finely stippled or smooth chromatin containing one or more distinct or indistinct nucleoli. The N : C ratio is generally high, and the cytoplasm varies from lightly to darkly basophilic. Similarities in the appearance of different types of blast cells can make a specific diagnosis difficult or impossible based on routinely stained blood and bone marrow smears. Despite this problem, the morphologic appearance of the blast cells can be helpful in reaching a presumptive diagnosis. Blast cells may also be tentatively identified by the company they keep. Consequently the types of easily identifiable cells that are increased in blood may be helpful in reaching a diagnosis (e.g., increased monocytes in acute monocytic or acute myelomonocytic leukemias and increased nucleated erythrocytes in erythroleukemia). Specific diagnosis often requires special histochemical stains, immunophenotyping, and/or assays for clonal rearrangements of lymphocyte antigen receptor genes.[71,193,451,475,497]

Lymphoblasts

Lymphoblasts are larger than the normal small lymphocytes present in blood. The nucleus is generally round but may be indented or convoluted. The chromatin is usually finely stippled but may be coarsely granular. One or more nucleoli are present in the nucleus, but they are often difficult to see in routinely stained blood films (Fig. 5-60, *A*). The cytoplasm is more basophilic than is seen in most blood lymphocytes and sometimes contains vacuoles. Rare lymphoblasts may be observed in disorders with increased antigenic stimulation; but when several of these cells are found during a differential count, lymphoid neoplasia is suspected.

ALL originates from the bone marrow, and lymphoblasts are generally although not invariably present in blood from animals with ALL (Fig. 5-60, *A,B*; Fig. 5-61).[29,275,330,471] Lymphoblasts are also released into blood in some animals with lymphoma (Fig. 5-60, *C,D*; Figs. 5-62, 5-63).[91,226,324,388] When present in blood, this pattern is sometimes called leukemic lymphoma or lymphosarcoma cell leukemia. The morphology of the neoplastic lymphoid cells in blood from animals with lymphoma is quite variable. One or more morphologic features that may be present include exceptionally large size, abundant cytoplasm, monocytoid appearance (see Fig. 5-62), and heavily vacuolated cytoplasm, as shown from a dog diagnosed with intravascular lymphoma (Fig. 5-60, *E*). Cells present in leukemic lymphoma in cattle often appear monocytoid (Fig. 5-64).[91,471] Nuclei may be especially convoluted (cerebriform) in the blood of dogs and cats with T lymphocyte epitheliotropic cutaneous lymphoma.[299] When these neoplastic cells with convoluted nuclei are present in blood, they have been referred to as Sézary cells, and this rare variant of epitheliotropic cutaneous lymphoma with leukemia has been referred to as the Sézary syndrome.* Lymphoblasts may lyse during blood film preparation, making it difficult to characterize them morphologically (Fig. 5-65, *A,B*).

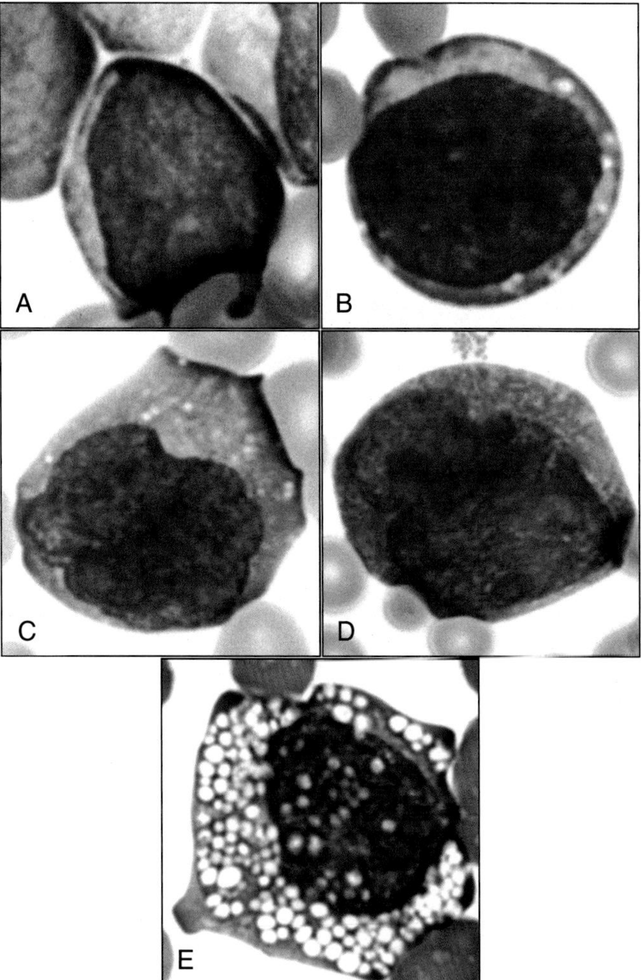

FIGURE 5-60

Lymphoblasts in blood. **A,** Lymphoblast in blood from a dog with acute lymphoblastic leukemia (ALL). Wright-Giemsa stain. **B,** Lymphoblast in blood from a cat with ALL. Wright-Giemsa stain. **C,** Large lymphoblast in blood from a dog with lymphoma. Wright-Giemsa stain. **D,** Large lymphoblast in blood from a cow with lymphoma. Wright-Giemsa stain. **E,** Large heavily vacuolated neoplastic cell in blood from a dog with intravascular lymphoma. The cell type is uncertain; however, it was considered most likely to be of NK cell origin. Aqueous Romanowsky stain.

E, Photograph of a stained blood film from a 2009 ASVCP slide review case submitted by L. V. Devai, R. W. Allison, T. R. Rizzi, A. W. Stern, T. A. Snider, and W. Vernau.

*References 149, 150, 333, 336, 409, 457, 502.

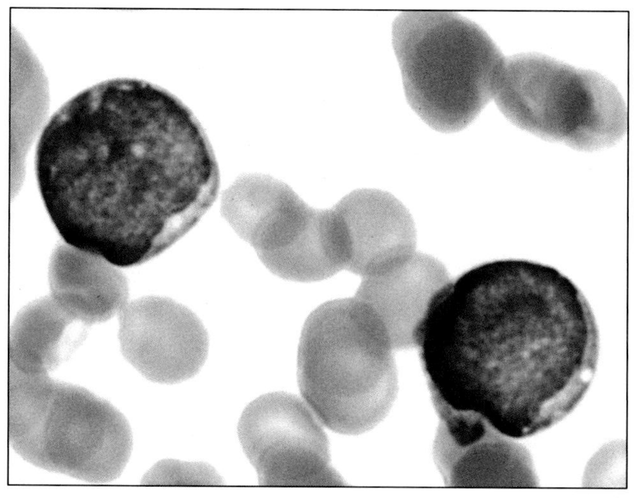

FIGURE 5-61
Lymphoblasts in blood from a dog with acute lymphoblastic leukemia (ALL). Wright-Giemsa stain.

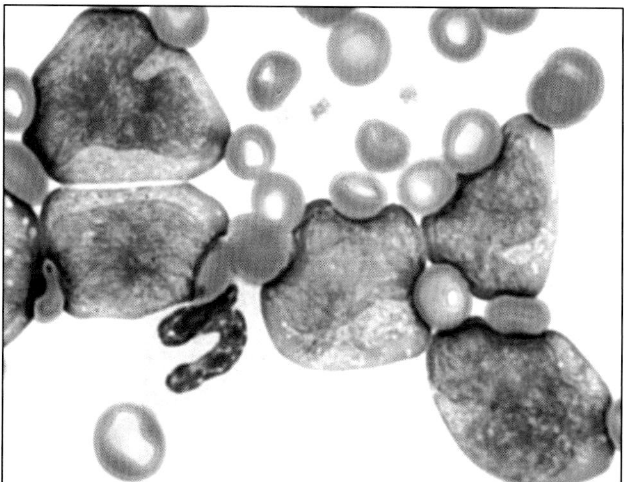

FIGURE 5-62
Pleomorphic lymphoblasts in blood from a dog with a T lymphocyte lymphoma. Wright-Giemsa stain.

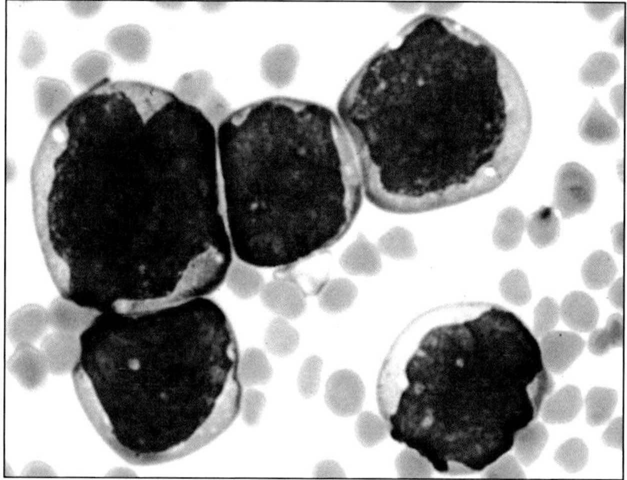

FIGURE 5-63
Lymphoblasts in blood from a goat with metastatic lymphoma. Wright-Giemsa stain.

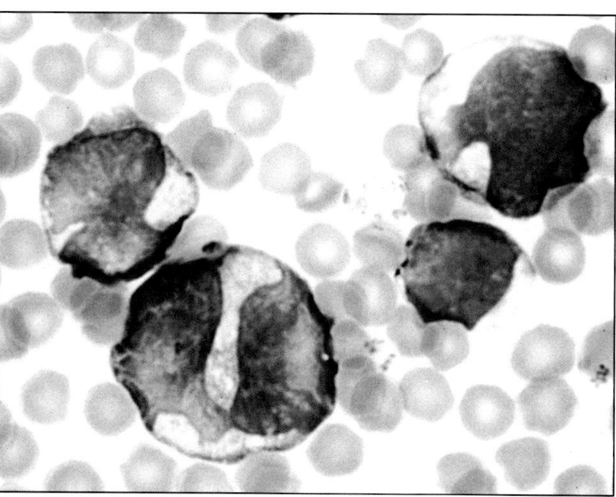

FIGURE 5-64
A small normal-appearing lymphocyte and three large monocytoid neoplastic lymphocytes in blood from a cow with metastatic lymphoma. Wright-Giemsa stain.

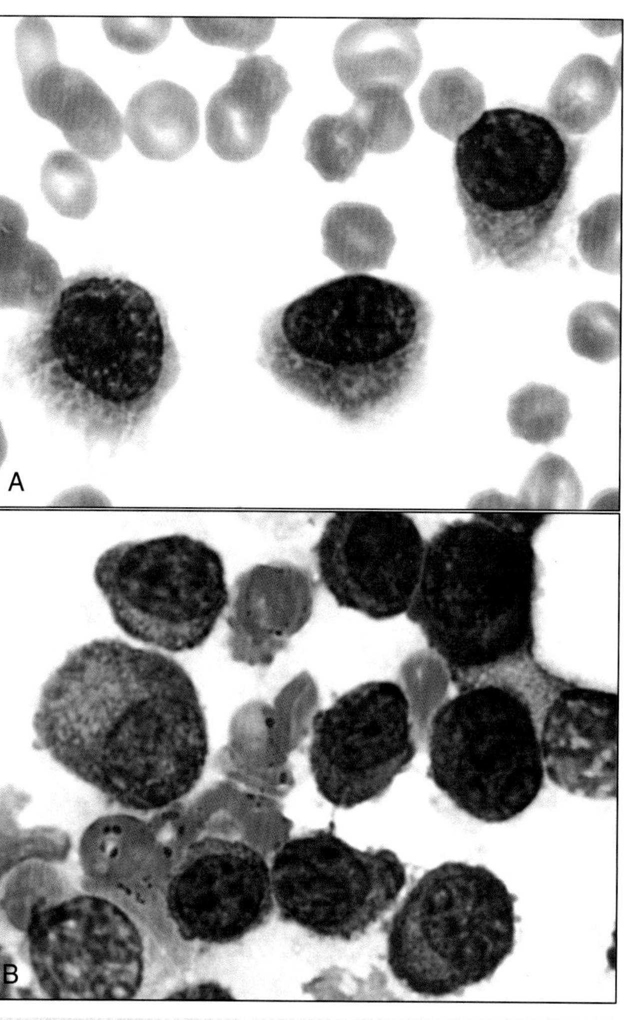

FIGURE 5-65
Plasmacytoid lymphoma in a dog. **A,** Blast cells in the blood tended to lyse, making morphologic identification difficult. **B,** Lymph node aspirate smear demonstrating the plasmacytoid appearance of the neoplastic cells. Wright-Giemsa stain.

FIGURE 5-66 **Nonlymphoid blast cells in blood**

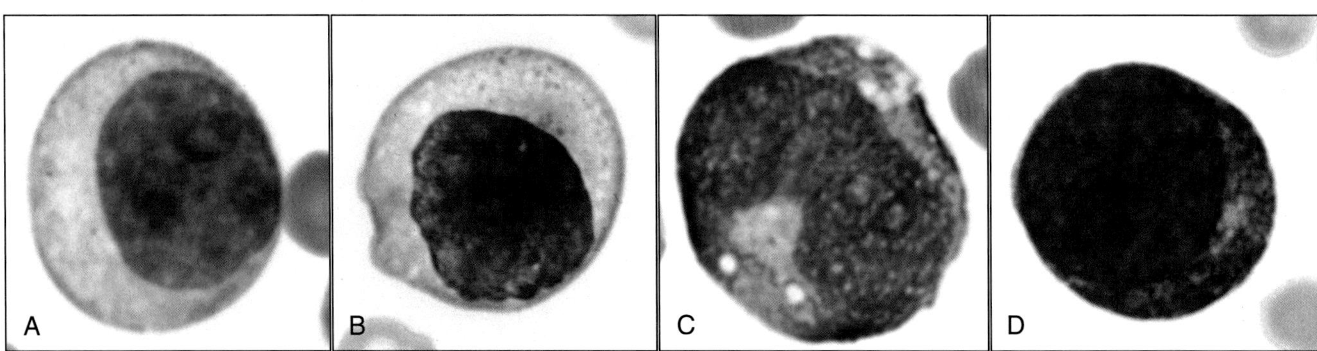

A, Myeloblast in blood from a cat with erythroleukemia (AML-M6). This neoplastic cell has a round nucleus and gray-blue cytoplasm. Two nucleoli are visible in the right side of the nucleus. Wright-Giemsa stain. **B,** Myeloblast in blood from a dog with myeloblastic leukemia (AML-M2). This cell may be classified as a type II myeloblast because it contains a few small magenta-staining granules in the gray-blue cytoplasm near the top of the cell. Wright-Giemsa stain. **C,** Monoblast in blood from a dog with acute myelomonocytic leukemia (AML-M4). The nucleus is more irregular than typically seen in myeloblasts. Wright-Giemsa stain. **D,** Rubriblast in blood from a cat with erythroleukemia (AML-M6Er). This neoplastic cell has a remarkably round nucleus with intensely basophilic cytoplasm. Wright-Giemsa stain.

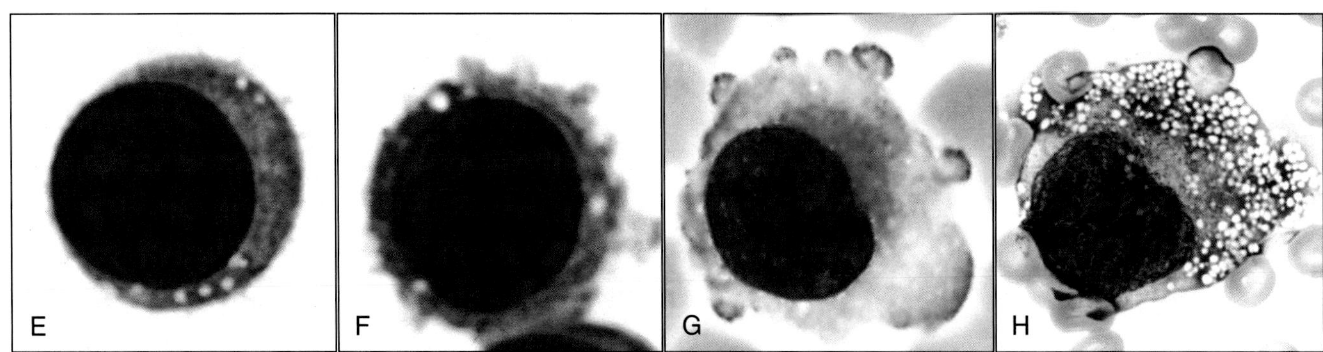

E, Megakaryoblast in blood from a dog with megakaryoblastic leukemia (AML-M7). The neoplastic cell has a remarkably round nucleus with cytoplasm that contains almost imperceptible pink granules and vacuoles. Wright-Giemsa stain. **F,** Megakaryoblast in blood from a dog with AML-M7. The neoplastic cell has a remarkably round nucleus with pinkish cytoplasm that contains vacuoles and has surface projections. Wright-Giemsa stain. **G,** Neoplastic dendritic cell in blood from a dog with dendritic cell leukemia. Wright stain. **H,** Giant nonhematopoietic neoplastic cell in blood from a dog with widespread metastasis. Although this tumor was highly anaplastic, a pancreatic carcinoma was considered the likely tumor type based on necropsy findings. Wright-Giemsa stain.

G, From Allison RW, Brunker JD, Breshears MA, et al. Dendritic cell leukemia in a golden retriever. Vet Clin Pathol. *2008;37:190-197.*

Myeloblasts

Type I myeloblasts appear as large round cells with round to oval nuclei that are generally centrally located in the cell. The N:C ratio is high (more than 1.5), and the nuclear outline is usually regular and smooth (Fig. 5-66, *A*). Nuclear chromatin is finely stippled, containing one or more nucleoli or nucleolar rings. The cytoplasm is generally moderately basophilic but not as dark as rubriblasts. Some myeloblasts may contain a few (less than 15) small magenta-staining granules in the cytoplasm and may be classified as type II myeloblasts (Fig. 5-66, *B*).[1] Myeloblasts with numerous magenta-staining granules are classified as type III myeloblasts.[194,227,471] Myeloblasts may be present in blood in low numbers in CML (Fig. 5-67). They are more often present in blood with various forms of AML, including myeloblastic leukemia (AML-M1 and AML-M2) (Fig. 5-68), acute myelomonocytic leukemia (AML-M4), and erythroleukemia (AML-M6) (Fig. 5-69).[194,227,316,471] Myeloblasts, promyelocytes, and myelocytes in blood all have round nuclei and resemble lymphoid cells, but cytochemical stains and/or recognition of surface markers can help differentiate these cell types in leukemic animals.[2,193]

Monoblasts

Monoblasts resemble myeloblasts except that their nuclear shape is irregularly round or convoluted in appearance (Fig. 5-66, *C*). A clear area in the cytoplasm, representing the Golgi

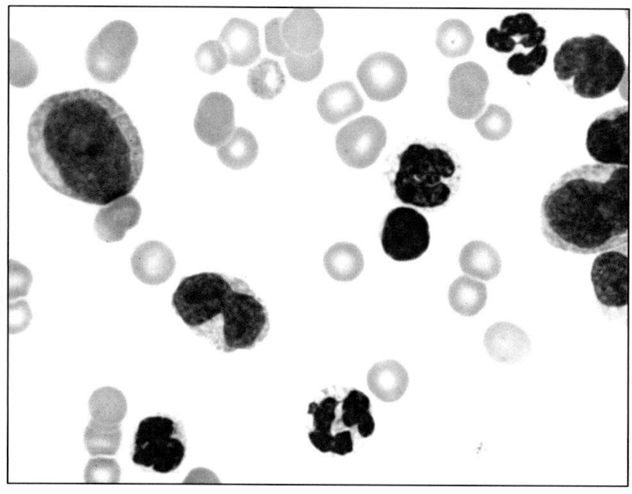

FIGURE 5-67
Blood from a cat with a presumptive diagnosis of chronic myeloid leukemia (CML) exhibiting marked neutrophilia with a prominent left shift. A bone marrow biopsy was not done to confirm the diagnosis. Rare myeloblasts *(top left)* were seen in the blood film. Wright-Giemsa stain.

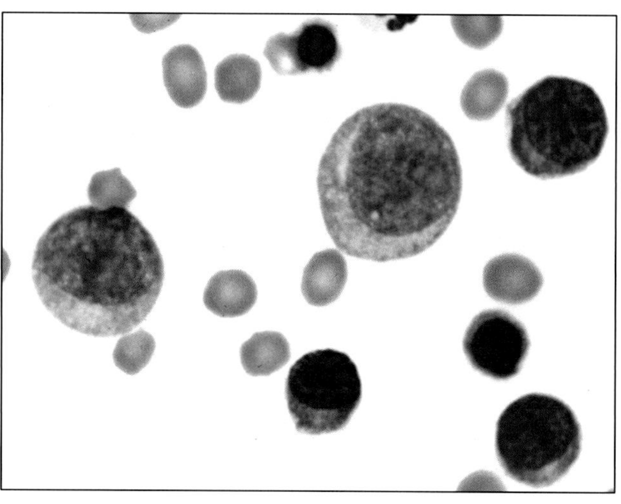

FIGURE 5-69
Blood from a cat with erythroleukemia (AML-M6). The two largest cells with pale-blue cytoplasm are myeloblasts. The smaller round cells are all erythroid precursors. Wright-Giemsa stain.

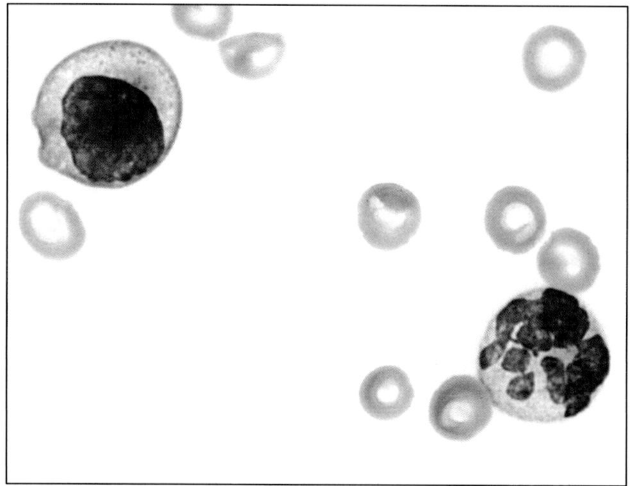

FIGURE 5-68
Type II myeloblast *(left)* and a hypersegmented neutrophil *(right)* in blood from a dog with myeloblastic leukemia (AML-M2). Wright-Giemsa stain.

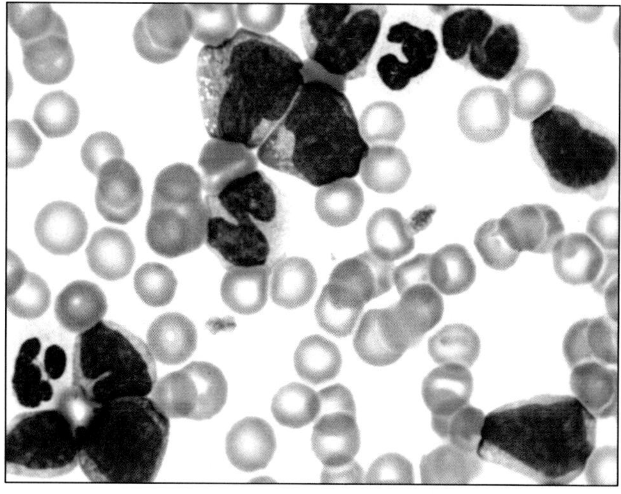

FIGURE 5-70
Blood from a dog with acute myelomonocytic leukemia (AML-M4). A mixture of neutrophils, monocytes, and precursors of both cell types are present. Wright-Giemsa stain.

zone, is often observed, especially near the site of nuclear indentation. The N:C ratio is high but may be somewhat lower than that in myeloblasts.[227] Monoblasts may be present in blood in animals with acute myelomonocytic leukemia (AML-M4) (Fig. 5-70) and acute monocytic leukemia (AML-M5) (Fig. 5-71).[194,225,316] Although rare, most horses reported with AML have had either AML-M4 or AML-M5.[313]

Rubriblasts

Rubriblasts have more basophilic cytoplasm than myeloblasts, monoblasts, and most lymphoblasts (Fig. 5-66, *D*). Although the other blasts mentioned have nuclei that are generally round in shape, the nucleus of a rubriblast is usually nearly perfectly round. The chromatin is generally finely granular, with one or more nucleoli. Rubriblasts are not usually seen in the blood of animals with regenerative anemia. They may be present in variable numbers in the blood of animals with erythroleukemia (AML-M6 or AML-M6Er) (Figs. 5-69, 5-72).[194,316,471]

Megakaryoblasts

Megakaryoblasts occur in the blood of animals with megakaryoblastic leukemia (AML-M7). Nuclei of megakaryoblasts are nearly as round as rubriblast nuclei, but their cytoplasm is typically less basophilic and may contain magenta-staining granules (see Fig. 5-66, *E,F*). Unique features present in some

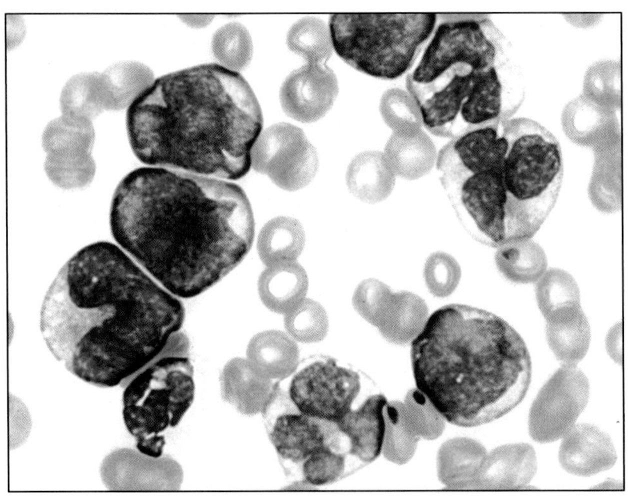

FIGURE 5-71
Blood from a dog with acute monocytic leukemia (AML-M5). All cells present, except a neutrophil *(bottom left)* are monocyte precursors or mature monocytes. Wright-Giemsa stain.

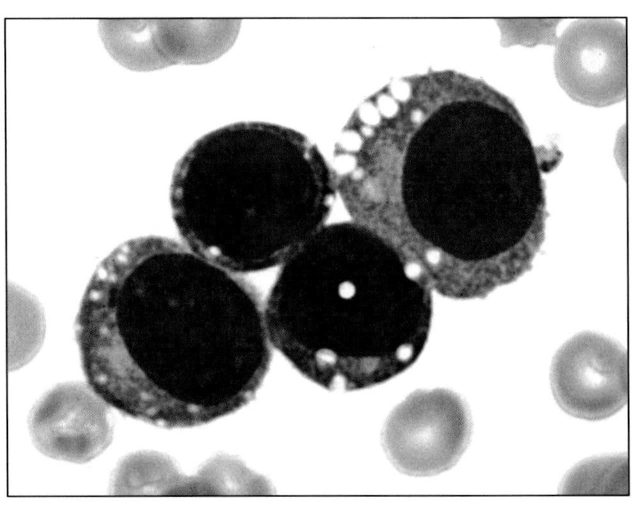

FIGURE 5-73
Blood from a dog with megakaryoblastic leukemia (AML-M7). Four neoplastic megakaryoblasts with prominent cytoplasmic vacuoles are present. Wright-Giemsa stain.

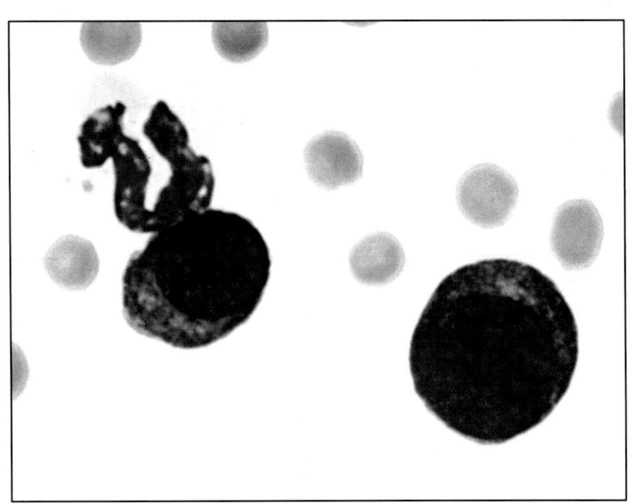

FIGURE 5-72
Blood from a cat with erythroleukemia (AML-M6Er). A neutrophil and two rubriblasts with basophilic cytoplasm are present. Wright-Giemsa stain.

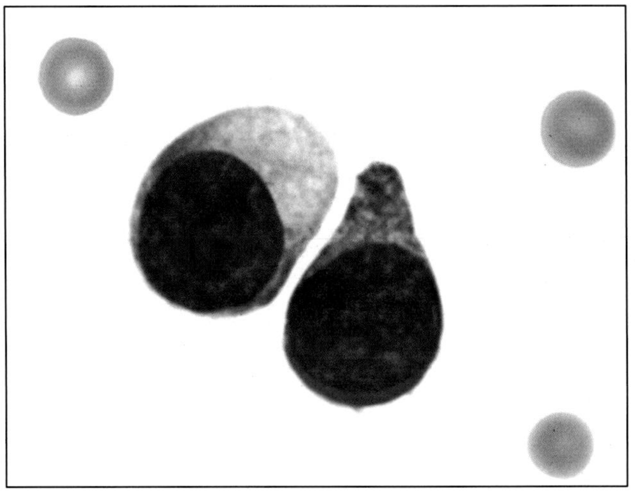

FIGURE 5-74
Blood from a cat with acute unclassified leukemia (AUL). Two unclassified neoplastic cells are present. Wright-Giemsa stain.

of these cells include multiple discrete vacuoles (Fig. 5-73) and cytoplasmic projections (see Fig. 5-66, *F*).[13,327,446,471]

Neoplastic Dendritic Cells

Dendritic cell leukemia has been described in a dog (see Fig. 5-66, *G*).[8] The neoplastic dendritic cells in this case were larger than neutrophils; they had round to oval nuclei with coarsely stippled to granular chromatin. Indistinct nucleoli were visible in some cells. The cytoplasm was blue, moderately abundant, and sometimes contained vacuoles. Cytoplasmic borders were often ruffled and indistinct.[8]

Unclassified Blast Cells

Primitive cells that cannot be classified with certainty are listed as unclassified during differential cell counts. When unclassified cells predominate in bone marrow (and sometimes blood), a diagnosis of acute unclassified leukemia (AUL) is made (Fig. 5-74).[227]

Metastatic Blast Cells

Although metastasis of tumors from nonhematopoietic organs is common, these neoplastic cells are rarely recognized in blood (except for malignant mast cells). When present, these blast cells are typically much larger than hematopoietic blast cells (see Fig. 5-66, *H*).

REFERENCES

1. Abraham G, Allersmeier M, Gottschalk J, et al. Effects of dermal dexamethasone application on ACTH and both basal and ACTH-stimulated cortisol concentration in normal horses. *J Vet Pharmacol Ther.* 2009;32:379-387.
2. Adam F, Villiers E, Watson S, et al. Clinical pathological and epidemiological assessment of morphologically and immunologically confirmed canine leukaemia. *Vet Comp Oncol.* 2009;7:181-195.
3. Allan FJ, Thompson KG, Jones BR, et al. Neutropenia with a probable hereditary basis in Border Collies. *N Z Vet J.* 1996;44:67-72.
4. Allan GS, Watson AD, Duff BC, et al. Disseminated mastocytoma and mastocytemia in a dog. *J Am Vet Med Assoc.* 1974;165:346-349.
5. Alleman AR, Wamsley HL: An update on anaplasmosis in dogs. *Vet Med.* 2008;103:212-220.
6. Allen KE, Li Y, Kaltenboeck B, et al. Diversity of *Hepatozoon* species in naturally infected dogs in the southern United States. *Vet Parasitol.* 2008;154:220-225.
7. Allison R, Williams P, Lansdowne J, et al. Fatal hepatic sarcocystosis in a puppy with eosinophilia and eosinophilic peritoneal effusion. *Vet Clin Pathol.* 2006;35:353-357.
8. Allison RW, Brunker JD, Breshears MA, et al. Dendritic cell leukemia in a golden retriever. *Vet Clin Pathol.* 2008;37:190-197.
9. Allison RW, Fielder SE, Meinkoth JH. What is your diagnosis? Blood film from an icteric cat. *Vet Clin Pathol.* 2010;39:125-126.
10. Allison RW, Velguth KE. Appearance of granulated cells in blood films stained by automated aqueous versus methanolic Romanowsky methods. *Vet Clin Pathol.* 2010;39:99-104.
11. Alroy J, Freden GO, Goyal V, et al. Morphology of leukocytes from cats affected with α-mannosidosis and mucopolysaccharidosis VI (MPS VI). *Vet Pathol.* 1989;26:294-302.
12. Alroy J, Orgad U, Ucci AA, et al. Neurovisceral and skeletal GM1-gangliosidosis in dogs with beta-galactosidase deficiency. *Science.* 1985;229:470-472.
13. Ameri M, Wilkerson MJ, Stockham SL, et al. Acute megakaryoblastic leukemia in a German Shepherd dog. *Vet Clin Pathol.* 2010;39:39-45.
14. Ammersbach MA, Kruth SA, Sears W, et al. The effect of glucocorticoids on canine lymphocyte marker expression and apoptosis. *J Vet Intern Med.* 2006;20:1166-1171.
15. Anane LH, Edwards KM, Burns VE, et al. Mobilization of gamma delta T lymphocytes in response to psychological stress, exercise, and beta-agonist infusion. *Brain Behav Immun.* 2009;23:823-829.
16. Anderson BH, Watson DL, Colditz IG. The effect of dexamethasone on some immunological parameters in cattle. *Vet Res Commun.* 1999;23:399-413.
17. Anderson DE, Constable PD, St Jean G, et al. Small-intestinal volvulus in cattle: 35 cases (1967-1992). *J Am Vet Med Assoc.* 1993;203:1178-1183.
18. Andreasen CB, Roth JA. Neutrophil functional defects. In: Feldman BF, Zinkl JG, Jain NC, eds. *Schalm's Veterinary Hematology.* 5th ed. Philadelphia: Lippincott Williams & Wilkins; 2000:356-365.
19. Andrews RG, Briddell RA, Appelbaum FR, et al. Stimulation of hematopoiesis in vivo by stem cell factor. *Curr Opin Hematol.* 1994;1:187-196.
20. Antognoni MT, Spaterna A, Lepri E, et al. Characteristic clinical, haematological and histopathological findings in feline mastocytoma. *Vet Res Commun.* 2003;27(Suppl 1):727-730.
21. Arjona A, Escolar E, Soto I, et al. Seroepidemiological survey of infection by feline leukemia virus and immunodeficiency virus in Madrid and correlation with some clinical aspects. *J Clin Microbiol.* 2000;38:3448-3449.
22. Aroch I, Klement E, Segev G. Clinical, biochemical, and hematological characteristics, disease prevalence, and prognosis of dogs presenting with neutrophil cytoplasmic toxicity. *J Vet Intern Med.* 2005;19:64-73.
23. Aroch I, Ofri R, Aizenberg I. Haematological, ocular and skeletal abnormalities in a Samoyed family. *J Small Anim Pract.* 1996;37:333-339.
24. Aroch I, Perl S, Markovics A. Disseminated eosinophilic disease resembling idiopathic hypereosinophilic syndrome in a dog. *Vet Rec.* 2001;149:386-389.
25. Atkins CE, DeFrancesco TC, Coats JR, et al. Heartworm infection in cats: 50 cases (1985-1997). *J Am Vet Med Assoc.* 2000;217:355-358.
26. Atkins CE, DeFrancesco TC, Miller MW, et al. Prevalence of heartworm infection in cats with signs of cardiorespiratory abnormalities. *J Am Vet Med Assoc.* 1998;212:517-520.
27. Auffray C, Sieweke MH, Geissmann F. Blood monocytes: development, heterogeneity, and relationship with dendritic cells. *Annu Rev Immunol.* 2009;27:669-692.
28. Aulitzky WE, Tilg H, Vogel W, et al. Acute hematologic effects of interferon alpha, interferon gamma, tumor necrosis factor alpha and interleukin 2. *Ann Hematol.* 1991;62:25-31.
29. Avery AC, Avery PR. Determining the significance of persistent lymphocytosis. *Vet Clin North Am Small Anim Pract.* 2007;37:267-282, vi.
30. Ayers JR, Leipold HW, Padgett GA. Lesions in Brangus cattle with Chediak-Higashi syndrome. *Vet Pathol.* 1988;25:432-436.
31. Bain BJ. Relationship between idiopathic hypereosinophilic syndrome, eosinophilic leukemia, and systemic mastocytosis. *Am J Hematol.* 2004;77:82-85.
32. Bain PJ, Alleman AR, Sheppard BJ, et al. What is your diagnosis? An 18-month-old spayed female boxer dog. *Vet Clin Pathol.* 1997;26:55.
33. Baird SM. Morphology of lymphocytes and plasma cells. In: Lichtman MA, Beutler E, Kipps TJ, et al, eds. *Williams Hematology.* 7th ed. New York: McGraw-Hill; 2006:1023-1030.
34. Baneth G. Feline hepatozoonosis. In: Greene CE, ed. *Infectious Diseases of the Dog and Cat.* 3rd ed. Philadelphia: Saunders Elsevier; 2006:705.
35. Baneth G, Aroch I, Tal N, et al. *Hepatozoon* species infection in domestic cats: a retrospective study. *Vet Parasitol.* 1998;79:123-133.
36. Barlough JE, Madigan JE, Turoff DR, et al. An *Ehrlichia* strain from a llama (*Lama glama*) and llama-associated ticks (*Ixodes pacificus*). *J Clin Microbiol.* 1997;35:1005-1007.
37. Barr SC, Gossett KA, Klei TR. Clinical, clinicopathologic, and parasitologic observations of trypanosomiasis in dogs infected with North American *Trypanosoma cruzi* isolates. *Am J Vet Res.* 1991;52:954-960.
38. Barrs VR, Beatty JA, McCandlish IA, et al. Hypereosinophilic paraneoplastic syndrome in a cat with intestinal T cell lymphosarcoma. *J Small Anim Pract.* 2002;43:401-405.
39. Barton AD. T-cell lymphocytosis associated with lymphocyte-rich thymoma. *Cancer.* 1997;80:1409-1417.
40. Batista FD, Harwood NE. The who, how and where of antigen presentation to B cells. *Nat Rev Immunol.* 2009;9:15-27.
41. Beale KM, Altman D, Clemmons RR, et al. Systemic toxicosis associated with azathioprine administration in domestic cats. *Am J Vet Res.* 1992;53:1236-1240.
42. Bell SA, Drew CP, Wilson WD, et al. Idiopathic chronic eosinophilic pneumonia in 7 horses. *J Vet Intern Med.* 2008;22:648-653.
43. Benschop RJ, Rodriguez-Feuerhahn M, Schedlowski M. Catecholamine-induced leukocytosis: early observations, current research, and future directions. *Brain Behav Immun.* 1996;10:77-91.
44. Berger J. The segmentation of nuclei in circulating neutrophils of laboratory rats. *Folia Haematol Int Mag Klin Morphol Blutforsch.* 1982;109:602-607.
45. Bernard SL, Leathers CW, Brobst DF, et al. Estrogen-induced bone marrow depression in ferrets. *Am J Vet Res.* 1983;44:657-661.
46. Berryessa NA, Marks SL, Pesavento PA, et al. Gastrointestinal pythiosis in 10 dogs from California. *J Vet Intern Med.* 2008;22:1065-1069.
47. Bessis M. *Living Blood Cells and Their Ultrastructure.* New York: Springer-Verlag; 1973.
48. Bienzle D. Monocytes and macrophages. In: Feldman BF, Zinkl JG, Jain NC, eds. *Schalm's Veterinary Hematology.* 5th ed. Philadelphia: Lippincott Williams & Wilkins; 2000:318-325.
49. Biermann H, Pietz B, Dreier R, et al. Murine leukocytes with ring-shaped nuclei include granulocytes, monocytes, and their precursors. *J Leukoc Biol.* 1999;65:217-231.
50. Bimczok D, Rothkotter HJ. Lymphocyte migration studies. *Vet Res.* 2006;37:325-338.
51. Binns RM, Whyte A, Licence ST. Constitutive and inflammatory lymphocyte trafficking. *Vet Immunol Immunopathol.* 1996;54:97-104.
52. Blanchard PC, Ridpath JF, Walker JB, et al. An outbreak of late-term abortions, premature births, and congenital deformities associated with a bovine viral diarrhea virus 1 subtype b that induces thrombocytopenia. *J Vet Diagn Invest.* 2010;22:128-131.
53. Blischok D, Bender H. What is your diagnosis? 15-year-old male domestic shorthair cat [disseminated histoplasmosis]. *Vet Clin Pathol.* 1996;25:113, 152.
54. Bloemena E, Weinreich S, Schellekens PTA. The influence of prednisolone on the recirculation of peripheral blood lymphocytes in vivo. *Clin Exp Immunol.* 1990;80:460-466.
55. Blue JT. Myelodysplasia: differentiating neoplastic from nonneoplastic syndromes of ineffective hematopoiesis in dogs. *Toxicol Pathol.* 2003;31(Suppl):44-48.
56. Bohn G, Welte K, Klein C. Severe congenital neutropenia: new genes explain an old disease. *Curr Opin Rheumatol.* 2007;19:644-650.
57. Bookbinder PF, Butt MT, Harvey HJ. Determination of the number of mast cells in lymph node, bone marrow, and buffy coat cytologic specimens from dogs. *J Am Vet Med Assoc.* 1992;200:1648-1650.
58. Borregaard N, Beutler E. Disorders of neutrophil function. In: Lichtman MA, Beutler E, Kipps TJ, et al, eds. *Williams Hematology.* 7th ed. New York: McGraw-Hill; 2006:921-957.

59. Bortnowski HB, Rosenthal RC. Gastrointestinal mast cell tumors and eosinophilia in two cats. *J Am Anim Hosp Assoc.* 1992;28:271-275.
60. Boudreaux MK, Wardrop KJ, Kiklevich V, et al. A mutation in the canine Kindlin-3 gene associated with increased bleeding risk and susceptibility to infections. *Thromb Haemost.* 2010;103:475-477.
61. Bowman DD, Frongillo MK, Johnson RC, et al. Evaluation of praziquantel for treatment of experimentally induced paragonimiasis in dogs and cats. *Am J Vet Res.* 1991;52:68-71.
62. Brain JD, Molina RM, DeCamp MM, et al. Pulmonary intravascular macrophages: their contribution to the mononuclear phagocyte system in 13 species. *Am J Physiol.* 1999;276:L146-L154.
63. Breitschwerdt EB. Feline bartonellosis and cat scratch disease. *Vet Immunol Immunopathol.* 2008;123:167-171.
64. Breitschwerdt EB, Brown TT, De Buysscher EV, et al. Rhinitis, pneumonia, and defective neutrophil function in the doberman pinscher. *Am J Vet Res.* 1987;48:1054-1062.
65. Brenner I, Shek PN, Zamecnik J, et al. Stress hormones and the immunological responses to heat and exercise. *Int J Sports Med.* 1998;19:130-143.
66. Brewer BD, Harvey JW, Mayhew IG, et al. Ehrlichiosis in a Florida horse. *J Am Vet Med Assoc.* 1984;185:446-447.
67. Brock KV, Jones JB, Shull RM, et al. Effect of canine parvovirus on erythroid progenitors in phenylhydrazine-induced regenerative hemolytic anemia in dogs. *Am J Vet Res.* 1989;50:965-969.
68. Brown DE, Thrall MA, Walkley SU, et al. Feline Niemann-Pick disease type C. *Am J Pathol.* 1994;144:1412-1415.
69. Brown MR, Rogers KS. Neutropenia in dogs and cats: a retrospective study of 261 cases. *J Am Anim Hosp Assoc.* 2001;37:131-139.
70. Bunch SE, Easley JR, Cullen JM. Hematologic values and plasma and tissue folate concentrations in dogs given phenytoin on a long-term basis. *Am J Vet Res.* 1990;51:1865-1868.
71. Burnett RC, Vernau W, Modiano JF, et al. Diagnosis of canine lymphoid neoplasia using clonal rearrangements of antigen receptor genes. *Vet Pathol.* 2003;40:32-41.
72. Calvert CA, Mahaffey MB, Lappin MR, et al. Pulmonary and disseminated eosinophilic granulomatosis in dogs. *J Am Anim Hosp Assoc.* 1988;24:311-320.
73. Campbell LJ, Maher DW, Tay DL, et al. Marrow proliferation and the appearance of giant neutrophils in response to recombinant human granulocyte colony stimulating factor (rhG-CSF). *Br J Haematol.* 1992;80:298-304.
74. Campbell TW, Ellis CK. *Avian and Exotic Animal Hematology and Cytology.* 3rd ed. Ames, IA: Blackwell Publishing; 2007.
75. Carakostas MC, Moore WE, Smith JE. Intravascular neutrophilic granulocyte kinetics in horses. *Am J Vet Res.* 1981;42:623-625.
76. Caramori G, Adcock I. Anti-inflammatory mechanisms of glucocorticoids targeting granulocytes. *Curr Drug Targets Inflamm Allergy.* 2005;4:455-463.
77. Carlson GP, Kaneko JJ. Influence of prednisolone on intravascular granulocyte kinetics of calves under nonsteady state conditions. *Am J Vet Res.* 1976;37:149-151.
78. Caro-Vadillo A, Martinez-Merlo E, Garcia-Real I, et al. Verminous pneumonia due to *Filaroides hirthi* in a Scottish terrier in Spain. *Vet Rec.* 2005;157:586-589.
79. Carrade DD, Foley JE, Borjesson DL, et al. Canine granulocytic anaplasmosis: a review. *J Vet Intern Med.* 2009;23:1129-1141.
80. Cayatte SM, McManus PM, Miller WHJ, et al. Identification of mast cells in buffy coat preparations from dogs with inflammatory skin diseases. *J Am Vet Med Assoc.* 1995;206:325-326.
81. Cello RM, Moulton JE, McFarland S. The occurrence of inclusion bodies in the circulating neutrophils of dogs with canine distemper. *Cornell Vet.* 1959;49:127-146.
82. Center SA, Randolph JF, Erb HN, et al. Eosinophilia in the cat: a retrospective study of 312 cases (1975 to 1986). *J Am Anim Hosp Assoc.* 1990;26:349-358.
83. Chatta GS, Price TH, Stratton JR, et al. Aging and marrow neutrophil reserves. *J Am Geriatr Soc.* 1994;42:77-81.
84. Chirico G, Gasparoni A, Ciardelli L, et al. Leukocyte counts in relation to the method of delivery during the first five days of life. *Biol Neonate.* 1999;75:294-299.
85. Chuammitri P, Ostojic J, Andreasen CB, et al. Chicken heterophil extracellular traps (HETs): novel defense mechanism of chicken heterophils. *Vet Immunol Immunopathol.* 2009;129:126-131.
86. Chusid MJ, Bujak JS, Dale DC. Defective polymorphonuclear leukocyte metabolism and function in canine cyclic neutropenia. *Blood.* 1975;46:921-930.
87. Clercx C, Peeters D, Snaps F, et al. Eosinophilic bronchopneumopathy in dogs. *J Vet Intern Med.* 2000;14:282-291.
88. Clinkenbeard KD, Cowell RL, Tyler RD. Disseminated histoplasmosis in cats: 12 cases (1981-1986). *J Am Vet Med Assoc.* 1987;190:1445-1448.
89. Clinkenbeard KD, Cowell RL, Tyler RD. Identification of *Histoplasma* organisms in circulating eosinophils of a dog. *J Am Vet Med Assoc.* 1988;192:217-218.
90. Clinkenbeard KD, Wolf AM, Cowell RL, et al. Feline disseminated histoplasmosis. *J Am Anim Hosp Assoc.* 1989;11:1223-1233.
91. Cockerell GL, Reyes RA. Bovine leukemia virus-associated lymphoproliferative disorders. In: Feldman BF, Zinkl JG, Jain NC, eds. *Schalm's Veterinary Hematology.* 5th ed. Philadelphia: Lippincott Williams & Wilkins; 2000.
92. Codner EC, Farris Smith LL. Characterization of the subclinical phase of ehrlichiosis in dogs. *J Am Vet Med Assoc.* 1986;189:47-50.
93. Collins MT, Suarez-Guemes F. Effect of hydrocortisone on circulating lymphocyte numbers and their mitogen-induced blastogenesis in lambs. *Am J Vet Res.* 1985;46:836-840.
94. Corcoran BM, Foster DJ, Fuentes VL. Feline asthma syndrome: a retrospective study of the clinical presentation in 29 cats. *J Small Anim Pract.* 1995;36:481-488.
95. Cornbleet PJ. Clinical utility of the band count. *Clin Lab Med.* 2002;22:101-136.
96. Corthay A. How do regulatory T cells work? *Scand J Immunol.* 2009;70:326-336.
97. Couto CG, Krakowka S, Johnson G, et al. In vitro immunologic features of Weimaraner dogs with neutrophil abnormalities and recurrent infections. *Vet Immunol Immunopathol.* 1989;23:103-112.
98. Cowell KR, Jezyk PF, Haskins ME, et al. Mucopolysaccharidosis in a cat. *J Am Vet Med Assoc.* 1976;169:334-339.
99. Cowell RL, Decker LS. Interpretation of feline leukocyte responses. In: Feldman BF, Zinkl JG, Jain NC, eds. *Schalm's Veterinary Hematology.* 5th ed. Philadelphia: Lippincott Williams & Wilkins; 2000:382-390.
100. Cowgill E, Neel J. Pleural fluid from a dog with marked eosinophilia. *Vet Clin Pathol.* 2003;32:147-149.
101. Cowles BE, Meyers KM, Wardrop KJ, et al. Prolonged bleeding time of Chediak-Higashi cats corrected by platelet transfusion. *Thromb Haemost.* 1992;67:708-712.
102. Crampton SP, Voynova E, Bolland S. Innate pathways to B-cell activation and tolerance. *Ann N Y Acad Sci.* 2010;1183:58-68.
103. Criado-Fornelio A, Buling A, Pingret JL, et al. Hemoprotozoa of domestic animals in France: prevalence and molecular characterization. *Vet Parasitol.* 2009;159:73-76.
104. Criado-Fornelio A, Ruas JL, Casado N, et al. New molecular data on mammalian *Hepatozoon* species (Apicomplexa: Adeleorina) from Brazil and Spain. *J Parasitol.* 2006;92:93-99.
105. Cunningham JM, Patnaik MM, Hammerschmidt DE, et al. Historical perspective and clinical implications of the Pelger-Huët cell. *Am J Hematol.* 2009;84:116-119.
106. Dale DC, Boxer L, Liles WC. The phagocytes: neutrophils and monocytes. *Blood.* 2008;112:935-945.
107. Darbès J, Majzoub M, Breuer W, et al. Large granular lymphocytic leukemia/lymphoma in six cats. *Vet Pathol.* 1998;35:370-379.
108. Darrah PA, Hondalus MK, Chen Q, et al. Cooperation between reactive oxygen and nitrogen intermediates in killing of *Rhodococcus equi* by activated macrophages. *Infect Immun.* 2000;68:3587-3593.
109. Dascanio JJ, Zhang CH, Antczak DF, et al. Differentiation of chronic lymphocytic leukemia in the horse. A report of two cases. *J Vet Intern Med.* 1992;6:225-229.
110. Davies AP, Hayden DW, Klausner JS, et al. Noncutaneous systemic mastocytosis and mast cell leukemia in a dog: case report and literature review. *J Am Anim Hosp Assoc.* 1981;17:361-368.
111. Davis JM, Albert JD, Tracy KJ, et al. Increased neutrophil mobilization and decreased chemotaxis during cortisol and epinephrine infusions. *J Trauma.* 1991;31:725-731.
112. Dawson JE, Abeygunawardena I, Holland CJ, et al. Susceptibility of cats to infection with *Ehrlichia risticii*, causative agent of equine monocytic ehrlichiosis. *Am J Vet Res.* 1988;49:2096-2100.
113. Dawson JE, Ewing SA. Susceptibility of dogs to infection with *Ehrlichia chaffeensis*, causative agent of human ehrlichiosis. *Am J Vet Res.* 1992;53:1322-1327.
114. Debacq C, Asquith B, Kerkhofs P, et al. Increased cell proliferation, but not reduced cell death, induces lymphocytosis in bovine leukemia virus-infected sheep. *Proc Natl Acad Sci USA.* 2002;99:10048-10053.
115. Decaro N, Campolo M, Lorusso A, et al. Experimental infection of dogs with a novel strain of canine coronavirus causing systemic disease and lymphopenia. *Vet Microbiol.* 2008;128:253-260.
116. Deubelbeiss KA, Dancey JT, Harker LA, et al. Neutrophil kinetics in the dog. *J Clin Invest.* 1975;55:833-839.
117. Di Santo JP. Natural killer cells: diversity in search of a niche. *Nat Immunol.* 2008;9:473-475.
118. Dial SM, Mitchell TW, LeCouteur RA, et al. GM_1-gangliosidosis (Type II) in three cats. *J Am Anim Hosp Assoc.* 1994;30:355-359.
119. Dieringer TM, Brown SA, Rogers KS, et al. Effects of lithium carbonate administration to healthy cats. *Am J Vet Res.* 1992;53:721-726.
120. Dillon AR, Brawner AR Jr, Robertson-Plouch CK, et al. Feline heartworm disease: correlations of clinical signs, serology, and other diagnostics–results of a multicenter study. *Vet Ther.* 2000;1:176-182.
121. Doerschuk CM, Downey GP, Doherty DE, et al. Leukocyte and platelet margination within microvasculature of rabbit lungs. *J Appl Physiol.* 1990;68:1956-1961.
122. Douglass TG, Driggers L, Zhang JG, et al. Macrophage colony stimulating factor: not just for macrophages anymore! A gateway into complex biologies. *Int Immunopharmacol.* 2008;8:1354-1376.

123. Duckett WM, Matthews HK. Hypereosinophilia in a horse with intestinal lymphosarcoma. *Can Vet J.* 1997;38:719-720.
124. Dumler JS, Barbet AF, Bekker CP, et al. Reorganization of genera in the families Rickettsiaceae and Anaplasmataceae in the order Rickettsiales: unification of some species of *Ehrlichia* with *Anaplasma, Cowdria* with *Ehrlichia* and *Ehrlichia* with *Neorickettsia*, descriptions of six new species combinations and designation of *Ehrlichia equi* and "HGE agent" as subjective synonyms of *Ehrlichia phagocytophila. Int J Syst Evol Microbiol.* 2001;51:2145-2165.
125. Dunn JK, Heath MF, Jefferies AR, et al. Diagnosis and hematologic features of probable essential thrombocythemia in two dogs. *Vet Clin Pathol.* 1999;28:131-138.
126. Dutta SK, Penney BE, Myrup AC, et al. Disease features in horses with induced equine monocytic ehrlichiosis (Potomac horse fever). *Am J Vet Res.* 1988;49:1747-1751.
127. Dykstra MJ, Sharp NJ, Olivry T, et al. A description of cutaneous-subcutaneous pythiosis in fifteen dogs. *Med Mycol.* 1999;37:427-433.
128. East LM, Savage CJ, Traub-Dargatz JL, et al. Enterocolitis associated with *Clostridium perfringens* infection in neonatal foals: 54 cases (1988-1997). *J Am Vet Med Assoc.* 1998;212:1751-1756.
129. Edwards DF, Parker JW, Wilkinson JE, et al. Plasma cell myeloma in the horse. A case report and literature review. *J Vet Intern Med.* 1993;7:169-176.
130. Egenvall A, Bjoersdorff A, Lilliehook I, et al. Early manifestations of granulocytic ehrlichiosis in dogs inoculated experimentally with a Swedish *Ehrlichia* species isolate. *Vet Rec.* 1998;143:412-417.
131. Eichacker P, Lawrence C. Steroid-induced hypersegmentation in neutrophils. *Am J Hematol.* 1985;18:41-45.
132. Ellis GS, Carlson DE, Hester L, et al. G-CSF, but not corticosterone, mediates circulating neutrophilia induced by febrile-range hyperthermia. *J Appl Physiol.* 2005;98:1799-1804.
133. Elsas PX, Neto HA, Cheraim AB, et al. Induction of bone-marrow eosinophilia in mice submitted to surgery is dependent on stress-induced secretion of glucocorticoids. *Br J Pharmacol.* 2004;143:541-548.
134. Endicott MM, Charney SC, McKnight JA, et al. Clinicopathological findings and results of bone marrow aspiration in dogs with cutaneous mast cell tumours: 157 cases (1999-2002). *Vet Comp Oncol.* 2007;5:31-37.
135. Erdman SE, Kanki PJ, Moore FM, et al. Clusters of lymphoma in ferrets. *Cancer Invest.* 1996;14:225-230.
136. Erdman SE, Reimann KA, Moore FM, et al. Transmission of a chronic lymphoproliferative syndrome in ferrets. *Lab Invest.* 1995;72:539-546.
137. Eyles JL, Hickey MJ, Norman MU, et al. A key role for G-CSF-induced neutrophil production and trafficking during inflammatory arthritis. *Blood.* 2008;112:5193-5201.
138. Fagbemi BO, Otesile EB, Makinde MO, et al. The relationship between dietary energy levels and the severity of *Trypanosoma brucei* infection in growing pigs. *Vet Parasitol.* 1990;35:29-42.
139. Faldyna M, Laznicka A, Toman M. Immunosuppression in bitches with pyometra. *J Small Anim Pract.* 2001;42:5-10.
140. Farstad IN, Norstein J, Brandtzaeg P. Phenotypes of B and T cells in human intestinal and mesenteric lymph. *Gastroenterology.* 1997;112:163-173.
141. Favier RP, van Leeuwen M, Teske E. Essential thrombocythaemia in two dogs. *Tijdschr Diergeneeskd.* 2004;129:360-364.
142. Ferrer JF, Marshak RR, Abt DA, et al. Relationship between lymphosarcoma and persistent lymphocytosis in cattle: a review. *J Am Vet Med Assoc.* 1979;175:705-708.
143. Fews D, Scase TJ, Battersby IA. Leiomyosarcoma of the pericardium, with epicardial metastases and peripheral eosinophilia in a dog. *J Comp Pathol.* 2008;138:224-228.
144. Fietta P, Delsante G. The effector T helper cell triade. *Riv Biol.* 2009;102:61-74.
145. Fine DM, Tvedten H. Chronic granulocytic leukemia in a dog. *J Am Vet Med Assoc.* 1999;214:1809-1812.
146. Flatland B, Fry MM, Baek SJ, et al. May-Hegglin anomaly in a Pug dog. *Vet Clin Pathol.* 2011;40:207-214.
147. Florins A, Gillet N, Asquith B, et al. Cell dynamics and immune response to BLV infection: a unifying model. *Front Biosci.* 2007;12:1520-1531.
148. Foley J, Nieto NC, Madigan J, et al. Possible differential host tropism in *Anaplasma phagocytophilum* strains in the Western United States. *Ann N Y Acad Sci.* 2008;1149:94-97.
149. Fontaine J, Bovens C, Bettenay S, et al. Canine cutaneous epitheliotropic T-cell lymphoma: a review. *Vet Comp Oncol.* 2009;7:1-14.
150. Foster AP, Evans E, Kerlin RL, et al. Cutaneous T-cell lymphoma with Sezary syndrome in a dog. *Vet Clin Pathol.* 1997;26:188-192.
151. Fox LE, Ford S, Alleman AR, et al. Aplastic anemia associated with prolonged high-dose trimethoprim-sulfadiazine administration in two dogs. *Vet Clin Pathol.* 1993;22:89-92.
152. Franks PT, Harvey JW, Mays MC, et al. Feline large granular lymphoma. *Vet Pathol.* 1986;23:200-202.
153. Franzen P, Aspan A, Egenvall A, et al. Acute clinical, hematologic, serologic, and polymerase chain reaction findings in horses experimentally infected with a European strain of *Anaplasma phagocytophilum. J Vet Intern Med.* 2005;19:232-239.
154. Franzen P, Berg AL, Aspan A, et al. Death of a horse infected experimentally with *Anaplasma phagocytophilum. Vet Rec.* 2007;160:122-125.
155. Frauenfelder HC, Fessler JF, Moore AB, et al. Effects of dexamethasone on endotoxin shock in the anesthetized pony: hematologic, blood gas, and coagulation changes. *Am J Vet Res.* 1982;43:405-411.
156. Frenais R, Rosenberg D, Burgaud S, et al. Clinical efficacy and safety of a once-daily formulation of carbimazole in cats with hyperthyroidism. *J Small Anim Pract.* 2009;50:510-515.
157. Fry MM, Forman MA. 5-fluorouracil toxicity with severe bone marrow suppression in a dog. *Vet Hum Toxicol.* 2004;46:178-180.
158. Fuchs TA, Abed U, Goosmann C, et al. Novel cell death program leads to neutrophil extracellular traps. *J Cell Biol.* 2007;176:231-241.
159. Fujino Y, Horiuchi H, Mizukoshi F, et al. Prevalence of hematological abnormalities and detection of infected bone marrow cells in asymptomatic cats with feline immunodeficiency virus infection. *Vet Microbiol.* 2009;136:217-225.
160. Fujiwara N, Kobayashi K. Macrophages in inflammation. *Curr Drug Targets Inflamm Allergy.* 2005;4:281-286.
161. Fulton R, Gasper PW, Ogilvie GK, et al. Effect of recombinant human granulocyte colony-stimulating factor on hematopoiesis in normal cats. *Exp Hematol.* 1991;19:759-767.
162. Furze RC, Rankin SM. The role of the bone marrow in neutrophil clearance under homeostatic conditions in the mouse. *FASEB J.* 2008;22:3111-3119.
163. Fyfe JC, Giger U, Hall CA, et al. Inherited selective intestinal cobalamin malabsorption and cobalamin deficiency in dogs. *Pediatr Res.* 1991;29:24-31.
164. Galli SJ, Metcalfe DD, Arber DA, et al. Basophils and mast cells and their disorders. In: Lichtman MA, Beutler E, Kipps TJ, et al, eds. *Williams Hematology.* 7th ed. New York: McGraw-Hill; 2006:879-897.
165. Ganz T, Lehrer RI. Production, distribution, and fate of monocytes and macrophages. In: Lichtman MA, Beutler E, Kipps TJ, et al, eds. *Williams Hematology.* 7th ed. New York: McGraw-Hill; 2006:979-986.
166. Garrett LD, Craig CL, Szladovits B, et al. Evaluation of buffy coat smears for circulating mast cells in healthy cats and ill cats without mast cell tumor-related disease. *J Am Vet Med Assoc.* 2007;231:1685-1687.
167. Gary AT, Kerl ME, Wiedmeyer CE, et al. Bone marrow hypoplasia associated with fenbendazole administration in a dog. *J Am Anim Hosp Assoc.* 2004;40:224-229.
168. Gaspar-Elsas MI, Queto T, Vasconcelos Z, et al. Evidence for a regulatory role of alpha 4-integrins in the maturation of eosinophils generated from the bone marrow in the presence of dexamethasone. *Clin Exp Allergy.* 2009;39:1187-1198.
169. Gaunt SD, Baker DC. Hemosiderin in leukocytes of dogs with immune-mediated hemolytic anemia. *Vet Clin Pathol.* 1986;15(2):8-10.
170. Geissmann F, Manz MG, Jung S, et al. Development of monocytes, macrophages, and dendritic cells. *Science.* 2010;327:656-661.
171. Gelain ME, Antoniazzi E, Bertazzolo W, et al. Chronic eosinophilic leukemia in a cat: cytochemical and immunophenotypical features. *Vet Clin Pathol.* 2006;35:454-459.
172. Gerner W, Kaser T, Saalmuller A. Porcine T lymphocytes and NK cells–an update. *Dev Comp Immunol.* 2009;33:310-320.
173. Gieg J, Rikihisa Y, Wellman M. Diagnosis of *Ehrlichia ewingii* infection by PCR in a puppy from Ohio. *Vet Clin Pathol.* 2009;38:406-410.
174. Gilbert RO, Rebhun WC, Kim CA, et al. Clinical manifestations of leukocyte adhesion deficiency in cattle: 14 cases (1977-1991). *J Am Vet Med Assoc.* 1993;202:445-449.
175. Gill AF, Gaunt S, Sirninger J. Congenital Pelger-Huët anomaly in a horse. *Vet Clin Pathol.* 2006;35:460-462.
176. Gingerich K, Guptill L. Canine and feline histoplasmosis: a review of a widespread fungus. *Vet Med.* 2008;103:248-264.
177. Gitzelmann R, Bosshard NU, Superti-Furga A, et al. Feline mucopolysaccharidosis VII due to β-glucuronidase deficiency. *Vet Pathol.* 1994;31:435-443.
178. Gleich S, Hartmann K. Hematology and serum biochemistry of feline immunodeficiency virus-infected and feline leukemia virus-infected cats. *J Vet Intern Med.* 2009;23:552-558.
179. Gommeren K, Duchateau L, Paepe D, et al. Investigation of physiologic leukopenia in Belgian Tervuren dogs. *J Vet Intern Med.* 2006;20:1340-1343.
180. Gossett KA. Anemias associated with drugs and chemicals. In: Feldman BF, Zinkl JG, Jain NC, eds. *Schalm's Veterinary Hematology.* 5th ed. Philadelphia: Lippincott Williams & Wilkins; 2000:185-189.
181. Gossett KA, Carakostas MC. Effect of EDTA on morphology of neutrophils of healthy dogs and dogs with inflammation. *Vet Clin Pathol.* 1984;13:22-25.
182. Gossett KA, MacWilliams PS. Ultrastructure of canine toxic neutrophils. *Am J Vet Res.* 1982;43:1634-1637.
183. Gossett KA, MacWilliams PS, Cleghorn B. Sequential morphological and quantitative changes in blood and bone marrow neutrophils in dogs with acute inflammation. *Can J Comp Med.* 1985;49:291-297.

184. Gossett KA, MacWilliams PS, Fulton RW. Viral inclusions in hematopoietic precursors in a dog with distemper. *J Am Vet Med Assoc.* 1982;181:387-388.
185. Goto Y, Hogg JC, Suwa T, et al. A novel method to quantify the turnover and release of monocytes from the bone marrow using the thymidine analog 5'-bromo-2'-deoxyuridine. *Am J Physiol Cell Physiol.* 2003;285:C253-C259.
186. Greenfield CL, Messick JB, Solter PF, et al. Results of hematologic analyses and prevalence of physiologic leukopenia in Belgian Tervuren. *J Am Vet Med Assoc.* 2000;216:866-871.
187. Gregoire C, Chasson L, Luci C, et al. The trafficking of natural killer cells. *Immunol Rev.* 2007;220:169-182.
188. Greig B, Armstrong PJ. Canine granulocytotropic anaplasmosis (*A. phagocytophilum* infection). In: Greene CE, ed. *Infectious Diseases of the Dog and Cat.* 3rd ed. St. Louis: Saunders Elsevier; 2006:219-224.
189. Greig B, Breitschwerdt E, Armstrong J. Canine granulocytotropic ehrlichiosis (*E. ewingii* infections). In: Greene CE, ed. *Infectious Diseases of the Dog and Cat.* 3rd ed. St. Louis: Saunders Elsevier; 2006:217-218.
190. Greiner M, Wolf G, Hartmann K. A retrospective study of the clinical presentation of 140 dogs and 39 cats with bacteraemia. *J Small Anim Pract.* 2008;49:378-383.
191. Griebel PJ, Qualtiere L, Davis WC, et al. Bovine peripheral blood leukocyte subpopulation dynamics following a primary bovine herpesvirus-1 infection. *Viral Immunol.* 1987;1:267-286.
192. Grinberg N, Elazar S, Rosenshine I, et al. Beta-hydroxybutyrate abrogates formation of bovine neutrophil extracellular traps and bactericidal activity against mammary pathogenic *Escherichia coli. Infect Immun.* 2008;76:2802-2807.
193. Grindem CB. Blood cell markers. *Vet Clin North Am Small Anim Pract.* 1996;26: 1043-1064.
194. Grindem CB. Acute myeloid leukemia. In: Feldman BF, Zinkl JG, Jain NC, eds. *Schalm's Veterinary Hematology.* 5th ed. Philadelphia: Lippincott Williams & Wilkins; 2000:717-726.
195. Grindem CB, Stevens JB, Brost DR, et al. Chronic myelogenous leukaemia with meningeal infiltration in a dog. *Comp Haematol Int.* 1992;2:170-174.
196. Grondin TM, Dewitt SF, Keeton KS. Pelger-Huët anomaly in an Arabian horse. *Vet Clin Pathol.* 2007;36:306-310.
197. Gustafson BW. Ivermectin in the treatment of *Physaloptera preputialis* in two cats. *J Am Anim Hosp Assoc.* 1995;31:416-418.
198. Hammer RF, Weber AF. Ultrastructure of agranular leukocytes in peripheral blood of normal cows. *Am J Vet Res.* 1974;35:527-536.
199. Hammond WP, Csiba E, Canin A, et al. Chronic neutropenia. A new canine model induced by human granulocyte colony-stimulating factor. *J Clin Invest.* 1991;87: 704-710.
200. Harvey JW. Hematology tip—stains for distemper inclusions. *Vet Clin Pathol.* 1982;11:12.
201. Harvey JW, Asquith RL, McNulty PK, et al. Haematology of foals up to one year old. *Equine Vet J.* 1984;16:347-353.
202. Harvey JW, Gaskin JM. Experimental feline haemobartonellosis. *J Am Anim Hosp Assoc.* 1977;13:28-38.
203. Harvey JW, Harr KE, Murphy D, et al. Hematology of healthy Florida manatees (*Trichechus manatus*). *Vet Clin Pathol.* 2009;38;183-193.
204. Haskins M, Giger U. Lysosomal storage diseases. In: Kaneko JJ, Harvey JW, Bruss ML, eds. *Clinical Biochemistry of Domestic Animals.* 6th ed. San Diego: Academic Press; 2008:731-749.
205. Haskins ME, Aguirre GD, Jezyk PF, et al. Mucopolysaccharidosis type VII (Sly syndrome): beta-glucuronidase-deficient. *Am J Physiol.* 1991;138:1553-1555.
206. Haskins ME, Desnick RJ, DiFerrante N, et al. β-glucuronidase deficiency in a dog: a model of human mucopolysaccharidosis VII. *Pediatr Res.* 1984;18:980-984.
207. Hatano Y, Taniuchi S, Masuda M, et al. Phagocytosis of heat-killed *Staphylococcus aureus* by eosinophils: comparison with neutrophils. *APMIS.* 2009;117:115-123.
208. Heinemann A, Sturm GJ, Ofner M, et al. Stem cell factor stimulates the chemotaxis, integrin upregulation, and survival of human basophils. *J Allergy Clin Immunol.* 2005;116:820-826.
209. Helfand SC, Soergel SA, MacWilliams PS, et al. Clinical and immunological effects of human recombinant interleukin-2 given by repetitive weekly infusion to normal dogs. *Cancer Immunol Immunother.* 1994;39:84-92.
210. Helton KA, Nesbitt GH, Caciolo PL. Griseofulvin toxicity in cats: literature and report of seven cases. *J Am Anim Hosp Assoc.* 1986;22:453-458.
211. Henningson JN, Topliff CL, Gil LH, et al. Effect of the viral protein N(pro) on virulence of bovine viral diarrhea virus and induction of interferon type I in calves. *Am J Vet Res.* 2009;70:1117-1123.
212. Henson JB, McGuire TC, Kobayashi K, et al. The diagnosis of equine infectious anemia using the complement-fixation test, siderocyte counts, hepatic biopsies, and serum protein alterations. *J Am Vet Med Assoc.* 1967;151:1830-1839.
213. Henson KL, Alleman AR, Fox LE, et al. Diagnosis of disseminated adenocarcinoma by bone marrow aspiration in a dog with leukoerythroblastosis and fever of unknown origin. *Vet Clin Pathol.* 1998;27:80-84.
214. Hess PR, English RV, Hegarty BC, et al. Experimental *Ehrlichia canis* infection in the dog does not cause immunosuppression. *Vet Immunol Immunopathol.* 2006;109:117-125.
215. Hess RS, Saunders HM, Van Winkle TJ, et al. Clinical, clinicopathologic, radiographic, and ultrasonographic abnormalities in dogs with fatal acute pancreatitis: 70 cases (1986-1995). *J Am Vet Med Assoc.* 1998;213:665-670.
216. Hikasa Y, Morita T, Futaoka Y, et al. Connective tissue-type mast cell leukemia in a dog. *J Vet Med Sci.* 2000;62:187-190.
217. Hirsch VM, Cunningham TA. Hereditary anomaly of neutrophil granulation in Birman cats. *Am J Vet Res.* 1984;45:2170-2174.
218. Hoffmann K, Sperling K, Olins AL, et al. The granulocyte nucleus and lamin B receptor: avoiding the ovoid. *Chromosoma.* 2007;116:227-235.
219. Hopper PE, Mandell CP, Turrel JM, et al. Probable essential thrombocythemia in a dog. *J Vet Intern Med.* 1989;3:79-85.
220. Horwitz MS, Duan Z, Korkmaz B, et al. Neutrophil elastase in cyclic and severe congenital neutropenia. *Blood.* 2007;109:1817-1824.
221. Huibregtse BA, Turner JL. Hypereosinophilic syndrome and eosinophilic leukemia: a comparison of 22 hypereosinophilic cats. *J Am Anim Hosp Assoc.* 1994;30:591-599.
222. Huizing M, Helip-Wooley A, Westbroek W, et al. Disorders of lysosome-related organelle biogenesis: clinical and molecular genetics. *Annu Rev Genomics Hum Genet.* 2008;9:359-386.
223. Jacobs G, Calvert C, Kaufman A. Neutropenia and thrombocytopenia in three dogs treated with anticonvulsants. *J Am Vet Med Assoc.* 1998;212:681-684.
224. Jain NC. *Schalm's Veterinary Hematology.* 4th ed. Philadelphia: Lea & Febiger; 1986.
225. Jain NC. Classification of myeloproliferative disorders in cats using criteria proposed by the animal leukaemia study group: a retrospective study of 181 cases (1969-1992). *Comp Haematol Int.* 1993;3:125-134.
226. Jain NC. *Essentials of Veterinary Hematology.* Philadelphia: Lea & Febiger; 1993.
227. Jain NC, Blue JT, Grindem CB, et al. Proposed criteria for classification of acute myeloid leukemia in dogs and cats. *Vet Clin Pathol.* 1991;20:63-82.
228. James FE, Mansfield CS. Clinical remission of idiopathic hypereosinophilic syndrome in a Rottweiler. *Aust Vet J.* 2009;87:330-333.
229. Johnson LR, Herrgesell EJ, Davidson AP, et al. Clinical, clinicopathologic, and radiographic findings in dogs with coccidioidomycosis: 24 cases (1995-2000). *J Am Vet Med Assoc.* 2003;222:461-466.
230. Johnsrude JD, Alleman AR, Schumacher J, et al. Cytologic findings in cerebrospinal fluid from two animals with GM_2-gangliosidosis. *Vet Clin Pathol.* 1996;25:80-83.
231. Joosten SA, Ottenhoff TH. Human CD4 and CD8 regulatory T cells in infectious diseases and vaccination. *Hum Immunol.* 2008;69:760-770.
232. Jordan HL, Cohn LA, Armstrong PJ. Disseminated *Mycobacterium avium* complex infection in three Siamese cats. *J Am Vet Med Assoc.* 1994;204:90-93.
233. Kakoma I, Hansen RD, Anderson BE, et al. Cultural, molecular, and immunological characterization of the etiologic agent for atypical canine ehrlichiosis. *J Clin Microbiol.* 1994;32:170-175.
234. Kamphuis E, Junt T, Waibler Z, et al. Type I interferons directly regulate lymphocyte recirculation and cause transient blood lymphopenia. *Blood.* 2006;108:3253-3261.
235. Kaname H, Mori Y, Sumida Y, et al. Changes in the leukocyte distribution and surface expression of adhesion molecules induced by hypothalamic stimulation in the cat. *Brain Behav Immun.* 2002;16:351-367.
236. Kankaanranta H, Moilanen E, Zhang X. Pharmacological regulation of human eosinophil apoptosis. *Curr Drug Targets Inflamm Allergy.* 2005;4:433-445.
237. Kaplan J, De Domenico I, Ward DM. et al. Chediak-Higashi syndrome. *Curr Opin Hematol.* 2008;15:22-29.
238. Kariya K, Konno A, Ishida T. Perforin-like immunoreactivity in four cases of lymphoma of large granular lymphocytes in the cat. *Vet Pathol.* 1997;34:156-159.
239. Karni RJ, Wangh LJ, Sanchez JA. Nonrandom location and orientation of the inactive X chromosome in human neutrophil nuclei. *Chromosoma.* 2001;110:267-274.
240. Katunguka-Rwakishaya E, Murray M, Holmes PH. The pathophysiology of ovine trypanosomosis: haematological and blood biochemical changes. *Vet Parasitol.* 1992;45:17-32.
241. Kaufman J. Diseases of the adrenal cortex of dogs and cats. *Mod Vet Pract.* 1984;65:429-434.
242. Kelemen E, Gergely P, Lehoczky D, et al. Permanent large granular lymphocytosis in the blood of splenectomized individuals without concomitant increase of in vitro natural killer cell cytotoxicity. *Clin Exp Immunol.* 1986;63:696-702.
243. Keller CB, Lamarre J. Inherited lysosomal storage disease in an English Springer Spaniel. *J Am Vet Med Assoc.* 1992;200:194-195.
244. Khoutorsky A, Bruchim Y. Transient leucopenia, thrombocytopenia and anaemia associated with severe acute phenobarbital intoxication in a dog. *J Small Anim Pract.* 2008;49:367-369.
245. Kijas JM, Bauer TR Jr, Gafvert S, et al. A missense mutation in the beta-2 integrin gene (ITGB2) causes canine leukocyte adhesion deficiency. *Genomics.* 1999;61:101-107.

246. Kirpensteijn J, Fingland RB. Cutaneous actinomycosis and nocardiosis in dogs: 48 cases (1980-1990). *J Am Vet Med Assoc.* 1992;201:917-920.
247. Kirpensteijn J, Fingland RB, Ulrich T, et al. Cholelithiasis in dogs: 29 cases (1980-1990). *J Am Vet Med Assoc.* 1993;202:1137-1142.
248. Kitoh K, Kitagawa H, Sasaki Y. Pathologic findings in dogs with shock induced by intravenous administration of heartworm extract. *Am J Vet Res.* 1998;59:1417-1422.
249. Knowles TG, Edwards JE, Bazeley KJ, et al. Changes in the blood biochemical and haematological profile of neonatal calves with age. *Vet Rec.* 2000;147:593-598.
250. Kodama A, Sakai H, Kobayashi K, et al. B-cell intestinal lymphoma with Mott cell differentiation in a 1-year-old miniature Dachshund. *Vet Clin Pathol.* 2008;37:409-415.
251. Kogan DA, Johnson LR, Jandrey KE, et al. Clinical, clinicopathologic, and radiographic findings in dogs with aspiration pneumonia: 88 cases (2004-2006). *J Am Vet Med Assoc.* 2008;233:1742-1747.
252. Kohn B, Arnold P, Kaser-Hotz B, et al. Malignant histiocytosis of the dog: 26 cases (1989-1992). *Kleintierpraxis.* 1993;38:409-424.
253. Kohn B, Goldschmidt MH, Hohenhaus AE, et al. Anemia, splenomegaly, and increased osmotic fragility of erythrocytes in Abyssinian and Somali cats. *J Am Vet Med Assoc.* 2000;217:1483-1491.
254. Kohn B, Weingart C, Eckmann V, et al. Primary immune-mediated hemolytic anemia in 19 cats: diagnosis, therapy, and outcome (1998-2004). *J Vet Intern Med.* 2006;20:159-166.
255. Kohn CW, Swardson C, Provost P, et al. Myeloid and megakaryocytic hypoplasia in related standardbreds. *J Vet Intern Med.* 1995;9:315-323.
256. Kosanke SD, Pierce KR, Bay WW. Clinical and biochemical abnormalities in porcine GM_2-gangliosidosis. *Vet Pathol.* 1978;15:685-699.
257. Kouro T, Takatsu K. IL-5- and eosinophil-mediated inflammation: from discovery to therapy. *Int Immunol.* 2009;21:1303-1309.
258. Kramer J, Tornquist S, Erfle J, et al. Large granular lymphocyte leukemia in a horse. *Vet Clin Pathol.* 1993;22:126-128.
259. Kringel H, Roepstorff A. *Trichuris suis* population dynamics following a primary experimental infection. *Vet Parasitol.* 2006;139:132-139.
260. Kubo H, Doyle NA, Graham L, et al. L- and P-selectin and CD11/CD18 in intracapillary neutrophil sequestration in rabbit lungs. *Am J Respir Crit Care Med.* 1999;159:267-274.
261. Kueck BD, Smith RE, Parkin J, et al. Eosinophilic leukemia: a myeloproliferative disorder distinct from the hypereosinophilic syndrome. *Hematol Pathol.* 1991;5:195-205.
262. La Perle KM, Piercy RJ, Long JF, et al. Multisystemic, eosinophilic, epitheliotropic disease with intestinal lymphosarcoma in a horse. *Vet Pathol.* 1998;35:144-146.
263. Lan NT, Yamaguchi R, Furuya Y, et al. Pathogenesis and phylogenetic analyses of canine distemper virus strain 007Lm, a new isolate in dogs. *Vet Microbiol.* 2005;110:197-207.
264. Lanevschi A, Daminet S, Niemeyer GP, et al. Granulocyte colony-stimulating factor deficiency in a rottweiler with chronic idiopathic neutropenia. *J Vet Intern Med.* 1999;13:72-75.
265. Langheinrich KA, Nielsen SW. Histopathology of feline panleukopenia: a report of 65 cases. *J Am Vet Med Assoc.* 1971;158:863-872.
266. Larsen S, Flagstad A, Aalbaek B. Experimental panleukopenia in the conventional cat. *Vet Pathol.* 1976;13:216-240.
267. Lascola K, Vandis M, Bain P, et al. Concurrent infection with *Anaplasma phagocytophilum* and *Mycoplasma haemolamae* in a young Alpaca. *J Vet Intern Med.* 2009;23:379-382.
268. Latimer KS. Pelger-Huët anomaly. In: Feldman BF, Zinkl JG, Jain NC, eds. *Schalm's Veterinary Hematology.* 5th ed. Philadelphia: Lippincott Williams & Wilkins; 2000:976-983.
269. Latimer KS, Bounous DI, Collatos C, et al. Extreme eosinophilia with disseminated eosinophilic granulomatous disease in a horse. *Vet Clin Pathol.* 1996;25:23-26.
270. Latimer KS, Campagnoli RP, Danilenko DM. Pelger-Huët anomaly in Australian shepherds: 87 cases (1991-1997). *Comp Haematol Int.* 2000;10:9-13.
271. Latimer KS, Jameson PH, Crowell WA, et al. Disseminated *Mycobacterium avium* complex infection in a cat: presumptive diagnosis by blood smear examination. *Vet Clin Pathol.* 1997;26:85-89.
272. Latimer KS, Robertson SL. Inherited leukocyte disorders. In: August JR, ed. *Consultations in Feline Internal Medicine 2,* Philadelphia: W.B. Saunders Co.; 1994:503-507.
273. Leifer CE, Matus RE, Patnaik AK, et al. Chronic myelogenous leukemia in the dog. *J Am Vet Med Assoc.* 1983;183:686-689.
274. Lepidi H, Bunnell JE, Martin ME, et al. Comparative pathology, and immunohistology associated with clinical illness after *Ehrlichia phagocytophila*-group infections. *Am J Trop Med Hyg.* 2000;62:29-37.
275. Lester GD, Alleman AR, Raskin RE, et al. Pancytopenia secondary to lymphoid leukemia in three horses. *J Vet Intern Med.* 1993;7:360-363.
276. Lewis GEJ, Huxsoll DL, Ristic M, et al. Experimentally induced infection of dogs, cats, and nonhuman primates with *Ehrlichia equi*, etiologic agent of equine ehrlichiosis. *Am J Vet Res.* 1975;36:85-88.
277. Ley K, Laudanna C, Cybulsky MI, et al. Getting to the site of inflammation: the leukocyte adhesion cascade updated. *Nat Rev Immunol.* 2007;7:678-689.
278. Lilliehook I, Gunnarsson L, Zakrisson G, et al. Diseases associated with pronounced eosinophilia: a study of 105 dogs in Sweden. *J Small Anim Pract.* 2000;41:248-253.
279. Lilliehook I, Tvedten H. Investigation of hypereosinophilia and potential treatments. *Vet Clin North Am Small Anim Pract.* 2003;33:1359-1378.
280. Lindbom L, Werr J. Integrin-dependent neutrophil migration in extravascular tissue. *Semin Immunol.* 2002;14:115-121.
281. Ling GV, Stabenfeldt GH, Comer KM, et al. Canine hyperadrenocorticism: pretreatment clinical and laboratory evaluation of 117 cases. *J Am Vet Med Assoc.* 1979;174:1211-1215.
282. Linterman MA, Vinuesa CG. Signals that influence T follicular helper cell differentiation and function. *Semin Immunopathol.* 2010;32:183-196.
283. Little SE, Allen KE, Johnson EM, et al. New developments in canine hepatozoonosis in North America: a review. *Parasit Vectors.* 2009;2(Suppl 1):S5.
284. Liu K, Waskow C, Liu X, et al. Origin of dendritic cells in peripheral lymphoid organs of mice. *Nat Immunol.* 2007;8:578-583.
285. Lofstedt J, Dohoo IR, Duizer G. Model to predict septicemia in diarrheic calves. *J Vet Intern Med.* 1999;13:81-88.
286. Lorente C, Sainz A, Tesouro MA. Immunophenotype of dogs with subclinical ehrlichiosis. *Ann N Y Acad Sci.* 2008;1149:114-117.
287. Losco PE. Local and peripheral eosinophilia in a dog with anaplastic mammary carcinoma. *Vet Pathol.* 1986;23:536-538.
288. Lowe AD, Campbell KL, Barger A, et al. Clinical, clinicopathological and histological changes observed in 14 cats treated with glucocorticoids. *Vet Rec.* 2008;162:777-783.
289. Lucroy MD, Madewell BR. Clinical outcome and associated diseases in dogs with leukocytosis and neutrophilia: 118 cases (1996-1998). *J Am Vet Med Assoc.* 1999;214:805-807.
290. Lucroy MD, Madewell BR. Clinical outcome and diseases associated with extreme neutrophilic leukocytosis in cats: 104 cases (1991-1999). *J Am Vet Med Assoc.* 2001;218:736-739.
291. Lund JE, Brown PK. Hypersegmented megakaryocytes and megakaryocytes with multiple separate nuclei in dogs treated with PNU-100592, an oxazolidinone antibiotic. *Toxicol Pathol.* 1997;25:339-343.
292. Lyles SE, Panciera DL, Saunders GK, et al. Idiopathic eosinophilic masses of the gastrointestinal tract in dogs. *J Vet Intern Med.* 2009;23:818-823.
293. Macallan DC, Wallace DL, Zhang Y, et al. B-cell kinetics in humans: rapid turnover of peripheral blood memory cells. *Blood.* 2005;105:3633-3640.
294. Macdonald D, Gordon AA, Kajitani H, et al. Interleukin-2 treatment-associated eosinophilia is mediated by interleukin-5 production. *Br J Haematol.* 1990;76:168-173.
295. MacEwen EG, Drazner FH, McClelland AJ, et al. Treatment of basophilic leukemia in a dog. *J Am Vet Med Assoc.* 1975;166:376-380.
296. Macintire DK, Vincent-Johnson N, Dillon AR, et al. Hepatozoonosis in dogs: 22 cases (1989-1994). *J Am Vet Med Assoc.* 1997;210:916-922.
297. Maddison JE, Hoff B, Johnson RP. Steroid responsive neutropenia in a dog. *J Am Anim Hosp Assoc.* 1982;19:881-886.
298. Madewell BR, Gunn C, Gribble DH. Mast cell phagocytosis of red blood cells in a cat. *Vet Pathol.* 1983;20:638-640.
299. Madewell BR, Munn RJ. Canine lymphoproliferative disorders. An ultrastructural study of 18 cases. *J Vet Intern Med.* 1990;4:63-70.
300. Madewell BR, Munn RJ, Phillips LP. Endocytosis of erythrocytes *in vivo* and particulate substances *in vitro* by feline neoplastic mast cells. *Can J Vet Res.* 1987;51:517-520.
301. Madewell BR, Wilson DW, Hornof WJ, et al. Leukemoid blood response and bone infarcts in a dog with renal tubular adenocarcinoma. *J Am Vet Med Assoc.* 1990;197:1623-1625.
302. Madigan JE, Gribble D. Equine ehrlichiosis in northern California: 49 cases (1968-1981). *J Am Vet Med Assoc.* 1987;190:445-448.
303. Madigan JE, Pusterla N. Ehrlichial diseases. *Vet Clin North Am Equine Pract.* 2000;16:487-499, ix.
304. Maeda K, Sakonju I, Kanda A, et al. Priming effects of lipopolysaccharide and inflammatory cytokines on canine granulocytes. *J Vet Med Sci.* 2010;72:55-60.
305. Mahaffey EA, Brown TP, Duncan JR, et al. Basophilic leukaemia in a dog. *J Comp Pathol.* 1987;97:393-399.
306. Mair TS, Hillyer MH, Taylor FG. Peritonitis in adult horses: a review of 21 cases. *Vet Rec.* 1990;126:567-570.
307. Marchetti V, Benetti C, Citi S, et al. Paraneoplastic hypereosinophilia in a dog with intestinal T-cell lymphoma. *Vet Clin Pathol.* 2005;34:259-263.
308. Marcos R, Santos M, Malhao F, et al. Pancytopenia in a cat with visceral leishmaniasis. *Vet Clin Pathol.* 2009;38:201-205.

309. Martin BA, Wiggs BR, Lee S, et al. Regional differences in neutrophil margination in dog lungs. *J Appl Physiol.* 1987;63:1253-1261.
310. Mason KV, Evans AG. Mosquito bite-caused eosinophilic dermatitis in cats. *J Am Vet Med Assoc.* 1991;198:2086-2088.
311. Matthews S, Dart AJ, Dowling BA, et al. Peritonitis associated with *Actinobacillus equuli* in horses: 51 cases. *Aust Vet J.* 2001;79:536-539.
312. McCauley I, Hartmann PE. Changes in piglet leucocytes, B lymphocytes and plasma cortisol from birth to three weeks after weaning. *Res Vet Sci.* 1984;37:234-241.
313. McClure JT. Leukoproliferative disorders in horses. *Vet Clin North Am Equine Pract.* 2000;16:165-182.
314. McLaughlin BG, Adams PS, Cornell WD, et al. Canine distemper viral inclusions in blood cells of four vaccinated dogs. *Can Vet J.* 1985;26:368-372.
315. McManus PM. Frequency and severity of mastocytemia in dogs with and without mast cell tumors: 120 cases (1995-1997). *J Am Vet Med Assoc.* 1999;215: 355-357.
316. McManus PM. Classification of myeloid neoplasms: a comparative review. *Vet Clin Pathol.* 2005;34:189-212.
317. McManus PM, Craig LE. Correlation between leukocytosis and necropsy findings in dogs with immune-mediated hemolytic anemia: 34 cases (1994-1999). *J Am Vet Med Assoc.* 2001;218:1308-1313.
318. McManus PM, Litwin C, Barber L. Immune-mediated neutropenia in 2 dogs. *J Vet Intern Med.* 1999;13:372-374.
319. Mdurvwa EG, Ogunbiyi PO, Gakou HS, et al. Pathogenic mechanisms of caprine arthritis-encephalitis virus. *Vet Res Commun.* 1994;18:483-490.
320. Mears EA, Raskin RE, Legendre AM. Basophilic leukemia in a dog. *J Vet Intern Med.* 1997;11:92-94.
321. Meng R, Bridgman R, Toivio-Kinnucan M, et al. Neutrophil elastase-processing defect in cyclic hematopoietic dogs. *Exp Hematol.* 2010;38:104-115.
322. Merad M, Manz MG, Karsunky H, et al. Langerhans cells renew in the skin throughout life under steady-state conditions. *Nat Immunol.* 2002;3:1135-1141.
323. Messick JB. Chronic myeloid leukemias. In: Feldman BF, Zinkl JG, Jain NC, eds. *Schalm's Veterinary Hematology.* 5th ed. Philadelphia: Lippincott Williams & Wilkins; 2000:733-739.
324. Meyer J, Delay J, Bienzle D. Clinical, laboratory, and histopathologic features of equine lymphoma. *Vet Pathol.* 2006;43:914-924.
325. Meyers KM. Chediak-Higashi syndrome. In: Feldman BF, Zinkl JG, Jain NC, eds. *Schalm's Veterinary Hematology.* 5th ed. Philadelphia: Lippincott Williams & Wilkins; 2000:971-975.
326. Meyers-Wallen VN, Haskins ME, Patterson DF. Hematologic values in healthy neonatal, weanling, and juvenile kittens. *Am J Vet Res.* 1984;45:1322-1327.
327. Michel RL, O'Handley P, Dade AW. Megakaryocytic myelosis in a cat. *J Am Vet Med Assoc.* 1976;168:1021-1025.
328. Michlewska S, Dransfield I, Megson IL, et al. Macrophage phagocytosis of apoptotic neutrophils is critically regulated by the opposing actions of pro-inflammatory and anti-inflammatory agents: key role for TNF-alpha. *FASEB J.* 2009;23:844-854.
329. Mizukoshi T, Fujino Y, Yasukawa K, et al. Essential thrombocythemia in a dog. *J Vet Med Sci.* 2006;68:1203-1206.
330. Modiano JF, Helfand SC. Acute lymphocytic leukemia. In: Feldman BF, Zinkl JG, Jain NC, eds. *Schalm's Veterinary Hematology.* 5th ed. Philadelphia: Lippincott Williams & Wilkins; 2000:631-637.
331. Mohri M, Sharifi K, Eidi S. Hematology and serum biochemistry of Holstein dairy calves: age related changes and comparison with blood composition in adults. *Res Vet Sci.* 2007;83:30-39.
332. Montella L, Masci AM, Merkabaoui G, et al. B-cell lymphopenia and hypogammaglobulinemia in thymoma patients. *Ann Hematol.* 2003;82:343-347.
333. Moore PF, Affolter VK, Graham PS, et al. Canine epitheliotropic cutaneous T-cell lymphoma: an investigation of T-cell receptor immunophenotype, lesion topography and molecular clonality. *Vet Dermatol.* 2009;20:569-576.
334. Mori A, Lee P, Izawa T, et al. Assessing the immune state of dogs suffering from pituitary gland dependent hyperadrenocorticism by determining changes in peripheral lymphocyte subsets. *Vet Res Commun.* 2009;33:757-769.
335. Mori Y, Iwasaki H, Kohno K, et al. Identification of the human eosinophil lineage-committed progenitor: revision of phenotypic definition of the human common myeloid progenitor. *J Exp Med.* 2009;206:183-193.
336. Moriello KA. Cutaneous lymphoma and variants. In: Feldman BF, Zinkl JG, Jain NC, eds. *Schalm's Veterinary Hematology.* 5th ed. Philadelphia: Lippincott Williams & Wilkins; 2000:648-653.
337. Morris DD, Bloom JC, Roby KA, et al. Eosinophilic myeloproliferative disorder in a horse. *J Am Vet Med Assoc.* 1984;185:993-996.
338. Morris DD, Moore JN. Tumor necrosis factor activity in serum from neonatal foals with presumed septicemia. *J Am Vet Med Assoc.* 1991;199:1584-1589.
339. Moser K, Tokoyoda K, Radbruch A, et al. Stromal niches, plasma cell differentiation and survival. *Curr Opin Immunol.* 2006;18:265-270.
340. Mukae H, Zamfir D, English D, et al. Polymorphonuclear leukocytes released from the bone marrow by granulocyte colony-stimulating factor: intravascular behavior. *Hematol J.* 2000;1:159-171.
341. Mukbel RM, Patten C Jr, Gibson K, et al. Macrophage killing of *Leishmania amazonensis* amastigotes requires both nitric oxide and superoxide. *Am J Trop Med Hyg.* 2007;76:669-675.
342. Muller G, Alldinger S, Moritz A, et al. GM_1-gangliosidosis in Alaskan huskies: clinical and pathologic findings. *Vet Pathol.* 2001;38:281-290.
343. Murray MJ. Salmonellosis in horses. *J Am Vet Med Assoc.* 1996;209:558-560.
344. Myers S, Wiks K, Giger U. Macrocytic anemia caused by naturally occurring folate deficiency in the cat (abstract). *Vet Clin Pathol.* 1996;25:30.
345. Mylonakis ME, Day MJ, Siarkou V, et al. Absence of myelofibrosis in dogs with myelosuppression induced by *Ehrlichia canis* infection. *J Comp Pathol* 2009;142:328-331.
346. Nair MG, Guild KJ, Artis D. Novel effector molecules in type 2 inflammation: lessons drawn from helminth infection and allergy. *J Immunol.* 2006;177:1393-1399.
347. Nash RA, Schuening F, Appelbaum F, et al. Molecular cloning and in vivo evaluation of canine granulocyte-macrophage colony-stimulating factor. *Blood.* 1991;78: 930-937.
348. Ndikuwera J, Smith DA, Obwolo MJ, et al. Chronic granulocytic leukaemia/eosinophilic leukaemia in a dog? *J Small Anim Pract.* 1992;33:553-557.
349. Neer TM, Dial SM, Pechman R, et al. Mucopolysaccharidosis VI in a miniature Pinscher. *J Vet Intern Med.* 1995;9:429-433.
350. Neuwelt EA, Johnson WG, Blank NK, et al. Characterization of a new model of G_{M2}-gangliosidosis (Sandloff's disease) in Korat cats. *J Clin Invest.* 1985;76: 482-490.
351. Neves JS, Weller PF. Functional extracellular eosinophil granules: novel implications in eosinophil immunobiology. *Curr Opin Immunol.* 2009;21:694-699.
352. Nfon CK, Toka FN, Kenney M, et al. Loss of plasmacytoid dendritic cell function coincides with lymphopenia and viremia during foot-and-mouth disease virus infection. *Viral Immunol.* 2010;23:29-41.
353. Nielsen HB, Secher NH, Kristensen JH, et al. Splenectomy impairs lymphocytosis during maximal exercise. *Am J Physiol.* 1997;272:R1847-R1852.
354. Niemeyer GP, Lothrop CD Jr. Cyclic hematopoiesis. In: Feldman BF, Zinkl JG, Jain NC, eds. *Schalm's Veterinary Hematology.* 5th ed. Philadelphia: Lippincott Williams & Wilkins; 2000:960-964.
355. O'Connor CR, Schraeder PL, Kurland AH, et al. Evaluation of the mechanisms of antiepileptic drug-related chronic leukopenia. *Epilepsia.* 1994;35:149-154.
356. O'Keefe DA, Couto CG, Burke-Schwartz C, et al. Systemic mastocytosis in 16 dogs. *J Vet Intern Med.* 1987;1:75-80.
357. Obradovich JE, Ogilvie GK, Powers BE, et al. Evaluation of recombinant canine granulocyte colony-stimulating factor as an inducer of granulopoiesis. *J Vet Intern Med.* 1991;5:75-79.
358. Ogawa H, Tu CH, Kagamizono H, et al. Clinical, morphologic, and biochemical characteristics of Chediak-Higashi syndrome in fifty-six Japanese black cattle. *Am J Vet Res.* 1997;58:1221-1226.
359. Oguma K, Kano R, Hasegawa A. In vitro study of neutrophil apoptosis in dogs. *Vet Immunol Immunopathol.* 2000;76:157-162.
360. Oguma K, Sano J, Kano R, et al. In vitro effect of recombinant human granulocyte colony-stimulating factor on canine neutrophil apoptosis. *Vet Immunol Immunopathol.* 2005;108:307-314.
361. Ohnmacht C, Voehringer D. Basophils protect against reinfection with hookworms independently of mast cells and memory Th2 cells. *J Immunol.* 2010;184:344-350.
362. Okada K, Nakae N, Kuramochi K, et al. Bovine leukemia virus high tax molecular clone experimentally induces leukemia/lymphoma in sheep. *J Vet Med Sci.* 2005;67:1231-1235.
363. Osbaldiston GW, Greve T. Estimating adrenal cortical function in dogs with ACTH. *Cornell Vet.* 1978;68:308-309.
364. Ozmen O, Sahinduran S, Haligur M, et al. Clinicopathologic observations on *Coenurus cerebralis* in naturally infected sheep. *Schweiz Arch Tierheilkd.* 2005;147:129-134.
365. Palic D, Ostojic J, Andreasen CB, et al. Fish cast NETs: neutrophil extracellular traps are released from fish neutrophils. *Dev Comp Immunol.* 2007;31:805-816.
366. Paltrinieri S, Cammarata MP, Cammarata G, et al. Some aspects of humoral and cellular immunity in naturally occurring feline infectious peritonitis. *Vet Immunol Immunopathol.* 1998;65:205-220.
367. Pardanani A, Verstovsek S. Hypereosinophilic syndrome, chronic eosinophilic leukemia, and mast cell disease. *Cancer J.* 2007;13:384-391.
368. Park YM, Bochner BS. Eosinophil survival and apoptosis in health and disease. *Allergy Asthma Immunol Res.* 2010;2:87-101.
369. Patel RT, Caceres A, French AF, et al. Multiple myeloma in 16 cats: a retrospective study. *Vet Clin Pathol.* 2005;34:341-352.
370. Paul AL, Shaw SP, Bandt C. Aplastic anemia in two kittens following a prescription error. *J Am Anim Hosp Assoc.* 2008;44:25-31.

371. Pearce RD, Callahan JW, Little PB, et al. Caprine β-D-mannosidosis: Characterization of a model lysosomal storage disorder. *Can J Vet Res.* 1990;54:22-29.
372. Perkins G, Ainsworth DM, Erb HN, et al. Clinical, haematological and biochemical findings in foals with neonatal equine herpesvirus-1 infection compared with septic and premature foals. *Equine Vet J.* 1999;31:422-426.
373. Perkins MC, Canfield P, Churcher RK, et al. Immune-mediated neutropenia suspected in five dogs. *Aust Vet J.* 2004;82:52-57.
374. Perryman LE. Molecular pathology of severe combined immunodeficiency in mice, horses, and dogs. *Vet Pathol.* 2004;41:95-100.
375. Peterson ME, Kintzer PP, Cavanaugh PG, et al. Feline hyperthyroidism : pretreatment clinical and laboratory evaluation of 131 cases. *J Am Vet Med Assoc.* 1983;183:103-110.
376. Peterson ME, Kintzer PP, Hurvitz AI. Methimazole treatment of 262 cats with hyperthyroidism. *J Vet Intern Med.* 1988;2:150-157.
377. Phillips B. Severe, prolonged bone marrow hypoplasia secondary to the use of carboplatin in an azotemic dog. *J Am Vet Med Assoc.* 1999;215:1250-1252.
378. Postorino NC, Wheeler SL, Park RD, et al. A syndrome resembling lymphomatoid granulomatosis in the dog. *J Vet Intern Med.* 1989;3:15-19.
379. Potgieter LN, Jones JB, Patton CS, et al. Experimental parvovirus infection in dogs. *Can J Comp Med.* 1981;45:212-216.
380. Potter TM, Macintire DK. *Hepatozoon americanum*: an emerging disease in the south-central/southeastern United States. *J Vet Emerg Crit Care (San Antonio).* 2010;20:70-76.
381. Poulsen LK, Hummelshoj L. Triggers of IgE class switching and allergy development. *Ann Med.* 2007;39:440-456.
382. Prasse KW, George LW, Whitlock RH. Idiopathic hypersegmentation of neutrophils in a horse. *J Am Vet Med Assoc.* 1981;178:303-305.
383. Prasse KW, Kaeberle ML, Ramsey FK. Blood neutrophil granulocyte kinetics in cats. *Am J Vet Res.* 1973;34:1021-1025.
384. Prieur DJ, Collier LL. Neutropenia in cats with the Chediak-Higashi syndrome. *Can J Vet Res.* 1987;51:407-408.
385. Raisis AL, Hodgson JL, Hodgson DR. Equine neonatal septicaemia: 24 cases. *Aust Vet J.* 1996;73:137-140.
386. Ramaiah SK, Harvey JW, Giguère S, et al. Intravascular hemolysis associated with liver disease in a horse with marked neutrophil hypersegmentation. *J Vet Intern Med.* 2003;17:360-363.
387. Raskin RE, Krehbiel JD. Myelodysplastic changes in a cat with myelomonocytic leukemia. *J Am Vet Med Assoc.* 1985;187:171-174.
388. Raskin RE, Krehbiel JD. Prevalence of leukemic blood and bone marrow in dogs with multicentric lymphoma. *J Am Vet Med Assoc.* 1989;194:1427-1429.
389. Rawlings CA, Prestwood AK, Beck BB. Eosinophilia and basophilia in *Dirofilaria immitis* and *Dipetalonema reconditum* infections. *J Am Anim Hosp Assoc.* 1980;16:699-704.
390. Reagan WJ. A review of myelofibrosis in dogs. *Toxicol Pathol.* 1993;21:164-169.
391. Reagan WJ, Murphy D, Battaglino M, et al. Antibodies to canine granulocyte colony-stimulating factor induce persistent neutropenia. *Vet Pathol.* 1995;32:374-378.
392. Redman TK, Rudolph K, Barr EB, et al. Pulmonary immunity to ragweed in a Beagle dog model of allergic asthma. *Exp Lung Res.* 2001;27:433-451.
393. Reese TA, Liang HE, Tager AM, et al. Chitin induces accumulation in tissue of innate immune cells associated with allergy. *Nature.* 2007;447:92-96.
394. Renshaw HW, Davis WC. Canine granulocytopathy syndrome: an inherited disorder of leukocyte function. *Am J Pathol.* 1979;95:731-744.
395. Renson P, Blanchard Y, Le Dimna M, et al. Acute induction of cell death-related IFN stimulated genes (ISG) differentiates highly from moderately virulent CSFV strains. *Vet Res.* 2010;41:7.
396. Reppas GP, Canfield PJ. Malignant mast cell neoplasia with local metastasis in a horse. *N Z Vet J.* 1996;44:22-25.
397. Reyers F, Leisewitz AL, Lobetti RG, et al. Canine babesiosis in South Africa: more than one disease. Does this serve as a model for falciparum malaria? *Ann Trop Med Parasitol.* 1998;92:503-511.
398. Ristic M, Dawson J, Holland CJ, et al. Susceptibility of dogs to infection with *Ehrlichia risticii*, causative agent of equine monocytic ehrlichiosis (Potomac horse fever). *Am J Vet Res.* 1988;49:1497-1500.
399. Robertson JM, MacLeod M, Marsden VS, et al. Not all CD4+ memory T cells are long lived. *Immunol Rev.* 2006;211:49-57.
400. Rose RJ, Allen JR, Hodgson DR, et al. Responses to submaximal treadmill exercise and training in the horse: changes in haematology, arterial blood gas and acid-base measurements, plasma biochemical values and heart rate. *Vet Rec.* 1983;113: 612-618.
401. Rossi G, Gelain ME, Foroni S, et al. Extreme monocytosis in a dog with chronic monocytic leukaemia. *Vet Rec.* 2009;165:54-56.
402. Rossof AH, Fehir KM, Budd HS, et al. Lithium carbonate enhances granulopoiesis and attenuates cyclophosphamide-induced injury in the dog. *Adv Exp Med Biol.* 1980; 127:155-166.
403. Rothenbacher HJ, Ishida K, Barner RD. Equine infectious anemia–part II. The sidero-leukocyte test as an aid in the clinical diagnosis. *Vet Med.* 1962;57:886-890.
404. Ruiz-Gopegui R, Espada Y. What is your diagnosis. Peripheral blood and abdominal fluid from a dog with abdominal distention [leishmaniasis]. *Vet Clin Pathol.* 1998;27:64,67.
405. Sakuma M, Nakahara Y, Suzuki H, et al. A case report: a dog with acute onset of *Hepatozoon canis* infection. *J Vet Med Sci.* 2009;71:835-838.
406. Salles II, Feys HB, Iserbyt BF, et al. Inherited traits affecting platelet function. *Blood Rev.* 2008;22:155-172.
407. Santos M, Marcos R, Assuncao M, et al. Polyarthritis associated with visceral leishmaniasis in a juvenile dog. *Vet Parasitol.* 2006;141:340-344.
408. Santos RL, Tsolis RM, Baumler AJ, et al. Hematologic and serum biochemical changes in *Salmonella* ser *Typhimurium*-infected calves. *Am J Vet Res.* 2002;63:1145-1150.
409. Schick RO, Murphy GF, Goldschmidt MH. Cutaneous lymphosarcoma and leukemia in a cat. *J Am Vet Med Assoc.* 1993;203:1155-1158.
410. Schmidlin H, Diehl SA, Blom B. New insights into the regulation of human B-cell differentiation. *Trends Immunol.* 2009;30:277-285.
411. Schroeder JT. Basophils beyond effector cells of allergic inflammation. *Adv Immunol.* 2009;101:123-161.
412. Schultze AE. Interpretation of canine leukograms. In: Feldman BF, Zinkl JG, Jain NC, eds. *Schalm's Veterinary Hematology.* 5th ed. Philadelphia: Lippincott Williams & Wilkins; 2000:366-381.
413. Schwartz I, Bensaid A, Polack B, et al. In vivo leukocyte tropism of bovine leukemia virus in sheep and cattle. *J Virol.* 1994;68:4589-4596.
414. Searcy GP, Orr JP. Chronic granulocytic leukemia in a horse. *Can Vet J.* 1981;22: 148-151.
415. Segev G, Klement E, Aroch I. Toxic neutrophils in cats: clinical and clinicopathologic features, and disease prevalence and outcome—a retrospective case control study. *J Vet Intern Med.* 2006;20:20-31.
416. Sellon RK, Rottman JB, Jordan HL, et al. Hypereosinophilia associated with transitional cell carcinoma in a cat. *J Am Vet Med Assoc.* 1992;201:591-593.
417. Sharifi H, Nassiri SM, Esmaelli H, et al. Eosinophilic leukaemia in a cat. *J Feline Med Surg.* 2007;9:514-517.
418. Sharkey LC, Rosol IJ, Gröne A, et al. Production of granulocyte colony-stimulating factor and granulocyte-macrophage colony-stimulating factor by carcinomas in a dog and a cat with paraneoplastic leukocytosis. *J Vet Intern Med.* 1996;10:405-408.
419. Sheikh J, Weller PF. Clinical overview of hypereosinophilic syndromes. *Immunol Allergy Clin North Am.* 2007;27:333-355.
420. Shelton GH, Linenberger ML. Hematologic abnormalities associated with retroviral infections in the cat. *Semin Vet Med Surg (Small Anim).* 1995;10:220-233.
421. Sheridan WP, Hunt P, Simonet S, et al. Hematologic effects of cytokines. In: Remick DG, Friedland JS, eds. *Cytokines in Health and Disease.* 2nd ed. New York: Marcel Dekker, Inc.; 1997:487-505.
422. Shi J, Gilbert GE, Kokubo Y, et al. Role of the liver in regulating numbers of circulating neutrophils. *Blood.* 2001;98:1226-1230.
423. Shidham VB, Swami VK. Evaluation of apoptotic leukocytes in peripheral blood smears. *Arch Pathol Lab Med.* 2000;124:1291-1294.
424. Shimizu T, Kawamura T, Miyaji C, et al. Resistance of extrathymic T cells to stress and the role of endogenous glucocorticoids in stress associated immunosuppression. *Scand J Immunol.* 2000;51:285-292.
425. Shimoda T, Shiranaga N, Mashita T, et al. A hematological study on thirteen cats with myelodysplastic syndrome. *J Vet Med Sci.* 2000;62:59-64.
426. Shimoda T, Shiranaga N, Mashita T, et al. Chronic myelomonocytic leukemia in a cat. *J Vet Med Sci.* 2000;62:195-197.
427. Shull RM, Powell D. Acquired hyposegmentation of granulocytes (pseudo-Pelger-Huët anomaly) in a dog. *Cornell Vet.* 1979;69:241-247.
428. Sigmundsdottir H, Butcher EC. Environmental cues, dendritic cells and the programming of tissue-selective lymphocyte trafficking. *Nat Immunol.* 2008;9:981-987.
429. Silverstein D, Carmichael KP, Wang P, et al. Mucopolysaccharidosis type VII in a German Shepherd dog. *J Am Vet Med Assoc.* 2004;224:553.
430. Singh B, Pearce JW, Gamage LN, et al. Depletion of pulmonary intravascular macrophages inhibits acute lung inflammation. *Am J Physiol Lung Cell Mol Physiol.* 2004;286:L363-L372.
431. Siracusa MC, Perrigoue JG, Comeau MR, et al. New paradigms in basophil development, regulation and function. *Immunol Cell Biol.* 2010;88:275-284.
432. Smith CW. Composition of neutrophils. In: Lichtman MA, Beutler E, Kipps TJ, et al, eds. *Williams Hematology.* 7th ed. New York: McGraw-Hill; 2006:847-854.
433. Smith CW. Production, distribution, and fate of neutrophils. In: Lichtman MA, Beutler E, Kipps TJ, et al, eds. *Williams Hematology.* 7th ed. New York: McGraw-Hill; 2006:855-861.
434. Smith GP, Perkins SL, Segal GH, et al. T-cell lymphocytosis associated with invasive thymomas. *Am J Clin Pathol.* 1994;102:447-453.
435. Smith GS. Neutrophils. In: Feldman BF, Zinkl JG, Jain NC, eds. *Schalm's Veterinary Hematology.* 5th ed. Philadelphia: Lippincott Williams & Wilkins; 2000:281-296.

436. Smith JE, Erickson HH, DeBowes RM, et al. Changes in circulating equine erythrocytes induced by brief, high-speed exercise. *Equine Vet J.* 1989;21:444-446.
437. Sontas HB, Dokuzeylu B, Turna O, et al. Estrogen-induced myelotoxicity in dogs: a review. *Can Vet J.* 2009;50:1054-1058.
438. Spencer LA, Weller PF. Eosinophils and Th2 immunity: contemporary insights. *Immunol Cell Biol.* 2010;88:250-256.
439. Stacy NI, Nabity MB, Hackendahl N, et al. B-cell lymphoma with Mott cell differentiation in two young adult dogs. *Vet Clin Pathol.* 2009;38:113-120.
440. Steinbach KH, Schick P, Trepel F, et al. Estimation of kinetic parameters of neutrophilic, eosinophilic, and basophilic granulocytes in human blood. *Blut.* 1979;39: 27-38.
441. Stephens L, Milne L, Hawkins P. Moving towards a better understanding of chemotaxis. *Curr Biol.* 2008;18:R485-R494.
442. Stockham SL, Basel DL, Schmidt DA. Mastocytemia in dogs with acute inflammatory diseases. *Vet Clin Pathol.* 1986;15(1):16-21.
443. Stockham SL, Schmidt DA, Curtis KS, et al. Evaluation of granulocytic ehrlichiosis in dogs of Missouri, including serologic status to *Ehrlichia canis, Ehrlichia equi,* and *Borrelia burgdorferi. Am J Vet Res.* 1992;53:63-68.
444. Stockham SL, Tyler JW, Schmidt DA, et al. Experimental transmission of granulocytic ehrlichial organisms in dogs. *Vet Clin Pathol.* 1990;19:99-104.
445. Summers C, Rankin SM, Condliffe AM, et al. Neutrophil kinetics in health and disease. *Trends Immunol.* 2010;31:318-324.
446. Suter SE, Vernau W, Fry MM, et al. CD34+, CD41+ acute megakaryoblastic leukemia in a dog. *Vet Clin Pathol.* 2007;36:288-292.
447. Sykes JE, Weiss DJ, Buoen LC, et al. Idiopathic hypereosinophilic syndrome in 3 Rottweilers. *J Vet Intern Med.* 2001;15:162-166.
448. Takahashi T, Kadosawa T, Nagase M, et al. Visceral mast cell tumors in dogs: 10 cases (1982-1997). *J Am Vet Med Assoc.* 2000;216:222-226.
449. Takeuchi Y, Matsuura S, Fujino Y, et al. Hypereosinophilic syndrome in two cats. *J Vet Med Sci.* 2008;70:1085-1089.
450. Tarrant JM, Stokol T, Blue JT, et al. Diagnosis of chronic myelogenous leukemia in a dog using morphologic, cytochemical, and flow cytometric techniques. *Vet Clin Pathol.* 2001;30:19-24.
451. Tasca S, Carli E, Caldin M, et al. Hematologic abnormalities and flow cytometric immunophenotyping results in dogs with hematopoietic neoplasia: 210 cases (2002-2006). *Vet Clin Pathol.* 2009;38:2-12.
452. Taylor JA. Leukocyte responses in ruminants. In: Feldman BF, Zinkl JG, Jain NC, eds. *Schalm's Veterinary Hematology.* 5th ed. Philadelphia: Lippincott Williams & Wilkins; 2000:391-404.
453. Thamsborg SM, Leifsson PS, Grondahl C, et al. Impact of mixed strongyle infections in foals after one month on pasture. *Equine Vet J.* 1998;30:240-245.
454. Thoday KL, Mooney CT. Historical, clinical and laboratory features of 126 hyperthyroid cats. *Vet Rec.* 1992;131:257-264.
455. Thommasen HV, Martin BA, Wiggs BR, et al. Effect of pulmonary blood flow on leukocyte uptake and release by dog lung. *J Appl Physiol.* 1984;56:966-974.
456. Thompson JP, Christopher MM, Ellison GW, et al. Paraneoplastic leukocytosis associated with a rectal adenomatous polyp in a dog. *J Am Vet Med Assoc.* 1992;201:737-738.
457. Thrall MA, Macy DW, Snyder SP, et al. Cutaneous lymphosarcoma and leukemia in a dog resembling Sezary syndrome in man. *Vet Pathol.* 1984;21:182-186.
458. Tizard IR. *Veterinary Immunology. An Introduction.* 8th ed. Philadelphia: Saunders Elsevier; 2009:1-527.
459. Toft P, Lillevang ST, Tonnesen E, et al. Redistribution of lymphocytes following *E. coli* sepsis. *Scand J Immunol.* 1993;38:541-545.
460. Toman M, Faldyna M, Knotigova P, et al. Postnatal development of leukocyte subset composition and activity in dogs. *Vet Immunol Immunopathol.* 2002;87: 321-326.
461. Topham NJ, Hewitt EW. Natural killer cell cytotoxicity: how do they pull the trigger? *Immunology.* 2009;128:7-15.
462. Toth SR, Nash AS, McEwan AM, et al. Chronic eosinophilic leukaemia in blast crises in a cat negative for feline leukaemia virus. *Vet Rec.* 1985;117:471-472.
463. Trowald-Wigh G, Ekman S, Hansson K, et al. Clinical, radiological and pathological features of 12 Irish setters with canine leucocyte adhesion deficiency. *J Small Anim Pract.* 2000;41:211-217.
464. Tsuchiya R, Kyotani K, Scott MA, et al. Role of platelet activating factor in development of thrombocytopenia and neutropenia in dogs with endotoxemia. *Am J Vet Res.* 1999;60:216-221.
465. Tvedten H, Riihimaki M. Hypersegmentation of equine neutrophils. *Vet Clin Pathol.* 2007;36:4-5.
466. Ulich TR, del Castillo J, Busser K, et al. Acute in vivo effects of IL-3 alone and in combination with IL-6 on the blood cells of the circulation and bone marrow. *Am J Pathol.* 1989;135:663-670.
467. Ulich TR, del Castillo J, Ni RX, et al. Hematologic interactions of endotoxin, tumor necrosis factor alpha (TNF alpha), interleukin 1, and adrenal hormones and the hematologic effects of TNF alpha in Corynebacterium parvum-primed rats. *J Leukoc Biol.* 1989;45:546-557.
468. Ulich TR, del CJ, Souza L. Kinetics and mechanisms of recombinant human granulocyte-colony stimulating factor-induced neutrophilia. *Am J Pathol.* 1988;133:630-638.
469. Unterer S, Deplazes P, Arnold P, et al. Spontaneous *Crenosoma vulpis* infection in 10 dogs: laboratory, radiographic and endoscopic findings. *Schweiz Arch Tierheilkd.* 2002;144:174-179.
470. Valent P, Dahinden CA. Role of interleukins in the regulation of basophil development and secretion. *Curr Opin Hematol.* 2010;17:60-66.
471. Valli VE. *Veterinary Comparative Hematopathology.* Ames, IA: Blackwell Publishing; 2007:119-456.
472. van Miert AS, van Duin CT, Wensing T. Fever and acute phase response induced in dwarf goats by endotoxin and bovine and human recombinant tumour necrosis factor alpha. *J Vet Pharmacol Ther.* 1992;15:332-342.
473. Vargo CL, Taylor SM, Haines DM. Immune mediated neutropenia and thrombocytopenia in 3 giant schnauzers. *Can Vet J.* 2007;48:1159-1163.
474. Vernau W, Moore PF. An immunophenotypic study of canine leukemias and preliminary assessment of clonality by polymerase chain reaction. *Vet Immunol Immunopathol.* 1999;69:145-164.
475. Villiers E, Baines S, Law AM, et al. Identification of acute myeloid leukemia in dogs using flow cytometry with myeloperoxidase, MAC387, and a canine neutrophil-specific antibody. *Vet Clin Pathol.* 2006;35:55-71.
476. Voehringer D. The role of basophils in helminth infection. *Trends Parasitol.* 2009;25:551-556.
477. Wardini AB, Guimaraes-Costa AB, Nascimento MT, et al. Characterization of neutrophil extracellular traps in cats naturally infected with feline leukemia virus. *J Gen Virol.* 2010;91:259-264.
478. Wardlaw A. Eosinophils and their disorders. In: Lichtman MA, Beutler E, Kipps TJ, et al, eds. *Williams Hematology.* 7th ed. New York: McGraw-Hill; 2006:863-878.
479. Watson AD, Wilson JT, Turner DM, et al. Phenylbutazone-induced blood dyscrasias suspected in three dogs. *Vet Rec.* 1980;107:239-241.
480. Watson ADJ, Wright RG. The ultrastructure of inclusions in blood cells of dogs with distemper. *J Comp Pathol.* 1974;84:417-427.
481. Weaver BMQ, Staddon GE, Pearson MRB. Tissue blood content in anaesthetised sheep and horses. *Comp Biochem Physiol [A].* 1989;94A:401-404.
482. Weiner LM, Li W, Holmes M, et al. Phase I trial of recombinant macrophage colony-stimulating factor and recombinant gamma-interferon: toxicity, monocytosis, and clinical effects. *Cancer Res.* 1994;54:4084-4090.
483. Weiser MG, Thrall MA, Fulton R, et al. Granular lymphocytosis and hyperproteinemia in dogs with chronic ehrlichiosis. *J Am Anim Hosp Assoc.* 1991;27:84-88.
484. Weisman JL, Woldemeskel M, Smith KD, et al. Blood smear from a pregnant cat that died shortly after partial abortion. *Vet Clin Pathol.* 2007;36:209-211.
485. Weiss DJ. Leukocyte response to toxic injury. *Toxicol Pathol.* 1993;21:135-140.
486. Weiss DJ. Aplastic anemia. In: Feldman BF, Zinkl JG, Jain NC, eds. *Schalm's Veterinary Hematology.* 5th ed. Philadelphia: Lippincott Williams & Wilkins; 2000: 212-215.
487. Weiss DJ. Bone marrow necrosis in dogs: 34 cases (1996-2004). *J Am Vet Med Assoc.* 2005;227:263-267.
488. Weiss DJ. Recognition and classification of dysmyelopoiesis in the dog: a review. *J Vet Intern Med.* 2005;19:147-154.
489. Weiss DJ. Evaluation of dysmyelopoiesis in cats: 34 cases (1996-2005). *J Am Vet Med Assoc.* 2006;228:893-897.
490. Weiss DJ, Aird B. Cytologic evaluation of primary and secondary myelodysplastic syndromes in the dog. *Vet Clin Pathol.* 2001;30:67-75.
491. Weiss DJ, Henson M. Pure white cell aplasia in a dog. *Vet Clin Pathol.* 2007;36:373-375.
492. Weiss DJ, Lulich J. Myelodysplastic syndrome with sideroblastic differentiation in a dog. *Vet Clin Pathol.* 1999;28:59-63.
493. Welles EG. Clinical interpretation of equine leukograms. In: Feldman BF, Zinkl JG, Jain NC, eds. *Schalm's Veterinary Hematology.* 5th ed. Philadelphia: Lippincott Williams & Wilkins; 2000:405-410.
494. Wellman ML. Lymphoproliferative disorders of large granular lymphocytes. Lake Buena Vista, FL, Proc 15th ACVIM Forum, 1997:20-21.
495. Westermann J, Schwinzer R, Jecker P, et al. Lymphocyte subsets in the blood. The influence of splenectomy, splenic autotransplantation, ageing, and the site of blood sampling on the number of B, T, CD4+, and CD8+ lymphocytes in the rat. *Scand J Immunol.* 1990;31:327-334.
496. Wilcox A, Russell KE. Hematologic changes associated with Adderall toxicity in a dog. *Vet Clin Pathol.* 2008;37:184-189.
497. Wilkerson MJ, Dolce K, Koopman T, et al. Lineage differentiation of canine lymphoma/leukemias and aberrant expression of CD molecules. *Vet Immunol Immunopathol.* 2005;106:179-196.

498. Willesen JL, Jensen AL, Kristensen AT, et al. Haematological and biochemical changes in dogs naturally infected with *Angiostrongylus vasorum* before and after treatment. *Vet J.* 2009;180:106-111.
499. Wolach B, van der Laan LJ, Maianski NA, et al. Growth factors G-CSF and GM-CSF differentially preserve chemotaxis of neutrophils aging in vitro. *Exp Hematol.* 2007;35:541-550.
500. Woldehiwet Z. *Anaplasma phagocytophilum* in ruminants in Europe. *Ann N Y Acad Sci.* 2006;1078:446-460.
501. Woldehiwet Z. The natural history of *Anaplasma phagocytophilum. Vet Parasitol.* 2010;167:108-122.
502. Wood C, Almes K, Bagladi-Swanson M, et al. Sezary syndrome in a cat. *J Am Anim Hosp Assoc.* 2008;44:144-148.
503. Workman HC, Vernau W. Chronic lymphocytic leukemia in dogs and cats: the veterinary perspective. *Vet Clin North Am Small Anim Pract.* 2003;33:1379-1399.
504. Yabsley MJ. Natural history of *Ehrlichia chaffeensis*: vertebrate hosts and tick vectors from the United States and evidence for endemic transmission in other countries. *Vet Parasitol.* 2010;167:136-148.
505. Yamada R, Tsuchida S, Hara Y, et al. Apoptotic lymphocytes induced by surgical trauma in dogs. *J Anesth.* 2002;16:131-137.
506. Yona S, Jung S. Monocytes: subsets, origins, fates and functions. *Curr Opin Hematol.* 2010;17:53-59.
507. Young AJ, Marston WL, Dudler L. Subset-specific regulation of the lymphatic exit of recirculating lymphocytes in vivo. *J Immunol.* 2000;165:3168-3174.
508. Young KM. Eosinophils. In: Feldman BF, Zinkl JG, Jain NC, eds. *Schalm's Veterinary Hematology.* 5th ed. Philadelphia: Lippincott Williams & Wilkins; 2000:297-307.
509. Yousefi S, Mihalache C, Kozlowski E, et al. Viable neutrophils release mitochondrial DNA to form neutrophil extracellular traps. *Cell Death Differ.* 2009;16:1438-1444.
510. Zarbock A, Ley K. Neutrophil adhesion and activation under flow. *Microcirculation.* 2009;16:31-42.
511. Zarbock A, Muller H, Kuwano Y, et al. PSGL-1-dependent myeloid leukocyte activation. *J Leukoc Biol.* 2009;86:1119-1124.
512. Zhang XF, Zhang JZ, Long SW, et al. Experimental *Ehrlichia chaffeensis* infection in beagles. *J Med Microbiol.* 2003;52:1021-1026.
513. Zhang Y, Wallace DL, de Lara CM, et al. In vivo kinetics of human natural killer cells: the effects of ageing and acute and chronic viral infection. *Immunology.* 2007;121:258-265.
514. Zhu J, Paul WE. Heterogeneity and plasticity of T helper cells. *Cell Res.* 2010;20:4-12.
515. Ziemer EL, Whitlock RH, Palmer JE, et al. Clinical and hematologic variables in ponies with experimentally induced equine ehrlichial colitis (Potomac horse fever). *Am J Vet Res.* 1987;48:63-67.
516. Zygner W, Gojska O, Rapacka G, et al. Hematological changes during the course of canine babesiosis caused by large *Babesia* in domestic dogs in Warsaw (Poland). *Vet Parasitol.* 2007;145:146-151.

CHAPTER

6

IMMUNOHEMATOLOGY

IMMUNE SYSTEM

The immune system is an integrated network composed of various cell types, numerous cytokines, and certain plasma proteins that work in synergy to eliminate infectious agents, parasites, and noxious antigens. Consequently defects in the immune response result in increased susceptibility to these foreign invaders. However, inappropriate or exaggerated immune responses can result in immune-mediated tissue injury. Because a thorough review of immunology is beyond the scope of this text, the reader is referred to current immunology textbooks for more detailed information.[140]

Innate Immunity

The innate immune system responds immediately once an invading organism is detected, but it lacks any form of memory and responds in a similar manner and time frame to a repeated challenge by an invading organism. Innate immunity (nonspecific immunity) is possible because chemical compositions of invading microorganisms differ from those of normal body components. Innate immunity involves neutrophils, eosinophils, basophils, macrophages, mast cells, and natural killer (NK) cells, along with the complement system, enzymes such as lysozyme, and carbohydrate-binding proteins that can promote microbial destruction. These cells express microbial pattern-recognition receptors that recognize pathogen-associated molecular patterns (PAMP) on invading microorganisms. Following activation, the cells release components that can result in microbial destruction. Activated cells also produce various cytokines that result in inflammation and the recruitment of additional cells that can attack and destroy invaders. The production and function of these various cell types are discussed in Chapters 3 and 5, respectively.[140]

Acquired Immunity

Acquired immunity, also known as specific immunity or adaptive immunity, is a more recent evolutionary development than innate immunity. It is distinguished by its specificity for an invading organism and for its ability to remember an encounter with an invader so that a more rapid and intense response can occur the second time the same invader is encountered. Lymphocytes are immunocompetent cells that respond to specific foreign antigens. The production and function of lymphocyte types are discussed in Chapters 3 and 5, respectively. B lymphocytes are primarily responsible for immunoglobulin (antibody) production. In contrast to B lymphocytes, which produce immunoglobulins carried in the blood (humoral immunity) to the site of a foreign antigen, T lymphocytes migrate to the site of a foreign antigen (cellular immunity). T lymphocytes are involved in immune regulation, cytotoxicity, delayed-type hypersensitivity, and graft-versus-host reactions. Helper T ($CD4^+$, $CD8^-$) lymphocytes secrete cytokines that influence immune responses, and cytotoxic T ($CD4^-$, $CD8^+$) lymphocytes play pivotal roles in cell-mediated immunity directed at fungi, protozoan organisms, and neoplastic cells. Regulatory T lymphocytes function to maintain a balance between activation of the immune system and prevention of autoimmunity.[30,81,140]

TESTS FOR IMMUNE-MEDIATED DISORDERS

Tests for Antierythrocyte Antibodies

Tests for antierythrocyte antibodies are done when autoagglutination is absent but immune-mediated hemolytic anemia is still suspected.

Direct Antiglobulin Test or Coombs' Test

The direct antiglobulin test (DAT) utilizes washed erythrocytes from the patient and species-specific antisera against IgG, IgM, and the third component of complement (C_3) to detect the presence of one or more of these factors on the surface of erythrocytes (Fig. 6-1). Blood should be collected in EDTA to avoid in vitro uptake of complement by erythrocytes.[146] The DAT may be done in either tubes or microtiter plates.[106] Unless clinical evidence of cold-agglutinin disease is present, this test is usually conducted only at 37°C, because a substantial number of healthy animals exhibit positive test results when the test is run at cold temperatures. In addition to primary immune-mediated hemolytic anemia (IMHA), neonatal isoerythrolysis, and blood transfusion reactions, the

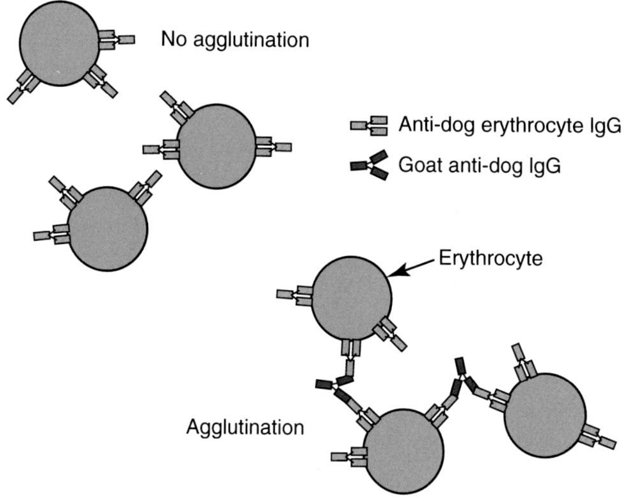

FIGURE 6-1

Direct antiglobulin test (Coombs' test). The addition of anti-dog IgG antibody results in the agglutination of erythrocytes coated with dog IgG.

DAT may be positive in association with various infectious, parasitic, neoplastic, inflammatory, and other secondary immune-mediated diseases. If a drug-induced immune-mediated disorder is suspected, the offending drug should be included in the assay system.[146]

A negative DAT does not rule out an IMHA. A false-negative test may occur if there are insufficient quantities of antibody or complement on erythrocytes, the ratio of antiglobulin in the reagent to antibody or complement on erythrocytes is not appropriate, the test is performed with an incorrect species-specific reagent or at an improper temperature, the antibodies and/or complement elute from erythrocytes because the assay is delayed, the washing of erythrocytes is not adequate, the pH of the washing solution is too low, the centrifugation of the sample is not sufficient or there is excessive agitation in reading the tube test, or the drug was not added to the test for an animal with a drug-induced immune-mediated hemolytic anemia.[146]

False-positive tests may occur if clots are present (resulting in complement activation), blood is collected through infusion lines used to administer dextrose containing solutions, cryptantigens are exposed by the actions of bacterial enzymes on erythrocytes in septicemic patients, naturally occurring cold autoantibodies result in complement binding to erythrocytes, hypergammaglobulinemia is present, glassware or saline is contaminated, or if excessive centrifugation of tubes or misreading of results occurs.[146]

Direct Immunofluorescence Flow Cytometry Assay

Fluorescein isothiocyanate (FITC)-labeled antibodies against immunoglobulins of the species being evaluated are used to label erythrocyte-bound immunoglobulins, which are subsequently detected using flow cytometry. The direct immunofluorescence flow assay has greater sensitivity but somewhat lower specificity than the DAT assay when used to evaluate IMHA in dogs.[121,146,155] The specificity is improved by setting a cutoff limit of greater than 5% positive cells before a test is considered positive. This should largely exclude low-level binding of immunoglobulin to normal (presumably aged) erythrocytes.[104]

Direct Enzyme-Linked Antiglobulin Test

The direct enzyme-linked antiglobulin test (DELAT) is an enzyme-linked immunosorbent assay (ELISA) that has been developed and evaluated for use in dogs. Regardless of the cause of the anemia, a majority of anemic dogs have increased erythrocyte-bound immunoglobulin and/or complement when the DELAT is used. This test has high sensitivity but low specificity for the diagnosis of primary IMHA. It is also time consuming and is typically used as a research tool and not in a clinical setting.[7,146]

Blood Typing

Large numbers of protein and complex carbohydrate antigens occur on the external surface of erythrocytes. Some antigens are present on erythrocytes from all members of a species and others (including blood group antigens) segregate genetically, appearing in some but not all members of a species. When an antigen is present in some members of the same species but is not common to all members of that species, it is called an alloantigen (also an isoantigen). If an alloantigen is presented to a member of the same species that does not have the alloantigen, it will be recognized as foreign and antibodies called alloantibodies (isoantibodies) will be produced against it.[71]

Blood group alloantigens are detected serologically on the surface of erythrocytes using agglutination and/or hemolysis tests. Blood groups have individual chromosomal loci and each locus has from two to many allelic genes. Most blood groups derive their antigenicity from the carbohydrate composition of membrane-associated glycolipids and glycoproteins. Most alloantigens are produced by erythroid cells, but some—such as the J group in cattle, the DEA-7 (Tr) group in dogs, the R group in sheep, and the A and O groups in pigs—are produced by other tissues and adsorbed from plasma.[1,110]

Blood groups in domestic animals have been reviewed.[1,13,110] They have been most extensively characterized in horses and cattle, in which blood typing was routinely used for animal identification and parentage testing. Blood typing for these purposes is being phased out in favor of assays based on DNA sequences. Blood group alloantigens of clinical significance are discussed subsequently under "Transfusion Reactions" and "Neonatal Isoerythrolysis," below.

Ideally, blood typing of donor and recipient animals for clinically significant erythrocyte alloantigens should be performed prior to all blood transfusions, as occurs in human medicine. Point-of-care card and gel typing tests are available for DEA 1.1 in dogs and types A and B in cats.[141] In addition, blood samples from potential donors can be sent to a limited number of commercial laboratories for blood typing, and blood donors can be selected that are negative for clinically significant erythrocyte alloantigens, including DEA 1.1 in dogs and Aa and Qa in horses. The use of blood from these donors, coupled with cross-matching of donor and recipient samples, will minimize the likelihood of severe transfusion reactions.[71]

Blood typing of animals may be done prior to mating to identify animals with the same blood types and to minimize the possibility of subsequent hemolytic reactions (neonatal isoerythrolysis) in newborn animals. This is most frequently done in mares that have previously given birth to foals that developed neonatal isoerythrolysis. It may also be considered in certain breeds of cats where type B blood is common (Table 6-1).[1,57,59,64]

Blood Cross-Match Tests

Blood cross-match tests are used to detect the presence of hemagglutinating and hemolyzing antibodies in the serum of donor and recipient animals. Suspensions of washed erythrocytes are incubated with serum samples, centrifuged, and examined for the presence of hemolysis and gross and microscopic agglutination. The major cross-match is used to detect antibodies in the recipient's serum that are directed against the donor's erythrocytes. The minor cross-match is used to detect antibodies in the donor's serum that are directed against the recipient's erythrocytes. Autoagglutination or severe hemolysis in the patient's blood sample precludes the accurate performance of cross-match tests.[141]

The absence of agglutination or hemolysis in cross-match tests does not indicate that animals have similar blood types. It indicates only that preexisting antibodies were not detected and that an acute hemolytic transfusion reaction is highly unlikely. A delayed transfusion reaction can still occur if important alloantigen differences are present. The benefit of the transfusion is short-lived in delayed transfusion reactions because antibodies made against the donor's erythrocytes result in phagocytosis and removal of these erythrocytes within a few days.[141] Additionally there can be reactions to transfused leukocyte or plasma protein antigens, with adverse reactions varying from urticaria to anaphylactic shock.[77,157]

Tests for Antinuclear Antibodies

The presence of circulating antinuclear antibodies (ANAs) is associated with various autoimmune diseases in humans and animals. ANAs are most often measured in dogs suspected of having systemic lupus erythematosus (SLE). Studies indicate that ANAs in dogs are primarily of the IgG type. Canine ANAs are heterogeneous and may be directed against various histone and nonhistone extractable antigen components of the nucleus but not against native double-stranded DNA.[37]

ANA Test

An indirect immunofluorescent antibody (IFA) technique is most widely used for ANA testing (Fig. 6-2). Typically a dilution of a patient's serum is placed on a glass slide with tissue cells fixed to the surface. After allowing time for the ANAs present in the patient's serum to become bound to the nuclei, the slides are rinsed and fluorescein-labeled antibodies directed against immunoglobulins of the same species as the patient's are added. The slides are again rinsed and the absence or presence of nuclear fluorescence (which occurs when ANAs are present) is determined using a fluorescent microscope. Alternatively, an immunoperoxidase method may be used in place of the immunofluorescent one described. Frozen rodent liver sections have been used most frequently as the substrate in veterinary medicine, but a human epithelial cell line (HEp-2) appears to be a superior ANA substrate because of its low reactivity with normal serum and the ease of reading the fluorescence pattern. Titers above 1/25 and 1/100 are considered

TABLE 6-1

Frequency of Blood Type B in Purebred Cats in the United States[a]

Type B Frequency	Breeds
25%-50%	Exotic shorthair, British shorthair, Cornish Rex, Devon Rex
5%-25%	Abyssinian, Birman, Persian, Himalayan, Somali, Sphynx, Scottish fold, Japanese bobtail
Less than 5%	Main Coon cat, Norwegian forest cat, domestic shorthair, domestic longhair
None	Siamese, Burmese, Tonkinese, Russian Blue, Oriental shorthair, American shorthair, Ocicat

[a]Type A frequency is determined by subtracting type B frequency from 100% because type AB is extremely rare. The table is modified from Andrews[1] and based on data published by Urs Giger and coworkers.[57,59,64]

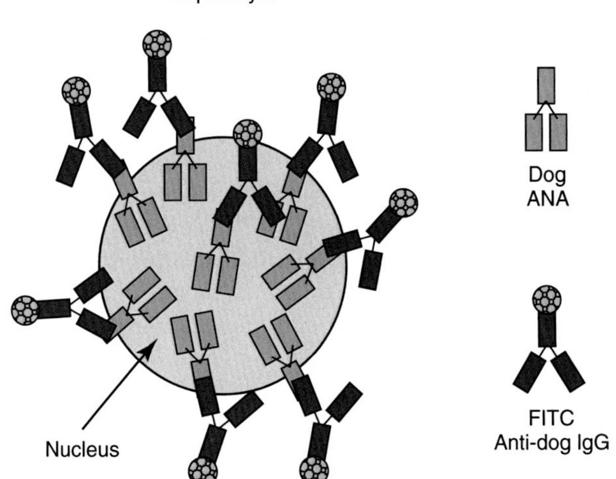

FIGURE 6-2
Antinuclear antibodies (ANA) test. Sections of liver are incubated with test serum and, following washing, the presence of ANA is demonstrated using fluorescein isothiocyanate (FITC)-labeled antibodies against immunoglobulins of the species being tested.

positive in dogs when HEp-2 and rat liver substrates, respectively, are used.[67]

Systemic autoimmune diseases are characterized by high serum ANA titers. This heterogeneous group of disorders may be subclassified as SLE or SLE-related diseases (called mixed connective tissue disease in humans). Two different nuclear staining patterns are recognized using HEp-2 cells as substrate in dogs. Dogs with homogeneous nuclear staining and positive chromosomal staining in mitotic cells are more likely to have SLE, and dogs with speckled nuclear staining and lack of chromosomal staining in mitotic cells are more likely to have SLE-related diseases.[69]

Propylthiouracil (PTU) treatment in cats can produce an immune-mediated disease syndrome characterized by anorexia, lymphadenopathy, weight loss, Coombs'-positive hemolytic anemia, thrombocytopenia, and a positive ANA serum test.[3,115] Chronic experimental hydralazine treatment induced ANA formation in the serum of some Beagle dogs.[4] The serum ANA test is positive in about one-third of Gordon setters with symmetrical lupoid onychodystrophy and black-hair follicular dysplasia, suggesting these may be immune-mediated disorders with a common genetic predisposition.[107] ANAs may also be present in serum from animals with chronic inflammatory, infectious, and neoplastic diseases; however, titers are usually low. In addition, some healthy cats and dogs are weakly ANA-positive.[12,37,60,108,136]

Lupus Erythematosus Cell Test

A lupus erythematosus (LE) cell is a leukocyte (usually a neutrophil) with a single large reddish-purple amorphous inclusion that nearly fills the cytoplasm of the cell (Fig. 6-3). This inclusion represents the nucleus of a damaged leukocyte that has been opsonized by ANA and complement and phagocytized by an intact leukocyte. LE cells occasionally form in vitro in stored anticoagulated blood, bone marrow, and joint fluids. The LE cell test is performed by promoting the formation of LE cells by rupturing leukocytes to expose their nuclear material either by forcing clotted blood through a sieve or by mixing anticoagulated blood vigorously with glass beads. After the leukocytes have been ruptured, the samples are incubated to allow time for LE cell formation. Buffy-coat smears are made, stained, and examined for the presence of LE cells. The finding of a single LE cell is considered a positive test result. With the ready availability of the ANA test, which is more sensitive and less labor-intensive to perform than the LE cell test, the latter test is now seldom done in veterinary laboratories. The advantage of the LE cell test is that it does not require species-specific reagents.[37]

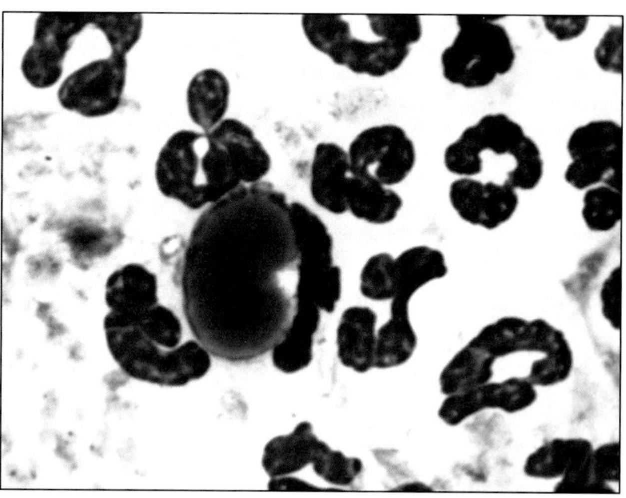

FIGURE 6-3
Lupus erythematosus (LE) cell. Buffy coat smear of an LE cell test demonstrating a LE cell that is a neutrophil containing phagocytized homogeneous nuclear material.

Tests for Antiplatelet Antibodies

A number of tests have been developed to detect antiplatelet antibodies. These include a direct immunofluorescence test using labeled antibodies bound to megakaryocytes and various ways of detecting immunoglobulin bound to platelet surfaces. The microscopic detection of immunofluorescence of megakaryocytes is a subjective test requiring that a bone marrow aspirate be done to obtain megakaryocytes.[90]

Increased platelet-bound immunoglobulins can be detected by flow cytometry,[84,100,156] immunoradiometric,[132] ELISA,[92] and microscopic platelet immunofluorescence asssays.[87] Most antiplatelet antibody in blood is bound to platelets; consequently direct assays of the patient's platelets are more sensitive than indirect assays using the patient's serum and platelets from a healthy control animal.[92] Unfortunately direct assays of platelets should be done within 24 hours after blood sample collection. Platelets naturally have some immunoglobulin adsorbed to their surfaces. The amount of platelet-bound immunoglobulin can increase with time after sample collection; consequently false-positive tests can be a significant problem with these assays.[156] Positive test results may also occur when immune complexes are adsorbed to platelets. False-negative tests may occur if antibodies have eluted from platelets during processing. Since these assays are generally designed to identify IgG on platelets, a false-negative test may result if IgM rather than IgG antibodies are bound to platelets.[132] False-negative tests may occur if assays are done after immunosuppressive therapy is initiated.[120] At this time none of the tests for antiplatelet antibodies are as readily available and as cost-effective as the DAT for antierythrocyte antibodies.

PRIMARY IMMUNE-MEDIATED DISORDERS

Some degree of immune-mediated cellular destruction occurs in many infectious, parasitic, neoplastic, inflammatory, and drug-induced diseases.[104] Disorders presented in this section do not appear to be secondary to other diseases but represent primary immune-mediated disorders.

Transfusion Reactions

Alloantigens vary in their potential to cause hemolytic transfusion reactions when mismatched blood is given. Many alloantigens are weak (do not induce antibodies of high titer) or induce antibodies that do not act at normal body temperature. Fortunately only a few alloantigens appear to be important in producing hemolytic disease in animals.

DEA 1.1 antibody-antigen interactions result in most of the acute hemolytic transfusion reactions in dogs,[1] but transfusion reactions have been reported against DEA 1.2,[65] DEA 4,[103] and an unclassified common antigen[23] on dog erythrocytes. A blood type termed *Dal* has been reported to be lacking in some Dalmatian dogs but is present in a high percentage of dogs other than Dalmatians. Dalmatians lacking the *Dal* antigen are likely at risk of delayed, and possibly acute hemolytic transfusion reactions if transfused with *Dal* antigen-positive blood.[150]

Incompatibilities in the AB blood group of cats has been recognized to cause transfusion reactions.[55,56,76] The A and B alloantigens (blood types) result from the expression of two different alleles at the same gene locus, with A being dominant over B.[1] Cats rarely express both type A and type B antigens (type AB) on erythrocytes. The frequency of blood types varies with location and breed of cat. From 0.3% (Northeast) to 4.7% (West Coast) of domestic short- and long-hair cats in the United States are type B, but up to 50% of purebred cats of certain breeds in the United States are type B.[1] A blood group antigen termed *Mik* has been reported in domestic shorthair cats that is capable of inducing a hemolytic transfusion reaction when *Mik*-positive RBCs are transfused into a *Mik*-negative recipient cat that has naturally occurring anti-*Mik* alloantibodies in its plasma.[150]

Aa and Qa are the most immunogenic alloantigens in horses and presumably the most likely to cause a hemolytic transfusion reaction.[133] A-negative pigs exhibit intravascular hemolysis when transfused with A-positive blood.[110]

For most blood groups in animals, antibody formation occurs only following prior exposure to different erythrocyte alloantigens via transfusion, pregnancy, or vaccination with products containing blood group antigens.[71] Consequently adverse transfusion reactions to unmatched erythrocytes generally do not occur at the time of the first blood transfusion. However, the AB and *Mik* groups in cats and the A group in pigs are characterized by "naturally occurring" antibodies (i.e., antibodies that occur in plasma in the absence of prior exposure to blood from another individual).[140] In these cases, hemolytic transfusion reactions can occur at the time of the first blood transfusion. This is especially true in the case of B-positive cats, which have naturally occurring anti-A antibodies of high hemolytic titer. In contrast, cats with type A blood have weak anti-B antibodies in their blood. Type B blood transfusions given to type A cats do not result in severe intravascular hemolysis, but the transfusion is not efficacious because the transfused erythrocytes are phagocytized and removed within a few days.[19]

Neonatal Isoerythrolysis

Animals with neonatal isoerythrolysis (NI) are healthy at birth but develop hemolytic anemia within a few hours to a few days after they ingest colostrum. Historically, Aa and Qa have been the most common antigens associated with neonatal isoerythrolysis in foals. Mares negative for one of these antigens develop antibodies against them and transfer these antibodies to their foals through colostrum. Hemolysis occurs when the foal inherits the respective antigen from the sire.[13] The dams become sensitized to these foreign erythrocyte antigens from leakage of fetal erythrocytes through the placenta during pregnancy or from exposure to fetal erythrocytes of the same blood type during a previous parturition. Generally the first foal born is unaffected, but subsequent foals carrying the same foreign antigen(s) will likely develop hemolytic anemia. Other alloantigens associated with neonatal isoerythrolysis in foals include Db, Dg, Pa, Qb, Qc, and a combination of Qa, Qb, and Qc.[14,96] Neonatal isoerythrolysis has been reported in mule foals because of an erythrocyte antigen not found in horses but present in some donkeys and mules.[14,143]

NI can occur in type A kittens born to primiparous type B queens because all adult type B cats naturally have high anti-A antibody titers. NI appears to be an important cause of neonatal death ("fading kitten syndrome") in purebred cats from breeds with high frequencies of type B blood (see Table 6-1).[18,58] Clinical signs that may be present include hemoglobinuria, pale mucous membranes, icterus, lethargy, weakness, tachypnea, tachycardia, collapse, and death. Tail-tip necrosis may occur in surviving kittens as a result of cold-acting IgM antibodies or localized thrombus formation.[15]

NI has been recognized in pigs, with antibodies usually directed against alloantigens of the E blood group.[140] Naturally occurring neonatal isoerythrolysis has not been reported in cattle, but it occurs in some calves born to cows previously vaccinated for anaplasmosis or other vaccines of bovine origin containing erythrocyte membranes.[95]

Blood typing of prospective breeding animals can be done to minimize the possibility of NI in offspring. The possibility of offspring developing NI can be evaluated by cross-matching the sire's erythrocytes with the dam's serum during pregnancy. If the potential for NI is identified prior to parturition, colostrum can be withheld from the offspring until a cross-match can be done between the erythrocytes of the offspring and the serum of the mother. If an incompatibility is present, the neonatal animal can be foster-fed for 2 days, allowing it to nurse from the mother after antibodies can no longer be absorbed as a result of gut closure.[6]

Primary Immune-Mediated Hemolytic Anemia

The binding of antibodies and/or complement to erythrocyte surfaces can result in phagocytosis by macrophages and in some case, complement activation and intravascular hemolysis. IMHA may be primary (also called autoimmune hemolytic anemia) or it may occur secondarily to rickettsial, bacterial, protozoal, viral, or hemoplasma infections; neoplasia (especially lymphomas); and toxin or drug exposure.[78,98,104] Vaccination with combination vaccines has been incriminated as a trigger of IMHA in dogs,[43] but subsequent studies were not able to verify this association.[22,24] In an autoimmune response, antibodies are directed against self antigens on erythrocytes. In secondary immune-mediated disorders, the immune response is directed against foreign antigens or altered self antigens, with inadvertent erythrocyte injury.

A diagnosis of IMHA is made if autoagglutination (persisting after saline washing of erythrocytes) is present, a positive DAT test is measured, or flow cytometry for erythrocyte surface immunoglobulin is positive.[104] A diagnosis of primary IMHA is reached by ruling out other disorders known to have concomitant IMHA.

About two-thirds of dogs with IMHA appear to have primary IMHA.[5,125] In contrast, IMHA in noncanine species is usually a secondary, rather than a primary, disorder.[98] Feline leukemia virus (FeLV) and *Mycoplasma haemofelis* are most commonly associated with IMHA in cats.[42,85]

Results from multiple studies of many dogs with primary IMHA have been summarized.* Primary IMHA is typically seen in middle-aged dogs (average age 6 years), with intact and neutered female dogs, neutered male dogs, and cocker spaniel dogs being overrepresented. Autoagglutination is reported to occur in about 60% and the DAT is positive in about 70% of dogs with primary IMHA. Spherocytosis is also present in about 75% of dogs with primary IMHA. Although the presence of spherocytosis strongly suggests that an immune-mediated process is present, other causes of spherocytosis—including exposure to venoms, zinc toxicity, transfusion of stored blood, and hereditary disorders—must be ruled out. Spherocytes are accurately recognized only in dogs because the degree of central pallor is naturally less in other domestic animals.

Anemia in IMHA is often severe, with a mean hematocrit value of about 15%. About two-thirds of dogs with primary IMHA have an absolute reticulocytosis. However, a regenerative response to this hemolytic anemia may be lacking if the onset of anemia is acute or if antibodies and/or complement are directed against reticulocytes or bone marrow precursor cells.[98] Hyperbilirubinemia is present in about 75% of cases and bilirubinuria is present in nearly all cases. Intravascular hemolysis, as evidenced by hemoglobinemia with hemoglobinuria, generally occurs in less than 20% of cases. In most cases of primary IMHA in dogs, increased IgG antibodies are bound to the erythrocytes, but in some cases IgM and/or complement are also bound to the erythrocytes. IgM antibodies and/or complement are most likely involved if autoagglutination or intravascular hemolysis is present.[98]

A leukocytosis (mean total leukocyte count about 32 × $10^3/\mu L$) is present in more than 80% of dogs with primary IMHA. This increase in total leukocyte count is primarily the result of neutrophilia (often with a left shift), but a monocytosis may also be present. Moderate to marked leukocytosis with a left shift indicates probable ischemic necrosis within tissues—including liver, kidney, heart, lung, and spleen—attributable to thromboembolic disease or anemic hypoxia.[101]

*References 22, 24, 78, 83, 97, 116, 125, 149.

Thrombocytopenia is present in about 60% of dogs with this disorder, but only about one-fourth have platelet counts below 50 × $10^3/\mu L$. The thrombocytopenia generally appears to result from increased platelet utilization. The prothrombin time (PT) is prolonged in about one-third of cases, and the activated partial thromboplastin time (APTT) is prolonged in about half of the cases. In addition, fibrin degradation products are often increased in plasma. It appears that many dogs with primary IMHA are in a hypercoagulable state at the time of diagnosis, with disseminated intravascular coagulation (DIC) and multiorgan venous thrombosis (especially pulmonary thrombosis) being common sequelae, which may result in death.

In some instances the concurrent thrombocytopenia also appears to be autoimmune in origin (Evans syndrome).[78] Primary IMHA may also be part of SLE, a multisystemic autoimmune disease.[53,140]

Primary IMHA is much less common in cats than in dogs. Kohn et al.[85] have reported findings from 19 cats with primary IMHA. Affected cats were typically young (median age 2 years). The anemia was generally severe (median hematocrit 12%) and often macrocytic (median MCV 56 fL). An absolute reticulocytosis was reported in less than half of the cases. In contrast to dogs, a leukocytosis was present in only 10% of cats, and about 30% of cats exhibited a lymphocytosis. Thrombocytopenia occurred in about 40% of the cats with primary IMHA, and PT and/or APTT times were prolonged in 30% of the cats evaluated. Hyperbilirubinemia occurred in nearly 70% of cats, with hyperglobulinemia reported in about half of the cats with primary IMHA.

Primary Immune-Mediated Thrombocytopenia

Immune-mediated thrombocytopenia (IMT) occurs when immunoglobulin (primarily IgG) is bound to the surface of platelets, resulting in the premature removal of platelets by macrophages. The presence of IMT is detected by measuring immunoglobulin bound to the patient's platelets (direct assays) or by measuring immunoglobulin in a patient's serum that is capable of binding to platelets collected from a healthy animal of the same species (indirect assay). Direct assays are more sensitive than indirect assays for detecting IMT (see "Tests for Antiplatelet Antibodies," above).

IMT may be primary (autoimmune), or it may occur secondarily to bacterial, viral, protozoal, or helminth infections; neoplasia; or drug administration.* In primary IMT, autoantibodies react to normal platelet antigens. Glycoprotein (GP) IIb and/or IIIa have been recognized as target antigens in some dogs.[91] The GP IIb/IIIa complex is the fibrinogen

*References 10, 26, 29, 35, 40, 63, 72, 88, 92, 123.

receptor essential for normal platelet aggregation. This may help explain the platelet dysfunction that has been measured in dogs with primary IMT.[86] Secondary IMT can occur if immune complexes are absorbed by platelets, if antibodies are produced against a foreign antigen bound to platelets, or if antibodies are reacting to platelet antigens altered in the course of the disease.[120]

Neonatal alloimmune thrombocytopenia has been reported in newborn horses,[20] mules,[122] and pigs.[50] In this disorder, thrombocytopenia develops in the neonate following the ingestion of colostrum containing antibodies against the newborn's platelets. A syndrome of ulcerative dermatitis, thrombocytopenia, and neutropenia has been described in neonatal foals under 4 days of age. Although the etiology was not determined, the authors suggested a possible relationship between colostral antibodies or some other factor in the colostrum and the abnormalities present.[112]

A diagnosis of primary IMT is made after ruling out other potential causes of IMT. In the absence of an antiplatelet antibody test, a presumptive diagnosis of primary IMT is often confirmed by a positive response to glucocorticoid therapy alone or in combination with immunosuppressant drugs (including vincristine, azathioprine, cyclophosphamide) or following splenectomy.[45,75,90] Primary IMT may occur in association with primary IMHA in what has been termed Evans syndrome in the human literature.[62,78,94,120] However, it is important to recognize that animals with IMHA may have accompanying thrombosis or DIC, which may account for the concomitant thrombocytopenia.[24] Primary IMT may also be a component of SLE, to be discussed subsequently.[88]

Although uncommon in animals, primary IMT is diagnosed most often in dogs, in which it occurs about twice as often in females as in males. It can occur at any age but is seen most commonly in middle-aged dogs, with an increased incidence reported most often in cocker spaniels, miniature and toy poodles, Old English sheep dogs, golden retrievers, and German shepherds.[90] Many dogs present with bleeding problems in the absence of other signs of illness, but some animals present with lethargy and weakness attributable to anemia. Gingival bleeding, cutaneous and mucosal petechial and ecchymotic hemorrhages, hematochezia or melena, epistaxis, hematuria, and ocular hemorrhages are common types of hemorrhage observed. Fever occurs in a low percentage of cases, and lymphadenopathy is uncommon, but splenomegaly may be recognized in about half of the cases.[120] Platelet counts in primary IMT (less than $30 \times 10^3/\mu L$ in 80% of cases) are generally lower than counts measured in secondary IMT.[120] Thrombocytopenia may be the only abnormal finding in the complete blood count (CBC), but about half of the dogs with primary IMT have an anemia (median HCT 31%) and 40% of cases have a leukocytosis (median total leukocytes $19 \times 10^3/\mu L$), with a neutrophilia (sometimes with a left shift) and monocytosis. PT and APTT tests are normal.[120]

Primary IMT is less often recognized in cats than in dogs. Cats have generally presented with evidence of hemorrhage including gingival bleeding, cutaneous and mucosal petechial and ecchymotic hemorrhages, epistaxis, hematuria, and hemoptysis. Lethargy is common. Thrombocytopenia is generally marked, and moderate to severe anemia is also generally present.[9,158]

Megakaryocyte numbers are usually increased in the bone marrow in response to the thrombocytopenia,[9] but rare cases of amegakaryocytic thrombocytopenia have been reported in dogs and cats that were believed to be immune-mediated.[52,89,159]

Primary Immune-Mediated Neutropenia

Primary (also termed idiopathic) immune-mediated neutropenia (IMN) appears to be uncommon in dogs and rare in cats.[16,17,31,47,113] This diagnosis is usually made by excluding other causes of neutropenia. Animals may present with fever and lethargy or may be asymptomatic. In these latter cases, neutropenia may be identified during a routine hematologic evaluation as part of an annual physical examination or prior to anesthesia. Some animals may also exhibit other evidence of immune-mediated disease including nonseptic meningitis, nonerosive polyarthritis, vascultitis, and thrombocytopenia.[31,145] Neutropenia is often severe (less than 500 neutrophils per microliter) without toxic cytoplasm in asymptomatic dogs.[16] A lymphocytosis may be present in cats with IMN.[31] Granulocytic hyperplasia with few mature neutrophils is most likely to be present in the bone marrow, but granulocytic hypoplasia or aplasia may occur when antigens on early neutrophil precursors are targeted.[31,152]

A number of diagnostic tests (including flow cytometry, immunofluorescence, leukoagglutination, and radioimmunoasssay) have been developed to detect increased antineutrophil antibodies.[151] Unfortunately these tests are not readily available and need further study to demonstrate their clinical usefulness. Consequently a diagnosis of IMN is generally made by excluding other causes of neutropenia. A substantial increase in neutrophil numbers in blood within 1 to 3 days after beginning immunosuppressive treatments with corticosteroids provides retrospective evidence for an IMN.

Systemic Lupus Erythematosus

Systemic autoimmune diseases are characterized by high serum ANA titers. This heterogeneous group of disorders may be subclassified as SLE or SLE-related diseases (called mixed connective tissue disease in humans). This latter category is largely characterized by musculoskeletal disorders, lethargy, and/or fever. Dogs with SLE also often exhibit polyarthritis but are more likely to have glomerulonephritis and hematologic disorders than are dogs with SLE-related diseases.[69] ANA-positive musculoskeletal disorders described in German shepherd and Nova Scotia duck-tolling retriever dogs may be considered SLE-related diseases.[68,69] Criteria for these subclassifications are not clearly established in animals. Proposed criteria for a diagnosis of SLE are given in Box 6-1.[135,138]

SLE is a chronic autoimmune disease characterized by the production of a variety of autoantibodies (especially antinuclear antibodies) that result in immune-mediated injury of

BOX 6-1 Diagnostic Criteria for Systemic Lupus Erythematosus (SLE)[a]

Major signs
Polyarthritis
Glomerulonephritis
Skin lesions
Polymyositis
Thrombocytopenia
Hemolytic anemia
Leukopenia

Minor signs
Fever of unknown origin
Central nervous system signs, seizures
Oral ulcerations
Lymphadenopathy
Pericarditis
Pleuritis

[a]SLE is diagnosed if two major signs are present with a high ANA titer (e.g., equal to or greater than 160) or one major sign and two minor signs are present with a high ANA titer. SLE is considered possible if one major sign and a high ANA titer is present or if two major signs are present but the ANA titer is low (<160).[135,138]

multiple organs. Abnormal T lymphocyte activation appears to prompt B lymphocytes to produce excessive amounts of autoantibodies. However, the exact mechanisms for the development of SLE remain unclear because the pathogenesis is a complex multifactorial event, with many abnormalities measured in the immune system of humans.[33]

SLE is fairly common in dogs but rare in cats and horses.[37] Possible manifestations of SLE are persistent or recurring fever, nonerosive polyarthritis, renal disorders, facial or mucocutaneous dermatitis, lymphadenopathy and/or splenomegaly, leukopenia, anemia (often DAT-positive), thrombocytopenia, polymyositis, and pleuropericarditis.[37] A diagnosis of SLE should be considered when several of these inflammatory processes are recognized in a patient that has a high serum ANA titer (see "Tests for Antinuclear Antibodies," above).

TESTS FOR IMMUNE DEFICIENCY DISORDERS

Neutrophil Function Tests

Numerous steps are required for neutrophil adhesion, chemotaxis, phagocytosis, and killing of bacteria; consequently a variety of tests are needed to fully assess neutrophil function.[27,153] These tests are not available in most commercial laboratories but are done in a limited number of research laboratories. Adhesion assays measure the ability of neutrophils to adhere to inorganic materials, including polysaccharides or nylon fibers, or biological structures, such as cultured endothelial cells. Chemotaxis assays measure the ability of neutrophils to migrate in the direction of various chemoattractants. The ability to phagocytize microbes can be determined microscopically. Microbial phagocytosis and killing can be assayed by bacterial culture after bacteria, serum, and neutrophils are incubated together. Lysosomal enzymes can be assayed following neutrophil lysis. The nitroblue tetrazolium (NBT) reduction test and the chemiluminescence test detect the presence of the oxidant burst needed for normal bacterial killing.

In addition to the classic assays discussed above, many assays using flow cytometry have been developed. These assays include measurement of increased F-actin as evidence of neutrophil activation, measurement of surface adhesion molecules using adhesion molecule-specific monoclonal antibodies, phagocytosis of fluorescently conjugated particles, and measurement of reactive oxygen molecules such as the dichlorofluorescein (DCF) assay.[27] The tests discussed are screening tests. More specialized tests are required to demonstrate specific molecular defects.

Lymphocyte Assays

A majority of circulating lymphocytes are T lymphocytes. Consequently the presence of a normal absolute blood lymphocyte count tends to rule out a generalized defect in T lymphocyte production. Lymphocyte blastogenic assays are used to determine the responsiveness of lymphocytes to various mitogens, which variably stimulate different lymphocyte subsets. T lymphocyte function may also be assessed in vitro using leukocyte migration inhibition assays, cytokine release assays, and cytotoxicity assays. Subpopulations of lymphocytes can be quantified using fluorescence labeling of surface molecules and flow cytometry.[140] For example, using flow cytometry, cats with feline immunodeficiency virus (FIV) infection have been shown to have reduced populations of $CD4^+$ T lymphocytes.[38]

Serum Immunoglobulin Assays

A variety of methods may be used to determine whether immunoglobulin deficiencies are present. Routine serum protein electrophoresis may be used as a screening test because immunoglobulins account for all of the protein that migrates in the γ region and some of the protein that migrates in the β region of electrophoretic gels (Fig. 6-4). A low γ-globulin concentration points to an immunoglobulin (usually IgG) deficiency. Various immunoelectrophoretic techniques can be used to make qualitative and quantitative serum immunoglobulin measurements. Specific immunoglobulin classes may be quantified using various methods, including immunofixation electrophoresis, radial immunodiffusion, ELISA, and turbidometric assays.[2,54,140] Reference intervals are generally established using adult animals. Consequently it is important not to overemphasize seemingly low serum immunoglobulin values in young animals. In dogs, for example, serum IgM concentrations may not reach adult reference intervals until several months after birth; serum IgG and IgA values may not reach adult reference values until such animals are 1 year of age or older (in the case of IgA).[46] Several semiquantitative

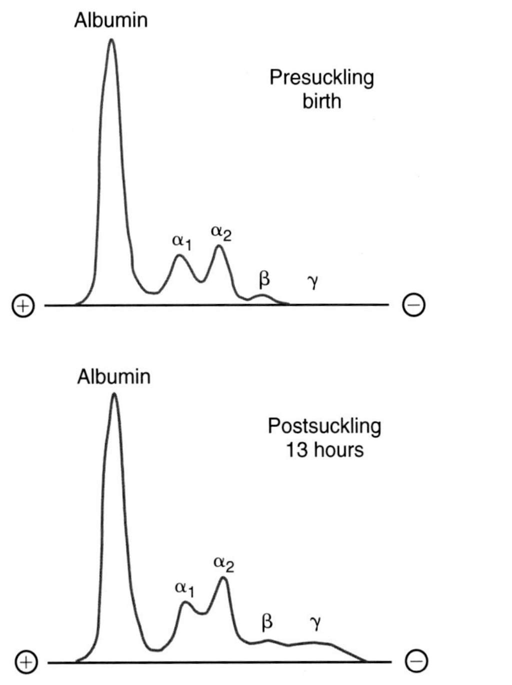

FIGURE 6-4

Serum protein electrophoretograms for a foal before and after suckling. The serum IgG concentration was less than 200 mg/dL before suckling and greater than 800 mg/dL after suckling.

tests—including zinc sulfate turbidity, glutaraldehyde coagulation, sodium sulfite precipitation, and immunoassays—have been used to screen for the failure of the passive transfer of immunity via colostrum in neonatal animals.[34,148]

IMMUNODEFICIENCY DISORDERS

Clinical Signs

Animals with immunodeficiencies generally suffer from recurrent and chronic infections. Common conditions that may be present include respiratory infections, diarrhea, dermatitis, pyoderma, otitis, and growth retardation. Infections with opportunistic organisms, such as *Pneumocystis* and *Cryptosporidium* species, also suggest the presence of an immunodeficiency. Animals with B lymphocyte defects generally have increased susceptibility to bacterial infections, and animals with T lymphocyte defects typically have increased susceptibility to viral, fungal, and protozoal infections. Animals with neutrophil defects generally have cutaneous and systemic infections with pyogenic bacteria.[46]

Inherited Neutrophil Defects

A number of inherited defects of neutrophils have been described. These include the Chédiak-Higashi syndrome in several animal species, β_2-integrin adhesion molecule deficiencies in dogs and cattle, bactericidal defects in dogs, and cyclic hematopoiesis in gray collie dogs. These disorders are discussed in Chapter 5.

Severe Combined Immunodeficiency

The production of T and B lymphocytes is deficient in severe combined immunodeficiency (SCID) syndromes.

Severe Combined Immunodeficiency Syndrome in Arabian Foals

SCID is transmitted as an autosomal recessive trait in Arabian foals. Affected foals have few or no circulating lymphocytes, hypoplasia of the primary and secondary lymphoid organs, and an inability to produce antibodies due to the absence of mature T and B lymphocytes. Failure to produce mature lymphocytes results from a mutation in the gene that encodes for the catalytic subunit of DNA-dependent protein kinase (DNA-PKCS). This enzyme is required for the gene rearrangement process that produces the antigen receptors on T and B lymphocytes. NK cell function is normal. The serum of foals collected prior to suckling normally contains some IgM, but this is not the case in SCID foals.[118] If affected foals suckle successfully shortly after birth, they acquire immunoglobulins from the mare and generally appear healthy. Once maternal immunoglobulins are catabolized, SCID foals become susceptible to a variety of overwhelming infections by pathogens, including equine adenovirus, *Rhodococcus equi*, *Pneumocystis carinii*, and *Cryptosporidium parvum*. They generally die by 2 to 5 months of age.[114,139,154]

Severe Combined Immunodeficiency Syndrome in Jack Russell Terriers

Like Arabian foals, affected Jack Russell pups also have a defect in the *DNA-PKCS* gene that appears to be transmitted as an autosomal recessive trait. Affected pups have profound lymphopenia, decreased serum immunoglobulins, and hypoplasia of all lymphoid organs. These SCID dogs generally die between 8 and 14 weeks of age.[8,102]

X-linked Severe Combined Immunodeficiency Syndrome in Dogs

An X-linked SCID syndrome has been recognized in Basset Hound and Cardigan Welsh Corgi dogs.[79,119] Affected male dogs fail to thrive; exhibit increased susceptibilities to bacterial, viral, and protozoal pathogens; lack palpable peripheral lymph nodes; and generally die by 5 to 6 months of age unless they are housed in a germ-free environment.[139] Absolute blood lymphocyte counts are generally decreased or in the low-normal range because T lymphocyte numbers are low. NK cell production is also reduced, but B lymphocyte counts may be increased in blood. B lymphocytes are unresponsive to T lymphocyte-dependent mitogens but respond to T lymphocyte-independent mitogens. B lymphocytes exhibit normal IgM production, but isotype class switching does not occur; consequently IgG and IgA concentrations are markedly reduced in blood.[70] Mutations of the common γ-chain gene that encodes for essential components of interleukin (IL)-2, IL-4, IL-7, IL-9, and IL-15 receptors have been shown to cause X-linked SCID syndrome in dogs.[73,139]

Serum Immunoglobulin Deficiencies

A heterogeneous group of disorders can result in reduced serum immunoglobulins in humans and animals. The specific defect that produces these abnormalities in animals is generally unknown.

Common Variable Immunodeficiency

Common variable immunodeficiency (CVID) in humans is characterized by reduced immunoglobulin (IgG, IgA, and/or IgM) concentrations in serum and increased susceptibility to infection. Several genetic defects have been reported to result in this phenotype in humans. Each defect disrupts B lymphocyte differentiation, maturation, and/or function.[28] Symptoms generally do not develop until young adulthood, but they may develop in children as young as 5 years old.[61]

CVID has been reported in adult horses (mean age about 11 years) with fever, persistent, multifocal bacterial infections (including pneumonia, meningitis, and septicemia), markedly decreased concentrations of IgM, moderately to markedly decreased concentrations of IgG, and variably decreased concentrations of IgA in serum resulting from markedly reduced numbers of B lymphocytes in lymphoid organs and blood.[48,109] Hematology findings included variable or persistent lymphopenia and frequent neutrophilia and hyperfibrinogenemia associated with infections. Lymphocyte proliferation assays generally revealed decreased responses to both B and T lymphocyte mitogens. The etiology of equine CVID is unknown.

A late-onset immunodeficiency has been reported in Sharpei dogs that is similar to CVID in humans. Increased susceptibility to infection beginning at about 3 years of age is reported. Serum IgA and IgM concentrations are low in most dogs, and serum IgG concentration is low in some. Abnormalities in T as well as B lymphocyte function are demonstrated in some dogs.[126]

CVID has been reported in seven young (less than 1 year old) miniature dachshund dogs with *Pneumocystis carinii* pneumonia. Abnormal findings included a lack of B lymphocytes in lymph nodes, decreased serum concentrations of all immunoglobulins measured, and abnormal responses of blood lymphocytes to mitogens.[93]

Fell Pony Syndrome

A primary immunodeficiency syndrome has been described in Fell ponies. Affected foals typically become ill at 2 to 4 weeks of age. They lose body mass and develop chronic infections with multiple systemic signs, including fever, diarrhea, mucopurulent ocular and/or nasal discharges, and bronchopneumonia. Lymphopenia and severe normocytic normochromic anemia with marrow erythroid hypoplasia are typically present.[131] Serum IgA and IgM concentrations are consistently low and serum IgG concentration is sometimes low. B lymphocyte numbers are markedly reduced in blood, lymph nodes, spleen, and bone marrow.

Selective Immunoglobulin Deficiencies

A number of selective immunoglobulin deficiencies have been described in domestic animals. These include IgM deficiency in horses and dogs,[46,117] IgA deficiency in dogs,[36,46] IgG deficiency in a foal,[21] and IgG_2 deficiency in cattle.[51]

Immunodeficiency in Cavalier King Charles Spaniels

Adult Cavalier King Charles spaniels with *Pneumocystis* pneumonia have been described with low (about 40% of normal) serum IgG concentration, normal serum IgA concentrations, and increased serum IgM concentrations. The authors speculate that a defect might exist in the ability of antigen-activated B lymphocytes to switch immunoglobulin class from IgM to IgG.[147]

X-linked Agammaglobulinemia in Foals

A possible X-linked agammaglobulinemia has been described in thoroughbred and standard-bred foals that have no identifiable B lymphocytes in blood. IgG, IgM, and IgA are low or absent, but T lymphocyte function appears to be normal.[46]

Immunodeficiency in Weimaraner Dogs

A poorly defined immunodeficiency disorder has been described in young (median age 4 months) Weimaraner dogs that is characterized by chronic, recurrent inflammation in various tissues, including bowel, skin, and the central nervous system. Metaphyseal osteopathy is also often present. Low concentrations of immunoglobulin (primarily IgG and less often IgM and/or IgA) are present, and some studies suggest a concomitant neutrophil function defect.[32,49,66]

Transient Hypogammaglobulinemia in Neonates

Transient hypogammaglobulinemia may occur in young animals if the onset of IgG and IgA production by the neonate is delayed following the disappearance of maternal antibodies at about 2 months of age. Deficient animals are susceptible to bacterial infections until their immune systems become fully functional at about 6 months of age.[46]

T Lymphocyte Immunodeficiency

T Lymphocyte Immunodeficiency in Growth Hormone-Deficient Dogs

An inbred family of Weimaraner dogs has been described with a fatal wasting syndrome, retarded growth, persistent infections, and anemia beginning at about 6 weeks of age. These pups had abnormalities in growth hormone metabolism and in thymus-dependent immune function. The thymus was small and depleted of T lymphocytes. B lymphocyte function appeared to be normal, with serum immunoglobulin concentrations within reference intervals.[128,129]

Hypotrichosis with Thymic Aplasia in Cats

This autosomal recessive disease results in lack of hair growth (nude kittens), lack of thymic development, and profound immunodeficiency in Birman kittens. Kittens fail to thrive, succumb to infections, and die within a few weeks.[25]

Lethal Acrodermatitis in English Bull Terriers

Acrodermatitis in English bull terriers is an autosomal recessive disease that is reported to result from impaired absorption and/or metabolism of zinc. Affected dogs have growth retardation and develop hyperkeratosis, parakeratosis, skin infections, diarrhea, and pneumonia. T lymphocyte function is impaired and there is lymphocyte depletion in the T lymphocyte area within lymphoid tissues. Serum zinc and copper concentrations are usually low, but zinc supplementation is not effective and the dogs generally die within 15 months of age.[80,99,144]

Complement Deficiency in Brittany Spaniel Dogs

An inherited deficiency of the third component of complement (C3) has been reported as an autosomal recessive trait in Brittany spaniel dogs. Homozygous affected animals suffer from recurrent sepsis, pneumonia, pyometra, and renal disease. Humoral immune responses to both T lymphocyte-dependent and T lymphocyte-independent antigens are defective in affected dogs.[11]

Viral Immune Deficiency Disorders

A number of viral immune deficiency disorders have been recognized in animals, a few of which are listed here. Feline acquired immunodeficiency syndrome (AIDS) is caused by FIV. Infected cats may be asymptomatic for months to years before signs of severe chronic inflammatory or neoplastic diseases are observed.[134] Increased susceptibility to infectious agents is associated with neutropenia and/or lymphopenia and decreased numbers of $CD4^+$ T lymphocytes.[137,142] A similar syndrome has been reported in primates with simian immunodeficiency virus (SIV) infections.[41]

FeLV is a potent immunosuppressive virus. There is an early loss of T_H lymphocyte function followed by a progressive depletion of $CD4^+$ T lymphocytes and eventually panlymphoid depletion.[39] Lymphopenia is generally not present in healthy infected cats[74,124] but is often present when animals become ill with FeLV-induced AIDS.[105] FeLV-positive cats are predisposed to a variety of secondary infections.

Other infectious diseases found to induce secondary immune deficiencies of T and/or B lymphocytes include canine distemper virus,[130] fetal equine herpesvirus I infection,[111] and bovine viral diarrhea virus in calves.[82]

Failure of Passive Transfer of Immunoglobulins

Failure of passive transfer of immunoglobulins is an acquired immunodeficiency disorder. Prior to suckling, newborn domestic animals have extremely low amounts of immunoglobulin in their plasma. Colostrum is rich in IgG and IgA but also contains some IgM and IgE. Colostral immunoglobulins (especially IgG) can be absorbed intact through an animal's small intestine during the first day of life.[140] If insufficient or poor-quality colostrum is produced, the intake of colostrum is inadequate, or if there is a failure of intestinal absorption, the neonate may not obtain sufficient antibodies to provide the necessary protection against bacterial infections (especially septicemia).[44,127,140] The reader may refer to "Serum Immunoglobulin Assays," above, for tests used to detect the failure of passive transfer. Reference values for plasma IgG in neonatal animals vary depending on the species being analyzed and the method used. In general, serum IgG concentrations below 400 mg/dL are considered inadequate, concentrations from 400 to 800 mg/dL are considered marginal, and concentrations above 800 mg/dL are considered sufficient when measured in foals 1 to 2 days after birth. Serum IgG concentration is considered adequate in calves if serum IgG concentrations exceed 1000 mg/dL.[140]

REFERENCES

1. Andrews GA. Red blood cell antigens and blood groups in the dog and cat. In: Feldman BF, Zinkl JG, Jain NC, eds. *Schalm's Veterinary Hematology.* 5th ed. Philadelphia: Lippincott Williams & Wilkins; 2000:767-773.
2. Attaelmannan M, Levinson SS. Understanding and identifying monoclonal gammopathies. *Clin Chem.* 2000;46:1230-1238.
3. Aucoin DP, Rubin RL, Peterson ME, et al. Dose-dependent induction of anti-native DNA antibodies in cats by propylthiouracil. *Arthritis Rheum.* 1988;31:688-692.
4. Balazs T, Robinson CJ, Balter N. Hydralazine-induced antinuclear antibodies in beagle dogs. *Toxicol Appl Pharmacol.* 1981;57:452-456.
5. Balch A, Mackin A. Canine immune-mediated hemolytic anemia: pathophysiology, clinical signs, and diagnosis. *Compend Contin Educ Vet.* 2007;29:217-225.
6. Barker RN. Anemia associated with immune responses. In: Feldman BF, Zinkl JG, Jain NC, eds. *Schalm's Veterinary Hematology.* 5th ed. Philadelphia: Lippincott Williams & Wilkins; 2000:169-177.
7. Barker RN, Gruffydd-Jones TJ, Elson CJ. Red cell-bound immunoglobulins and complement measured by an enzyme-linked antiglobulin test in dogs with autoimmune haemolysis or other anaemias. *Res Vet Sci.* 1993;54:170-178.
8. Bell TG, Butler KL, Sill HB, et al. Autosomal recessive severe combined immunodeficiency of Jack Russell terriers. *J Vet Diagn Invest.* 2002;14:194-204.
9. Bianco D, Armstrong PJ, Washabau RJ. Presumed primary immune-mediated thrombocytopenia in four cats. *J Feline Med Surg.* 2008;10:495-500.
10. Bloom JC, Thiem PA, Sellers TS, et al. Cephalosporin-induced immune cytopenia in the dog: demonstration of erythrocyte-, neutrophil-, and platelet-associated IgG following treatment with cefazedone. *Am J Hematol.* 1988;28:71-78.
11. Blum JR, Cork LC, Morris JM, et al. The clinical manifestations of a genetically determined deficiency of the third component of complement in the dog. *Clin Immunol Immunopathol.* 1985;34:304-315.
12. Bohnhorst JO, Hanssen I, Moen T. Immune-mediated fever in the dog. Occurrence of antinuclear antibodies, rheumatoid factor, tumor necrosis factor and interleukin-6 in serum. *Acta Vet Scand.* 2002;43:165-171.
13. Bowling AT. Red blood cell antigens and blood groups in the horse. In: Feldman BF, Zinkl JG, Jain NC, eds. *Schalm's Veterinary Hematology.* 5th ed. Philadelphia: Lippincott Williams & Wilkins; 2000:774-777.
14. Boyle AG, Magdesian KG, Ruby RE. Neonatal isoerythrolysis in horse foals and a mule foal: 18 cases (1988-2003). *J Am Vet Med Assoc.* 2005;227:1276-1283.
15. Bridle KH, Littlewood JD. Tail tip necrosis in two litters of Birman kittens. *J Small Anim Pract.* 1998;39:88-89.
16. Brown CD, Parnell NK, Schulman RL, et al. Evaluation of clinicopathologic features, response to treatment, and risk factors associated with idiopathic neutropenia in dogs: 11 cases (1990-2002). *J Am Vet Med Assoc.* 2006;229:87-91.
17. Brown MR, Rogers KS. Neutropenia in dogs and cats: a retrospective study of 261 cases. *J Am Anim Hosp Assoc.* 2001;37:131-139.
18. Bücheler J. Fading kitten syndrome and neonatal isoerythrolysis. *Vet Clin North Am Small Anim Pract.* 1999;29:853-870.
19. Bücheler J, Giger U. Alloantibodies against A and B blood types in cats. *Vet Immunol Immunopathol.* 1993;38:283-295.
20. Buechner-Maxwell V, Scott MA, Godber L, et al. Neonatal alloimmune thrombocytopenia in a quarter horse foal. *J Vet Intern Med.* 1997;11:304-308.
21. Buntain B. IgG immunodeficiency in a half-Arabian foal with salmonellosis. *Vet Med Small Anim Clin.* 1981;76:231-234.
22. Burgess K, Moore A, Rand W, et al. Treatment of immune-mediated hemolytic anemia in dogs with cyclophosphamide. *J Vet Intern Med.* 2000;14:456-462.

23. Callan MB, Jones LT, Giger U. Hemolytic transfusion reactions in a dog with an alloantibody to a common antigen. *J Vet Intern Med.* 1995;9:277-279.
24. Carr AP, Panciera DL, Kidd L. Prognostic factors for mortality and thromboembolism in canine immune-mediated hemolytic anemia: a retrospective study of 72 dogs. *J Vet Intern Med.* 2002;16:504-509.
25. Casal ML, Straumann U, Sigg C, et al. Congenital hypotrichosis with thymic aplasia in nine birman kittens. *J Am Anim Hosp Assoc.* 1994;30:600-602.
26. Clabough DL, Gebhard D, Flaherty MT, et al. Immune-mediated thrombocytopenia in horses infected with equine infectious anemia virus. *J Virol.* 1991;65:6242-6251.
27. Comazzi S. Evaluation of neutrophil function. In: Weiss DJ, Wardrop KJ, eds. *Schalm's Veterinary Hematology.* 6th ed. Ames, IA: Wiley-Blackwell; 2010:1114-1122.
28. Conley ME, Dobbs AK, Farmer DM, et al. Primary B cell immunodeficiencies: comparisons and contrasts. *Annu Rev Immunol.* 2009;27:199-227.
29. Cortese L, Sica M, Piantedosi D, et al. Secondary immune-mediated thrombocytopenia in dogs naturally infected by *Leishmania infantum. Vet Rec.* 2009;164:778-782.
30. Corthay A. How do regulatory T cells work? *Scand J Immunol.* 2009;70:326-336.
31. Couto CG. Immune-mediated neutropenia. In: Feldman BF, Zinkl JG, Jain NC, eds. *Schalm's Veterinary Hematology.* 5th ed. Philadelphia: Lippincott Williams & Wilkins; 2000:815-818.
32. Couto CG, Krakowka S, Johnson G, et al. In vitro immunologic features of Weimaraner dogs with neutrophil abnormalities and recurrent infections. *Vet Immunol Immunopathol.* 1989;23:103-112.
33. Crispin JC, Liossis SN, Kis-Toth K, et al. Pathogenesis of human systemic lupus erythematosus: recent advances. *Trends Mol Med.* 2010;16:47-57.
34. Davis R, Giguère S. Evaluation of five commercially available assays and measurement of serum total protein concentration via refractometry for the diagnosis of failure of passive transfer of immunity in foals. *J Am Vet Med Assoc.* 2005;227:1640-1645.
35. Davis WM. Hapten-induced immune-mediated thrombocytopenia in a dog. *J Am Vet Med Assoc.* 1984;184:976-977.
36. Day MJ. Possible immunodeficiency in related rottweiler dogs. *J Small Anim Pract.* 1999;40:561-568.
37. Day MJ. Systemic lupus erythematosus. In: Feldman BF, Zinkl JG, Jain NC, eds. *Schalm's Veterinary Hematology.* 5th ed. Philadelphia: Lippincott Williams & Wilkins; 2000:819-826.
38. de Parseval A, Chatterji U, Sun P, et al. Feline immunodeficiency virus targets activated CD4+ T cells by using CD134 as a binding receptor. *Proc Natl Acad Sci U S A.* 2004;101:13044-13049.
39. Diehl LJ, Hoover EA. Early and progressive helper T-cell dysfunction in feline leukemia virus-induced immunodeficiency. *J Acquir Immune Defic Syndr.* 1992;5:1188-1194.
40. Dircks BH, Schuberth HJ, Mischke R. Underlying diseases and clinicopathologic variables of thrombocytopenic dogs with and without platelet-bound antibodies detected by use of a flow cytometric assay: 83 cases (2004-2006). *J Am Vet Med Assoc.* 2009;235:960-966.
41. Dua N, Reubel G, Moore PF, et al. An experimental study of primary feline immunodeficiency virus infection in cats and a historical comparison to acute simian and human immunodeficiency virus diseases. *Vet Immunol Immunopathol.* 1994; 43:337-355.
42. Dunn JK, Searcy GP, Hirsch VM. The diagnostic significance of a positive direct antiglobulin test in anemic cats. *Can J Comp Med.* 1984;48:349-353.
43. Duval D, Giger U. Vaccine-associated immune-mediated hemolytic anemia in the dog. *J Vet Intern Med.* 1996;10:290-295.
44. Fecteau G, Smith BP, George LW. Septicemia and meningitis in the newborn calf. *Vet Clin North Am Food Anim Pract.* 2009;25:195-208.
45. Feldman BF, Handagama P, Lubberink AA. Splenectomy as adjunctive therapy for immune-mediated thrombocytopenia and hemolytic anemia in the dog. *J Am Vet Med Assoc.* 1985;187:617-619.
46. Felsburg PJ. T cell, immunoglobulin, and complement immunodeficiency disorders. In Weiss DJ, Wardrop KJ, eds. *Schalm's Veterinary Hematology.* 6th ed. Ames, IA: Wiley-Blackwell; 2010:400-405.
47. Fidel JL, Pargass IS, Dark MJ, et al. Granulocytopenia associated with thymoma in a domestic shorthaired cat. *J Am Anim Hosp Assoc.* 2008;44:210-217.
48. Flaminio MJ, Tallmadge RL, Salles-Gomes CO, et al. Common variable immunodeficiency in horses is characterized by B cell depletion in primary and secondary lymphoid tissues. *J Clin Immunol.* 2009;29:107-116.
49. Foale RD, Herrtage ME, Day MJ. Retrospective study of 25 young weimaraners with low serum immunoglobulin concentrations and inflammatory disease. *Vet Rec.* 2003;153:553-558.
50. Forster LM. Neonatal alloimmune thrombocytopenia, purpura, and anemia in 6 neonatal piglets. *Can Vet J.* 2007;48:855-857.
51. Francoz D, Lapointe JM, Wellemans V, et al. Immunoglobulin G2 deficiency with transient hypogammaglobulinemia and chronic respiratory disease in a 6-month-old Holstein heifer. *J Vet Diagn Invest.* 2004;16:432-435.
52. Gaschen FP, Smith Meyer B, Harvey JW. Amegakaryocytic thrombocytopenia and immune-mediated haemolytic anaemia in a cat. *Comp Haematol Int.* 1992;2: 175-178.
53. Gershwin LJ. Antinuclear antibodies in domestic animals. *Ann N Y Acad Sci.* 2005;1050:364-370.
54. Gershwin LJ. Bovine immunoglobulin E. *Vet Immunol Immunopathol.* 2009;132: 2-6.
55. Giger U, Akol KG. Acute hemolytic transfusion reaction in an Abyssinian cat with blood group type B. *J Vet Intern Med.* 1990;4:315-316.
56. Giger U, Bücheler J. Transfusion of type-A and type-B blood to cats. *J Am Vet Med Assoc.* 1991;198:411-418.
57. Giger U, Bücheler J, Patterson DF. Frequency and inheritance of A and B blood types in feline breeds of the United States. *J Hered.* 1991;82:15-20.
58. Giger U, Casal ML. Feline colostrum–friend or foe: maternal antibodies in queens and kittens. *J Reprod Fertil Suppl.* 1997;51:313-316.
59. Giger U, Griot-Wenk M, Bücheler J, et al. Geographical variation of the feline blood type frequencies in the United States. *Feline Pract.* 1991;19:21-27.
60. Ginel PJ, Lucena R. Investigation of antinuclear antibodies in canine atopic dermatitis. *J Vet Med A Physiol Pathol Clin Med.* 2001;48:193-198.
61. Glocker E, Ehl S, Grimbacher B. Common variable immunodeficiency in children. *Curr Opin Pediatr.* 2007;19:685-692.
62. Goggs R, Boag AK, Chan DL. Concurrent immune-mediated haemolytic anaemia and severe thrombocytopenia in 21 dogs. *Vet Rec.* 2008;163:323-327.
63. Gould SM, McInnes EL. Immune-mediated thrombocytopenia associated with *Angiostrongylus vasorum* infection in a dog. *J Small Anim Pract.* 1999;40:227-232.
64. Griot-Wenk ME, Giger U. Feline transfusion medicine–Blood types and their clinical importance. *Vet Clin North Am Small Anim Pract.* 1995;25:1305-1322.
65. Hale AS. Canine blood groups and their importance in veterinary transfusion medicine. *Vet Clin North Am Small Anim Pract.* 1995;25:1323-1332.
66. Hansen P, Clercx C, Henroteaux M, et al. Neutrophil phagocyte dysfunction in a weimaraner with recurrent infections. *J Small Anim Pract.* 1995;36:128-131.
67. Hansson H, Trowald-Wigh G, Karlsson-Parra A. Detection of antinuclear antibodies by indirect immunofluorescence in dog sera: comparison of rat liver tissue and human epithelial-2 cells as antigenic substrate. *J Vet Intern Med.* 1996;10:199-203.
68. Hansson-Hamlin H, Lilliehook I. A possible systemic rheumatic disorder in the Nova Scotia duck tolling retriever. *Acta Vet Scand.* 2009;51:16.
69. Hansson-Hamlin H, Lilliehook I, Trowald-Wigh G. Subgroups of canine antinuclear antibodies in relation to laboratory and clinical findings in immune-mediated disease. *Vet Clin Pathol.* 2006;35:397-404.
70. Hartnett BJ, Somberg RL, Krakowka S, et al. B-cell function in canine X-linked severe combined immunodeficiency. *Vet Immunol Immunopathol.* 2000;75:121-134.
71. Harvey JW. The erythrocyte: physiology, metabolism and biochemical disorders. In: Kaneko JJ, Harvey JW, Bruss ML, eds. *Clinical Biochemistry of Domestic Animals.* 6th ed. San Diego, CA: Academic Press; 2008:173-240.
72. Helfand SC. Neoplasia and immune-mediated thrombocytopenia. *Vet Clin North Am Small Anim Pract.* 1988;18:267-270.
73. Henthorn PS, Somberg RL, Fimiani VM, et al. IL-2R gamma gene microdeletion demonstrates that canine X-linked severe combined immunodeficiency is a homologue of the human disease. *Genomics.* 1994;23:69-74.
74. Hofmann-Lehmann R, Holznagel E, Ossent P, et al. Parameters of disease progression in long-term experimental feline retrovirus (feline immunodeficiency virus and feline leukemia virus) infections: hematology, clinical chemistry, and lymphocyte subsets. *Clin Diagn Lab Immunol.* 1997;4:33-42.
75. Hoyt PG, Gill MS, Angel KL, et al. Corticosteroid-responsive thrombocytopenia in two beef cows. *J Am Vet Med Assoc.* 2000;217:717-720.
76. Hubler M, Kaelin S, Hagen A, et al. Feline neonatal isoerythrolysis in two litters. *J Small Anim Pract.* 1987;28:833-838.
77. Hurcombe SD, Mudge MC, Hinchcliff KW. Clinical and clinicopathologic variables in adult horses receiving blood transfusions: 31 cases (1999-2005). *J Am Vet Med Assoc.* 2007;231:267-274.
78. Jackson ML, Kruth SA. Immune-mediated hemolytic anemia and thrombocytopenia in the dog: a retrospective study of 55 cases diagnosed from 1979 through 1983 at the Western College of Veterinary Medicine. *Can Vet J.* 1985;26:245-250.
79. Jezyk PF, Felsburg PJ, Haskins ME, et al. X-linked severe combined immunodeficiency in the dog. *Clin Immunol Immunopathol.* 1989;52:173-189.
80. Jezyk PF, Haskins ME, Kay-Smith WE, et al. Lethal acrodermatitis in bull terriers. *J Am Vet Med Assoc.* 1986;188:833-839.
81. Joosten SA, Ottenhoff TH. Human CD4 and CD8 regulatory T cells in infectious diseases and vaccination. *Hum Immunol.* 2008;69:760-770.
82. Kelling CL, Steffen DJ, Topliff CL, et al. Comparative virulence of isolates of bovine viral diarrhea virus type II in experimentally inoculated six- to nine-month-old calves. *Am J Vet Res.* 2002;63:1379-1384.
83. Klag AR, Giger U, Shofer FS. Idiopathic immune-mediated hemolytic anemia in dogs: 42 cases (1986-1990). *J Am Vet Med Assoc.* 1993;202:783-788.

84. Kohn B, Linden T, Leibold W. Platelet-bound antibodies detected by a flow cytometric assay in cats with thrombocytopenia. *J Feline Med Surg.* 2006;8:254-260.
85. Kohn B, Weingart C, Eckmann V, et al. Primary immune-mediated hemolytic anemia in 19 cats: diagnosis, therapy, and outcome (1998-2004). *J Vet Intern Med.* 2006;20:159-166.
86. Kristensen AT, Weiss DJ, Klausner JS. Platelet dysfunction associated with immune-mediated thrombocytopenia in dogs. *J Vet Intern Med.* 1994;8:323-327.
87. Kristensen AT, Weiss DJ, Klausner JS, et al. Comparison of microscopic and flow cytometric detection of platelet antibody in dogs suspected of having immune-mediated thrombocytopenia. *Am J Vet Res.* 1994;55:1111-1114.
88. Kristensen AT, Weiss DJ, Klausner JS, et al. Detection of antiplatelet antibody with a platelet immunofluorescence assay. *J Vet Intern Med.* 1994;8:36-39.
89. Lachowicz JL, Post GS, Moroff SD, et al. Acquired amegakaryocytic thrombocytopenia–four cases and a literature review. *J Small Anim Pract.* 2004;45:507-514.
90. Lewis DC. Immune-mediated thrombocytopenia. In: Feldman BF, Zinkl JG, Jain NC, eds. *Schalm's Veterinary Hematology.* 5th ed. Philadelphia: Lippincott Williams & Wilkins; 2000:807-814.
91. Lewis DC, Meyers KM. Studies of platelet-bound and serum platelet-bindable immunoglobulins in dogs with idiopathic thrombocytopenia purpura. *Exp Hematol.* 1996;24:696-701.
92. Lewis DC, Meyers KM, Callan MB, et al. Detection of platelet-bound and serum platelet-bindable antibodies for diagnosis of idiopathic thrombocytopenic purpura in dogs. *J Am Vet Med Assoc.* 1995;206:47-52.
93. Lobetti R. Common variable immunodeficiency in miniature dachshunds affected with *Pneumonocystis carinii* pneumonia. *J Vet Diagn Invest.* 2000;12:39-45.
94. Lubas G, Ciattini F, Gavazza A. Immune-mediated thrombocytopenia and hemolytic anemia (Evans' syndrome) in a horse. *Equine Pract.* 1997;19:27-32.
95. Luther DG, Cox HU, Nelson WO. Screening for neonatal isohemolytic anemia in calves. *Am J Vet Res.* 1985;46:1078-1079.
96. MacLeay JM. Neonatal isoerythrolysis involving the Qc and Db antigens in a foal. *J Am Vet Med Assoc.* 2001;219:79-81, 50.
97. McAlees TJ. Immune-mediated haemolytic anaemia in 110 dogs in Victoria, Australia. *Aust Vet J.* 2010;88:25-28.
98. McCullough S. Immune-mediated hemolytic anemia: understanding the nemesis. *Vet Clin North Am Small Anim Pract.* 2003;33:1295-1315.
99. McEwan NA, McNeil PE, Thompson H, et al. Diagnostic features, confirmation and disease progression in 28 cases of lethal acrodermatitis of bull terriers. *J Small Anim Pract.* 2000;41:501-507.
100. McGurrin MK, Arroyo LG, Bienzle D. Flow cytometric detection of platelet-bound antibody in three horses with immune-mediated thrombocytopenia. *J Am Vet Med Assoc.* 2004;224:83-87, 53.
101. McManus PM, Craig LE. Correlation between leukocytosis and necropsy findings in dogs with immune-mediated hemolytic anemia: 34 cases (1994-1999). *J Am Vet Med Assoc.* 2001;218:1308-1313.
102. Meek K, Kienker L, Dallas C, et al. SCID in Jack Russell terriers: a new animal model of DNA-PKcs deficiency. *J Immunol.* 2001;167:2142-2150.
103. Melzer KJ, Wardrop KJ, Hale AS, et al. A hemolytic transfusion reaction due to DEA 4 alloantibodies in a dog. *J Vet Intern Med.* 2003;17:931-933.
104. Morley P, Mathes M, Guth A, et al. Anti-erythrocyte antibodies and disease associations in anemic and nonanemic dogs. *J Vet Intern Med.* 2008;22:886-892.
105. Ogilvie GK, Tompkins MB, Tompkins WA. Clinical and immunologic aspects of FeLV-induced immunosuppression. *Vet Microbiol.* 1988;17:287-296.
106. Overmann JA, Sharkey LC, Weiss DJ, et al. Performance of 2 microtiter canine Coombs' tests. *Vet Clin Pathol.* 2007;36:179-183.
107. Ovrebo BJ, Hanssen I, Moen T. Antinuclear antibodies (ANA) in Gordon setters with symmetrical lupoid onychodystrophy and black hair follicular dysplasia. *Acta Vet Scand.* 2001;42:323-329.
108. Pedersen NC. A review of immunologic diseases of the dog. *Vet Immunol Immunopathol.* 1999;69:251-342.
109. Pellegrini-Masini A, Bentz AI, Johns IC, et al. Common variable immunodeficiency in three horses with presumptive bacterial meningitis. *J Am Vet Med Assoc.* 2005;227:114-122, 87.
110. Penedo MCT. Red blood cell antigens and blood groups in the cow, pig, sheep, goat, and llama. In: Feldman BF, Zinkl JG, Jain NC, eds. *Schalm's Veterinary Hematology.* 5th ed. Philadelphia: Lippincott Williams & Wilkins; 2000:778-782.
111. Perkins G, Ainsworth DM, Erb HN, et al. Clinical, haematological and biochemical findings in foals with neonatal equine herpesvirus-1 infection compared with septic and premature foals. *Equine Vet J.* 1999;31:422-426.
112. Perkins GA, Miller WH, Divers TJ, et al. Ulcerative dermatitis, thrombocytopenia, and neutropenia in neonatal foals. *J Vet Intern Med.* 2005;19:211-216.
113. Perkins MC, Canfield P, Churcher RK, et al. Immune-mediated neutropenia suspected in five dogs. *Aust Vet J.* 2004;82:52-57.
114. Perryman LE, McGuire TC, Crawford TB. Maintenance of foals with combined immunodeficiency: causes and control of secondary infections. *Am J Vet Res.* 1978;39:1043-1047.
115. Peterson ME, Hurvitz AI, Leib MS, et al. Propylthiouracil-associated hemolytic anemia, thrombocytopenia, and antinuclear antibodies in cats with hyperthyroidism. *J Am Vet Med Assoc.* 1984;184:806-808.
116. Piek CJ, Junius G, Dekker A, et al. Idiopathic immune-mediated hemolytic anemia: treatment outcome and prognostic factors in 149 dogs. *J Vet Intern Med.* 2008;22:366-373.
117. Plechner AJ. IgM deficiency in 2 Doberman Pinschers. *Mod Vet Pract.* 1979;60:150.
118. Poppie MJ, McGuire TC. Combined immunodeficiency with failure of colostral immunoglobulins transfer in foals. *Vet Rec.* 1976;99:44-46.
119. Pullen RP, Somberg RL, Felsburg PJ, et al. X-linked severe combined immunodeficiency in a family of Cardigan Welsh corgis. *J Am Anim Hosp Assoc.* 1997;33:494-499.
120. Putsche JC, Kohn B. Primary immune-mediated thrombocytopenia in 30 dogs (1997-2003). *J Am Anim Hosp Assoc.* 2008;44:250-257.
121. Quigley KA, Chelack BJ, Haines DM, et al. Application of a direct flow cytometric erythrocyte immunofluorescence assay in dogs with immune-mediated hemolytic anemia and comparison to the direct antiglobulin test. *J Vet Diagn Invest.* 2001;13:297-300.
122. Ramirez S, Gaunt SD, McClure JJ, et al. Detection and effects on platelet function of anti-platelet antibody in mule foals with experimentally induced neonatal alloimmune thrombocytopenia. *J Vet Intern Med.* 1999;13:534-539.
123. Reef VB, Dyson SS, Beech J. Lymphosarcoma and associated immune-mediated hemolytic anemia and thrombocytopenia in horses. *J Am Vet Med Assoc.* 1984;184:313-317.
124. Reimann KA, Bull RW, Crow SE, et al. Immunologic profiles of cats with persistent, naturally acquired feline leukemia virus infection. *Am J Vet Res.* 1986;47:1935-1939.
125. Reimer ME, Troy GC, Warnick LD. Immune-mediated hemolytic anemia: 70 cases (1988-1996). *J Am Anim Hosp Assoc.* 1999;35:384-391.
126. Rivas AL, Tintle L, Argentieri D, et al. A primary immunodeficiency syndrome in Shar-Pei dogs. *Clin Immunol Immunopathol.* 1995;74:243-251.
127. Robinson JA, Allen GK, Green EM, et al. A prospective study of septicaemia in colostrum-deprived foals. *Equine Vet J.* 1993;25:214-219.
128. Roth JA, Kaeberle ML, Grier RL, et al. Improvement in clinical condition and thymus morphologic features associated with growth hormone treatment of immunodeficient dwarf dogs. *Am J Vet Res.* 1984;45:1151-1155.
129. Roth JA, Lomax LG, Altszuler N, et al. Thymic abnormalities and growth hormone deficiency in dogs. *Am J Vet Res.* 1980;41:1256-1262.
130. Schobesberger M, Summerfield A, Doherr MG, et al. Canine distemper virus-induced depletion of uninfected lymphocytes is associated with apoptosis. *Vet Immunol Immunopathol.* 2005;104:33-44.
131. Scholes SF, Holliman A, May PD, et al. A syndrome of anaemia, immunodeficiency and peripheral ganglionopathy in Fell pony foals. *Vet Rec.* 1998;142:128-134.
132. Scott MA, Kaiser L, Davis JM, et al. Development of a sensitive immunoradiometric assay for the detection of platelet surface-associated immunoglobulins in thrombocytopenic dogs. *Am J Vet Res.* 2002;63:124-129.
133. Sellon DC. Blood transfusions in large animals. In: Feldman BF, Zinkl JG, Jain NC, eds. *Schalm's Veterinary Hematology.* 5th ed. Philadelphia: Lippincott Williams & Wilkins; 2000:849-854.
134. Shelton GH, Linenberger ML, Persik MT, et al. Prospective hematologic and clinicopathologic study of asymptomatic cats with naturally acquired feline immunodeficiency virus infection. *J Vet Intern Med.* 1995;9:133-140.
135. Smee NM, Harkin KR, Wilkerson MJ. Measurement of serum antinuclear antibody titer in dogs with and without systemic lupus erythematosus: 120 cases (1997-2005). *J Am Vet Med Assoc.* 2007;230:1180-1183.
136. Smith BE, Tompkins MB, Breitschwerdt EB. Antinuclear antibodies can be detected in dog sera reactive to Bartonella vinsonii subsp. berkhoffii, Ehrlichia canis, or Leishmania infantum antigens. *J Vet Intern Med.* 2004;18:47-51.
137. Sparkes AH, Hopper CD, Millard WG, et al. Feline immunodeficiency virus infection. Clinicopathologic findings in 90 naturally occurring cases. *J Vet Intern Med.* 1993;7:85-90.
138. Stull JW, Evason M, Carr AP, et al. Canine immune-mediated polyarthritis: clinical and laboratory findings in 83 cases in western Canada (1991-2001). *Can Vet J.* 2008;49:1195-1203.
139. Suter SE. Severe combined immunodeficiency. In: Weiss DJ, Wardrop KJ, eds. *Schalm's Veterinary Hematology.* 6th ed. Ames, IA: Wiley-Blackwell; 2010.
140. Tizard IR. *Veterinary Immunology. An Introduction.* 8th ed. Philadelphia: Saunders Elsevier; 2009.
141. Tocci LJ, Ewing PJ. Increasing patient safety in veterinary transfusion medicine: an overview of pretransfusion testing. *J Vet Emerg Crit Care (San Antonio).* 2009;19:66-73.
142. Tompkins MB, Nelson PD, English RV, et al. Early events in the immunopathogenesis of feline retrovirus infections. *J Am Vet Med Assoc.* 1991;199:1311-1315.
143. Traub-Dargatz JL, McClure JJ, Koch C, et al. Neonatal isoerythrolysis in mule foals. *J Am Vet Med Assoc.* 1995;206:67-70.

144. Uchida Y, Moon-Fanelli AA, Dodman NH, et al. Serum concentrations of zinc and copper in bull terriers with lethal acrodermatitis and tail-chasing behavior. *Am J Vet Res.* 1997;58:808-810.
145. Vargo CL, Taylor SM, Haines DM. Immune mediated neutropenia and thrombocytopenia in 3 giant schnauzers. *Can Vet J.* 2007;48:1159-1163.
146. Wardrop KJ. The Coombs' test in veterinary medicine: past, present, future. *Vet Clin Pathol.* 2005;34:325-334.
147. Watson PJ, Wotton P, Eastwood J, et al. Immunoglobulin deficiency in Cavalier King Charles Spaniels with *Pneumocystis* pneumonia. *J Vet Intern Med.* 2006;20:523-527.
148. Weaver DM, Tyler JW, VanMetre DC, et al. Passive transfer of colostral immunoglobulins in calves. *J Vet Intern Med.* 2000;14:569-577.
149. Weinkle TK, Center SA, Randolph JF, et al. Evaluation of prognostic factors, survival rates, and treatment protocols for immune-mediated hemolytic anemia in dogs: 151 cases (1993-2002). *J Am Vet Med Assoc.* 2005;226:1869-1880.
150. Weinstein NM, Blais MC, Harris K, et al. A newly recognized blood group in domestic shorthair cats: the Mik red cell antigen. *J Vet Intern Med.* 2007;21:287-292.
151. Weiss DJ. Evaluation of antineutrophil IgG antibodies in persistently neutropenic dogs. *J Vet Intern Med.* 2007;21:440-444.
152. Weiss DJ, Henson M. Pure white cell aplasia in a dog. *Vet Clin Pathol.* 2007;36:373-375.
153. Weiss DJ, Walcheck B. Neutrophil function. In: Kaneko JJ, Harvey JW, Bruss ML, eds. *Clinical Biochemistry of Domestic Animals.* 6th ed. San Diego, CA: Academic Press; 2008:331-350.
154. Wiler R, Leber R, Moore BB, et al. Equine severe combined immunodeficiency: a defect in V(D)J recombination and DNA-dependent protein kinase activity. *Proc Natl Acad Sci U S A.* 1995;92:11485-11489.
155. Wilkerson MJ, Davis E, Shuman W, et al. Isotype-specific antibodies in horses and dogs with immune-mediated hemolytic anemia. *J Vet Intern Med.* 2000;14:190-196.
156. Wilkerson MJ, Shuman W. Alterations in normal canine platelets during storage in EDTA anticoagulated blood. *Vet Clin Pathol.* 2001;30:107-113.
157. Wilson EM, Holcombe SJ, Lamar A, et al. Incidence of transfusion reactions and retention of procoagulant and anticoagulant factor activities in equine plasma. *J Vet Intern Med.* 2009;23:323-328.
158. Wondratschek C, Weingart C, Kohn B. Primary immune-mediated thrombocytopenia in cats. *J Am Anim Hosp Assoc.* 2010;46:12-19.
159. Zini E, Hauser B, Meli ML, et al. Immune-mediated erythroid and megakaryocytic aplasia in a cat. *J Am Vet Med Assoc.* 2007;230:1024-1027.

CHAPTER

7

EVALUATION OF HEMOSTASIS: COAGULATION AND PLATELET DISORDERS

Hemostasis depends on vascular integrity, platelet numbers and function, and coagulation. Vascular integrity is determined in large measure by the health of endothelial cells and their extracellular matrix. Damage to vessel walls can result in hemorrhage and/or activation of platelets and coagulation. When arteries are severed, there is a transient reflex vasoconstriction that slows the loss of blood and allows some time for the platelet plug to begin forming and coagulation to commence, which eventually result in the formation of a stable thrombus.

BLOOD PLATELETS (THROMBOCYTES)

Normal Morphology

Blood platelets (thrombocytes) in mammals are small round-to-oval anucleated cell fragments (thin discs when unstimulated) that form from proplatelet cylinders of megakaryocyte cytoplasm (see Chapter 3). Platelet cytoplasm appears light blue, with many small reddish-purple granules when visualized using routine blood stains (Fig. 7-1, *A,B*). Equine platelets often stain poorly with Wright-Giemsa stain (Fig. 7-1, *C*), but they generally stain better with Diff-Quik (Fig. 7-1, *D*).

Domestic cats (and other members of the Felidae family) normally exhibit greater variation in platelet size (2 to 6 μm or larger) than seen in other domestic animals or humans (2 to 4 μm). This size variability in cats may be related to an altered M-loop region in β1-tubulin compared with other mammals.[49] The presence of these larger platelets (Fig. 7-1, *E*) results in higher mean platelet volumes (MPVs) in healthy cats than in other domestic animals. Feline platelets appear especially sensitive to activation during blood sample collection and handling, resulting in degranulated platelet aggregates, which may be overlooked by an inexperienced observer (Fig. 7-2, *A*). Some of the precipitated cryoglobulin recognized in blood from a cat with a monoclonal cryoglobulinemia has also been found to resemble aggregates of degranulated platelets (Fig. 7-2, *B*).[237] Platelets typically stain uniformly purple with the new methylene blue wet preparation (Fig. 7-3).

Newly formed platelets have higher RNA content and have been termed reticulated platelets. They cannot be quantified by morphology but can be counted using flow cytometry following labeling of RNA with a fluorescent dye.[400,442,542]

Thrombocytes in nonmammalian species have nuclei and are much larger than those of mammals. They have a high nuclear-to-cytoplasmic (N:C) ratio and are often oval or elongated with light blue or nearly colorless cytoplasm in stained blood films (Figs 7-4, *A,* 7-5). Cytoplasmic vacuoles may be present at one or both ends of a cell. Granules are usually not apparent. When thrombocytes are more round in shape, they can be difficult to differentiate from lymphocytes. Like mammalian platelets, thrombocytes appear clumped on blood films when they are activated (Fig. 7-4, *B*).

Platelet Life Span and Counts in Blood

Mean platelet life spans of 4 to 6 days have been reported in dogs, cats, horses, and cattle.[121,231,257,470] The platelet life span increased from a mean of 5.5 days to a mean of 8 days after splenectomy in dogs, suggesting that the spleen is especially adept at recognizing and removing aged platelets in dogs.[124,319] Platelet senescence is associated with changes that have characteristics of apoptosis, including increased surface phosphatidylserine (PS), which may promote their removal from circulation by macrophages.[409]

Normal platelet counts vary depending on the species, with minimal reference values as low as $100 \times 10^3/\mu L$ in horses and maximal reference values as high as $800 \times 10^3/\mu L$ in several domestic animal species.[260] The numbers normally present in blood greatly exceed those needed for adequate hemostasis. Thrombocyte counts are much lower in nonmammalian species than they are in mammals. In most avian species, thrombocyte counts range between $20 \times 10^3/\mu L$ and $30 \times 10^3/\mu L$.[221]

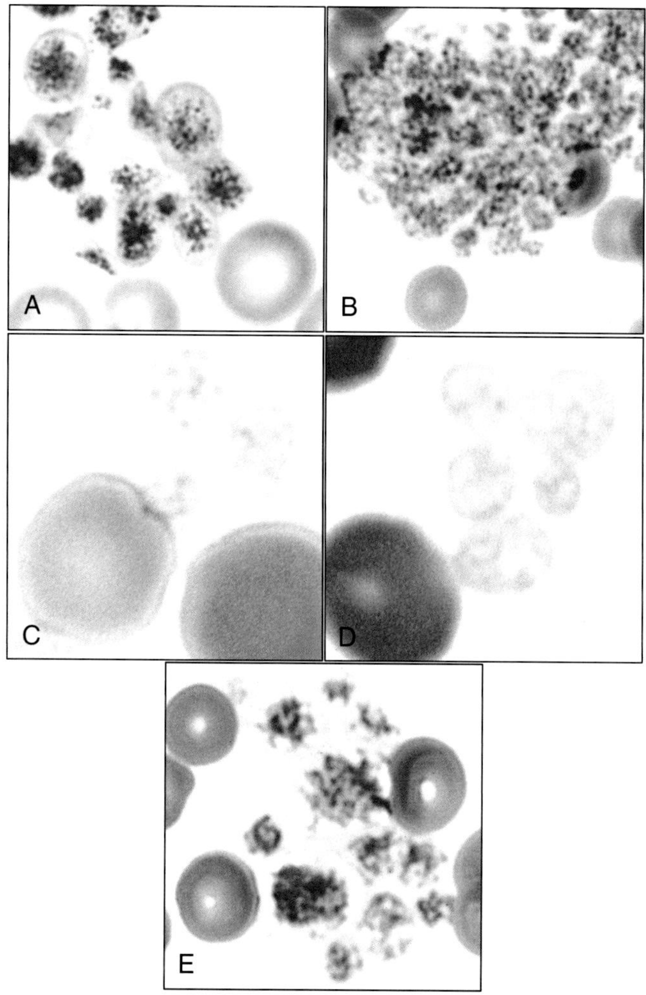

FIGURE 7-1

Normal platelet morphology in stained blood films from domestic animals. **A,** Aggregate of platelets in blood from a dog. Wright-Giemsa stain. **B,** Aggregate of platelets in blood from a cow. Wright-Giemsa stain. **C,** Three pale-staining platelets in blood from a horse. Wright-Giemsa stain. **D,** Five platelets in blood from a horse. Diff-Quik stain. **E,** Aggregate of platelets in blood from a cat demonstrating the presence of large platelets and the variation in platelet size that is characteristic of this species. Wright-Giemsa stain.

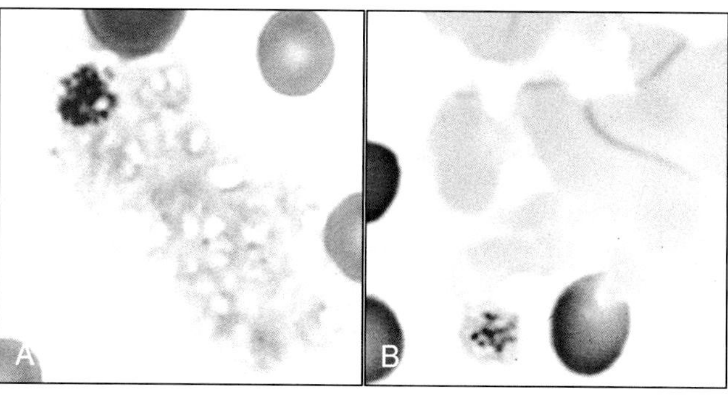

FIGURE 7-2

Degranulated platelet aggregate versus cryoglobulin globules in stained blood films. **A,** Aggregate of activated and degranulated platelets in blood from a cat. Only a single platelet in the upper left of the aggregate still contains visible granules. Wright-Giemsa stain. **B,** Blue-staining homogeneous globules of cryoglobulin in blood from an American domestic shorthaired cat with multiple myeloma and an IgG monoclonal cryoglobulinemia. The precipitated globules sometimes mimic the appearance of an aggregate of degranulated platelets. A single platelet is present at the bottom between two erythrocytes. Wright stain.

B, Photograph of a stained blood film from a 1999 ASVCP slide review case submitted by T. Stokol, J. Blue, F. Hickford, Y. von Gessel, and J. Billings.

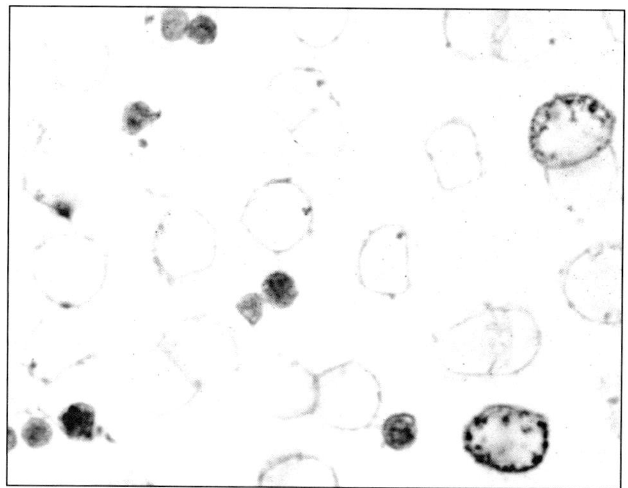

FIGURE 7-3

Mild thrombocytosis following splenectomy in blood from a dog. Platelets appear as small purple cells and erythrocytes appear as unstained ghosts. Single small Heinz bodies in many erythrocytes appear as basophilic "dots." Reticulocytes are present at top right and bottom right. An *Anaplasma platys* morula is present in a platelet in the bottom left part of the image. New methylene blue wet mount stain.

Platelet Metabolism

As in other blood cells, glucose is the major energy source for platelets. In contrast to anucleated erythrocytes, platelets have mitochondria and consequently utilize the Krebs cycle and oxidative phosphorylation. Little of the pyruvate produced by glycolysis is metabolized through the Krebs cycle in resting platelets, but oxidative metabolism, as well as glycolytic metabolism, is markedly increased when platelets are activated to meet increased needs for adenosine triphosphate (ATP) production. Biochemically, platelets have often been compared with white skeletal muscle. They have active anaerobic glycolysis and synthesize and utilize large amounts of glycogen.[402] Platelets have a dense tubular system analogous to the calcium ion (Ca^{2+}) sequestering sarcoplasmic reticulum present in skeletal muscle (Fig. 7-6). Except for ruminants and horses, domestic mammals have a well-developed canalicular system that is continuous with the surface membrane (Fig. 7-7).[46] Microtubules and microfilaments are present and composed of a variety of contractile proteins including actin, myosin, and related proteins. Microtubular coils help to maintain the discoid shape of resting platelets.[46] Changes in actin filament conformation and the organization of associated proteins are required for platelet shape change, spreading, aggregation, secretion, and clot retraction.[46]

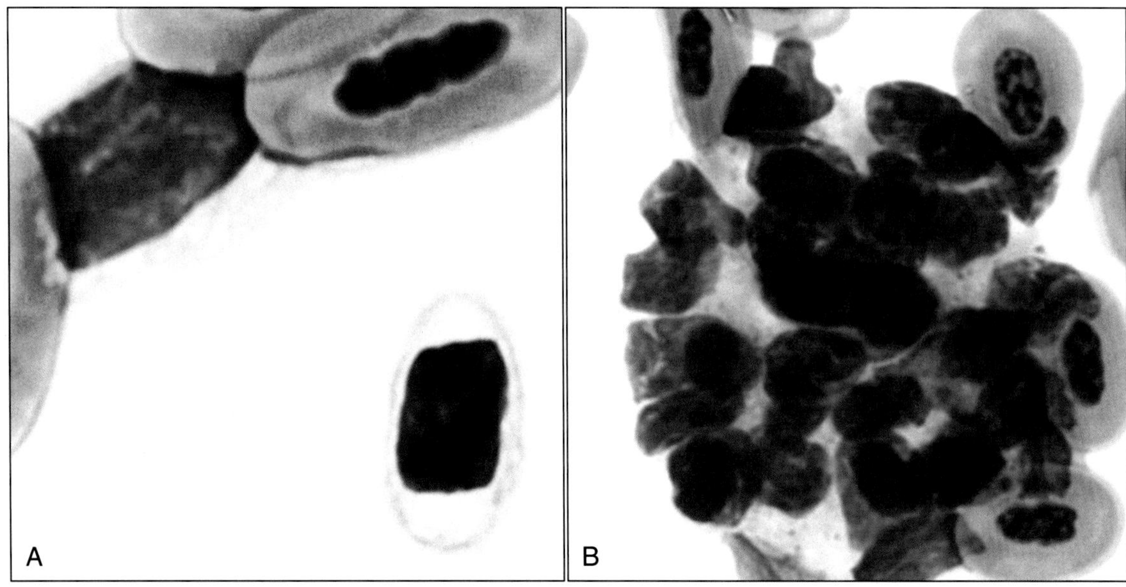

FIGURE 7-4
Morphology of thrombocytes in bird blood films. **A,** Lymphocyte *(top left)* and thrombocyte *(bottom right)* in blood from an Amazon parrot. **B,** Aggregate of thrombocytes in blood from a macaw. Wright-Giemsa stain.

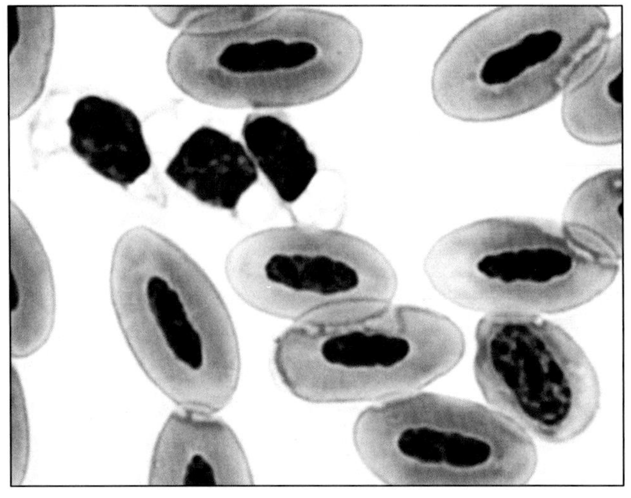

FIGURE 7-5
Three thrombocytes *(top left)* and a polychromatophilic erythrocyte *(bottom right)* in blood from an Amazon parrot. Wright-Giemsa stain.

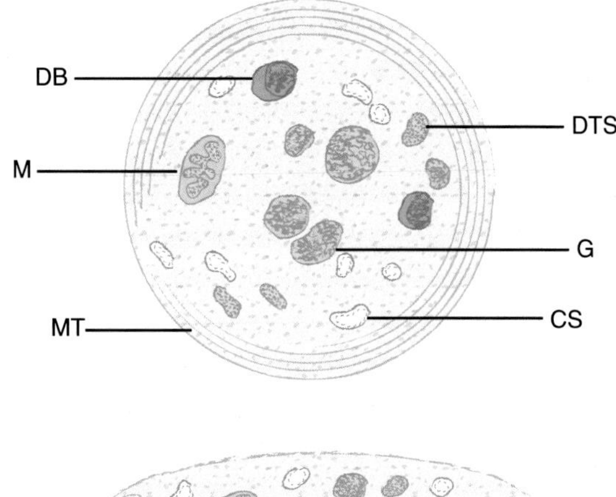

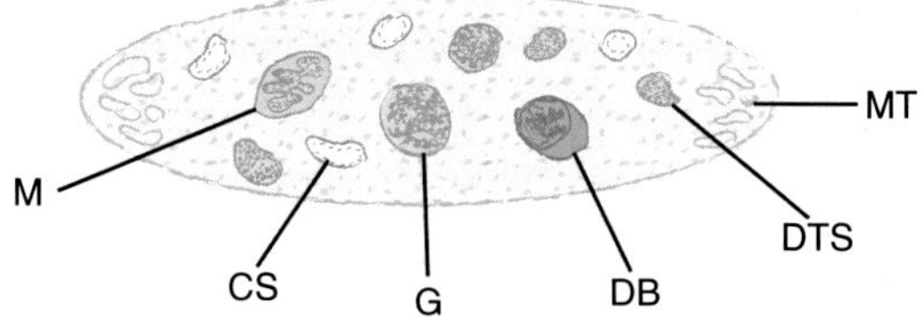

FIGURE 7-6
Platelet ultrastructure. DB, dense bodies; M, mitochondria; MT, microtubules; DTS, dense tubular system; G, granules; CS, canalicular system.

Adenine nucleotides are present in metabolic and storage pools within platelets. As in other cells, ATP accounts for most of the adenine nucleotide in the metabolic pool. The ATP in this pool provides energy for cell functions. In addition to energy needed for normal homeostatic processes, platelets expend large amounts of energy during the release reaction and aggregation, to be discussed later. The storage pool of adenine nucleotides is contained within dense granules (also called dense bodies or δ-granules), which contain about two-thirds of the total adenine nucleotides in the cell. In contrast to the cytoplasm, where ATP predominates, the ADP/ATP ratio is about 1.5 in dense granules. In addition to adenine nucleotides, these dense bodies contain considerable amounts of serotonin, Ca^{2+}, inorganic polyphosphates, and smaller amounts of other molecules, which are all secreted outside the platelets during the release reaction (degranulation).[427] The contents of α-granules and some of the contents of lysosomes are also secreted when platelets are activated. Some of the contents of α-granules are synthesized by

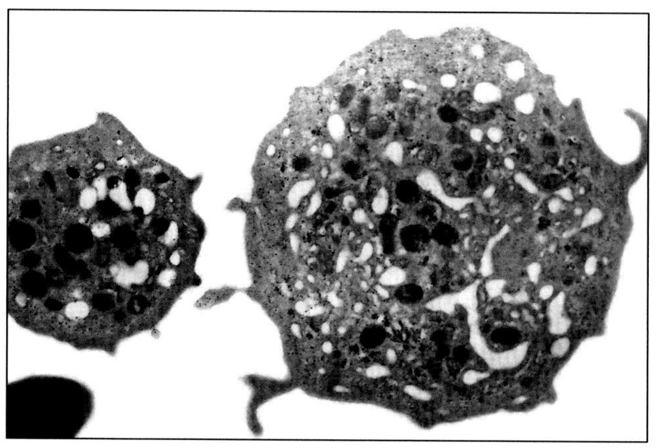

FIGURE 7-7
Transmission electron photomicrograph of a small and a large platelet from the blood of a healthy cat collected into EDTA. Granules and an extensive canalicular system are visible.

Courtesy of Charles F. Simpson.

megakaryocytes and others are taken up from the plasma. Although α-granule content varies by species, a partial list might include adhesive proteins (von Willebrand factor [vWF], fibrinogen, fibronectin, thrombospondin), coagulation factors (factors V, VII, XI and XIII), protease inhibitors (plasminogen activator inhibitor, tissue factor pathway inhibitor, α_2-antiplasmin), CXC chemokines (platelet factor 4 [PF4] and β-thromboglobulin), P-selectin (CD62P), glycoprotein (GP) receptors GPIb/IX/V (CD42) and GPIIb/IIIa (CD41/CD61), and other components, including chemotactic, mitogenic, and vascular permeability factors. Platelets also contain lysozyme granules, which contain hydrolytic enzymes.[46,57,427]

Platelets express various glycoprotein molecules on their surfaces that are needed for normal adhesion (platelet to extracellular matrix) and aggregation (platelet-to-platelet binding). The glycoprotein complex GPIb/IX/V is especially important for the adhesion of platelets to vWF that is bound to the subendothelial matrix. The GPIIb/IIIa complex ($\alpha_{IIb}\beta_3$ integrin) is essential for normal platelet aggregation, which is mediated largely by fibrinogen.[271]

Platelets have several functions in hemostasis. The first is the formation of a platelet plug at the site of vessel injury. Formation of a platelet plug alone is sufficient to stop bleeding from an injury to a small vessel. Second, platelet activation results in the translocation of negatively charged phospholipids (primarily PS) from the inner surfaces to the outer surfaces of platelets. These aminophospholipids bind certain coagulation factors in close proximity on platelet surfaces, thereby accelerating coagulation.[271] Third, activated platelets secrete PF4 (CXCL4) from their α-granules, which binds to heparin-like molecules on endothelial surfaces near the activated platelets. This binding displaces antithrombin (also called antithrombin III), which also binds to these heparin-like molecules, thereby inhibiting local antithrombin activity and promoting coagulation.[7]

Finally, the presence of platelets helps maintain normal vascular integrity in some manner. Vascular endothelium is thin, fragile, and leaky in animals with low platelet counts (thrombocytopenia).[284] Platelets help protect vessels from bleeding during inflammation in a way that is not dependent on the formation of a platelet plug.[194] The relationship between platelets and endothelial cells is complex and poorly understood, but platelet granules have a variety of vasoactive molecules that might promote the integrity of the endothelial barrier. Sphingosine-1 phosphate, a phospholipid product of platelets, is one substance that appears to be an important mediator protecting the vascular barrier.[451]

PRIMARY HEMOSTASIS

Vascular Phase

Primary hemostasis consists of a vascular phase and a platelet phase. Following the severing of vessels, a reflex vasoconstriction temporarily retards blood flow, allowing time for formation of the platelet plug to begin and coagulation to commence. The damage or removal of endothelial cells exposes the subcellular matrix, resulting in platelet adhesion. Following vessel injury, tissue factor (TF) on subendothelial adventitial cells activates coagulation.[468] Although platelet plug formation and coagulation are discussed below in separate sections, it is important to realize that these processes are interrelated. Thrombin generated during coagulation is one of the agonists that activates platelets, and coagulation occurs on the surface of activated platelets in vivo, which greatly accelerates the coagulation process.[271]

Platelet Phase

In response to vessel wall injury or exposure to foreign surfaces, platelets rapidly undergo the processes of adhesion, shape change, secretion, and aggregation through a complex series of coordinated processes that culminate in the formation of a precisely located platelet plug. Because of the rapidity of intracellular responses and synergy between secondary messenger systems, it is not possible to organize the various effector systems into a clearly defined temporal sequence. Reciprocal activation of effector systems also makes it difficult to define a clear sequence of events.[271]

Platelet Adhesion

Optimal platelet adhesion requires the binding of the platelet surface glycoprotein GPIb/IX/V complex to vWF molecules on the surface of the subendothelium. The GPIb/IX/V complex does not bind circulating vWF; it binds only vWF molecules that have been immobilized within the extracellular matrix, where vWF is bound primarily to collagen. It appears that the conformation of vWF changes upon binding to the extracellular matrix, so that it readily binds to the GPIb subunit of the GPIb/IX/V complex on platelets, especially when shear force is applied, as occurs when flowing blood is exposed to the subendothelial surface (Fig. 7-8).[271]

vWF is a component of the factor VIII:vWF macromolecular complex (Fig. 7-9). It circulates as a series of disulfide-bonded polymers with a molecular weight of up to 20 × 10^3 kDa in blood. vWF polymers bind to factor VIII (FVIII), a smaller protein (molecular weight 285 kDa) that functions as a procoagulant.[79] In humans, about 1 molecule of FVIII binds per 50 monomers of vWF. Binding of FVIII to vWF prolongs the circulation time of FVIII.[513] These two factors are controlled by different genes and are synthesized independently. vWF, previously referred to as factor VIII:R (related antigen), is encoded by an autosomal gene and synthesized by endothelial cells and megakaryocytes (in some species). FVIII, also referred to as antihemophilic factor, is an X-linked gene product that is synthesized primarily in the liver (probably by hepatocytes).[309] The binding of vWF to the extracellular matrix is associated with decreased binding of FVIII.[513]

Although vWF appears to be the most important factor in the extravascular matrix for platelet adhesion under flow conditions, other factors can promote platelet adhesion. Thrombospondin-1 is an alternate substrate to vWF for binding to platelet GPIb under high shear conditions. Under static conditions with low shear, platelets adhere directly to collagen in the subendothelium using GPVI and $\alpha_2\beta_1$ (GPIa-IIa) receptors.[271]

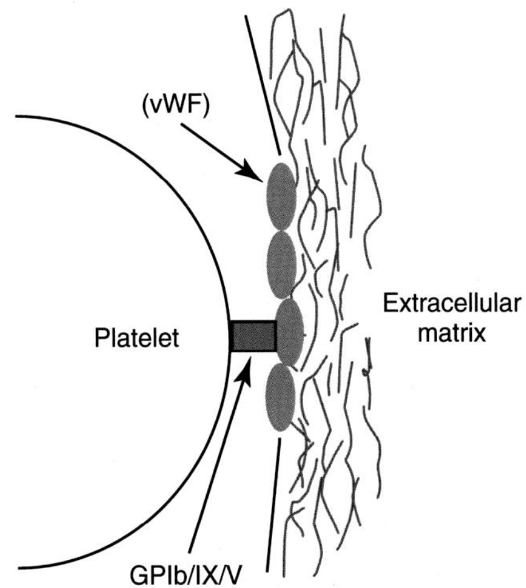

FIGURE 7-8
von Willebrand factor (vWF) is needed for optimal adhesion of platelets to the subendothelial matrix under flow conditions. vWF binds to a glycoprotein complex GPIb/IX/V receptor on the platelet surface.

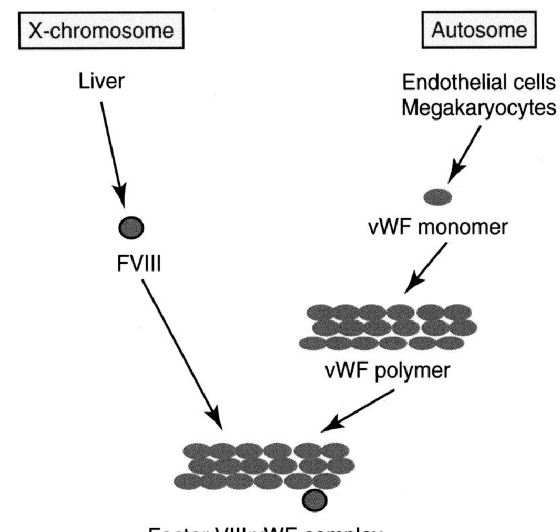

FIGURE 7-9
Factor VIII (FVIII) and vWF are produced by different genes and circulate bound together as a high-molecular-weight complex. vWF monomers are produced by endothelial cells and megakaryocytes and assemble into polymers, which bind about 1 FVIII molecule per 50 vWF monomers.

Platelet Activation

The adhesion of platelets to the extracellular matrix under shear conditions and their binding to collagen and other strong agonists, including thrombin generated during coagulation, result in the activation of phospholipase C (PLC) in the platelet membrane (Fig. 7-10). PLC cleaves a unique membrane phospholipid, phosphatidylinositol, 4,5-bisphosphate (PIP_2), into inositol triphosphate (IP_3) and 1,2-diacylglycerol (DAG). IP_3 diffuses through the cytoplasm and binds to a calcium channel receptor in the dense tubular system, which stimulates the release of calcium ions.[271] The rise in the cytosolic concentration of calcium results in a cascade of intracellular changes and activity. Calcium ions and DAG bind to and activates calcium diacylglycerol guanine nucleotide exchange factor I (CalDAG-GEFI), which activates the Rap1b GTPase through the exchange of bound

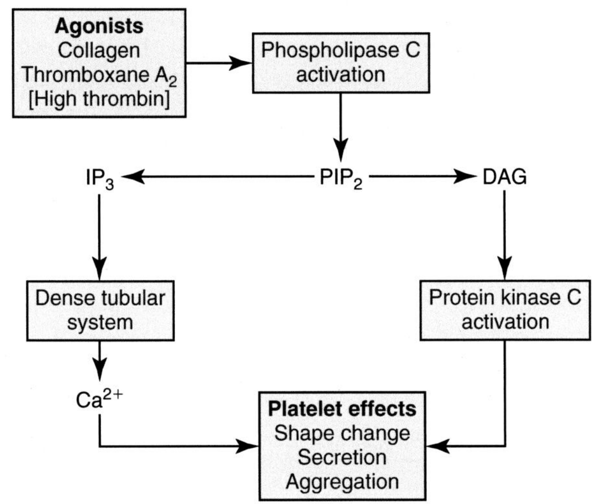

FIGURE 7-10
Overview of the activation of phospholipase C and the resultant platelet effects. PIP_2, phospholipid phosphatidylinositol 4,5-bisphosphate; IP_3, inositol triphosphate; DAG, 1,2-diacylglycerol; Ca^{2+}, calcium ions. (See text for more details.)

GDP for GTP. Activated Rap1b promotes the conformational change and activation of the GPIIb/IIIa integrin, so that it binds fibrinogen. CalDAG-GEFI also appears to link increases in intracellular calcium ions to signaling pathways that regulate the synthesis of thromboxane A_2 (TxA_2) and release of granules.[33] Inherited defects in CalDAG-GEFI lead to defects in platelet function and to bleeding in affected dogs and cattle.[44] Intracellular calcium ions and DAG together work to activate protein kinase C isoforms, which phosphorylate other molecules. Taken together, these reactions and others, including phosphatidylinositol-3 kinase (PI3K), stimulate platelets in various ways, resulting in TxA_2 synthesis, shape change, integrin activation, secretion, aggregation, and platelet procoagulant activity.[66,191,220]

Phospholipase A_2 is also activated, which stimulates the hydrolysis of phospholipids (especially phosphatidylcholine) from the dense tubular system, causing the release of arachidonic acid. Arachidonic acid is subsequently metabolized to TxA_2 by the cyclooxygenase enzyme pathway (Fig. 7-11).[271] Phospholipase A_2 (in conjunction with an acetyltransferase) is also involved in generating platelet-activating factor (PAF, 1-alkyl-2-acetyl-*sn*-glycero-3-phosphocholine), another agonist that induces platelet aggregation.[66,102] PAF can be produced not only by activated platelets but also by activated endothelial cells and leukocytes.[113,298,533] PAF is an important proinflammatory mediator that has multiple effects beyond platelet activation.[218,298,314]

Epinephrine does not function as an agonist by itself but potentiates platelet activation and secretion induced by other agonists. Platelets from some dogs do not respond to TxA_2 in vitro owing to impaired TxA_2-G protein coupling, but this defect is normalized by pretreatment with epinephrine.[44]

Platelet activation is inhibited by prostacyclin (prostaglandin I_2, or PGI_2). When stimulated by agonists including thrombin and PAF, endothelial cells produce increased amounts of PGI_2 as a product of arachidonic acid metabolism (see Fig. 7-11).[234,406] This antagonist has an antiaggregatory effect by stimulating cyclic adenosine monophosphate (cAMP) synthesis in platelets. Agonists tend to counteract this effect by lowering platelet cAMP concentrations.[264,271] Activated endothelial cells also suppress platelet reactivity by increasing the rate of nitric oxide (NO) synthesis. NO inhibits platelet activation by activating intracellular guanylate cyclase, which leads to the formation of cyclic guanosine monophosphate (cGMP).[271] NO and PGI_2 also function as potent vasodilators.[264,356]

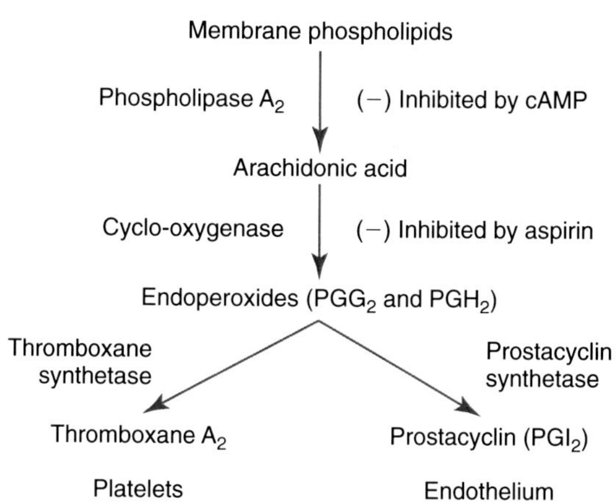

FIGURE 7-11
Activation of phospholipase A_2 and the generation of thromboxane A_2 (TxA_2) in platelets and prostacyclin in endothelial cells.

Change in Platelet Shape

The discoid shape of resting platelets is maintained by circumferential bundles of microtubules beneath the platelet membrane and an extensive network of short actin filaments, forming a membrane skeleton. Following binding to vWF and collagen, platelets are activated, the microtubular coils reorganize into linear arrays, and actin disassembles and reassembles as platelets form filopodia and spread.[46,271] Negatively charged phospholipids and glycoprotein receptors are also exposed on the surface. Platelets have surface receptors for various subendothelial components including collagen, fibronectin, laminin, and thrombospondin.[31] The collagen receptor ($\alpha_2\beta_1$ integrin) functions both in adhesion and as an agonist receptor that activates platelets.[46]

Platelet Secretion

Platelet secretion (release or degranulation) requires energy-dependent contractile mechanisms. Granules are crushed together (fusion and dissolution) by a surrounding web of microtubules and microfilaments. The contents of dense bodies and granules are discharged into the open canalicular system, which is continuous with the platelet surface.[427] Ruminant, equine, and elephant platelets have minimal canalicular systems; granules and dense bodies primarily discharge their contents by fusing with the external platelet membrane.[46,145] Contraction of individual platelets and the platelet aggregate facilitates the discharge of material into surrounding plasma. ADP, serotonin, and calcium released from dense bodies promote platelet aggregation.[427]

Platelet Aggregation

ADP, TxA_2, thrombin, and PAF are important agonists that promote platelet aggregation. Serotonin is also an important agonist in some species. Optimal platelet aggregation requires fibrinogen and Ca^{2+}. The actions of these agonists result in the increased exposure and activation of GPIIb/IIIa, a β_3-integrin platelet surface receptor that binds to fibrinogen (Fig. 7-12). Aggregation occurs when symmetric fibrinogen molecules bind to exposed receptors on adjacent platelets. vWF also promotes platelet aggregation when shear forces are high in flowing blood.[271,462] The resultant platelet plug may be sufficient to stop bleeding from small vessels. As discussed further on, the bleeding-time test, which measures the time needed to form the platelet plug, is dependent on platelet numbers and function.

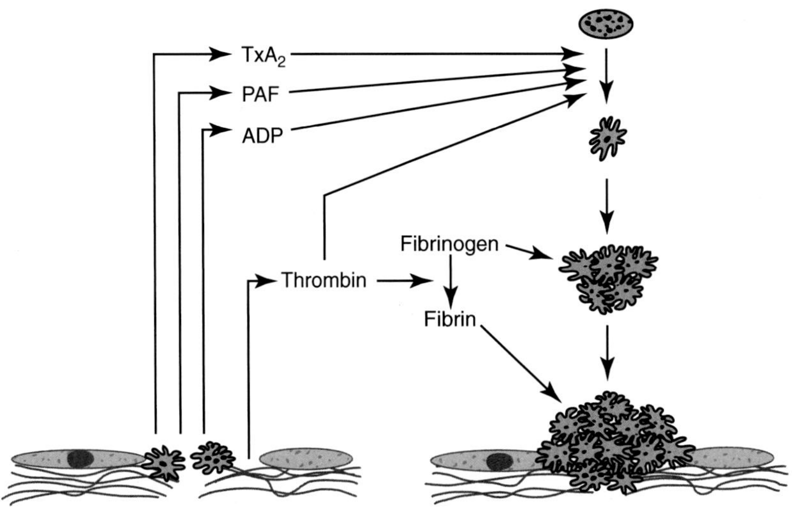

FIGURE 7-12

Primary factors involved in platelet aggregation. TxA_2, thromboxane A_2; PAF, platelet activating factor; ADP, adenosine diphosphate.

Platelet Procoagulant Activity

Phospholipids are asymmetrically located in the plasma membrane of resting cells, including platelets, because of the presence of the Mg-ATP-dependent enzymes flippase and floppase. Negatively charged aminophospholipids are concentrated more in the inner leaflet of the platelet membrane because of an inward-directed pump for PS and phosphatidylethanolamine known as aminophospholipid translocase or flippase. Neutral phospholipids, including phosphatidylcholine and sphingomyelin, are transported to the outer membrane leaflet of platelets by floppase activity.[77]

The activation of platelets by agonists results in the calcium-dependent activation of scramblase (an enzyme that promotes unspecific bidirectional redistribution of phospholipids across the bilayer) and inhibition of flippase activities. The net result is that negatively charged phospholipid (primarily PS) is translocated from the internal leaflet to the external leaflet of the plasma membrane.[173,279] Negatively charged aminophospholipids on the surface of activated platelets have been termed "platelet factor 3" or "platelet procoagulant activity." The translocation of PS to the surface of activated platelets accelerates coagulation because positively charged Ca^{2+} binds to the negatively charged phospholipids and to the negatively charged carboxyl groups of coagulation factors. Binding of coagulation factors to platelets not only brings them together to enhance interactions but also helps to protect them from inhibitors.[271]

Platelet activation results not only in enhanced reactivity toward other platelets—forming platelet aggregates (Fig. 7-13) and prompting enhanced reactivity toward leukocytes, thus forming platelet-leukocyte aggregates—but also in the shedding of microparticles (microvesicles) from the platelet surface.[365,545] These microparticles have procoagulant activity, expressing PS, activation-dependent adhesion molecules, and possibly TF on their surfaces.[279,381] Platelet microparticles bind to and activate leukocytes and endothelial cells, which may promote thrombosis and inflammation.[77,187] Platelet activation ultimately results in platelet changes that appear to be proinflammatory and broadly consistent with cell necrosis.[255]

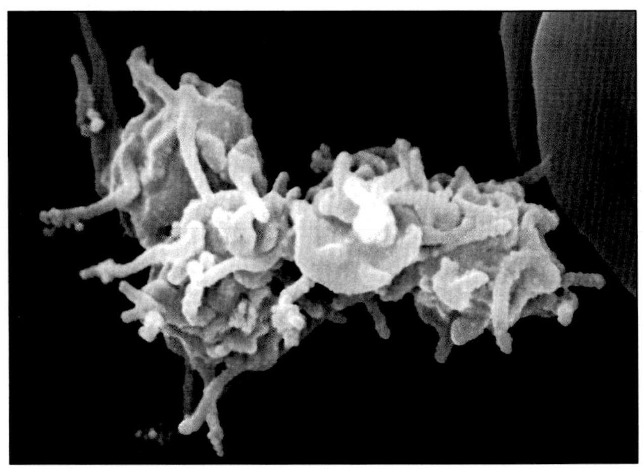

FIGURE 7-13

Scanning electron photomicrograph of a small aggregate of platelets exhibiting prominent filopodia formation.

PS is also exposed on the surface of platelets undergoing apoptosis via a pathway different from that for platelet activation. This PS exposure presumably promotes platelet clearance under steady-state conditions. Whether this has any relevance to thrombin generation in vivo remains to be determined.[255]

SECONDARY HEMOSTASIS

Overview

Secondary hemostasis is composed of coagulation and consolidation of the temporary hemostatic platelet plug into a definitive hemostatic plug. Coagulation is an enzymatic process involving the conversion of proenzymes to active enzymes. Some activated coagulation factors are themselves enzymes, and others (factors V and VIII) are cofactors that combine in complexes to generate specific enzymatic activities. A series of enzymatic reactions, each producing active enzymes, results in an amplification of the original stimulus to initiate coagulation. Ca^{2+} ions are required for multiple reactions in coagulation. The final product of coagulation is the formation of cross-linked fibrin strands around and, to a lesser extent, through the platelet plug, making it stronger and decreasing the likelihood that rebleeding will occur.

Coagulation has classically been divided into intrinsic and extrinsic coagulation pathways (Fig 7-14), with both utilizing a common pathway beginning with factor X (FX). This presentation of coagulation events is useful in dividing coagulation into components in order to study their relationships and interpret diagnostic test results, but it is not accurate from a physiologic point of view. The classic presentation implies that coagulation can be induced by either the extrinsic or the intrinsic pathway. It does not show the importance of the extrinsic pathway in activating the intrinsic pathway or that coagulation is a cellular or at least membrane-bound event.[368]

Coagulation factors have been given one or more names and also assigned a Roman numeral. Fibrinogen (factor I), prothrombin (factor II), TF or tissue thromboplastin (factor III), and Ca^{2+} (factor IV) are usually referred to by their names. Other factors are more often referred to by their numbers. There is no factor VI. All factors except Ca^{2+} are proteins, most of which are synthesized in the liver. All factors except TF are normally present in the circulation.

Vitamin K is required for the synthesis of functional factors II, VII, IX, and X, as well as protein C and protein S. Following synthesis of the protein molecules in the liver, a vitamin K-dependent carboxylation (via γ-glutamyl carboxylase) of glutamic acid residues on these molecules is required for them to bind Ca^{2+} and become functional (Fig. 7-15). Cats and sheep that have γ-glutamyl carboxylase deficiencies have bleeding episodes because of low vitamin K-dependent coagulant factor activities.[267,473] Dicumarol-type anticoagulant drugs, including warfarin and brodifacoum, inhibit the vitamin K epoxide (or oxido) reductase (VKOR) enzyme complex needed to recycle vitamin K, resulting in the production of inactive coagulation proteins.[105,477]

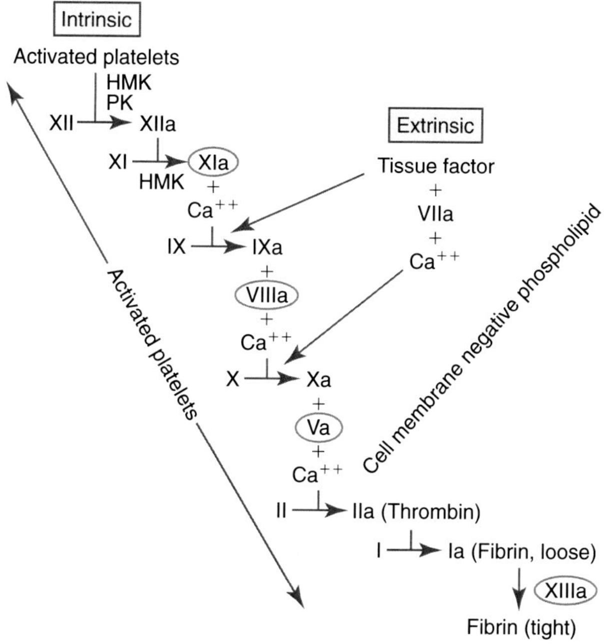

FIGURE 7-14

A diagram of the classical coagulation cascade. HMK, high-molecular-weight kininogen; PK, prekallikrein; VIII, coagulant component of the FVIII complex; Ca^{2+}, calcium ions. Roman numerals refer to coagulation factors with these numbers, and an associated "a" indicates that the factor is activated. The circled coagulation factors are activated by thrombin. Activated platelets express negatively charged phospholipids (primarily phosphatidylserine) on their surfaces.

Initiation of Coagulation (Activation of the Extrinsic Pathway or Tissue Factor Pathway)

A small amount (about 1%) of factor VII (FVII) in blood is activated (FVIIa). Coagulation is initiated in vivo when blood containing FVIIa comes in contact with TF on the surface of cells or cell membranes (i.e., microparticles from cells) (Fig. 7-16).[77] TF is a glycoprotein that depends on its association

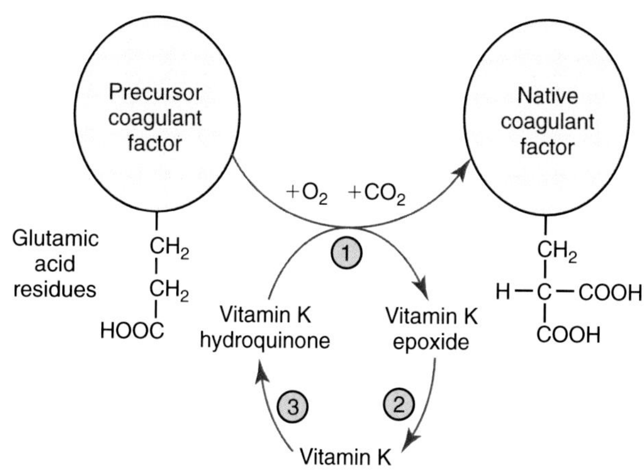

FIGURE 7-15

Vitamin K cycle resulting in the γ-carboxylation of glutamic acid residues in coagulation proteins. Enzymes include vitamin K γ-glutamyl carboxylase (1) and vitamin K epoxide reductase (2) and (3). Dicumarol-type anticoagulant drugs, including warfarin and brodifacoum, inhibit the vitamin K epoxide reductase, resulting in inactive coagulation proteins.

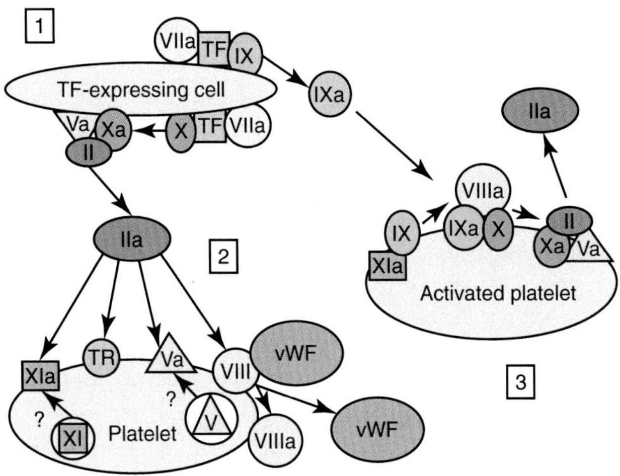

FIGURE 7-16

Cell-based model of coagulation. Roman numerals refer to coagulation factors with these numbers, and an associated "a" indicates that the factor is activated. (1) Initiation of coagulation begins on tissue factor (TF)-bearing cells such as subendothelial fibroblasts exposed by vessel injury. Reactions shown on the surface of this TF-bearing cell generate small amounts of thrombin (IIa) and activated factor IX (IXa) that diffuse away from the cell. (2) Amplification of coagulation results from thrombin's activation of platelets and coagulation factors. Thrombin activates platelets near TF-bearing cells by binding to thrombin receptors (TR) on the surface of platelets. Platelets can also be activated by binding to collagen and von Willebrand factor (vWF) in the extracellular matrix in the area of the TF-bearing cells *(not shown)*. Factors V and XI from plasma, or possibly from platelet granules (shown with "?" in the figure), bind to the surface of activated platelets and are activated to Va and XIa by thrombin. The action of thrombin also results in dissociation of factor VIII from vWF and activation of factor VIII to VIIIa. (3) Propagation of coagulation occurs when activated factors generated in the initiation and amplification phases of coagulation assemble in complexes on the surfaces of activated platelets, which have phosphatidylserine expressed on their surfaces. The activation of factor XII may also contribute to the activation of factor XI on the surface of activated platelets (not shown). Factor XIa activates factor IX to IXa, and some IXa may also diffuse to activated platelets from TF-bearing cells. Factor IXa combines with factor VIIIa to activate factor X, and Xa combines with Va to form a complex that cleaves prothrombin (II) to generate a burst of thrombin that converts fibrinogen to fibrin *(not shown)*.

with negatively charged phospholipid (most notably PS) to bind FVII/FVIIa. TF is not expressed on unstimulated blood or endothelial cells but it is constitutively expressed on the surface of many other cell types that are not normally in contact with the circulation. This includes cell types surrounding vessels as well as parenchymal cells in a variety of tissues, such as brain, heart, lung, and kidney.[405]

Following vessel injury, TF on subendothelial adventitial cells—such as adventitial fibroblasts, pericytes, and smooth muscle cells—activates coagulation. TF expression can also be induced in blood monocytes and possibly endothelial cells by endotoxin and/or inflammatory cytokines. TF has been reported on activated platelets; but, if present, this may come from the transfer of microparticles from activated monocytes or other cells to platelets.[173,397]

The TF-FVIIa complex on membrane surfaces activates additional amounts of FVII to FVIIa, which generates larger amounts of the TF-FVIIa complex on membranes. This complex activates factor IX (FIX) and FX to FIXa and FXa respectively. Although not optimal, FXa can directly activate some factor V (FV) to FVa, and the combination of FXa with cofactor FVa forms a complex called prothrombinase on the surfaces of TF-bearing cells, which converts prothrombin to thrombin. The activation of this tissue factor pathway in vivo functions to rapidly generate trace amounts of thrombin; however, the small amount of thrombin generated results in minimal fibrin formation. Coagulation generally begins on the surface of TF-bearing perivascular cells, but it is completed on the surface of activated platelets.[467]

Amplification of Coagulation

Following vessel injury, platelets bind via vWF to the subendothelial extracellular matrix near the TF-bearing cells that activate coagulation. Platelets are activated by this binding under shear conditions. Thrombin produced by activation of the tissue factor pathway also activates platelets by binding to thrombin receptors (see Fig. 7-16), including protease-activated receptors (PARs) and GPIb/IX/V.[44] Following activation, platelets produce agonists—including TxA_2, PAF, and ADP—which, together with thrombin, induce platelet aggregation and platelet plug formation. Platelet activation also results in the exposure of negative phospholipids (platelet procoagulant) on the platelets' surfaces. Some coagulation factors in platelet granules (including FV and FXI, at least in some species) are also deposited on platelet surfaces after platelet activation and secretion.

The vWF/FVIII complex binds to activated platelets, and thrombin cleaves a portion of the FVIII molecule to form activated FVIIIa. FVIII activation results in the dissociation of this molecule from vWF.[375] FVIIIa remains bound to platelets because activated platelets express distinct binding sites for FVIIIa (see Fig. 7-16). Thrombin also activates FV to FVa. This cofactor not only circulates in blood but may also be present in platelet granules and may be deposited on activated platelet surfaces following granule secretion.[244] Finally, thrombin activates FXI to FXIa, which is also bound to the surfaces of activated platelets.[79,137] At the end of the amplification phase of coagulation, activated platelets have negatively charged phospholipids, FVa, FVIIIa, and FXIa, present on their surfaces, priming them for rapid propagation of coagulation (see Fig. 7-16).[243]

Propagation of Coagulation (Activity of the Intrinsic Pathway)

Factor XII Activation of Factor XI

A long-held consensus mechanism for the activation of coagulation in vitro (contact activation) is shown in Figure 7-17.[182,514] In this model, factor XII (FXII) comes in contact with an anionic, wettable surface (including blood collection tubes made of glass) and undergoes autoactivation, which generates a small amount of active FXII (FXIIa). FXIIa may

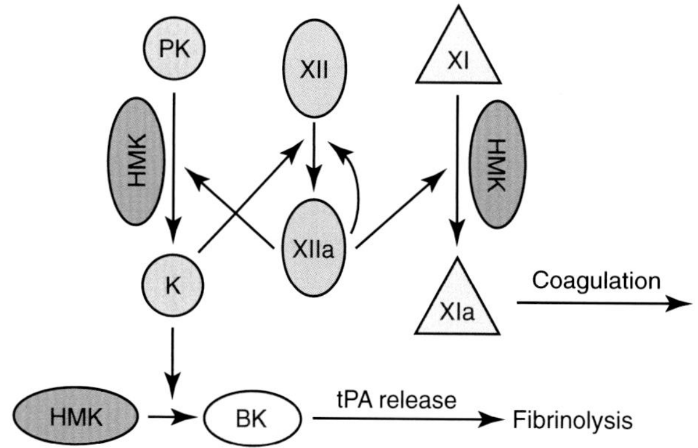

FIGURE 7-17

Contact activation of coagulation occurs in vitro when factor XII (FXII) comes in contact with foreign surfaces (such as the glass of blood collection tubes). FXII autoactivates to active FXII (FXIIa), and FXIIa may autohydrolyze additional FXII to FXIIa. FXIIa also interacts with prekallikrein (PK), which is bound to high-molecular-weight kininogen (HMK). Reciprocal interactions with FXIIa and prekallikrein generate a FXIIa fragment and kallikrein (K) respectively. FXIIa also activates factor XI (FXI), which is bound to HMK. Factor XIa then activates Factor IX *(not shown)*, which propagates the intrinsic pathway of coagulation. Kallikrein generates bradykinin (BK) from HMK and BK stimulates the release of tissue plasminogen activator (tPA) from endothelial cells, which activates fibrinolysis. Contact activation is also believed to occur on activated platelets that have secreted negatively charged polyphosphates on their surfaces.

autohydrolyze FXII to produce more FXIIa. In addition, FXIIa interacts with prekallikrein, which is bound to high-molecular-weight kininogen (HMK). Reciprocal interactions between FXIIa and prekallikrein generate an active fragment of FXIIa (FXIIf) and kallikrein respectively. FXIIa activates factor XI (FXI), which is also bound to HMK, which propagates the intrinsic pathway of coagulation.[182] Some aspects of this model of contact activation (especially the interactions of these proteins with foreign surfaces) have been challenged.[514]

Because people, cats, and dogs with FXII deficiency exhibit no hemorrhagic tendencies and some marine mammals, birds, and reptiles naturally lack this factor, it has generally been accepted that FXII activation is of little importance to normal hemostasis in vivo.[185] However, FXII is acknowledged to be important in the plasma kallikrein-kinin system. FXIIf-generated kallikrein converts HMK to bradykinin, which causes vasodilation, increased vascular permeability, and prompts an inflammatory response.[265] Bradykinin also stimulates the release of tissue plasminogen activator (tPA) from endothelial cells, which promotes fibrinolysis, as discussed further on.[182] FXIIf activates complement (C1r) in addition to generating kallikrein.[275]

Although FXII is apparently not essential for normal hemostasis, it may play a role in the growth of thrombi under pathologic conditions.[100,428] The activation of human platelets results in the secretion of dense granule contents, which include polyphosphates. FXII appears to be activated following binding to polyphosphates on the surfaces of platelets. This FXII activation promotes both coagulation and the generation of bradykinin.[265] Secreted polyphosphates may have additional effects on coagulation. Polyphosphates are reported to enhance thrombin-mediated FV activation, and their incorporation into fibrin fibers is reported to make them more resistant to lysis.[80]

Thrombin Activation of FXI

FXI binds to activated platelets via HMK and is believed to primarily be activated in vivo by thrombin initially generated by the activation of the tissue factor pathway. However, some FXI activation may also occur as a result of FXIIa on activated platelets, and FXI may be autoactivated by FXIa.[80,154] Because FXI deficiency results in only mild bleeding in animals and humans (compared with the severe bleeding that occurs with FIX and FVIII deficiencies[185]) FXI does not appear to have a major role in early fibrin generation. FXIa is postulated to be part of a positive feedback loop that sustains thrombin generation through FIX activation to subsequently generate large amounts of fibrin.[154] In addition, some FIXa generated on TF-bearing cells can detach and bind to nearby activated platelets and promote coagulation on platelet surfaces (see Fig. 7-16).[271] Thus FIX is activated by both FXIa and the TF-FVIIa complex. In contrast, little of the FXa generated by TF-bearing cells becomes bound to activated platelets, because FXa that dissociates from the TF-binding cells is rapidly inactivated by the antithrombin and tissue factor pathway inhibitor (TFPI) present in blood. FIXa is not inactivated by TFPI and only slowly inactivated by antithrombin.[467]

FIXa combines with cofactor FVIIIa on activated platelet surfaces to form a complex sometimes called tenase that activates FX (Figs. 7-16, 7-18).[185] FVa that is bound to platelet surfaces functions as a cofactor for FXa and forms a complex called prothrombinase on the surfaces of activated platelets. This complex converts large amounts of prothrombin to thrombin. The thrombin thus formed is released from platelets and converts fibrinogen to fibrin monomers; these polymerize spontaneously by hydrogen bonding to form unstable non-cross-linked fibrin polymers around the platelet plug (see Fig. 7-18).

Stabilization of the Thrombus

The last step in fibrin polymerization involves the formation of covalent cross-links between fibrin monomers. Factor XIII (FXIII, fibrin stabilizing factor) is activated by thrombin. The FXIIIa formed is a Ca^{2+}-dependent transglutaminase that catalyzes the formation of covalent bonds between lysine and glutamine residues of different monomers. Cross-linked fibrin is an insoluble protein polymer that stabilizes the platelet plug.[185] Thrombin also activates a thrombin-activatable fibrinolysis inhibitor (TAFI) that makes the fibrin formed more resistant to lysis (see "Fibrinolysis," below).[328] Finally, the incorporation of polyphosphates from the dense granules secreted by platelets into fibrin fibers is reported also to make fibrin more resistant to lysis.[80]

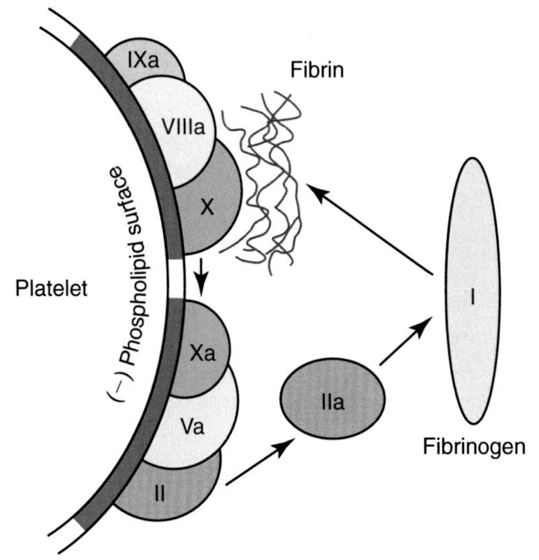

FIGURE 7-18

Assembly of coagulation factors on an activated platelet surface, primarily binding to phosphatidylserine, the negatively charged phospholipid. Roman numerals refer to coagulation factors with these numbers, and an associated "a" indicates that the factor is activated. The fibrin that is formed is deposited on the activated platelet.

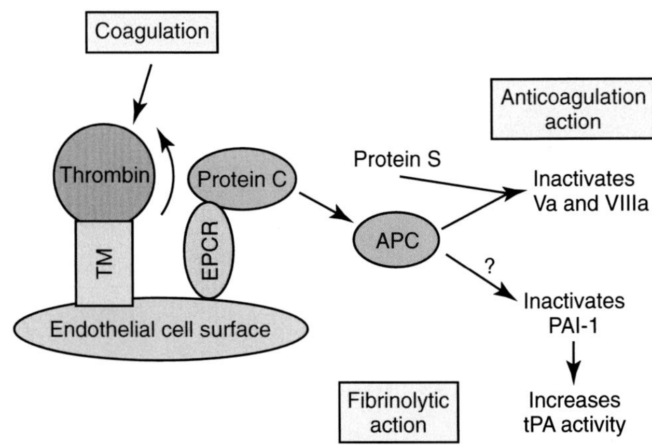

FIGURE 7-19

Actions involving protein C. Roman numerals refer to coagulation factors with these numbers, and an associated "a" indicates that the factor is activated. TM, thrombomodulin; EPCR, endothelial protein C receptor; APC, activated protein C; PAI-1, plasminogen activator inhibitor 1; tPA, tissue plasminogen activator.

Inhibitors of Thrombus Formation

Once a thrombus composed of platelets and fibrin is formed over an area of vascular injury, the coagulation process must be terminated to prevent thrombotic occlusion of normal areas of the vasculature adjacent to the injury. Endothelial cells are especially important in limiting, by various mechanisms, thrombus formation to the site of injury. Unstimulated platelets do not adhere to the surface of healthy vascular endothelial cells because these endothelial cells possess thromboresistant properties.

Inhibition of Platelet Aggregation

Endothelial cells synthesize and release PGI_2 and NO, powerful vasodilators that inhibit platelet aggregation. Endothelial cells also inhibit platelet function by virtue of an ectoenzyme (Ecto-ADPase/CD39/NTPDase) that has adenosine diphosphatase (ADPase) activity and can degrade ADP released from activated platelets.[264]

Antithrombin

Endothelial cells synthesize heparan sulfate proteoglycans, which are tightly associated with the endothelium and accelerate the inactivation of coagulation factors by antithrombin, the major thrombin inhibitor.[461] In addition to thrombin, antithrombin inhibits other proteases, including factors IXa, Xa, XIa, and XIIa.[185]

Protein C Anticoagulant Pathway

Endothelial cells express the membrane protein thrombomodulin on their surfaces (Fig. 7-19). Thrombin binds to thrombomodulin, which inhibits thrombin's procoagulant activity. This 1:1 thrombin:thrombomodulin complex activates both protein C and TAFI, discussed under "Fibrinolysis," below. Protein C is a vitamin K-dependent plasma protein that circulates in an inactive form. It binds to an endothelial protein C receptor (EPCR), which enhances its activation by the thrombin:thrombomodulin complex. Activated protein C dissociates from EPCR and interacts with protein S (a vitamin K-dependent cofactor) to inhibit coagulation by proteolytically degrading FVa and FVIIIa on the surfaces of activated platelets. Although the physiologic significance of its effect is unclear, activated protein C can also promote fibrinolysis by inactivating the plasminogen activator inhibitor 1 (PAI-1).[156,157]

Tissue Factor Pathway Inhibitor

TFPI is synthesized by endothelial cells, and most TFPI is associated with the endothelium. FXa and the TF-VIIa complex are inhibited by the bivalent TFPI formerly called the lipoprotein-associated coagulation inhibitor.[137] Protein S is a cofactor for the TFPI system, in addition to the protein C anticoagulant pathway.[92]

Platelet-Secreted Inhibitors

In addition to their potent roles in promoting coagulation, platelets secrete coagulation inhibitors, including protease nexin-1 (inhibits thrombin), protease nexin-2 (inhibits FXIa), and TFPI from α-granules. These factors may help to prevent the propagation of thrombosis beyond a site of injury.[516]

Additional Coagulation Inhibitors

α_1-Protease inhibitor (α_1-antitrypsin), C1-esterase inhibitor, and α_2-macroglobulin are less important inhibitors of thrombus formation.

FIBRINOLYSIS

Fibrinolysis is activated by the release of tPA from damaged endothelium. The amount of tPA available to stimulate fibrinolysis may be increased by activated protein C inactivating PAI-1.[156] Plasminogen coprecipitates with fibrin as a thrombus forms. Conversion of plasminogen to plasmin by tPA is accelerated in the presence of fibrin (Fig. 7-20).[377] Plasmin is not a highly specific enzyme, but its affinity for fibrin helps to limit its action. Plasmin-catalyzed hydrolysis of fibrin results in the formation of fibrin degradation products (fibrin split products), which have antihemostatic properties.[185]

Inhibitors of fibrinolysis also occur in plasma. Endothelial cells produce PAI-1, which inhibits tPA. TAFI is activated by the thrombin-thrombospondin complex. It removes carboxy-terminal lysine groups from fibrin, resulting in decreased binding of plasminogen and tPA to fibrin and consequently decreased generation of plasmin. This slows but does not eliminate fibrinolysis.[328,553] Thrombin's central role in coagulation and fibrinolysis is summarized in Figure 7-21.

α_2-Antiplasmin inhibits free plasmin, but plasmin bound to fibrin is protected. α_2-Macroglobulin inhibits activated protein C and may inhibit plasmin to some extent. It also inhibits some activated coagulation factors.

Fibrinolysis occurs more readily in capillaries than in the systemic circulation. A much higher density of endothelial cells is found in capillaries. Consequently thrombomodulin-mediated protein C activation and thrombin clearance are greater in capillaries than in large vessels.[444] In addition, tPA release is greater in capillaries, and there may be less antiplasmin available to inhibit fibrinolysis. Rapid fibrinolysis of thrombi in large vessels could be life-threatening, but fibrinolysis is likely important in maintaining the integrity of capillary beds.

ANTICOAGULANTS

Coagulation is prevented in blood samples by using either Ca^{2+} chelators (ethylenediaminetetraacetate [EDTA] and citrate) or heparin in blood collection tubes. EDTA is the preferred anticoagulant for complete blood count (CBC) determinations in most species. Minimal sample dilution occurs following mixing with EDTA, and blood films prepared by using this anticoagulant exhibit optimal staining with routine blood stains. Blood from nonmammals has often been collected for hematology studies using heparin (rather than EDTA) as an anticoagulant because the blood of some birds (ratites) and some reptiles (chelonians) has been reported to hemolyze when collected with EDTA. This is clearly not a universal problem in birds and reptiles.[222] The disadvantage of heparin is that leukocytes do not stain as well and platelets (thrombocytes) usually clump more than in blood collected with EDTA.

Sodium citrate has generally been the preferred anticoagulant for collecting plasma for coagulation tests and for collecting platelets for platelet function tests.[84,363] However, hirudin (a leech-derived direct thrombin inhibitor) performed better than citrate as an anticoagulant in a whole-blood impedance aggregometer.[25] Samples collected in citrate solution are diluted by 10%. If platelet counts are done, they must be corrected for this dilution. However, platelet aggregates form more readily in dog blood collected in citrate, resulting in lower automated platelet counts than in blood collected in EDTA.[485] Citrate is also the anticoagulant typically used in solutions for blood collection and storage for transfusions.[371]

The binding of heparin to antithrombin greatly accelerates the inhibition of thrombin by antithrombin, thereby inhibiting coagulation. FIXa, FXa, and the VIIa-TF complex also appear to be inhibited by the antithrombin-heparin complex.

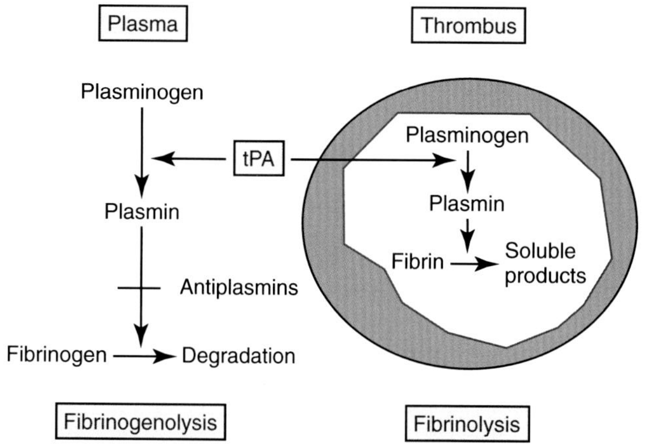

Plasma
Plasminogen
tPA
Plasmin
Antiplasmins
Fibrinogen → Degradation
Fibrinogenolysis
Thrombus
Plasminogen
Plasmin
Fibrin → Soluble products
Fibrinolysis

FIGURE 7-20
Actions of tissue plasminogen activator (tPA) and plasmin.

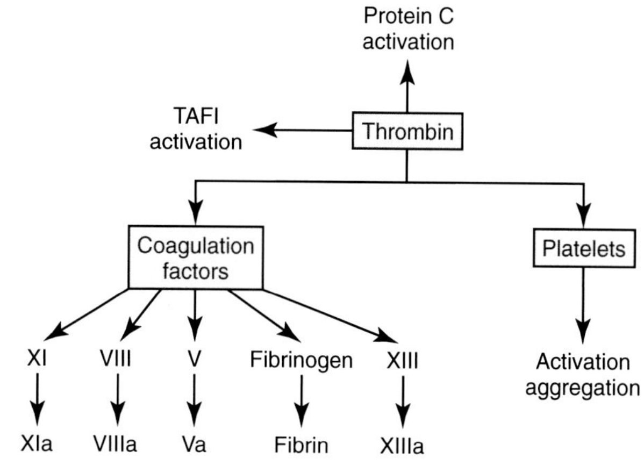

FIGURE 7-21
Actions of thrombin. Roman numerals refer to coagulation factors with these numbers, and an associated "a" indicates that the factor is activated. TAFI, thrombin-activatable fibrinolysis inhibitor.

Heparin is used as an anticoagulant for CBCs in species where EDTA results in hemolysis. Lithium heparin is utilized as an anticoagulant when plasma (rather than serum) is used for clinical chemistry profiles. Heparin is often added to isotonic salt solutions used to flush intravenous lines and may be injected to inhibit blood coagulation in vivo. Heparin is not recommended for platelet counts because platelets tend to clump when blood is collected in heparin.[281]

SCREENING TESTS FOR HEMOSTATIC DISORDERS

No single diagnostic test evaluates all hemostatic components. Consequently several hemostatic tests are usually done to determine the nature of a hemostatic disorder.

Platelet Count

Platelet counts are usually performed using blood collected with EDTA as the anticoagulant. The presence of platelet clumps can result in erroneously low platelet counts. Stained blood films should be examined each time platelet counts are done to verify that low platelet counts, determined manually or by machine, are valid. Factors used to estimate platelet numbers vary depending on the microscope used, method of blood film preparation, and area of the film examined; however, the formula given below generally provides a reasonable platelet estimate.

$$\text{Platelets per microliter} = \text{number of platelets per } 100\times \text{ oil field} \times 20{,}000$$

Cat platelets are larger than those of the other domestic animals; consequently it is not possible for impedance counters (such as the Coulter Counter S+4 and the Abbott Cell-Dyne 3500) to accurately separate cat platelets from erythrocytes by size.[383] Cell counters that count platelets using laser flow cytometry (such as the Siemens Advia 120) are able to count cat platelets more accurately in whole blood. Unfortunately platelet aggregates form readily during blood collection in cats; as a result, spuriously low automated platelet counts will often be present. Platelet aggregate formation is decreased in cat blood collected in citrate, theophylline, adenosine, and dipyridamole (CTAD) vacuum tubes (BD Diagnostics, Franklin Lakes, NJ) containing platelet inhibitors.[382]

Platelet counts in healthy greyhounds, Polish Ogar dogs, and Cavalier King Charles spaniels are generally lower than those measured in other dog breeds. The mean platelet count in Polish Ogar dogs was $167 \times 10^3/\mu L$, compared with $344 \times 10^3/\mu L$ for dogs of other breeds in Poland.[345] Using an impedance counter (Abbott Cell-Dyne 3500), the reference interval (mean ± 2 standard deviations) determined for platelet counts in Greyhounds was 90,000 to 290,000/µL, compared with a reference interval of 140,000 to 380,000/µL for dogs of other breeds.[448] The lower limit of the reference interval for platelet counts in Cavalier King Charles spaniels has been difficult to determine with certainty because there is a high incidence of an asymptomatic inherited thrombocytopenia with macrothrombocytes in this breed. Although overlap occurs, platelet counts below $100 \times 10^3/\mu L$ suggest the homozygous state, with intermediate counts (about $200 \times 10^3/\mu L$) expected in the heterozygous state and platelet counts above $250 \times 10^3/\mu L$ generally present in unaffected dogs.[127] Platelet counts determined using impedance counters are erroneously low in Cavalier King Charles spaniels with macrothrombocytes because these counters cannot differentiate large platelets from small erythrocytes.[394]

Mean Platelet Volume

The mean platelet volume (MPV) is the average volume of a single platelet recorded in femtoliters (fL). Within the normal ranges of platelet counts and MPVs, there is an inverse correlation between platelet count and MPV and a direct correlation between MPV and megakaryocyte ploidy (i.e., larger megakaryocytes) in healthy humans.[34,35] An inverse correlation between platelet counts and MPVs has also been reported in cats and dogs but not in horses, cattle, or goats.[48]

MPV determinations vary considerably with the instrument and anticoagulant used for the assay.[424] Impedance cell counters can accurately determine the MPV in whole blood from dogs and horses but not in whole blood from cats. Cell counters that count and size platelets using laser flow cytometry may be able to accurately measure the MPV in whole blood of cats, but platelet aggregates often form during blood collection in cats, resulting in spuriously high MPV values.[551] Of domestic animal species, cats had the highest MPVs (mean 11 fL), followed by dogs (mean 7.2 fL), horses (mean 5.0 fL), cattle (mean 4.8 fL), and goats (mean 4.2 fL) when blood was collected with sodium citrate and assayed using the same automated analyzer (Series 810, Baker Instruments Corp., Allentown, PA).[48] These values would be somewhat different if EDTA were used as the anticoagulant or if a different analyzer were used for the assays.

Results from studies on the effects of anticoagulants and storage conditions on MPV are contradictory. The MPV was reported to be higher when dog blood was collected with EDTA versus citrate as the anticoagulant in an early study,[217] but the MPV was reported to be lower when dog blood was collected with EDTA versus citrate as the anticoagulant in a more recent study.[485] No change in MPV was found in EDTA-anticoagulated dog blood stored for a day in one study,[520] but increases in MPV have been reported with storage of EDTA-anticoagulated dog blood in other studies.[179,217] Discrepancies in the effect of temperature on MPV during storage have also been reported.[179] These differences may be explained by the variable effects of anticoagulants on platelet activation and shape and by the various ways in which automated analyzers size platelets.[424,551]

A high MPV value suggests the presence of increased thrombopoiesis.[112,311] Interestingly, the MPV increased in mice within 8 hours after the production of thrombocytopenia, but 40 hours were required before increased megakaryocyte ploidy was observed. The MPV has been reported to be increased in some dogs with nonimmune-mediated regenerative thrombocytopenia[143] as well as in inflammatory conditions that result in enhanced platelet utilization/destruction.[366,548] However, the MPV can also be high in animals with myeloid neoplasms and, in cats, with feline leukemia virus (FeLV)-induced thrombocytopenia.[54,147] Cavalier King Charles spaniel dogs with inherited macrothrombocytopenia have higher MPV values because of the occurrence of a population of macrothrombocytes.[127] A macrothrombocytopenia has also been reported in a pug dog with the May-Hegglin anomaly (see Fig. 5-24), as discussed in Chapter 5.[164]

Although the MPV is expected to be increased in response to thrombocytopenia, normal or even decreased MPVs have been associated with dogs and humans with immune-mediated thrombocytopenia (IMT), presumably because of the presence of platelet fragments (as opposed to the formation of small platelets).[143,280,385] Consequently a normal MPV does not rule out enhanced thrombopoiesis, especially in primary IMT in dogs.[143] In fact, most dogs with an increased reticulated platelet count do not have an increased MPV.[400]

MPVs have been reported to be slightly higher in hyperthyroid cats and slightly lower in hypothyroid dogs than in euthyroid animals.[490] Dogs with phosphofructokinase deficiency of erythrocytes and skeletal muscle have mildly increased MPVs with normal platelet counts.

Bleeding Time

The buccal mucosal bleeding time test consists of penetration of the buccal mucosa with a sharp blade, which results in a free flow of blood and measurement of the time required for the bleeding to stop.[223,327] The incision is standardized by using a disposable spring-loaded lancet. The buccal mucosal bleeding time is done to evaluate platelet function in animals with normal or near-normal platelet counts. Since this test is expected to be prolonged in animals with low platelet counts, it provides no additional information in animals already known to have severe thrombocytopenia.[263] Platelet function abnormalities include inherited and acquired abnormalities of the platelets themselves, as well as deficiencies in the proteins required for normal platelet adherence (vWF) and aggregation (fibrinogen).[67,540] Bleeding times are normal when coagulation defects are present as long as platelet numbers and function are normal.[67] If left undisturbed, bleeding will usually stop in less than 4 minutes in healthy dogs and less than 3 minutes in healthy cats.[223,403,449] The test is imprecise, with repeat bleeding times varying by as much as 2 minutes.[449] Bleeding times may be longer in animals with prominent anemia, resulting in low blood viscosity.[39,58] The template bleeding time in horses has poor reproducibility and may be as long as 14 minutes in healthy horses.[454]

Activated Clotting Time

The activated clotting time (ACT) test evaluates the intrinsic and common coagulation pathways (Fig. 7-22). It must be done in close proximity to the animal being evaluated. The ACT requires a special collection tube containing siliceous earth and a method to maintain collection tubes at 37°C. Blood is collected into prewarmed tubes and maintained at 37°C until clotting has occurred. With the use of an automated coagulation timer, the ACT is usually less than 200 seconds in horses, less than 180 seconds in cattle,[430] less than 165 seconds in cats,[27] and less than 95 seconds in dogs.[188,504] Investigators using MAX-ACT tubes (Helena Laboratories, Beaumont, TX) indicate that the ACT in normal cats and dogs should be less than 85 seconds.[453] A positive correlation has been reported between ACT and C-reactive protein in dogs; consequently the investigators suggested that the ACT might be used as a screening test to access underlying inflammation as well as to determine hemostasis in the dog.[101]

Activated Partial Thromboplastin Time

The activated partial thromboplastin time (APTT) test is also used to evaluate the intrinsic and common pathways (see Fig. 7-22). It is usually measured using plasma prepared from blood collected with 3.2% sodium citrate as the anticoagulant in a 9:1 blood to citrate mixture. Assays should generally be done within an hour of sample collection, although the samples are stable for at least 6 hours when kept refrigerated.[91,96] However, some reports suggest that even longer storage times are possible.[178] Point-of-care analyzers are available that measure APTT using nonanticoagulated whole blood or citrate-anticoagulated whole blood.[504] Reference intervals vary with the methods used.[24,183] The APTT from a healthy animal of the same species can be measured at the

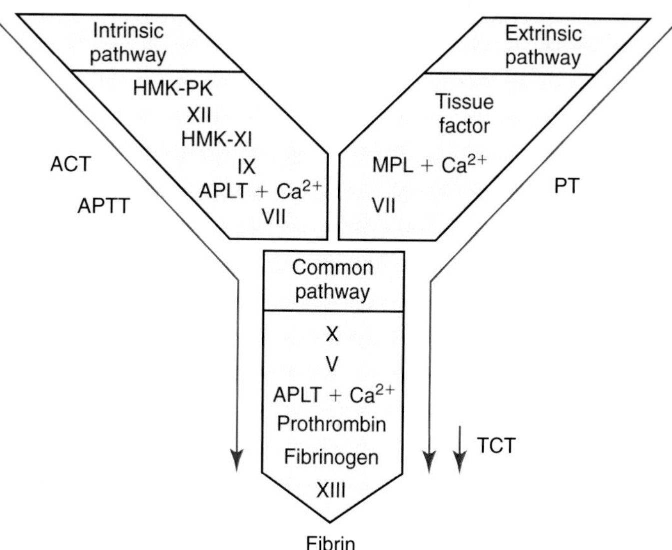

FIGURE 7-22
Components of the classical coagulation cascade as evaluated using activated clotting time (ACT), activated partial thromboplastin time (APTT), prothrombin time (PT), and thrombin clotting time (TCT) tests. Roman numerals refer to coagulation factors with these numbers. HMK, high-molecular-weight kininogen; PK, prekallikrein; Ca^{2+}, calcium ions; APLT, activated platelets.

same time as that of a control. The APTT is likely to be prolonged if the patient's time is 30% longer than the control's time.

The presence of an antiphospholipid antibody (lupus anticoagulant) can cause prolonged APTTs. This appears to account for the longer APTTs reported in healthy Bernese Mountain dogs compared with other breeds.[376,378] Antiphospholipid antibodies are discussed under "Acquired Coagulation Disorders," below.

The APTT is artifactually prolonged if the plasma-to-anticoagulant ratio is inappropriately low, as occurs if insufficient blood is collected into a vacuum tube containing premeasured citrate solution or if erythrocytosis (e.g., severe dehydration) is present. The APTT may be shortened somewhat in inflammatory conditions with a high fibrinogen concentration because the addition of fibrinogen to citrated plasma in dogs resulted in a slight but significant shortening of the APTT.[301]

Prothrombin Time

The prothrombin time (PT) test is used to evaluate the extrinsic and common pathways (see Fig. 7-22). It is usually measured using plasma prepared from blood collected with 3.2% sodium citrate as the anticoagulant in a 9:1 blood to citrate mixture. Assays should generally be done within an hour of sample collection, but they are stable for at least 6 hours when kept refrigerated.[91,96] However, some reports suggest that longer storage times are possible.[178] Point-of-care analyzers are available that measure PT using nonanticoagulated whole blood or citrate-anticoagulated whole blood.[504] Reference intervals vary with the methods used.[24,183] The PT from a healthy animal of the same species can be measured at the same time as that of a control. The PT is likely to be prolonged if the patient's time is 30% longer than the control's time. The PT may be shortened somewhat in inflammatory conditions with a high fibrinogen concentration because the addition of fibrinogen to citrated plasma in dogs resulted in a slight but significant shortening of the PT.[301]

Thrombin Clotting Time

The thrombin clotting time (TCT) test is initiated by adding thrombin. It is used as an assay for quantitative and/or qualitative fibrinogen disorders. The TCT utilizes citrated plasma, like the PT and APTT tests, and sample handling is similar to that for those tests. As expected, the addition of fibrinogen to citrated plasma in dogs and rats resulted in a substantial shortening of the TCT.[301] The TCT reference interval will depend on the method used.[24]

Fibrinogen

Fibrinogen is needed for normal platelet-to-platelet binding during platelet aggregation, and it is the precursor of fibrin in blood coagulation. Fibrin deposited in tissues provides scaffolding for inflammatory cells, fibroblasts, and endothelial cells. Plasma fibrinogen is an acute-phase protein, which increases with inflammatory diseases in all species[148]; but this increase seems to be most consistent in ruminants and horses.[43,149,258,494,500] Fibrinogen is increased with hyperadrenocorticism,[259] pregnancy,[507,510] and nephrotic syndrome in dogs.[1]

Fibrinogen concentrations may be low, normal, or high in animals with disseminated intravascular coagulation (DIC).[23,144,482] Although fibrinogen is consumed in forming thrombi, conditions that cause DIC may also stimulate increased fibrinogen synthesis.[252,349] Hypofibrinogenemia has been reported in some horses and dogs with hemangiosarcoma.[219,266] It is unclear whether this is related to localized coagulation or DIC.

Fibrinogen is synthesized in the liver; consequently plasma fibrinogen may be low in some animals with liver failure. The venoms of pit vipers, including rattlesnakes, have thrombin-like activities that cleave fibrinogen and produce a defibrinogenation syndrome where blood collected for analysis in the laboratory does not clot. [250,283] More information is given under "Snake Venoms," below. Afibrinogenemia has been described in a Bichon Frise dog. This condition was believed to have been acquired as a result of an antifibrinogen antibody that may have been acquired via multiple blood transfusions.[540] Inherited fibrinogen deficiencies have been reported in dogs, cats, goats, and a lamb.[68,162]

The heat precipitation test is a practical test for the estimation of fibrinogen (see Chapter 2), but it is not sensitive enough to differentiate low-normal from low fibrinogen values when determinations are made by subtraction of total protein values measured with a refractometer. More accurate values can be obtained by ocular micrometry (Millar's technique), but somewhat more time is required and a microscope with a calibrated ocular micrometer is needed.[37] The Millar technique has been automated in a hematology analyzer (QBC Vet Autoreader IDEXX) and results compare favorably to a thrombin-initiated clotting time assay in horses.[494]

Fibrinogen is most accurately measured using coagulation-based assays, the most common of which is a thrombin-initiated clotting rate assay (Clauss clotting method).[24,320,486] This method involves measuring the rate of fibrinogen-to-fibrin conversion in diluted samples in the presence of excess thrombin. Under these conditions, the fibrinogen content in plasma is rate-limiting, and the fibrinogen concentration is inversely proportional to the clotting time. Consequently the clotting time is used to measure fibrinogen concentration by comparing the patient's clotting time with a standard curve of clotting time versus fibrinogen concentration. Hemolysis and lipemia result in falsely decreased fibrinogen concentrations,[24] as do high concentrations of fibrin degradation products (as occurs in DIC).[353]

Fibrin(ogen) Degradation Products and D-Dimer Assays

FDP Assays

The fibrin(ogen) degradation products (FDP) tests provide evidence of fibrinolysis in vivo. FDPs produced by fibrinolysis have antihemostatic properties that promote hemorrhage,[201,355] which may occur as a sequela to DIC, especially in dogs.[480]

Antibody-based kits for the measurement of FDPs in human serum and plasma have been developed.[42] Fortunately several assays have sufficient cross-reactivity to be used for domestic animals, but test results can vary depending on the kit used. Positive FDP tests occur in animals with fibrinolysis secondary to thromboembolism (localized thrombosis) and DIC and in those with fibrinogenolysis (e.g., Eastern diamondback rattlesnake envenomation).[30,206] Increased plasma FDP values have also been reported in dogs with naturally occurring internal hemorrhage,[206,457] but increased FDP concentrations could not be reproduced by experimental injection of blood in dogs.[333] The half-life of FDPs in the circulation in humans is about 5 hours; consequently a positive FDP test indicates recent or ongoing fibrinolysis or fibrinogenolysis.[65]

In addition to DIC and thromboembolism, a plasma FDP test was sometimes positive in dogs with a variety of conditions, including neoplasia, immune-mediated hemolytic anemia, pancreatitis, gastric dilatation-volvulus, heat stroke, severe trauma, sepsis, protein-losing nephropathy, liver disease, hyperadrenocorticism, and chronic heart failure.[42] Somewhat increased FDP values have been associated with intense exercise and pregnancy in humans.[286,491] False-positive results may be due to improper collection and handling of samples. This has especially been a problem with serum assays. Neither plasma nor serum FDP assays appear to be sensitive enough to be used as diagnostic tests for DIC in horses.[486]

D-Dimer Assays

When plasmin cleaves soluble fibrin (or fibrinogen), FDP fragments X, Y, D, and E are produced. When plasmin cleaves cross-linked fibrin, different degradation products are produced. These cross-linked oligomers (X-oligomers) vary in molecular weight. They contain a D-dimer epitope, which is produced by FXIIIa–mediated cross-linking of fibrin and exposed by plasmin cleavage.[479] The D-dimer tests utilize monoclonal antibodies against a human D-dimer epitope. Traditional FDP assays cannot distinguish between fibrinolysis and fibrinogenolysis. A positive D-dimer test indicates the presence of fibrinolysis. This test is not affected by hemolysis and is stable for at least 2 days at room temperature and at least 1 month with frozen samples.[52]

Compared to FDP assays, the latex agglutination D-dimer assay is reported to have similar or slightly better sensitivity and specificity for the diagnosis of DIC and thromboembolism in dogs.[206,479,484] In addition to thromboembolism and DIC, plasma D-dimer values are increased with a variety of disorders in dogs, including neoplasia, immune-mediated disease, inflammation, liver disease, renal failure, postoperative states, and internal hemorrhage.[131,140,206,374] Positive tests in animals with internal hemorrhage presumably result from fibrinolysis of clots that form after bleeding has occurred. Although DIC or thromboembolism may have also been present in some of these disorders, it is important to recognize that the D-dimer test is specific for fibrinolysis. It is not specific for DIC or localized thromboembolism.

Healthy horses are reported to have D-dimer values of 551 to 875 μg/L of plasma when measured by enzyme-linked immunosorbent assay (ELISA). In contrast, dogs and humans generally have values below 250 μg/L. Consequently higher cutoff concentrations (e.g., greater than 1000 μg/L) are required in horses before a positive test result is reported.[486] Although the sensitivity of the D-dimer test was only about 50% for horses with colic-associated DIC, it was better than sensitivities determined for FDP assays.[486] The D-dimer test was positively associated with a diagnosis of sepsis in foals but was not considered a good predictor of DIC in these animals.[8] The D-dimer test was also positively associated with enteritis or peritonitis in adult horses with colic, and nonsurvivors had significantly higher D-dimer values than did survivors.[97]

The D-dimer test has not been adequately evaluated in cats.[29,480] An immunoturbidimetric assay did not appear to accurately measure D-dimers in cat plasma.[59] When D-dimer concentrations were measured in plasma using a semiquantitative latex agglutination test (Accuclot D-Dimer, Sigma Diagnostics), 8 of 12 cats with DIC and 16 of 36 sick cats without DIC were positive. Based on these findings, this D-dimer test was considered to be of limited value for the diagnosis of DIC in cats.[497]

Thromboelastography

Thromboelastography (TEG) utilizes special analyzers to detect and continuously display changes in viscoelastic properties of citrated whole blood as it clots (Fig. 7-23).[292,320] Instruments measure the initiation time (R, or clot time) in minutes for the amplitude of the tracings to go from 0 to 2 mm, clot kinetics (K, or clot formation time) in minutes for the tracing to go from 2 to 20 mm amplitude, the slope (α angle) between 2 and 20 mm amplitude in the tracings,

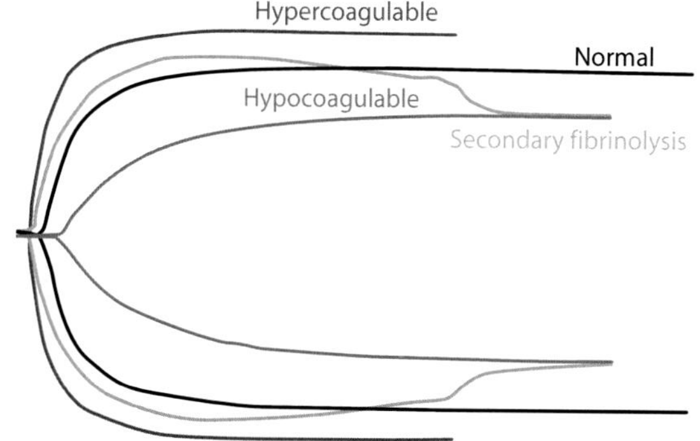

FIGURE 7-23

Thromboelastograph tracings using canine kaolin-activated blood and a Haemoscope TEG instrument. Tracings of normocoagulable, hypocoagulable, hypercoagulable, and secondary fibrinolytic states are shown.

Redrawn from Kol A, Borjesson DL. Application of thromboelastography/thromboelastometry to veterinary medicine. Vet Clin Pathol. *2010; 39:405–416.*

maximal amplitude (MA) in mm, and clot lysis (%) at 30 and 60 minutes. TEG studies the combined effects of soluble and cellular components of coagulation, which provides a more global evaluation of hemostasis than occurs when components of coagulation are studied independently. In light of the complexity of this system, it is not surprising that a number of factors can influence test results. Preanalytic variables include venipuncture technique, storage time, storage temperature, and in vitro hemolysis. Platelet counts, fibrinogen concentration, and HCT can produce changes in TEG tracings.[292,301] High HCTs result in TEG tracings indicating that a hypocoagulable state is present, as has been reported for greyhounds.[512] Conversely, low HCTs result in TEG tracings indicating that a hypercoagulable state is present. It is unclear whether these are simply in vitro artifacts or truly reflect an effect of erythrocyte numbers or blood viscosity on hemostasis in vivo.[292]

With standardized methods, care to minimize preanalytic variables and knowledge of the factors that can influence results, TEG may be a sensitive procedure that can supplement information gained from other hemostatic tests. Its greatest potential appears to be in recognizing hypercoagulable and hypocoagulable states, which may result in more timely and effective treatments.[292,537,538] TEG can also provide evidence of hyperfibrinolysis, but so far D-dimer concentrations have correlated poorly with TEG clot lysis results in veterinary medicine.[292]

SPECIALIZED TESTS FOR HEMOSTATIC DISORDERS

von Willebrand Factor

von Willebrand Factor (vWF) is a glycoprotein composed of polymers of various molecular weights. This factor is required for normal platelet adhesion; consequently it is assayed when a defect in platelet function is suspected. Inherited vWF deficiency (von Willebrand disease) is especially common in certain dog breeds (e.g., Doberman pinschers). Thus this factor may be measured prior to surgery or in the reproduction of dogs from breeds in which the disease is prevalent.[69] Some investigators have indicated that hypothyroidism may result in decreased vWF concentrations in the plasma of dogs,[14] but others have been unable to confirm this relationship.[399] In addition, thyroid treatment did not increase plasma vWF in euthyroid dogs with von Willebrand disease.[236] vWF is increased by interleukin-6 (IL-6) injection in dogs and may increase in plasma as an acute-phase protein during inflammation.[78] Increased concentrations have been reported in dogs with pregnancy,[320] endotoxemia,[386] sepsis,[437] and after exercise and epinephrine infusion.[344] IL-11 also promotes vWF synthesis in dogs.[393] Desmopressin (1-deamino-8-D-arginine vasopressin [DDAVP]) treatment transiently increases vWF concentration in plasma by stimulating the release of vWF stored in endothelial Weibel-Palade bodies.[344]

vWF antigen concentration in plasma is generally quantified using ELISAs, but this may also be done using immunoturbidometric methods.[76,320] Results are reported as percent of control mean. Dogs with vWF antigen less than 50% are generally considered positive and dogs with vWF antigen greater than 70% are generally considered negative, with intermediate values being unclassified; however, these values can differ based on the tests used.[76] There is substantial temporal variation in individual dogs, making identification of carrier animals difficult.[369] Consequently repeated tests of the same animal may be necessary to obtain a reliable estimate of vWF concentration. High-molecular-weight vWF polymers are required for normal platelet adhesion. Polymeric distribution of vWF is determined by protein immunoelectrophoresis and labeling with anti-vWF probes.[69]

Antithrombin

Plasma antithrombin can be measured using chromogen assays.[320] It may be decreased in hypercoagulable states (e.g., equine colic and hyperadrenocortism in dogs),[146,259] DIC,[23,357,532] protein-losing nephropathies and enteropathies,[203] chronic hepatitis with cirrhosis,[416] and sepsis.[22,132] Antithrombin is increased in cats with various disease conditions, suggesting that it behaves as an acute-phase protein in this species.[59]

PIVKA (Proteins Induced by Vitamin K Absence or Antagonism)

The PIVKA test (Thrombotest, Accurate Chemical and Scientific Corp., Westbury, NY) is a simple, sensitive coagulation test that was developed to monitor humans treated with warfarin; it has been recommended for use in the diagnosis of anticoagulant toxicity in dogs.[370] It is essentially a modified PT test that utilizes a particular tissue thromboplastin and diluted plasma to result in longer clotting times than the standard PT test. The PIVKA test is not specific for vitamin K deficiency. It may be prolonged with various defects in the extrinsic and/or common pathways.[95,440] The PIVKA test does not offer any advantage over the PT test in the diagnosis of rodenticide toxicities, because PT tests are consistently markedly prolonged in these disorders.[190] However, the PIVKA test might be helpful in identifying subtle coagulation abnormalities of the extrinsic or common pathways, because PT tests designed for humans may lack sensitivity for the detection of coagulopathies in certain animal species.[95]

Reticulated Platelet Count

Reticulated platelets are newly formed platelets (less than 1 day old in dogs) that contain increased amounts of ribonucleic acid (RNA).[123] Reticulated platelets have enhanced responses to agonists, which may promote the maintenance of hemostasis in regenerative thrombocytopenias.[407,432] Humans with thrombocytosis and high reticulated platelet counts were more likely to develop thrombosis than were individuals with thrombocytosis and normal reticulated platelet counts.[431] It is not clear whether the high reticulated platelet count enhances the likelihood of thrombus formation or simply reflects enhanced platelet turnover in these patients.

Reticulated platelets have been quantified by detecting fluorescence in thiazole orange-stained platelets using a flow cytometer. Unfortunately this assay is not usually available in clinical settings. Reference intervals vary considerably depending on the methods and equipment used for the assays.[329,400] Reticulated platelets have been measured in dogs using the PLT-O channel of a Sysmex XT2000iV hematology analyzer (Sysmex, Kobe, Japan).[400] A negative proportional bias was found with this instrument compared with flow cytometry using a FACS scan cytometer (BD Biosciences). Reticulated platelet counts determined with both methods were increased in a population of thrombocytopenic dogs that did not have increased MPVs, indicating that reticulated platelet counts are more sensitive in identifying increased thrombopoiesis than are MPVs.

Analogous to the use of reticulocyte counts in determining the cause of an anemia, an increased percentage of reticulated platelets in a thrombocytopenic animal suggests that the thrombocytopenia results from increased platelet destruction or consumption and not from decreased platelet production.[329,442] The percentage of reticulated platelets is generally within the reference interval in animals with thrombocytopenia resulting from decreased platelet production.[529]

In contrast to regenerative anemias, in which increases in absolute reticulocyte counts are expected, absolute reticulated platelet counts (reticulated platelets per microliter) are not typically increased in regenerative thrombocytopenias, especially when platelet counts are below $50 \times 10^3/\mu L$.[329,529,542] This lack of an increase in the absolute reticulated platelet count in blood may be explained if reticulated platelets are destroyed or consumed at the same rate as nonreticulated platelets. Absolute reticulated platelet counts may be increased in reactive thrombocytosis, as has been demonstrated in dogs given IL-6 experimentally.[408]

Samples should be assayed on the same day they are collected. Surprisingly, the percentage of reticulated platelets increases after 24 hours of storage in the refrigerator or at room temperature.[400,466]

Platelet Function

The bleeding time test, discussed earlier in this chapter, is an in vivo platelet function test. Specialized platelet function tests are typically done in specialized diagnostic hemostasis laboratories or research laboratories.

Flow Cytometry

Platelet activation can be measured using flow cytometry. Annexin V has specific binding affinity for aminophospholipids (primarily PS) on activated platelets; consequently, increased annexin V binding on platelets indicates platelet activation. An increase of P-selectin (CD62P) or fibrinogen on the surface of platelets as well as the presence of platelet-leukocyte aggregates and platelet microparticles have also been used to identify platelet activation.[271,282,388,527,545] The formation of platelet-leukocyte aggregates correlates with enhanced reactivity of platelets toward neutrophils as well as toward other platelets.[298] In addition, the measurement of a decrease in mean platelet component (MPC) concentration using automated hematology analyzers suggests platelet activation.[366,455,551]

Platelet Function Analyzer

A platelet function analyzer (PFA-100) has been validated for use in animals. It is essentially an in vitro modified bleeding time test that uses citrated plasma and depends on platelet adhesion, secretion, and aggregation. Blood is drawn at a high shear rate through an aperture coated with agonists. The closure time is recorded as the time required for the aperture to be occluded with platelet aggregates and for the blood flow to stop.[495] The closure time is prolonged in dogs with thrombocytopenia, with longer times occurring in animals with lower platelet counts. The closure time is also prolonged in dogs with von Willebrand disease and inherited platelet function defects.[83] It is prolonged in dogs treated with aspirin but not in those with coagulopathies (coumarin toxicity and FVIII deficiency).[351] Like the buccal mucosal bleeding time,[39,58] the closure time is longer in dogs with lower HCTs. A decrease of HCT from 40% to 30% resulted in a significant prolongation of the closure time, which was prolonged even more with further decreases in HCT. This effect of HCT limits the clinical applicability of the PFA-100 in anemic animals.[351]

Platelet Aggregation

Platelet aggregation is evaluated in aggregometers following the addition of various agonists (e.g., ADP, thrombin, and collagen). Optical platelet aggregation or light-transmission aggregation is measured in platelet-rich plasma using a spectrophotometer. As platelets aggregate, the sample becomes less opaque and increased light transmission is graphed using a recorder attached to the spectrophotometer. Whole-blood platelet aggregation is measured using electrical impedance. As activated platelets aggregate to two electrodes, the impedance increases.[495]

Platelet Secretion

Platelet secretion is examined by measuring the release of contents from dense granules after agonist stimulation.[342] The Whole Blood Lumi-Aggregometer (Chrono-Log Corporation, Havertown, PA) has been validated for use in dogs.[273] It measures the platelet aggregation and secretion of ATP simultaneously. Assays are time-sensitive. Whole-blood samples must stand 60 minutes at room temperature after blood collection for platelets to become responsive, and assays should be completed within 3 hours of blood collection.[273]

Antiplatelet Antibody

Increased platelet-bound immunoglobulins are most often detected in animals using flow cytometry.[290,337,541] Most antiplatelet antibody in blood is bound to platelets; consequently direct assays of the patient's platelets are more sensitive than indirect assays using serum from the patient and platelets from a healthy control animal.[313] Unfortunately, direct assays of platelets should be done within 24 hours after blood sample collection. Platelets naturally have some immunoglobulin adsorbed to their surfaces. The amount of platelet-bound immunoglobulin can increase with time after sample collection; consequently false-positive tests can be a significant problem with these assays.[541] Positive test results may occur when immune complexes are adsorbed to platelets as well as when antiplatelet antibodies are present. Refer to Chapter 6 for more information concerning antiplatelet antibodies.

Specific Coagulation Factors

The measurement of fibrinogen is discussed earlier in this chapter. Assays for other specific coagulation factors are done in a few specialized diagnostic and hemostasis research laboratories including the Comparative Coagulation Laboratory, Animal Health Diagnostic Center, College of Veterinary Medicine, Cornell University, Ithaca, New York. Plasma samples from humans or animals with known coagulation factor deficiencies are used in modified PT and APTT assays.[348,350] The degree of correction of the long clotting times of factor-deficient plasma by the plasma being tested is proportional to the activity of the specific factor being analyzed for in the test sample. Chromogenic assays are also available for some coagulation factors.[320]

CLINICAL SIGNS OF HEMOSTATIC DISORDERS

If bleeding is excessive or unexplained, a defect in one or more of the components of hemostasis may be present. The type of hemorrhage observed may give some clue about the nature of the defect or defects present. Diffuse cutaneous or mucosal discoloration, resulting from hemorrhage and edema, suggests the presence of a vascular defect, as may occur with vasculitis.[418] Petechial and ecchymotic cutaneous and/or mucosal hemorrhages and epistaxis are suggestive of thrombocytopenia. Spontaneous bleeding due to uncomplicated thrombocytopenia occurs less often in cats than in dogs. Unless there is a concomitant platelet function abnormality, coagulopathy, or vasculopathy, spontaneous bleeding seldom occurs in cats with platelet counts above $30 \times 10^3/\mu L$, and it may not occur in cats with counts as low as $15 \times 10^3/\mu L$.[270,290] Bleeding is more likely to occur in thrombocytopenic animals if trauma or inflammation is present.[194] The presence of an inherited platelet defect is suspected in a young animal with epistaxis, mucosal bleeding, unexplained petechial and ecchymotic hemorrhages, or when excessive bleeding occurs when teeth are shed.[44] Mucosal hemorrhage, cutaneous bruising, and prolonged bleeding from surgical or traumatic wounds are typically seen in dogs with vWD, but petechiae do not appear to be a sign of vWD in dogs. Sites of mucosal bleeding include gingival hemorrhage, gastrointestinal hemorrhage, hematuria, prolonged estral bleeding, and epistaxis.[69]

Spontaneous hematomas and hemorrhage into body cavities, including hemarthrosis, are more likely to result from coagulation defects than from vascular defects or platelet abnormalities.[72] Acute hemothorax, hemoabdomen, or both have been reported in aged (more than 15 years old) horses treated with phenylephrine for nephrosplenic entrapment of the large colon. Vessel rupture may have occurred because of drug-induced hypertension combined with reduced vessel compliance or elasticity in the aged horse.[168] Acute hemoabdomen and acute hemorrhage in other tumor sites may occur in dogs with hemangiosarcomas that rupture spontaneously.

Some greyhounds bleed excessively after surgery, but the cause has not been identified. Defects in primary and secondary hemostasis have not been identified, but alterations in fibrinolysis may be present.[305]

PLATELET DISORDERS

Abnormal Platelet Morphology

Macrothrombocytes

Platelets that are as large as erythrocytes or larger in diameter are called macrothrombocytes or macroplatelets (Fig. 7-24, *A-E*). Cats have large, variably sized platelets, with some in normal cats as large as erythrocytes (see Fig. 7-1, *E*).[49] The presence of frequent macrothrombocytes in a thrombocytopenic animal suggests that enhanced thrombopoiesis is present (Fig. 7-24, *A-C*), but macrothrombocytes may also be present in thrombocytopenic animals with myeloid neoplasms (Fig. 7-24, *D-E*).[225] Macrothrombocytes develop in cats with FeLV infections.[54] Macrothrombocytes may be present in nonthrombocytopenic animals that have recently recovered from thrombocytopenia (Fig. 7-25, *A,B*).

Macrothrombocytes are present in Cavalier King Charles spaniel dogs with inherited macrothrombocytopenia (Fig. 7-26), discussed later in this chapter.[74,127] A second inherited disorder with macrothrombocytes (see Fig. 5-24) and thrombocytopenia has also been described in a pug dog with the May-Hegglin anomaly (see Chapter 5 and later in this chapter for more information).[164]

Activated Platelets

Partially activated platelets are no longer discs (Fig. 7-27, *A*) but have thin cytoplasmic processes extending from a spherical cell body (Fig. 7-27, *B*). When platelets are more fully activated, their granules are crushed together by a surrounding web of microtubules and microfilaments (Fig. 7-27, *C*). This central aggregate of platelet granules may be mistaken for a nucleus (Fig. 7-24, *C;* Fig. 7-27, *C*). Platelet aggregates often form following platelet activation in vitro. If degranulation occurs, aggregates may be difficult to recognize as platelets, appearing as light-blue material on stained blood films (Fig. 7-2, *A;* Fig. 7-28). The presence of platelet aggregates should be recorded because the platelet count may be erroneously decreased.

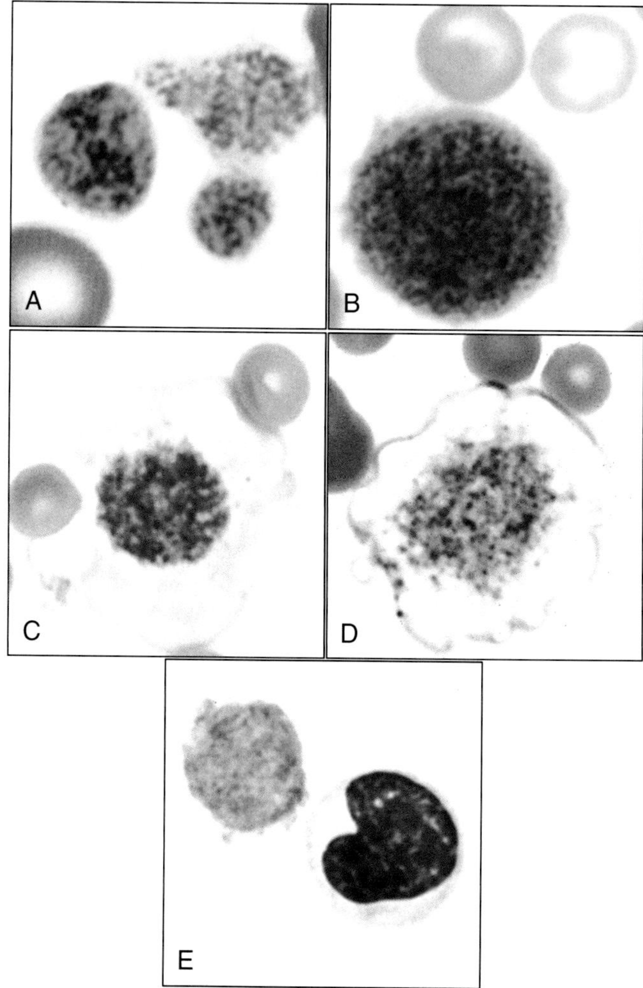

FIGURE 7-24
Macrothrombocytes in stained blood films. **A,** Macrothrombocytes in blood from a dog with a regenerative immune-mediated thrombocytopenia. The intense basophilia suggests that these may be reticulated platelets. **B,** Macrothrombocyte in blood from a dog with a thrombocytosis associated with chronic iron-deficiency anemia. **C,** Macrothrombocyte with aggregated granules, which may be mistaken for a nucleus in blood, from a cat with an abdominal abscess and toxic left shift in the blood. **D,** Macrothrombocyte with centrally located granules in blood from a cat with myelodysplastic syndrome. **E,** Macrothrombocyte *(left)* and metamyeloctye *(right)* in blood from a dog with chronic myeloid leukemia. Wright-Giemsa stain.

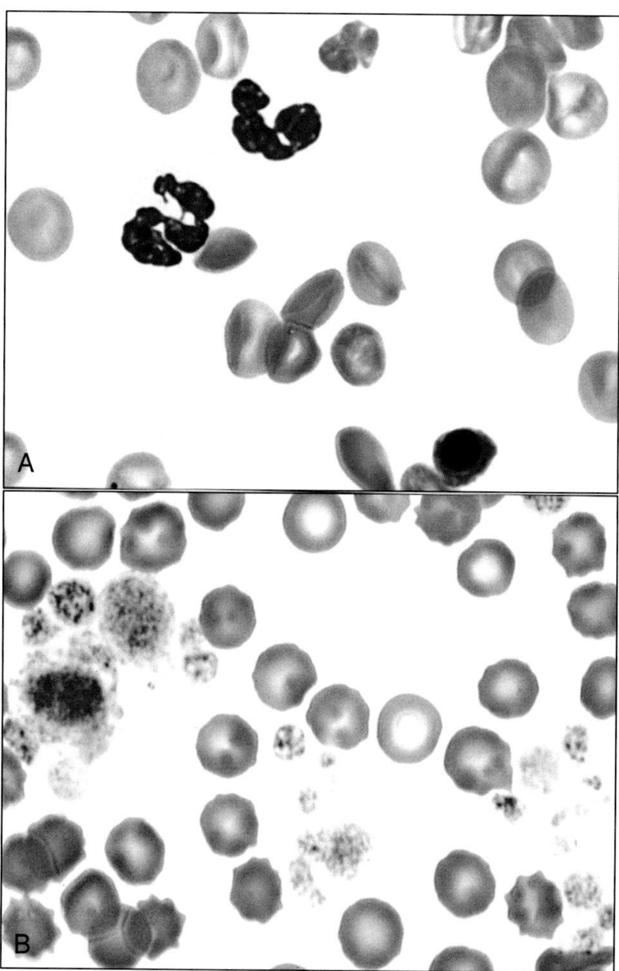

FIGURE 7-25
Rebound thrombocytosis after therapy in a dog with immune-mediated thrombocytopenia. **A,** Thrombocytopenia (platelets = $20 \times 10^3/\mu L$) and regenerative anemia prior to therapy. Polychromatophilic erythrocytes, a metarubricyte *(bottom),* and two neutrophils are present. **B,** Thrombocytosis (platelets = $950 \times 10^3/\mu L$) with several macrothrombocytes in blood a week after beginning prednisone therapy. Wright-Giemsa stain.

Hypogranular Platelets

Hypogranular platelets may result from platelet activation and secretion, but they have also been seen in animals with myeloid neoplasms (Fig. 7-29, *A-C*).[81,225] Hypogranular platelets must be differentiated from cytoplasmic fragments from other cells, as may occur with leukemic lymphomas (Fig. 7-30).[523]

Anaplasma platys *Infection*

Anaplasma platys (previously *Ehrlichia platys*) is a rickettsial parasite that specifically infects platelets and causes infectious cyclic thrombocytopenia in dogs.[227] This agent is unique in that it is the only intracellular infectious agent described in humans or animals to specifically infect platelets. *A. platys* organisms appear as blue inclusions in platelets when blood films are stained with Wright-Giemsa or new methylene blue (Fig. 7-31, *A-D*). Similar-appearing inclusions have been seen in platelets from a cat.[447]

Ultrastructurally, organisms range from 350 to 1250 nm in diameter; are round, oval, or bean-shaped; and are surrounded by a double membrane. Infected platelets may contain one to three single membrane-lined vacuoles with 1 to 15 organisms per vacuole (Fig. 7-32, *A-B*).[12,229] Organisms appear to enter platelets by adhering to the platelet surface followed by endocytosis. Therefore the vacuolar membrane is probably derived from the external platelet membrane. Repeated binary fission of organisms within the vacuole results in the formation of a morula.[229]

The prepatent period is 1 to 2 weeks following experimental injection with infected blood. Cyclic parasitemia and concomitant thrombocytopenia occur at 1 to 2 week intervals (Fig. 7-33). Parasitized platelets are easily found during the initial parasitemia, but subsequent parasitemias have decreasing percentages of parasitized platelets, making the recognition of morulae within platelets difficult. Platelet counts usually remain below 20,000/µL for only 1 or 2 days, before rapidly increasing.[227] Mild normocytic normochromic anemia may also be present. Based on serum iron and bone marrow studies, decreases in the hematocrit may be attributed to the anemia of inflammatory disease. Slight to moderate increases in acute-phase proteins and immunoglobulins and slightly decreased albumin may be present in serum samples.[16]

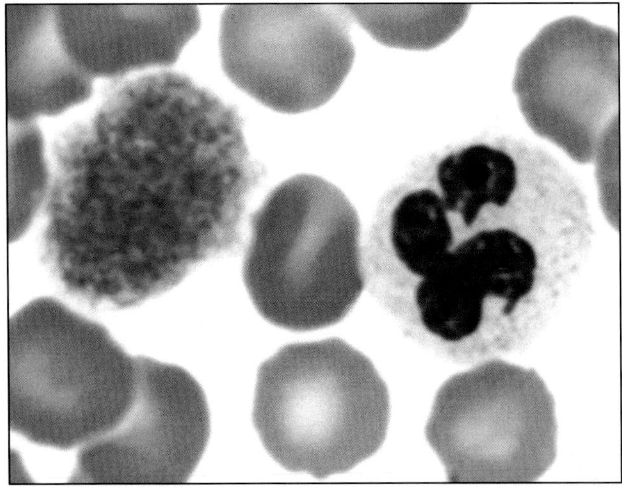

FIGURE 7-26
Macrothrombocyte *(left)* and a neutrophil *(right)* in a blood film from a Cavalier King Charles spaniel with inherited macrothrombocytopenia. Wright-Giemsa stain.

Infected dogs in the United States usually do not exhibit evidence of illness. Mild fever may occur at the time of the initial parasitemia. Minimal or no evidence of hemorrhage is present in most cases, but epistaxis, petechiae, and ecchymosis of the mucous membranes have been reported. Prominent uveitis has also been reported in one case. Although infection with U.S. isolates of *A. platys* seldom results in serious disease, significant clinical signs have been reported in infected dogs outside the United States.[227]

Diagnosis of infection with this agent can be made by observing organisms within platelets, but this is difficult unless daily samples are taken, and even then, less than 1% of platelets may be infected. An IFA test for antibodies against *A. platys* has been developed, but it probably cross-reacts to some degree with other rickettsial (especially *Anaplasma* species) organisms. The Snap 4Dx (IDEXX Laboratories, Inc., MA) has a component to identify dogs previously exposed to *A. phagocytophilum,* which cross-reacts with *A. platys*. These *Anaplasma* species can be differentiated using PCR and *16S rRNA* gene sequencing.[227]

Thrombocytopenia

Thrombocytopenia denotes decreased numbers of blood platelets. Primary causes of thrombocytopenia include decreased production, increased platelet utilization in thrombus formation, and increased destruction. The distinction between these causes is not always clear and the pathogenesis of thrombocytopenia associated with infectious agents (viral, rickettsial, bacterial, and protozoal) appears to be multifactorial. Less likely causes of thrombocytopenia include sequestration and acute massive external hemorrhage. Bone marrow examination can be helpful in the differential diagnosis of

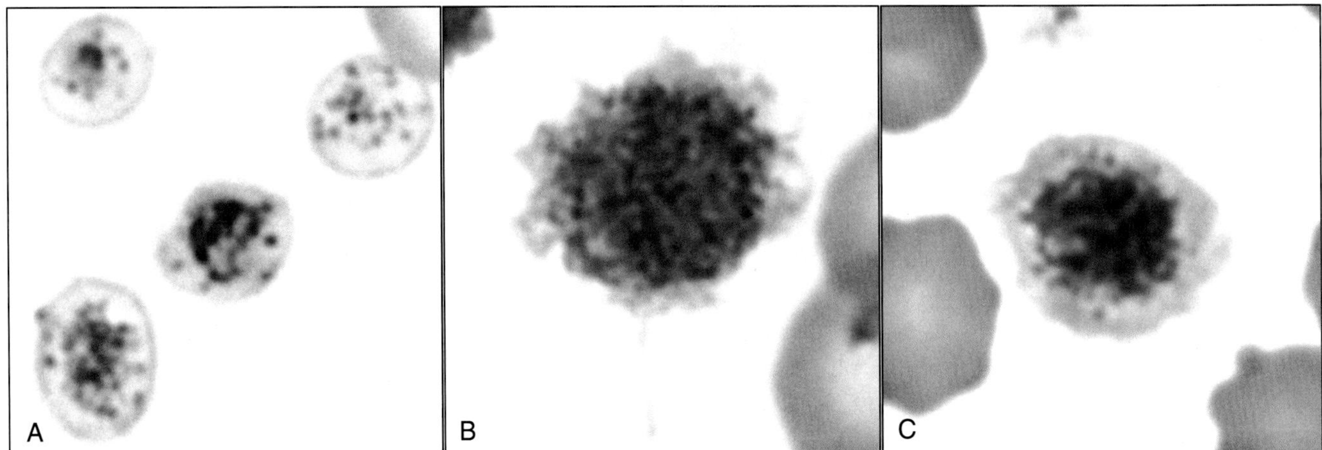

FIGURE 7-27
Resting versus activated platelet morphology in stained blood films. **A,** Unstimulated platelet morphology in blood from a dog. Platelets appear as round to oval discs without filopodia formation or centralized granules. **B,** Activated platelet in blood from a dog with prominent filopodia formation. **C,** Activated platelet in blood from a cat with centralized granules and filopodia formation.

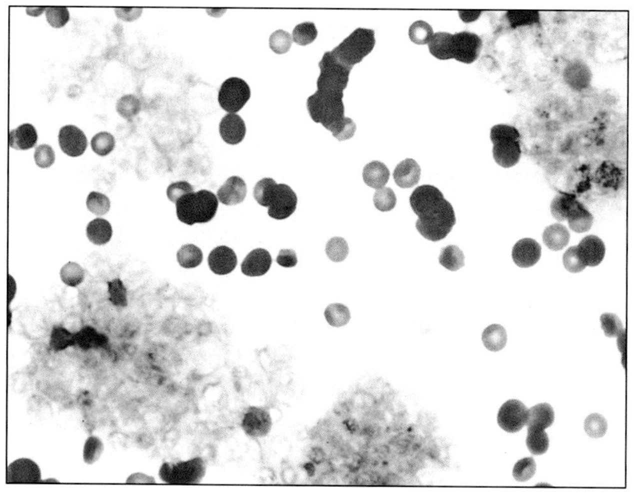

FIGURE 7-28

Thrombocytosis in blood from a cat with large aggregates of degranulated platelets, which resulted in a spuriously high total leukocyte count when assayed using an impedance hematology analyzer. Wright-Giemsa stain.

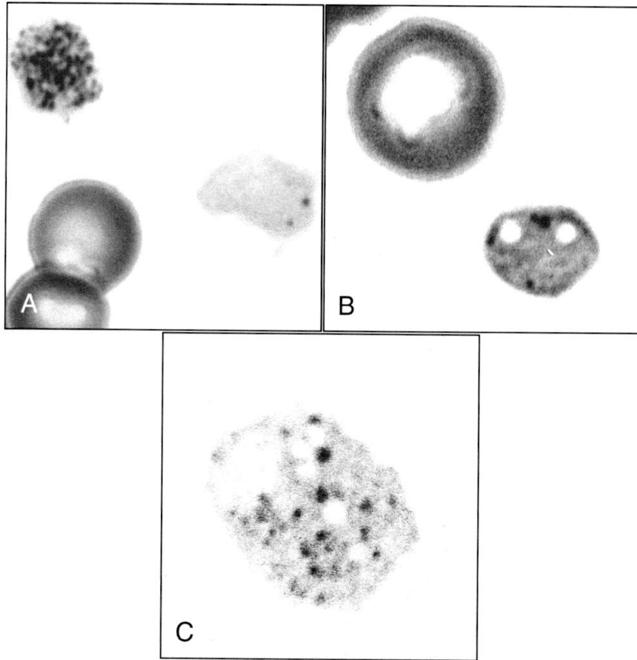

FIGURE 7-29

Hypogranular platelets in stained blood films. **A,** Platelet with granules *(top left)* and a hypogranular platelet *(right)* in blood from a dog with chronic myeloid leukemia. **B,** Hypogranular platelet in blood from a dog with erythroleukemia (AML-M6Er). **C,** Hypogranular macrothrombocyte in blood from a dog with chronic myeloid leukemia. Wright-Giemsa stain.

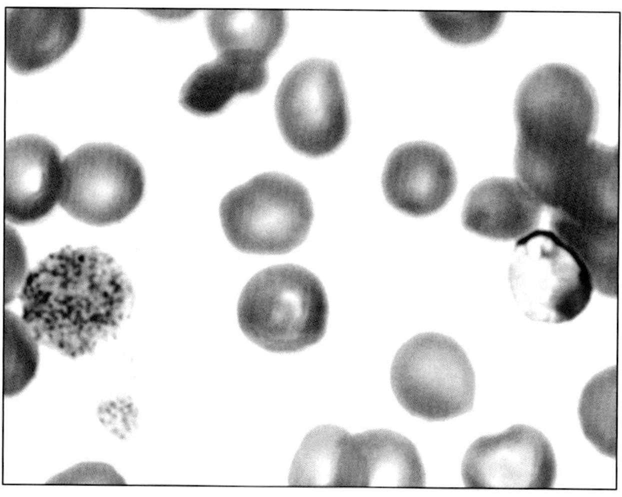

FIGURE 7-30

Basophilic cytoplasmic fragment *(far right)* and macrothrombocyte *(far left)* in blood from a dog with acute lymphoblastic leukemia. The fragment might be confused with a hypogranular platelet. Wright-Giemsa stain.

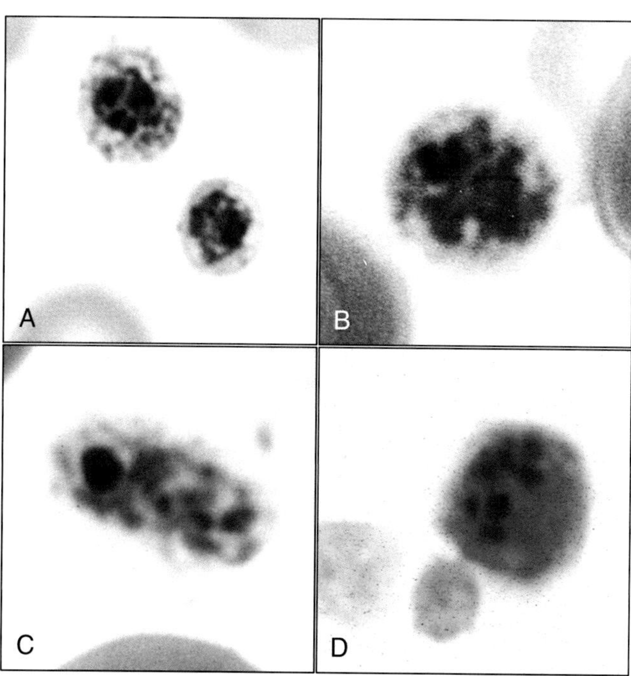

FIGURE 7-31

Anaplasma platys morulae in platelets from dogs. **A-C,** Platelets each containing an *A. platys* morula, which stain dark-blue, in contrast to the normal magenta-staining granules. Wright-Giemsa stain. **D,** Platelet containing an *A. platys* morula, with multiple subunits visible. New methylene blue wet mount preparation.

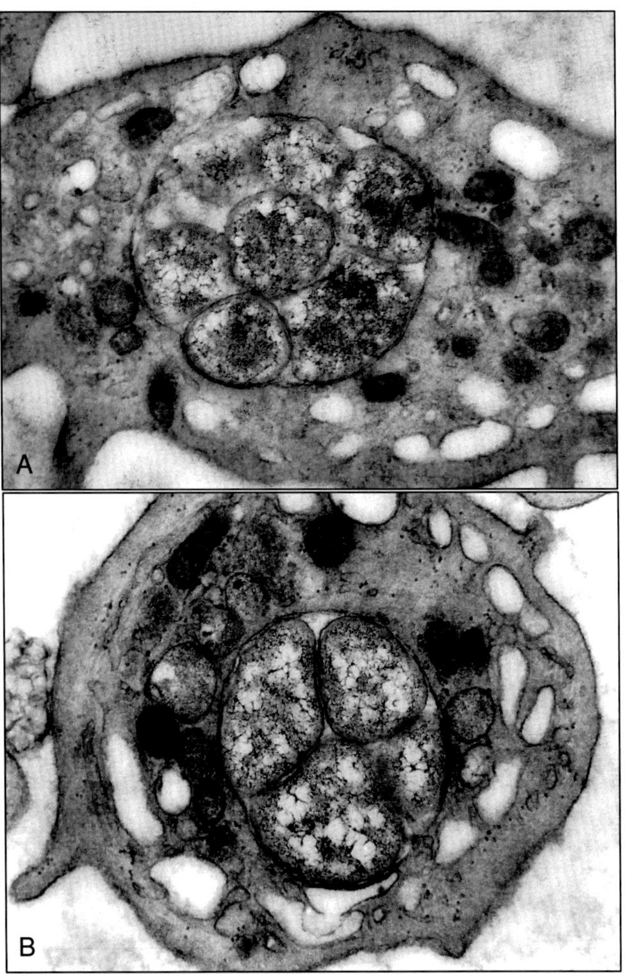

FIGURE 7-32

Transmission electron photomicrographs of dog platelets each containing an *A. platys* morula. Platelet granules and canalicular system are also visible. **A,** Platelet with a membrane-lined vacuole containing seven visible organisms. **B,** Platelet with a membrane-lined vacuole containing four visible organisms.

From Harvey JW, Simpson CF, Gaskin JM. Cyclic thrombocytopenia induced by a Rickettsia-like agent in dogs. J Infect Dis. *1978;137:182-188.*

thrombocytopenia, especially in the absence of accompanying coagulation abnormalities.

Decreased Platelet Production

Thrombocytopenia is a consistent finding with hypoplastic and aplastic bone marrow. It is also often present in myelophthisic disorders characterized by the replacement of normal hematopoietic cells with abnormal ones. Examples include myeloid neoplasms, lymphoid neoplasms, and multiple myeloma. Thrombocytopenia may also sometimes be present secondary to the extensive metastasis of lymphomas, carcinomas, and mast cell tumors (see Chapters 4 and 9 for more details concerning these disorders).

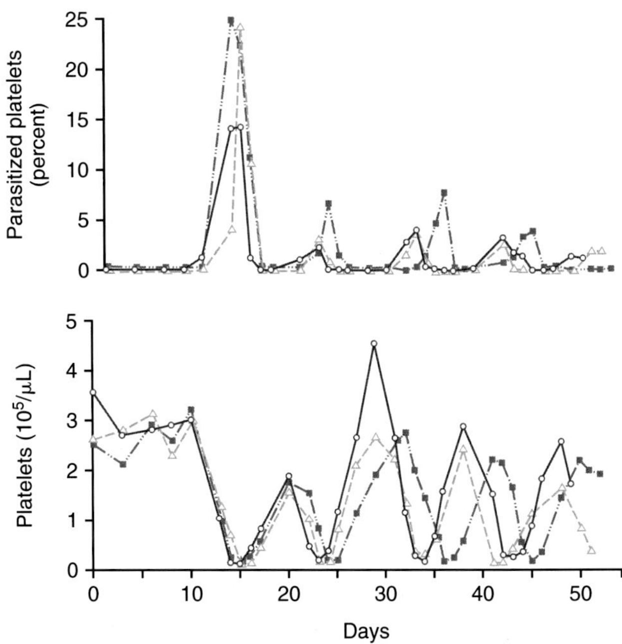

FIGURE 7-33

Parasitemic and thrombocytopenic episodes in three young dogs infected intravenously with *Anaplasma platys* organisms at time 0.

Thrombocytopenia is often recognized in cats infected with FeLV and less often in those infected with feline immunodeficiency virus (FIV).[54,177,193,270] Examination of bone marrow generally reveals the presence of a myelodysplastic syndrome or less often leukemia.[177,524]

The replication of viruses in megakaryocytes may contribute to the development of thrombocytopenia in some viral infections.[15,26,152,177] Platelet production is also decreased in horses infected with equine infectious anemia virus, but the mechanism has not been determined.[121]

Most IMTs result from increased platelet destruction in the circulation, but rare cases of amegakaryocytic thrombocytopenia that were believed to be immune-mediated have been reported in dogs and cats.[181,303,552] The long-term use of a recombinant human thrombopoietin (TPO) can result in a persistent thrombocytopenia in animals when antibodies made against the recombinant TPO also neutralize the endogenous TPO of the species receiving treatment. The subsequent lack of endogenous TPO results in decreased platelet production.[122]

Platelet counts cycle in gray collie dogs with inherited cyclic hematopoiesis because of intermittently decreased platelet production. However, thrombocytopenia is minimal, if present at all, because the decreased production is short relative to platelet life spans.[216]

Increased Platelet Utilization

Increased platelet utilization (consumption) occurs in association with DIC and thromboembolism (discussed later), with hemangiosarcoma in dogs with or without DIC,[215] and with vascular lesions including vasculitis.[103,118,325,358] In addition to vascular injury associated with certain inflammatory conditions, some inflammatory cytokines, most notably PAF, promote platelet aggregation.[380,505]

Thrombocytopenia may be present following envenomation by poisonous snakes, especially vipers.[9,142,317,543] Components of venom may directly induce platelet activation and aggregation. Platelet activation and aggregation may also occur in response to vessel injury induced by components of venom.[438] The hematologic effects are discussed under "Snake Venoms," later in this chapter.

Increased Platelet Destruction

The presence of increased immunoglobulin on the surfaces of platelets can result in increased phagocytosis of platelets and subsequent thrombocytopenia. IMT can be either primary or secondary. Autoantibodies are directed against platelet-specific epitopes in primary IMT, which has also been called autoimmune thrombocytopenia or idiopathic thrombocytopenia purpura (ITP). Primary IMT is uncommon in dogs and rare in other species (see Chapter 6 for more information about primary IMT).

Neonatal alloimmune thrombocytopenia has rarely been reported in newborn horses,[75] mules,[422] and pigs.[166] Analogous to neonatal isoerythrolysis, this disorder occurs when maternal antibodies against paternal epitopes on the surface of neonatal platelets are passively transferred to the neonate in colostrum.

Secondary IMT results from the exposure of hidden or altered antigens on platelet surfaces, the binding of external antigens to platelets (e.g., drugs), or the adsorption of antigen-antibody complexes to the platelet surface.[89,419] Secondary IMT may occur in association with various drugs,[40,129] infectious agents,* neoplasia,[143,232,295,426] and other immune-mediated disorders, such as systemic lupus erythematosus (SLE).[143,295]

The intravenous infusion of unfractionated heparin induces a mild thrombocytopenia in some horses.[359,361] In contrast, platelet counts did not decrease following the intravenous administration of low-molecular-weight heparin.[359] The mechanism has not been determined in horses, but heparin-induced thrombocytopenia (HIT) appears to be immune-mediated in humans. In humans, platelet activation results in the release of PF4/CXCL4, which binds to endothelial cells, displacing antithrombin bound to heparan sulfate. The administration of heparin results in the displacement of PF4 into the circulation, where it forms large multimolecular complexes with heparin. These PF4/heparin complexes elicit antibody formation in a small percentage of patients receiving ongoing heparin therapy. The antibody-PF4-heparin complex binds to Fc receptors on the platelet surface and induces platelet activation, aggregation, and the release of procoagulant microparticles, which may lead to thrombosis in humans.[7]

*References 106, 116, 143, 202, 209, 313.

The administration of granulocyte-monocyte colony-stimulating factor (GM-CSF) and macrophage colony-stimulating factor (M-CSF) to dogs results in a shortened platelet life span and thrombocytopenia, apparently by activating the monocyte/macrophage system.[2,19,167,372,396] Monocyte and/or macrophage activation may be a mechanism of increased platelet destruction observed in a variety of inflammatory diseases in which these endogenous cytokine concentrations in plasma are increased.

In addition to increased erythrocyte phagocytosis, increased phagocytosis of platelets may occur with the hemophagocytic syndrome (macrophage activation syndrome), which is characterized by greater than 2% hemophagocytic macrophages in bone marrow.[302,517] This syndrome develops secondary to some infectious, neoplastic, and immune-mediated conditions, but an underlying disease may not always be identified.[517,525] Thrombocytopenia is often present in dogs and cats with hemophagocytic histiocytic sarcoma, where phagocytosis of platelets may occur along with erythrocytes.*

Sequestration of Platelets

Sequestration of platelets in an enlarged spleen may result in thrombocytopenia. Platelet counts decreased in dogs when intravenous PGI_2 was used to cause splenic enlargement.[379] Causes of splenomegaly include hereditary hemolytic anemias, immune-mediated diseases, infections, inflammation, splenic congestion (including use of anesthetics or tranquilizers), splenic torsion, and infiltrative diseases.[304,476] Increased platelet utilization or destruction also contributes to the development of thrombocytopenia in some of these disorders. When splenomegaly results in increased removal of platelets and/or other blood cells by the spleen, the term *hypersplenism* may be used.[297,458,526] Blood platelet counts decrease in dogs during hypothermia, and this decrease has been attributed to sequestration of platelets in the liver.[414]

Massive External Hemorrhage

Because of platelet storage in the spleen and/or lungs, acute hemorrhage usually causes minimal decreases in blood platelet counts. Platelet counts seldom decrease below $100 \times 10^3/\mu L$ because of acute hemorrhage alone, although counts have decreased to as low as $30 \times 10^3/\mu L$ in dogs with massive hemorrhage secondary to anticoagulant rodenticide toxicity.[312,457] It may be that these platelets aggregated at sites of hemorrhage. If so, platelet utilization could have contributed to the development of thrombocytopenia in addition to platelet loss in blood. Thrombocytopenia may be accentuated in animals with hemorrhage if a large transfusion of packed erythrocytes or stored blood is given.[272] These platelet-poor transfusions can have a dilution effect on platelet numbers in blood. Platelet counts may be increased in animals with chronic hemorrhage, especially when it results in iron-deficiency anemia.[226]

*References 117, 170, 174, 251, 289, 362.

Infections and Thrombocytopenia

Thrombocytopenia often occurs in association with infectious agents, especially those present in blood. The pathogenesis of thrombocytopenia may be multifactorial and is not always understood. Vascular injury and/or adsorption of immune complexes to platelet surfaces may be involved with some infectious agents.[15] Direct effects on platelets have been suggested with some organisms.[6,229] Some viruses and chronic *Ehrlichia canis* infections decrease platelet production, although immune-mediated platelet destruction also contributes to the thrombocytopenia in ehrlichiosis.[209,519]

A variety of cytokines are released in response to infectious agents and some of them have effects on circulating platelet numbers.[93,134,460] IL-6 promotes platelet production and enhances platelet responsiveness to thrombin.[277,408] In contrast, IL-10 and IFN-α inhibit platelet production.[472] PAF promotes platelet aggregation, which results in thrombocytopenia.[380,505] M-CSF and GM-CSF appear to produce thrombocytopenia by activating macrophages and enhancing their phagocytosis of platelets.[2,19,167,372,396]

Thrombocytopenia is usually present with acute protozoal (*Babesia, Theileria, Cytauxzoon* species) infections of erythrocytes, but thrombocytopenia is not generally present with hemotrophic *Mycoplasma* or *Anaplasma* infections of erythrocytes (see Chapter 4 for more information). Thrombocytopenia is a common finding in rickettsial (*Ehrlichia, Anaplasma,* and *Neorickettsia*) infections of leukocytes (see Chapter 5 for more information). *Rickettsia rickettsii* invades and replicates within endothelial cells, resulting in vessel damage and vasculitis, followed by activation of platelets and coagulation; however, overt DIC rarely occurs.[205] Increased amounts of immunoglobulin bound to platelets suggest an immune-mediated component of the thrombocytopenia in *R. rickettsii* infections.[209] *A. platys* specifically infects dog platelets and causes a cyclic thrombocytopenia (see previous discussion above under "*Anaplasma platys* Infection"). Whereas an initial thrombocytopenia may develop primarily as a consequence of direct injury to platelets by replicating organisms, immune-mediated mechanisms of platelet removal may be more important during subsequent thrombocytopenic episodes.[172]

Infections with various African *Trypanosoma* species consistently cause thrombocytopenia during parasitemias.[128,395] Thrombocytopenia has been associated with *Sarcocystis* species in pigs,[21] cattle,[171] and a dog.[5] Accompanying coagulopathies in pigs and cattle indicated the presence of DIC.

Thrombocytopenia is commonly recognized in dogs with leishmaniasis. The presence of platelet-bound IgG and IgM in thrombocytopenic dogs suggests that a secondary IMT is present.[116] However, some dogs with leishmaniasis have accompanying coagulopathies consistent with DIC.[508] Thrombocytopenia is recognized in about one-third of the dogs with *Hepatozoon canis* infection,[20] but platelet counts are more often increased in *Hepatozoon americanum* infections.[322]

Thrombocytopenia occurs in association with various viral infections. The thrombocytopenia has been attributed to decreased platelet production with some viral infections, including parvovirus in dogs and cats,[503,549] FIV,[177,193] and FeLV.[193,459]

Evidence of decreased marrow production plus evidence of increased platelet utilization or destruction has been provided for canine distemper virus,[15] equine infectious anemia (EIA) virus,[106,121,443] classic swine fever (hog cholera),[197,387,446] African swine fever virus,[26,151] and bovine viral diarrhea (BVD) virus.[475,518] Transient thrombocytopenia has been reported within 2 days of dogs being vaccinated with vaccines containing a modified distemper virus.[332,415]

Bluetongue virus causes thrombocytopenia in sheep, but the mechanism has not been described.[334] The thrombocytopenia in equine viral arteritis may be in response to endothelial cell damage.[135,136] The African horse sickness virus,[465] feline infectious peritonitis virus,[531] and infectious canine hepatitis virus[535] appear to produce thrombocytopenia in association with DIC.

Thrombocytopenia is common in association with bacterial infections, especially when bacteria and/or endotoxin are present in blood.* Thrombocytopenia is common in dogs with infective endocarditis,[493] and thrombocytopenia may occur in dogs and cats with *Bartonella* species bacteremia.[61,198] Thrombocytopenia has been reported with hepatic abscesses in dogs,[160] leptospirosis in dogs,[196] tularemia in cats,[546] and spirochetemia in dogs infected with relapsing fever spirochetes.[62,478,534] These *Borrelia* organisms may react directly with platelets and contribute to the production of thrombocytopenia.[6]

Thrombocytopenia may also occur secondary to disseminated fungal infections, especially with histoplasmosis.[107,108,463]

Drug- and Chemical-Induced Thrombocytopenia

Most drug- and chemical-induced thrombocytopenias result from either toxic effects on the bone marrow or the ability of the compounds to function as haptens, inducing secondary immune-mediated destruction of platelets. Drugs and chemicals that have been reported to cause thrombocytopenia—and often also leukopenia and/or anemia—include cancer chemotherapeutic agents (carboplatin, cisplatin, cyclophosphamide, lomustine, fluorouracil, deoxycoformycin, doxorubicin),† antimicrobials (cephalosporins, sulfonamides, dapsone, griseofulvin),[40,308,502,526] nonsteroidal anti-inflammatory drugs (phenylbutazone, carprofen),[339,522] antihelminthics (albendazole, levamisole),[13,487] antithyroid drugs (methimazole, propylthiouracil),[412,526] immunosuppressive azathioprine,[28] exogenous or endogenous estrogens (dogs and ferrets),[287,471] the psychostimulant dextroamphetamine and amphetamine (Adderall),[539] phenobarbital,[256] the antiviral drug ribavirin,[530] the antipsoriasis cream calcipotriol,[159] the angiotensin-converting enzyme inhibitor captopril,[247] and various toxins (phenol, fluoroacetate, *Macrozamia* seeds, trichothecenes, and bracken fern).[109,189,347,401,410]

*References 32, 55, 60, 64, 110, 180, 207, 505, 526.
†References 176, 212, 213, 360, 436, 528.

Neoplasia and Thrombocytopenia

The pathogenesis of thrombocytopenia associated with neoplasia varies and cannot always be identified.[103,208] Thrombocytopenia occurs with a variety of tumor types but is most common in lymphomas and hemangiosarcomas in dogs and in animals with tumors being treated with chemotherapy.[103,208] There is a lack of production of platelets in primary neoplasia of bone marrow, including myelodysplastic syndrome (MDS), acute myeloid leukemia (AML), acute lymphoblastic leukemia (ALL), and multiple myeloma.[3,241,310,404,528] Thrombocytopenia and neutropenia are less common in chronic lymphocytic leukemia (CLL) than in ALL, at least in part because bone marrow is not typically replaced by neoplastic cells in CLL to the extent that occurs in ALL.[496] Metastatic lymphomas and mast cell tumors can sometimes have substantial bone marrow infiltrates that might result in decreased platelet production.[326,341,496] Decreased platelet production also occurs with estrogen-secreting tumors in dogs.[471]

Platelets may be consumed within some tumors, including hemangiosarcoma and hemophagocytic histiosarcoma,[174,215,362,474,528] although the latter neoplasm may also have significant bone marrow infiltrates, which could result in decreased platelet production. Tumors generate prothrombotic environments capable of the activation of platelets and coagulation by expressing TF, releasing procoagulant microparticles, and secreting cytokines that make the endothelium prothrombotic.[242] Hyperactive platelets that might promote thrombus formation have been described in canine lymphoma.[498] The sluggish blood flow and contorted vessels in tumors may also enhance the thrombogenic environment of tumors.[242] Not surprisingly, thrombosis and DIC are common sequelae to neoplasia in animals.[158,163,208,384]

Immune-mediated platelet destruction has been reported with some tumors, especially lymphomas.* Immune-mediated platelet destruction might account for the greater prevalence of thrombocytopenia in dogs with leukemic T lymphocyte high-grade lymphomas versus those with leukemic B lymphocyte high-grade lymphomas. Alternatively, these T lymphocyte neoplasms might have more pronounced bone marrow infiltrates than B lymphocyte neoplasms.[496]

Platelets may be lost through tumor-induced hemorrhage. However, the platelet count is not generally significantly reduced unless there is an acute, severe hemorrhage, as may occur when hemangiosarcomas rupture.[103]

Inherited Thrombocytopenia

Macrothrombocytes are present in Cavalier King Charles spaniel dogs with inherited macrothrombocytopenia (see Fig. 7-26).[74] Dogs with this defect do not exhibit increased bleeding tendencies, presumably because the total platelet mass in blood is not decreased.[506] A mutation in β-1 tubulin has been identified in these dogs; it was suggested that this could result in unstable α-β-tubulin dimers within protofilaments, leading to abnormal proplatelet formation.[127] The identification of the genetic defect allows for a separation of Cavalier King Charles dogs clear of the defect (platelet count $336 \pm 148 \times 10^3/\mu L$, MPV 12 ± 2 fL, mean ± SD) from heterozygous affected (platelet count $196 \pm 64 \times 10^3/\mu L$, MPV 16 ± 3 fL, mean ± SD) dogs and homozygous affected (platelet count $74 \pm 36 \times 10^3/\mu L$, MPV 28 ± 6 fL, mean ± SD) dogs.[127]

Macrothrombocytopenia has been described in a pug dog with the May-Hegglin anomaly, which is characterized by a triad of leukocyte inclusions (see Chapter 5 for discussion), thrombocytopenia, and macrothrombocytes (see Fig. 5-24). It results from a mutation in the *MYH9* gene, which encodes for the heavy chain of nonmuscle myosin IIA. The presence of macrothrombocytes is most likely associated with defective fragmentation of proplatelets formed by megakaryocyte cytoplasmic projections.[164]

Pseudothrombocytopenia

It is essential that a blood film estimation of platelet numbers be done as a quality control measure for each automated platelet count. The presence of platelet aggregates can result in erroneously low platelet counts. Platelet aggregates usually form when platelets are activated during the collection and handling of blood samples. EDTA-dependent pseudothrombocytopenia, resulting from platelet aggregation, has been reported in dogs, horses, and pigs.[240,421,544] When EDTA-dependent pseudothrombocytopenia is present, such platelet aggregation may be prevented by the collection of blood samples using citrate instead of EDTA as the anticoagulant. However, citrate should not replace EDTA as the preferred anticoagulant for platelet counts, at least in dogs, because platelet aggregates form more readily in blood from dogs collected in citrate, resulting in lower automated platelet counts than in blood collected in EDTA.[485] Pseudothrombocytopenias may be reported in cats if whole blood platelet counts are performed using electronic cell counters because cat platelets are large and difficult to separate from erythrocytes based on cell volumes.

Some healthy Cavalier King Charles spaniels and a pug dog with the May-Hegglin anomaly have macrothrombocytopenia. Platelet counts are low when manual platelet counts are done, but they are generally even lower when they are determined with electronic cell counters because some of the macrothrombocytes are too large to be counted as platelets by automated cell counters.[164,394]

Abnormalities in Platelet Function

Acquired Defects in Platelet Function

In addition to causing thrombocytopenia, antiplatelet antibodies may reduce platelet function.[294] This reduced function may be explained by the finding that GPIIb/IIIa (fibrinogen receptor) and GPIb-IX (part of vWF receptor complex) are the most frequently targeted antigens in IMT in humans.[338] This reduced function could also explain why thrombocytopenic cats with platelet-bound antibodies appear more likely to bleed at a given platelet count than thrombocytopenic cats without platelet-bound antibodies.[290]

*References 143, 232, 278, 290, 295, 426.

FDPs released during fibrinolysis may reduce platelet function by antagonizing fibrinogen binding to GPIIb/IIIa.[201] Human patients with markedly elevated immunoglobulins (paraproteins)—as occurs with multiple myeloma, Waldenstrom's macroglobulinemia, and benign monoclonal gammopathy—have increased tendencies to bleed. Although the mechanisms are poorly understood, defects in platelet function may contribute to this bleeding diathesis.[130,192,200] Defects resulting in reduced platelet function may occur in association with uremia and liver disease.[58,354,445] Bile acids inhibit platelet aggregation and may contribute to the reduced platelet function reported in liver disease.[53]

Decreased platelet function can also occur following the administration of nonsteroidal anti-inflammatory drugs, such as aspirin and phenylbutazone, which inhibit TxA_2 synthesis.[85,254,343,445] New platelet inhibitor drugs continue to be developed in humans that may also be used for treating thrombotic disorders in animals.[56,175,245] In addition, a large number of drugs—including antihistamines, calcium channel blockers, halothane, isoflurane, some barbiturates, and certain antibiotics—may interact with platelets and interfere with normal platelet aggregation.[38,165,175,390] Platelet function may also be reduced in various myeloid neoplasms with abnormal platelet formation. Decreased platelet function has been reported in association with some infectious agents.[175] This might be explained if platelets are activated in vivo and become hypofunctional when tested in vitro.

Inherited Platelet Function Defects

Several inherited platelet defects (termed thrombopathy or thrombopathia) have been reported in animals; these can cause excessive mucosal bleeding, epistaxis, petechial and ecchymotic hemorrhages, and excessive bleeding following minor trauma or when shedding of teeth occurs. Animals with these disorders usually have normal platelet counts and normal platelet morphology.

Deficiencies in the GPIIb subunit of the GPIIb/IIIa fibrinogen receptor on the surface of platelets result in bleeding diatheses in Great Pyrenees and Otterhound dogs and in thoroughbred, quarter horse, Peruvian Paso, and Oldenbourg horses. These defects appear to be homologous to Glanzmann's thrombasthenia in humans.[44] A defect in the ADP receptor P2Y12 has recently been reported in a Greater Swiss Mountain dog that had life-threatening hemorrhage following elective surgery.[45]

Not only does a deficiency in the amount of the GPIIb/IIIa on platelets impair platelet function, but defects in the signaling pathway or pathways that activate this integrin molecule also result in platelet function defects. This includes mutations in the gene encoding calcium diacylglycerol guanine nucleotide exchange factor I (CalDAG-GEFI), which have resulted in thrombopathies in Basset hounds, Spitz dogs, Landseer (European-Continental type) dogs, and Simmental cattle.[47,50]

A mutation in the *Kindlin-3* gene in a German shepherd dog resulted in increased susceptibility to infection and life-threatening hemorrhage (see Chapter 5 for more information).[51] The Kindlin-3 protein is critical in the pathway of β-integrin activation in both leukocytes and platelets. A deficiency of Kindlin-3 prevents GPIIb/IIIa integrin activation in platelets, which results in impaired platelet aggregation and a prolonged buccal bleeding time.[51]

Several platelet storage-pool disorders have been reported to result in bleeding tendencies in animals. Platelet-dense granule defects have been reported in pigs and American cocker spaniel dogs.[82,420] Platelet-dense granule deficiency also occurs in Persian cats, three breeds of cattle, blue foxes, killer whales, and Aleutian mink as part of the inherited Chédiak-Higashi syndrome. Animals with Chédiak-Higashi syndrome have partial albinism with defects in the granules of several tissues including skin, leukocytes, and platelets (see Chapter 5 for more information).[120] A mutation in the *CHS1/LYST* gene is responsible for Chédiak-Higashi syndrome in Japanese black cattle.[300] Platelets from gray collie dogs with cyclic hematopoiesis appear to have storage-pool and signal-transduction defects, but bleeding is not of clinical significance in this disorder. Cyclic hematopoiesis in dogs results from a mutation in the *AP3B1* gene (see Chapter 5 for more information).[340]

Activated platelets normally translocate PS to their surfaces (platelet procoagulant), which greatly accelerates coagulation in vivo. A family of German shepherd dogs has been recognized with intramuscular hemorrhage, hyphema, epistaxis, and prolonged bleeding with cutaneous bruising after surgery. Although platelet phospholipid content was normal, platelets from these dogs had diminished PS exposure on their surfaces and a failure of microvesiculation when stimulated by platelet agonists.[73] These are the characteristics of Scott syndrome in humans; however, the molecular defect or defects are unknown.[71] Although this is a platelet defect, the nature of the bleeding, especially the deep muscle bleeding, is more suggestive of a coagulopathy. This clinical presentation can be attributed to the inability of the platelets to support coagulation. Platelet function tests (including bleeding time) were normal because increased negative phospholipids on the surface of platelets is not required for platelet adhesion and aggregation. Routine coagulation tests (including PT and APTT) were also normal because these tests are performed in citrate plasma without platelets.[70] The phospholipid needed for these coagulation tests is included in the reagents used for the assays. Neither the PFA-100 analyzer nor a TEG analyzer could identify this defect. These dogs exhibited decreased activated platelet microparticle release by flow cytometry in fresh blood, but this assay cannot be used as a screening test in day-old blood because platelet activation artifacts preclude overnight storage for next-day analysis.[73]

von Willebrand Disease

Von Willebrand disease (vWD) is a heterogeneous inherited bleeding disorder resulting from quantitative and/or qualitative defects of vWF. It is by far the most common bleeding disorder in dogs, having been recognized in more than 50 breeds. vWD is classified into three general types, based on vWF concentration in plasma, the multimeric structure of vWF, and clinical severity. Type 1 vWD has a low vWF concentration (less than 50% of normal) in plasma, but the multimeric structure of vWF is normal. Type 1 vWD appears to be transmitted as an autosomal dominant trait with variable penetrance. Mildly affected dogs may exhibit no bleeding tendency. Most type 1 dogs that bleed have less than 20% of normal vWF concentration in plasma. Type 2A (the only type 2 subtype described in animals to date) vWD dogs have low plasma vWF concentrations, with a disproportionate loss of high-molecular-weight polymers. Type 3 vWD dogs have virtually no vWF in plasma. In addition, FVIII in plasma may be mildly decreased in dogs with type 3 vWD. Dogs with types 2 and 3 vWD have severe bleeding tendencies. Types 2 and 3 vWD are transmitted as autosomal recessive traits.[69]

Type 1 vWD is common in several breeds—including the Doberman pinscher, German shepherd, golden retriever, poodle, Pembroke Welsh corgi, and Shetland sheepdog—but additional breeds are also affected. Type 2A vWD has been reported in the German short-haired pointer and German wire-haired pointer. Type 3 vWD has been reported in Dutch Kooikers, Scottish terriers, and Shetland sheepdogs, with sporadic cases in other breeds. vWD has also been found in pigs (type 3), a Himalayan cat (type 3), an Arabian horse (type 1), a quarter horse (type 2A), thoroughbreds (type 2A), and a Simmental calf (type 2A).[69] Animals with vWD have prolonged bleeding times because vWF is needed for normal platelet adhesion to the subendothelium. The ADP/collagen closure time is also prolonged when tested with a platelet function analyzer (PFA-100, Dade-Behring).[352] Decreased vWF concentrations may result in decreased FVIII activity because the binding of FVIII to vWF prolongs the half-life of FVIII in the circulation. However, the decrease in FVIII is usually not sufficient to result in a significant prolongation of the APTT.[69,423]

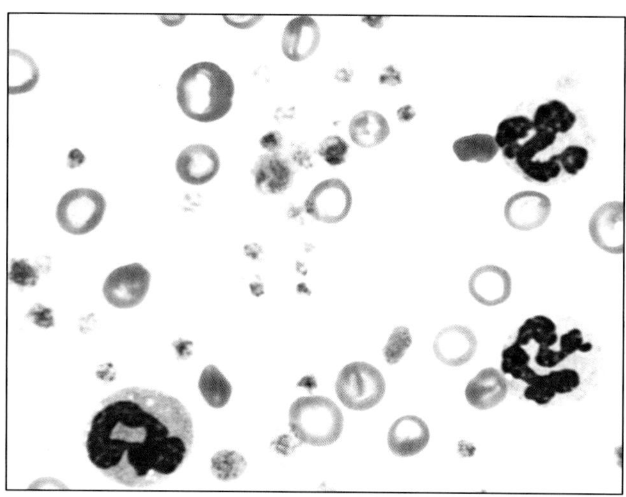

FIGURE 7-34
Thrombocytosis in blood from a dog with chronic iron-deficiency anemia. Smaller hypochromic erythrocytes and several larger polychromatophilic erythrocytes are present. A monocyte *(bottom)* and two neutrophils are also present. Wright-Giemsa stain.

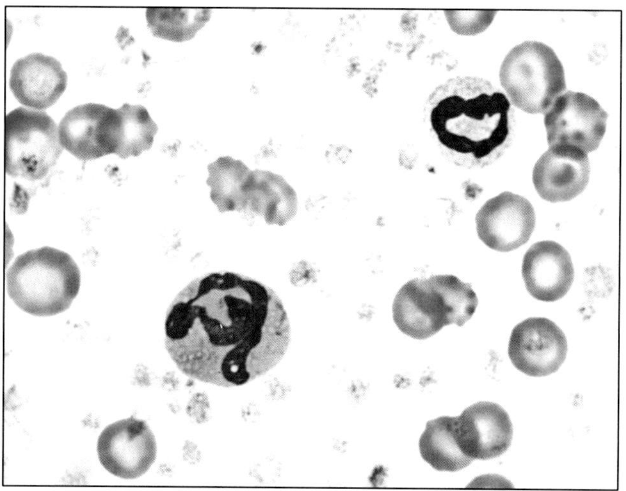

FIGURE 7-35
Marked thrombocytosis in blood from a dog diagnosed with essential thrombocythemia. A basophil *(bottom)* and neutrophil *(top right)* are also present. Wright stain.

Photograph of a stained blood film from a 1987 ASVCP slide review case submitted by C. P. Mandell, N. C. Jain, and J. G. Zinkl.

Thrombocytosis

Thrombocytosis refers to the presence of platelet counts above the reference interval (Fig. 7-34). When a high platelet count results from a clonal proliferation of megakaryocytes, it is called essential thrombocythemia (Fig. 7-35).

The spleen stores about one-third of the total platelet mass in humans, and splenic contraction results in increased blood platelet counts.[153,450] Some studies have reported increased platelet counts following α-adrenergic stimulation or exercise in animals,[169,316] and other studies have not.[269,364,391] Splenectomy can also result in a thrombocytosis, which can last for several months.[429,515]

Reactive thrombocytosis may occur when TPO concentrations are increased.[262] Thrombocytosis is seen in association with various inflammatory and neoplastic conditions in animals.[214,434,456,481] Although a number of cytokines—such as IL-1, IL-3, GM-CSF, and IL-11—might be involved, IL-6 appears to be the main mediator of inflammation-induced thrombocytosis.[4,125,155,262,408] IL-6 appears to stimulate thrombopoiesis by increasing TPO synthesis and release into plasma.[277]

Thrombocytosis may also occur in association with acute anemia.[253] Recombinant erythropoietin induces thrombocytosis in cats, dogs, and humans.[119,511] Thrombocytosis as well as erythrocytosis was reported in a horse with a hepatoblastoma and increased plasma erythropoietin concentration.[195]

Plasma TPO has been reported to be increased in humans with hepatoblastoma,[293] but TPO was not measured in the equine case. Thrombocytosis has also been reported in two cats with erythrocytosis secondary to a unilateral renal adenocarcinoma.[285] Plasma erythropoietin values were within reference intervals but considered inappropriately high in view of the increased erythrocyte mass. Both the erythrocytosis and the thrombocytosis resolved following surgical removal of the affected kidney.

Thrombocytosis is often present in animals with chronic hemorrhage resulting in iron-deficiency anemia (see Fig. 7-34).[226,228] The platelet increase in iron-deficiency anemia may in part be related to stimulation of megakaryopoiesis by a high erythropoietin concentration in plasma,[318] but the mechanism has not been clearly defined.[274]

A single intravenous injection of vincristine in experimental dogs induced a transient mild decrease in platelet counts followed by a moderate increase in counts, with peak platelet counts observed 8 days after drug administration.[323] Other antineoplastic drugs, including doxorubicin, have been reported to cause both thrombocytopenia and thrombocytosis.[214,389] It is unclear if these findings reflect differences in drug dosage or a rebound thrombocytosis to an earlier thrombocytopenia or whether they are attributable to other, unknown factors.[214,481] Thrombocytosis has been reported in dogs with hyperadrenocorticism,[214] but the administration of glucocorticoids does not appear to cause a consistent thrombocytosis in dogs.[481] Thrombocytosis has been reported in hyperthyroid cats in one study,[434] while no hyperthyroid cats were reported to have a thrombocytosis in another study.[490]

Platelet counts may be spuriously elevated if erythrocyte fragments, cytoplasmic fragments of nucleated cells, lipemia, bacteria, cryoglobulins, or technical difficulties are present.[550] Thus it is important that stained blood films be examined to determine if a true thrombocytosis is present.

Thrombocytosis may be present in animals with myeloid neoplasms, including essential thrombocythemia, acute megakaryoblastic leukemia, CML, and possibly primary erythrocytosis (polycythemia vera) in cats.[434,481] Essential thrombocythemia has been diagnosed in animals with persistent markedly elevated platelet counts, typically in excess of $1 \times 10^6/\mu L$ (see Fig. 7-35), for which a cause for a reactive thrombocytosis could not be identified. Platelet morphology is typically normal; however, increased MPVs have been reported in two dogs believed to have thrombocythemia.[147] Essential thrombocythemia may be viewed as the platelet counterpart of primary erythrocytosis (see Chapter 9 for more information).

COAGULATION DISORDERS

Acquired Coagulation Disorders

Hypercoagulable State

The increased tendency for coagulation to occur without clinical signs or laboratory evidence of thrombosis is termed a hypercoagulable state. An increased risk of thrombosis may also be described as thrombophilia or a prethrombotic state.[320] Platelet hyperreactivity (e.g., increased IL-6 and PAF generation during inflammatory conditions),[90,261,407] increased concentrations of coagulation factors (e.g., hyperfibrinogenemia in response to inflammation),[211] decreased concentrations of coagulation inhibitors (e.g., decreased antithrombin secondary to nephrotic syndrome),[203,433] hypofibrinolysis (e.g., increased plasminogen activator inhibitor, as an acute-phase response to inflammation),[22] or combinations thereof may produce a hypercoagulable state. Acquired and inherited protein C deficiency appears to enhance coagulation in horses.[22,150] Although not available as a routine diagnostic test, the finding of increased thrombin-antithrombin complexes is an indirect measure of thrombin generation and provides evidence of a hypercoagulable state.[483,499]

Dogs with hyperadrenocorticism tend to be in a hypercoagulable state. Levels of coagulation factors II, V, VII, IX, X, XII, fibrinogen, and thrombin-antithrombin complexes were significantly increased, and antithrombin was significantly decreased in plasma from dogs with hyperadrenocorticism compared with plasma from control dogs.[259] Dogs have been classified as hypercoagulable using TEG. This has included about 50% of dogs with malignant neoplasia,[296] a majority of dogs with IMHA,[464]and dogs with parvovirus enteritis.[398]

Septic foals are often hypercoagulable with a strong likelihood of developing DIC.[8] Horses with colic resulting from ischemic or inflammatory gastrointestinal disease may develop a hypercoagulable state as evidenced by decreased antithrombin and protein C levels and increased thrombin-antithrombin complexes in plasma.[499] However, TEG failed to identify a similar group of horses with colic as hypercoagulable even though conventional coagulation tests supported that classification.[146] Nearly half of the cats with hypertrophic cardiomyopathy were classified as hypercoagulable based on conventional laboratory tests.[29,483]

Hypercoagulable animals may develop localized thrombosis or DIC. There is overlap in laboratory test results from animals with these disorders. Consequently it can be difficult to determine, using laboratory tests alone, whether an animal is prethrombotic or has already progressed to a thrombotic state. Physical findings and diagnostic imaging are especially important in diagnosing localized thrombosis.[211] Several hemostatic test abnormalities are required to make a diagnosis of DIC (see subsequent discussion).

Thromboembolism (Localized Thrombosis)

The pathogenesis of thrombosis may involve endothelial activation or injury; altered blood flow (turbulence or stasis); changes in coagulation factors, fibrinolytic factors, or their inhibitors; and platelet activation. Large-vessel thrombosis may occur in association with immune-mediated, infectious, and traumatic vascular injury[135]; neoplasia (especially hemangiosarcoma in dogs); sepsis; endotoxemia (primarily horses); immune-mediated hemolytic anemia (common in dogs)[88]; protein-losing nephropathy or enteropathy[111,141]; hyperadrenocorticism; glucocorticoid therapy; acute pancreatic necrosis;

BOX 7-1 Conditions That May Result in Disseminated Intravascular Coagulation

Septicemia (various Gram-negative and Gram-positive bacteria)
Viremia (infectious canine hepatitis, feline infectious peritonitis, African swine fever, hog cholera, African horse sickness)
Protozoal parasites (babesiosis, trypanosomiasis, sarcocystosis, leishmaniasis, and cytauxzoonosis)
Metazoal parasites (heartworms and lungworms)
Marked tissue injury (heatstroke, trauma, and surgical procedures)
Intravascular hemolysis
Obstetric complications
Malignancy (hemangiosarcoma, disseminated carcinomas, leukemia, lymphoma)
Traumatic shock
Liver disease
Pancreatitis
Gastric dilatation-volvulus and abomasal displacement
Toxins (snake and insect venoms, aflatoxin, and insecticides)

thrombocytosis[246]; heart disease (vegetative endocarditis, dirofilariasis, cardiomyopathy)[126,306,493]; hyperthyroidism (cats)[469]; liver disease (cats); and indwelling intravenous catheters.*

When thrombus formation is localized, platelet counts, coagulation tests, and FDP values may be normal. Several studies suggest the D-dimer test is more sensitive than FDP tests (especially serum-based tests) for the diagnosis of thromboembolism in dogs.[374,479] While the D-dimer test does not have sufficiently high positive predictive value to rule in thromboembolism or DIC in dogs, its high sensitivity results in a sufficiently high negative predictive value to help rule out thromboembolism and DIC when the test is negative.[374]

Disseminated Intravascular Coagulation

DIC is a syndrome in which diffuse thrombosis and secondary fibrinolysis occur in small vessels. It is not a primary disorder but rather a sequela to other diseases. DIC may occur with disorders where TF is exposed on cell surfaces, widespread vascular injury is present, widespread platelet activation occurs, blood flow is reduced, or there is impaired removal of activated coagulation factors by the liver. Conditions that may induce DIC are shown in Box 7-1.[480] Undoubtedly other disorders can be added to this list.

DIC is generally initiated by the disseminated presentation of TF in blood. This may involve widespread tissue injury, especially endothelial injury, that results in the exposure of TF on subendothelial cells and parenchymal cells. Proinflammatory cytokines produced in various infectious and noninfectious inflammatory disorders may stimulate the exposure of TF on blood monocytes and possibly on endothelial cells. Some neoplastic cells also express TF, which can promote DIC when these cells are in contact with blood.[480] Thrombin generated by the TF pathway also activates platelets, which results in the translocation of negative phospholipids to platelet surfaces and platelet aggregation. Increased numbers of microparticles (microvesicles) released by stimulated platelets, monocytes, endothelial cells, tumor cells, and apoptotic cells promote widespread thrombosis, because they express procoagulant PS and sometimes also TF on their surfaces. Microparticles from platelets appear to be especially important in promoting coagulation.[173]

*References 206, 211, 268, 307, 374, 384, 452.

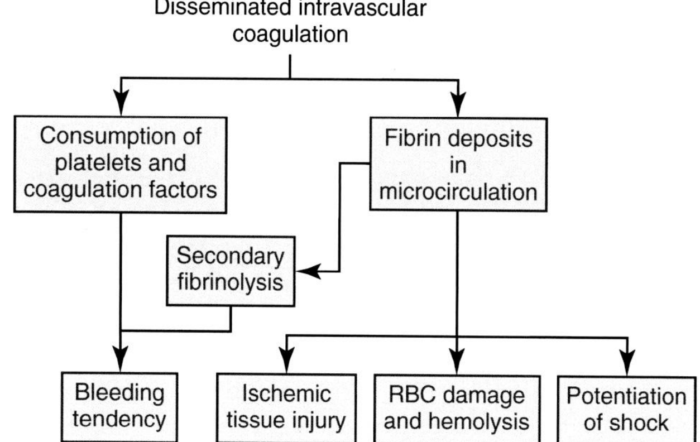

FIGURE 7-36
Pathophysiology of disseminated intravascular coagulation. RBC, red blood cell.

The formation of thrombi in vessels can result in tissue hypoxia and organ damage (Fig. 7-36). The consumption of coagulation factors and platelets in the formation of these thrombi create a tendency for hemorrhage. This propensity to bleed is increased by subsequent fibrinolysis, which not only breaks down thrombi but also produces FDPs that interfere with normal platelet aggregation and fibrin polymerization.[201,355] Hemorrhage occurs in some dogs with DIC but is uncommon in horses and cats.[480] DIC can result in shock, and shock can potentiate DIC, resulting in a vicious cycle of events. DIC often occurs as a life-threatening event causing organ failure and/or hemorrhage, but it may also occur in a chronic form without severe clinical signs.

There are no uniformly accepted criteria for the diagnosis of DIC. Traditional criteria for diagnosing DIC in animals include the finding of two or more of the following abnormalities: thrombocytopenia, prolonged coagulation time (PT or APTT), hypofibrinogenemia, decreased antithrombin activity, and increased D-dimer or FDP concentrations.[480] Others have recommended finding at least three abnormal hemostatic parameters including thrombocytopenia, prolonged PT, prolonged APTT, hypofibrinogenemia, increased D-dimers, and erythrocyte fragmentation.[536] A multiple logistic regression model has been developed to diagnose DIC in dogs using results from PT, APTT, D-dimer, and fibrinogen assays.[536]

The APTT is more often prolonged than is the PT in DIC. Mild to moderate thrombocytopenia is a consistent finding in dogs but a less consistent finding in cats and horses with DIC.[480,486] Fibrinogen is an acute-phase protein; consequently, the fibrinogen concentration may be normal or increased in DIC when underlying inflammation is present. Antithrombin is generally low in dogs and horses with DIC.[480] Antithrombin may also be low in some cats with DIC, but it is often normal or even increased because it appears to be an acute-phase protein in cats.[59] D-dimer concentration is a sensitive test for DIC in dogs (75%-100% positive); but it is a less sensitive test for DIC in horses (about 50%).[480] About two-thirds of the cats with DIC had positive D-dimer tests in a small study.[497] The D-dimer test appears to be more sensitive than FDP tests in the diagnosis of DIC in dogs and horses.[479,486] Extensive local intravascular coagulation may occur in some dogs with hemangiosarcoma. Laboratory findings in these cases are similar to those seen in DIC, making differentiation of DIC from local intravascular coagulation difficult.

Schistocytes may be seen with DIC, where they can be formed by the impact of erythrocytes with fibrin strands in flowing blood (see Fig. 4-53).[425] Schistocytes are most often seen in dogs but can also be seen in other species with DIC.[252,497]

When animals with DIC are assayed using TEG, they may appear hypercoagulable, normocoagulable, or hypocoagulable. The hypocoagulable state presumably develops when consumption of platelets and fibrinogen limits additional coagulation. Hypocoagulable dogs with DIC are more likely to die than hypercoagulable dogs.[537]

Hemolytic-Uremic Syndrome

Hemolytic-uremic syndrome (HUS) is a thrombotic microangiopathy consisting of thrombocytopenia, microangiopathic hemolytic anemia, and acute renal failure. In humans, HUS is classified as either typical (diarrhea-associated) or atypical (nondiarrheal) HUS.

The typical form accounts for more than 90% of the human cases. It occurs most commonly in children and follows gastrointestinal infections with enterohemorrhagic *Escherichia coli* (predominantly serotype O157:H7), which produces Shiga toxin. Shiga toxin is also produced by *Shigella dysenteriae* type 1. These organisms colonize the intestinal tract and release Shiga toxin into the blood; it then disseminates throughout the body and binds to receptors on endothelial cells. Bacteremia is rarely recognized. Shiga toxin is internalized by receptor-mediated endocytosis. It activates and damages endothelial cells, which then triggers platelet adhesion, thrombus formation, and leukocyte-dependent inflammation. Microthrombi are found most often in renal glomeruli, the intestinal tract, the brain, and the pancreas.[276] Children with *E. coli* O157:H7 infection appeared to be in a hypercoagulable state prior to developing HUS, indicating that accelerated thrombogenesis and inhibition of fibrinolysis precede renal injury and presumably cause acute renal failure.[98] A non-O157:H7 strain of *E. coli*, which caused HUS and death in a child, was inoculated orally into 40-day-old dogs, where it resulted in watery and slightly hemorrhagic diarrhea, followed by death in 5 or 6 days. These pups had necrotic lesions in the liver and bacterial emboli in the kidney at necropsy. The primary cause of death was microvascular thrombosis caused by the bacteria, leading to renal and multiple organ failure. Urine output was reported to be decreased and serum urea nitrogen was increased prior to death, but unfortunately CBCs were not performed.[521]

The atypical form of HUS in humans occurs secondary to various diseases including pneumococcal pneumonia, human immunodeficiency virus infection, chemotherapeutic and immunosuppressive drugs, malignancy, SLE, and antiphospholipid syndrome. Atypical HUS involves complement dysregulation.[161]

HUS has rarely been reported in animals. Several cases in dogs appear similar to the typical HUS reported in humans.[99,138,248] A similar condition but without gastrointestinal signs has been observed in greyhounds.[118] The disorder is characterized by thrombocytopenia, anemia, azotemia, and a cutaneous vasculopathy in addition to a renal glomerular vasculopathy. Skin lesions were characterized by hemorrhages, fibrinoid arteritis, and thrombosis. Renal lesions included peracute glomerular necrosis particularly involving afferent arterioles, with intravascular coagulation in glomerular capillaries.[87] Ultrastructural examination of glomerular capillaries from affected greyhounds revealed endothelial swelling, detachment, and necrosis, with platelet adhesion, platelet aggregation, and fibrin deposition. No etiologic agents or electron-dense deposits typical of immune complexes were observed.[235] The feeding of raw beef contaminated with *E. coli* has been suggested as a possible cause.[87,118,235] A similar cutaneous and renal vasculopathy syndrome has been reported in a Great Dane dog.[439]

HUS—characterized by hemolysis, thrombocytopenia, azotemia, oliguria, and thrombotic microangiopathy involving glomeruli—was diagnosed in a postpartum mare with endometritis. An *E. coli* 0103:H2 was isolated from the mare's uterus and gastrointestinal tract. A similar presentation has also been diagnosed in a postpartum cow with severe suppurative endometritis.[435] A disorder resembling the renal component of the HUS was diagnosed in two horses with acute renal failure and necrotizing vascuolpathy with marked fibrin deposition in the renal glomeruli.[367] Atypical HUS was also considered a possibility in three cats treated with cyclosporine after renal transplants.[11]

Antiphospholipid Antibody

Healthy Bernese Mountain dogs are reported to have prolonged APTTs compared with other breeds. This appears to result from a high prevalence of an antiphospholipid antibody (lupus anticoagulant) in the plasma of these dogs.[376] The presence of antiphospholipid antibodies (antibodies against phospholipids, phospholipid-binding proteins, and phospholipid-protein complexes) is associated with an increased risk of thrombosis in humans (antiphospholipid syndrome). The presence of antiphospholipid antibodies appears to prime platelets and endothelial cells for activation, but a triggering event such as an infection, trauma, or surgery may be required for thrombosis to occur.[413] The importance of antiphospholipid antibodies in promoting thrombosis in animals requires further study. The presence of a lupus-type anticoagulant has been reported in a dog with nephrotic syndrome, pulmonary thromboembolism, and hemolysis.[488]

Liver Disease

The liver is the primary site for the synthesis of coagulation factors. Consequently, generalized liver disease may result in prolonged PT and APTT and an increased bleeding tendency due to decreased circulating coagulation factors.* Because of these synthetic functions and the vascular nature of the liver, coagulation screening tests are generally done prior to performing liver biopsies. Liver disorders may also contribute to the development of DIC, as has been reported in infectious canine hepatitis and aflatoxin B1 toxicity.[204,535] The coagulation defect of aflatoxicosis is primarily due to reduced hepatic synthesis of coagulation factors except when hepatic necrosis is severe enough to initiate DIC.[17,139,204] The presence of endotoxemia augments aflatoxin B1 toxicity, with the combined substances more likely to initiate DIC than aflatoxin B1 alone.[321]

Vitamin K Deficiency

Vitamin K is essential in a carboxylation reaction that results in the formation of active coagulation factors II, VII, IX, and X as well as protein C and protein S (Fig. 7-15).[105] Vitamin K deficiency may occur in malabsorptive syndromes, including bile duct obstruction, or from sterilization of the intestine by prolonged use of antibiotics.[72,373] Vitamin K deficiency appears to be present in at least some cats with hepatic lipidosis, severe inflammatory bowel disease, and severe inflammatory bowel disease associated with cholangiohepatitis, because these animals had prolonged coagulation tests that shortened following vitamin K therapy.[95] Bilirubin cholelithiasis and extrahepatic bile duct obstruction have resulted in prolonged coagulation times in pyruvate kinase-deficient cats,[224,509] at least in part related to decreased vitamin K absorption. Vitamin K deficiency resulting in hemorrhage and death has been reported in cats fed commercial canned diets high in salmon or tuna.[489]

Sweet clover and sweet vernal grasses contain coumarin, which is converted to the toxin dicumarol by the action of several mold species when the grasses are improperly processed under high moisture conditions. Dicumarol in these moldy feedstuffs inhibits VKOR, which provides vitamin K hydroquinone for the carboxylation of select glutamic acid residues of the vitamin K-dependent proteins.[477] Consequently dicumarol toxicity can result in hemorrhage in cattle and other species consuming moldy sweet clover and sweet vernal grass hay.[417,441] The discovery of dicumarol toxicity led to the development of warfarin and related compounds that are now used as rodenticides and as therapeutic anticoagulants. Animals that consume anticoagulant rodenticides develop life-threatening bleeding disorders characterized by markedly prolonged PT and APTT tests but a normal TCT.[291,312,335,370,547] The PT test is generally reported to be more sensitive than the APTT test in the recognition of early anticoagulant rodenticide toxicity because of the short half-life of FVII in the circulation,[72] but the APTT was prolonged earlier and was more pronounced than the PT in horses with experimental brodifacoum toxicity.[41]

Vitamin K-deficient animals and humans developed further reduction in the vitamin K-dependent coagulation factors when treated with vitamin E. Studies suggest that vitamin E interferes at the vitamin K-dependent carboxylation step in active coagulation factor synthesis.[114,115] Certain β-lactam antibiotics and salicylate may also interfere with vitamin K metabolism.[238,331]

A 4-week-old standardbred colt presented with life-threatening bleeding and vitamin K-dependent coagulation factor deficiencies. The colt responded to vitamin K therapy with a return of coagulation tests to normal, but the foal failed to thrive and was euthanized at 9 weeks of age.[336] It was not determined if this was an inherited or a noninherited congenital vitamin K deficiency, as occurs in some human infants.[492]

Snake Venoms

Elapid snakes—including coral snakes, cobras, mambas, sea snakes, and kraits—have primarily neurotoxic venom.[104] In contrast, vipers—including rattlesnakes, copperheads, and cottonmouths—have primarily hemotoxic venom. However, these characterizations of venoms by type of snake are not consistent. For example, some elapid snakes have hemotoxins as components of their venom.[233,249] Hemotoxic venom damages the circulatory system and muscle tissue and causes swelling, hemorrhage, and necrosis. Viper venoms contain various components that can promote or inhibit hemostatic mechanisms, including coagulation, fibrinolysis, platelet function, and vascular integrity.[438] The venoms of many species of snakes contain one or more components that induce hemorrhage (hemorrhagins) through damage to vessel walls.[250]

Some snakes have venom that can induce DIC, which is followed by bleeding.[10] Several snakes have venom that activates prothrombin. Other snakes have venom that activates FX and/or FV.[250]

The venoms of pit vipers (subfamily Crotalidae) have thrombin-like activities that can clot fibrinogen in vitro, but these enzymes do not exhibit all of the effects of thrombin. They generally cleave only fibrinopeptide A from fibrinogen (a few, like the water moccasin, cleave only fibrinopeptide B), and they do not activate FXIII, so cross-linking of fibrin does not occur.[250] These friable clots are rapidly dissolved following release of tPA from endothelial cells and activation of the fibrinolytic system in vivo. This rapid fibrinolysis is associated

*References 36, 94, 299, 315, 411, 416, 501.

with a massive production of circulating fibrin degradation products.[133,543] This defibrinogenation syndrome results in blood that remains unclottable for as long as 3 days in human patients who do not receive antivenom after being bitten by eastern diamondback rattlesnakes.[283]

Thrombocytopenia may also be present after pit viper envenomation because some venoms activate platelets and because platelets may be activated in response to damage to the endothelium.[142,210,438,543]

Some snakes have components in their venoms that appear to have anticoagulant properties by preventing the formation of the prothrombinase complex on activated platelet surfaces. Several snake venoms (including the southern copperhead) activate protein C, which inhibits coagulation and promotes fibrinolysis. The venom of some snakes may indirectly stimulate fibrinolysis by blocking fibrinolytic inhibitors, such as α_2-antiplasmin and α_2-macroglobulin. Many snake venoms have components that can either induce or inhibit platelet aggregation, including phospholipases, which are ubiquitous in snake venoms.[250]

Hereditary Coagulation Disorders

An inherited coagulation factor deficiency is considered when unexplained hemorrhage occurs or hemorrhage is protracted after surgery. Although rare, hereditary coagulation defects are recognized much more often in dogs than in other domestic animal species. The likelihood that a coagulation defect will result in clinically significant hemorrhage varies with the nature of the defect.[68]

Factor XII and Prekallikrein Deficiencies

FXII deficiency occurs most often in cats (domestic short-haired, domestic long-haired, Siamese, Himalayan) but has also been recognized in dogs (miniature poodle, Chinese Shar Pei).[68] Animals with FXII deficiency have markedly prolonged APTT and ACT tests, but they do not have a bleeding disorder. Although FXII is not essential for normal hemostasis, it may play a role in the growth of thrombi under pathologic conditions.[100,428]

Like animals with FXII deficiency, dogs (Chinese Shar Pei, German shorthaired pointer, Shih Tzu), horses (Belgian horses, miniature horses), and cattle with prekallikrein deficiency have prolonged APTTs but generally do not exhibit an increased bleeding tendency.[68,288,392] Excessive hemorrhage was reported after castration of a Belgian horse with prekallikrein deficiency.[186] However, it is possible that the bleeding episode was not caused by this deficiency but simply prompted hemostatic testing of an otherwise asymptomatic deficiency because two prekallikrein-deficient siblings of this animal did not have histories of bleeding.

Factor XI Deficiency

Hemorrhage associated with this deficiency in cattle (Holstein, Japanese black cattle), dogs (Kerry blue terrier, English springer spaniel), and cats (domestic shorthaired) is generally mild until a deficient animal is subjected to trauma or surgery, at which time major bleeding can occur. Different genetic defects have been recognized in Holstein and Japanese black cattle.[68,185]

Factor IX and Factor VIII Deficiencies

Both of these deficiencies result in severe bleeding disorders and are transmitted as X chromosome-linked recessive traits; consequently, these disorders are usually recognized in male animals. FIX deficiency (hemophilia B) has been identified in many breeds of dogs and in British short hair, Siamese-cross, and domestic shorthaired cats.[68,199] FVIII deficiency (hemophilia A, classical hemophilia) has been recognized in many breeds of dogs, cats, and horses, as well as in Hereford cattle and a newborn alpaca.[68,185,230,346]

Factor VII Deficiency

FVII deficiency has been recognized in multiple breeds of dogs but appears most commonly in laboratory beagles, where inadvertent propagation of the deficiency has occurred.[86,185] FVII deficiency is usually discovered fortuitously when coagulation screening reveals a prolonged PT. Affected dogs generally do not have a history of bleeding, but they may experience bruising or prolonged bleeding following surgery or postpartum. This mild bleeding tendency with FVII deficiency (one affected dog had only 0.4% normal activity) seems paradoxical given the importance of the factor in initiating coagulation, but apparently little activity is required to initiate coagulation.[184]

Defects in the Common Coagulation Pathway

FX deficiency results in severe bleeding episodes in dogs. It has been reported in American cocker spaniels, a Jack Russell terrier, and a domestic shorthaired cat. In American cocker spaniels, this deficiency results in stillborn pups or fatal bleeding episodes in the neonatal period.[185]

Prothrombin (factor II) deficiency has been reported in English cocker spaniel and boxer dogs.[68,239] Bleeding episodes are generally mild.

Fibrinogen (factor I) deficiency causes mild to severe bleeding episodes. Inherited deficiencies have been reported in dogs, cats, goats, and a lamb.[68,162] FV and FXIII deficiencies have not been reported in animals.

Vitamin K-Dependent Coagulopathies

Vitamin K-dependent coagulopathies have been recognized in Devon Rex cats, Rambouillet sheep, a Labrador retriever dog, and a 4-week-old standardbred colt.* Affected cats and sheep are deficient in the enzyme γ-glutamyl carboxylase (see Fig. 7-15), resulting in reduction in the activities of prothrombin, FVII, FIX, and FX. Some animals exhibit minimal bleeding tendencies, but fatal hemorrhagic episodes have occurred in some affected cats. Periparturient hemorrhage and death generally occur in lambs with this disorder. Although a

*References 18, 267, 324, 330, 336, 473.

hereditary defect was suspected in the Labrador dog, a specific cause was not determined. Either a deficiency in γ-glutamyl carboxylase or a deficiency in the VKOR complex would be consistent with the clinical and laboratory findings in this dog.[63] It is unknown whether the colt had an acquired neonatal vitamin K deficiency or a hereditary defect in vitamin K recycling.[336]

INTERPRETATION OF HEMOSTATIC TEST PROFILES

The utilization of a number of hemostatic tests concomitantly helps differentiate causes of hemorrhage, including simple thrombocytopenia; DIC; vWD; vasculitis; rodenticide toxicity; liver disease; and inherited defects of the intrinsic, extrinsic, and common coagulation pathways. Examples of hemostatic test profiles and their interpretations are given below.

1. *Thrombocytopenia with normal APTT, PT, and FDP tests.* Thrombocytopenias without abnormalities in coagulation tests generally result from lack of production or enhanced platelet destruction. Bone marrow biopsies are needed to determine whether there is an abnormality in platelet production by megakaryocytes. Generalized marrow hypoplasia and aplasia are more common than pure amegakaryocytic thrombocytopenias, which are rare in animals. Myelophthisis resulting from marrow neoplasia can also result in thrombocytopenia. Enhanced platelet destruction is the most common cause of thrombocytopenia, occurring as a result of a primary or secondary immune-mediated process.
2. *Thrombocytopenia with prolonged APTT and PT test results and a positive FDP test.* This profile suggests a consumption of both platelets and coagulation factors, as occurs in DIC. Plasma antithrombin concentration is generally low when measured. All four abnormalities listed will not be present in every animal with DIC. Of these assays, the PT test is most likely to be normal.
3. *Normal platelet count, prolonged APTT and PT test results, and a negative FDP test.* This profile suggests either multiple coagulation defects, as can occur in rodenticide toxicity and liver disease, or much less likely, an inherited defect in the common pathway. Platelet counts may be decreased in animals subsequent to marked blood loss associated with rodenticide toxicity. Inexplicably, serum FDP concentrations have been reported to be increased in some dogs with anticoagulant rodenticide toxicity. Collection of blood from a heparinized IV line should also be considered as a factitious cause of this hemostatic profile.
4. *Normal platelet count and PT, prolonged APTT, and a negative FDP test.* This profile suggests an inherited defect in the intrinsic pathway, an inappropriately low plasma to anticoagulant ratio, or hemoconcentration.
5. *Normal platelet count and APTT, prolonged PT, and a negative FDP test.* This profile suggests an inherited defect in the extrinsic pathway (i.e., FVII deficiency), or early anticoagulant rodenticide toxicity in some species.
6. *Normal platelet count, APTT, and PT with a negative FDP test in the presence of a bleeding diathesis.* This profile suggests a platelet function defect or vascular injury. A concomitant prolonged bleeding time suggests a platelet function abnormality is present. Inherited platelet abnormalities or vWD could be present. vWD is diagnosed by measuring vWF in plasma by specialized laboratories. Some cases with severe vWF deficiency exhibit slightly prolonged APTT test results due to decreased FVIII in plasma.

REFERENCES

1. Abdullah R. Hemostatic abnormalities in nephrotic syndrome. *Vet Clin North Am Small Anim Pract.* 1988;18:105-113.
2. Abrams K, Yunusov MY, Slichter S, et al. Recombinant human macrophage colony-stimulating factor-induced thrombocytopenia in dogs. *Br J Haematol.* 2003;121:614-622.
3. Adam F, Villiers E, Watson S, et al. Clinical pathological and epidemiological assessment of morphologically and immunologically confirmed canine leukaemia. *Vet Comp Oncol.* 2009;7:181-195.
4. Alexandrakis MG, Passam FH, Moschandrea IA, et al. Levels of serum cytokines and acute phase proteins in patients with essential and cancer-related thrombocytosis. *Am J Clin Oncol.* 2003;26:135-140.
5. Allison R, Williams P, Lansdowne J, et al. Fatal hepatic sarcocystosis in a puppy with eosinophilia and eosinophilic peritoneal effusion. *Vet Clin Pathol.* 2006;35:353-357.
6. Alugupalli KR, Michelson AD, Joris I, et al. Spirochete-platelet attachment and thrombocytopenia in murine relapsing fever borreliosis. *Blood.* 2003;102:2843-2850.
7. Arepally GM, Ortel TL. Heparin-induced thrombocytopenia. *Annu Rev Med.* 2010;61:77-90.
8. Armengou L, Monreal L, Tarancon I, et al. Plasma D-dimer concentration in sick newborn foals. *J Vet Intern Med.* 2008;22:411-417.
9. Aroch I, Harrus S. Retrospective study of the epidemiological, clinical, haematological and biochemical findings in 109 dogs poisoned by *Vipera xanthina palestinae. Vet Rec.* 1999;144:532-535.
10. Aroch I, Segev G, Klement E, et al. Fatal *Vipera xanthina palestinae* envenomation in 16 dogs. *Vet Hum Toxicol.* 2004;46:268-272.
11. Aronson LR, Gregory C. Possible hemolytic uremic syndrome in three cats after renal transplantation and cyclosporine therapy. *Vet Surg.* 1999;28:135-140.
12. Arraga-Alvarado C, Palmar M, Parra O, et al. *Ehrlichia platys* (*Anaplasma platys*) in dogs from Maracaibo, Venezuela: an ultrastructural study of experimental and natural infections. *Vet Pathol.* 2003;40:149-156.
13. Atwell RB, Thornton JR, Odlum J. Suspected drug-induced thrombocytopenia associated with levamisole therapy in a dog. *Aust Vet J.* 1981;57:91-93.
14. Avgeris S, Lothrop CD Jr, McDonald TP. Plasma von Willebrand factor concentration and thyroid function in dogs. *J Am Vet Med Assoc.* 1990;196:921-924.
15. Axthelm MK, Krakowka S. Canine distemper virus-induced thrombocytopenia. *Am J Vet Res.* 1987;48:1269-1275.
16. Baker DC, Gaunt SD, Babin SS. Anemia of inflammation in dogs infected with *Ehrlichia platys. Am J Vet Res.* 1988;49:1014-1016.
17. Baker DC, Green RA. Coagulation defects of aflatoxin intoxicated rabbits. *Vet Pathol.* 1987;24:62-70.
18. Baker DC, Robbe SL, Jacobson L, et al. Hereditary deficiency of vitamin-K-dependent coagulation factors in Rambouillet sheep. *Blood Coagul Fibrinolysis.* 1999;10:75-80.
19. Baker GR, Levin J. Transient thrombocytopenia produced by administration of macrophage colony-stimulating factor: investigations of the mechanism. *Blood.* 1998;91:89-99.
20. Baneth G. *Hepatozoon canis* infection. In: Greene CE, ed. *Infectious Diseases of the Dog and Cat.* 3rd ed. St. Louis: Saunders Elsevier; 2006:698-705.
21. Barrows PL, Prestwood AK, Green CE. Experimental *Sarcocystis suicanis* infections: disease in growing pigs. *Am J Vet Res.* 1982;43:1409-1412.
22. Barton MH, Morris DD, Norton N, et al. Hemostatic and fibrinolytic indices in neonatal foals with presumed septicemia. *J Vet Intern Med.* 1998;12:26-35.
23. Bateman SW, Mathews KA, Abrams-Ogg AC, et al. Diagnosis of disseminated intravascular coagulation in dogs admitted to an intensive care unit. *J Am Vet Med Assoc.* 1999;215:798-804.

24. Bauer N, Eralp O, Moritz A. Reference intervals and method optimization for variables reflecting hypocoagulatory and hypercoagulatory states in dogs using the STA Compact automated analyzer. *J Vet Diagn Invest.* 2009;21:803-814.
25. Baumgarten A, Wilhelmi M, Kalbantner K, et al. Measurement of platelet aggregation in ovine blood using a new impedance aggregometer. *Vet Clin Pathol.* 2010; 39:149-156.
26. Bautista MJ, Gomez-Villamandos JC, Carrasco L, et al. Ultrastructural pathology of the bone marrow in pigs inoculated with a moderately virulent strain (DR'78) of African swine fever virus. *Histol Histopathol.* 1998;13:713-720.
27. Bay JD, Scott MA, Hans JE. Reference values for activated coagulation time in cats. *Am J Vet Res.* 2000;61:750-753.
28. Beale KM, Altman D, Clemmons RR, et al. Systemic toxicosis associated with azathioprine administration in domestic cats. *Am J Vet Res.* 1992;53:1236-1240.
29. Bedard C, Lanevschi-Pietersma A, Dunn M. Evaluation of coagulation markers in the plasma of healthy cats and cats with asymptomatic hypertrophic cardiomyopathy. *Vet Clin Pathol.* 2007;36:167-172.
30. Bell WR Jr. Defibrinogenating enzymes. *Drugs.* 1997;54(Suppl 3):18-30.
31. Bennett JS, Berger BW, Billings PC. The structure and function of platelet integrins. *J Thromb Haemost.* 2009;7(Suppl 1):200-205.
32. Bentz AI, Wilkins PA, MacGillivray KC, et al. Severe thrombocytopenia in 2 thoroughbred foals with sepsis and neonatal encephalopathy. *J Vet Intern Med.* 2002; 16:494-497.
33. Bergmeier W, Stefanini L. Novel molecules in calcium signaling in platelets. *J Thromb Haemost.* 2009;7(Suppl 1):187-190.
34. Bessman JD. The relation of megakaryocyte ploidy to platelet volume. *Am J Hematol.* 1984;16:161-170.
35. Bessman JD, Williams LJ, Gilmer PR Jr. The inverse relation of platelet size and count in normal subjects, and an artifact of other particles. *Am J Clin Pathol.* 1981;76:289-293.
36. Biourge V, MacDonald MJ, King L. Feline hepatic lipidosis: pathogenesis and nutritional management. *Comp Cont Ed Pract Vet.* 1990;12:1244-1258.
37. Blaisdell FS, Dodds WJ. Evaluation of two microhematocrit methods for quantitating plasma fibrinogen. *J Am Vet Med Assoc.* 1977;171:340-342.
38. Blaise GA, Parent M, Laurin S, et al. Platelet-induced vasomotion of isolated canine coronary artery in the presence of halothane or isoflurane. *J Cardiothorac Vasc Anesth.* 1994;8:175-181.
39. Blajchman MA, Bordin JO, Bardossy L, et al. The contribution of the haematocrit to thrombocytopenic bleeding in experimental animals. *Br J Haematol.* 1994;86:347-350.
40. Bloom JC, Thiem PA, Sellers TS, et al. Cephalosporin-induced immune cytopenia in the dog: demonstration of erythrocyte-, neutrophil-, and platelet-associated IgG following treatment with cefazedone. *Am J Hematol.* 1988;28:71-78.
41. Boermans HJ, Johnstone I, Black WD, et al. Clinical signs, laboratory changes and toxicokinetics of brodifacoum in the horse. *Can J Vet Res.* 1991;55:21-27.
42. Boisvert AM, Swenson CL, Haines CJ. Serum and plasma latex agglutination tests for detection of fibrin(ogen) degradation products in clinically ill dogs. *Vet Clin Pathol.* 2001;30:133-140.
43. Borges AS, Divers TJ, Stokol T, et al. Serum iron and plasma fibrinogen concentrations as indicators of systemic inflammatory diseases in horses. *J Vet Intern Med.* 2007;21:489-494.
44. Boudreaux MK. Inherited intrinsic platelet disorders. In: Weiss DJ, Wardrop KJ, eds. *Schalm's Veterinary Hematology.* 6th ed. Ames: Wiley-Blackwell; 2010: 619-625.
45. Boudreaux MK. P2Y12 receptor gene mutation in a Greater Swiss Mountain dog (abstract). *Vet Clin Pathol.* 2010;39:557.
46. Boudreaux MK. Platelet structure. In: Weiss DJ, Wardrop KJ, eds. *Schalm's Veterinary Hematology.* 6th ed. Ames, IA: Wiley-Blackwell; 2010:561-568.
47. Boudreaux MK, Catalfamo JL, Klok M. Calcium-diacylglycerol guanine nucleotide exchange factor I gene mutations associated with loss of function in canine platelets. *Transl Res.* 2007;150:81-92.
48. Boudreaux MK, Ebbe S. Comparison of platelet number, mean platelet volume and platelet mass in five mammalian species. *Comp Haematol Int.* 1998;8:16-20.
49. Boudreaux MK, Osborne CD, Herre AC, et al. Unique structure of the M loop region of beta1-tubulin may contribute to size variability of platelets in the family felidae. *Vet Clin Pathol.* 2010;39:417-423.
50. Boudreaux MK, Schmutz SM, French PS. Calcium diacylglycerol guanine nucleotide exchange factor I (CalDAG-GEFI) gene mutations in a thrombopathic Simmental calf. *Vet Pathol.* 2007;44:932-935.
51. Boudreaux MK, Wardrop KJ, Kiklevich V, et al. A mutation in the canine Kindlin-3 gene associated with increased bleeding risk and susceptibility to infections. *Thromb Haemost.* 2010;103:475-477.
52. Boutet P, Heath F, Archer J, et al. Comparison of quantitative immunoturbidimetric and semiquantitative latex-agglutination assays for D-dimer measurement in canine plasma. *Vet Clin Pathol.* 2009;38:78-82.
53. Bowen DJ, Clemmons RM, Meyer DJ, et al. Platelet functional changes secondary to hepatocholestasis and elevation of serum bile acids. *Thromb Res.* 1988;52:649-654.
54. Boyce JT, Kociba GJ, Jacobs RM, et al. Feline leukemia virus-induced thrombocytopenia and macrothrombocytosis in cats. *Vet Pathol.* 1986;23:16-20.
55. Brady CA, Otto CM, Van Winkle TJ, et al. Severe sepsis in cats: 29 cases (1986-1998). *J Am Vet Med Assoc.* 2000;217:531-535.
56. Brainard BM, Epstein KL, Lobato D, et al. Effects of clopidogrel and aspirin on platelet aggregation, thromboxane production, and serotonin secretion in horses. *J Vet Intern Med*; 2011;25:116-122.
57. Brandt E, Ludwig A, Petersen F, et al. Platelet-derived CXC chemokines: old players in new games. *Immunol Rev.* 2000;177:204-216.
58. Brassard JA, Meyers KM, Person M, et al. Experimentally induced renal failure in the dog as an animal model of uremic bleeding. *J Lab Clin Med.* 1994;124:48-54.
59. Brazzell JL, Borjesson DL. Evaluation of plasma antithrombin activity and D-dimer concentration in populations of healthy cats, clinically ill cats, and cats with cardiomyopathy. *Vet Clin Pathol.* 2007;36:79-84.
60. Breitschwerdt EB. Infectious thrombocytopenia in dogs. Comp *Cont Ed Pract Vet.* 1988;10:1177-1190.
61. Breitschwerdt EB. Feline bartonellosis and cat scratch disease. *Vet Immunol Immunopathol.* 2008;123:167-171.
62. Breitschwerdt EB, Nicholson WL, Kiehl AR, et al. Natural infections with *Borrelia* spirochetes in two dogs in Florida. *J Clin Microbiol.* 1994;32:352-357.
63. Brenner B, Kuperman AA, Watzka M, et al. Vitamin K-dependent coagulation factors deficiency. *Semin Thromb Hemost.* 2009;35:439-446.
64. Brianceau P, Divers TJ. Acute thrombosis of limb arteries in horses with sepsis: five cases (1988-1998). *Equine Vet J.* 2001;33:105-109.
65. Brommer EJP, Engbers J, Laarse AVD, et al. Survival of fibrinogen degradation products in the circulation after thrombolytic therapy for acute myocardial infarction. *Fibrinolysis.* 1987;1:149-153.
66. Brooks AC, Menzies-Gow NJ, Wheeler-Jones CP, et al. Regulation of platelet activating factor-induced equine platelet activation by intracellular kinases. *J Vet Pharmacol Ther.* 2009;32:189-196.
67. Brooks M, Catalfamo J. Buccal mucosa bleeding time is prolonged in canine models of primary hemostatic disorders. *Thromb Haemost.* 1993;70:777-780.
68. Brooks MB. Hereditary coagulopathies. In: Weiss DJ, Wardrop KJ, eds. *Schalm's Veterinary Hematology.* 6th ed. Ames, IA: Wiley-Blackwell; 2010:661-667.
69. Brooks MB, Catalfamo JL. Von Willebrand disease. In: Weiss DJ, Wardrop KJ, eds. *Schalm's Veterinary Hematology.* 6th ed. Ames, IA: Wiley-Blackwell; 2010:612-618.
70. Brooks MB, Catalfamo JL, Brown HA, et al. A hereditary bleeding disorder of dogs caused by a lack of platelet procoagulant activity. *Blood.* 2002;99:2434-2441.
71. Brooks MB, Catalfamo JL, Etter K, et al. Exclusion of ABCA-1 as a candidate gene for canine Scott syndrome. *J Thromb Haemost.* 2008;6:1608-1610.
72. Brooks MB, De Laforcade A. Acquired coagulopathies. In: Weiss DJ, Wardrop KJ, eds. *Schalm's Veterinary Hematology.* 6th ed. Ames, IA: Wiley-Blackwell; 2010:654-660.
73. Brooks MB, Randolph J, Warner K, et al. Evaluation of platelet function screening tests to detect platelet procoagulant deficiency in dogs with Scott syndrome. *Vet Clin Pathol.* 2009;38:306-315.
74. Brown SJ, Simpson KW, Baker S, et al. Macrothrombocytosis in cavalier King Charles spaniels. *Vet Rec.* 1994;135:281-283.
75. Buechner-Maxwell V, Scott MA, Godber L, et al. Neonatal alloimmune thrombocytopenia in a quarter horse foal. *J Vet Intern Med.* 1997;11:304-308.
76. Burgess H, Wood D. Validation of a von Willebrand factor antigen enzyme-linked immunosorbent assay and newly developed collagen-binding assay. *Can J Vet Res.* 2008;72:420-427.
77. Burnier L, Fontana P, Kwak BR, et al. Cell-derived microparticles in haemostasis and vascular medicine. *Thromb Haemost.* 2009;101:439-451.
78. Burstein SA, Peng J, Friese P, et al. Cytokine-induced alteration of platelet and hemostatic function. *Stem Cells.* 1996;14(Suppl 1):154-162.
79. Butenas S, Mann KG. Blood coagulation. *Biochemistry (Mosc).* 2002;67:3-12.
80. Caen J, Wu Q. Hageman factor, platelets and polyphosphates: early history and recent connection. *J Thromb Haemost.* 2010;8:1670-1674.
81. Cain GR, Feldman BF, Kawakami TG, et al. Platelet dysplasia associated with megakaryoblastic leukemia in a dog. *J Am Vet Med Assoc.* 1986;188:529-530.
82. Callan MB, Bennett JS, Phillips DK, et al. Inherited platelet δ-storage pool disease in dogs causing severe bleeding: An animal model for a specific ADP deficiency. *Thromb Haemostas.* 1995;74:949-953.
83. Callan MB, Giger U. Assessment of a point-of-care instrument for identification of primary hemostatic disorders in dogs. *Am J Vet Res.* 2001;62:652-658.
84. Callan MB, Shofer FS, Catalfamo JL. Effects of anticoagulant on pH, ionized calcium concentration, and agonist-induced platelet aggregation in canine platelet-rich plasma. *Am J Vet Res.* 2009;70:472-477.
85. Cambridge H, Lees P, Hooke RE, et al. Antithrombotic actions of aspirin in the horse. *Equine Vet J.* 1991;23:123-127.

86. Carlstrom LP, Jens JK, Dobyns ME, et al. Inadvertent propagation of factor VII deficiency in a canine mucopolysaccharidosis type I research breeding colony. *Comp Med.* 2009;59:378-382.
87. Carpenter JL, Andelman NC, Moore FM, et al. Idiopathic cutaneous and renal glomerular vasculopathy of greyhounds. *Vet Pathol.* 1988;25:401-407.
88. Carr AP, Panciera DL, Kidd L. Prognostic factors for mortality and thromboembolism in canine immune-mediated hemolytic anemia: a retrospective study of 72 dogs. *J Vet Intern Med.* 2002;16:504-509.
89. Carrasco L, Madsen LW, Salguero FJ, et al. Immune complex-associated thrombocytopenic purpura syndrome in sexually mature Gottingen minipigs. *J Comp Pathol.* 2003;128:25-32.
90. Carrick JB, Morris DD, Moore JN. Administration of a receptor antagonist for platelet-activating factor during equine endotoxaemia. *Equine Vet J.* 1993;25:152-157.
91. Casella S, Giannetto C, Fazio F, et al. Assessment of prothrombin time, activated partial thromboplastin time, and fibrinogen concentration on equine plasma samples following different storage conditions. *J Vet Diagn Invest.* 2009;21:674-678.
92. Castoldi E, Hackeng TM. Regulation of coagulation by protein S. *Curr Opin Hematol.* 2008;15:529-536.
93. Cavaillon JM. Cytokines and macrophages. *Biomed Pharmacother.* 1994; 48:445-453.
94. Center SA, Elston TH, Rowland PH, et al. Fulminant hepatic failure associated with oral administration of diazepam in 11 cats. *J Am Vet Med Assoc.* 1996;209:618-625.
95. Center SA, Warner K, Corbett J, et al. Proteins invoked by vitamin K absence and clotting times in clinically ill cats. *J Vet Intern Med.* 2000;14:292-297.
96. Ceron JJ, Carli E, Tasca S, et al. Evaluation of EDTA hematology tubes for collection of blood samples for tests of secondary hemostasis in dogs. *Am J Vet Res.* 2008;69:1141-1147.
97. Cesarini C, Monreal L, Armengou L, et al. Association of admission plasma D-dimer concentration with diagnosis and outcome in horses with colic. *J Vet Intern Med.* 2010;24:1490-1497.
98. Chandler WL, Jelacic S, Boster DR, et al. Prothrombotic coagulation abnormalities preceding the hemolytic-uremic syndrome. *N Engl J Med.* 2002;346:23-32.
99. Chantrey J, Chapman PS, Patterson-Kan JC. Haemolytic-uraemic syndrome in a dog. *J Vet Med A Physiol Pathol Clin Med.* 2002;49:470-472.
100. Cheng Q, Tucker EI, Pine MS, et al. A role for factor XIIa-mediated factor XI activation in thrombus formation in vivo. *Blood.* 2010;116:3981-3989.
101. Cheng T, Mathews KA, Abrams-Ogg AC, et al. Relationship between assays of inflammation and coagulation: a novel interpretation of the canine activated clotting time. *Can J Vet Res.* 2009;73:97-102.
102. Chilton FH, Cluzel M, Triggiani M. Recent advances in our understanding of the biochemical interactions between platelet-activating factor and arachidonic acid. *Lipids.* 1991;26:1021-1027.
103. Chisholm-Chait A. Mechanisms of thrombocytopenia in dogs with cancer. *Comp Cont Ed Pract Vet.* 2000;22:1006-1012.
104. Chrisman CL, Hopkins AL, Ford SL, et al. Acute, flaccid quadriplegia in three cats with suspected coral snake envenomation. *J Am Anim Hosp Assoc.* 1996;32:343-349.
105. Chu PH, Huang TY, Williams J, et al. Purified vitamin K epoxide reductase alone is sufficient for conversion of vitamin K epoxide to vitamin K and vitamin K to vitamin KH2. *Proc Natl Acad Sci U S A.* 2006;103:19308-19313.
106. Clabough DL, Gebhard D, Flaherty MT, et al. Immune-mediated thrombocytopenia in horses infected with equine infectious anemia virus. *J Virol.* 1991;65:6242-6251.
107. Clinkenbeard KD, Cowell RL, Tyler RD. Disseminated histoplasmosis in cats: 12 cases (1981-1986). *J Am Vet Med Assoc.* 1987;190:1445-1448.
108. Clinkenbeard KD, Cowell RL, Tyler RD. Disseminated histoplasmosis in dogs: 12 cases (1981-1986). *J Am Vet Med Assoc.* 1988;193:1443-1447.
109. Collicchio-Zuanaze R, Sakate M, Langrafe L, et al. Hematological and biochemical profiles and histopathological evaluation of experimental intoxication by sodium fluoroacetate in cats. *Hum Exp Toxicol.* 2010;29:903-913.
110. Constable PD, Schmall LM, Muir WW III, et al. Respiratory, renal, hematologic, and serum biochemical effects of hypertonic saline solution in endotoxemic calves. *Am J Vet Res.* 1991;52:990-998.
111. Cook AK, Cowgill LD. Clinical and pathological features of protein-losing glomerular disease in the dog: a review of 137 cases (1985-1992). *J Am Anim Hosp Assoc.* 1996;32:313-322.
112. Corash L, Chen HY, Levin J, et al. Regulation of thrombopoiesis: effects of the degree of thrombocytopenia on megakaryocyte ploidy and platelet volume. *Blood.* 1987;70:177-185.
113. Corl CM, Gandy JC, Sordillo LM. Platelet activating factor production and proinflammatory gene expression in endotoxin-challenged bovine mammary endothelial cells. *J Dairy Sci.* 2008;91:3067-3078.
114. Corrigan JJ Jr. Coagulation problems relating to vitamin E. *Am J Pediatr Hematol Oncol.* 1979;1:169-173.
115. Corrigan JJ Jr. The effect of vitamin E on warfarin-induced vitamin K deficiency. *Ann N Y Acad Sci.* 1982;393:361-368.
116. Cortese L, Sica M, Piantedosi D, et al. Secondary immune-mediated thrombocytopenia in dogs naturally infected by *Leishmania infantum*. *Vet Rec.* 2009;164: 778-782.
117. Court EA, Earnest-Koons KA, Barr SC, et al. Malignant histiocytosis in a cat. *J Am Vet Med Assoc.* 1993;203:1300-1302.
118. Cowan LA, Hertzke DM, Fenwick BW, et al. Clinical and clinicopathologic abnormalities in Greyhounds with cutaneous and renal glomerular vasculopathy: 18 cases (1992-1994). *J Am Vet Med Assoc.* 1997;210:789-793.
119. Cowgill LD, James KM, Levy JK, et al. Use of recombinant human erythropoietin for management of anemia in dogs and cats with renal failure. *J Am Vet Med Assoc.* 1998;212:521-528.
120. Cowles BE, Meyers KM, Wardrop KJ, et al. Prolonged bleeding time of Chediak-Higashi cats corrected by platelet transfusion. *Thromb Haemost.* 1992;67:708-712.
121. Crawford TB, Wardrop KJ, Tornquist SJ, et al. A primary production deficit in the thrombocytopenia of equine infectious anemia. *J Virol.* 1996;70:7842-7850.
122. Dale DC, Nichol JL, Rich DA, et al. Chronic thrombocytopenia is induced in dogs by development of cross-reacting antibodies to the MpL ligand. *Blood.* 1997;90:3456-3461.
123. Dale GL, Friese P, Hynes LA, et al. Demonstration that thiazole-orange-positive platelets in the dog are less than 24 hours old. *Blood.* 1995;85:1822-1825.
124. Dale GL, Wolf RF, Hynes LA, et al. Quantitation of platelet life span in splenectomized dogs. *Exp Hematol.* 1996;24:518-523.
125. Dan K, Gomi S, Inokuchi K, et al. Effects of interleukin-1 and tumor necrosis factor on megakaryocytopoiesis: mechanism of reactive thrombocytosis. *Acta Haematol.* 1995;93:67-72.
126. Davidson BL, Rozanski EA, Tidwell AS, et al. Pulmonary thromboembolism in a heartworm-positive cat. *J Vet Intern Med.* 2006;20:1037-1041.
127. Davis B, Toivio-Kinnucan M, Schuller S, et al. Mutation in beta1-tubulin correlates with macrothrombocytopenia in Cavalier King Charles Spaniels. *J Vet Intern Med.* 2008;22:540-545.
128. Davis CE. Thrombocytopenia: a uniform complication of African trypanosomiasis. *Acta Trop.* 1982;39:123-133.
129. Davis WM. Hapten-induced immune-mediated thrombocytopenia in a dog. *J Am Vet Med Assoc.* 1984;184:976-977.
130. De Gopegui RR, Espada Y, Vilafranca M, et al. Paraprotein-induced defective haemostasis in a dog with IgA (kappa-light chain) forming myeloma. *Vet Clin Pathol.* 1994;23:70-71.
131. de Laforcade AM, Freeman LM, Shaw SP, et al. Hemostatic changes in dogs with naturally occurring sepsis. *J Vet Intern Med.* 2003;17:674-679.
132. de Laforcade AM, Rozanski EA, Freeman LM, et al. Serial evaluation of protein C and antithrombin in dogs with sepsis. *J Vet Intern Med.* 2008;22:26-30.
133. de Sousa-e-Silva MC, Tomy SC, Tavares FL, et al. Hematological, hemostatic and clinical chemistry disturbances induced by *Crotalus durissus terrificus* snake venom in dogs. *Hum Exp Toxicol.* 2003;22:491-500.
134. Deitschel SJ, Kerl ME, Chang CH, et al. Age-associated changes to pathogen-associated molecular pattern-induced inflammatory mediator production in dogs. *J Vet Emerg Crit Care (San Antonio).* 2010;20:494-502.
135. Del Piero F. Equine viral arteritis. *Vet Pathol.* 2000;37:287-296.
136. Del Piero F, Wilkins PA, Lopez JW, et al. Equine viral arteritis in newborn foals: clinical, pathological, serological, microbiological and immunohistochemical observations. *Equine Vet J.* 1997;29:178-185.
137. DelGiudice LA, White GA. The role of tissue factor and tissue factor pathway inhibitor in health and disease states. *J Vet Emerg Crit Care (San Antonio).* 2009;19:23-29.
138. Dell'Orco M, Bertazzolo W, Pagliaro L, et al. Hemolytic-uremic syndrome in a dog. *Vet Clin Pathol.* 2005;34:264-269.
139. Dereszynski DM, Center SA, Randolph JF, et al. Clinical and clinicopathologic features of dogs that consumed foodborne hepatotoxic aflatoxins: 72 cases (2005-2006). *J Am Vet Med Assoc.* 2008;232:1329-1337.
140. Dewhurst E, Cue S, Crawford E, et al. A retrospective study of canine D-dimer concentrations measured using an immunometric "Point-of-Care" test. *J Small Anim Pract.* 2008;49:344-348.
141. DiBartola SP, Tarr MJ, Parker AT, et al. Clinicopathologic findings in dogs with renal amyloidosis: 59 cases (1976-1986). *J Am Vet Med Assoc.* 1989;195:358-364.
142. Dickinson CE, Traub-Dargatz JL, Dargatz DA, et al. Rattlesnake venom poisoning in horses: 32 cases (1973-1993). *J Am Vet Med Assoc.* 1996;208:1866-1871.
143. Dircks BH, Schuberth HJ, Mischke R. Underlying diseases and clinicopathologic variables of thrombocytopenic dogs with and without platelet-bound antibodies detected by use of a flow cytometric assay: 83 cases (2004-2006). *J Am Vet Med Assoc.* 2009;235:960-966.
144. Dolente BA, Wilkins PA, Boston RC. Clinicopathologic evidence of disseminated intravascular coagulation in horses with acute colitis. *J Am Vet Med Assoc.* 2002; 220:1034-1038.

145. Du Plessis L, Stevens K. Blood platelets of the African elephant. *J Comp Pathol.* 2002;127:208-210.
146. Dunkel B, Chan DL, Boston R, et al. Association between hypercoagulability and decreased survival in horses with ischemic or inflammatory gastrointestinal disease. *J Vet Intern Med.* 2010;24:1467-1474.
147. Dunn JK, Heath MF, Jefferies AR, et al. Diagnosis and hematologic features of probable essential thrombocythemia in two dogs. *Vet Clin Pathol.* 1999;28:131-138.
148. Eckersall PD. Proteins, proteomics, and the dysproteinemias. In: Kaneko JJ, Harvey JW, Bruss ML, eds. *Clinical Biochemistry of Domestic Animals.* 6th ed. San Diego, CA: Academic Press; 2008:117-155.
149. Eckersall PD, Conner JG. Bovine and canine acute phase proteins. *Vet Res Commun.* 1988;12:169-178.
150. Edens LM, Morris DD, Prasse KW, et al. Hypercoaguable state associated with a deficiency of protein C in a thoroughbred colt. *J Vet Intern Med.* 1993;7:190-193.
151. Edwards JF, Dodds WJ, Slauson DO. Coagulation changes in African swine fever virus infection. *Am J Vet Res.* 1984;45:2414-2420.
152. Edwards JF, Dodds WJ, Slauson DO. Megakaryocytic infection and thrombocytopenia in African swine fever. *Vet Pathol.* 1985;22:171-176.
153. el-Sayed MS. Effects of exercise on blood coagulation, fibrinolysis and platelet aggregation. *Sports Med.* 1996;22:282-298.
154. Emsley J, McEwan PA, Gailani D. Structure and function of factor XI. *Blood.* 2010;115:2569-2577.
155. Ertenli I, Kiraz S, Ozturk MA, et al. Pathologic thrombopoiesis of rheumatoid arthritis. *Rheumatol Int.* 2003;23:49-60.
156. Esmon CT. Protein C pathway in sepsis. *Ann Med.* 2002;34:598-605.
157. Esmon CT. Inflammation and the activated protein C anticoagulant pathway. *Semin Thromb Hemost.* 2006;32(Suppl 1):49-60.
158. Estrin MA, Wehausen CE, Jessen CR, et al. Disseminated intravascular coagulation in cats. *J Vet Intern Med.* 2006;20:1334-1339.
159. Fan TM, Simpson KW, Trasti S, et al. Calcipotriol toxicity in a dog. *J Small Anim Pract.* 1998;39:581-586.
160. Farrar ET, Washabau RJ, Saunders HM. Hepatic abscesses in dogs: 14 cases (1982-1994). *J Am Vet Med Assoc.* 1996;208:243-247.
161. Favaloro EJ. Hemolytic uremic syndrome. *Semin Thromb Hemost.* 2010;36:573-574.
162. Fecteau G, Zinkl JG, Smith BP, et al. Dysfibrinogenemia or afibrinogenemia in a Border Leicester lamb. *Can Vet J.* 1997;38:443-444.
163. Feldman BF, Madewell BR, O'Neill S. Disseminated intravascular coagulation: antithrombin, plasminogen, and coagulation abnormalities in 41 dogs. *J Am Vet Med Assoc.* 1981;179:151-154.
164. Flatland B, Fry MM, Baek SJ, et al. May-Hegglin anomaly in a Pug dog. *Vet Clin Pathol.* 2011;40:207-214.
165. Folts JD. Inhibition of platelet activity in vivo by amlodipine alone and combined with aspirin. *Int J Cardiol.* 1997;62(Suppl 2):S111-S117.
166. Forster LM. Neonatal alloimmune thrombocytopenia, purpura, and anemia in 6 neonatal piglets. *Can Vet J.* 2007;48:855-857.
167. Francois B, Trimoreau F, Vignon P, et al. Thrombocytopenia in the sepsis syndrome: role of hemophagocytosis and macrophage colony-stimulating factor. *Am J Med.* 1997;103:114-120.
168. Frederick J, Giguère S, Butterworth K, et al. Severe phenylephrine-associated hemorrhage in five aged horses. *J Am Vet Med Assoc.* 2010;237:830-834.
169. Freedman ML, Karpatkin S. Heterogeneity of rabbit platelets. V. Preferential splenic sequestration of megathrombocytes. *Br J Haematol.* 1975;31:255-262.
170. Freeman L, Stevens J, Loughman C, et al. Malignant histiocytosis in a cat. *J Vet Intern Med.* 1995;9:171-173.
171. Frelier PF, Lewis RM. Hematologic and coagulation abnormalities in acute bovine sarcocystosis. *Am J Vet Res.* 1984;45:40-48.
172. French TW, Harvey JW. Canine infectious cyclic thrombocytopenia (*Ehrlichia platys* infection in dogs). In: Woldehiwet Z, Ristic M, eds. *Rickettsial and Chlamydial Diseases of Domestic Animals.* New York: Pergamon Press; 1993:195-208.
173. Freyssinet JM, Toti F. Formation of procoagulant microparticles and properties. *Thromb Res.* 2010;125(Suppl 1):S46-S48.
174. Friedrichs KR, Young KM. Histiocytic sarcoma of macrophage origin in a cat: case report with a literature review of feline histiocytic malignancies and comparison with canine hemophagocytic histiocytic sarcoma. *Vet Clin Pathol.* 2008;37:121-128.
175. Fry MM. Acquired platelet dysfunction. In: Weiss DJ, Wardrop KJ, eds. *Schalm's Veterinary Hematology.* 6th ed. Ames, IA: Wiley-Blackwell; 2010:626-631.
176. Fry MM, Forman MA. 5-Fuorouracil toxicity with severe bone marrow suppression in a dog. *Vet Hum Toxicol.* 2004;46:178-180.
177. Fujino Y, Horiuchi H, Mizukoshi F, et al. Prevalence of hematological abnormalities and detection of infected bone marrow cells in asymptomatic cats with feline immunodeficiency virus infection. *Vet Microbiol.* 2009;136:217-225.
178. Furlanello T, Caldin M, Stocco A, et al. Stability of stored canine plasma for hemostasis testing. *Vet Clin Pathol.* 2006;35:204-207.
179. Furlanello T, Tasca S, Caldin M, et al. Artifactual changes in canine blood following storage, detected using the ADVIA 120 hematology analyzer. *Vet Clin Pathol.* 2006;35:42-46.
180. Galarneau JR, Fortin M, Lapointe JM, et al. *Citrobacter freundii* septicemia in two dogs. *J Vet Diagn Invest.* 2003;15:297-299.
181. Gaschen FP, Smith Meyer B, Harvey JW. Amegakaryocytic thrombocytopenia and immune-mediated haemolytic anaemia in a cat. *Comp Haematol Int.* 1992;2:175-178.
182. Gebbink MF, Bouma B, Maas C, et al. Physiological responses to protein aggregates: fibrinolysis, coagulation and inflammation (new roles for old factors). *FEBS Lett.* 2009;583:2691-2699.
183. Geffre A, Grollier S, Hanot C, et al. Canine reference intervals for coagulation markers using the STA Satellite(R) and the STA-R Evolution(R) analyzers. *J Vet Diagn Invest.* 2010;22:690-695.
184. Gentry PA. Comparative aspects of blood coagulation. *Vet J.* 2004;168:238-251.
185. Gentry PA, Burgess H, Wood D. Hemostasis. In: Kaneko JJ, Harvey JW, Bruss ML, eds. *Clinical Biochemistry of Domestic Animals.* 6th ed. San Diego, CA: Academic Press; 2008:287-330.
186. Geor RJ, Jackson ML, Lewis KD, et al. Prekallikrein deficiency in a family of Belgian horses. *J Am Vet Med Assoc.* 1990;197:741-745.
187. George FD. Microparticles in vascular diseases. *Thromb Res.* 2008;122(Suppl 1): S55-S59.
188. Gerber B, Taboada J, Lothrop CD Jr, et al. Determination of normal values using an automated coagulation timer for activated coagulation time and its application in dogs with hemophilia. *J Vet Intern Med.* 1999;13:433-436.
189. Gieger TL, Correa SS, Taboada J, et al. Phenol poisoning in three dogs. *J Am Anim Hosp Assoc.* 2000;36:317-321.
190. Giger U. Differing opinions on value of PIVKA test. *J Am Vet Med Assoc.* 2003;222:1070-1071.
191. Gilio K, Munnix IC, Mangin P, et al. Non-redundant roles of phosphoinositide 3-kinase isoforms alpha and beta in glycoprotein VI-induced platelet signaling and thrombus formation. *J Biol Chem.* 2009;284:33750-33762.
192. Glaspy JA. Hemostatic abnormalities in multiple myeloma and related disorders. *Hematol Oncol Clin North Am.* 1992;6:1301-1314.
193. Gleich S, Hartmann K. Hematology and serum biochemistry of feline immunodeficiency virus-infected and feline leukemia virus-infected cats. *J Vet Intern Med.* 2009;23:552-558.
194. Goerge T, Ho-Tin-Noe B, Carbo C, et al. Inflammation induces hemorrhage in thrombocytopenia. *Blood.* 2008;111:4958-4964.
195. Gold JR, Warren AL, French TW, et al. What is your diagnosis? Biopsy impression smear of a hepatic mass in a yearling Thoroughbred filly. *Vet Clin Pathol.* 2008;37:339-343.
196. Goldstein RE, Lin RC, Langston CE, et al. Influence of infecting serogroup on clinical features of leptospirosis in dogs. *J Vet Intern Med.* 2006;20:489-494.
197. Gomez-Villamandos JC, Salguero FJ, Ruiz-Villamor E, et al. Classical swine fever: pathology of bone marrow. *Vet Pathol.* 2003;40:157-163.
198. Goodman RA, Breitschwerdt EB. Clinicopathologic findings in dogs seroreactive to *Bartonella henselae* antigens. *Am J Vet Res.* 2005;66:2060-2064.
199. Goree M, Catalfamo JL, Aber S, et al. Characterization of the mutations causing hemophilia B in 2 domestic cats. *J Vet Intern Med.* 2005;19:200-204.
200. Gorski J, Luka K, Czestochowska E. Platelet function and survival in multiple myeloma. *Haematologia (Budap).* 1993;25:131-135.
201. Gouin I, Lecompte T, Morel MC, et al. *In vitro* effect of plasmin on human platelet function in plasma. Inhibition of aggregation caused by fibrinogenolysis. *Circulation.* 1992;85:935-941.
202. Gould SM, McInnes EL. Immune-mediated thrombocytopenia associated with *Angiostrongylus vasorum* infection in a dog. *J Small Anim Pract.* 1999;40:227-232.
203. Green RA, Kabel AL. Hypercoagulable state in three dogs with nephrotic syndrome: role of acquired antithrombin III deficiency. *J Am Vet Med Assoc.* 1982; 181:914-917.
204. Greene CE, Barsanti JA, Jones BD. Disseminated intravascular coagulation complicating aflatoxicosis in dogs. *Cornell Vet.* 1977;67:29-49.
205. Greene CE, Breitschwerdt EB. Rocky Mountain spotted fever, murine typhuslike disease, rickettsialpox, and Q fever. In: Greene CE, ed. *Infectious Diseases of the Dog and Cat.* 3rd ed. St. Louis: Saunders Elsevier; 2006:232-245.
206. Griffin A, Callan MB, Shofer FS, et al. Evaluation of a canine D-dimer point-of-care test kit for use in samples obtained from dogs with disseminated intravascular coagulation, thromboembolic disease, and hemorrhage. *Am J Vet Res.* 2003;64:1562-1569.
207. Grindem CB, Breitschwerdt EB, Corbett WT, et al. Epidemiologic survey of thrombocytopenia in dogs: a report on 987 cases. *Vet Clin Pathol.* 1991;20:38-43.
208. Grindem CB, Breitschwerdt EB, Corbett WT, et al. Thrombocytopenia associated with neoplasia in dogs. *J Vet Intern Med.* 1994;8:400-405.

209. Grindem CB, Breitschwerdt EB, Perkins PC, et al. Platelet-associated immunoglobulin (antiplatelet antibody) in canine Rocky Mountain spotted fever and ehrlichiosis. *J Am Anim Hosp Assoc.* 1999;35:56-61.
210. Hackett TB, Wingfield WE, Mazzaferro EM, et al. Clinical findings associated with prairie rattlesnake bites in dogs: 100 cases (1989-1998). *J Am Vet Med Assoc.* 2002;220:1675-1680.
211. Hackner SG, Schaer BD. Thrombotic disorders. In: Weiss DJ, Wardrop KJ, eds. *Schalm's Veterinary Hematology.* 6th ed. Ames, IA: Wiley-Blackwell; 2010:668-678.
212. Hahn KA, McEntee MF, Daniel GB, et al. Hematologic and systemic toxicoses associated with carboplatin administration in cats. *Am J Vet Res.* 1997;58:677-679.
213. Hahn KA, Rohrbach BW, Legendre AM, et al. Hematologic changes associated with weekly low-dose cisplatin administration in dogs. *Vet Clin Pathol.* 1997;26:29-31.
214. Hammer AS. Thrombocytosis in dogs and cats: a retrospective study. *Comp Haematol Int.* 1991;1:181-186.
215. Hammer AS, Couto CG, Swardson C, et al. Hemostatic abnormalities in dogs with hemangiosarcoma. *J Vet Intern Med.* 1991;5:11-14.
216. Hammond WP, Dale DC. Lithium therapy of canine cyclic hematopoiesis. *Blood.* 1980;55:26-28.
217. Handagama P, Feldman BF, Kono CS, et al. Mean platelet volume artifacts: the effect of anticoagulants and temperature on canine platelets. *Vet Clin Pathol.* 1986;15(4):13-17.
218. Hardie EM, Kruse-Elliott K. Endotoxic shock. Part I: A review of causes. *J Vet Intern Med.* 1990;4:258-266.
219. Hargis AM, Feldman BF. Evaluation of hemostatic defects secondary to vascular tumors in dogs: 11 cases (1983-1988). *J Am Vet Med Assoc.* 1991;198:891-894.
220. Harper MT, Poole AW. Diverse functions of protein kinase C isoforms in platelet activation and thrombus formation. *J Thromb Haemost.* 2010;8:454-462.
221. Harr KE. Overview of avian hemostasis. In: Weiss DJ, Wardrop KJ, eds. *Schalm's Veterinary Hematology.* 6th ed. Ames, IA: Wiley-Blackwell; 2010:703-707.
222. Harr KE, Raskin RE, Heard DJ. Temporal effects of 3 commonly used anticoagulants on hematologic and biochemical variables in blood samples from macaws and Burmese pythons. *Vet Clin Pathol.* 2005;34:383-388.
223. Harrell K. Bleeding time. In: Vaden SL, Knoll JS, Smith FWK, et al, eds. *Blackwell's Five-Minute Veterinary Consult: Laboratory Tests and Diagnostic Procedures.* Ames, IA: Wiley-Blackwell; 2009:98-100.
224. Harvey AM, Holt PE, Barr FJ, et al. Treatment and long-term follow-up of extrahepatic biliary obstruction with bilirubin cholelithiasis in a Somali cat with pyruvate kinase deficiency. *J Feline Med Surg.* 2007;9:424-431.
225. Harvey JW. Myeloproliferative disorders in dogs and cats. *Vet Clin North Am Small Anim Pract.* 1981;11:349-381.
226. Harvey JW. Iron metabolism and its disorders. In: Kaneko JJ, Harvey JW, Bruss ML, eds. *Clinical Biochemistry of Domestic Animals.* 6th ed. San Diego, CA: Academic Press; 2008:259-285.
227. Harvey JW. Thrombocytotropic anaplasmosis (*A. platys* [*E. platys*] infection). In: Greene CE, ed. *Infectious Diseases of the Dog and Cat.* 4th ed. St. Louis: Saunders Elsevier; 2011: in press.
228. Harvey JW, French TW, Meyer DJ. Chronic iron deficiency anemia in dogs. *J Am Anim Hosp Assoc.* 1982;18:946-960.
229. Harvey JW, Simpson CF, Gaskin JM. Cyclic thrombocytopenia induced by a Rickettsia-like agent in dogs. *J Infect Dis.* 1978;137:182-188.
230. Healy PJ, Sewell CA, Exner T, et al. Haemophilia in Hereford cattle: factor VIII deficiency. *Aust Vet J.* 1984;61:132-133.
231. Heilmann E, Friese P, Anderson S, et al. Biotinylated platelets: a new approach to the measurement of platelet life span. *Br J Haematol.* 1993;85:729-735.
232. Helfand SC. Neoplasia and immune-mediated thrombocytopenia. *Vet Clin North Am Small Anim Pract.* 1988;18:267-270.
233. Heller J, Mellor DJ, Hodgson JL, et al. Elapid snake envenomation in dogs in New South Wales: a review. *Aust Vet J.* 2007;85:469-479.
234. Hermán F, Magyar K, Filep JG. In vivo antiaggregatory action of platelet-activating factor in beagle dogs: role for prostacyclin. *Thromb Haemos.* 1991; 65:296-299.
235. Hertzke DM, Cowan LA, Schoning P, et al. Glomerular ultrastructural lesions of idiopathic cutaneous and renal glomerular vasculopathy of greyhounds. *Vet Pathol.* 1995;32:451-459.
236. Heseltine JC, Panciera DL, Troy GC, et al. Effect of levothyroxine administration on hemostatic analytes in Doberman Pinschers with von Willebrand disease. *J Vet Intern Med.* 2005;19:523-527.
237. Hickford FH, Stokol T, VanGessel YA, et al. Monoclonal immunoglobulin G cryoglobulinemia and multiple myeloma in a domestic shorthair cat. *J Am Vet Med Assoc.* 2000;217:1029-1033.
238. Hildebrandt E, Suttie JW. Indirect inhibition of vitamin K epoxide reduction by salicylate. *J Pharm Pharmacol.* 1984;36:586-591.
239. Hill BL, Zenoble RD, Dodds WJ. Prothrombin deficiency in a cocker spaniel. *J Am Vet Med Assoc.* 1982;181:262-263.
240. Hinchcliff KW, Kociba GJ, Mitten LA. Diagnosis of EDTA-dependent pseudothrombocytopenia in a horse. *J Am Vet Med Assoc.* 1993;203:1715-1716.
241. Hisasue M, Okayama H, Okayama T, et al. Hematologic abnormalities and outcome of 16 cats with myelodysplastic syndromes. *J Vet Intern Med.* 2001;15:471-477.
242. Ho-Tin-Noe B, Goerge T, Wagner DD. Platelets: guardians of tumor vasculature. *Cancer Res.* 2009;69:5623-5626.
243. Hoffman M. A cell-based model of coagulation and the role of factor VIIa. *Blood Rev.* 2003;17(Suppl 1):S1-S5.
244. Hoffman M, Monroe DM III: A cell-based model of hemostasis. *Thromb Haemost.* 2001;85:958-965.
245. Hogan DF, Andrews DA, Green HW, et al. Antiplatelet effects and pharmacodynamics of clopidogrel in cats. *J Am Vet Med Assoc.* 2004;225:1406-1411.
246. Hogan DF, Dhaliwal RS, Sisson DD, et al. Paraneoplastic thrombocytosis-induced systemic thromboembolism in a cat. *J Am Anim Hosp Assoc.* 1999;35: 483-486.
247. Holland M, Stobie D, Shapiro W. Pancytopenia associated with administration of captopril to a dog. *J Am Vet Med Assoc.* 1996;208:1683-1686.
248. Holloway S, Senior D, Roth L, et al. Hemolytic uremic syndrome in dogs. *J Vet Intern Med.* 1993;7:220-227.
249. Holloway SA, Parry BW. Observations on blood coagulation after snakebite in dogs and cats. *Aust Vet J.* 1989;66:364-366.
250. Hutton RA, Warrell DA. Action of snake venom components on the haemostatic system. *Blood Rev.* 1993;7:176-189.
251. Ide K, Setoguchi-Mukai A, Nakagawa T, et al. Disseminated histiocytic sarcoma with excessive hemophagocytosis in a cat. *J Vet Med Sci.* 2009;71:817-820.
252. Irmak K, Sen I, Col R, et al. The evaluation of coagulation profiles in calves with suspected septic shock. *Vet Res Commun.* 2006;30:497-503.
253. Jackson CW, Simone JV, Edwards CC. The relationship of anemia and thrombocytosis. *J Lab Clin Med.* 1974;84:357-368.
254. Jackson ML, Searcy GP, Olexson DW. The effect of oral phenylbutazone on whole blood platelet aggregation in the dog. *Can J Comp Med.* 1985;49:271-277.
255. Jackson SP, Schoenwaelder SM. Procoagulant platelets: are they necrotic? *Blood.* 2010;116:2011-2018.
256. Jacobs G, Calvert C, Kaufman A. Neutropenia and thrombocytopenia in three dogs treated with anticonvulsants. *J Am Vet Med Assoc.* 1998;212:681-684.
257. Jacobs RM, Boyce JT, Kociba GJ. Flow cytometric and radioisotopic determination of platelet survival time in normal cats and feline leukemia virus-infected cats. *Cytometry.* 1986;7:64-69.
258. Jacobsen S, Nielsen JV, Kjelgaard-Hansen M, et al. Acute phase response to surgery of varying intensity in horses: a preliminary study. *Vet Surg.* 2009;38:762-769.
259. Jacoby RC, Owings JT, Ortega T, et al. Biochemical basis for the hypercoagulable state seen in Cushing syndrome. *Arch Surg.* 2001;136:1003-1006.
260. Jain NC. *Essentials of Veterinary Hematology.* Philadelphia: Lea & Febiger; 1993.
261. Jarvis GE, Evans RJ. Endotoxin-induced platelet aggregation in heparinised equine whole blood in vitro. *Res Vet Sci.* 1994;57:317-324.
262. Jelkmann W. The role of the liver in the production of thrombopoietin compared with erythropoietin. *Eur J Gastroenterol Hepatol.* 2001;13:791-801.
263. Jergens AE, Turrentine MA, Kraus KH, et al. Buccal mucosa bleeding times of healthy dogs and of dogs in various pathologic states, including thrombocytopenia, uremia, and von Willebrand's disease. *Am J Vet Res.* 1987;48:1337-1342.
264. Jin RC, Voetsch B, Loscalzo J. Endogenous mechanisms of inhibition of platelet function. *Microcirculation.* 2005;12:247-258.
265. Johne J, Blume C, Benz PM, et al. Platelets promote coagulation factor XII-mediated proteolytic cascade systems in plasma. *Biol Chem.* 2006;387:173-178.
266. Johns I, Stephen JO, Del PF, et al. Hemangiosarcoma in 11 young horses. *J Vet Intern Med.* 2005;19:564-570.
267. Johnson JS, Soute BA, Olver CS, et al. Defective gamma-glutamyl carboxylase activity and bleeding in Rambouillet sheep. *Vet Pathol.* 2006;43:726-732.
268. Johnson LR, Lappin MR, Baker DC. Pulmonary thromboembolism in 29 dogs: 1985-1995. *J Vet Intern Med.* 1999;13:338-345.
269. Johnstone IB, Viel L, Crane S, et al. Hemostatic studies in racing standardbred horses with exercise-induced pulmonary hemorrhage. Hemostatic parameters at rest and after moderate exercise. *Can J Vet Res.* 1991;55:101-106.
270. Jordan HL, Grindem CB, Breitschwerdt EB. Thrombocytopenia in cats: a retrospective study of 41 cases. *J Vet Intern Med.* 1993;7:261-265.
271. Jurk K, Kehrel BE. Platelets: physiology and biochemistry. *Semin Thromb Hemost.* 2005;31:381-392.
272. Jutkowitz LA, Rozanski EA, Moreau JA, et al. Massive transfusion in dogs: 15 cases (1997-2001). *J Am Vet Med Assoc.* 2002;220:1664-1669.
273. Juttner C, Rodriguez M, Fragio C. Optimal conditions for simultaneous measurement of platelet aggregation and ATP secretion in canine whole blood. *Res Vet Sci.* 2000;68:27-32.
274. Kadikoylu G, Yavasoglu I, Bolaman Z, et al. Platelet parameters in women with iron deficiency anemia. *J Natl Med Assoc.* 2006;98:398-402.

275. Kaplan AP. Enzymatic pathways in the pathogenesis of hereditary angioedema: the role of C1 inhibitor therapy. *J Allergy Clin Immunol.* 2010;126:918-925.
276. Karpman D, Sartz L, Johnson S. Pathophysiology of typical hemolytic uremic syndrome. *Semin Thromb Hemost.* 2010;36:575-585.
277. Kaser A, Brandacher G, Steurer W, et al. Interleukin-6 stimulates thrombopoiesis through thrombopoietin: role in inflammatory thrombocytosis. *Blood.* 2001;98: 2720-2725.
278. Keller ET. Immune-mediated disease as a risk factor for canine lymphoma. *Cancer.* 1992;70:2334-2337.
279. Key NS. Analysis of tissue factor positive microparticles. *Thromb Res.* 2010;125 (Suppl 1):S42-S45.
280. Khan I, Zucker-Franklin D, Karpatkin S. Microthrombocytosis and platelet fragmentation associated with idiopathic/autoimmune thrombocytopenia. *Br J Haematol.* 1975; 31:449-460.
281. Kingston JK, Bayly WM, Sellon DC, et al. Effects of sodium citrate, low molecular weight heparin, and prostaglandin E1 on aggregation, fibrinogen binding, and enumeration of equine platelets. *Am J Vet Res.* 2001;62:547-554.
282. Kingston JK, Bayly WM, Sellon DC, et al. Measurement of the activation of equine platelets by use of fluorescent-labeled annexin V, anti-human fibrinogen antibody, and anti-human thrombospondin antibody. *Am J Vet Res.* 2002;63:513-519.
283. Kitchens CS. From ETOH to FAB: the medicalization of therapy for pit viper envenomation. *Trans Am Clin Climatol Assoc.* 2001;112:117-135.
284. Kitchens CS, Weiss L. Ultrastructural changes of endothelium associated with thrombocytopenia. *Blood.* 1975;46:567-578.
285. Klainbart S, Segev G, Loeb E, et al. Resolution of renal adenocarcinoma-induced secondary inappropriate polycythaemia after nephrectomy in two cats. *J Feline Med Surg.* 2008;10:264-268.
286. Kline JA, Williams GW, Hernandez-Nino J. D-dimer concentrations in normal pregnancy: new diagnostic thresholds are needed. *Clin Chem.* 2005;51:825-829.
287. Kociba GJ, Caputo CA. Aplastic anemia associated with estrus in pet ferrets. *J Am Vet Med Assoc.* 1981;178:1293-1294.
288. Kociba GJ, Ratnoff OD, Loeb WF, et al. Bovine plasma thromboplastin antecedent (Factor XI) deficiency. *J Lab Clin Med.* 1969;74:37-41.
289. Kohn B, Arnold P, Kaser-Hotz B, et al. Malignant histiocytosis of the dog: 26 cases (1989-1992). *Kleintierpraxis.* 1993;38:409-424.
290. Kohn B, Linden T, Leibold W. Platelet-bound antibodies detected by a flow cytometric assay in cats with thrombocytopenia. *J Feline Med Surg.* 2006;8:254-260.
291. Kohn B, Weingart C, Giger U. Haemorrhage in seven cats with suspected anticoagulant rodenticide intoxication. *J Feline Med Surg.* 2003;5:295-304.
292. Kol A, Borjesson DL. Application of thromboelastography/thromboelastometry to veterinary medicine. *Vet Clin Pathol.* 2010;39:405-416.
293. Komura E, Matsumura T, Kato T, et al. Thrombopoietin in patients with hepatoblastoma. *Stem Cells.* 1998;16:329-333.
294. Kristensen AT, Weiss DJ, Klausner JS. Platelet dysfunction associated with immune-mediated thrombocytopenia in dogs. *J Vet Intern Med.* 1994;8:323-327.
295. Kristensen AT, Weiss DJ, Klausner JS, et al. Detection of antiplatelet antibody with a platelet immunofluorescence assay. *J Vet Intern Med.* 1994;8:36-39.
296. Kristensen AT, Wiinberg B, Jessen LR, et al. Evaluation of human recombinant tissue factor-activated thromboelastography in 49 dogs with neoplasia. *J Vet Intern Med.* 2008;22:140-147.
297. Kuehn NF, Gaunt SD. Hypocellular marrow and extramedullary hematopoiesis in a dog: hematologic recovery after splenectomy. *J Am Vet Med Assoc.* 1986; 188:1313-1315.
298. Kulkarni S, Woollard KJ, Thomas S, et al. Conversion of platelets from a proaggregatory to a proinflammatory adhesive phenotype: role of PAF in spatially regulating neutrophil adhesion and spreading. *Blood.* 2007;110:1879-1886.
299. Kummeling A, Teske E, Rothuizen J, et al. Coagulation profiles in dogs with congenital portosystemic shunts before and after surgical attenuation. *J Vet Intern Med.* 2006;20:1319-1326.
300. Kunieda T, Ide H, Nakagiri M, et al. Localization of the locus responsible for Chediak-Higashi syndrome in cattle to bovine chromosome 28. *Anim Genet.* 2000;31: 87-90.
301. Kurata M, Sasayama Y, Yamasaki N, et al. Mechanism for shortening PT and APTT in dogs and rats–effect of fibrinogen on PT and APTT. *J Toxicol Sci.* 2003;28:439-443.
302. Kuzmanova SI. The macrophage activation syndrome: a new entity, a potentially fatal complication of rheumatic disorders. *Folia Med (Plovdiv).* 2005;47:21-25.
303. Lachowicz JL, Post GS, Moroff SD, et al. Acquired amegakaryocytic thrombocytopenia–four cases and a literature review. *J Small Anim Pract.* 2004;45:507-514.
304. Lander H, Lloyd JV, Schultz BG. Studies of platelet survival and behavior in sheep. *J Lab Clin Med.* 1965;66:887.
305. Lara-Garcia A, Couto CG, Iazbik MC, et al. Postoperative bleeding in retired racing greyhounds. *J Vet Intern Med.* 2008;22:525-533.
306. Laste NJ, Harpster NK. A retrospective study of 100 cases of feline distal aortic thromboembolism: 1977-1993. *J Am Anim Hosp Assoc.* 1995;31:492-500.
307. Laurenson MP, Hopper K, Herrera MA, et al. Concurrent diseases and conditions in dogs with splenic vein thrombosis. *J Vet Intern Med.* 2010;24:1298-1304.
308. Lees GE, McKeever PJ, Ruth GR. Fatal thrombocytopenic hemorrhagic diathesis associated with dapsone administration to a dog. *J Am Vet Med Assoc.* 1979;175:49-52.
309. Lenting PJ, Van Mourik JA, Mertens K. The life cycle of coagulation factor VIII in view of its structure and function. *Blood.* 1998;92:3983-3996.
310. Lester GD, Alleman AR, Raskin RE, et al. Pancytopenia secondary to lymphoid leukemia in three horses. *J Vet Intern Med.* 1993;7:360-363.
311. Levin J, Levin FC, Hull DF III, et al. The effects of thrombopoietin on megakaryocyte-CFC, megakaryocytes, and thrombopoiesis: with studies of ploidy and platelet size. *Blood.* 1982;60:989-998.
312. Lewis DC, Bruyette DS, Kellerman DL, et al. Thrombocytopenia in dogs with anticoagulant rodenticide-induced hemorrhage: eight cases (1990-1995). *J Am Anim Hosp Assoc.* 1997;33:417-422.
313. Lewis DC, Meyers KM, Callan MB, et al. Detection of platelet-bound and serum platelet-bindable antibodies for diagnosis of idiopathic thrombocytopenic purpura in dogs. *J Am Vet Med Assoc.* 1995;206:47-52.
314. Lien DC, Worthen GS, Henson PM, et al. Platelet-activating factor causes neutrophil accumulation and neutrophil-mediated increased vascular permeability in canine trachea. *Am Rev Respir Dis.* 1992;145:693-700.
315. Lisciandro SC, Hohenhaus A, Brooks M. Coagulation abnormalities in 22 cats with naturally occurring liver disease. *J Vet Intern Med.* 1998;12:71-75.
316. Ljungqvist U. Platelet response to adrenalin infusion in splenectomised and non-splenectomised dogs. *Acta Chir Scand.* 1971;137:291-297.
317. Lobetti RG, Joubert K. Retrospective study of snake envenomation in 155 dogs from the Onderstepoort area of South Africa. *J S Afr Vet Assoc.* 2004;75:169-172.
318. Loo M, Beguin Y. The effect of recombinant human erythropoietin on platelet counts is strongly modulated by the adequacy of iron supply. *Blood.* 1999;93: 3286-3293.
319. Lotter MG, Badenhorst PN, Heyns AD, et al. Kinetics, distribution, and sites of destruction of canine blood platelets with In-111 oxine. *J Nucl Med.* 1980;21: 36-40.
320. Lubas G, Caldin M, Wiinberg B, et al. Laboratory testing of coagulation disorders. In: Weiss DJ, Wardrop KJ, eds. *Schalm's Veterinary Hematology.* 6th ed. Ames, IA: Wiley-Blackwell; 2010:1082-1100.
321. Luyendyk JP, Copple BL, Barton CC, et al. Augmentation of aflatoxin B1 hepatotoxicity by endotoxin: involvement of endothelium and the coagulation system. *Toxicol Sci.* 2003;72:171-181.
322. Macintire DK, Vincent-Johnson NA, Craig TM. *Hepatozoon americanum* infection. In: Greene CE, ed. *Infectious Diseases of the Dog and Cat.* 3rd ed. St. Louis: Saunders Elsevier; 2006:705-711.
323. Mackin AJ, Allen DG, Johnston IB. Effects of vincristine and prednisone on platelet numbers and function in clinically normal dogs. *Am J Vet Res.* 1995;56: 100-108.
324. Maddison JE, Watson ADJ, Eade IG, et al. Vitamin K-dependent multifactor coagulopathy in Devon Rex cats. *J Am Vet Med Assoc.* 1990;197:1495-1497.
325. Maratea KA, Snyder PW, Stevenson GW. Vascular lesions in nine Gottingen minipigs with thrombocytopenic purpura syndrome. *Vet Pathol.* 2006;43:447-454.
326. Marconato L, Bettini G, Giacoboni C, et al. Clinicopathological features and outcome for dogs with mast cell tumors and bone marrow involvement. *J Vet Intern Med.* 2008;22:1001-1007.
327. Marks SL. The buccal mucosal bleeding time. *J Am Anim Hosp Assoc.* 2000;36:289-290.
328. Martinelli I, Bucciarelli P, Mannucci PM. Thrombotic risk factors: basic pathophysiology. *Crit Care Med.* 2010;38:S3-S9.
329. Maruyama H, Yamagami H, Watari T, et al. Reticulated platelet levels in whole blood and platelet-rich plasma of dogs with various platelet counts measured by flow cytometry. *J Vet Med Sci.* 2009;71:195-197.
330. Mason DJ, Abrams-Ogg A, Allen D, et al. Vitamin K-dependent coagulopathy in a black Labrador Retriever. *J Vet Intern Med.* 2002;16:485-488.
331. Matsubara T, Touchi A, Harauchi T, et al. Depression of liver microsomal vitamin K epoxide reductase activity associated with antibiotic-induced coagulopathy. *Biochem Pharmacol.* 1989;38:2693-2701.
332. McAnulty JF, Rudd RG. Thrombocytopenia associated with vaccination of a dog with a modified-live paramyxovirus vaccine. *J Am Vet Med Assoc.* 1985;186: 1217-1219.
333. McCaw DL, Jergens AE, Turrentine MA, et al. Effect of internal hemorrhage on fibrin(ogen) degradation products in canine blood. *Am J Vet Res.* 1986;47: 1620-1621.
334. McColl KA, Gould AR. Bluetongue virus infection in sheep: haematological changes and detection by polymerase chain reaction. *Aust Vet J.* 1994;71:97-101.
335. McConnico RS, Copedge K, Bischoff KL. Brodifacoum toxicosis in two horses. *J Am Vet Med Assoc.* 1997;211:882-886.

336. McGorum BC, Henderson IS, Stirling D, et al. Vitamin K deficiency bleeding in a Standardbred colt. *J Vet Intern Med.* 2009;23:1307-1310.
337. McGurrin MK, Arroyo LG, Bienzle D. Flow cytometric detection of platelet-bound antibody in three horses with immune-mediated thrombocytopenia. *J Am Vet Med Assoc.* 2004;224:83-87, 53.
338. McMillan R. The pathogenesis of chronic immune thrombocytopenic purpura. *Semin Hematol.* 2007;44:S3-S11.
339. Mellor PJ, Roulois AJ, Day MJ, et al. Neutrophilic dermatitis and immune-mediated haematological disorders in a dog: suspected adverse reaction to carprofen. *J Small Anim Pract.* 2005;46:237-242.
340. Meng R, Bridgman R, Toivio-Kinnucan M, et al. Neutrophil elastase-processing defect in cyclic hematopoietic dogs. *Exp Hematol.* 2010;38:104-115.
341. Meyer J, Delay J, Bienzle D. Clinical, laboratory, and histopathologic features of equine lymphoma. *Vet Pathol.* 2006;43:914-924.
342. Meyers KM, Holmsen H, Seachord CL. Comparative study of platelet dense granule constituents. *Am J Physiol.* 1982;243:R454-R461.
343. Meyers KM, Lindner C, Katz J, et al. Phenylbutazone inhibition of equine platelet function. *Am J Vet Res.* 1979;40:265-270.
344. Meyers KM, Wardrop KJ, Dodds WJ, et al. Effect of exercise, DDAVP, and epinephrine on the factor VIII:C/von Willebrand factor complex in normal dogs and von Willebrand factor deficient Doberman pinscher dogs. *Thromb Res.* 1990;57:97-108.
345. Micun J, Sobczak-Filipiak M, Winnicka A, et al. Thrombocytopenia as a characteristic trait in the Polish ogar dog. *Pol J Vet Sci.* 2009;12:523-525.
346. Miesner MD, Anderson DE. Factor-VIII deficiency in a newborn alpaca. *J Vet Intern Med.* 2006;20:1248-1250.
347. Mills JN, Lawley MJ, Thomas J. *Macrozamia* toxicosis in a dog. *Aust Vet J.* 1996;73:69-72.
348. Mischke R. Optimization of coagulometric tests that incorporate human plasma for determination of coagulation factor activities in canine plasma. *Am J Vet Res.* 2001;62:625-629.
349. Mischke R. Acute haemostatic changes in accidentally traumatised dogs. *Vet J.* 2005;169:60-64.
350. Mischke R, Junker J, Deegen E. Sensitivity of commercial prothrombin time reagents to detect coagulation factor deficiencies in equine plasma. *Vet J.* 2006;171:114-119.
351. Mischke R, Keidel A. Influence of platelet count, acetylsalicylic acid, von Willebrand's disease, coagulopathies, and haematocrit on results obtained using a platelet function analyser in dogs. *Vet J.* 2003;165:43-52.
352. Mischke R, Keidel A. Influence of platelet count, acetylsalicylic acid, von Willebrand's disease, coagulopathies, and haematocrit on results obtained using a platelet function analyser in dogs. *Vet J.* 2003;165:43-52.
353. Mischke R, Menzel D, Wolling H. Comparison of different methods to measure fibrinogen concentration in canine plasma with respect to their sensitivity towards the fibrinogen degradation products X, Y and D. *Haemostasis.* 2000;30:131-138.
354. Mischke R, Schulze U. Studies on platelet aggregation using the Born method in normal and uraemic dogs. *Vet J.* 2004;168:270-275.
355. Mischke R, Wolling H, Nolte I. Detection of anticoagulant activities of isolated canine fibrinogen degradation products X, Y, D and E using resonance thrombography. *Blood Coagul Fibrinolysis.* 2004;15:81-88.
356. Mitchell JA, Ali F, Bailey L, et al. Role of nitric oxide and prostacyclin as vasoactive hormones released by the endothelium. *Exp Physiol.* 2008;93:141-147.
357. Monreal L, Angles A, Espada Y, et al. Hypercoagulation and hypofibrinolysis in horses with colic and DIC. *Equine Vet J Suppl.* 2000;32:19-24.
358. Monreal L, Villatoro AJ, Hooghuis H, et al. Clinical features of the 1992 outbreak of equine viral arteritis in Spain. *Equine Vet J.* 1995;27:301-304.
359. Monreal L, Villatoro AJ, Monreal M, et al. Comparison of the effects of low-molecular-weight and unfractioned heparin in horses. *Am J Vet Res.* 1995;56:1281-1285.
360. Moore AS, London CA, Wood CA, et al. Lomustine (CCNU) for the treatment of resistant lymphoma in dogs. *J Vet Intern Med.* 1999;13:395-398.
361. Moore BR, Hinchcliff KW. Heparin: a review of its pharmacology and therapeutic use in horses. *J Vet Intern Med.* 1994;8:26-35.
362. Moore PF, Affolter VK, Vernau W. Canine hemophagocytic histiocytic sarcoma: a proliferative disorder of CD11d+ macrophages. *Vet Pathol.* 2006;43:632-645.
363. Morales F, Couto CG, Iazbik MC. Effects of 2 concentrations of sodium citrate on coagulation test results, von Willebrand factor concentration, and platelet function in dogs. *J Vet Intern Med.* 2007;21:472-475.
364. Moritz A, Walcheck BK, Deye J, et al. Effects of short-term racing activity on platelet and neutrophil activation in dogs. *Am J Vet Res.* 2003;64:855-859.
365. Moritz A, Walcheck BK, Weiss DJ. Flow cytometric detection of activated platelets in the dog. *Vet Clin Pathol.* 2003;32:6-12.
366. Moritz A, Walcheck BK, Weiss DJ. Evaluation of flow cytometric and automated methods for detection of activated platelets in dogs with inflammatory disease. *Am J Vet Res.* 2005;66:325-329.
367. Morris CF, Robertson JL, Mann PC, et al. Hemolytic uremic-like syndrome in two horses. *J Am Vet Med Assoc.* 1987;191:1453-1454.
368. Morrissey JH, Pureza V, Davis-Harrison RL, et al. Blood clotting reactions on nanoscale phospholipid bilayers. *Thromb Res.* 2008;122(Suppl 1):S23-S26.
369. Moser J, Meyers KM, Meinkoth JH, et al. Temporal variation and factors affecting measurement of canine von Willebrand factor. *Am J Vet Res.* 1996;57:1288-1293.
370. Mount ME, Kim BU, Kass PH. Use of a test for proteins induced by vitamin K absence or antagonism in diagnosis of anticoagulant poisoning in dogs: 325 cases (1987-1997). *J Am Vet Med Assoc.* 2003;222:194-198.
371. Mudge MC, MacDonald MH, Owens SD, et al. Comparison of 4 blood storage methods in a protocol for equine pre-operative autologous donation. *Vet Surg.* 2004;33:475-486.
372. Nash RA, Burstein SA, Storb R, et al. Thrombocytopenia in dogs induced by granulocyte-macrophage colony-stimulating factor: increased destruction of circulating platelets. *Blood.* 1995;86:1765-1775.
373. Neer TM, Hedlund CS. Vitamin K-dependent coagulopathy in a dog with bile and cystic duct obstructions. *J Am Anim Hosp Assoc.* 1989;25:461-464.
374. Nelson OL, Andreasen C. The utility of plasma D-dimer to identify thromboembolic disease in dogs. *J Vet Intern Med.* 2003;17:830-834.
375. Nesheim M, Pittman DD, Giles AR, et al. The effect of plasma von Willebrand factor on the binding of human factor VIII to thrombin-activated human platelets. *J Biol Chem.* 1991;266:17815-17820.
376. Nielsen L, Wiinberg B, Kjelgaard-Hansen M, et al. The presence of antiphospholipid antibodies in healthy adult Bernese Mountain dogs (abstract). *Vet Clin Pathol.* 2010;39:546.
377. Nieuwenhuizen W. Fibrin-mediated plasminogen activation. *Ann N Y Acad Sci.* 2001;936:237-246.
378. Nikolic NL, Wiinberg B, Kjelgaard HM, et al. Prolonged activated prothromboplastin time and breed specific variation in haemostatic analytes in healthy adult Bernese Mountain dogs. *Vet J.* 2011; in press.
379. Noguchi K, Matsuzaki T, Ojiri Y, et al. Prostacyclin causes splenic dilation and haematological change in dogs. *Clin Exp Pharmacol Physiol.* 2006;33:81-88.
380. Noguchi K, Matsuzaki T, Shiroma N, et al. Involvement of nitric oxide and eicosanoids in platelet-activating factor-induced haemodynamic and haematological effects in dogs. *Br J Pharmacol.* 1996;118:941-950.
381. Nomura S, Ozaki Y, Ikeda Y. Function and role of microparticles in various clinical settings. *Thromb Res.* 2008;123:8-23.
382. Norman EJ, Barron RC, Nash AS, et al. Evaluation of a citrate-based anticoagulant with platelet inhibitory activity for feline blood cell counts. *Vet Clin Pathol.* 2001;30:124-132.
383. Norman EJ, Barron RC, Nash AS, et al. Prevalence of low automated platelet counts in cats: comparison with prevalence of thrombocytopenia based on blood smear estimation. *Vet Clin Pathol.* 2001;30:137-140.
384. Norris CR, Griffey SM, Samii VF. Pulmonary thromboembolism in cats: 29 cases (1987-1997). *J Am Vet Med Assoc.* 1999;215:1650-1654.
385. Northern J Jr, Tvedten HW. Diagnosis of microthrombocytosis and immune-mediated thrombocytopenia in dogs with thrombocytopenia: 68 cases (1987-1989). *J Am Vet Med Assoc.* 1992;200:368-372.
386. Novotny MJ, Turrentine MA, Johnson GS, et al. Experimental endotoxemia increases plasma von Willebrand factor antigen concentrations in dogs with and without free-radical scavenger therapy. *Circ Shock.* 1987;23:205-213.
387. Nunez A, Gomez-Villamandos JC, Sanchez-Cordon PJ, et al. Expression of proinflammatory cytokines by hepatic macrophages in acute classical swine fever. *J Comp Pathol.* 2005;133:23-32.
388. Nylander S, Mattsson C, Lindahl TL. Characterisation of species differences in the platelet ADP and thrombin response. *Thromb Res.* 2006;117:543-549.
389. O'Keefe DA, Schaeffer DJ. Hematologic toxicosis associated with doxorubicin administration in cats. *J Vet Intern Med.* 1992;6:276-282.
390. O'Rourke ST, Folts JD, Albrecht RM. Inhibition of canine platelet aggregation by barbiturates. *J Lab Clin Med.* 1986;108:206-212.
391. Ojiri Y, Noguchi K, Shiroma N, et al. Uneven changes in circulating blood cell counts with adrenergic stimulation to the canine spleen. *Clin Exp Pharmacol Physiol.* 2002;29:53-59.
392. Okawa T, Yanase T, Shimokawa MT, et al. Prekallikrein deficiency in a dog. *J Vet Med Sci.* 2011;73:107-111.
393. Olsen EH, McCain AS, Merricks EP, et al. Comparative response of plasma VWF in dogs to up-regulation of VWF mRNA by interleukin-11 versus Weibel-Palade body release by desmopressin (DDAVP). *Blood.* 2003;102:436-441.
394. Olsen LH, Kristensen AT, Qvortrup K, et al. Comparison of manual and automated methods for determining platelet counts in dogs with macrothrombocytopenia. *J Vet Diagn Invest.* 2004;16:167-170.
395. Omotainse SO, Anosa VO. Leucocyte and thrombocyte responses in dogs experimentally infected with *Trypanosoma brucei. Rev Elev Med Vet Pays Trop.* 1995;48:254-258.
396. Oren H, Duman N, Abacioglu H, et al. Association between serum macrophage colony-stimulating factor levels and monocyte and thrombocyte counts in healthy, hypoxic, and septic term neonates. *Pediatrics.* 2001;108:329-332.

397. Osterud B. Tissue factor expression in blood cells. *Thromb Res.* 2010;125(Suppl 1):S31-S34.
398. Otto CM, Rieser TM, Brooks MB, et al. Evidence of hypercoagulability in dogs with parvoviral enteritis. *J Am Vet Med Assoc.* 2000;217:1500-1504.
399. Panciera DL, Johnson GS. Plasma von Willebrand factor antigen concentration and buccal mucosal bleeding time in dogs with experimental hypothyroidism. *J Vet Intern Med.* 1996;10:60-64.
400. Pankraz A, Bauer N, Moritz A. Comparison of flow cytometry with the Sysmex XT2000iV automated analyzer for the detection of reticulated platelets in dogs. *Vet Clin Pathol.* 2009;38:30-38.
401. Parent-Massin D. Haematotoxicity of trichothecenes. *Toxicol Lett.* 2004;153:75-81.
402. Parise LV, Smyth SS, Shet AS, et al. Platelet morphology, biochemistry, and function. In: Lichtman MA, Beutler E, Kipps TJ, et al, eds. *Williams Hematology.* 7th ed. New York: McGraw-Hill; 2006:1587-1663.
403. Parker MT, Collier LL, Kier AB, et al. Oral mucosal bleeding times of normal cats and cats with Chediak-Higashi syndrome or Hageman trait (factor XII deficiency). *Vet Clin Pathol.* 1988;17(1):9-12.
404. Patel RT, Caceres A, French AF, et al. Multiple myeloma in 16 cats: a retrospective study. *Vet Clin Pathol.* 2005;34:341-352.
405. Pawlinski R, Mackman N. Cellular sources of tissue factor in endotoxemia and sepsis. *Thromb Res.* 2010;125(Suppl 1):S70-S73.
406. Pearson JD. The control of production and release of haemostatic factors in the endothelial cell. *Baillieres Clin Haematol.* 1993;6:629-651.
407. Peng J, Friese P, Heilmann E, et al. Aged platelets have an impaired response to thrombin as quantitated by P-selectin expression. *Blood.* 1994;83:161-166.
408. Peng J, Friese P, Wolf RF, et al. Relative reactivity of platelets from thrombopoietin- and interleukin-6-treated dogs. *Blood.* 1996;87:4158-4163.
409. Pereira J, Soto M, Palomo I, et al. Platelet aging in vivo is associated with activation of apoptotic pathways: studies in a model of suppressed thrombopoiesis in dogs. *Thromb Haemost.* 2002;87:905-909.
410. Perez-Alenza MD, Blanco J, Sardon D, et al. Clinico-pathological findings in cattle exposed to chronic bracken fern toxicity. *N Z Vet J.* 2006;54:185-192.
411. Peterson JL, Couto CG, Wellman ML. Hemostatic disorders in cats: a retrospective study and review of the literature. *J Vet Intern Med.* 1995;9:298-303.
412. Peterson ME, Hurvitz AI, Leib MS, et al. Propylthiouracil-associated hemolytic anemia, thrombocytopenia, and antinuclear antibodies in cats with hyperthyroidism. *J Am Vet Med Assoc.* 1984;184:806-808.
413. Pierangeli SS, Chen PP, Raschi E, et al. Antiphospholipid antibodies and the antiphospholipid syndrome: pathogenic mechanisms. *Semin Thromb Hemost.* 2008;34:236-250.
414. Pina-Cabral JM, Ribeiro-da-Silva A, Meida-Dias A. Platelet sequestration during hypothermia in dogs treated with sulphinpyrazone and ticlopidine–reversibility accelerated after intra-abdominal rewarming. *Thromb Haemost.* 1985;54:838-841.
415. Pineau S, Belbeck LW, Moore S. Levamisole reduces the thrombocytopenia associated with myxovirus vaccination. *Can Vet J.* 1980;21:82-84.
416. Prins M, Schellens CJ, van Leeuwen MW, et al. Coagulation disorders in dogs with hepatic disease. *Vet J.* 2010;185:163-168.
417. Puschner B, Galey FD, Holstege DM, et al. Sweet clover poisoning in dairy cattle in California. *J Am Vet Med Assoc.* 1998;212:857-859.
418. Pusterla N, Watson JL, Affolter VK, et al. Purpura haemorrhagica in 53 horses. *Vet Rec.* 2003;153:118-121.
419. Putsche JC, Kohn B. Primary immune-mediated thrombocytopenia in 30 dogs (1997-2003). *J Am Anim Hosp Assoc.* 2008;44:250-257.
420. Radvanyi-Hofmann H, Roussi J, Launay JM, et al. Characterization of a thrombopathy (type delta storage pool disease) affecting a pig colony. *Nouv Rev Fr Hematol.* 1992;34:133-140.
421. Ragan HA. Platelet agglutination induced by ethylenediaminetetraacetic acid in blood samples from a miniature pig. *Am J Vet Res.* 1972;33:2601-2603.
422. Ramirez S, Gaunt SD, McClure JJ, et al. Detection and effects on platelet function of anti-platelet antibody in mule foals with experimentally induced neonatal alloimmune thrombocytopenia. *J Vet Intern Med.* 1999;13:534-539.
423. Rathgeber RA, Brooks MB, Bain FT, et al. Clinical vignette. Von Willebrand disease in a Thoroughbred mare and foal. *J Vet Intern Med.* 2001;15:63-66.
424. Reardon DM, Hutchinson D, Preston FE, et al. The routine measurement of platelet volume: a comparison of aperture-impedance and flow cytometric systems. *Clin Lab Haematol.* 1985;7:251-257.
425. Rebar AH, Lewis HB, DeNicola DB, et al. Red cell fragmentation in the dog: an editorial review. *Vet Pathol.* 1981;18:415-426.
426. Reef VB, Dyson SS, Beech J. Lymphosarcoma and associated immune-mediated hemolytic anemia and thrombocytopenia in horses. *J Am Vet Med Assoc.* 1984;184:313-317.
427. Rendu F, Brohard-Bohn B. The platelet release reaction: granules' constituents, secretion and functions. *Platelets.* 2001;12:261-273.
428. Renne T, Gailani D. Role of Factor XII in hemostasis and thrombosis: clinical implications. *Expert Rev Cardiovasc Ther.* 2007;5:733-741.
429. Richardson EF, Brown NO. Hematological and biochemical changes and results of aerobic bacteriological culturing in dogs undergoing splenectomy. *J Am Anim Hosp Assoc.* 1996;32:199-210.
430. Riley JH, Lassen ED. Activated coagulation times in normal cows. *Vet Clin Pathol.* 1979;8:31-33.
431. Rinder HM, Schuster JE, Rinder CS, et al. Correlation of thrombosis with increased platelet turnover in thrombocytosis. *Blood.* 1998;91:1288-1294.
432. Rinder HM, Tracey JB, Recht M, et al. Differences in platelet alpha-granule release between normals and immune thrombocytopenic patients and between young and old platelets. *Thromb Haemost.* 1998;80:457-462.
433. Ritt MG, Rogers KS, Thomas JS. Nephrotic syndrome resulting in thromboembolic disease and disseminated intravascular coagulation in a dog. *J Am Anim Hosp Assoc.* 1997;33:385-391.
434. Rizzo F, Tappin SW, Tasker S. Thrombocytosis in cats: a retrospective study of 51 cases (2000-2005). *J Feline Med Surg.* 2007;9:319-325.
435. Roby KA, Bloom JC, Becht JL. Postpartum hemolytic-uremic syndrome in a cow. *J Am Vet Med Assoc.* 1987;190:187-190.
436. Rodman LE, Farnell DR, Coyne JM, et al. Toxicity of cordycepin in combination with the adenosine deaminase inhibitor 2'-deoxycoformycin in beagle dogs. *Toxicol Appl Pharmacol.* 1997;147:39-45.
437. Rogers CL, Rozanski EA. Von Willebrand factor antigen concentration in dogs with sepsis. *J Vet Intern Med.* 2010;24:229-230.
438. Rojnuckarin P. Snake venom and haemostasis; an overview. *Asia-Pacific Oncology & Haematology.* 2008;1:93-96.
439. Rotermund A, Peters M, Hewicker-Trautwein M, et al. Cutaneous and renal glomerular vasculopathy in a great dane resembling 'Alabama rot' of greyhounds. *Vet Rec.* 2002;151:510-512.
440. Rozanski EA, Drobatz KJ, Hugher D, et al. Thrombotest (PIVKA) test results in 25 dogs with acquired and hereditary coagulopathies. *J Vet Emerg Crit Care (San Antonio).* 1999;9:73-78.
441. Runciman DJ, Lee AM, Reed KF, et al. Dicoumarol toxicity in cattle associated with ingestion of silage containing sweet vernal grass (*Anthoxanthum odoratum*). *Aust Vet J.* 2002;80:28-32.
442. Russell KE, Perkins PC, Grindem CB, et al. Flow cytometric method for detecting thiazole orange-positive (reticulated) platelets in thrombocytopenic horses. *Am J Vet Res.* 1997;58:1092-1096.
443. Russell KE, Perkins PC, Hoffman MR, et al. Platelets from thrombocytopenic ponies acutely infected with equine infectious anemia virus are activated in vivo and hypofunctional. *Virology.* 1999;259:7-19.
444. Sagripanti A, Carpi A. Antithrombotic and prothrombotic activities of the vascular endothelium. *Biomed Pharmacother.* 2000;54:107-111.
445. Sakai M, Watari T, Miura T, et al. Effects of DDAVP administrated subcutaneously in dogs with aspirin-induced platelet dysfunction and hemostatic impairment due to chronic liver diseases. *J Vet Med Sci.* 2003;65:83-86.
446. Sanchez-Cordon PJ, Nunez A, Salguero FJ, et al. Lymphocyte apoptosis and thrombocytopenia in spleen during classical swine fever: role of macrophages and cytokines. *Vet Pathol.* 2005;42:477-488.
447. Santarém VA, Laposy CB, Farias MR. *Ehrlichia platys*-like inclusions and morulae in platelets of a cat (abstract). *Brazilian J Vet Sci.* 2000;7:130.
448. Santoro SK, Garrett LD, Wilkerson M. Platelet concentrations and platelet-associated IgG in greyhounds. *J Vet Intern Med.* 2007;21:107-112.
449. Sato I, Anderson GA, Parry BW. An interobserver and intraobserver study of buccal mucosal bleeding time in Greyhounds. *Res Vet Sci.* 2000;68:41-45.
450. Schaffner A, Augustiny N, Otto RC, et al. The hypersplenic spleen. A contractile reservoir of granulocytes and platelets. *Arch Intern Med.* 1985;145:651-654.
451. Schaphorst KL, Chiang E, Jacobs KN, et al. Role of sphingosine-1 phosphate in the enhancement of endothelial barrier integrity by platelet-released products. *Am J Physiol Lung Cell Mol Physiol.* 2003;285:L258-L267.
452. Schermerhorn T, Pembleton-Corbett JR, Kornreich B. Pulmonary thromboembolism in cats. *J Vet Intern Med.* 2004;18:533-535.
453. See AM, Swindells KL, Sharman MJ, et al. Activated coagulation times in normal cats and dogs using MAX-ACT tubes. *Aust Vet J.* 2009;87:292-295.
454. Segura D, Monreal L. Poor reproducibility of template bleeding time in horses. *J Vet Intern Med.* 2008;22:238-241.
455. Segura D, Monreal L, Armengou L, et al. Mean platelet component as an indicator of platelet activation in foals and adult horses. *J Vet Intern Med.* 2007;21:1076-1082.
456. Sellon DC, Levine JF, Palmer K, et al. Thrombocytosis in 24 horses (1989-1994). *J Vet Intern Med.* 1997;11:24-29.
457. Sheafor SE, Couto CG. Anticoagulant rodenticide toxicity in 21 dogs. *J Am Anim Hosp Assoc.* 1999;35:38-46.
458. Shelly SM. Causes of canine pancytopenia. *Comp Cont Ed Pract Vet.* 1988;10:9-16.
459. Shelton GH, Linenberger ML. Hematologic abnormalities associated with retroviral infections in the cat. *Semin Vet Med Surg (Small Anim).* 1995;10:220-233.

460. Sheridan WP, Hunt P, Simonet S, et al. Hematologic effects of cytokines. In: Remick DG, Friedland JS, eds. *Cytokines in Health and Disease.* 2nd ed. New York: Marcel Dekker, Inc.; 1997:487-505.
461. Shimada K, Kobayashi M, Kimura S, et al. Anticoagulant heparin-like glycosaminoglycans on endothelial cell surface. *Jpn Circ J.* 1991;55:1016-1021.
462. Shinozaki K, Kawasaki T, Kambayashi J, et al. Species differences in platelet aggregation induced by platelet-activating factor (PAF). *Methods Find Exp Clin Pharmacol.* 1992;14:663-665.
463. Singh K, Flood J, Welsh RD, et al. Fatal systemic phaeohyphomycosis caused by *Ochroconis gallopavum* in a dog (*Canis familaris*). *Vet Pathol.* 2006;43:988-992.
464. Sinnott VB, Otto CM. Use of thromboelastography in dogs with immune-mediated hemolytic anemia: 39 cases (2000-2008). *J Vet Emerg Crit Care (San Antonio).* 2009;19:484-488.
465. Skowronek AJ, LaFranco L, Stone-Marschat MA, et al. Clinical pathology and hemostatic abnormalities in experimental African horsesickness. *Vet Pathol.* 1995;32:112-121.
466. Smith R III, Thomas JS. Quantitation of reticulated platelets in healthy dogs and in nonthrombocytopenic dogs with clinical disease. *Vet Clin Pathol.* 2002;31:26-32.
467. Smith SA. The cell-based model of coagulation. *J Vet Emerg Crit Care (San Antonio).* 2009;19:3-10.
468. Smith SA. Overview of hemostasis. In: Weiss DJ, Wardrop KJ, eds. *Schalm's Veterinary Hematology.* 6th ed. Ames, IA: Wiley-Blackwell; 2010:635-653.
469. Smith SA, Tobias AH, Jacob KA, et al. Arterial thromboembolism in cats: acute crisis in 127 cases (1992-2001) and long-term management with low-dose aspirin in 24 cases. *J Vet Intern Med.* 2003;17:73-83.
470. Snyder TA, Watach MJ, Litwak KN, et al. Platelet activation, aggregation, and life span in calves implanted with axial flow ventricular assist devices. *Ann Thorac Surg.* 2002;73:1933-1938.
471. Sontas HB, Dokuzeylu B, Turna O, et al. Estrogen-induced myelotoxicity in dogs: a review. *Can Vet J.* 2009;50:1054-1058.
472. Sosman JA, Verma A, Moss S, et al. Interleukin 10-induced thrombocytopenia in normal healthy adult volunteers: evidence for decreased platelet production. *Br J Haematol.* 2000;111:104-111.
473. Soute BA, Ulrich MM, Watson AD, et al. Congenital deficiency of all vitamin K-dependent blood coagulation factors due to a defective vitamin K-dependent carboxylase in Devon Rex cats. *Thromb Haemost.* 1992;68:521-525.
474. Southwood LL, Schott HC, Henry CJ, et al. Disseminated hemangiosarcoma in the horse: 35 cases. *J Vet Intern Med.* 2000;14:105-109.
475. Spagnuolo M, Kennedy S, Foster JC, et al. Bovine viral diarrhoea virus infection in bone marrow of experimentally infected calves. *J Comp Pathol.* 1997;116:97-100.
476. Spangler WL, Kass PH. Splenic myeloid metaplasia, histiocytosis, and hypersplenism in the dog (65 cases). *Vet Pathol.* 1999;36:583-593.
477. Stafford DW. The vitamin K cycle. *J Thromb Haemost.* 2005;3:1873-1878.
478. Stevenson C, Schwan T. *Borrelia hermsii* spirochetemia in a dog (abstract). *Vet Clin Pathol.* 2010;39:524.
479. Stokol T. Plasma D-dimer for the diagnosis of thromboembolic disorders in dogs. *Vet Clin North Am Small Anim Pract.* 2003;33:1419-1435.
480. Stokol T. Disseminated intravascular coagulation. In: Weiss DJ, Wardrop KJ, eds. *Schalm's Veterinary Hematology.* 6th ed. Ames, IA: Wiley-Blackwell; 2010:679-688.
481. Stokol T. Essential thrombocythemia and reactive thrombocytosis. In: Weiss DJ, Wardrop KJ, eds. *Schalm's Veterinary Hematology.* 6th ed. Ames, IA: Wiley-Blackwell; 2010:605-611.
482. Stokol T, Brooks M. Diagnosis of DIC in cats: is it time to go back to the basics? *J Vet Intern Med.* 2006;20:1289-1290.
483. Stokol T, Brooks M, Rush JE, et al. Hypercoagulability in cats with cardiomyopathy. *J Vet Intern Med.* 2008;22:546-552.
484. Stokol T, Brooks MB, Erb HN, et al. D-dimer concentrations in healthy dogs and dogs with disseminated intravascular coagulation. *Am J Vet Res.* 2000;61:393-398.
485. Stokol T, Erb HN. A comparison of platelet parameters in EDTA- and citrate-anticoagulated blood in dogs. *Vet Clin Pathol.* 2007;36:148-154.
486. Stokol T, Erb HN, De Wilde L, et al. Evaluation of latex agglutination kits for detection of fibrin(ogen) degradation products and D-dimer in healthy horses and horses with severe colic. *Vet Clin Pathol.* 2005;34:375-382.
487. Stokol T, Randolph JF, Nachbar S, et al. Development of bone marrow toxicosis after albendazole administration in a dog and cat. *J Am Vet Med Assoc.* 1997;210:1753-1756.
488. Stone MS, Johnstone IB, Brooks M, et al. Lupus-type "anticoagulant" in a dog with hemolysis and thrombosis. *J Vet Intern Med.* 1994;8:57-61.
489. Strieker MJ, Morris JG, Feldman BF, et al. Vitamin K deficiency in cats fed commercial fish-based diets. *J Small Anim Pract.* 1996;37:322-326.
490. Sullivan P, Gompf R, Schmeitzel L, et al. Altered platelet indices in dogs with hypothyroidism and cats with hyperthyroidism. *Am J Vet Res.* 1993;54:2004-2009.
491. Sumann G, Fries D, Griesmacher A, et al. Blood coagulation activation and fibrinolysis during a downhill marathon run. *Blood Coagul Fibrinolysis.* 2007;18:435-440.
492. Suzuki S, Iwata G, Sutor AH. Vitamin K deficiency during the perinatal and infantile period. *Semin Thromb Hemost.* 2001;27:93-98.
493. Sykes JE, Kittleson MD, Chomel BB, et al. Clinicopathologic findings and outcome in dogs with infective endocarditis: 71 cases (1992-2005). *J Am Vet Med Assoc.* 2006;228:1735-1747.
494. Tamzali Y, Guelfi JF, Braun JP. Plasma fibrinogen measurement in the horse: comparison of Millar's technique with a chronometric technique and the QBC-Vet Autoreader. *Res Vet Sci.* 2001;71:213-217.
495. Tarnow I, Kristensen AT. Evaluation of platelet function. In: Weiss DJ, Wardrop KJ, eds. *Schalm's Veterinary Hematology.* 6th ed. Ames, IA: Wiley-Blackwell; 2010:1123-1132.
496. Tasca S, Carli E, Caldin M, et al. Hematologic abnormalities and flow cytometric immunophenotyping results in dogs with hematopoietic neoplasia: 210 cases (2002-2006). *Vet Clin Pathol.* 2009;38:2-12.
497. Tholen I, Weingart C, Kohn B. Concentration of D-dimers in healthy cats and sick cats with and without disseminated intravascular coagulation (DIC). *J Feline Med Surg.* 2009;11:842-846.
498. Thomas JS, Rogers KS. Platelet aggregation and adenosine triphosphate secretion in dogs with untreated multicentric lymphoma. *J Vet Intern Med.* 1999;13:319-322.
499. Topper MJ, Prasse KW. Use of enzyme-linked immunosorbent assay to measure thrombin-antithrombin III complexes in horses with colic. *Am J Vet Res.* 1996;57:456-462.
500. Topper MJ, Prasse KW. Analysis of coagulation proteins as acute-phase reactants in horses with colic. *Am J Vet Res.* 1998;59:542-545.
501. Toulza O, Center SA, Brooks MB, et al. Evaluation of plasma protein C activity for detection of hepatobiliary disease and portosystemic shunting in dogs. *J Am Vet Med Assoc.* 2006;229:1761-1771.
502. Trepanier LA, Danhof R, Toll J, et al. Clinical findings in 40 dogs with hypersensitivity associated with administration of potentiated sulfonamides. *J Vet Intern Med.* 2003;17:647-652.
503. Truyen U, Addie D, Belak S, et al. Feline panleukopenia. ABCD guidelines on prevention and management. *J Feline Med Surg.* 2009;11:538-546.
504. Tseng LW, Hughes D, Giger U. Evaluation of a point-of-care coagulation analyzer for measurement of prothrombin time, activated partial thromboplastin time, and activated clotting time in dogs. *Am J Vet Res.* 2001;62:1455-1460.
505. Tsuchiya R, Kyotani K, Scott MA, et al. Role of platelet activating factor in development of thrombocytopenia and neutropenia in dogs with endotoxemia. *Am J Vet Res.* 1999;60:216-221.
506. Tvedten H, Lilliehook I, Hillstrom A, et al. Plateletcrit is superior to platelet count for assessing platelet status in Cavalier King Charles Spaniels. *Vet Clin Pathol.* 2008;37:266-271.
507. Ulutas PA, Musal B, Kiral F, et al. Acute phase protein levels in pregnancy and oestrus cycle in bitches. *Res Vet Sci.* 2009;86:373-376.
508. Valladares JE, Ruiz De Gopegui R, Riera C, et al. Study of haemostatic disorders in experimentally induced leishmaniasis in Beagle dogs. *Res Vet Sci.* 1998;64:195-198.
509. van GC, Savary-Bataille K, Chiers K, et al. Bilirubin cholelithiasis and haemosiderosis in an anaemic pyruvate kinase-deficient Somali cat. *J Small Anim Pract.* 2008;49:479-482.
510. Vannucchi CI, Mirandola RM, Oliveira CM. Acute-phase protein profile during gestation and diestrous: proposal for an early pregnancy test in bitches. *Anim Reprod Sci.* 2002;74:87-99.
511. Vaziri ND. Thrombocytosis in EPO-treated dialysis patients may be mediated by EPO rather than iron deficiency. *Am J Kidney Dis.* 2009;53:733-736.
512. Vilar P, Couto CG, Westendorf N, et al. Thromboelastographic tracings in retired racing greyhounds and in non-greyhound dogs. *J Vet Intern Med.* 2008;22:374-379.
513. Vlot AJ, Koppelman SJ, van den Berg MH, et al. The affinity and stoichiometry of binding of human factor VIII to von Willebrand factor. *Blood.* 1995;85:3150-3157.
514. Vogler EA, Siedlecki CA. Contact activation of blood-plasma coagulation. *Biomaterials.* 2009;30:1857-1869.
515. Waldmann TA, Weissman SM, Berlin N. The effect of splenectomy on erythropoiesis in the dog. *Blood.* 1960;15:873-883.
516. Walsh PN. Platelets: yin and yang. *Blood.* 2010;115:1-2.
517. Walton RM, Modiano JF, Thrall MA, et al. Bone marrow cytological findings in 4 dogs and a cat with hemophagocytic syndrome. *J Vet Intern Med.* 1996;10:7-14.
518. Walz PH, Steficek BA, Baker JC, et al. Effect of experimentally induced type II bovine viral diarrhea virus infection on platelet function in calves. *Am J Vet Res.* 1999;60:1396-1401.
519. Waner T, Leykin I, Shinitsky M, et al. Detection of platelet-bound antibodies in beagle dogs after artificial infection with *Ehrlichia canis.* *Vet Immunol Immunopathol.* 2000;77:145-150.
520. Waner T, Yuval D, Nyska A. Electronic measurement of canine mean platelet volume. *Vet Clin Pathol.* 1989;18:84-86.

521. Wang JY, Wang SS, Yin PZ. Haemolytic-uraemic syndrome caused by a non-O157: H7 *Escherichia coli* strain in experimentally inoculated dogs. *J Med Microbiol.* 2006;55:23-29.
522. Watson AD, Wilson JT, Turner DM, et al. Phenylbutazone-induced blood dyscrasias suspected in three dogs. *Vet Rec.* 1980;107:239-241.
523. Weiser MG, Cockerell GL, Smith JA, et al. Cytoplasmic fragmentation associated with lymphoid leukemia in ruminants: interference with electronic determination of platelet concentration. *Vet Pathol.* 1989;26:177-178.
524. Weiss DJ. New insights into the physiology and treatment of acquired myelodysplastic syndromes and aplastic pancytopenia. *Vet Clin North Am Small Anim Pract.* 2003;33:1317-1334.
525. Weiss DJ. Hemophagocytic syndrome in dogs: 24 cases (1996-2005). *J Am Vet Med Assoc.* 2007;230:697-701.
526. Weiss DJ, Evanson OA. A retrospective study of feline pancytopenia. *Comp Haematol Int.* 2000;10:50-55.
527. Weiss DJ, Evanson OA, McClenahan D, et al. Shear-induced platelet activation and platelet-neutrophil aggregate formation by equine platelets. *Am J Vet Res.* 1998;59:1243-1246.
528. Weiss DJ, Evanson OA, Sykes J. A retrospective study of canine pancytopenia. *Vet Clin Pathol.* 1999;28:83-88.
529. Weiss DJ, Townsend E. Evaluation of reticulated platelets in dogs. *Comp Haematol Int.* 1998;8:166-170.
530. Weiss RC, Cox NR, Boudreaux MK. Toxicologic effects of ribavirin in cats. *J Vet Pharmacol Therap.* 1993;16:301-316.
531. Weiss RC, Dodds WJ, Scott FW. Disseminated intravascular coagulation in experimentally induced feline infectious peritonitis. *Am J Vet Res.* 1980;41: 663-671.
532. Welch RD, Watkins JP, Taylor TS, et al. Disseminated intravascular coagulation associated with colic in 23 horses (1984-1989). *J Vet Intern Med.* 1992;6:29-35.
533. Whatley RE, Zimmerman GA, McIntyre TM, et al. Lipid metabolism and signal transduction in endothelial cells. *Prog Lipid Res.* 1990;29:45-63.
534. Whitney MS, Schwan TG, Sultemeier KB, et al. Spirochetemia caused by *Borrelia turicatae* infection in 3 dogs in Texas. *Vet Clin Pathol.* 2007;36:212-216.
535. Wigton DH, Kociba GJ, Hoover EA. Infectious canine hepatitis: animal model for viral-induced disseminated intravascular coagulation. *Blood.* 1976;47:287-296.
536. Wiinberg B, Jensen AL, Johansson PI, et al. Development of a model based scoring system for diagnosis of canine disseminated intravascular coagulation with independent assessment of sensitivity and specificity. *Vet J.* 2010;185:292-298.
537. Wiinberg B, Jensen AL, Johansson PI, et al. Thromboelastographic evaluation of hemostatic function in dogs with disseminated intravascular coagulation. *J Vet Intern Med.* 2008;22:357-365.
538. Wiinberg B, Jensen AL, Rozanski E, et al. Tissue factor activated thromboelastography correlates to clinical signs of bleeding in dogs. *Vet J.* 2009;179:121-129.
539. Wilcox A, Russell KE. Hematologic changes associated with Adderall toxicity in a dog. *Vet Clin Pathol.* 2008;37:184-189.
540. Wilkerson MJ, Johnson GS, Stockham S, et al. Afibrinogenemia and a circulating antibody against fibrinogen in a Bichon Frise dog. *Vet Clin Pathol.* 2005;34:148-155.
541. Wilkerson MJ, Shuman W. Alterations in normal canine platelets during storage in EDTA anticoagulated blood. *Vet Clin Pathol.* 2001;30:107-113.
542. Wilkerson MJ, Shuman W, Swist S, et al. Platelet size, platelet surface-associated IgG, and reticulated platelets in dogs with immune-mediated thrombocytopenia. *Vet Clin Pathol.* 2001;30:141-149.
543. Willey JR, Schaer M. Eastern diamondback rattlesnake (*Crotalus adamanteus*) envenomation of dogs: 31 cases (1982-2002). *J Am Anim Hosp Assoc.* 2005;41:22-33.
544. Wills TB, Wardrop KJ. Pseudothrombocytopenia secondary to the effects of EDTA in a dog. *J Am Anim Hosp Assoc.* 2008;44:95-97.
545. Wills TB, Wardrop KJ, Meyers KM. Detection of activated platelets in canine blood by use of flow cytometry. *Am J Vet Res.* 2006;67:56-63.
546. Woods JP, Crystal MA, Morton RJ, et al. Tularemia in two cats. *J Am Vet Med Assoc.* 1998;212:81-83.
547. Woody BJ, Murphy MJ, Ray AC, et al. Coagulopathic effects and therapy of brodifacoum toxicosis in dogs. *J Vet Intern Med.* 1992;6:23-28.
548. Yilmaz Z, Eralp O, Ilcol YO. Evaluation of platelet count and its association with plateletcrit, mean platelet volume, and platelet size distribution width in a canine model of endotoxemia. *Vet Clin Pathol.* 2008;37:159-163.
549. Yilmaz Z, Senturk S. Characterisation of lipid profiles in dogs with parvoviral enteritis. *J Small Anim Pract.* 2007;48:643-650.
550. Zandecki M, Genevieve F, Gerard J, et al. Spurious counts and spurious results on haematology analysers: a review. Part I: platelets. *Int J Lab Hematol.* 2007;29:4-20.
551. Zelmanovic D, Hetherington EJ. Automated analysis of feline platelets in whole blood, including platelet count, mean platelet volume, and activation state. *Vet Clin Pathol.* 1998;27:2-9.
552. Zini E, Hauser B, Meli ML, et al. Immune-mediated erythroid and megakaryocytic aplasia in a cat. *J Am Vet Med Assoc.* 2007;230:1024-1027.
553. Zorio E, Gilabert-Estelles J, Espana F, et al. Fibrinolysis: the key to new pathogenetic mechanisms. *Curr Med Chem.* 2008;15:923-929.

CHAPTER

8

Bone Marrow Examination

REASONS TO EXAMINE BONE MARROW

Bone marrow evaluation is indicated when peripheral blood abnormalities are detected. The most common indications are persistent neutropenia, unexplained thrombocytopenia, poorly regenerative anemia, or a combination thereof. Examples of proliferative abnormalities in which bone marrow examination may be indicated include persistent thrombocytosis or leukocytosis, abnormal blood cell morphology, or the unexplained presence of immature cells in blood (e.g., nucleated erythroid cells in the absence of polychromasia or a neutrophilic left shift in the absence of inflammation).

Bone marrow is sometimes examined to stage neoplastic conditions (lymphomas and mast-cell tumors); to estimate the adequacy of body iron stores; to evaluate lytic bone lesions; and to search for occult disease in animals with fever of unknown origin, unexplained weight loss, and unexplained malaise. Bone marrow examination can also be useful in determining the cause of a hyperproteinemia when it occurs secondarily to multiple myeloma, lymphoma, leishmaniasis, and systemic fungal diseases. It may also reveal the cause of a hypercalcemia when associated with lymphoid neoplasms, multiple myeloma, or metastatic neoplasms to bone.

In veterinary medicine, bone marrow aspirates are done more frequently than core biopsies. Aspirates are easier, faster, and less expensive to perform than are core biopsies. Bone marrow core biopsies require special needles that cut a solid core of material, which is then placed in fixative, decalcified, embedded, sectioned, stained, and examined microscopically by a pathologist. Core biopsy sections provide a more accurate way of evaluating marrow cellularity and examining for metastatic neoplasia than do aspirate smears, but cell morphology is more difficult to assess.

There are few contraindications for bone marrow aspirates and core biopsies. Restraint, sedation, and anesthesia (when used) generally pose more risks for the patient than the biopsy procedure itself. Postbiopsy hemorrhage is a potential complication in patients with hemostatic diatheses, but it rarely occurs. Hemorrhage may occur after the biopsy of animals with monoclonal hyperglobulinemias, but it is easily controlled by placing a suture in the skin incision and applying pressure over the biopsy site. Postbiopsy infection is also a potential complication, but it is highly unlikely to occur if proper techniques are used. The major contraindication to bone marrow aspiration and core biopsies is when they are unnecessary (e.g., the anemia is regenerative or the cause of the neutropenia is recognized to be sepsis).

SITES FOR BONE MARROW BIOPSY

Young animals have active (red) marrow throughout most skeletal bones. Active marrow recedes from long bones as adulthood is reached, because the bone marrow space expands faster than the blood volume as the animal grows.[53] Once animals stop growing, blood cell numbers must be maintained, but increased production to accommodate growth is no longer required. As hematopoietic cells disappear, the marrow space is replaced by fat (yellow marrow) and is in a resting state. Hematopoietic cells may expand back into long bones if needed, as might occur in response to anemia. Active marrow remains in the flat bones (vertebrae, sternum, ribs, and pelvis) and proximal ends of the humerus and femur in adults.[53]

Ilium

The iliac crest is often used as a site to aspirate/biopsy marrow in dogs and is sometimes used in cats.[29,53] The biopsy needle is positioned so that it enters the greatest prominence of the iliac crest, parallel to the long axis of the wing of the ilium (Fig. 8-1). The wing of the ilium may also be aspirated at its central depression, which is caudal and ventral to the iliac crest. The tuber coxae has been used as a site for bone marrow collection in young horses, but adequate marrow samples cannot be obtained from this site in adult horses because of a lack of active marrow.[58]

Proximal Femur

For small cats and toy breeds of dogs, in which the ilium is especially thin, the marrow may be aspirated from the head of the proximal femur by way of the trochanteric fossa (see

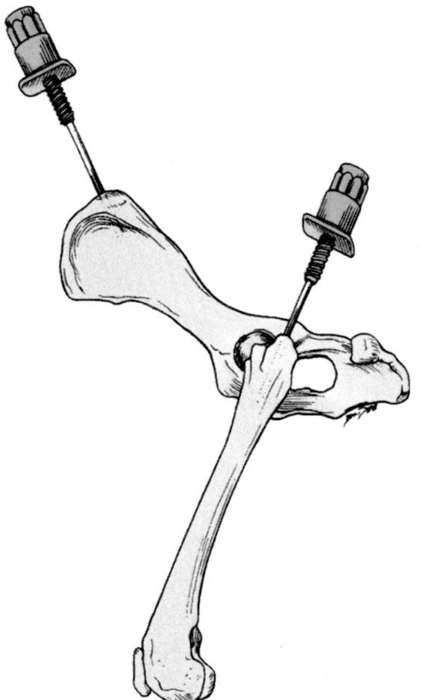

FIGURE 8-1

Bone marrow biopsy site for the iliac crest and proximal femur.

From Grindem CB. Bone marrow biopsy and evaluation. Vet Clin N Am Small Anim Pract. *1989:19:669-696, as modified from Harvey JW. Bone marrow aspiration biopsy.* NAVC Clinician's Brief. *2004;February: 44-47.*

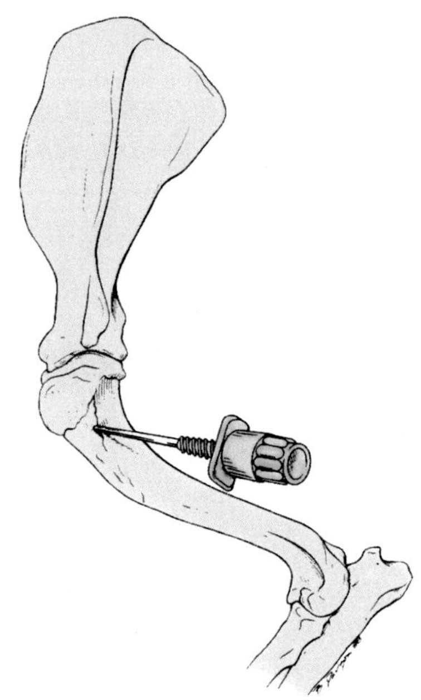

FIGURE 8-2

Bone marrow biopsy site for the proximal humerus.

From Grindem CB. Bone marrow biopsy and evaluation. Vet Clin N Am Small Anim Pract. *1989:19:669-696, as modified from Harvey JW. Bone marrow aspiration biopsy.* NAVC Clinician's Brief. *2004; February:44-47.*

Fig. 8-1).[29,53] This site is not suitable for obtaining a core biopsy.

Proximal Humerus

Aspiration of marrow from the cranial side of the proximal end of the humerus is also commonly done in small animals, especially in those that are obese.[29] This site has also been recommended for use in calves.[47] The greater tubercle is palpated, and the needle is inserted into the flat area on the craniolateral surface of the proximal humerus distal to the tubercle (Fig. 8-2).

Sternum

In large dogs, the third, fourth, or fifth sternebra can be aspirated/biopsied.[53] The collection of marrow from the sternum poses the risk of inadvertent penetration of the thorax and damage to structures in the thoracic cavity. A short biopsy needle (preferably with an adjustable guard) should be used, and care should be taken to remain in the center of these bones to minimize the risk of pneumothorax, uncontrolled hemorrhage, or cardiac laceration. Although there is also some risk to the person collecting sternal marrow from standing large animals, the sternum (third or fourth sternebra) is the preferred site for collecting high-quality aspirates/biopsies from adult horses, cattle, sheep, and llamas. Sternebrae are identified by palpating ribs to their articulations with the sternum.[47]

Proximal Ribs

The proximal (dorsal) ends of the ribs have been used for bone marrow aspirates in large animals, although the bone is difficult to penetrate with biopsy needles in adults and can severely damage the needles.[58,59] There is also a risk of pneumothorax or uncontrolled hemorrhage when ribs are biopsied.[5]

Other Sites

Aspirates/biopsies may be taken from other bone marrow sites if specific lesions are identified using diagnostic imaging. These are done to identify the nature of the lesion, rather than to evaluate hematopoiesis.

TECHNIQUE OF BONE MARROW ASPIRATION

The needle used to aspirate marrow must have a removable stylet, which remains in place until the marrow cavity is entered to prevent obstruction of the needle's lumen with cortical bone. A 16- or 18-gauge needle (Rosenthal, Illinois sternal, or Jamshidi) between 1 and 1.5 inches long is satisfactory (Fig. 8-3).

The usefulness of bone marrow aspirate cytology as a diagnostic aid depends on the proper collection of the bone marrow sample and preparation of high-quality marrow

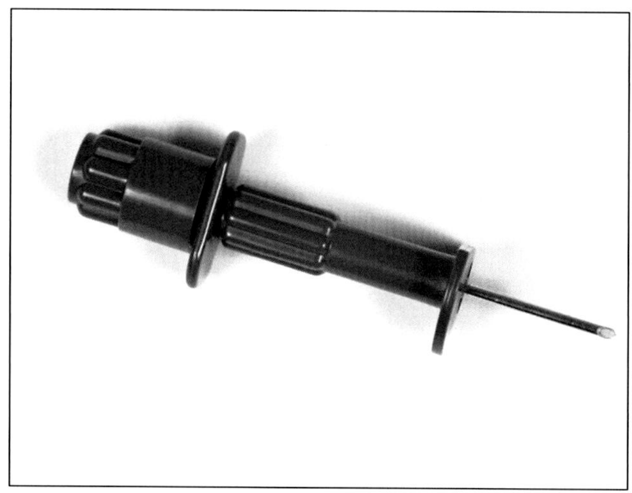

FIGURE 8-3
Bone marrow aspiration needle. An 18-gauge Illinois bone marrow aspiration needle with stylet in place and adjustable guard to limit the depth of penetration.

smears. In most cases with dogs and large animals, only local anesthesia is needed for aspiration biopsies. However, tranquilization is often used, especially in patients that resist positioning by manual restraint. Bone marrow aspirates are often done under light anesthesia in cats. Collection sites are prepared by clipping the hair and scrubbing the skin with antiseptic soap preparations (Fig. 8-4, *A*). A local anesthetic is injected under the skin and down to the periosteum overlying the site to be aspirated, and a small skin incision is made with a scalpel blade to facilitate passing the needle through the skin (Fig. 8-4, *B*). Sterile needles and gloves are always used, but the aspiration site is generally not draped. If general anesthesia is required for other procedures, bone marrow aspiration may be scheduled at the same time to minimize the stress on the animal.

To enter the marrow space, moderate pressure is applied to the needle (with the stylet locked in place) as the needle is rotated in an alternating clockwise-counterclockwise motion (Fig. 8-4, *C*). Once the needle is firmly embedded into the bone, it is usually within the marrow cavity. The stylet is then removed (Fig. 8-4, *D*) and a 10- to 20-mL syringe is attached to the needle (Fig. 8-4, *E*). Vigorous negative pressure should be applied by rapidly pulling the plunger back as far as possible. If no anticoagulant is added to the syringe, the negative pressure is released, and the complete assembly is rapidly removed for smear preparation as soon as a few drops appear in the syringe. If marrow does not appear in the syringe, the stylet is replaced and the needle is repositioned for another aspiration attempt.

If no anticoagulant is used, smears must be prepared within seconds after bone marrow collection, because bone marrow clots rapidly. Smears prepared once clotting begins cannot be evaluated, because most of the nucleated cells will be lysed during smear preparation. We prefer to collect bone marrow into a syringe that contains EDTA as an anticoagulant, because it reduces the chance of clotting before a smear is prepared and allows time to prepare multiple smears that may be needed for special stains. Additionally, the ability to collect bone marrow particles in anticoagulated samples, prior to smear preparation, increases the likelihood of getting sufficient particles to make an accurate interpretation of the aspirate smear. An EDTA-containing solution can be prepared by adding 0.35 mL of sterile saline to a 7-mL EDTA tube, which yields a 2.5% or 3% EDTA solution, depending on whether the tube contains dry EDTA or EDTA dissolved in water. About 0.5 mL of this EDTA solution is drawn into the syringe using a regular needle prior to attaching the syringe to the bone marrow aspiration needle.[30] Although smears need not be made immediately when collected with EDTA, they should be prepared within minutes after collection, because bone marrow cells (especially granulocytic cells) degenerate rapidly.

About 1 mL of marrow is aspirated into the syringe containing EDTA. Following mixing, the contents are expelled into a petri dish. It is important for accurate bone marrow evaluation that smears contain marrow particles (stroma and associated cells). Marrow particles appear as small white grains (flecks) in the blood-contaminated aspirate material. The particles tend to loosely adhere to the bottom of the petri dish when it is tilted. The particles are collected by pipette (Fig. 8-4, *F*) or a hematocrit capillary tube to use for smear preparation.

To concentrate particles in blood-contaminated aspirates, aspirated material can be placed on one end of a glass slide, which is then held vertically (Fig. 8-5, *A*). Particles tend to stick to the slide while blood runs off. A second glass slide is placed across the area of particle adherence, perpendicular to the first slide. After marrow spreads between the slides (Fig. 8-5, *B*), they are pulled apart in the horizontal plane.

Rather than use a perpendicular glass slide to spread the bone marrow particles, a square 22- by 22-mm 1.5-mm thick coverslip may be used in the same manner (Fig. 8-6, *A*). This produces both a coverslip and a glass slide preparation. Alternatively, one might consider using the two-coverslip method described for blood films in Chapter 2. The lighter weight of a top coverslip puts less pressure on particles than a top glass slide does. Consequently the use of coverslips may decrease the rupturing of nucleated cells, which happens more readily in samples collected with EDTA in saline compared with samples collected without an anticoagulant.[30] If a marrow aspirate contains particles without excessive blood contamination, one can place the aspirated material in the middle of a slide and place a second slide on top of it; the slides are then slid apart horizontally, as shown in Figure 8-6, *B*.

Bone marrow aspirate preparations from dead animals are usually of poor quality, even when collected soon after death. Once clots have formed, cells will be lysed during aspiration and smear preparation. If marrow is to be collected from an animal that is to be euthanized, it is recommended that the animal be anesthetized for marrow collection, followed by administration of the euthanasia solution.

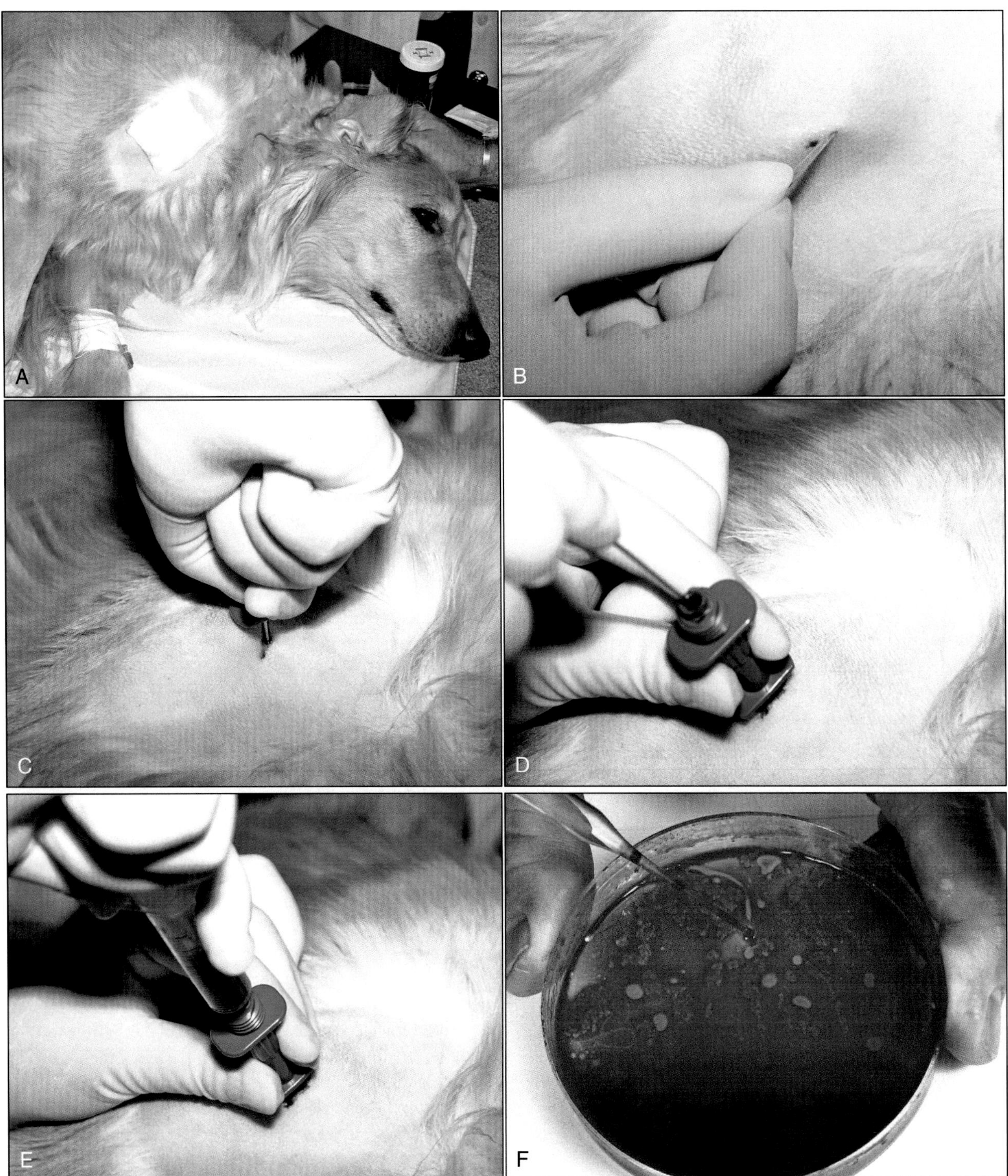

FIGURE 8-4

Bone marrow aspiration procedure. **A,** The biopsy site over the flat area on the craniolateral surface of the proximal humerus distal to the greater tubercle is prepared by clipping the hair and scrubbing the skin with antiseptic soap. **B,** A small skin incision is made with a scalpel blade to facilitate passing the needle through the skin. **C,** Moderate pressure is applied to the needle (with the stylet locked in place) as the needle is rotated in an alternating clockwise-counterclockwise motion. **D,** Once the needle is firmly embedded into the bone, the needle cap (if present) and stylet are removed. **E,** A syringe containing EDTA is attached to the needle and red marrow is aspirated into the syringe. **F,** Aspirated bone marrow containing anticoagulant is expelled into a petri dish. A pipette is then used to collect particles to be used in preparing smears.

All of the above from Harvey JW. Bone marrow aspiration biopsy. NAVC Clinician's Brief. *2004;February:44-47.*

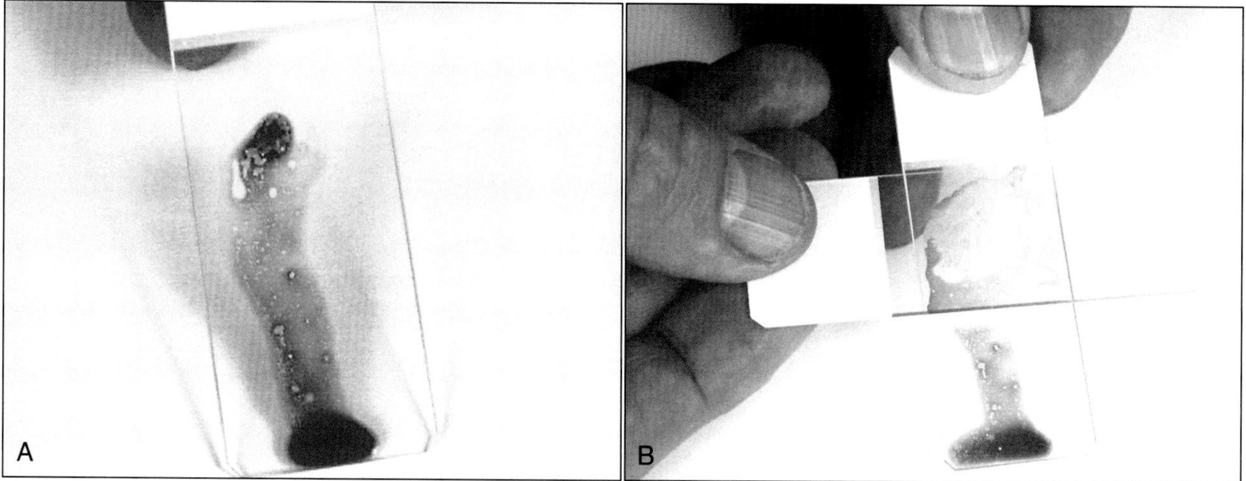

FIGURE 8-5
Technique for concentrating bone marrow particles prior to preparation of blood film. **A,** Blood-contaminated bone marrow aspirates are expelled onto one end of a glass slide that is then held vertically. Particles tend to stick to the slide while contaminating blood runs off and may be wicked away by absorbent material. **B,** A second glass slide is placed across the area of particle adherence, perpendicular to the first slide. The slides are held together, causing bone marrow to spread between them; then they are rapidly pulled apart in the horizontal plane and quickly air-dried.

If bone marrow is collected at necropsy, the marrow material should be mixed with a solution containing albumin before a smear is made to decrease cell lysis. One method recommends collecting bone marrow from an opened bone using a paintbrush and placing it on a piece of parafilm next to a drop of 22% bovine serum albumin solution. The paintbrush is then dipped in the albumin solution and mixed with the marrow material prior to smear preparation.[47] Another method recommends mixing marrow collected from the cadaver with a 5% solution of bovine serum albumin (prepared in physiologic saline), followed by smear preparation.[4]

Smears are stained with a Romanowsky-type blood stain such as Wright, Giemsa, or a combination thereof. Satisfactory results can usually be obtained with the Diff-Quik stain, a rapid modified Wright stain. The appropriate staining time(s) for the stain or stains being used is determined with experience. Thicker smears will require longer staining times. About twice the time is required for staining bone marrow smears compared to blood films. Smears containing marrow particles will have blue-staining material on them, which is visible grossly (Fig. 8-7). When examined microscopically, particles contain blood cell precursors and stromal elements (Fig. 8-8). Fat is dissolved away during alcohol fixation, but it is represented in particles by the presence of variably sized unstained circular areas.

If adequate smears are available, one smear should be stained using the Prussian blue procedure for iron. In contrast to other species, healthy cats typically lack stainable iron in their marrow aspirates. If leukemia is present, additional special stains may be needed to help differentiate the type of leukemia.

Bone marrow aspirate smears are often submitted for staining and evaluation by a clinical pathologist. Unfixed aspirate smears should not be mailed in a package that also contains tissue in formalin, because the formalin vapors will interfere with the staining quality of cells in the aspirate smears.

TECHNIQUE OF BONE MARROW CORE BIOPSY

Core biopsies are essential if there are repeated dry taps (e.g., failure to collect marrow particles by aspiration). Dry taps may be the result of technical error, but they can also occur when the marrow is packed with cells, as when a leukemia is present, and they usually occur when myelofibrosis is present. Dry taps or poor-quality samples are common when marrow aspirates are attempted on very young animals, even though the marrow is generally highly cellular. Core biopsy sections provide a more accurate way of evaluating marrow cellularity and examining for myelofibrosis, granulomatous diseases involving bone marrow, or metastatic neoplasia than do aspirate smears.[12,55] Core biopsies are also needed to diagnose vascular abnormalities (edema and hemorrhage) and acute inflammation (fibrin deposition and focal neutrophilic infiltrates).[74] To maximize information concerning bone marrow composition, we recommend collecting aspirate and core biopsy samples at the same time. Even when a core biopsy is not planned, it is advisable to have a core biopsy needle available in case a dry tap should occur.

Preparation of the animal and the site for a bone marrow core biopsy is the same as that described earlier for a marrow

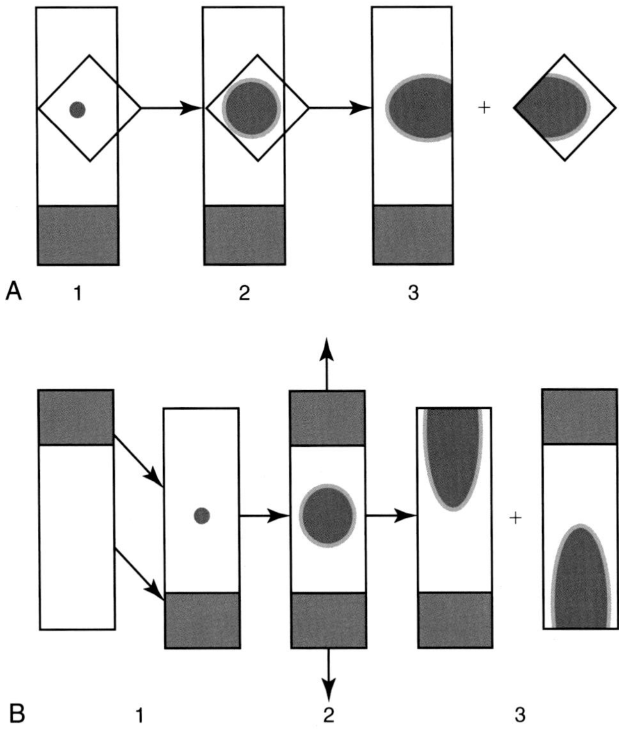

FIGURE 8-6
Bone marrow aspirate smear preparations. **A,** Assuming sufficient particles are present, a drop of aspirated material is placed on a glass slide and a coverslip is placed on top of the aspirated material at a right angle to the glass slide as shown. After the aspirate material spreads between the slide and coverslip, the coverslip is slid smoothly from the glass slide in a horizontal plane at a right angle to the glass slide, and both coverslip and glass slide are air-dried. This technique has been recommended for bone marrow aspirates collected with EDTA in saline because the lighter weight of a coverslip is less likely to result in cell lysis from frictional forces than the heavier weight of the glass slide. **B,** Assuming sufficient particles are present, a drop of aspirated material is placed in the center of a glass slide and a second glass slide is placed on top of the aspirated material on the first slide as shown. After the aspirated material spreads between the slides, they are quickly pulled apart in a horizontal plane, and both slides are rapidly air-dried.

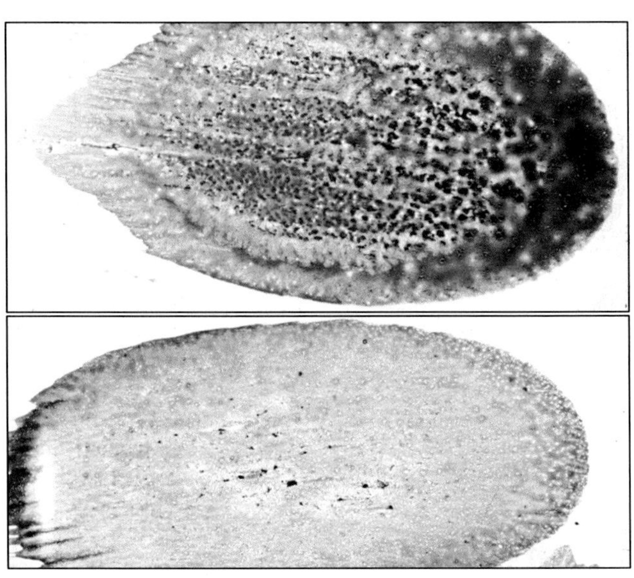

FIGURE 8-7
Two stained bone marrow smears are shown. The scant blue-staining material in the bottom smear indicates that only a few, small marrow particles are present. The abundant blue-staining material in the top smear indicates that a large amount of particulate bone marrow is present. Wright-Giemsa stain.

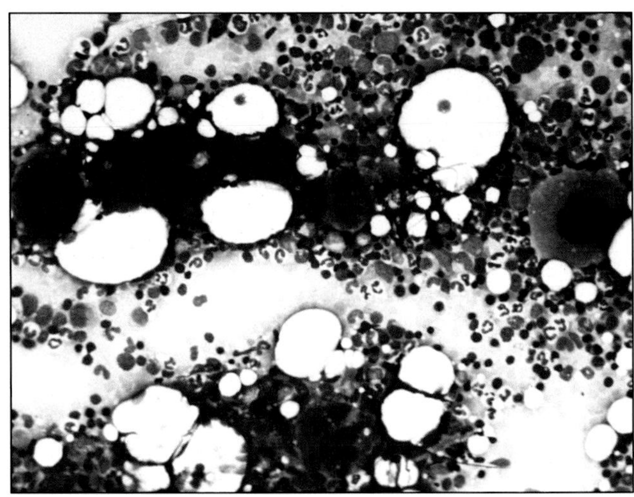

FIGURE 8-8
Normal bone marrow aspirate smear from a dog. Variably sized unstained circular areas indicate where fat was dissolved away during alcohol fixation. The large cells present are megakaryocytes. Wright-Giemsa stain.

aspirate. Core biopsies require the use of special needles designed to cut a solid core of material. Jamshidi bone marrow biopsy needles, 11 to 13 gauge and 3 to 4 inches long, are used in our veterinary hospital (Fig. 8-9). Depending on the species and size of the animal, core biopsies may be taken from the wing of the ilium, head of the humerus, or sternum. Core biopsies and aspirates should be taken from distantly located sites to ensure that one collection does not result in disruption of the area where the other sample is being collected. Collection from two separate sites should also increase the likelihood of identifying tumor metastasis.[12]

With the stylet locked in place, moderate pressure is applied to the needle as it is rotated in an alternating clockwise-counterclockwise motion (Fig. 8-10, *A*). Once the needle is firmly embedded into the bone, the stylet is removed (Fig. 8-10, *B*) and the needle is advanced using the same clockwise-counterclockwise motion (Fig. 8-10, *C*). If possible, the needle should be advanced 1 inch to get sufficient material for evaluation. Once the needle has been advanced to its maximal depth, several 360-degree twists are made and it is withdrawn. The core within the needle is pushed out using a wire, which accompanies the needle. This is done by placing the wire in the tip of the needle and forcing the core out of

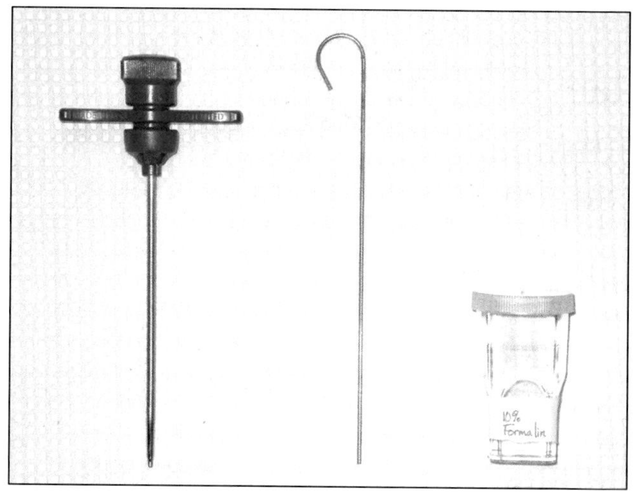

FIGURE 8-9

Bone marrow core biopsy needle. An 11-gauge Jamshidi core bone marrow biopsy needle with stylet in place, wire used to push the core biopsy from the needle, and container with formalin fixative.

Courtesy of Heather Wamsley.

the handle end of the needle (Fig. 8-10, *D*). Because the tip of the needle is tapered, pushing the core out through the tip would add crush artifacts to the core.

The head of the femur is not used for core biopsies because a core of material does not stay in the needle when it is withdrawn. Because core biopsy needles are larger than aspirate needles, the wing of the ilium in cats is generally too thin to allow for the collection of a core sample parallel to its long axis, as is typically done in dogs. However, core biopsies may be collected from the ilium in cats by making two or three perpendicular punch biopsies completely through the most dorsal aspect of the wing of the ilium. The short cores that are obtained have cortical bone on both ends. Multiple cores are needed to obtain sufficient material for evaluation.

If attempts to aspirate bone marrow have resulted in dry taps or poor-quality smears, the core biopsy may be gently rolled between two glass slides (Fig. 8-10, *E*) or across a single glass slide using the tip of the needle and then stained in the same manner as aspirate smears. These roll preparations are generally of lower quality than aspirate smears. In particular, the number of megakaryocytes and amount of stainable iron present is generally underrepresented. After one or more roll preparations are made, the core is placed in fixative (Fig. 8-10, *F*) and submitted to a surgical pathology service, where it is decalcified, embedded, sectioned, stained with hematoxylin and eosin (H&E) and possibly other stains, and examined microscopically by a pathologist (Fig. 8-11). Fixatives other than formalin are sometimes preferred; consequently the surgical pathology service should be consulted prior to sample collection. Unfixed aspirate smears, core roll preparations, or other exfoliative cytology preparations should not be mailed in the same package with formalin-fixed tissue because the formalin vapors will interfere with the staining quality of cells in the exfoliative cytology preparations.

MORPHOLOGIC IDENTIFICATION OF CELLS

This discussion focuses primarily on the morphologic appearance of cells in aspirate smears stained with Wright-Giemsa, but examples of core biopsy sections stained with H&E are also presented. Marrow particles appear as blue-staining areas in aspirate smears when viewed grossly (see Fig. 8-7). When examined microscopically, they contain blood cell precursors, vessels, reticular cells, macrophages, and plasma cells (see Fig. 8-8). Fat is dissolved away during alcohol fixation, but it is represented in particles by the presence of variably sized, unstained circular areas. Most particles in normal animals are composed of one-third to two-thirds cells (see Figs. 8-8, 8-11).

Megakaryocytic Series

Megakaryoblasts are the earliest recognizable cell in this series. They have a single nucleus and deeply basophilic cytoplasm (Fig. 8-12, *A*). This cell type is not recognized in most normal aspirate smears because it occurs in small numbers and is difficult to differentiate from other blast cells. Promegakaryocytes, which have two or four nuclei and deeply basophilic cytoplasm, are easily recognized (Fig. 8-12, *A*, *B*). These cells are much larger than leukocytes or nucleated erythroid precursor cells. Subsequent nuclear reduplications result in progressively larger basophilic megakaryocytes (Fig. 8-12, *C*). Nuclei in basophilic megakaryocytes are joined into a lobulated mass, making it difficult to count the number of nuclear reduplications that have occurred. The synthesis of magenta-staining cytoplasmic granules imparts a pink color to the cytoplasm characteristic of mature (granular) megakaryocytes (Fig. 8-12, *D*). Megakaryocytes are gigantic and vary from 50 to 200 μm in diameter, with larger cells having greater nuclear ploidy.

Erythrocytic Series

Morphologic changes that occur as cells of the erythroid series undergo maturation include diminution in size, decrease in nuclear-to-cytoplasmic (N:C) ratio, progressive nuclear condensation, and the appearance of red cytoplasmic color as hemoglobin is synthesized and accumulates within the cytoplasm (Fig. 8-13).

Rubriblasts

The earliest recognizable cell type in the erythroid series is the rubriblast. This is a relatively large cell with a high N:C ratio and intensely basophilic cytoplasm resulting from the presence of many polyribosomes. The nucleus of the rubriblast is usually almost perfectly round and the chromatin is finely granular, containing one or more pale blue to medium blue nucleoli (see Fig. 8-13, *A*).

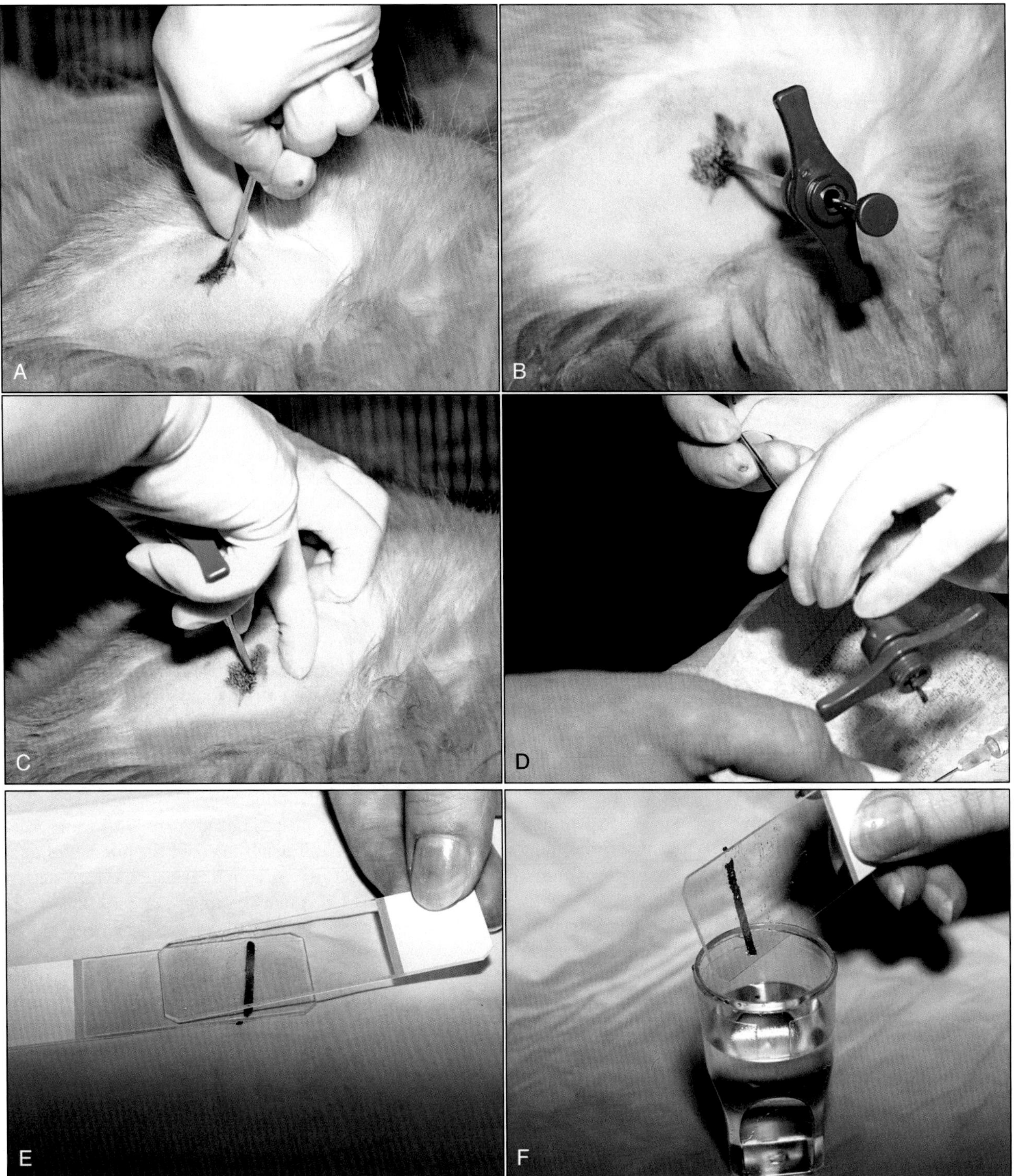

FIGURE 8-10

Core bone marrow biopsy procedure. **A,** Moderate pressure is applied to the needle (with the stylet locked in place) as the needle is rotated in an alternating clockwise-counterclockwise motion. **B,** Once the needle is firmly embedded into the bone, the needle cap (if present) and stylet are removed. **C,** The needle is again advanced using the same clockwise-counterclockwise motion. If possible, the needle should be advanced one inch to get sufficient material for evaluation. **D,** The core within the needle is pushed out onto a glass slide using a wire accompanying the needle. This is done by placing the wire in the tip of the needle and forcing the core out of the handle end of the needle. **E,** The core biopsy is gently rolled across a glass slide using a second glass slide. It will subsequently be stained with a routine blood stain such as Wright-Giemsa. **F,** After one or more roll preparations are made, the core is placed in fixative.

All of the above from Harvey JW. Bone marrow core biopsy. NAVC Clinician's Brief. *2004;October:32-35.*

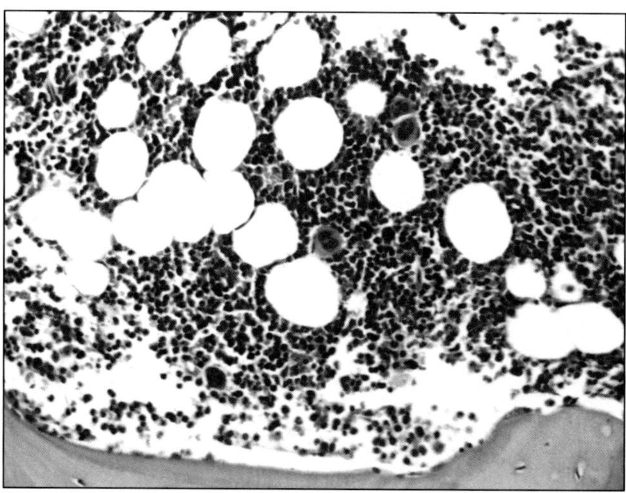

FIGURE 8-11
Low-power image of a normal bone marrow core biopsy from a dog. The bone marrow core biopsy has been fixed, decalcified, sectioned, and stained with hematoxylin and eosin (H&E). Pink-staining trabecular bone is present at the bottom. Variably sized unstained circular areas indicate where fat was dissolved away during fixation. The large cells present are megakaryocytes.

Prorubricytes
When nucleoli are no longer visible and slightly coarser chromatin clumping is present, the cell is classified as a prorubricyte (see Fig. 8-13, *B*). The N:C ratio is generally slightly less than in rubriblasts.

Basophilic Rubricytes
The next cell type in the erythroid series is the basophilic rubricyte. These cells still have blue cytoplasm but they are smaller than prorubricytes, have lower N:C ratios, and have nuclear condensation into light and dark areas, giving the nucleus a cartwheel appearance (see Fig. 8-13, *C*).

Polychromatophilic Rubricytes
The combined presence of hemoglobin (red) and ribosomes (blue) accounts for the reddish-blue cytoplasm characteristic of polychromatophilic rubricytes. They also tend to be smaller than basophilic rubricytes and have more nuclear condensation (see Fig. 8-13, *D*).

Metarubricytes
The most mature nucleated erythroid cell type is the small metarubricyte (see Fig. 8-13, *E*). Its nucleus is dark (pyknotic), with few or no clear areas; its cytoplasm is usually polychromatophilic but may be red (normochromic).

Polychromatophilic Erythrocytes (Reticulocytes)
When the metarubricyte nucleus is lost, a reticulocyte is formed. Reticulocytes formed from polychromatophilic metarubricytes will appear as polychromatophilic erythrocytes (see Fig. 8-13, *F*). Continued hemoglobin synthesis and loss of ribosomes results in the formation of mature erythrocytes with red-staining cytoplasm (see Fig. 8-13, *F*).

Granulocytic Series
Morphologic changes that occur as cells of the granulocytic series undergo maturation include slight diminution in size, decrease in N:C ratio, progressive nuclear condensation, changes in nuclear shape, and the appearance of cytoplasmic granules. The background (i.e., nongranular) cytoplasm's color changes from gray-blue to light blue to nearly colorless in the progression from myeloblasts to mature granulocytes (see Fig. 8-13).

Myeloblasts
The first recognizable cells in the granulocytic series are called myeloblasts. Type I myeloblasts appear as large round cells with round to oval nuclei, which are generally centrally located in the cell. The N:C ratio is high (greater than 1.5), and the nuclear outline is usually regular and smooth (see Fig. 8-13, *G*). Nuclear chromatin is finely stippled, containing one or more nucleoli or nucleolar rings. The cytoplasm is generally moderately basophilic (gray-blue in color) and not as dark as that of rubriblasts. Primary granules begin to form in late myeloblasts; consequently some of these cells may contain a few (typically less than 15) small magenta-staining granules in the cytoplasm. Such cells may be classified as type II myeloblasts. Myeloblasts with nucleoli and large numbers of magenta-staining granules have been classified as type III myeloblasts (Fig. 8-14, *A*).[37]

Promyelocytes (Progranulocytes)
Large numbers of magenta-staining primary granules are visible within the cytoplasm of promyelocytes, but nucleoli are no longer visible (see Fig. 8-13, *H*). Promyelocytes may be somewhat larger than myeloblasts because of their more abundant cytoplasm.

Myelocytes
Primary, magenta-staining granules characteristic of promyelocytes are no longer visualized in myelocytes; secondary granules that characterize neutrophils, eosinophils, and basophils appear at this stage. Myelocytes still have round nuclei, but they are generally smaller with more nuclear condensation and have lighter blue cytoplasm than promyelocytes. It is difficult to visualize the secondary granules within neutrophilic myelocytes because of their neutral staining characteristics (see Fig. 8-13, *I*). Eosinophilic myelocytes and basophilic myelocytes are identified by their characteristic granules (see Fig. 8-13, *M,Q*; Fig. 8-14, *B,C*). The large secondary granules in equine eosinophils may appear bluish before becoming bright red as the cell matures (see Fig. 8-14, *B*). Eosinophil granules are generally round in animals except cats, where they are rod-shaped. Cat basophilic myelocytes are also distinctive, having a mixture of dark-purple and light-lavender round to oval granules that typically fill the cytoplasm (see Fig. 8-14, *C*).

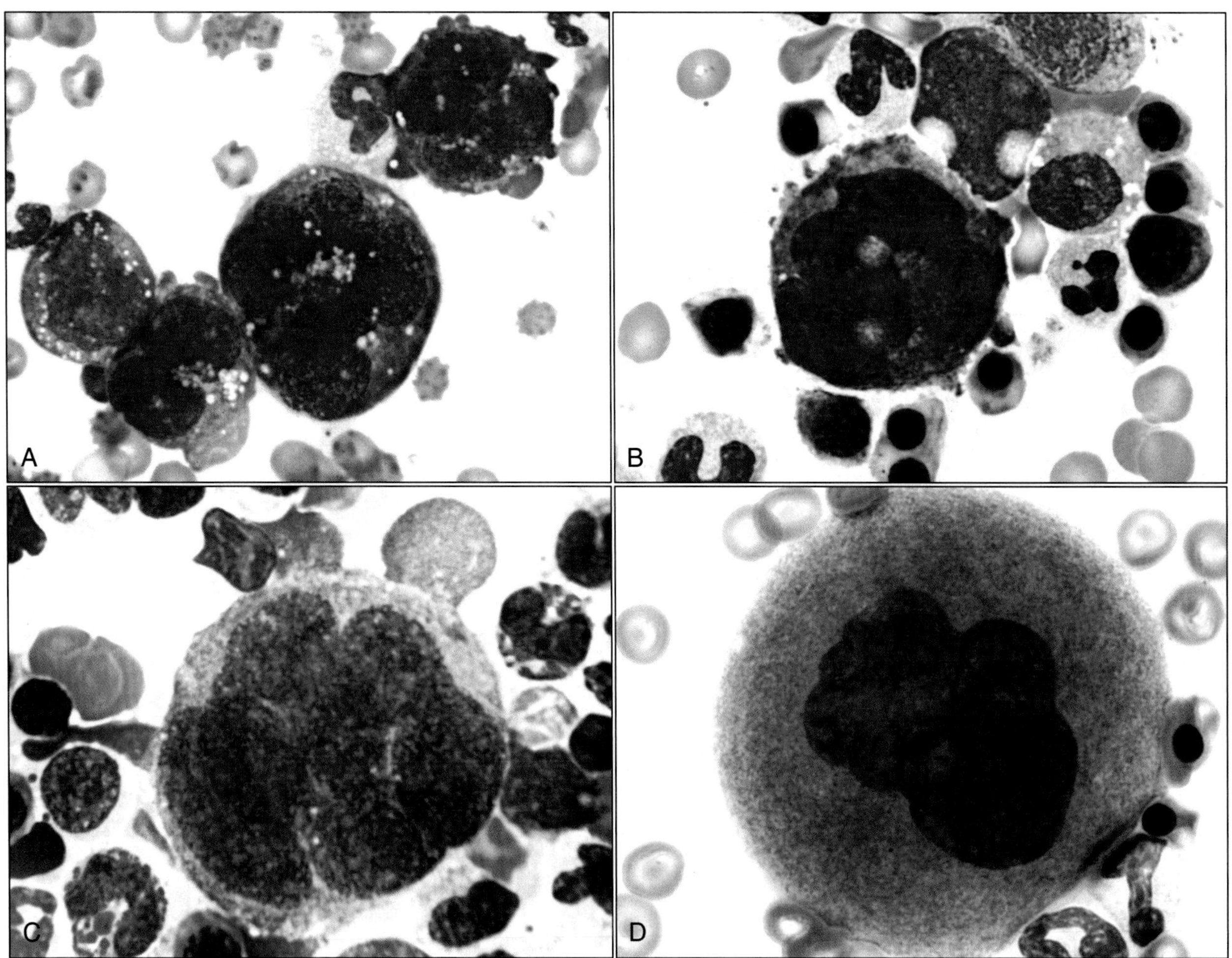

FIGURE 8-12

Megakaryocyte developmental stages in bone marrow aspirate smears from dogs. **A,** Megakaryoblast with single nucleus *(far left),* promegakaryocyte with two nuclei *(bottom left),* promegakaryocyte with four nuclei *(top right),* and a megakaryocytic cell with six nuclei that may be considered intermediate between a promegakaryocyte and a basophilic megakaryocyte. **B,** Promegakaryocyte with four nuclei surrounded by smaller myeloid and erythroid precursors. **C,** Basophilic megakaryocyte with blue cytoplasm and multiple fused nuclei. **D,** Mature megakaryocyte with magenta-staining granules in the cytoplasm. Multiple fused nuclei are present. All of the above are shown at the same magnification to demonstrate the enlargement that occurs as megakaryocytes develop. Wright-Giemsa stain.

Metamyelocytes

Once nuclear indentation and condensation become readily apparent, precursor cells are no longer capable of division. Precursors with kidney-shaped nuclei are called metamyelocytes. Nuclei with slight indentations extending less than 25% into the nucleus are still classified as myelocytes. Like myelocytes, the granules may be neutrophilic, eosinophilic, or basophilic in staining characteristics (see Fig. 8-13, *J,N,R*).

Band Cells

Cells with thinner rod-shaped nuclei with smooth parallel sides are called bands (see Fig. 8-13, *K,O,S*). No area of the nucleus has a diameter less than two-thirds the diameter of any other area of the nucleus. Band cell nuclei twist to conform to the space within the cytoplasm, and horseshoe or S-shaped nuclei are common.

Segmented Granulocytes

The final stage in granulocyte development is the segmented or mature granulocyte. The nuclear membrane is no longer smooth and the nuclear width becomes irregular and segments into two or more lobes in these cells. The nuclear chromatin is moderately to densely clumped, and the background cytoplasm is often colorless in neutrophils but may appear faintly blue or faintly pink (see Fig. 8-13, *L*). Nuclei of eosinophils and basophils are generally less segmented than the nuclei of neutrophils, and specific granules can be identified in their cytoplasm (see Fig. 8-13, *P,T*).

Monocytic Series

The monocytic series consists of monoblasts, promonocytes, and monocytes. They account for a small percentage of total marrow cells and cannot be reliably differentiated from early

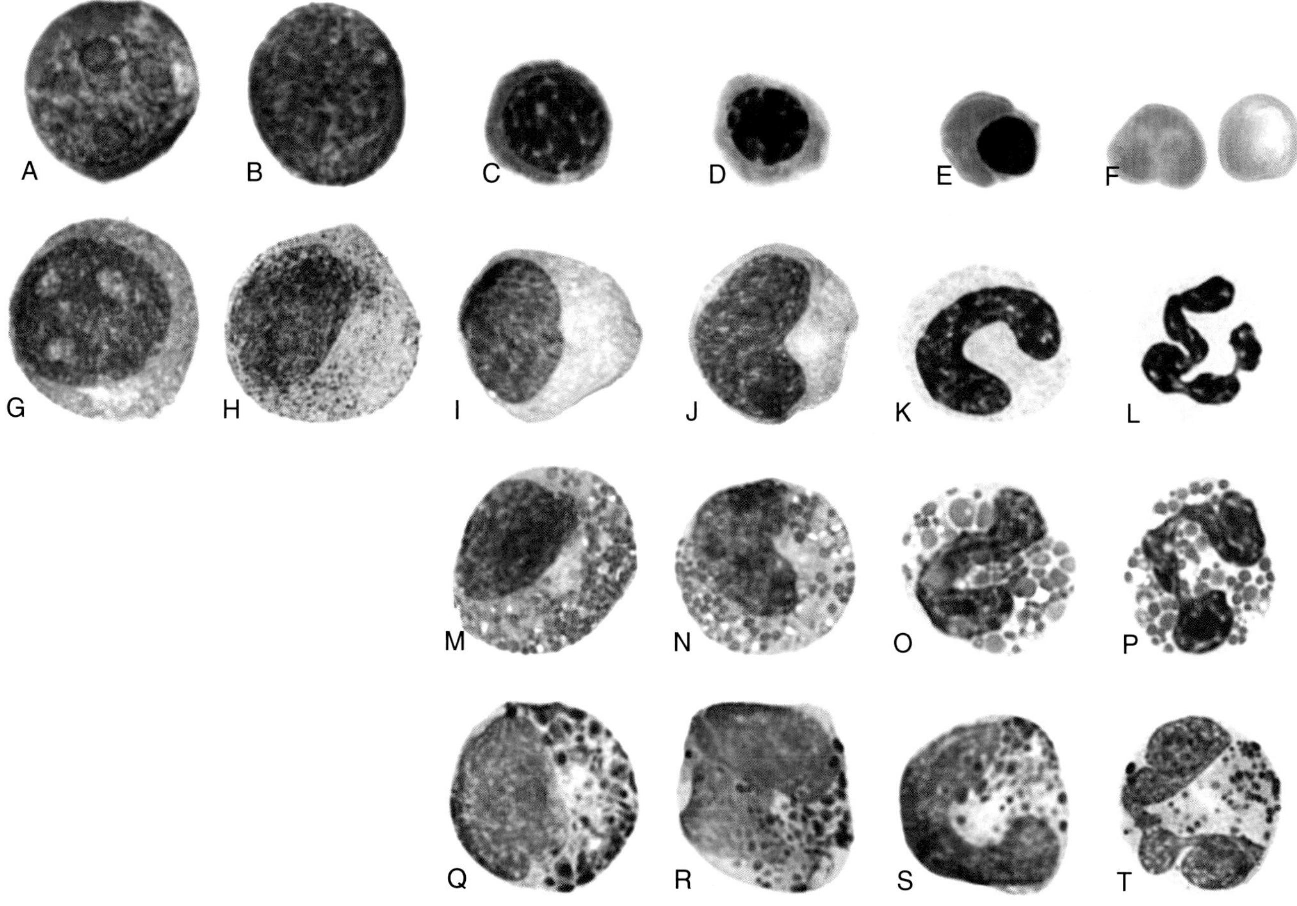

FIGURE 8-13

Maturation of erythroid and granulocytic cells in Wright-Giemsa-stained bone marrow aspirate smears from dogs. **A,** Rubriblast with intensely basophilic cytoplasm. The nucleus has finely clumped chromatin and contains at least three circular nucleoli. **B,** Prorubricyte with intensely basophilic cytoplasm and finely clumped nuclear chromatin. Nucleoli are not seen. **C,** Basophilic rubricyte with blue-staining cytoplasm and coarsely clumped nuclear chromatin. **D,** Polychromatophilic rubricyte with bluish-red (polychromatophilic) cytoplasm and coarsely clumped nuclear chromatin. **E,** Metarubricyte with polychromatophilic cytoplasm and a dark pyknotic nucleus. **F,** Polychromatophilic erythrocyte (reticulocyte) formed after nuclear extrusion *(left)* and a mature erythrocyte *(right).* **G,** Myeloblast with blue cytoplasm lacking clearly visible granules. The nucleus has finely clumped chromatin and contains three circular nucleoli. **H,** Promyelocyte with blue cytoplasm containing many magenta-staining granules. The nucleus has finely clumped chromatin without visible nucleoli. **I,** Neutrophilic myelocyte with light-blue cytoplasm and a round nucleus exhibiting moderately clumped chromatin. Neutrophilic granules do not stain. **J,** Neutrophilic metamyelocyte with light-blue cytoplasm and a kidney-shaped nucleus. **K,** Band neutrophil with light-pink cytoplasm. **L,** Mature neutrophil with segmented nucleus and nearly colorless cytoplasm. **M,** Eosinophilic myelocyte with a round nucleus and large numbers of eosinophilic granules in the cytoplasm. **N,** Eosinophilic metamyelocyte with a kidney-shaped nucleus and eosinophilic granules in the cytoplasm. **O,** Band eosinophil with eosinophilic granules in the cytoplasm. **P,** Mature eosinophil. **Q,** Basophilic myelocyte with a round nucleus and purple granules in the cytoplasm. **R,** Basophilic metamyelocyte with kidney-shaped nucleus and purple granules in the cytoplasm. **S,** Band basophil with purple granules in the cytoplasm. **T,** Mature basophil with segmented nucleus and purple granules in the cytoplasm. Wright-Giemsa stain.

granulocytic cells, except for promyelocytes, which have numerous magenta-staining granules. Monoblasts resemble myeloblasts except that their nuclear shape is irregularly round to convoluted in appearance (Fig. 8-15, *A*). Promonocytes are similar in appearance to myelocytes and metamyelocytes (Fig. 8-15, *B*). Monocytes in bone marrow are identical to those seen in peripheral blood (Fig. 8-15, *C*).

Macrophages

Macrophages are large cells with abundant cytoplasm and nuclei that are round to oval in shape with finely clumped chromatin (Fig. 8-16, *A*). The cytoplasm of macrophages generally contains vacuoles and phagocytized material such as pyknotic nuclear debris, hemosiderin, and, rarely, erythrocytes and leukocytes (Fig. 8-16, *B*). Hemosiderin in macrophages

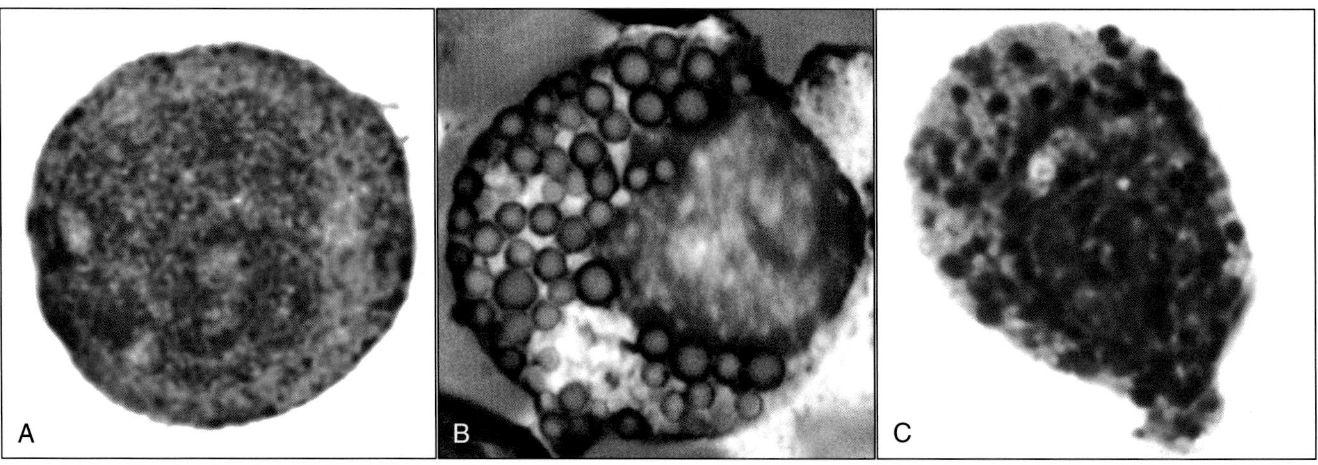

FIGURE 8-14

Myeloid precursor cells in bone marrow. **A,** Type III myeloblast from a dog containing numerous magenta-staining granules in the cytoplasm. Three nucleoli are visible within the nucleus. **B,** Eosinophilic myelocyte from a horse with a round nucleus and many large round granules in the cytoplasm. The granules stain bluish rather than having the bright red color that is characteristic of mature eosinophils. **C,** Basophilic myelocyte from a cat with a round nucleus and a mixture of purple and light lavender granules in the cytoplasm. Wright-Giemsa stain.

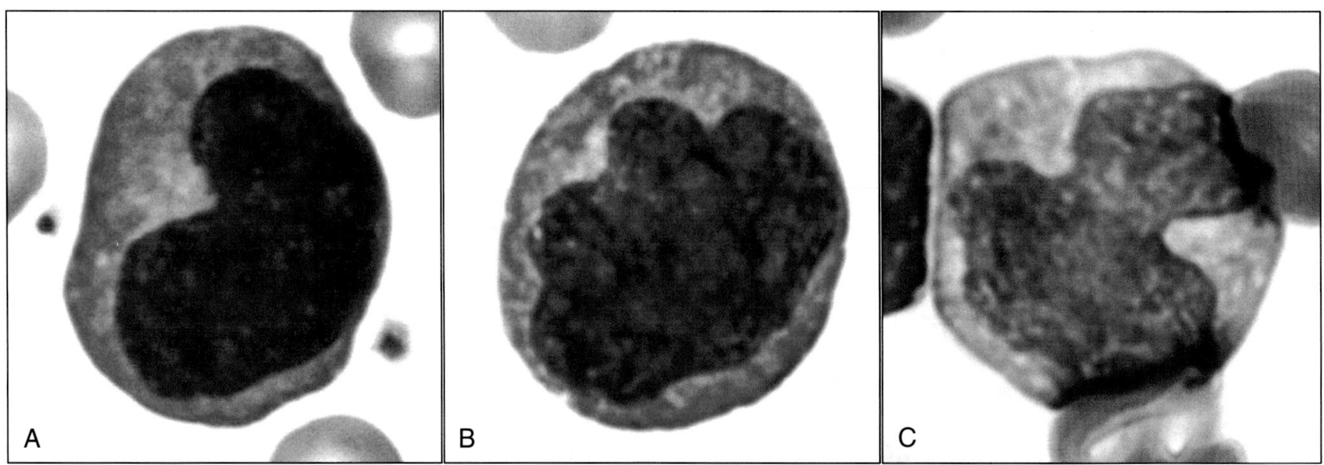

FIGURE 8-15

Monocyte development in dog bone marrow. **A,** Monoblast with basophilic cytoplasm and kidney-shaped nucleus containing nucleoli. **B,** Presumptive promonocyte with convoluted nucleus and basophilic cytoplasm. **C,** Monocyte with convoluted nucleus and lighter-blue cytoplasm. Wright-Giemsa stain.

appears gray to black when stained with routine blood stains. Although nucleated erythrocyte precursors develop around central macrophages in the marrow, these erythroid islands are rarely seen in aspirate smears (Fig. 8-17) because they are easily disrupted during aspiration and smear preparation.

Lymphocytes

Most bone marrow lymphocytes are small, with morphology identical to that seen in blood (Fig. 8-18, *A, B*). However, lymphopoiesis normally occurs in bone marrow; consequently, low numbers of lymphoblasts and prolymphocytes, as well as reactive lymphocytes, may be present (see Fig. 8-16, *A*).

Plasma Cells

Plasma cells are larger, have a lower N:C ratio, and have greater cytoplasmic basophilia than resting lymphocytes. The presence of a prominent Golgi apparatus may create a pale perinuclear area (Golgi zone) in the cytoplasm (see Fig. 8-18, *C*). They typically have eccentrically located nuclei with coarse chromatin clumping in a mosaic pattern. Plasma cells may

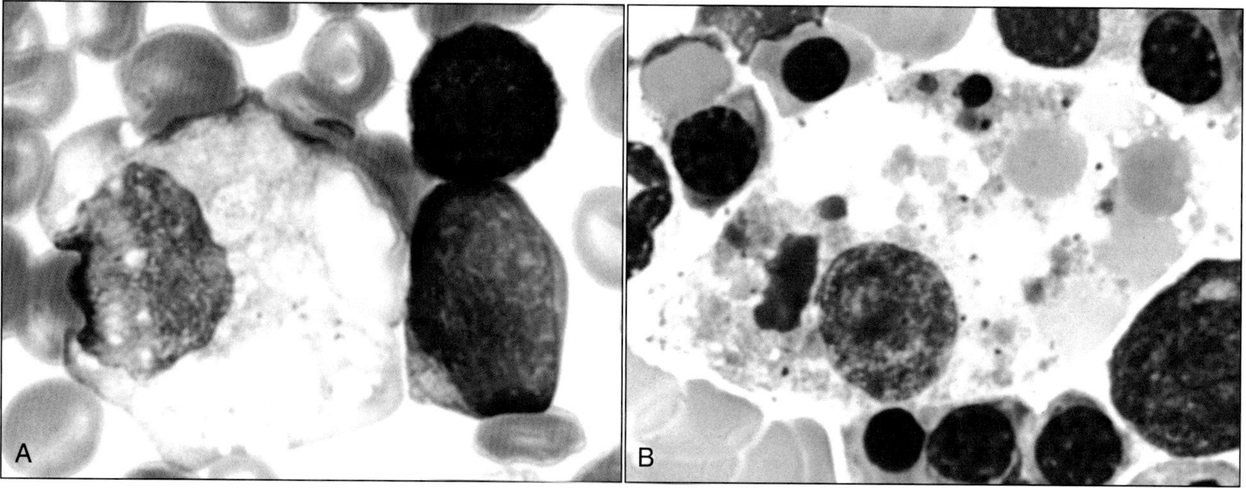

FIGURE 8-16
Macrophages in bone marrow aspirates from dogs. **A,** Foamy macrophage containing a lysed, phagocytized erythrocyte in the cytoplasm *(left)*, prolymphocyte or possible lymphoblast with a single nucleolus in the nucleus *(bottom right)*, and prorubricyte *(top right)*. **B,** Macrophage exhibiting erythrophagocytosis. The cytoplasm also contains nuclear debris and gray-staining material consistent with hemosiderin. Wright-Giemsa stain.

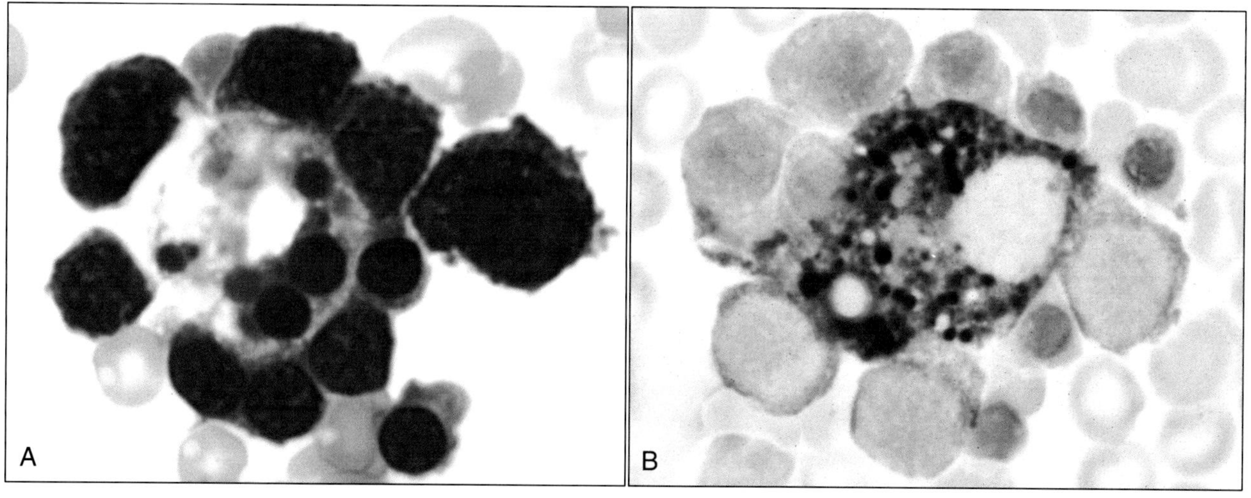

FIGURE 8-17
Erythroid islands in bone marrow aspirate smears. **A,** Erythroid island in bone marrow aspirate from a cat. A central macrophage with phagocytized material is surrounded by developing nucleated erythroid cells. Pale spots in some erythrocytes are Heinz bodies. Wright-Giemsa stain. **B,** Erythroid island in bone marrow aspirate from a dog. A central macrophage with phagocytized red-staining nuclear material is surrounded by developing nucleated erythroid cells. The cytoplasm of the macrophage stains dark blue, indicating the presence of large amounts of hemosiderin. Prussian blue stain.

rarely contain bluish or sometimes pinkish inclusions (Russell bodies) within the cytoplasm. These inclusions are usually round (see Fig. 8-18, *D, E*), but they may be needle-like (see Fig. 8-18, *F*) or appear to coalesce, filling the cytoplasm with material (see Fig. 8-18, *G*). These inclusions are composed of dilated rough endoplasmic reticulum containing immunoglobulin and other glycoproteins.[18,36] This appears to result from a defect in processing or transport of these proteins.[18] Plasma cells filled with Russell bodies have been called Mott cells. The cytoplasm of some plasma cells may stain reddish, especially at the periphery of the cell. These plasma cells have been called flame cells (see Fig. 8-18, *H*).[2,82]

FIGURE 8-18 **Lymphocytes and plasma cells from bone marrow aspirate smears from dogs**

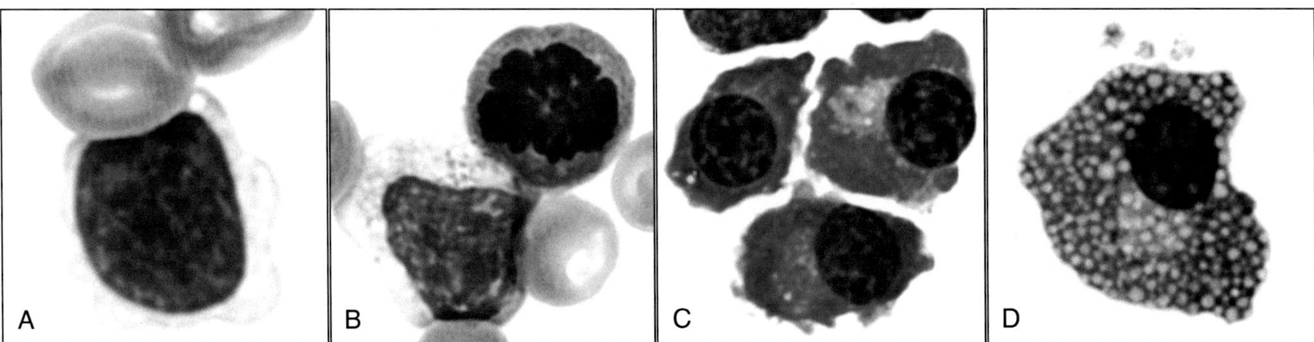

A, Small lymphocyte. **B,** Large granular lymphocyte *(bottom left)* and mitotic, polychromatophilic rubricyte *(top right).* **C,** Three plasma cells with voluminous, deeply basophilic cytoplasm, eccentric nuclei, and pale Golgi zones in their cytoplasm. The nuclei exhibit coarse chromatin clumping in a mosaic pattern. This image is of lower magnification than the other images in this figure. **D,** A plasma cell containing large numbers of small bluish inclusions (Russell bodies) within the cytoplasm.

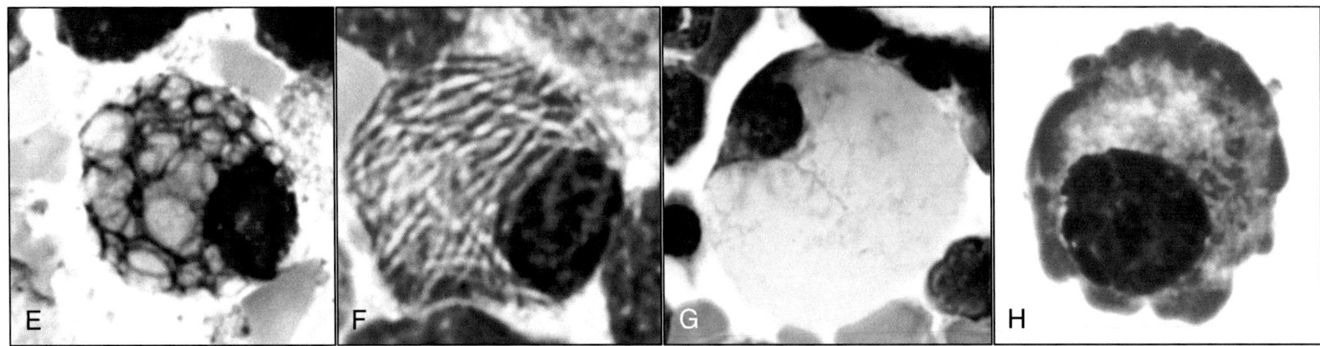

E, A plasma cell containing large bluish inclusions (Russell bodies) within the cytoplasm. **F,** A plasma cell with cytoplasm filled with blue-staining needle-like inclusions. **G,** A plasma cell with cytoplasm filled with turquoise-staining material. **H,** A plasma cell with cytoplasm that stained red at the periphery (flame cell). Wright-Giemsa stain.

Osteoclasts

Osteoclasts are multinucleated giant cells that phagocytize bone. They may be confused with megakaryocytes; however, the nuclei present in osteoclasts are clearly separate (Fig. 8-19, *A*), in contrast to the fused nuclear material present in megakaryocytes. The cytoplasm stains blue and often contains variably sized magenta-staining granular material associated with the removal and digestion of bone (Fig. 8-19, *B*). Osteoclasts are rarely seen in marrow aspirates from adult animals, but they may be present in disorders in which lysis of bone is increased, such as the hypercalcemia of malignancy.[49] When observed in histologic sections, they are located near bony surfaces (Fig. 8-20, *A*). Osteoclasts are consistently found in aspirates or in core biopsies from young growing animals in which bone remodeling is active (Fig. 8-20, *B*).

Osteoblasts

Osteoblasts are relatively large cells with eccentric nuclei and foamy basophilic cytoplasm (Fig. 8-21, *A,B*). A clear area (Golgi zone) may be visible in the central part of the cytoplasm. Superficially, osteoblasts appear similar to plasma cells, but they are larger and have less-condensed nuclear chromatin. Osteoblast nuclei are round to oval in shape, have reticular chromatin, and may have one or two nucleoli. Osteoblasts generally occur in groups lining trabecular surfaces (see Fig. 8-20, *A,B*) and tend to remain in small groups when present in aspirate smears (see Fig. 8-21, *A,B*).

Mitotic Figures

The bone marrow is actively producing new blood cells at all times, but mitosis itself is a brief part of the cell cycle. Consequently mitotic cells normally account for less than 2% of all nucleated cells in bone marrow (Figs. 8-18, *B;* 8-22, *A,B*). The origin of some mitotic cells may be identified by the characteristics of the cytoplasm—for example, the presence of hemoglobin or granules (see Fig. 8-22, *A, B*).

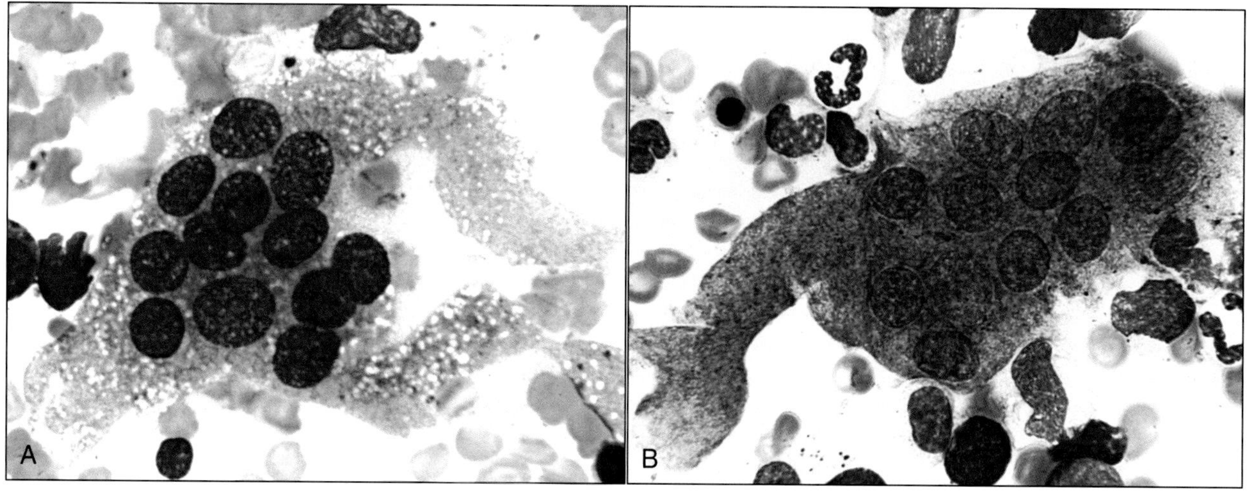

FIGURE 8-19
Osteoclasts in bone marrow from dogs. **A,** Multinucleated osteoclast in bone marrow aspirate. **B,** Multinucleated osteoclast in bone marrow aspirate. Wright-Giemsa stain.

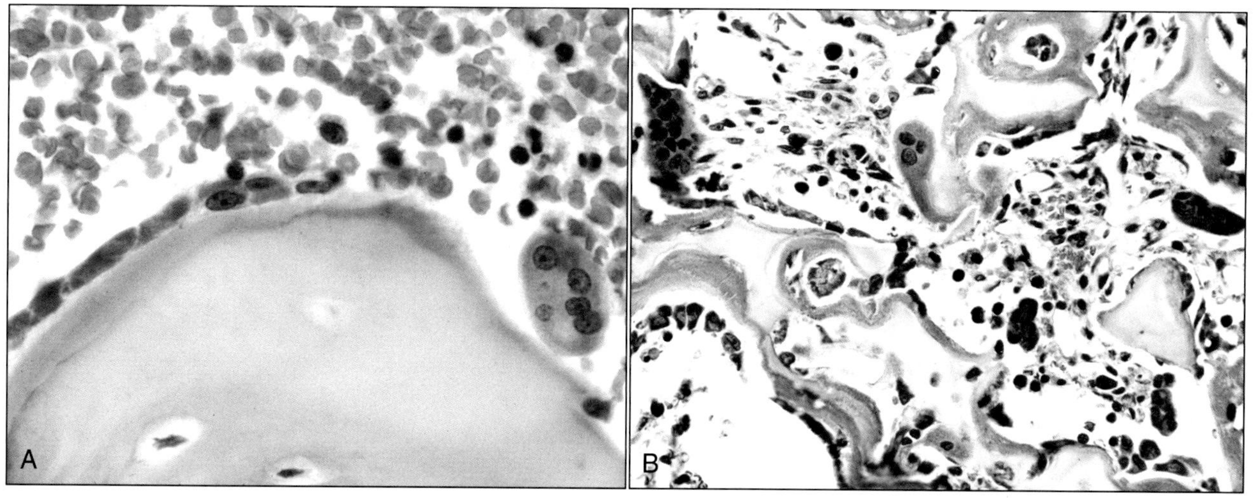

FIGURE 8-20
Osteoclasts and osteoblasts in bone marrow histopathology sections from dogs. **A,** Osteoclast *(multinucleated cell on right)* and osteoblasts *(line of adjacent cells on left)* along trabecular bone in a core bone marrow biopsy from a dog with generalized marrow hypoplasia secondary to severe chronic ehrlichiosis. **B,** Large multinucleated osteoclasts *(right, top left and top center)* and many osteoblasts lining the trabeculae in a young growing dog with ongoing ossification and bone remodeling. Bone and osteoid at the periphery of the trabeculae are pink, while the remaining central cartilage is pale. Decalcified bone, H&E stain.

***B,** Courtesy of Rose E. Raskin.*

Miscellaneous Cells and Free Nuclei

Vascular and connective tissue cells are usually ruptured during aspiration and smear preparation, although low numbers of intact cells may occasionally be seen (Fig. 8-23, *A,B*). Stromal cells are more obvious in aplastic bone marrow aspirates in which normal blood cell precursors are markedly reduced or absent (Fig. 8-24). Ruptured stromal cells account for some of the free nuclei found in bone marrow smears (see Fig. 8-22, *C-E*). Free nuclei also come from various other bone marrow cells, especially in smears made from clotted marrow, in thin smears, or in thin areas of smears where excess forces have destroyed the cells. Free nuclei from

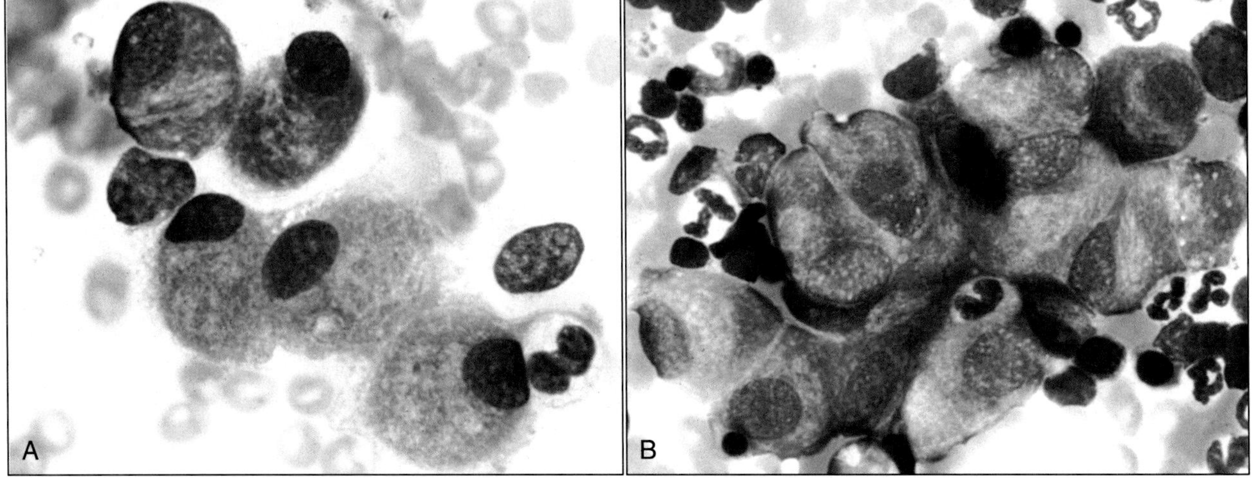

FIGURE 8-21

Clusters of osteoblasts in bone marrow aspirates from dogs. **A,** Five osteoblasts with eccentric nuclei and voluminous cytoplasm. **B,** Large clump of osteoblasts with eccentric nuclei and voluminous cytoplasm. Wright-Giemsa stain.

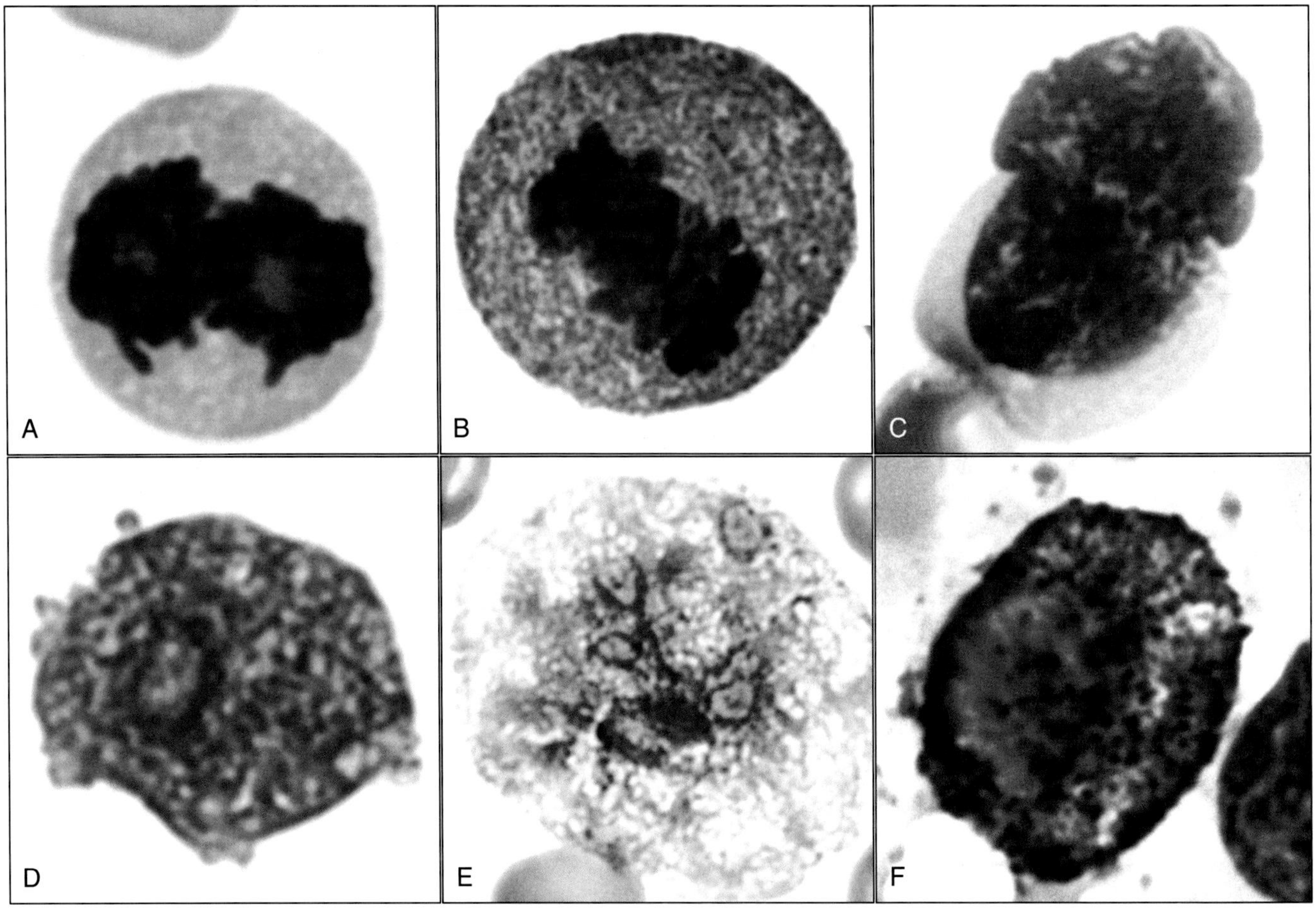

FIGURE 8-22

Mitotic cells, free nuclei, and a mast cell in bone marrow aspirates from dogs. **A,** Mitotic polychromatophilic rubricyte. **B,** Mitotic promyelocyte with numerous magenta-staining granules. **C,** Partially ruptured cell demonstrating the appearance of free nuclear material *(top right).* **D,** Reddish staining material is a free nucleus with some open spaces. The blue inclusion is a nucleolus. **E,** Reddish staining material is a free nucleus in which the chromatin is dispersed in a lacelike manner. This appearance has been called a basket cell even though it has no cytoplasm. **F,** Mast cell with round eccentric nucleus *(left part of cell)* and purple granules in the cytoplasm. Wright-Giemsa stain.

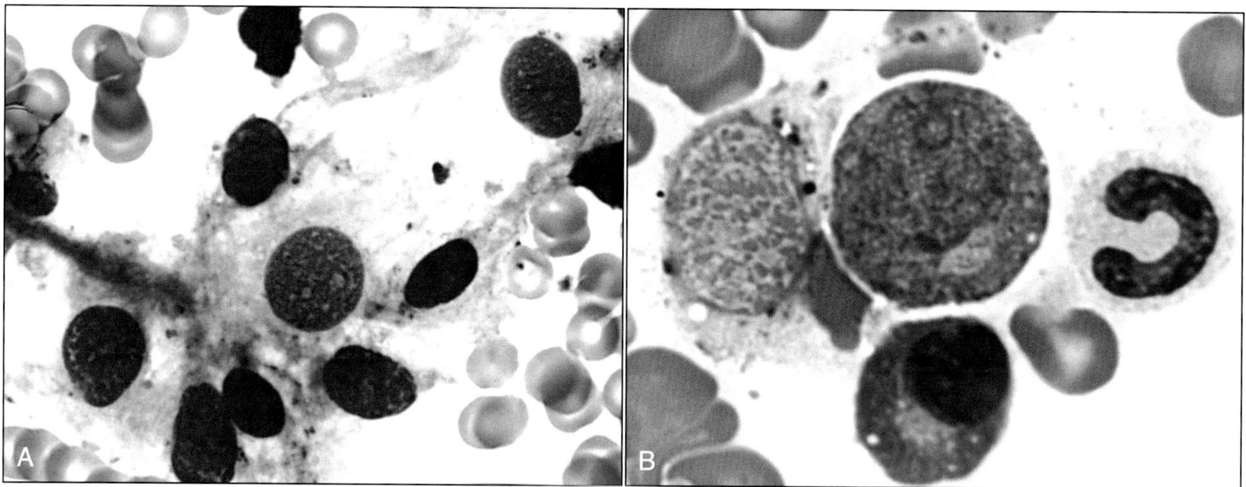

FIGURE 8-23
Stromal cells in bone marrow aspirate smears from dogs. **A,** Spindle-shaped stromal cells with "wispy" cytoplasm. **B,** An elongated stromal cell with "wispy" cytoplasm *(left),* a type III myeloblast with magenta-staining cytoplasmic granules and a single nucleolus in the nucleus *(center),* a band neutrophil *(right),* and a plasma cell *(bottom).* Wright-Giemsa stain.

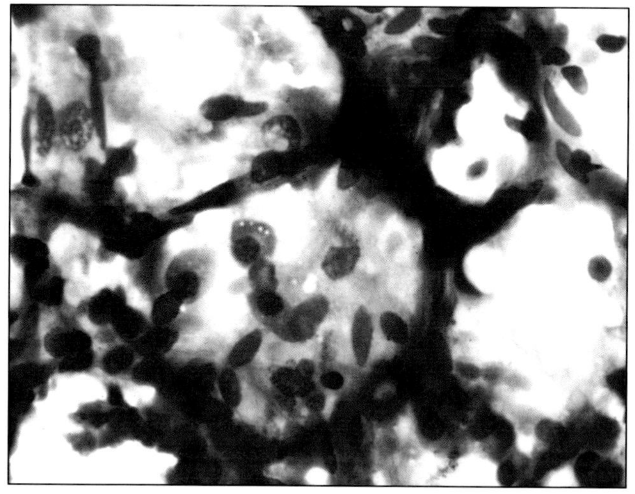

FIGURE 8-24
Residual stroma with three plasma cells *(below and left of center)* in bone marrow from a dog with aplastic anemia secondary to severe chronic ehrlichiosis. Variably sized unstained circular areas indicate where fat was dissolved away during alcohol fixation. The black-staining material is hemosiderin. Wright-Giemsa stain.

metarubricytes have been called hematogones. The term *basket cell* has been used to refer to free nuclei in which the chromatin is dispersed in a lacelike manner (see Fig. 8-22, *E*).

Adipocytes vary in size and number in bone marrow. Although normal marrow contains many adipocytes, these cells readily rupture during sample collection and smear preparation. Adipocytes appear as large vacuoles in marrow particles after the fat has been removed during smear fixation (see Figs. 8-8, 8-11).

Mast-cell precursors are produced in the bone marrow, but mature mast cells are seldom seen in normal bone marrow.[11] Mast cells are round cells with round nuclei. They typically have large numbers of purple granules in the cytoplasm (see Fig.8-22, *F*).

ORGANIZED APPROACH TO BONE MARROW EVALUATION

Smears and core biopsy sections should be scanned with low-power objectives to gain an appreciation of the overall cellularity and determine the adequacy of megakaryocyte numbers. Normal marrow appears heterogeneous. If some or all of a marrow smear or core section appears homogeneous, an abnormal population of cells is probably present. Regional infiltrates of neoplastic cells are more easily appreciated in core sections than in aspirate smears.

As a general rule, erythroid precursors are smaller, have more nearly spherical nuclei with more condensed nuclear chromatin, and have darker cytoplasm than do granulocyte precursors at similar maturational stages. Consequently smaller and darker cells, observed by scanning marrow smears at low power, are usually erythroid precursors unless lymphocytes are increased in numbers, and the larger, paler cells are usually granulocyte precursors. Identification of specific cell types is more difficult in core biopsy sections compared with aspirate smears; consequently sections may be stained with Giemsa and periodic acid-Schiff (PAS) in addition to H&E in an attempt to identify the cell types present.

Complete 500-cell differential cell counts from several normal domestic animal species are given in Table 8-1 to provide information concerning the normal distribution of

TABLE 8-1

Bone Marrow Differential Cell Counts in Some Domestic Animal Species

Cell Type	Dogs ($n = 6$)	Cats ($n = 7$)[a]	Horses ($n = 4$)[a]	Cattle ($n = 3$)[a]
Myeloblast	0.4-1.1	0-0.4	0.3-1.5	0-0.2
Promyelocyte	1.1-2.3	0-3.0	1.0-1.9	0-1.4
Neutrophilic myelocyte	3.1-6.1	0.6-8.0	1.9-3.2	2.8-3.4
Neutrophilic metamyelocyte	5.3-8.8	4.4-13.2	2.1-7.3	2.8-6.2
Neutrophilic band	12.7-17.2	12.8-16.6	6.8-14.7	4.6-8.4
Neutrophil	13.8-24.2	6.8-22.0	9.6-21.0	11.2-22.6
Total eosinophilic cells	1.8-5.6	0.8-3.2	2.8-6.8	2.8-3.8
Total basophilic cells	0-0.8	0-0.4	0-1.5	0-1.0
Rubriblast	0.2-1.1	0-0.8	0.6-1.1	0-0.2
Prorubricyte	0.9-2.2	0-1.6	1.0-2.0	0.4-1.2
Basophilic rubricyte	3.7-10.0	1.6-6.2	4.5-11.1	4.8-8.4
Polychromatophilic rubricyte	15.5-25.1	8.6-23.2	14.7-26.0	23.0-36.4
Metarubricyte	9.2-16.4	1.0-10.4	11.4-19.7	9.2-16.8
M:E ratio	0.9-1.76	1.21-2.16	0.52-1.45	0.61-0.97
Lymphocytes	1.7-4.9	11.6-21.6	1.8-6.7	3.6-6.0
Plasma cells	0.6-2.4	0.2-1.8	0.2-1.8	0.2-1.2
Monocytes	0.4-2.0	0.2-1.6	0-1.0	0.4-2.2
Macrophages	0-0.4	0-0.2	0	0-0.8

[a]Values for cats, horses and cattle from Jain, 1993.[36]
n = Number of animals evaluated.

cells. The time required to perform such counts (up to 1 hour) precludes their use in clinical practice. Either a modified differential count is performed or mental estimates concerning the distribution of cells may be made. Because veterinary students and residents are trained in our laboratory and information from our cases may be published, we routinely perform a modified differential, as shown in Appendix 1. Others may categorize cells into groups and use the values to calculate an erythroid maturation index (EMI) and myeloid maturation index (MMI).[33] Trained professionals, who regularly examine bone marrow aspirate smears, typically examine the bone marrow in a systematic manner, make a number of judgments based on their knowledge of the normal appearance of bone marrow, and record their finding in narrative form as presented here.

Cellularity

The cellularity of bone marrow is estimated by examining the proportion of cells versus fat present in particles. Normal cellularity varies between 25% and 75% cells, depending on the age of the animal (Fig. 8-25, *A,B*).[32] If the particles are composed of more than 75% cells, the marrow is interpreted as hypercellular (Fig. 8-26, *A,B*), and if the particles are composed of more than 75% fat, the marrow is interpreted as hypocellular (Fig. 8-27, *A,B*). Unfortunately the cellularity of the marrow is not uniform. Some marrow particles may have normal or high cellularity (Fig. 8-28, *A*) and others may have low cellularity (Fig. 8-28, *B*) in the same aspirate smear, because of patchy differences in cellularity (Fig. 8-29). Obviously the more particles one can evaluate, the more likely it will be that the estimate of overall marrow cellularity will be accurate. If few or no particles are present on smears, it is not possible to accurately estimate the marrow cellularity.

The overall cellularity of bone marrow decreases with age because of a loss of skeletal bone mass, resulting in increased marrow space.[57,66,81] The marrow is highly cellular in young growing animals, where cells must be produced not only to compensate for normal cell turnover, but also to respond to growth of the cardiovascular system. Marrow cellularity decreases with age because the ratio of bone marrow space to blood volume increases.

Marrow can become hypercellular when one or more cell types exhibit increased proliferation in response to peripheral needs, as occurs in response to anemia (erythroid hyperplasia) or purulent inflammation (granulocytic hyperplasia). The marrow may also become hypercellular secondary to dysplastic or neoplastic proliferations of marrow cells or from infiltration of neoplastic cells from peripheral tissues (e.g., a metastatic lymphoma). Defects in either the progenitor cells or the bone marrow microenvironment necessary for their survival and proliferation can result in hypocellular marrow (Fig. 8-27, *A,B*).

Megakaryocytes

The frequency and morphology of megakaryocytes should be evaluated by scanning areas of aspirate smears containing particles at low power using a 10× objective. Most large particles should have several associated megakaryocytes (Fig. 8-30), and normally 80% to 90% of megakaryocytes are of the granular, mature type.[45] Megakaryocytes are not evenly

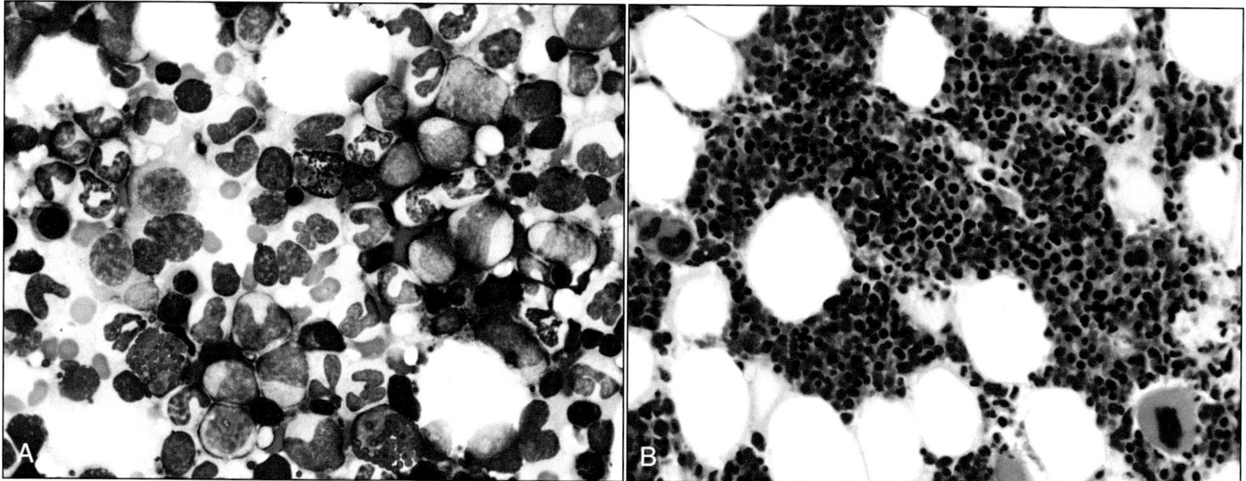

FIGURE 8-25
Normal cellularity in bone marrow from a horse. **A,** Bone marrow aspirate smear from a horse. No megakaryocytes are visible in this field. The unstained circular areas represent adipocytes dissolved away during alcohol fixation. Wright-Giemsa stain. **B,** Bone marrow section from a core biopsy collected from the same horse as the aspirate shown in **(A).** The unstained circular areas represent adipocytes dissolved away during fixation. Low magnification with H&E stain.

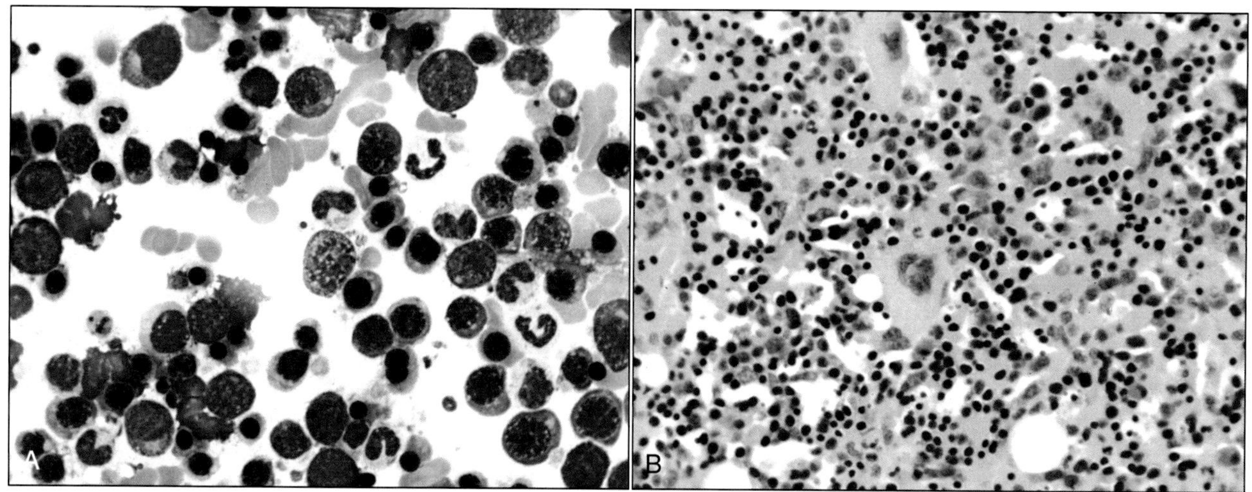

FIGURE 8-26
Increased cellularity in bone marrow from a horse with hemolytic anemia which may have been secondary to a lymphoid neoplasm. **A,** The increased cellularity visible in an aspirate smear resulted primarily from erythroid hyperplasia. The M:E ratio was 0.16. Wright-Giemsa stain. **B,** Bone marrow section from a core biopsy collected from the same horse as the aspirate shown in **(A).** The large cell near the center is a megakaryocyte. Clear areas indicate that a small amount of fat was present. Low magnification with H&E stain.

distributed in bone marrow; consequently it is difficult to estimate megakaryocyte numbers accurately in bone marrow aspirate smears. Multiple fields containing particles should be scanned to determine an average number of megakaryocytes per field. Examination of between 20 and 25 fields is required to achieve a coefficient of variation of 20%. According to one study, if less than 5 megakaryocytes are seen per low-power field using the 10× objective, megakaryocyte numbers are considered low. If 5 to 15 megakaryocytes are seen per low-power field, megakaryocyte numbers are likely normal; and if greater than 15 are seen per low-power field, megakaryocyte numbers are considered increased.[45] Others have suggested slightly different reference values, with less than 3 megakaryocytes per low-power field suggesting megakaryocytic hypoplasia and more than 10 to 20 megakaryocytes per low-power field suggesting megakaryocytic hyperplasia.[30] These guidelines apply only for particle-rich marrow aspirates because megakaryocytes tend to be associated with particles

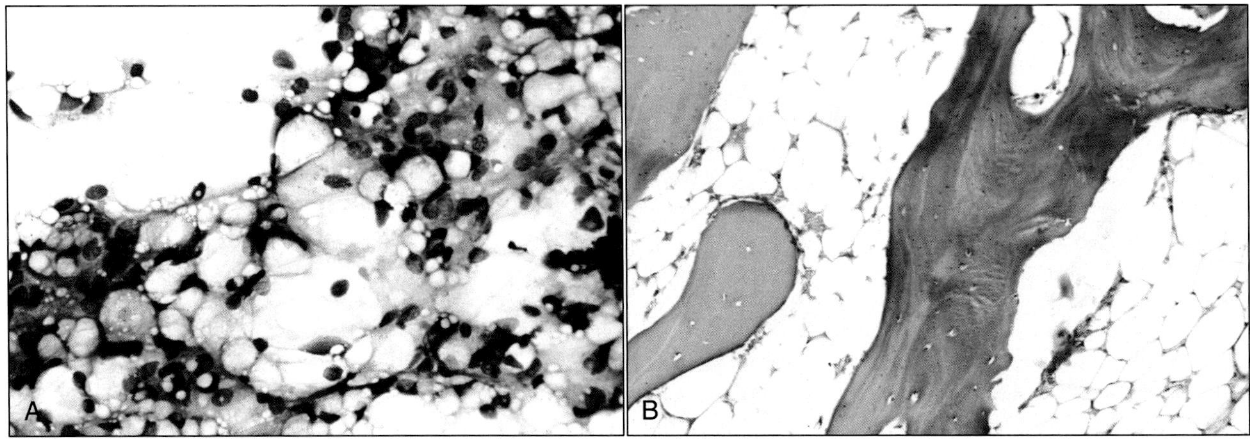

FIGURE 8-27

Low cellularity in bone marrow from a cat with aplastic anemia. **A,** Low cellularity in a bone marrow aspirate smear consisting primarily of stromal cells and fat, from a cat with an aplastic anemia following chemotherapy for an ocular lymphoma. Wright-Giemsa stain. **B,** Low cellularity in a bone marrow core biopsy section collected from the same cat as the aspirate shown in **(A).** The red-staining material is trabecular bone. Low magnification with H&E stain.

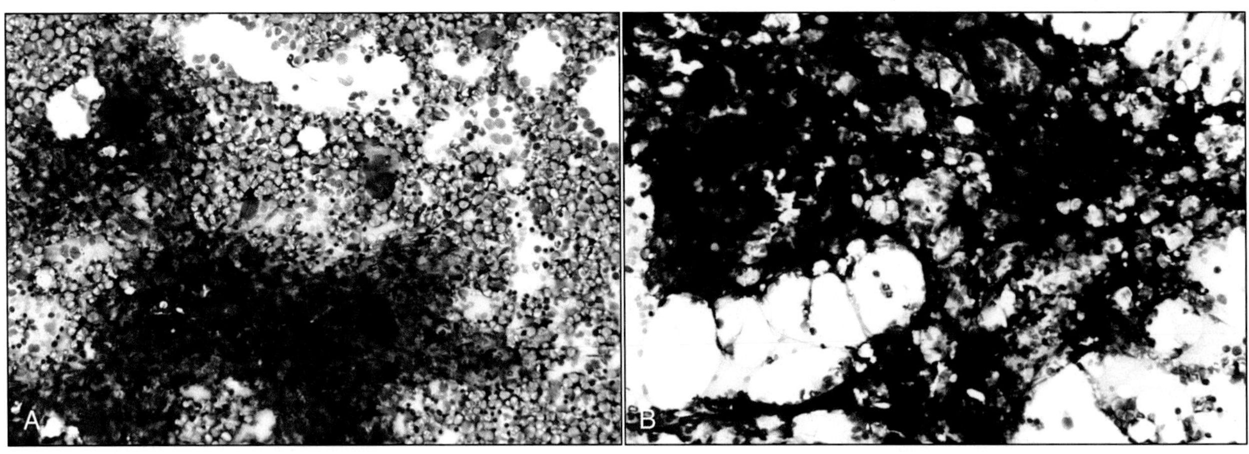

FIGURE 8-28

Variable cellularity in a bone marrow aspirate smear from a dog with *Ehrlichia canis* infection. **A,** High cellularity in one large marrow particle. **B,** Low cellularity in a different particle present in the same bone marrow aspirate smear as shown in **(A)**. Wright-Giemsa stain.

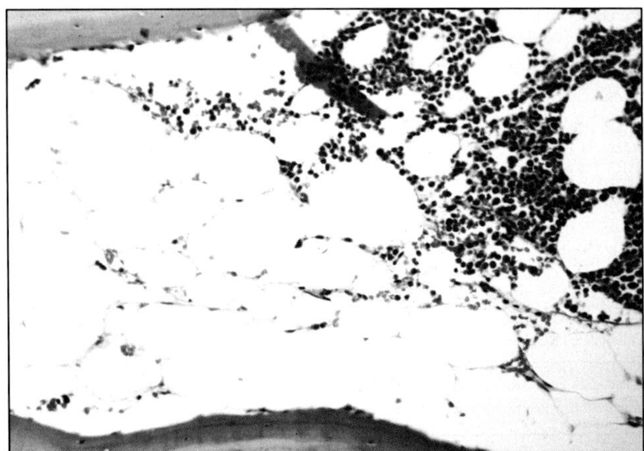

FIGURE 8-29

Variable cellularity in a section from a bone marrow core biopsy collected from the same dog as the aspirate particles shown in Figure 8-28 **(A)** and **(B)**. H&E stain.

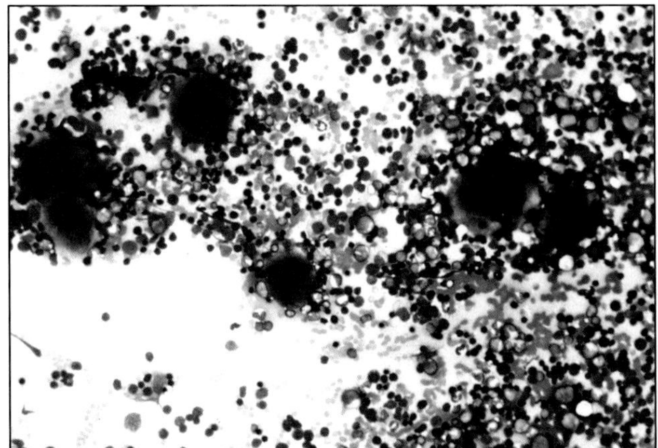

FIGURE 8-30

Five megakaryocytes are visible in a bone marrow aspirate particle from a dog. Wright-Giemsa stain.

in aspirate smears. Megakaryocyte numbers will be lower in marrow aspirates of poor quality. Abnormal megakaryocyte morphology (e.g., increased numbers of promegakaryocytes or the presence of dwarf megakaryocytes) should be noted when present.

Erythroid Cells

The maturation and morphology of the erythroid series should be evaluated to determine if it is complete (frequent polychromatophilic erythrocytes should be present) and orderly. There is generally a progressive increase in numbers with each stage of development, from low numbers of rubriblasts (generally less than 1%) to high numbers of polychromatophilic rubricytes, which may account for one quarter of all nucleated cells in the bone marrow.[36] Metarubricytes are numerous but generally not as numerous as polychromatophilic rubricytes.

Rubriblasts and prorubricytes usually do not exceed 5% of all nucleated cells. If the proportion of these immature cells is increased, this finding should be noted. An increase in mature as well as immature cells of the erythroid series is expected in response to anemia. If immature erythroid cells are increased and later stages are not, it suggests that a proliferative abnormality is present. Additional abnormal morphologic findings that should be recorded include megaloblastic cells, frequent binucleated cells, and pleomorphic nuclei.

Because reticulocytes are rarely released into blood in response to anemia in horses, reticulocyte counts can be done in bone marrow aspirates from horses to assist in the differential diagnosis of anemia. Greater than 5% reticulocytes suggests a regenerative response to anemia.[58]

Granulocytic Cells

The distribution of granulocytic cells should be evaluated to determine whether the series is complete (i.e., a normal number of mature granulocytes are present) and orderly. There is generally a progressive increase in numbers with each stage of development, from low numbers of myeloblasts (often less than 1%) to high numbers of mature neutrophils, which may account for nearly one-quarter of all nucleated cells in the bone marrow.[36] Myeloblasts and promyelocytes generally do not exceed 5% of all nucleated cells. If the proportion of these immature cells is increased, this finding should be noted. An increase in mature as well as immature cells of the myeloid series is expected in inflammatory disorders resulting in granulocytic hyperplasia. If immature granulocytic cells are increased and later stages are not, it indicates that either more mature cells have been depleted in the marrow granulocyte pool, as occurs in acute inflammation, or that a proliferative abnormality is present.[59] Morphologic abnormalities such as large cell size and vacuolated cytoplasm should be reported.

Total eosinophilic cells usually account for less than 6% of all nucleated cells in the marrow, with basophilic precursors generally accounting for less than 1% of all nucleated cells. Higher numbers of eosinophilic cells have been reported in llamas.[3] The increased representation of the eosinophilic or basophilic series should be recorded. An increase in one or both of these cell lines is usually associated with inflammatory conditions that result in increased numbers of eosinophils or basophils in blood and/or tissues. They may also be increased in association with some myeloid neoplasms.

TABLE 8-2

Normal Myeloid-to-Erythroid Ratios in Some Domestic Animal Species

Species	Range	Mean
Dog	0.75-2.53	1.25
Cat	1.21-2.16	1.63
Horse	0.50-1.50	0.93
Cow	0.31-1.85	0.71
Sheep	0.77-1.68	1.09
Pig	0.73-2.81	1.77

Values from Jain, 1993.[36]

Myeloid-to-Erythroid Ratio

A myeloid-to-erythroid (M:E) ratio (also referred to as a granulocytic-to-erythroid ratio) is calculated by examining 500 cells and dividing the number of granulocytic cells, including mature granulocytes, by the number of nucleated erythroid cells. Alternatively, this ratio may be estimated by experienced professionals. Normal M:E ratios in some domestic animals are given in Table 8-2. Dilution of a bone marrow aspirate with blood can result in a falsely high M:E ratio, especially if a substantial neutrophilia is present in blood.

Lymphocytes

Specific comments are in order regarding the number and morphology of lymphocytes. Small lymphocytes generally account for less than 10% of all nucleated cells in normal animals, but they may reach 14% in some healthy dogs[33,52] and 20% in some healthy cats.[36,66] Low numbers of lymphoblasts and prolymphocytes may be present, but they are difficult to differentiate from rubriblasts and prorubricytes. Small lymphoid follicles may be present in both normal and diseased animals examined by histopathology.[9,69]

Increased numbers of mature lymphocytes may be seen in bone marrow from animals with chronic lymphocytic leukemia (CLL), and increased numbers of small lymphocytes have been reported in the bone marrow of cats and dogs with erythroid aplasia and immune-mediated nonregenerative hemolytic anemia.[54,63,71,76] Increased numbers of small lymphocytes have also been reported in cats with a thymoma or cholangiohepatitis.[71] Lymphocytes in the bone marrow from cats with CLL tended to be somewhat larger, with cleaved or lobulated nuclei, compared with lymphocytes in bone marrow from cats with a reactive lymphocytosis. When examined by histopathology, lymphocytes tended to organize into lymphoid aggregates (primarily B lymphocytes) in cats with a reactive lymphocytosis. In contrast, proliferating lymphocytes (predominantly T lymphocytes) were diffusely distributed in the bone marrow of cats with a thymoma and cats and dogs with CLL.[54,71]

Increased numbers of prolymphocytes and/or lymphoblasts suggest the presence of either acute lymphoblastic leukemia or a metastatic lymphoma.[54] Glucocorticoid treatment results in the movement of recirculating lymphocytes from blood to bone marrow,[7,19] but the percentage of lymphocytes in the marrow does not appear to increase,[19,38] possibly because glucocorticoids can concomitantly decrease the population of proliferating lymphocytes normally present within the marrow.[19]

Plasma Cells

Plasma cells tend to be concentrated within particles on bone marrow smears. This uneven distribution prevents accurate counting. They are generally present in low numbers (less than 2% of all nucleated cells).[32] When plasma cells exceed 3% of total nucleated cells, they are considered to be increased. In addition to multiple myeloma,[51,73] increased numbers of plasma cells can occur in the bone marrow in dogs and cats with immune-mediated hemolytic anemia, immune-mediated thrombocytopenia, and erythroid aplasia.[72,76] Plasma cells are also increased in bone marrow in response to some infectious agents, including *E. canis* and visceral leishmaniasis (as high as 25% plasma cells) in dogs and feline infectious peritonitis in cats.[6,40] Increased plasma cells have been reported in rare cases of myelodysplasia in dogs.[79] Increased percentages of plasma cells have been described associated with estrogen-induced marrow damage in dogs[28]; however, it is unclear if the number of plasma cells is truly increased or if the percentage is only increased relative to the decreased number of hematopoietic cells.

Mononuclear Phagocytes

Monocytes and their precursors comprise a small portion (less than 3%) of bone marrow cells. They are difficult to differentiate from early granulocytic cells. Increased numbers of monocyte precursors may be present in response to inflammatory conditions, but the occurrence of high numbers of monoblasts indicates that a myeloid neoplasm is present.

Macrophages generally do not exceed 1% of total nucleated cells in the bone marrow of normal animals. Macrophages may be increased in the bone marrow with necrotic, granulomatous inflammatory, and neoplastic (histiocytic sarcoma) conditions.[24,46,70,77] Infectious agents may be present within macrophages in conditions such as leishmaniasis, histoplasmosis, mycobacteriosis, and cytauxzoonosis.[14,15,22,30]

Prominent phagocytosis of nucleated and/or anucleated erythrocytes by macrophages may occur in association with primary or secondary immune-mediated anemias,[76] blood parasites (e.g., *Babesia, Cytauxzoon, Leishmania, Trypanosoma,* and hemoplasma species),[22,30,42] hemophagocytic histiocytic sarcoma,[24,46] the hemophagocytic syndrome,[68,75] following blood transfusion,[30] and in acquired and congenital dyserythropoiesis.[13,34,80] Prominent leukophagocytosis is rare but may be seen in association with immune-mediated neutropenia or when increased marrow apoptosis is present, as occurs in myeloid neoplasms.[8,56] Phagocytized leukocytes may also be seen with the hemophagocytic syndrome.[75] Macrophages may contain phagocytized cellular debris in response to marrow necrosis.[20,61,70] Macrophages can phagocytize damaged or dead cells not coated with antibody or complement because of the presence of scavenger receptors on their surfaces that are capable of recognizing altered carbohydrate and/or phospholipid moieties.[64]

Other Cell Types

Comments should always be made concerning the cell types listed above, if only to report that they are present in normal numbers with normal morphology. Comments are generally made only concerning cell types listed below when they are present in increased numbers.

Mitotic figures are increased when the proportion of cells undergoing replication in the bone marrow is increased. Mitotic figures may be somewhat increased in myeloid or erythroid hyperplasia, but they are more consistently increased in acute myeloid and acute lymphoblastic leukemias. Dramatically increased numbers of mitotic erythroid cells occur within the first few hours after the administration of vincristine (Fig. 8-31),[1] and increased numbers of mitotic figures have been reported in animals with congenital dyserythropoiesis.[34,62]

Osteoclasts and osteoblasts are commonly seen in bone marrow aspirates of young growing animals but are rarely seen in normal adult animals. Increased numbers of osteoclasts and osteoblasts may be seen in adult animals when bone remodeling is increased, as in disorders with increased parathyroid concentrations, and in association with osteosarcomas.[16,43]

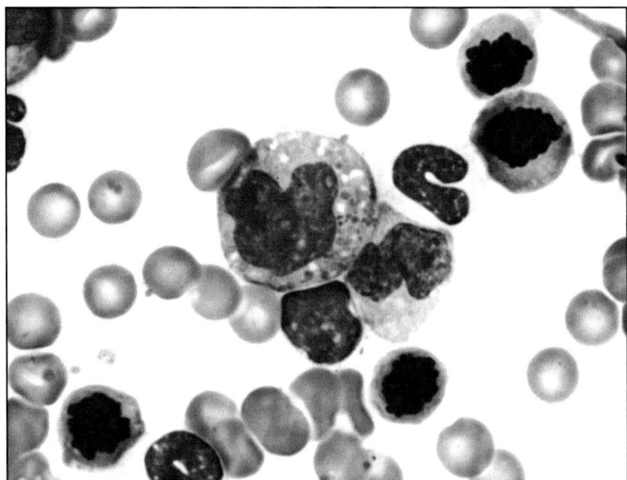

FIGURE 8-31
Four mitotic polychromatophilic erythroid cells are present in bone marrow from a dog 6 hours after an intravenous vincristine treatment. The largest cell in the center is an eosinophilic metamyelocyte. Wright-Giemsa stain.

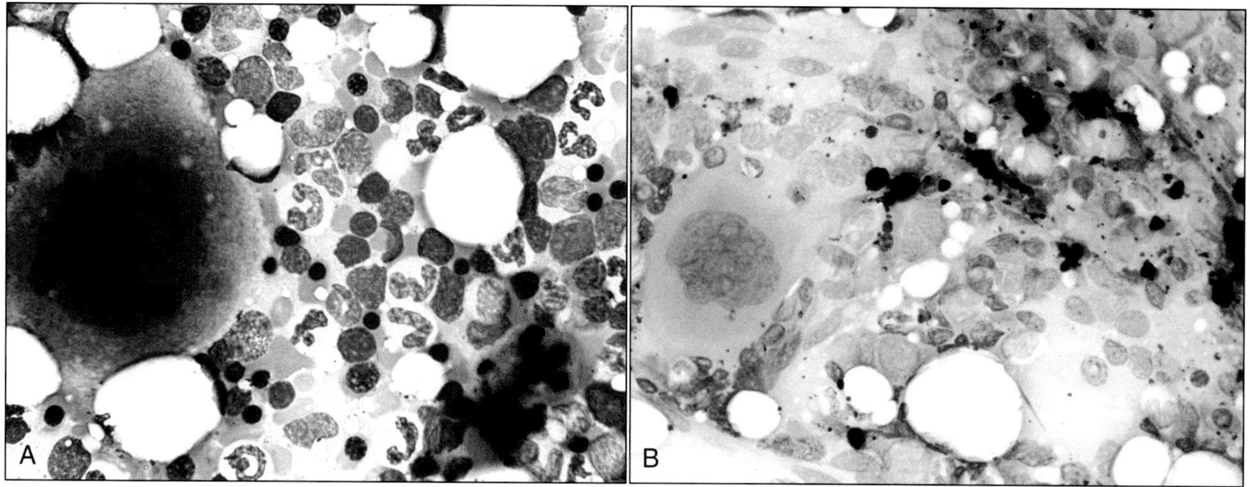

FIGURE 8-32
Bone marrow aspirate from a dog demonstrating the appearance of hemosiderin with Wright-Giemsa and Prussian blue stains. **A,** Hemosiderin is visible as black globules in the bottom right. A mature megakaryocyte is present at the left edge. Wright-Giemsa stain. **B,** Hemosiderin is visible as blue-staining material. A mature megakaryocyte is present at the left edge. Prussian blue stain.

Mast cells are rarely seen in the bone marrow from normal domestic animals, but they may occur in dogs with aplastic anemia of various etiologies.[11,48,67] They may also be present in some inflammatory conditions. The administration of interleukin-3 and interleukin-6 together, but neither factor alone, results in marrow mast-cell development in rats.[60] Mast cells may also occur in the marrow of animals with metastatic mast cell tumors.[44,50] Bone marrow involvement is especially likely in noncutaneous systemic mastocytosis, as occurs most frequently in cats.[17,27,39,41,50]

Increased numbers of reticular stromal cells suggest that stromal hyperplasia and/or myelofibrosis is present. A core biopsy is essential to confirm these suspicions.

Metastatic cells from nonhematopoietic sarcomas or carcinomas are rarely recognized in bone marrow biopsies but should be reported when present.[73]

Stainable Iron

Hemosiderin appears gray to black when stained with routine blood stains. It may be seen within macrophages or as free material from ruptured macrophages (Fig. 8-32, *A*). The Prussian blue stain is used to evaluate bone marrow hemosiderin stores. Smears may be sent to a commercial laboratory for this stain, or a stain kit can be purchased and applied in-house (Harleco Ferric Iron Histochemical Reaction Set, #6498693, EM Diagnostic Systems, Gibbstown, NJ). When this stain is applied, iron-positive material stains blue, in contrast to the dark pink color of the cells and background (Fig. 8-32, *B*). Stainable iron is easily found in normal marrow aspirates from most domestic mammals including llamas as long as particles are present.[3] Using the Prussian blue stain, a good-quality marrow aspirate smear with at least nine particles has been recommended to adequately access marrow hemosiderin stores in macrophages.[35]

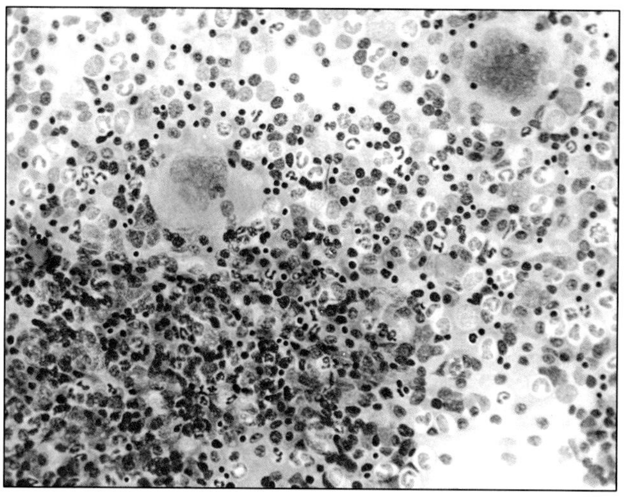

FIGURE 8-33
Lack of stainable iron (hemosiderin) in a bone marrow aspirate from a dog with chronic iron-deficiency anemia. Two megakaryocytes are visible in the upper portion of the image. Prussian blue stain.

Determination of stainable iron in bone marrow is used as a measure of total body iron stores. [10,23] A lack of stainable iron is consistent with iron deficiency (Fig. 8-33); however, negative iron staining is not necessarily predictive of iron deficiency.[26] Cats normally lack stainable iron in their marrow.[9,31] Stainable iron may be absent in dogs and humans with polycythemia vera.[65,69] In addition, some cattle (especially younger animals) lack stainable iron in the marrow even though marrow iron can be demonstrated by a chemical assay.[10] Cattle that lack stainable iron generally have lower marrow iron concentrations when these are measured chemically than cattle with a positive iron stain. Similarly, recently

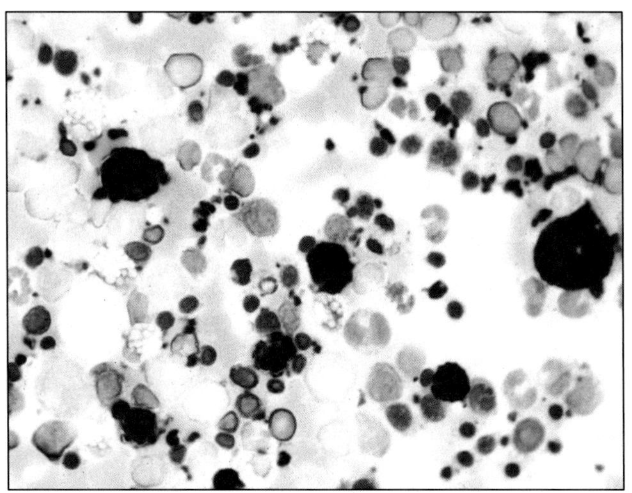

FIGURE 8-34

A large amount of stainable iron *(blue-staining material)* is present in a bone marrow aspirate from a normal aged horse. Prussian blue stain.

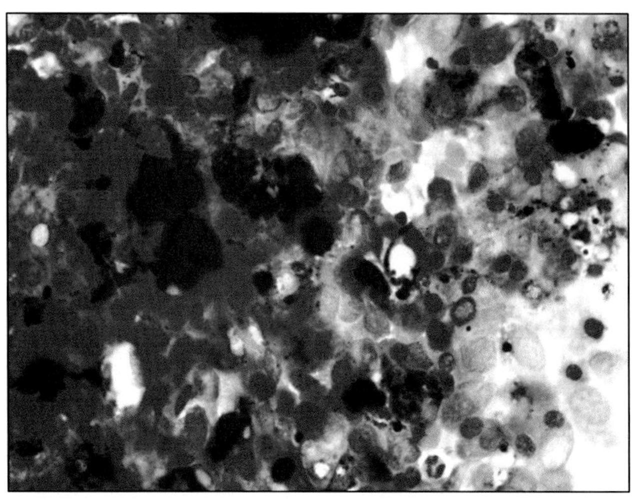

FIGURE 8-35

Increased stainable iron *(blue-staining material)* in a bone marrow aspirate from a dog with a hemolytic anemia. Prussian blue stain.

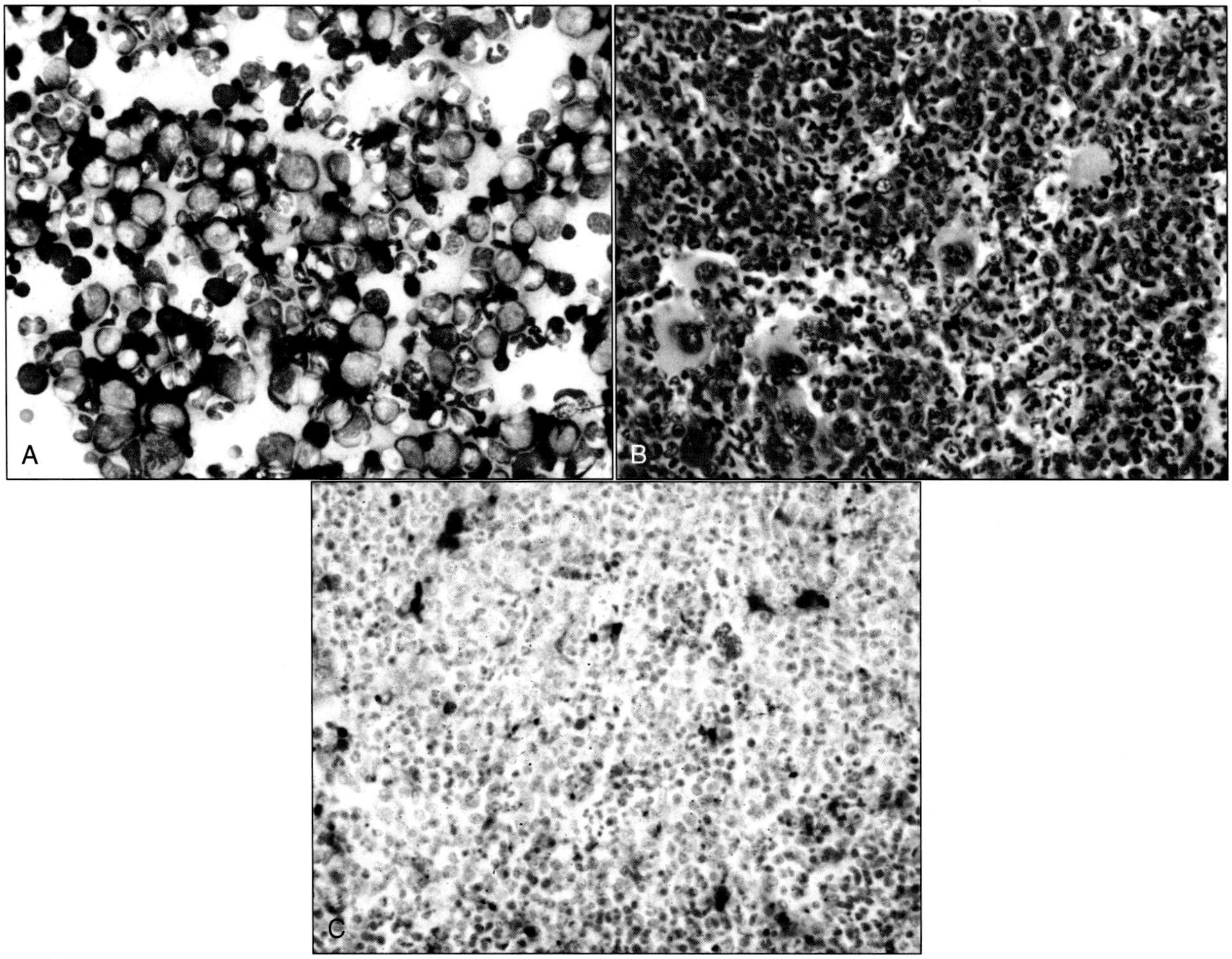

FIGURE 8-36

Generalized hypercellularity with increased hemosiderin in bone marrow from a cat with myelodysplastic syndrome (MDS). **A,** Aspirate smear of bone marrow from a cat with MDS. A left shift in both granulocytic and erythroid series is present. Wright-Giemsa stain. **B,** Postmortem bone marrow section from the same cat with MDS as presented in **(A).** Several megakaryocytes are present in the central area and in the lower left of the image. H&E stain. **C,** Prominent stainable iron (blue-staining material) in a postmortem bone marrow section collected from the same cat with MDS presented in **(A)** and **(B)**. Prussian blue stain.

weaned dogs have little or no stainable iron in their marrow, presumably reflecting low iron stores at the end of the nursing period.[25] Stainable iron in the marrow tends to increase with advancing age in humans, dogs, horses, and cattle.[10,23,33] This phenomenon appears to be especially prominent in old horses, which can have marked amounts of stainable iron present in the bone marrow (Fig. 8-34). Stainable iron in bone marrow is generally increased in animals with hemolytic anemia (Fig. 8-35) and dyserythropoiesis, in which phagocytosis of erythroid cells is increased,[13,34,62,78] and in animals with anemia resulting from decreased erythrocyte production, including the anemia of inflammatory disease.[21] The presence of stainable iron is considered an abnormal finding in cats and may be detected in some animals with myeloid neoplasms (Fig. 8-36, *A-C*), hemolytic anemias, or after blood transfusions.[9,31,63]

Interpretation

The final step in evaluating a bone marrow aspirate is to provide an interpretation of the cytologic findings in light of the history, clinical findings, CBC, and results from other diagnostic tests and procedures. For example, a high M:E ratio could indicate the presence of either increased granulocytic cells or decreased erythroid cells. Examination of CBC results from blood collected at the same time, as well as an estimate of the overall cellularity, usually allows the correct interpretation to be made. Bone marrow examination generally provides information concerning the pathogenesis of abnormalities recognized in blood, and sometimes a specific diagnosis can be made.

REFERENCES

1. Alleman AR, Harvey JW. The morphologic effects of vincristine sulfate on canine bone marrow cells. *Vet Clin Pathol.* 1993;22:36-41.
2. Altman DH, Meyer DJ, Thompson JP, et al. Canine IgG_{2c} myeloma with Mott and flame cells. *J Am Anim Hosp Assoc.* 1991;27:419-423.
3. Andreasen CB, Gerros TC, Lassen ED. Evaluation of bone marrow cytology and stainable iron content in healthy adult llamas. *Vet Clin Pathol.* 1994;23:38-42.
4. Andrews CM. The preparation of bone marrow smears from femurs obtained at autopsy. *Comp Haematol Int.* 1991;1:229-232.
5. Berggren PC. Aplastic anemia in a horse. *J Am Vet Med Assoc.* 1981;179:1400-1402.
6. Binhazim AA, Chapman WL Jr, Latimer KS, et al. Canine leishmaniasis caused by *Leishmania leishmania infantum* in two Labrador retrievers. *J Vet Diagn Invest.* 1992;4:299-305.
7. Bloemena E, Weinreich S, Schellekens PTA. The influence of prednisolone on the recirculation of peripheral blood lymphocytes *in vivo*. *Clin Exp Immunol.* 1990;80:460-466.
8. Bloom JC, Thiem PA, Sellers TS, et al. Cephalosporin-induced immune cytopenia in the dog: demonstration of erythrocyte-, neutrophil-, and platelet-associated IgG following treatment with cefazedone. *Am J Hematol.* 1988;28:71-78.
9. Blue JT. Myelofibrosis in cats with myelodysplastic syndrome and acute myelogenous leukemia. *Vet Pathol.* 1988;25:154-160.
10. Blum JW, Zuber U. Iron stores of liver, spleen and bone marrow, and serum iron concentrations in female dairy cattle in relationship to age. *Res Vet Sci.* 1975;18:294-298.
11. Bookbinder PF, Butt MT, Harvey HJ. Determination of the number of mast cells in lymph node, bone marrow, and buffy coat cytologic specimens from dogs. *J Am Vet Med Assoc.* 1992;200:1648-1650.
12. Brunning RD, Bloomfield CD, McKenna RW, et al. Bilateral trephine bone marrow biopsies in lymphoma and other neoplastic diseases. *Ann Intern Med.* 1975;82:365-366.
13. Canfield PJ, Watson ADJ, Ratcliffe RCC. Dyserythropoiesis, sideroblasts/siderocytes and hemoglobin crystallization in a dog. *Vet Clin Pathol.* 1987;16(1):21-28.
14. Clinkenbeard KD, Cowell RL, Tyler RD. Disseminated histoplasmosis in cats: 12 cases (1981-1986). *J Am Vet Med Assoc.* 1987;190:1445-1448.
15. Clinkenbeard KD, Cowell RL, Tyler RD. Disseminated histoplasmosis in dogs: 12 cases (1981-1986). *J Am Vet Med Assoc.* 1988;193:1443-1447.
16. Cook SD, Skinner HB, Haddad RJ. A quantitative histologic study of osteoporosis produced by nutritional secondary hyperparathyroidism in dogs. *Clin Orthop Relat Res.* 1983;105-120.
17. Davies AP, Hayden DW, Klausner JS, et al. Noncutaneous systemic mastocytosis and mast cell leukemia in a dog: case report and literature review. *J Am Anim Hosp Assoc.* 1981;17:361-368.
18. El-Okda M, Ko YH, Xie SS, et al. Russell bodies consist of heterogenous glycoproteins in B-cell lymphoma cells. *Am J Clin Pathol.* 1992;97:866-871.
19. Fauci AS. Mechanisms of corticosteroid action on lymphocyte subpopulations. I. Redistribution of circulating T and B lymphocytes to the bone marrow. *Immunology.* 1975;28:669-680.
20. Felchle LM, McPhee LA, Kerr ME, et al. Systemic lupus erythematosus and bone marrow necrosis in a dog. *Can Vet J.* 1996;37:742-744.
21. Feldman BF, Kaneko JJ, Farver TB. Anemia of inflammatory disease in the dog: ferrokinetics of adjuvant-induced anemia. *Am J Vet Res.* 1981;42:583-585.
22. Foglia MV, Restucci B, Pagano A, et al. Pathological changes in the bone marrow of dogs with leishmaniosis. *Vet Rec.* 2006;158:690-694.
23. Franken P, Wensing T, Schotman AJ. The concentration of iron in the liver, spleen and plasma, and the amount of iron in bone marrow of horses. *Zentralbl Veterinarmed A.* 1981;28:381-389.
24. Friedrichs KR, Young KM. Histiocytic sarcoma of macrophage origin in a cat: case report with a literature review of feline histiocytic malignancies and comparison with canine hemophagocytic histiocytic sarcoma. *Vet Clin Pathol.* 2008;37:121-128.
25. Fry MM, Kirk CA. Reticulocyte indices in a canine model of nutritional iron deficiency. *Vet Clin Pathol.* 2006;35:172-181.
26. Ganti AK, Moazzam N, Laroia S, et al. Predictive value of absent bone marrow iron stores in the clinical diagnosis of iron deficiency anemia. *In Vivo.* 2003;17:389-392.
27. Garner FM, Lingeman CH. Mast-cell neoplasms in the domestic cat. *Pathol Vet.* 1970;7:517-530.
28. Gaunt SD, Pierce KR. Effect of estradiol on hematopoietic and marrow adherent cells of dogs. *Am J Vet Res.* 1986;47:906-909.
29. Grindem CB. Bone marrow biopsy and evaluation. *Vet Clin North Am Small Anim Pract.* 1989;19:669-696.
30. Grindem CB, Tyler RD, Cowell RL. The bone marrow. In: Cowell RL, Tyler RD, Meinkoth JH, et al, eds. *Diagnostic Cytology and Hematology of the Dog and Cat.* 3rd ed. St. Louis: Mosby Elsevier; 2008:422-450.
31. Harvey JW. Myeloproliferative disorders in dogs and cats. *Vet Clin North Am Small Anim Pract.* 1981;11:349-381.
32. Harvey JW. Canine bone marrow: normal hematopoiesis, biopsy techniques, and cell identification and evaluation. *Comp Cont Ed Pract Vet.* 1984;6:909-926.
33. Hoff B, Lumsden JH, Valli VE. An appraisal of bone marrow biopsy in assessment of sick dogs. *Can J Comp Med.* 1985;49:34-42.
34. Holland CT, Canfield PJ, Watson ADJ, Allan GS. Dyserythropoiesis, polymyopathy, and cardiac disease in three related English springer spaniels. *J Vet Intern Med.* 1991;5:151-159.
35. Hughes DA, Stuart-Smith SE, Bain BJ. How should stainable iron in bone marrow films be assessed? *J Clin Pathol.* 2004;57:1038-1040.
36. Jain NC. *Essentials of Veterinary Hematology.* Philadelphia: Lea & Febiger; 1993.
37. Jain NC, Blue JT, Grindem CB, et al. Proposed criteria for classification of acute myeloid leukemia in dogs and cats. *Vet Clin Pathol.* 1991;20:63-82.
38. Jasper DE, Jain NC. The influence of adrenocorticotropic hormone and prednisolone upon marrow and circulating leukocytes in the dog. *Am J Vet Res.* 1965;26:844-850.
39. Khan KN, Sagartz JE, Koenig G, et al. Systemic mastocytosis in a goat. *Vet Pathol.* 1995;32:719-721.
40. Kuehn NF, Gaunt SD. Clinical and hematologic findings in canine ehrlichiosis. *J Am Vet Med Assoc.* 1985;186:355-358.
41. Liska WD, MacEwen EG, Zaki FA, et al. Feline systemic mastocytosis: a review and results of splenectomy in seven cases. *J Am Anim Hosp Assoc.* 1979;15:589-597.
42. Longan-Henfrey LL, Anosa VO, Wells CW. The role of the bone marrow in bovine trypanotolerance. II. Macrophage function in *Trypanosoma congolense*-infected cattle. *Comp Haematol Int.* 1999;9:208-218.
43. Malluche HH, Matthews C, Faugere MC, et al. 1,25-Dihydroxyvitamin D maintains bone cell activity, and parathyroid hormone modulates bone cell number in dogs. *Endocrinology.* 1986;119:1298-1304.
44. Marconato L, Bettini G, Giacoboni C, et al. Clinicopathological features and outcome for dogs with mast cell tumors and bone marrow involvement. *J Vet Intern Med.* 2008;22:1001-1007.

45. Mischke R, Busse L, Bartels D, et al. Quantification of thrombopoietic activity in bone marrow aspirates of dogs. *Vet J.* 2002;164:269-274.
46. Moore PF, Affolter VK, Vernau W. Canine hemophagocytic histiocytic sarcoma: a proliferative disorder of CD11d+ macrophages. *Vet Pathol.* 2006;43:632-645.
47. Moritz A, Bauer NB, Weiss DJ, et al. Evaluation of bone marrow. In: Weiss DJ, Wardrop KJ, eds. *Schalm's Veterinary Hematology.* 6th ed. Ames, IA: Wiley-Blackwell; 2010,
48. Mylonakis ME, Koutinas AF, Leontides LS. Bone marrow mastocytosis in dogs with myelosuppressive monocytic ehrlichiosis *(Ehrlichia canis)*: a retrospective study. *Vet Clin Pathol.* 2006;35:311-314.
49. Norrdin RW, Powers BE. Bone changes in hypercalcemia of malignancy in dogs. *J Am Vet Med Assoc.* 1983;183:441-444.
50. O'Keefe DA, Couto CG, Burke-Schwartz C, et al. Systemic mastocytosis in 16 dogs. *J Vet Intern Med.* 1987;1:75-80.
51. Patel RT, Caceres A, French AF, et al. Multiple myeloma in 16 cats: a retrospective study. *Vet Clin Pathol.* 2005;34:341-352.
52. Penny RH, Carlisle CH. The bone marrow of the dog: a comparative study of biopsy material obtained from the iliac crest, rib and sternum. *J Small Anim Pract.* 1970;11:727-734.
53. Perman V, Osborne CA, Stevens JB. Bone marrow biopsy. *Vet Clin North Am.* 1974;4:293-310.
54. Raskin RE, Krehbiel JD. Histopathology of canine bone marrow in malignant lymphoproliferative disorders. *Vet Pathol.* 1988;25:83-88.
55. Raskin RE, Krehbiel JD. Prevalence of leukemic blood and bone marrow in dogs with multicentric lymphoma. *J Am Vet Med Assoc.* 1989;194:1427-1429.
56. Raza A, Mundle S, Iftikhar A, et al. Simultaneous assessment of cell kinetics and programmed cell death in bone marrow biopsies of myelodysplastics reveals extensive apoptosis as the probable basis for ineffective hematopoiesis. *Am J Hematol.* 1995;48:143-154.
57. Rozman C, Reverter JC, Feliu E, et al. Variations of fat tissue fractions in abnormal human bone marrow depend both on size and number of adipocytes: a stereologic study. *Blood.* 1990;76:892-895.
58. Russell KE, Sellon DC, Grindem CB. Bone marrow in horses: indications, sample handling, and complications. *Comp Cont Ed Pract Vet.* 1994;16:1359-1365.
59. Schalm OW, Lasmanis J. Cytologic features of bone marrow in normal and mastitic cows. *Am J Vet Res.* 1976;37:359-363.
60. Sheridan WP, Hunt P, Simonet S, et al. Hematologic effects of cytokines. In: Remick DG, Friedland JS, eds. *Cytokines in Health and Disease.* 2nd ed. New York: Marcel Dekker; 1997:487-505.
61. Shimoda T, Shiranaga N, Mashita T, et al. Bone marrow necrosis in a cat infected with feline leukemia virus. *J Vet Med Sci.* 2000;62:113-115.
62. Steffen DJ, Elliott GS, Leipold HW, et al. Congenital dyserythropoiesis and progressive alopecia in Polled Hereford calves: hematologic, biochemical, bone marrow cytologic, electrophoretic, and flow cytometric findings. *J Vet Diagn Invest.* 1992;4:31-37.
63. Stokol T, Blue JT. Pure red cell aplasia in cats: 9 cases (1989-1997). *J Am Vet Med Assoc.* 1999;214:75-79.
64. Terpstra V, van Berkel TJC. Scavenger receptors on liver Kupffer cells mediate the in vivo uptake of oxidatively damaged red cells in mice. *Blood.* 2000;95:2157-2163.
65. Thiele J, Zankovich R, Schneider G, et al. Primary (essential) thrombocythemia versus polycythemia vera rubra. A histomorphometric analysis of bone marrow features in trephine biopsies. *Anal Quant Cytol Histol.* 1988;10:375-382.
66. Tyler RD, Cowell RL, Meador V. Bone marrow evaluation. In: August JR, ed. *Consultations in Feline Internal Medicine 2.* Philadelphia: Saunders; 1994:515-523.
67. Walker D, Cowell RL, Clinkenbeard KD, et al. Bone marrow mast cell hyperplasia in dogs with aplastic anemia. *Vet Clin Pathol.* 1997;26:106-111.
68. Walton RM, Modiano JF, Thrall MA, et al. Bone marrow cytological findings in 4 dogs and a cat with hemophagocytic syndrome. *J Vet Intern Med.* 1996;10:7-14.
69. Weiss DJ. Histopathology of canine nonneoplastic bone marrow. *Vet Clin Pathol.* 1986;15(2):7-11.
70. Weiss DJ. Bone marrow necrosis in dogs: 34 cases (1996-2004). *J Am Vet Med Assoc.* 2005;227:263-267.
71. Weiss DJ. Differentiating benign and malignant causes of lymphocytosis in feline bone marrow. *J Vet Intern Med.* 2005;19:855-859.
72. Weiss DJ. A retrospective study of the incidence and classification of bone marrow disorders in cats (1996-2004). *Comp Clin Pathol.* 2006;14:179-185.
73. Weiss DJ. A retrospective study of the incidence and the classification of bone marrow disorders in the dog at a veterinary teaching hospital (1996-2004). *J Vet Intern Med.* 2006;20:955-961.
74. Weiss DJ. Acute bone marrow stromal injury in the dog. *J Comp Pathol.* 2007;16:223-228.
75. Weiss DJ. Hemophagocytic syndrome in dogs: 24 cases (1996-2005). *J Am Vet Med Assoc.* 2007;230:697-701.
76. Weiss DJ. Bone marrow pathology in dogs and cats with non-regenerative immune-mediated haemolytic anaemia and pure red cell aplasia. *J Comp Pathol.* 2008;138:46-53.
77. Weiss DJ, Greig B, Aird B, et al. Inflammatory disorders of bone marrow. *Vet Clin Pathol.* 1992;21:79-84.
78. Weiss DJ, Lulich J. Myelodysplastic syndrome with sideroblastic differentiation in a dog. *Vet Clin Pathol.* 1999;28:59-63.
79. Weiss DJ, Raskin RE, Zerbe C. Myelodysplastic syndrome in two dogs. *J Am Vet Med Assoc.* 1985;187:1038-1040.
80. Weiss DJ, Reidarson TH. Idiopathic dyserythropoiesis in a dog. *Vet Clin Pathol.* 1989;18:43-46.
81. Williams EA, Kelly PJ. Age-related changes in bone in the dog: calcium homeostasis. *J Orthop Res.* 1984;2:8-14.
82. Zinkl JG, LeCouteur RA, Davis DC, et al. "Flaming" plasma cells in a dog with IgA multiple myeloma. *Vet Clin Pathol.* 1983;12(3):15-19.

CHAPTER

9

DISORDERS OF BONE MARROW

GENERALIZED INCREASES IN HEMATOPOIETIC CELLS

The marrow is highly cellular in young growing animals because cells must be produced in response to the growth of the cardiovascular system, as well as to compensate for normal cell turnover. Marrow cellularity decreases with age because the ratio of bone marrow space to blood volume increases.

Bone marrow is generally considered to be hypercellular when more than 75% of the space consists of hematopoietic cells.[168] This estimate is easily performed in core bone marrow biopsy specimens, but is more challenging in bone marrow aspirate smears that have variable amounts of blood contamination. In aspirate smears, the cellularity is generally determined by examining as many marrow particles (spicules) as possible and estimating the area occupied by cells versus the area occupied by fat.

Marrow can become hypercellular when one or more cell lines exhibit increased proliferation in response to peripheral needs or demands. For example, both erythrocytic and granulocytic cell lines may be increased in immune-mediated hemolytic anemia (IMHA) in dogs, in which animals often exhibit a regenerative anemia with accompanying leukocytosis and left shift.[409] Megakaryocytic hyperplasia can occur if immune-mediated thrombocytopenia (IMT) is present. In a retrospective study of dogs, panhyperplasia of bone marrow was observed most frequently in association with mast cell tumors, lymphomas, and blood loss anemia.[508] Hypercellularity was exhibited in bone marrow from a dog that had blood-loss iron deficiency anemia with an associated thrombocytosis (Fig. 9-1) and from a dog that had inherited erythrocyte phosphofructokinase deficiency with an accompanying neutrophilia (Fig. 9-2). Panhyperplasia has been reported in the bone marrow of cats with IMHA, IMT, and feline leukemia virus (FeLV)-associated anemia.[507] Although rare, generalized marrow hyperplasia may occur in response to cytopenias in blood resulting from hypersplenism.[423,523] Generalized hypercellular marrow may be present in some animals with myelodysplastic disorders, but abnormalities in cell morphology and/or distributions are present (see Fig. 8-36, *A-C*). Primary erythrocytosis (polycythemia vera) may sometimes exhibit a generalized marrow hyperplasia.[231,500]

GENERALIZED DECREASES IN HEMATOPOIETIC CELLS

Hypocellular/Aplastic Bone Marrow

Bone marrow is generally considered to be hypocellular when less than 25% of the space consists of hematopoietic cells.[168] This estimate is easily performed in core bone marrow biopsy specimens but is more challenging in bone marrow aspirate smears that have variable amounts of blood contamination. In aspirate smears, the cellularity is generally determined by examining as many marrow particles as possible and estimating the area occupied by hematopoietic cells versus the area occupied by fat. However, it should be recognized that fat may not have replaced hematopoietic cells in some disorders, including acute marrow injury with necrosis and edema, gelatinous transformation of bone marrow, and myelofibrosis.

When all hematopoietic cell types—erythrocytic, granulocytic, and megakaryocytic—are markedly reduced or absent, the marrow is said to be aplastic; anemic animals with generalized marrow aplasia are said to have an aplastic anemia (Fig. 9-3, *A,B*). Stromal cells (adipocytes, reticular cells, endothelial cells, and macrophages), plasma cells, and some lymphocytes are still present in aplastic bone marrow samples (Fig. 9-3, *C*). Macrophages typically contain increased amounts of hemosiderin because storage iron is not utilized for erythrocyte production (Fig. 9-3, *C,D*). Mast cells may also be present in moderate numbers in aplastic bone marrow samples in dogs (Fig. 9-3, *C*).[42,332,489] The peripheral blood is characterized by a nonregenerative anemia, neutropenia, and thrombocytopenia.

When only one cell line is reduced or absent, more restrictive terms, such as *granulocytic hypoplasia* or *erythroid aplasia,* are used to describe the abnormalities present. Hypocellular or aplastic bone marrow is associated with markedly reduced numbers of hematopoietic stem cells and progenitor cells. The

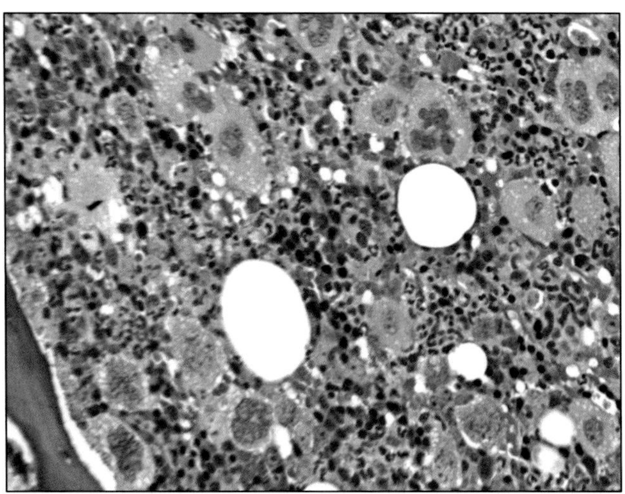

FIGURE 9-1
Hypercellular core bone marrow biopsy from a dog with iron-deficiency anemia. Megakaryocytic hyperplasia resulted in a peripheral thrombocytosis. H&E stain.

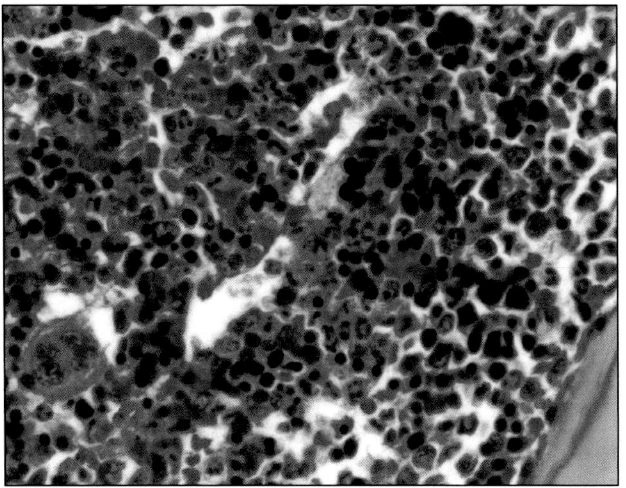

FIGURE 9-2
Hypercellular core bone marrow biopsy from a dog with erythrocyte phosphofructokinase deficiency. A megakaryocyte is present *(lower left)*. H&E stain.

nature of the abnormalities resulting in deficient stem cells and progenitor cells is usually unknown.

The majority of cases of aplastic anemia in humans are idiopathic; however, viruses, chemicals, and idiosyncratic reactions to certain drugs have been associated with some human cases.[228] Most cases of aplastic anemia in humans appear to be mediated by a T lymphocyte immune reaction against hematopoietic stem cells. A drug or virus may trigger the expansion of cytotoxic T lymphocytes, resulting in the destruction of hematopoietic stem cells. Interferons (especially interferon-γ) and tumor necrosis factor-α (TNF-α) produced by these cells can induce apoptosis in $CD34^+$ hematopoietic progenitor cells, which may contribute to hematopoietic suppression in humans with aplastic anemia.[550] A primary immune-mediated reaction directed against hematopoietic precursor cells has also been proposed as a cause of aplastic anemia in dogs.[489]

Drug-induced causes of aplastic anemia or generalized marrow hypoplasia in animals include estrogen toxicity in dogs[438]; phenylbutazone toxicity in dogs[498,527] and possibly a horse[104]; trimethoprim-sulfadiazine administration in dogs[130,515,527]; bracken fern poisoning in cattle and sheep[354,432]; trichloroethylene-extracted soybean meal in cattle[449]; albendazole administration in dogs, cats, and juvenile alpacas[159,448,522]; fenbendazole administration in a dog[142]; griseofulvin toxicity in cats and possibly a dog[47,178,402]; azathioprine toxicity[198,393,515]; various cancer chemotherapeutic agents[363,400,501,523]; and radiation.[339,417,418] Meclofenamic acid and quinidine have also been incriminated as potential causes of aplastic anemia in dogs.[527] Other drugs are believed to be myelosuppressive, causing multiple cytopenias, but bone marrow was not evaluated to demonstrate aplasia.[515]

Exogenous estrogen injections can result in aplastic anemia in dogs, as can high levels of endogenous estrogens produced by Sertoli cell, interstitial cell, and granulosa cell tumors.[302,325,427,450] Functional cystic ovaries also have the potential of inducing myelotoxicity in dogs.[55] Ferrets have induced ovulations and may remain in estrus for long periods of time when not bred. This prolonged exposure to high endogenous estrogen concentrations can result in aplastic anemia.[30,236]

Parvovirus infections can cause erythroid hypoplasia as well as myeloid hypoplasia in canine pups,[370,395] but the animals may not become anemic because of the long life spans of erythrocytes. Thrombocytopenia is mild or absent because megakaryocytes may still be present in the bone marrow (Fig. 9-4, *A,B*). Either affected pups die acutely or the bone marrow returns rapidly to normal before anemia can develop. In contrast to its effects in pups, parvovirus is reported to have a minimal effect on erythroid progenitors in adult dogs.[54] Only myeloid hypoplasia was reported during histologic examination of bone marrow from parvovirus-infected viremic cats in early studies[252,255]; however, in a later study, generalized marrow aplasia has been reported in naturally infected cats that died.[53]

Although some degree of marrow hypoplasia and/or dysplasia often occurs in cats with FeLV infections,[86] true aplastic anemia is not a well-documented sequela.[399] Hypocellular bone marrow has been reported in experimental cats coinfected with FeLV and feline parvovirus.[277]

Aplastic anemia with resultant pancytopenia and depletion of lymphoid tissues has been reported in neonatal calves in Europe. Prominent clinical signs included mucosal petechial hemorrhages, cutaneous bleeding, melena, and high fever. A viral etiology was suspected, but viral isolation was not successful. Polymerase chain reaction (PCR) assays for bovine viral diarrhea (BVD), bluetongue, and epizootic hemorrhagic disease virus were also negative.[352]

Dogs with acute *Ehrlichia canis* infections may recover spontaneously or develop chronic disease, which generally

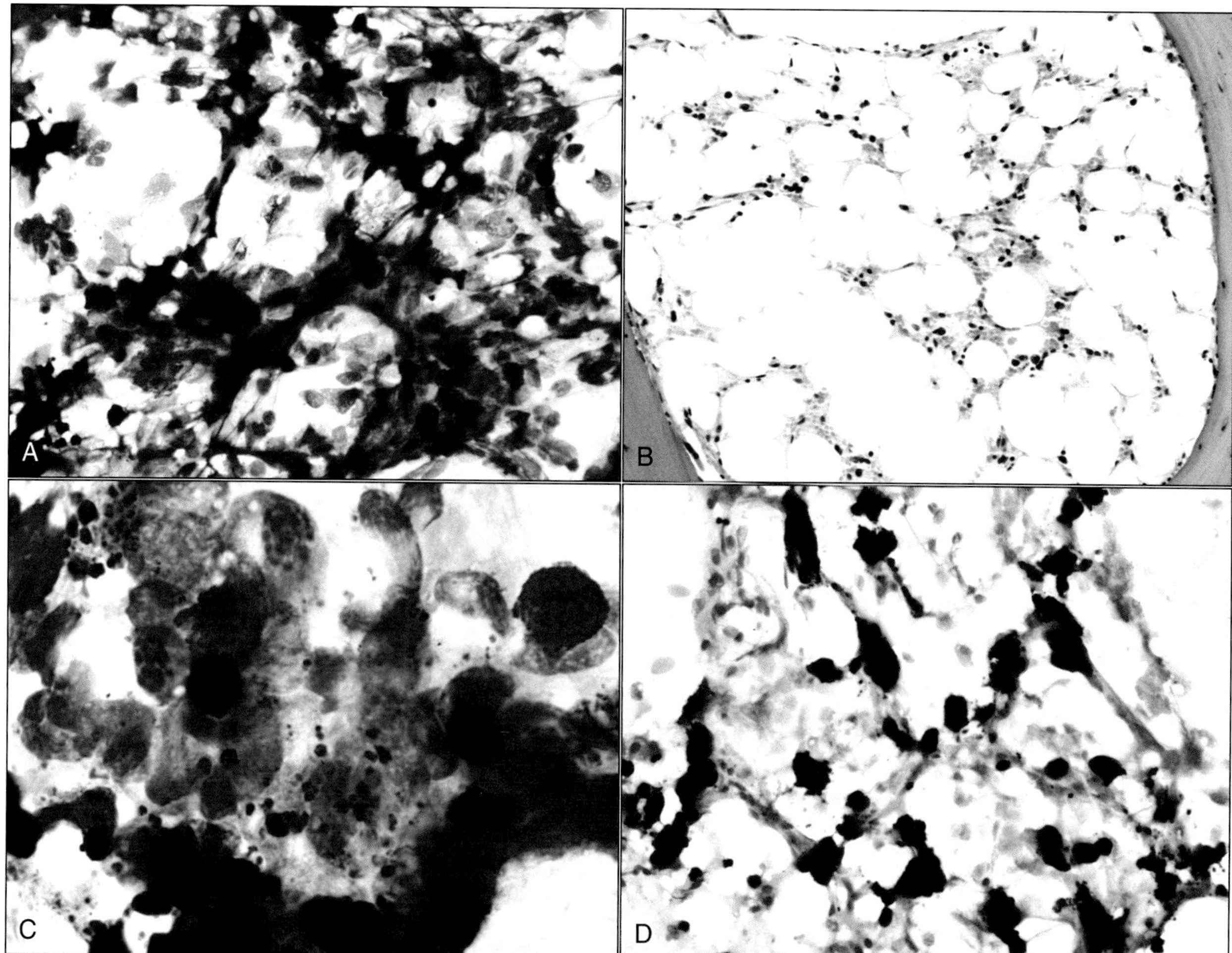

FIGURE 9-3

Hypocellular bone marrow aspirate smears and core biopsy sections from dogs. **A,** Generalized hypocellularity in an aspirate smear of bone marrow from a dog with estrogen-induced aplastic anemia. Stromal cells and fat predominate. The circular purple objects are mast cells and the black globular material is hemosiderin. Wright-Giemsa stain. **B,** Generalized hypocellularity in a section from a bone marrow core biopsy collected from a dog with an idiopathic aplastic anemia. H&E stain. **C,** Purple-staining mast cells *(top)* and brown- to black-staining hemosiderin in the same aspirate smear of bone marrow collected from the dog with estrogen-induced aplastic anemia presented in **(A)**. Wright-Giemsa stain. **D,** Blue-staining hemosiderin in an aspirate smear of bone marrow from the same dog with estrogen-induced aplastic anemia presented in **(A)** and **(C)**. Prussian blue stain.

involves some degree of marrow hypoplasia. Although rare, aplastic anemia may develop in association with severe chronic ehrlichiosis in dogs.[59,331] Erythroid and megakaryocytic hypoplasia has been reported in two cats with *E. canis*-like infections.[50]

Hypocellular bone marrow has been reported in a dog with splenomegaly and marked extramedullary hematopoiesis, which returned to normal after splenectomy.[244] It was speculated that the spleen might have produced cellular or humoral inhibitors of hematopoiesis in the bone marrow.

Congenital aplastic anemia, renal abnormalities, and skin lesions have been reported in newborn foals whose dams were treated for equine protozoal myeloencephalitis with sulfonamides, pyrimethamine, folic acid, and vitamin E during pregnancy.[468] Aplastic anemia was present at birth in a foal born to a mare that was treated with trimethoprim-sulfamethoxazole for severe placentitis for 1 to 2 months before she gave birth (Fig. 9-5). Aplastic anemia in a 14-day-old Holstein calf may have also developed in utero, although the calf was treated for diarrhea with sulfamethazine 5 days before examination.[10] An in utero toxic insult was suspected in a 9-week-old Clydesdale foal with aplastic anemia.[317]

Generalized bone marrow hypoplasia, with myeloid and megakaryocytic hypoplasia more prominent than erythroid hypoplasia, has been reported in eight young standardbred horses sired by the same stallion.[237] Genetic defects involving the marrow microenvironment, one or more growth factors, or pluripotent stem cells were suggested as possible causes. Hypocellular bone marrow has been reported in a Holstein calf with congenital chondrodysplastic dwarfism.[337]

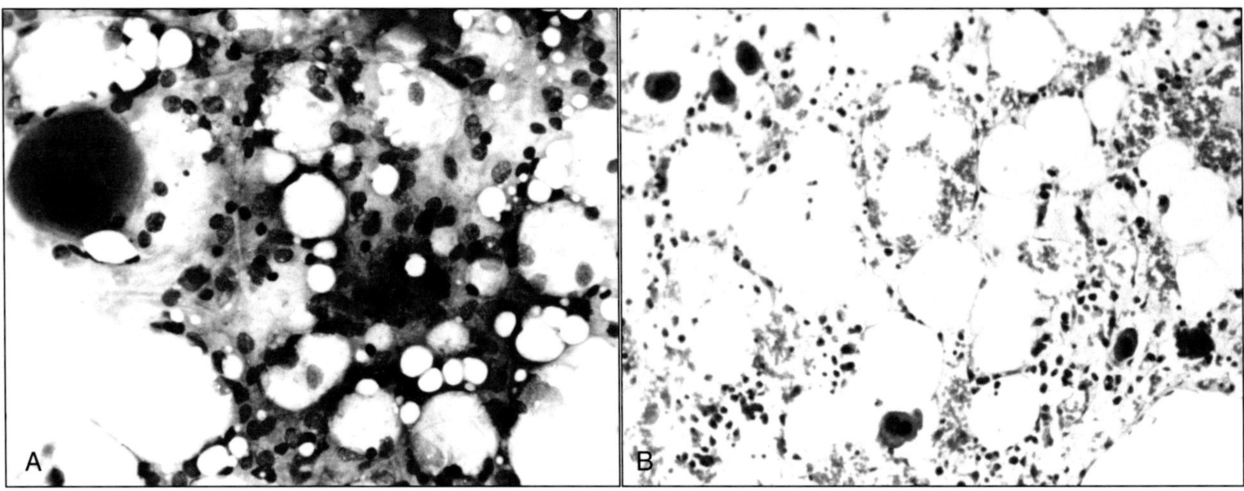

FIGURE 9-4

Hypocellular bone marrow aspirate smear and core bone marrow biopsy section from a leukopenic dog with acute parvovirus infection. **A,** Stromal cells and fat predominate in an aspirate smear, but a megakaryocyte is present *(upper left).* Wright-Giemsa stain. **B,** Although granulocytic and erythroid precursors are markedly reduced in the core bone marrow biopsy, normal numbers of megakaryocytes remain. H&E stain.

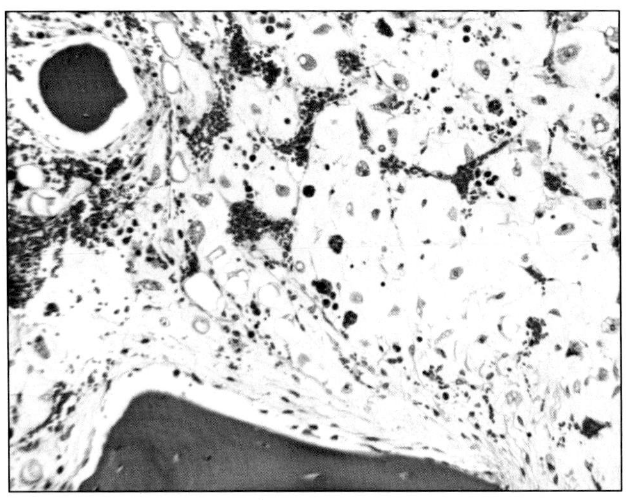

FIGURE 9-5

Bone marrow section from a 4-day-old foal with aplastic anemia that was pancytopenic (hematocrit, 11%; total leukocyte count, $0.4 \times 10^3/\mu L$; platelets, $85 \times 10^3/\mu L$) at birth. The dam was treated with trimethoprim-sulfamethoxazole for severe placentitis for 1 to 2 months before birth. Gelatinous transformation of bone marrow contains only rare hematopoietic cells (smaller, darker round cells), as well as a low number of macrophages containing brown pigment (hemosiderin) and lipid vacuoles. Red decalcified bone *(top left and bottom),* H&E stain.

Idiopathic aplastic anemia has also been reported in dogs,[111,489,521] cats,[507] and horses.[29,258,317] One case of erythroid and myeloid aplasia with normal megakaryocyte numbers has been reported in a horse; the etiology was unknown.[493]

Acute Bone Marrow Injury and Necrosis

Two major forms of cell death, necrosis and apoptosis, are recognized. Necrosis refers to a form of cell death and degeneration secondary to the inability of mitochondria to generate sufficient energy in the form of ATP. Cells swell and burst after losing their ability to regulate osmotic balance. A variable inflammatory response occurs secondary to the release of intracellular contents. In contrast, mitochondrial function is less affected and ATP concentrations are higher in cells undergoing apoptosis (physiologic cell death). The nuclear chromatin condenses, the nucleus rounds up into a single dense sphere (pyknosis) or fragments into multiple dense spheres (karyorrhexis), and the cell shrinks by as much as 30%. Soon after the process is begun, the cell is recognized and phagocytized by macrophages. Cytoplasmic contents are not shed externally; therefore, there is no release of proinflammatory mediators. A third form of cell death, called autophagy-associated cell death, occurs when cells do not receive sufficient nutrients for extended periods of time and therefore digest available internal substrates and die.[196]

Necrosis may be caused by ischemia resulting from damage or disruption of the microcirculation or by direct damage to the proliferating hematopoietic cells. Edema (amorphous proteinaceous material between hematopoietic cells), hemorrhage, and acute inflammation may also be present as a result of increased vascular permeability following vessel injury.[517] Necrosis may be recognized antemortem (Fig. 9-6, *A*), but it is most often recognized when histologic samples are examined postmortem (Figs. 9-6, *B,* and 9-7, *A*) because it is a transient event that often has a focal distribution.

The appearance of necrosis varies depending on the time course and cause.[195] When histologic sections are examined, initial lesions exhibit altered staining of hematopoietic cells with indistinct cellular outlines (see Fig. 9-6).[500] Hemorrhage and/or edema may also be present if vessels are injured.[195] Later, the areas of necrosis become hypocellular as the cells lyse and are replaced by amorphous granular eosinophilic debris. This stage of necrosis must be differentiated from

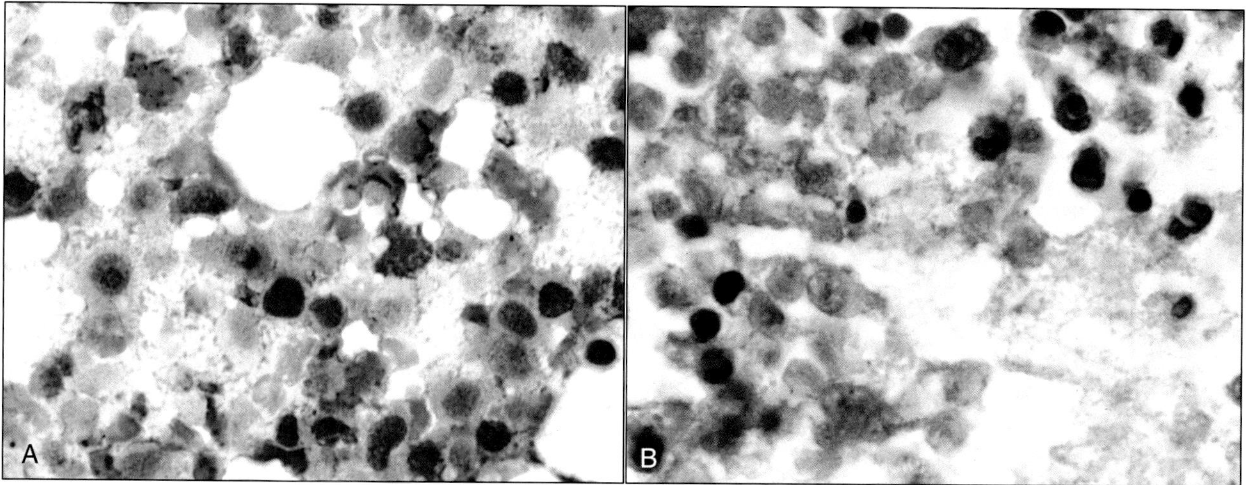

FIGURE 9-6
Necrosis in the bone marrow of a FeLV-negative pancytopenic cat. **A,** The background in an antemortem bone marrow aspirate smear appears granular and bluish to purple in color; the remaining cells are impossible to classify, because of degenerative changes. Wright-Giemsa stain. **B,** Necrosis in a postmortem bone marrow section. The circular pink areas represent necrotic cells in which the nucleus is no longer visible. Most remaining cells with visible nuclei appear to be granulocytic cells. H&E stain.

fibrin, edema, and collection artifact. A Fraser-Lendrum stain for fibrin can be helpful in this regard.[500] Macrophages, many of which contain phagocytized cellular debris, occur in increased numbers in necrotic marrow. Myelofibrosis occurs subsequently to necrosis, similar to the healing process that occurs in other damaged tissues.[188,195,513]

Aspirate smears from necrotic marrow may be confused with smears resulting from poor-quality sample collection or staining techniques. Marrow particles may appear elongated and "stringy."[520] The background appears granular and is bluish to purple in color. The remaining cells are difficult to classify because of morphologic changes caused by degeneration (see Fig. 9-6, *A*). Nuclei appear smudged and cytoplasmic margins are usually ill defined. When visible, the cytoplasm is basophilic and sometimes vacuolated.[188,391] Often only free nuclei or nuclear fragments are seen. Macrophages with phagocytized debris are commonly observed.[119,520]

Disorders that have been reported in association with marrow necrosis in animals include septicemia and/or endotoxemia,[503,520,523] feline infectious peritonitis,[53,510] FeLV infection,[430] acute parvovirus infection in dogs,[43] BVD,[112,415] *Ehrlichia canis* infection in dogs,[520] drug administration (including chemotherapeutic agents, estradiol [dogs], phenobarbital, mitotane, carprofen, metronidazole, colchicine, fenbendazole, and cephalosporin antibiotics),[36,188,199,503,517] neoplasia,[101,114,227,500,503] myelodysplastic syndrome,[507] nonregenerative IMHA,[512] systemic lupus erythematosus in dogs,[119,503] disseminated intravascular coagulation,[388,519,523] and chronic renal disease in cats treated with recombinant erythropoietin (EPO) or blood transfusions.[510] Multifocal bone marrow necrosis and fibrosis was recognized in a horse with an equine herpesvirus-2 infection (see Fig. 9-7). The cause of bone marrow necrosis may not always be identified.[120,188,503,507,529]

Gelatinous Transformation of Bone Marrow

Gelatinous transformation of bone marrow (mucoid degeneration, serous atrophy of fat) involves morphologic changes in bone marrow that combine the loss of hematopoietic cells and the atrophy of fat with the deposition of gelatinous substances in the marrow spaces. Aspirated bone marrow has a mucoid consistency, resulting from the extracellular matrix material present. This material appears as a pink background in bone marrow aspirate smears stained with routine blood stains (Fig. 9-8, *A*) and in histologic sections stained with H&E (Fig. 9-8, *B*). Although the composition may vary somewhat, the material is composed of acid mucopolysaccharides, mainly hyaluronic acid, which stain strongly with Alcian blue at pH 2.5 (Fig. 9-8, *C*). The Alcian blue-positive staining is lost when samples are pretreated with bovine testicular hyaluronidase.[40] Routine fixation in 10% neutral-buffered formalin is not ideal for staining acid mucopolysaccharides. Material is better preserved for optimal staining by fixation in 10% acid formalin with 70% alcohol.[28] Edema may resemble gelatinous transformation in H&E-stained sections, but edematous fluid does not stain with Alcian blue.[40]

Gelatinous transformation of bone marrow in humans is generally associated with severe malnutrition accompanying disorders such as neoplasia, alcoholism, anorexia nervosa, infectious diseases (including acquired immunodeficiency syndrome [AIDS]), maldigestion, chronic heart failure, and metabolic disorders. Long bones are more likely to exhibit gelatinous transformation than flat bones.[482] Widespread

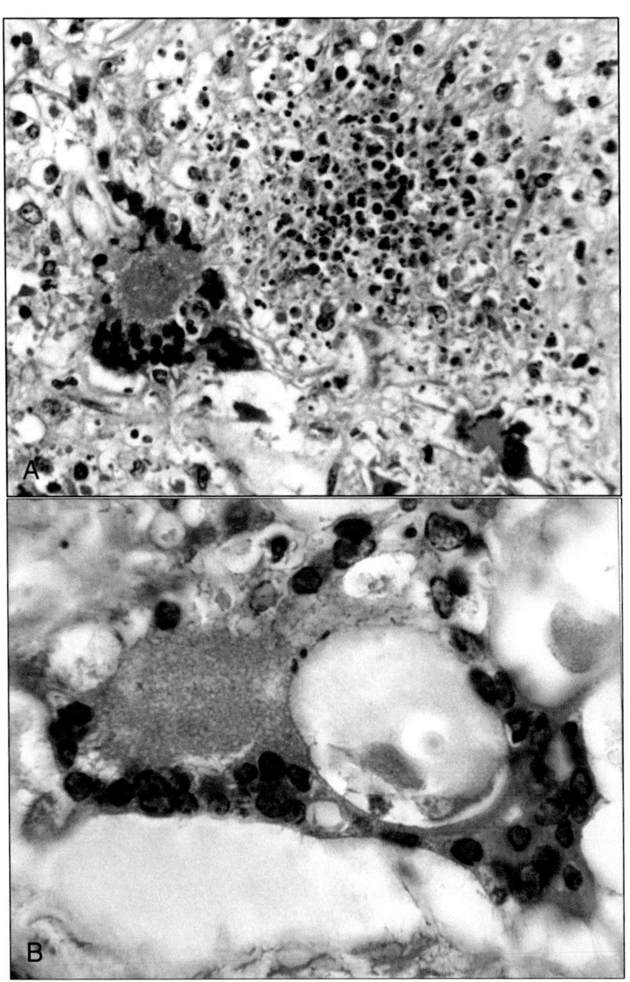

FIGURE 9-7

Bone marrow section from a 12-year-old Warmblood gelding with multifocal necrosis. **A,** A focus of necrosis in the marrow space, which is flanked by large syncytial cells. **B,** A multinucleated syncytial cell containing eosinophilic intranuclear inclusions. Similar cells with intranuclear inclusions were also present in the lungs, liver, and gastrointestinal tract during necropsy examination. Tissues collected at necropsy were positive for equine herpesvirus-2. H&E stain.

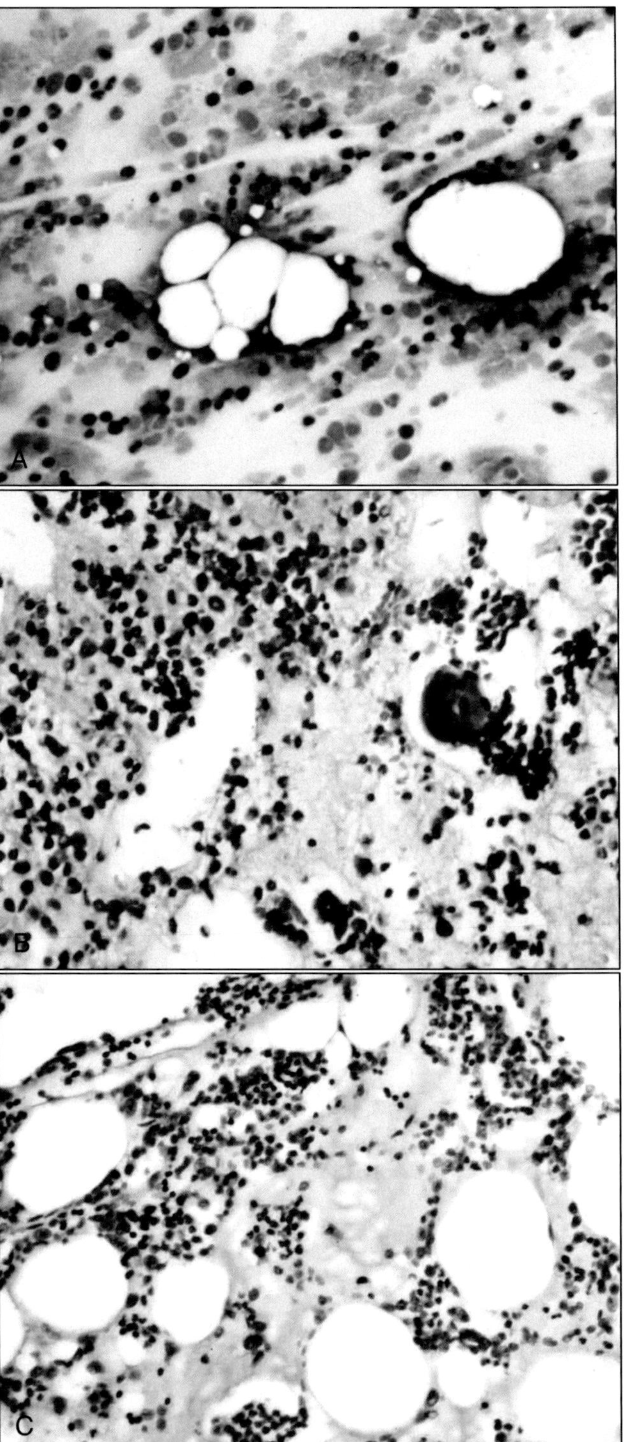

FIGURE 9-8

Gelatinous transformation of bone marrow from a cat with cancer-induced cachexia. **A,** Aspirate bone marrow smear containing gelatinous material. Wright stain. **B,** Bone marrow section. H&E stain. **C,** Bone marrow section. Alcian blue stain.

Courtesy of Julia Blue.

involvement may result in anemia, leukopenia, and less often thrombocytopenia.[28,482]

Gelatinous transformation of bone marrow has also been recognized in cachexic cats suffering from chronic diseases (including chronic renal disease and oral or gastric ulcers) and chronic anorexia.[513] Bone marrow from cats with gelatinous transformation may still contain fat (see Fig. 9-8). Other reports of gelatinous transformation of bone marrow in animals include starvation in reindeer,[218] fluoride intoxication in calves,[301] diet restriction in male Gottingen minipigs,[41] and an emaciated miniature horse.[28]

Myelofibrosis

Myelofibrosis is suspected when repeated attempts at marrow aspiration are unsuccessful or a poor-quality aspirate is obtained that contains some spindle-shaped cells (Fig. 9-9).

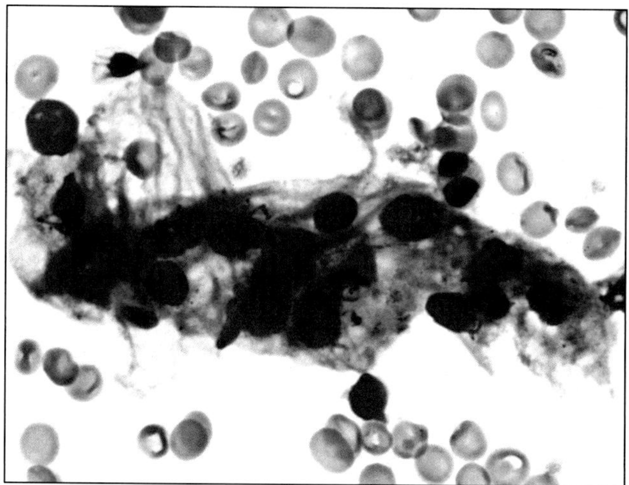

FIGURE 9-9
A cluster of stromal cells is present in a smear prepared from a bone marrow aspirate attempt from a dog with a nonregenerative anemia. The presence of a few stromal cells in a specimen acquired during an unsuccessful attempt to collect bone marrow particles by aspiration suggested the possibility of fibrosis, which was confirmed by core biopsy and histopathology. Wright-Giemsa stain.

A definitive diagnosis can be made only by examining histologic sections of bone marrow.

Fibrous tissue consists of variable amounts of actively proliferating fibroblasts, reticulin fibers, and dense collagenous connective tissue.[500] The term *myelofibrosis* is used when there is an apparent excess of reticulin/collagen fibers in bone marrow that is produced by activated and/or proliferating marrow reticular cells.[488] Low levels of myelofibrosis may be definitively recognized only by using special stains (Fig. 9-10, *A-C*).

Type I collagen forms thick fibrils, while type III collagen forms thin fibrils. Reticulin fibers are visible as argyrophilic fibers in histologic sections of tissues stained using silver impregnating methods, such as Gomori stain (see Fig. 9-10, *B*).[37] Reticulin fibers are primarily composed of individual type III collagen fibrils or small bundles of type III collagen fibrils that surround a core of type I fibrils. These fibrils are imbedded in a matrix of glycoproteins and glycosaminoglycans; silver stains appear to bind to this matrix rather than the collagen fibrils themselves.[247] When present in normal marrow, reticulin fibers are located primarily in perivascular and peritrabecular areas.[488] Larger collagen fibers composed primarily of type I collagen with less interfibrillar material are stained using a trichrome stain such as Masson trichrome (see Fig. 9-10, *C*). Few or no collagen fibers are visible using trichrome stains in normal bone marrow.[247,488] The term *reticulin fibrosis* is used when argyrophilic fibers are increased in number and size; and the term *collagen fibrosis* is used when trichrome-positive fibers are present. Some fibrotic marrows also have increased vascularization, which results in increased amounts of type IV collagen in basement membranes.[37] Reticulin fibrosis may be present without collagen fibrosis, but collagen

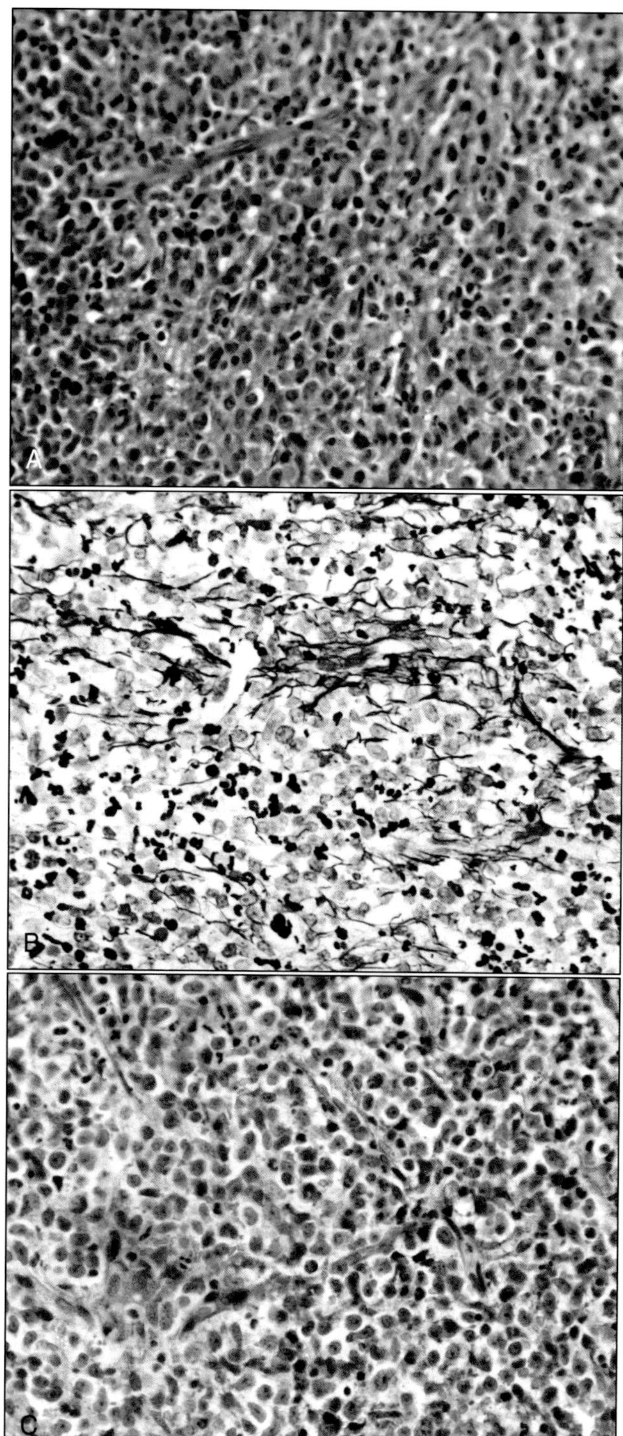

FIGURE 9-10
Myelofibrosis in a bone marrow core biopsy from a dog with ALL ($CD3^+$, $CD79^-$, $CD4^-$, $CD8^-$). Hematologic findings included a hematocrit of 44%, a total leukocyte count of $1.9 \times 10^3/\mu L$ with $0.8 \times 10^3/\mu L$ neutrophils, and a platelet count of $65 \times 10^3/\mu L$. Attempts to aspirate bone marrow resulted in dry taps. **A,** The marrow was hypercellular, and most of the cells were neoplastic lymphocytes. Cells appear to form lines, suggesting fibrosis. H&E stain. **B,** Black reticulin fibers are visible following staining of the section with Gomori stain. **C,** Bluish collagen fibers are visible following staining of the section with Masson trichrome stain.

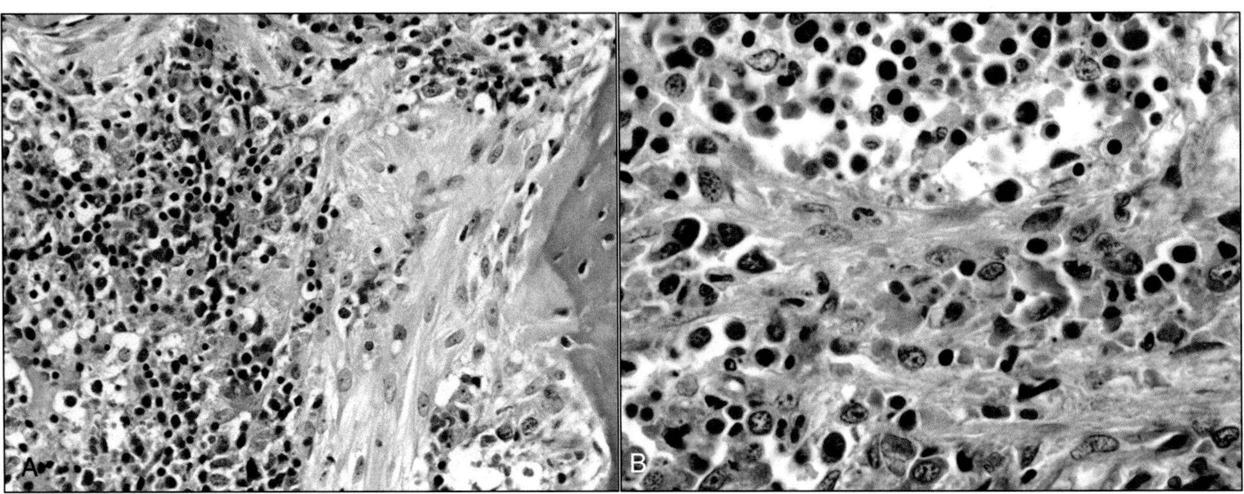

FIGURE 9-11

Myelofibrosis in bone marrow core biopsies from dogs. **A,** Myelofibrosis in a bone marrow section from a core biopsy collected from a dog with myelodysplastic syndrome (MDS). Reticular cells and collagen are readily visible at the top and to the right next to the darker pink trabecular bone. Hematopoietic cells (primarily erythroid precursors) are concentrated to the left. H&E stain. **B,** Myelofibrosis in a bone marrow section from a core biopsy collected from a dog with a poorly regenerative anemia. Hematopoietic cells are present in linear arrangements, separated by pale eosinophilic extracellular collagenous material at the bottom of the field. H&E stain.

fibrosis is almost never revealed by trichrome staining without increased reticulin.[247]

When myelofibrosis is extensive, it is recognized in sections stained with H&E (Fig. 9-11, *A,B;* Fig. 9-12, *A,B*). In these instances, marrow sections contain little or no fat. Hematopoietic cells may be present in linear arrangements, separated by palely eosinophilic extracellular collagenous material (see Fig. 9-11, *B*). Areas of marked myelofibrosis consist of fibroblasts and extracellular matrix, with no remaining hematopoietic cells (see Fig. 9-12). Increased hemosiderin is often present in bone marrow samples with prominent myelofibrosis (see Fig. 9-11, *B;* Fig. 9-12).[37,488]

Primary myelofibrosis (previously known as myelofibrosis with myeloid metaplasia or agnogenic myeloid metaplasia) in humans is a clonal myeloproliferative neoplasm. It is characterized by a proliferation of megakaryocytes and granulocytes, myelofibrosis, extramedullary hematopoiesis (especially in the spleen), and anemia with increased nucleated erythrocytes and immature neutrophils in blood (called leukoerythroblastic anemia in human hematology).[454] A similar syndrome has not been described in animals, although myelofibrosis may be present in animals with various myeloid neoplasms.

Myelofibrosis appears to be a sequela to marrow injury, including necrosis, vascular damage, inflammation, and neoplasia.[513] It is postulated that these disorders result in the direct or indirect production of cytokines capable of stimulating fibroblasts.[388] Transforming growth factor-β (TGF-β), which is produced by a number of cell types including megakaryocytes and platelets, may be the most important factor in this regard.[247]

Prominent myelofibrosis has been documented in animals with marrow necrosis,[519] myeloproliferative neoplasms,[37,52,64,167] lymphoproliferative neoplasms,[519] non-marrow-origin neoplasia,[519] drug treatment (phenobarbital, phenylbutazone, and colchicine),[515] nonregenerative IMHA in dogs and cats,[447,513] and dogs with inherited pyruvate kinase deficiency.[170,416] It has also been described as resulting from unknown causes.[13,190,388,488,519]

Marked myelofibrosis has been reported as a congenital (presumably inherited) disorder in young pygmy goats that also had megakaryocytic hyperplasia and dysplasia.[62] Myelofibrosis has been described in a family of poodles with laboratory and clinical findings similar to pyruvate kinase deficiency,[379] but definitive studies were not performed to eliminate the possibility that these animals had pyruvate kinase deficiency as well. It has been proposed that marrow fibrosis, like cirrhosis, occurs in response to damage caused by iron overload in pyruvate kinase-deficient dogs.[551] However, factors associated with marked erythropoiesis may contribute to the development of myelofibrosis. Extremely high pharmacologic doses of recombinant human EPO elicited both marked erythropoiesis and myelofibrosis in experimental dogs.[19]

With the exception of dogs with inherited hemolytic anemias, animals with myelofibrosis typically have nonregenerative anemia. Blood leukocyte counts and platelet counts are often normal or increased in idiopathic cases of myelofibrosis, but they may be decreased, especially when collagen fibrosis is extensive.[190,247] Multiple cytopenias are more likely to occur in animals with concomitant myeloid neoplasms.

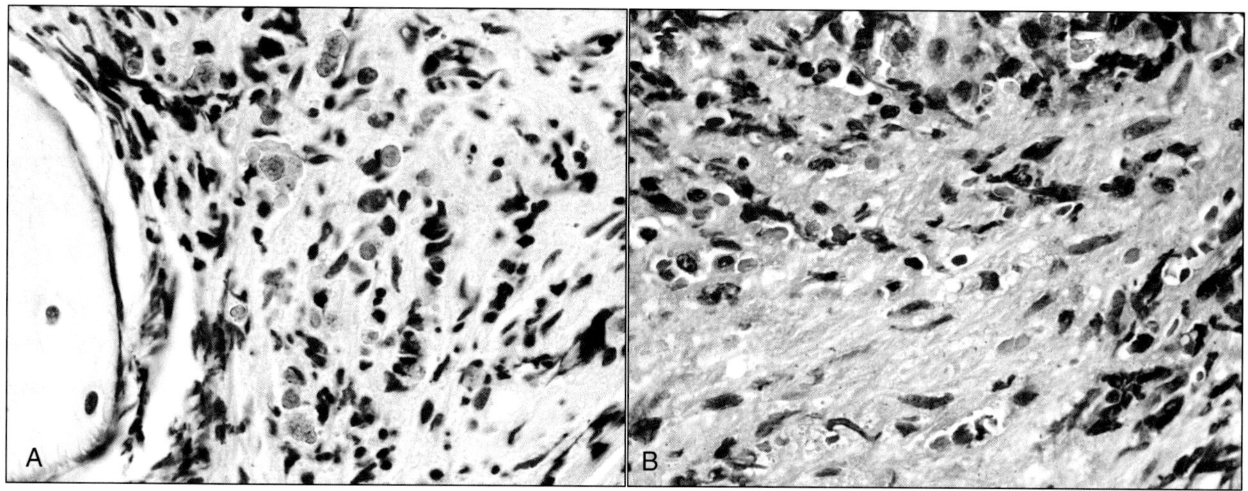

FIGURE 9-12
Myelofibrosis in a postmortem bone marrow section from a cat with chronic lymphocytic leukemia (CLL). **A,** Trabecular bone is located at the left edge. Reticular cells and collagen dominate the field although some hematopoietic precursors are present. The orange globular material is hemosiderin. H&E stain. **B,** Reticular cells and collagen (turquoise fibers) dominate the field, although some hematopoietic precursors are present. The orange globular material is hemosiderin. Masson trichrome stain.

Generalized Osteosclerosis/Hyperostosis

Osteosclerosis refers to a thickening of trabecular (spongy) bone, and *hyperostosis* refers to a widening of cortical (compact) bone from appositional growth of osseous tissue at endosteal and/or periosteal surfaces. Osteopetrosis is a form of osteosclerosis resulting from decreased bone resorption secondary to decreased numbers and/or abnormal function of osteoclasts.[315,536] As a result of osteosclerosis and sometimes hyperostosis, the space available for hematopoiesis decreases. The remaining marrow space may appear hypocellular or exhibit fibrosis. Anemia occurs more often than thrombocytopenia or leukopenia. A variety of inherited, metabolic, inflammatory, and neoplastic disorders have been reported to cause generalized osteosclerosis in humans.[536]

Generalized osteosclerosis/hyperostosis is suspected when increased difficulty is encountered in the manual advancement of biopsy needles into bone and marrow aspirates cannot be obtained. Osteosclerosis can potentially be recognized using core biopsies, but the presence of increased bone relative to marrow space may simply be reflective of the area of bone the needle has entered. Antemortem diagnosis of generalized osteosclerosis and/or hyperostosis is usually made using diagnostic imaging.

Osteopetrosis has been described in dogs, cats, and horses with mild to severe nonregenerative anemia.[31,241,262,341,344] Thrombocytopenia and neutropenia are less likely to be present.[262,344] Osteopetrosis, anemia, thrombocytopenia, and marrow necrosis have been reported in beef calves naturally infected with BVD virus.[414] Osteopetrosis occurs as an inherited disorder in Angus calves, which are typically aborted late in gestation.[265] A defect in the gene that produces the SLC4A2 osteoclast anion exchanger prevents bone resorption due to the lack of acidification of the resorption lacunae.[315]

Osteosclerosis and myelofibrosis have been described in a dog with erythroid hypoplasia.[105] Osteosclerosis and nonregenerative anemia have been reported in cats infected with FeLV, although it was suggested that these disorders occurred independently.[192] Osteosclerosis and myelofibrosis occur in dogs with erythrocyte pyruvate kinase deficiency and in poodles with clinical and laboratory findings similar to those in documented cases of pyruvate kinase deficiency.[372,379,416] The anemia in dogs with pyruvate kinase deficiency is regenerative, although the magnitude of the reticulocyte count may be lower as marrow pathology becomes more severe.[372,416]

ABNORMALITIES OF THE ERYTHROID SERIES

Erythroid Hyperplasia

Erythroid hyperplasia is reported when the bone marrow cellularity is normal or increased, the absolute neutrophil count is normal or increased, and the myeloid:erythroid (M:E) ratio is low (Fig. 9-13, *A-C*). If the marrow is hypocellular and/or the absolute neutrophil count is low, a low M:E ratio indicates that granulocytic hypoplasia is present.

Approximately 4 days are required from the time an experimental animal is made anemic by phlebotomy for a peak reticulocyte response to occur in blood because this is the time required for reticulocytes to be produced following stimulation of erythroid progenitor cells by EPO.[7,51,435] Early erythroid precursors can increase in bone marrow within 12 hours after EPO stimulation,[476] but several days are probably

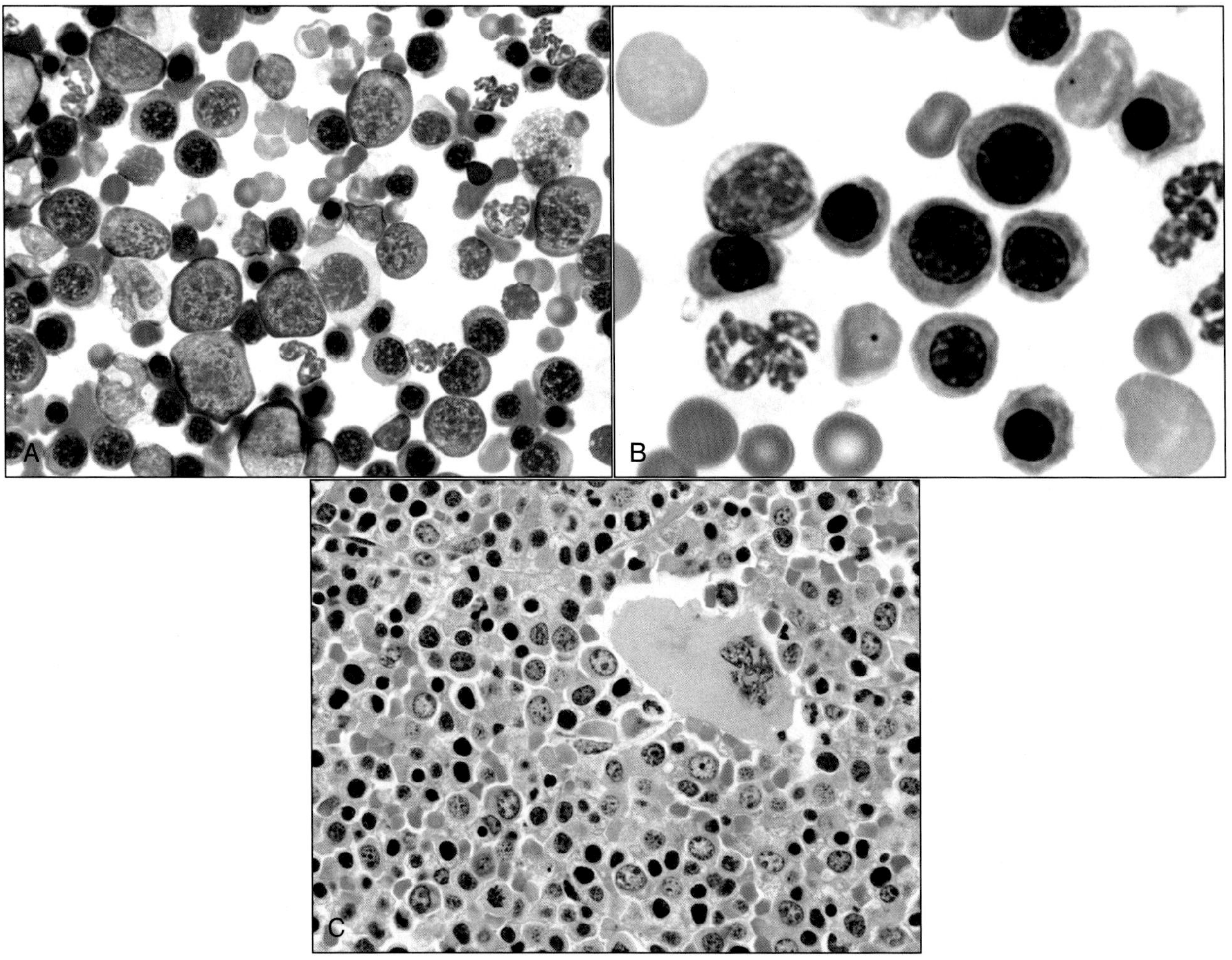

FIGURE 9-13

Erythroid hyperplasia in bone marrow from a horse with immune-mediated hemolytic anemia. **A,** The large cells with dark-blue cytoplasm in a bone marrow aspirate smear are early erythroid precursors. Wright-Giemsa stain. **B,** Higher magnification of a bone marrow aspirate smear with increased numbers of polychromatophilic erythrocytes (reticulocytes), indicating that the erythroid response is effective. Wright-Giemsa stain. **C,** Core bone marrow biopsy section. A large mature megakaryocyte is present near the center of the image. H&E stain.

required after hemorrhage or hemolysis has occurred before erythroid hyperplasia is prominent enough to result in a low M:E ratio. Bone marrow examination is generally not needed in anemic animals with an absolute reticulocytosis unless other cytopenias are also present.

Horses rarely release reticulocytes from the bone marrow even when an increased production of erythrocytes occurs. Consequently, bone marrow evaluation is often needed to determine whether an appropriate response to anemia is present in a horse. If the marrow cellularity is normal or increased and the neutrophil count is normal or increased, an M:E ratio below 0.5 suggests that a regenerative response to anemia is present (see Fig. 9-13).[404]

Erythroid hyperplasia may be effective (increasing hematocrit and/or reticulocytosis) or ineffective. Effective erythroid hyperplasia occurs in response to hemolytic or blood-loss anemia. It also occurs in response to primary or secondary erythrocytosis (polycythemia),[151,175,231,494] although the M:E ratio is often within the reference range.[306] Rubriblasts and prorubricytes are usually increased slightly in animals with effective erythroid hyperplasia; however, the predominant nucleated erythroid cells remain rubricytes and metarubricytes.[189] Many polychromatophilic erythrocytes (reticulocytes) should be present in bone marrow aspirates when the erythroid hyperplasia is effective (see Fig. 9-13, *B*). A reticulocyte count may be done in the bone marrow aspirate to assist in this assessment. Bone marrow reticulocyte counts above 5% provide evidence for an effective regenerative response in horses.[404]

Ineffective erythroid hyperplasia may occur in severe iron deficiency,[171] cobalamin deficiency in Border Collies (Fig. 9-14),[324] folate deficiency in a cat (Fig. 9-15),[330] certain myeloid neoplasms,[107,208,308,319] congenital dyserythropoiesis,[191,441] and in dogs and cats with nonregenerative IMHA

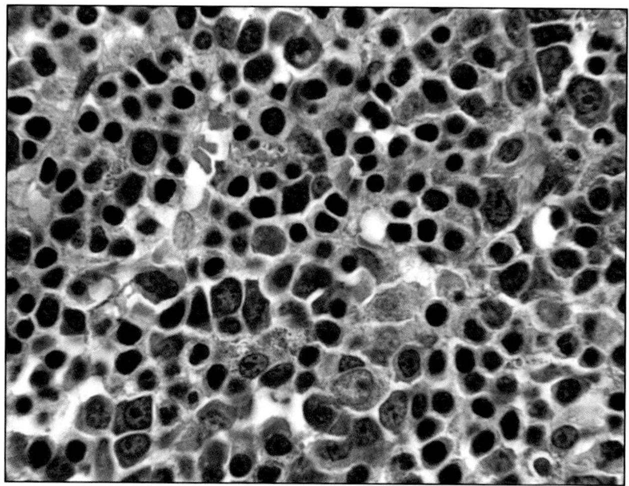

FIGURE 9-14
Hypercellular bone marrow core biopsy section with ineffective erythroid hyperplasia and increased hemosiderin (golden granules) from a Border Collie with cobalamin deficiency. H&E stain. Occasional binucleation and some oval nuclei and nuclear blebbing were seen in rubricytes and metarubricytes in a bone marrow aspirate smear *(not shown)*. The hematocrit was 22% with a metarubricytosis ($6.7 \times 10^3/\mu L$) and normal absolute reticulocyte count in blood.

Photograph of a bone marrow core biopsy section from a 2009 ASVCP slide review case submitted by C. Flint, C. McBrien, J. Fyfe, and M. Scott.

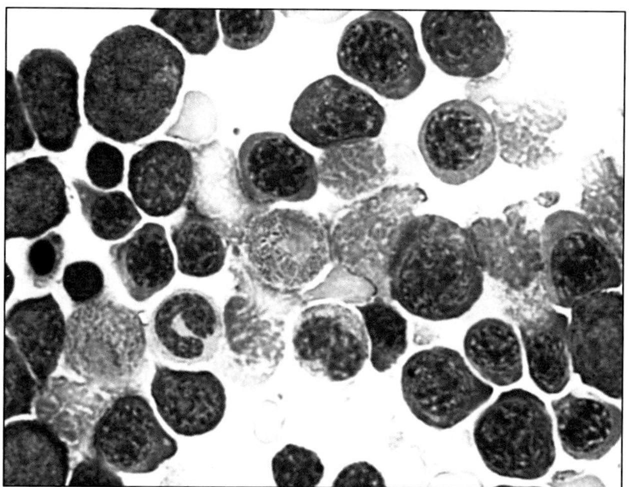

FIGURE 9-15
Erythroid hyperplasia with megaloblastic rubricytes in a bone marrow aspirate smear from a cat with folate deficiency. Wright stain.

Courtesy of Sherry Myers.

(Fig. 9-16).[216,447,512] The immune-mediated destruction of metarubricytes and reticulocytes, as well as other pathologic events that may be present (including vascular injury, inflammation, macrophage activation, myelodysplasia, myelofibrosis), apparently results in ineffective erythropoiesis.[447,512]

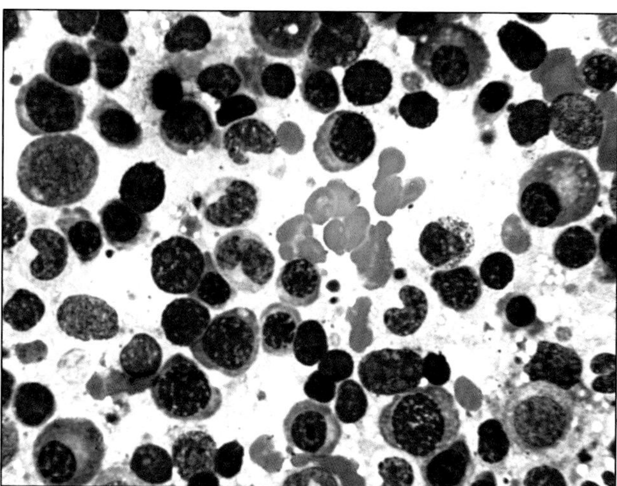

FIGURE 9-16
Erythroid hyperplasia in a bone marrow aspirate smear from a dog with a nonregenerative, immune-mediated hemolytic anemia. The presence of megaloblastic rubricytes in the absence of polychromasia is consistent with ineffective erythropoiesis. Wright-Giemsa stain.

Selective Erythroid Hypoplasia or Aplasia

Erythroid hypoplasia is reported when the bone marrow cellularity is normal or decreased, the absolute neutrophil count is normal or decreased, and the M:E ratio is high (Fig. 9-17). When the M:E ratio exceeds 75:1 and morphologic abnormalities are not present in other cell lines, the terms *selective erythroid aplasia* or *pure red cell aplasia* are used.[512] If the marrow is hypercellular and/or the absolute neutrophil count is high, a high M:E ratio indicates that granulocytic hyperplasia is present.

Selective erythroid aplasia occurs as either a congenital or acquired disorder in humans. Congenital erythroid aplasia in humans (Diamond-Blackfan anemia) appears to represent a heterogeneous group of genetic disorders.[73,271] Approximately 40% of cases are associated with other congenital defects, especially malformations of the head and upper limbs. Acquired erythroid aplasia in humans may occur in association with disorders including B-19 parvovirus infection, proliferative disorders involving large granular lymphocytes, anti-EPO antibodies (primarily from treatment with recombinant EPO), thymomas, and myelodysplastic syndrome (MDS). Erythroid aplasia has also been reported in humans in association with the administration of many drugs as well as with autoimmune diseases, various hematopoietic neoplasms, solid tumors, infections, vascular diseases, pregnancy, and severe renal failure.[408]

Acquired selective erythroid hypoplasia or selective erythroid aplasia occurs in dogs and cats when an immune response is directed against early erythroid precursor cells (Fig. 9-17, *A,B*).[447,512] This response may develop through antibody- or cell-mediated mechanisms that completely inhibit erythroid production or result in a maturation arrest at various stages of erythroid maturation (Fig. 9-18).

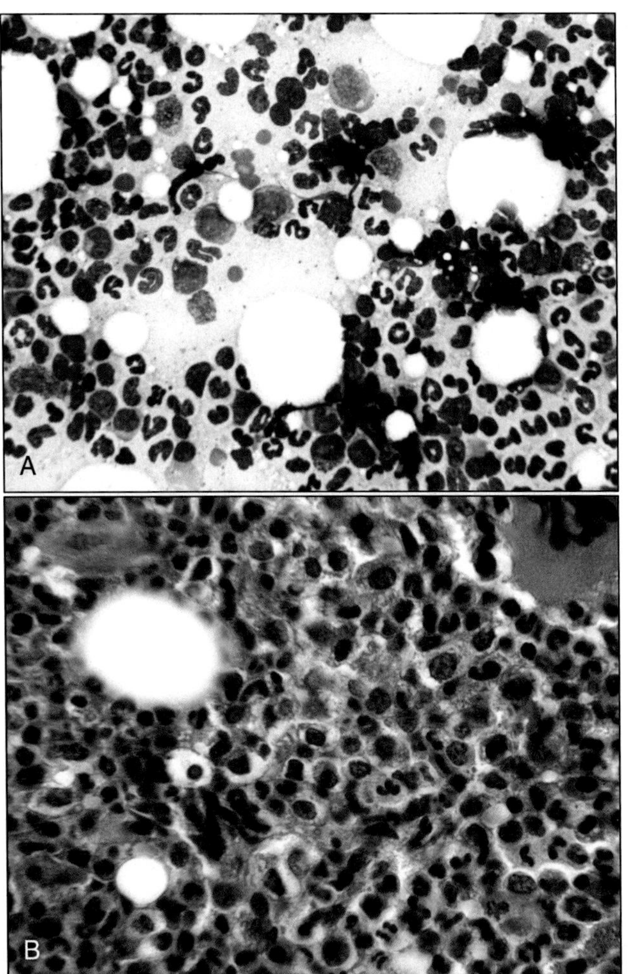

FIGURE 9-17

Erythroid aplasia in bone marrow from a dog. **A,** Bone marrow aspirate smear with a complete lack of erythroid precursors. Black material is hemosiderin. Wright-Giemsa stain. **B,** Bone marrow core biopsy lacking erythroid precursors. Part of a megakaryocyte is visible in the upper right corner. H&E stain.

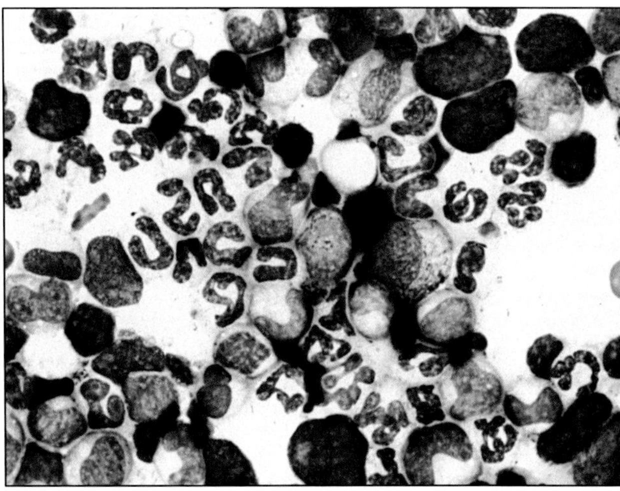

FIGURE 9-18

Erythroid maturation arrest in an aspirate smear of bone marrow from a dog with systemic lupus erythematosus, which included a Coombs-positive nonregenerative anemia. Most of the erythroid cells were rubriblasts or prorubricytes. Wright-Giemsa stain.

Phagocytosis of early erythroid precursor cells may sometimes be recognized in selective erythroid hypoplasia (Fig. 9-19, *A-C*). An immune-mediated attack might be targeted against a maturation-associated antigen, resulting only in the destruction of erythroid precursors in the marrow, or at a common antigen on precursors and mature erythrocytes, which would result in the destruction of precursors in the bone marrow and concurrent erythrocyte destruction in the circulation.[447] The classification of these disorders as being immune-mediated is largely based on positive responses to immunotherapy, but some animals have positive Coombs and/or antinuclear antibody (ANA) tests. In addition, antibodies in the serum of some dogs with selective erythroid aplasia have been reported to inhibit erythropoiesis in bone marrow cultures.[499] Finally, increased numbers of small lymphocytes in the bone marrow of cats (and some dogs) with selective erythroid hypoplasia and selective erythroid aplasia (Fig. 9-20) suggest that cell-mediated immune mechanisms may be important in the pathogenesis of these disorders.[446,447,512]

Erythroid hypoplasia or aplasia is a common finding in animals with MDS and acute myeloid leukemia (AML) that have prominent proliferative abnormalities in granulocytic and/or megakaryocytic cell lines.[436,516] Erythroid hypoplasia is reported to be a rare sequela to vaccination against parvovirus in dogs.[100] High doses of chloramphenicol cause reversible erythroid hypoplasia in some dogs[495] and erythroid aplasia in cats (Fig. 9-21).[497] Erythroid aplasia, together with megakaryocytic aplasia and neutrophilic hyperplasia, is seen in early estrogen toxicity in dogs.[423,501] A dog has been reported to have congenital erythroid aplasia based on histopathologic examination of bone marrow at necropsy, but the M:E ratio was normal when aspirate smears were examined several days prior to euthanasia.[197] Transient erythroid hypoplasia apparently occurs at regular intervals in gray Collie dogs with inherited cyclic hematopoiesis, but it does not cause anemia because it is of short duration and followed by a period of erythroid hyperplasia.[1,251,413]

Selective erythroid hypoplasia or aplasia occurs in cats infected with FeLV subgroup C but not in those infected only with subgroups A or B (Fig. 9-22, *A,B*).[398] The cell surface receptor for FeLV-C is called FLVCR. This receptor has been demonstrated to be a heme exporter.[376] Free heme is toxic to cells, and it appears that the binding of FeLV-C to FLVCR on rubriblasts inhibits heme export from these cells, resulting in their destruction.[226] This exporter can also export protoporphyrin IX and coproporphyrin and appears to be important in heme recycling by macrophages. The plasma protein hemopexin facilitates the export of heme from tissues and the transport of heme to the liver.[546]

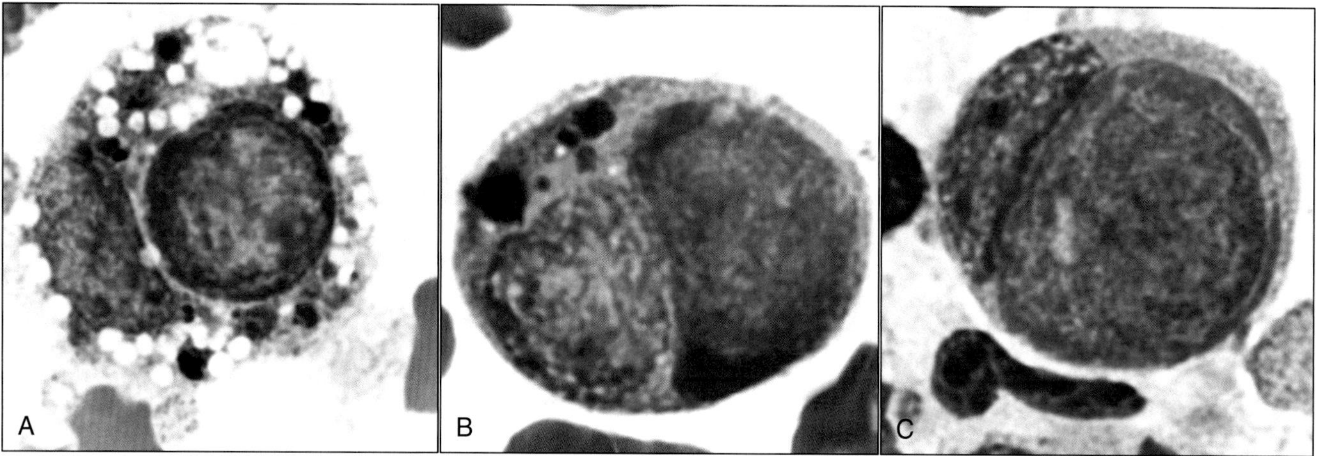

FIGURE 9-19
Phagocytosis of nucleated basophilic erythrocyte precursors in a bone marrow aspirate smear from a dog with nonregenerative immune-mediated hemolytic anemia. A maturation arrest was present, with few cells more mature than prorubricytes seen. **A,** Vacuolated macrophage containing a basophilic erythrocyte precursor, hemosiderin, and debris in the cytoplasm. **B,** Macrophage containing a phagocytized basophilic erythrocyte precursor in its cytoplasm *(right side)*. The nucleus of the macrophage is on the left side, and the dark material in the cytoplasm above the nucleus is hemosiderin. **C,** A phagocytized basophilic erythrocyte precursor has displaced the nucleus of the macrophage to the top left. Wright-Giemsa stain.

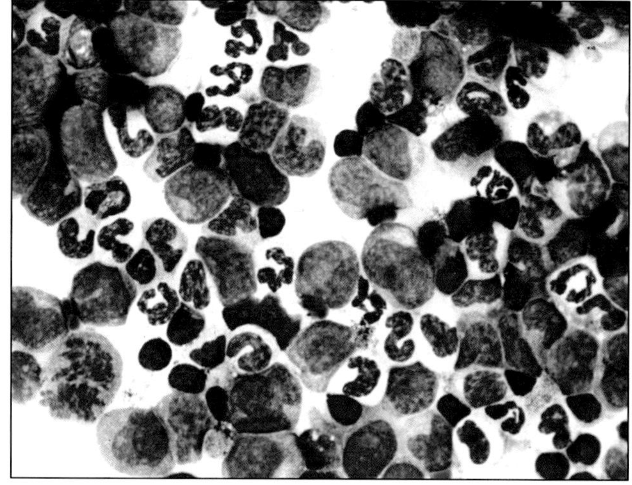

FIGURE 9-20
Selective erythroid aplasia in an aspirate smear of bone marrow from a Coombs-positive, 8-month-old Maltese dog. Small lymphocytes accounted for 15% of all nucleated cells. Wright-Giemsa stain.

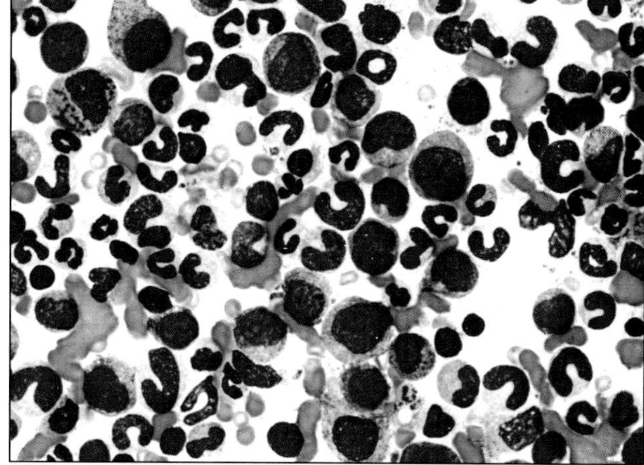

FIGURE 9-21
Selective erythroid aplasia in an aspirate smear of bone marrow from a cat given chloramphenicol at a high therapeutic dosage for 9 days. Wright-Giemsa stain.

Marked erythroid hypoplasia has been reported in dogs, cats, and horses given recombinant human EPO.[90,364,540] Antibodies made against this human recombinant glycoprotein apparently cross-react with the animals' endogenous EPO.

Erythroid production is reduced in chronic renal disease[189] and endocrine deficiencies (hypopituitarism, hypoadrenocorticism, hypothyroidism, and hypoandrogenism) but is not usually pronounced enough to result in an M:E ratio in the marrow that is increased above the reference interval.

A mild to moderate nonregenerative anemia often accompanies chronic inflammatory and neoplastic disorders. The cause of this anemia of inflammatory disease (anemia of chronic disease) is multifactorial and only partially understood. Abnormalities that can contribute to the anemia include the production of inflammatory mediators that directly or indirectly inhibit erythropoiesis, decreased serum iron, shortened erythrocyte life spans, and blunted EPO response to the anemia.[171] The M:E ratio is typically high in clinical cases of the anemia of inflammatory disease in dogs

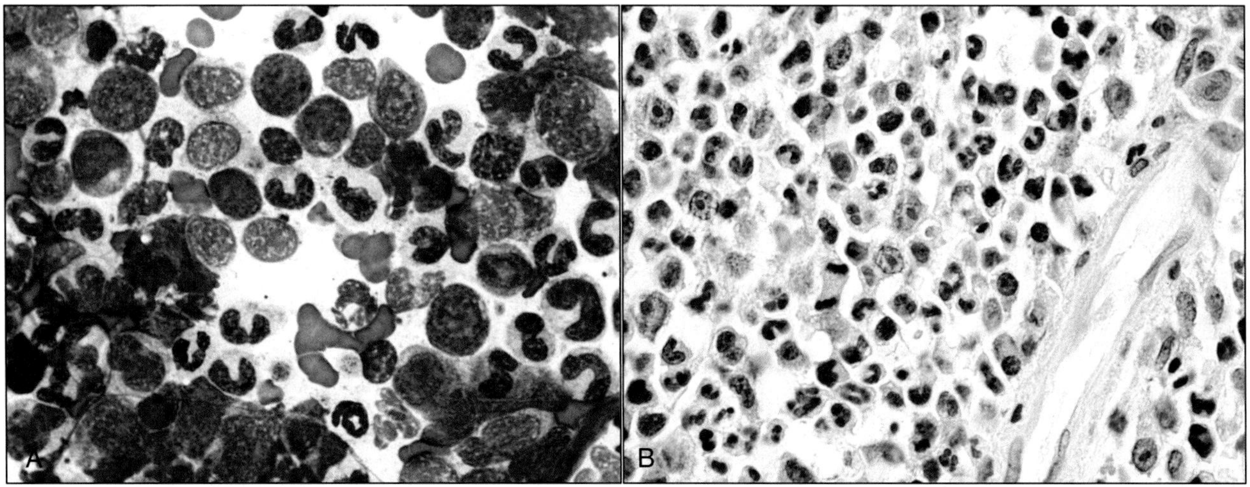

FIGURE 9-22

Marked erythroid hypoplasia in bone marrow from a FeLV-positive cat. **A,** A left shift in granulocytic cells with some giantism is also visible in a bone marrow aspirate smear. Wright-Giemsa stain. **B,** Megakaryocytic hypoplasia and erythroid hypoplasia are demonstrated in a bone marrow biopsy section. H&E stain.

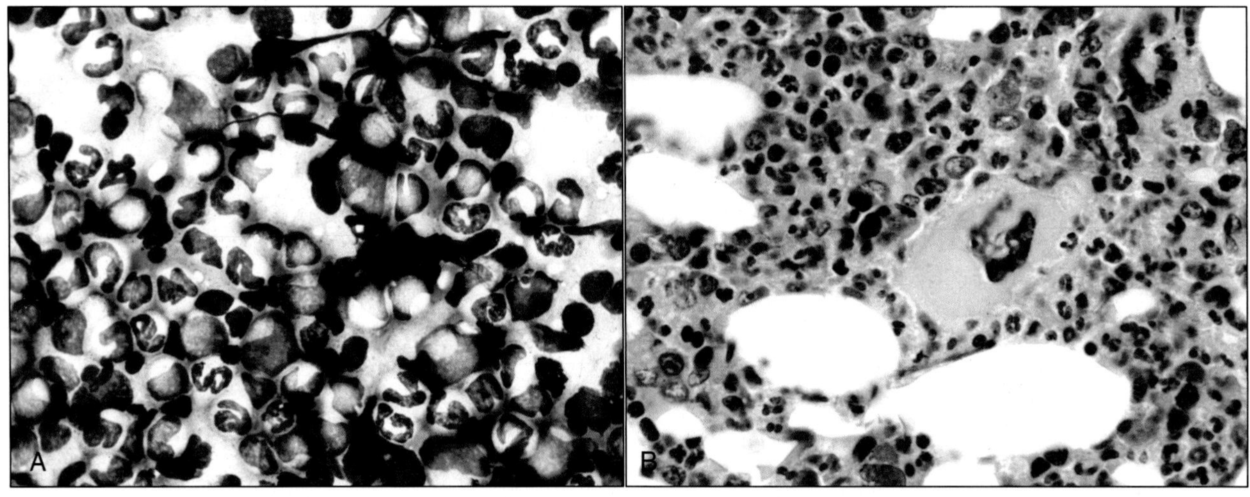

FIGURE 9-23

Erythroid hypoplasia in bone marrow from dogs with the anemia of inflammatory disease. **A,** Mild erythroid hypoplasia and granulocytic hyperplasia in an aspirate smear. Black-staining material near the center of the image is hemosiderin. Wright-Giemsa stain. **B,** Erythroid hypoplasia and increased hemosiderin (orange-staining material) in a bone marrow section from a core biopsy. Two mature megakaryocytes are present. H&E stain.

(Fig. 9-23, *A,B*),[189] not only because of deficient erythropoiesis but also because of concomitant granulocytic hyperplasia.[11]

Dyserythropoiesis

The term *dyserythropoiesis* is used to refer to various disorders in which abnormal erythrocyte maturation and/or morphology is associated with ineffective erythropoiesis. Erythroid abnormalities that may be present include megaloblastic cells, abnormal nuclear shapes, premature nuclear pyknosis, nuclear fragmentation, multinucleated cells, internuclear chromatin bridging, nuclear and cytoplasmic asynchrony, maturation arrest, and siderotic inclusions.

Megaloblastic erythroid cells are larger than normal, with a more stranded arrangement of chromatin and abundant parachromatin, giving a pronounced light and dark pattern to the nucleus (Fig. 9-24, *A-E*). The cytoplasm is generally abundant and hemoglobin synthesis may be present at earlier stages of development than typically seen (e.g., nuclear and cytoplasmic asynchrony). Rubricytes and metarubricytes may be macrocytic without prominent nuclear abnormalities (Fig.

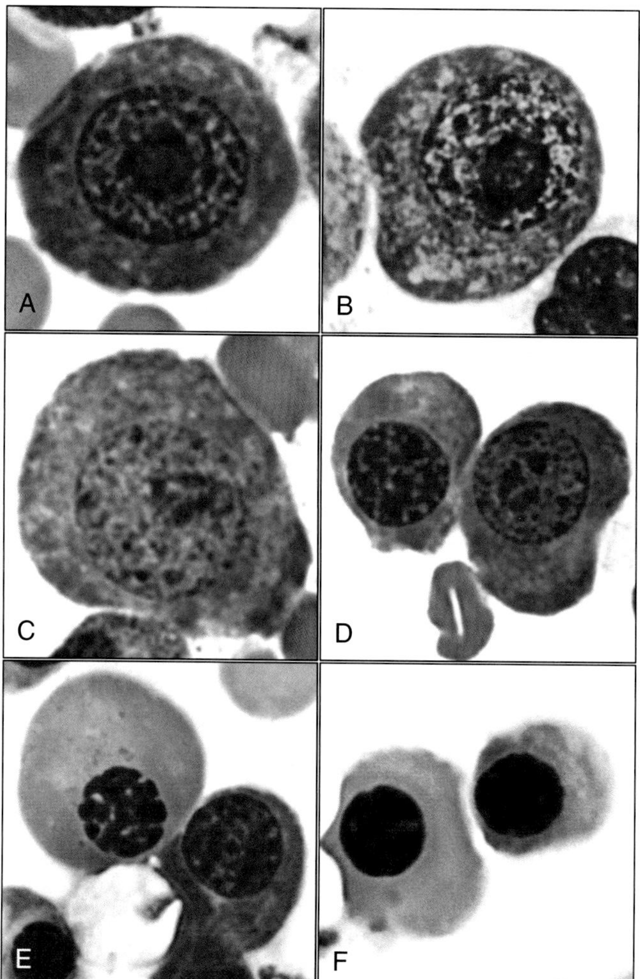

FIGURE 9-24

Megaloblastic erythroid cells in bone marrow aspirate smears. **A,** Megaloblastic erythroid precursor from a cat with erythroleukemia (AML-M6). **B,** Megaloblastic erythroid precursor from a cat with AML-M2. **C,** Megaloblastic erythroid precursor in an aspirate smear of bone marrow from a FeLV-positive cat with MDS. **D,** Megaloblastic erythroid precursor from a cat with MDS. **E,** Macrocytic polychromatophilic rubricyte *(top left)* and basophilic rubricyte *(right)* from a horse with MDS. **F,** Macrocytic orthochromatic metarubricyte *(left)* from a horse with MDS. Wright-Giemsa stain.

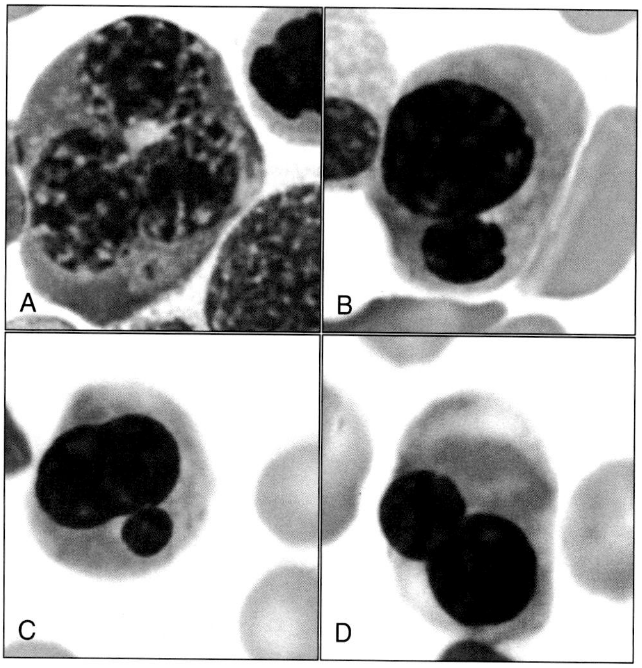

9-24, *F*). These morphologic abnormalities are most often seen in animals with myeloid neoplasms.* Megaloblastic erythropoiesis occurs most commonly in ill cats with FeLV infections, but it has also been reported in cats with feline immunodeficiency virus (FIV) infections.[426] Megaloblastic erythroid cells have been reported in the marrow of cats with natural and experimentally induced folate deficiency (see Fig. 9-15).[330,464] Finally, some miniature and toy poodles exhibit a nonanemic macrocytosis, metarubricytosis, and/or erythrocytes with multiple Howell-Jolly bodies and variable

*References 88, 107, 181, 185, 309, 319.

FIGURE 9-25

Trinucleation and nuclear lobulation in erythroid precursors in bone marrow aspirate smears from dogs. **A,** Trinucleation from a dog with lymphoma and mild dyserythropoiesis. Prior chemotherapy was not listed in the medical record. **B,** Lobulated nucleus in a polychromatophilic rubricyte from the same dog with mild dyserythropoiesis as presented in **(A)**. **C,** Lobulated nucleus in a polychromatophilic metarubricyte from a dog 1 day after treatment with vincristine. **D,** Lobulated nucleus in a polychromatophilic metarubricyte from the same vincristine-treated dog as presented in **(C)**.

megaloblastic abnormalities in the bone marrow. Serum folate and B_{12} values are normal in this hereditary poodle macrocytosis.[66,410,514]

Multinucleated erythroid cells (Fig. 9-25, *A*) have been reported in animals with myeloid neoplasms[209,309,319,530] and in those with acquired and congenital dyserythropoiesis.[275,441,531] Nuclear lobulations, pyknosis, and/or fragmentation may occur in animals with myeloid neoplasms,[88,426] acquired and congenital dyserythropoiesis,[185,191,441,531] and following treatment with drugs that interfere with DNA synthesis, including antimetabolites (e.g., azathioprine, hydroxyurea, cytosine arabinoside), alkylating agents (e.g., cyclophosphamide), folate antagonists (e.g., methotrexate), and plant alkaloids (e.g., vincristine) (Fig. 9-25, *B-D*).[5,38] Internuclear chromatin bridging has been reported in cattle with congenital dyserythropoiesis and in hereditary poodle macrocytosis.[441,514]

Maturational arrests at various stages of erythroid development, with a resultant lack of polychromatophilic erythrocytes, may occur in acquired myeloid neoplasms,[39] in congenital dyserythropoiesis,[441] and in some drug-induced disorders (e.g., cephalosporin antibiotics).[97] It is a common finding in nonregenerative IMHA, especially in dogs (see Fig. 9-16).[216,443,447] A nonregenerative immune-mediated anemia with erythroid maturation arrest has also been reported in a ferret.[291] Asynchrony of nuclear and cytoplasmic maturation, in which hemoglobinization precedes nuclear maturation, may occur in acquired myeloid neoplasms as well as in congenital dyserythropoiesis.[207,441]

Iron-positive basophilic stippling has been reported in rubricytes and metarubricytes (nucleated siderocytes) from animals with myeloid neoplasms,[39,88,185,528,530] dogs with idiopathic dyserythropoiesis (including inflammatory disorders),[67,172,506] and the use of drugs/chemicals, including chloramphenicol (Fig. 9-26, *A,B*), hydroxyzine, lead, zinc, and an oxazolidinone antibiotic.[169,174,276,365]

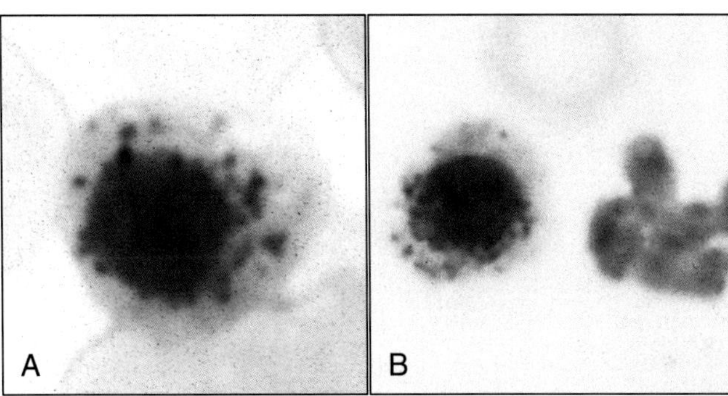

FIGURE 9-26

Siderotic (iron-positive) metarubricytes in an aspirate smear of bone marrow from a dog receiving chloramphenicol therapy. **A,** Blue granules in the cytoplasm indicate the presence of iron. **B,** Siderotic metarubricyte *(left)*. Because the iron-positive granules circle the nucleus, it may be called a ringed sideroblast in human hematology. Prussian blue stain.

ABNORMALITIES OF THE GRANULOCYTIC SERIES

Granulocytic Hyperplasia

Granulocytic hyperplasia is reported when the bone marrow cellularity is normal or increased, the hematocrit is normal or increased, and the M:E ratio is high. If the marrow is hypocellular and/or the hematocrit is low, a high M:E ratio suggests that erythroid hypoplasia is present. Because neutrophilic cells are usually much more numerous than eosinophilic or basophilic cells in bone marrow, the term *granulocytic hyperplasia* generally indicates the presence of neutrophilic hyperplasia. Eosinophilic and/or basophilic hyperplasia may accompany neutrophilic hyperplasia, but they rarely account for increased M:E ratios on their own.

Neutrophilic Hyperplasia

Neutrophilic hyperplasia may be effective or ineffective. Effective neutrophilic hyperplasia results in a peripheral neutrophilia, with or without a left shift. It occurs in response to various hematopoietic growth factors, with granulocyte-colony stimulating factor (G-CSF) being most important.[11] Two or more days are required from the time of growth factor stimulation until neutrophilic hyperplasia is prominent enough to increase the M:E ratio outside of the reference interval.[11,152]

Neutrophilic hyperplasia occurs most frequently in response to bacterial infections, but it may also occur in response to immune-mediated inflammatory disorders, necrosis, chemical and drug toxicities, and malignancy (Fig. 9-27, *A,B*).[123,207] The natural release or injection of recombinant G-CSF,

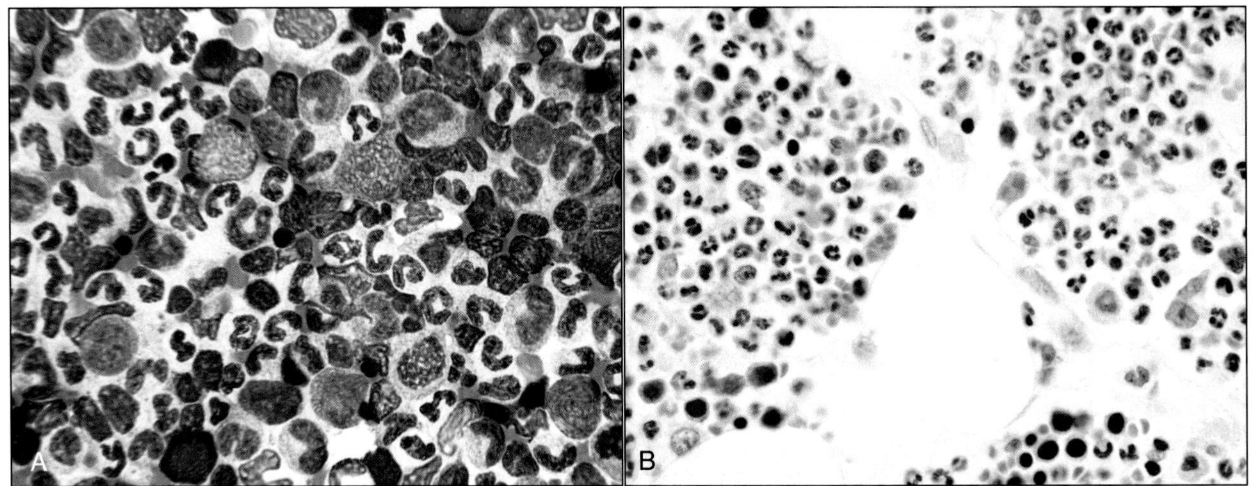

FIGURE 9-27

Neutrophilic hyperplasia in bone marrow. **A,** Neutrophilic hyperplasia in an aspirate smear of bone marrow from a dog with neutrophilia and nonregenerative anemia secondary to immune-mediated polyarthritis. Wright-Giemsa stain. **B,** Neutrophilic hyperplasia and erythroid hypoplasia in a bone marrow section from a core biopsy collected from a cat with marked mature neutrophilia and nonregenerative anemia, for which a cause was not determined. H&E stain.

granulocyte/macrophage-colony stimulating factor (GM-CSF), and interleukin (IL)-3 result in peripheral neutrophilia and neutrophilic hyperplasia in the bone marrow.[92,338,348,477,553] Extreme neutrophilic hyperplasia in bone marrow and peripheral neutrophilia have been reported as a paraneoplastic syndrome in dogs and cats with tumors that produce hematopoietic growth factors.[102,253,421,465]

The proportions of myeloblasts and promyelocytes are generally not increased out of proportion to more mature neutrophilic cells in animals with ongoing neutrophilic hyperplasia (Fig. 9-27, *A,B*). Myeloblasts did not exceed 6% of all nucleated cells in 14 cats with myeloid hyperplasia.[208] However, myeloblasts may be increased substantially following early and/or intense stimulation with growth factors, especially if there is a concomitant depletion of mature neutrophils (Fig. 9-28, *A,B*).[11,189,428,443,465] The proportion of mature granulocytes in bone marrow may be decreased in animals with inflammation and accompanying granulocytic hyperplasia because cytokines such as G-CSF, IL-1, and TNF-α (either directly or indirectly) result in increased release of neutrophils from the marrow, in addition to stimulating the proliferation of neutrophil precursors.[11] Evidence of cytoplasmic toxicity, including vacuolation of early neutrophilic precursors, may also be present (see Fig. 9-28, *A*).

Neutrophilic hyperplasia may be present in animals with inherited hematologic disorders.[335,475] Marked neutrophilia with or without a modest left shift is usually present in dogs and cattle with deficiencies in β_2 integrin adhesion molecules.[148,334] Granulocyte hyperplasia also follows cyclic episodes of neutrophilic hypoplasia in gray Collie dogs with cyclic hematopoiesis.[72,93]

Marked neutrophilic hyperplasia and concomitant erythroid and megakaryocytic aplasia occur during the first 3 weeks after the injection of a toxic dose of estrogen in dogs (Fig. 9-29).[501] This is followed by generalized hypoplasia or aplasia and death or slow recovery.

Neutrophilic hyperplasia is present in animals with chronic myeloid leukemia (CML). The percentage of immature neutrophilic cells is increased, but the percentage of myeloblasts does not exceed 20% of all nucleated cells. Dysplastic changes are also typically present in one or more marrow cell lines.[83,157,167,215,368]

Ineffective neutrophilic hyperplasia refers to the occurrence of a persistent neutropenia with neutrophilic hyperplasia in the bone marrow (Fig. 9-30). Increased numbers of immature granulocyte precursors and decreased numbers of mature neutrophils are typically present within the marrow. Ineffective neutrophilic hyperplasia frequently occurs in MDS and acute myeloid leukemia (AML).[39,167] It is especially common in neutropenic cats with FeLV and/or FIV infections.[27,39,293,426]

Immune-mediated neutropenia may result in secondary neutrophilic hyperplasia in response to the premature removal of blood neutrophils. Immune-mediated neutropenia in dogs has been characterized by having granulocytic hyperplasia with decreased numbers of band and segmented neutrophils and increased numbers of immature stages in bone marrow.[38,359]

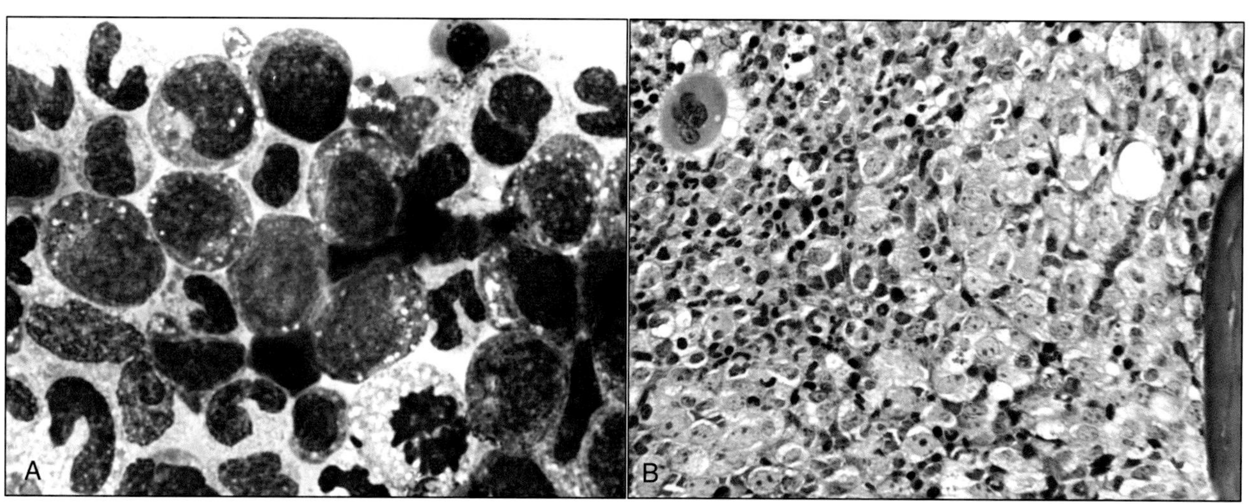

FIGURE 9-28

Neutrophilic hyperplasia with a toxic left shift in the neutrophilic cells in bone marrow from a dog with a severe leukopenia and neutropenia (1.4 and 0.2 × 10^3/μL, respectively) in blood. The M:E ratio (7.7:1) and frequency of plasma cells (18%) were increased. **A,** Toxic neutrophilic precursors in a bone marrow aspirate smear. Discrete cytoplasmic vacuoles were apparent in early neutrophilic precursors, and foamy (less distinct) vacuolation was present in metamyelocytes and band neutrophils. A single rubricyte *(top right of center),* a mitotic cell *(bottom right of center),* and a plasma cell *(center)* are present. Wright-Giemsa stain. **B,** Vacuolated neutrophilic precursors with marked left shift in a core bone marrow biopsy section from the dog presented in **(A).** Trabecular bone is located on the right and a megakaryocyte is present in the top left. H&E stain. Sepsis was considered likely and antibiotic therapy was initiated. The total leukocyte count and total neutrophil count were 7.3 and 5.1 × 10^3/μL, respectively, 2 days later.

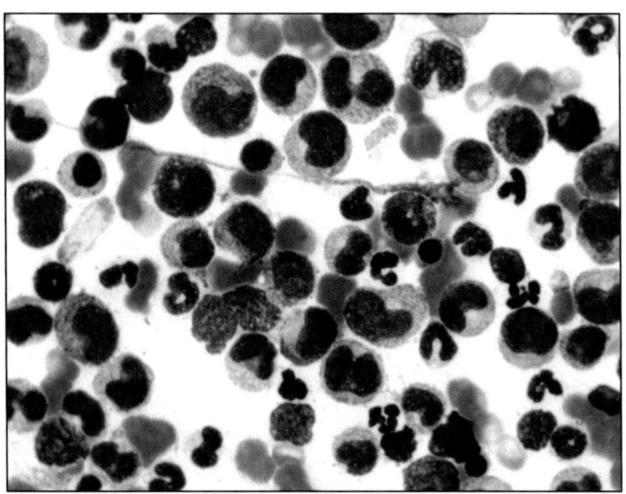

FIGURE 9-29

Neutrophilic hyperplasia and erythroid hypoplasia in an aspirate smear of bone marrow from a dog 13 days after an estradiol cypionate (ECP) injection for mismating. Wright-Giemsa stain.

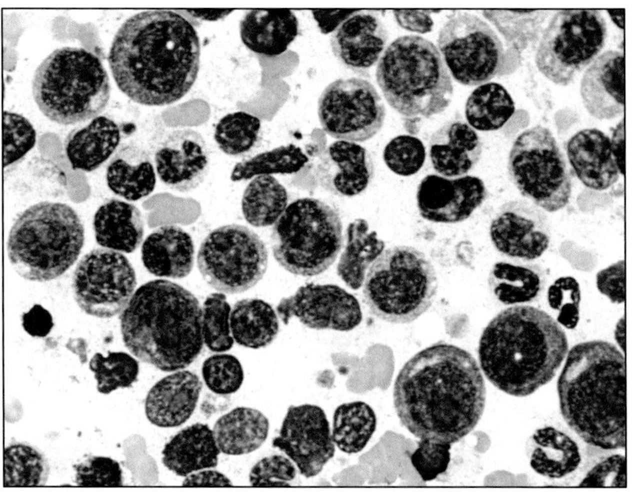

FIGURE 9-30

Ineffective neutrophilic hyperplasia and erythroid hypoplasia in an aspirate smear of bone marrow from a persistently leukopenic FIV-infected cat. Fewer band and mature neutrophils were present than normal. Wright-Giemsa stain.

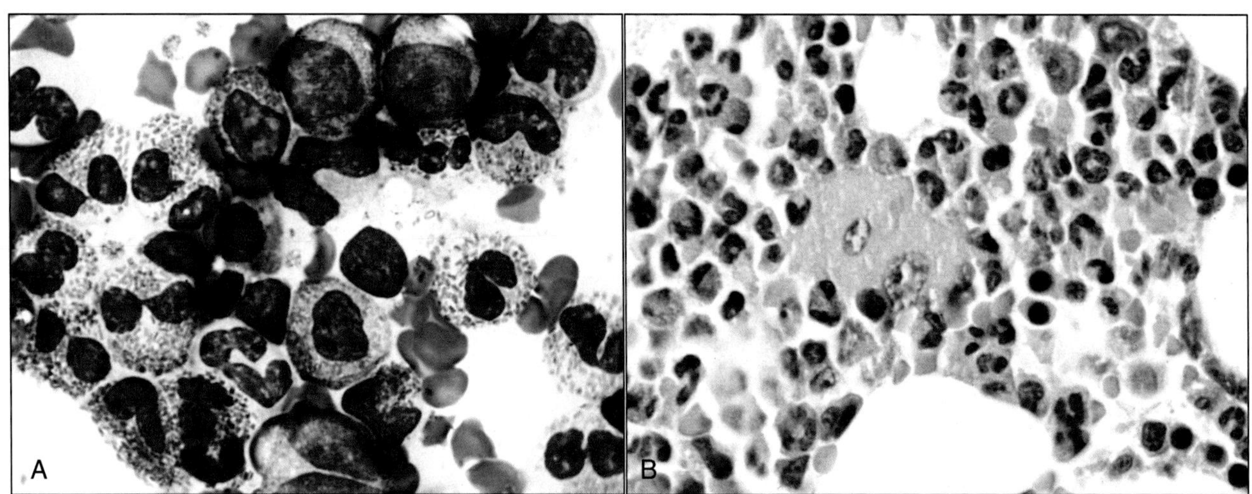

FIGURE 9-31

Eosinophilic hyperplasia in bone marrow from cats. **A,** Eosinophilic hyperplasia in an aspirate smear of bone marrow from a cat with marked peripheral eosinophilia, probably associated with a hypereosinophilic syndrome. Wright-Giemsa stain. **B,** Eosinophilic hyperplasia in a bone marrow core biopsy section collected from a cat with lymphocytic-plasmacytic gastritis and peripheral eosinophilia. H&E stain.

However, neutrophilic hypoplasia may be present when more immature neutrophilic precursors are eliminated.[310,359,483,526]

Neutropenia has been reported in dogs treated with anticonvulsants that had neutrophilic hyperplasia and orderly maturation in the marrow, suggesting a peripheral destruction of neutrophils.[204]

Eosinophilic Hyperplasia

Eosinophilic hyperplasia is generally present in bone marrow when eosinophilia is present in blood (Fig. 9-31, *A,B;* Fig. 9-32).[209,406] Eosinophilia occurs in disorders that result in increased IL-5 production.[238] The injection of recombinant IL-2 resulted in a peripheral eosinophilia in dogs and cats that was likely mediated by IL-5 production by T lymphocytes.[177,278,467]

Eosinophilia may accompany parasitic diseases, especially those caused by nematodes and flukes. It is more likely to be present when intestinal nematodes are migrating within the body than when they are only located within the intestine.[355] Eosinophilia may occur in association with inflammatory conditions of organs that normally contain numerous mast cells, such as the skin, lungs, intestine, and uterus. It may be present in animals with immunoglobulin E (IgE)-mediated

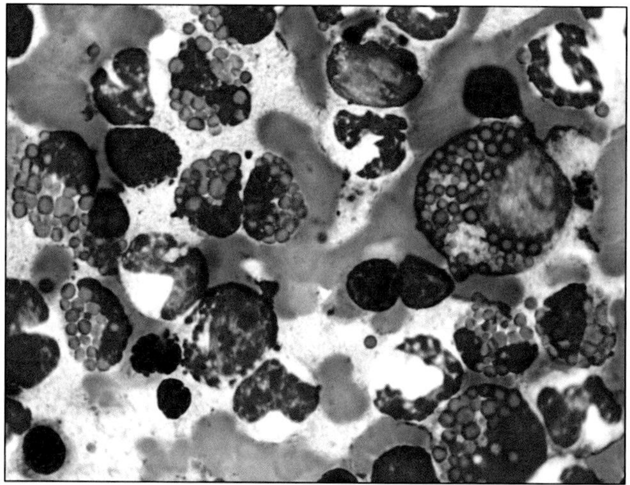

FIGURE 9-32
Eosinophilic hyperplasia in an aspirate smear of bone marrow from a horse with an abdominal mast cell tumor and marked peripheral eosinophilia. Some of the granules in the eosinophilic myelocytes stain bluish-red. Wright-Giemsa stain.

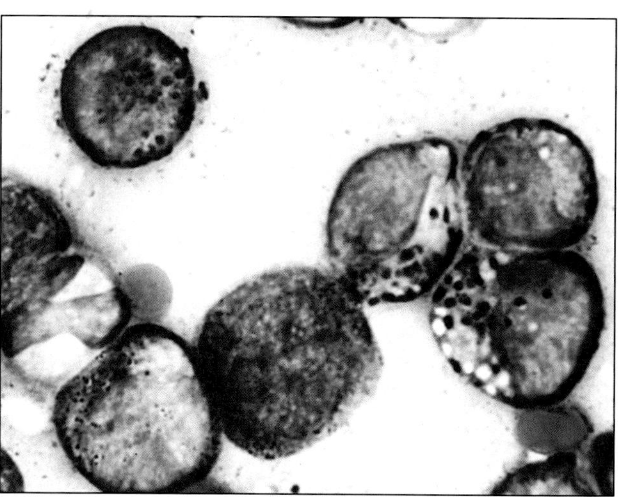

FIGURE 9-33
Basophilic hyperplasia in an aspirate smear of bone marrow from a cat with AML-M2. Four basophilic myelocytes *(one upper left, three right center)* are present. A type II myeloblast is present at bottom center and a promyelocyte is present at bottom left. Wright-Giemsa stain.

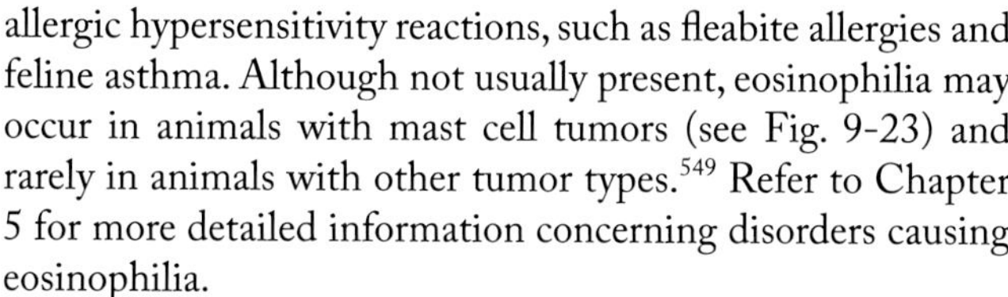

allergic hypersensitivity reactions, such as fleabite allergies and feline asthma. Although not usually present, eosinophilia may occur in animals with mast cell tumors (see Fig. 9-23) and rarely in animals with other tumor types.[549] Refer to Chapter 5 for more detailed information concerning disorders causing eosinophilia.

Marked eosinophilia with extensive eosinophilic organ infiltrates in animals (primarily cats) and humans has been classified as either a chronic eosinophilic leukemia or hypereosinophilic syndrome.* However, it has been difficult to separate this collection of heterogeneous disorders into two distinct entities. Prominent eosinophilic left shifts in bone marrow, blood, and organ infiltrates are more likely to occur in animals with eosinophilic leukemia[145,200,452,470]; however, some left shifting in eosinophil precursors within the bone marrow may occur in reactive disorders.[358]

With the use of new molecular and genetic diagnostic techniques, it appears that most human cases of hypereosinophilic syndrome are neoplastic rather than reactive disorders.[20,351,422] This same phenomenon may be recognized in veterinary medicine as additional molecular and genetic techniques become available.[145,420] However, an idiopathic hypereosinophilic syndrome in Rottweiler dogs was considered to be a reactive process, because mean serum IgE concentrations were markedly high, no karyotype abnormalities were identified on cytogenetic analysis, and one dog underwent spontaneous remission.[211,455]

Increased numbers of eosinophils may be present in bone marrow samples from cats with MDS and AML even in the absence of peripheral eosinophilia.[208,210,429] Eosinophilia may also be present in CML, where neutrophilia predominates,[124,167,264,368] and in essential thrombocythemia, a myeloproliferative neoplasm with marked thrombocytosis.[320]

Basophilic Hyperplasia

Basophilic hyperplasia is generally present in bone marrow when peripheral basophilia is present.[209] Basophilia usually accompanies eosinophilia, and like eosinophilia, basophilia is generally associated with IgE-mediated disorders, including parasitic infestations (especially with nematodes and flukes) and allergic conditions.[366] It is most commonly seen in dogs and cats with dirofilariasis in the southern United States.[17,386]

Basophilia may occur in some animals with mast cell tumors, primarily noncutaneous types,* and in dogs diagnosed with essential thrombocythemia.[106,118,194,320] It has also been reported in dogs with pulmonary lymphomatoid granulomatosis.[21,369] Chapter 5 offers more detailed information concerning disorders that cause basophilia.

A marked basophilic left shift is present in the blood and bone marrow of dogs with basophilic leukemia,[280,288,311] and increased numbers of basophilic precursors may rarely be present in the bone marrow of cats with myeloid neoplasms (Fig. 9-33).[46,208,210] Basophilic leukemia must be differentiated from mast cell neoplasia with mastocytemia (sometimes called mast cell leukemia). Mast cells have round nuclei and basophils have segmented nuclei.[14,96,180,456]

Granulocytic Hypoplasia

Granulocytic hypoplasia is reported when the bone marrow cellularity is normal or decreased, the hematocrit is normal or

*References 16, 145, 200, 212, 242, 256, 327, 342, 358, 420, 459, 538.

*References 4, 45, 96, 113, 345, 367.

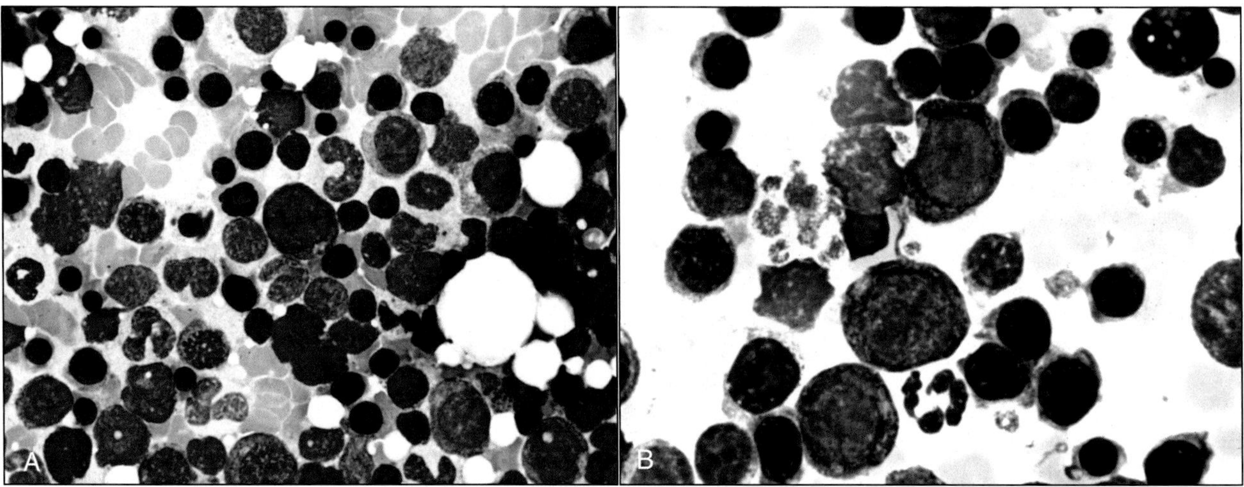

FIGURE 9-34

Granulocytic hypoplasia in bone marrow aspirate smears from cats. **A,** Granulocytic hypoplasia of unknown etiology in an aspirate smear of bone marrow from an FeLV-negative FIV-negative neutropenic cat with normal hematocrit and platelet count. **B,** Granulocytic hypoplasia of unknown etiology in an aspirate smear of bone marrow from a FeLV-negative cat with severe neutropenia. The hematocrit and platelet counts were normal. Most cells present are nucleated erythrocyte precursors. Wright-Giemsa stain.

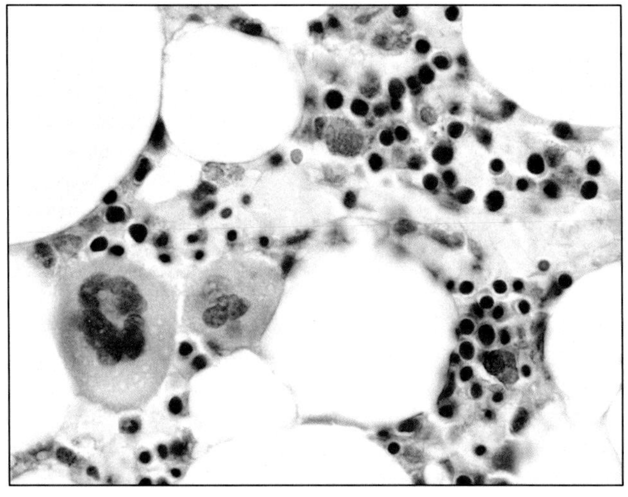

FIGURE 9-35

Granulocytic hypoplasia in a bone marrow core biopsy section collected from a dog 6 days after therapy with vincristine, L-asparaginase, and prednisone was initiated for a mediastinal tumor. Two megakaryocytes and many erythroid precursors are present. The orange-staining globular material is hemosiderin. H&E stain.

increased, and the M : E ratio is low. If the marrow is hypercellular and/or the hematocrit is low, a low M : E ratio indicates the presence of erythroid hyperplasia. Because neutrophilic cells are normally much more numerous than eosinophilic or basophilic cells in bone marrow, the term *granulocytic hypoplasia* indicates the presence of neutrophilic hypoplasia (Fig. 9-34, *A,B;* Fig. 9-35). Eosinophilic hypoplasia and/or basophilic hypoplasia may accompany neutrophilic hypoplasia, but few basophil precursors are normally present in bone marrow, making an interpretation of basophilic hypoplasia difficult.

Selective Neutrophilic Hypoplasia or Aplasia

Selective neutrophilic hypoplasia may be immune-mediated, drug-induced (which may be a secondary immune-mediated disorder), inherited, or idiopathic in humans.*

Ineffective neutrophil production is present in humans with chronic idiopathic neutropenia. The M : E ratio in the bone marrow is low and there is a prominent left shift in the granulocytic series. The presence of activated T lymphocytes—producing proapoptotic mediators including IFN-γ and Fas-ligand—is believed to contribute to the impaired survival of granulocytic progenitor cells in the bone marrow. The balance between prosurvival and proapoptotic mediators may be altered further by an increased local production of the hematopoietic inhibitors TNF-α and TGF-β1 and decreased levels of the anti-inflammatory cytokine IL-10.[350] A similar mechanism has been described in idiopathic aplastic anemia in humans.[297]

Most dogs with immune-mediated neutropenia have neutrophilic hyperplasia in the bone marrow; but some exhibit neutrophilic hypoplasia and two dogs had a complete lack of neutrophil precursors in the marrow (pure white cell aplasia).[56,310,359,483,526] Neutropenia that was believed to have been immune-mediated was described in a cat with a thymoma. A left shift was present, and the M : E ratio was approximately 1 : 1, which is slightly low for cats (see Table 8-2).[121] Neutrophilic hypoplasia with a maturational arrest in the neutrophilic series may occur when autoantibodies recognize antigenic determinants expressed not only by mature neutrophils but also by bone marrow granulocytic precursors.[74,165]

Cytotoxic drugs used to treat immune-mediated diseases and cancer typically result in generalized marrow injury, but in

*References 12, 32, 68, 75, 221, 350, 501.

some cases injury to the neutrophilic series is more severe than injury to the erythroid or megakaryocytic series. Azathioprine can produce neutropenia resulting from selective neutrophilic hypoplasia in some cats.[26] Experimental studies in cats have also demonstrated that doxorubicin can sometimes produce neutropenia without anemia or thrombocytopenia, but the investigators did not examine bone marrow to determine whether selective neutrophilic hypoplasia was present.[346]

Many drugs have been reported to cause neutropenia in humans, and neutrophilic hypoplasia is commonly present in bone marrow.[32] Griseofulvin is a fungistatic antibiotic that has been reported to cause neutropenia in cats with dermatophyte infections but not in experimental cats without dermatophyte infections (Fig. 9-36).[178,245] FIV-infected cats appear to have an increased risk of developing griseofulvin-induced toxicity.[424] In these cases, bone marrow evaluation has revealed evidence of neutrophilic hypoplasia. Methimazole treatment has been reported to cause neutropenia in hyperthyroid cats, but bone marrow findings were not given.[361] Transient methimazole-induced generalized marrow aplasia has been reported in humans.[323] Lithium carbonate can cause neutrophilic hypoplasia with maturational arrest and neutropenia in cats.[99]

Neutropenia has been reported in animals given recombinant G-CSF from another species.[162,389] This phenomenon apparently occurs because the recipient develops antibodies that react not only against the foreign recombinant protein but also against the recipient's endogenous G-CSF. Marked neutrophilic hypoplasia occurred when canine recombinant G-CSF was injected into rabbits[389] but not when recombinant human G-CSF was injected into dogs, although the dogs became neutropenic.[162] In the latter instance, the authors speculated that the antibody was bound to G-CSF on the surface of circulating neutrophils, resulting in an immune-mediated premature destruction of these cells.

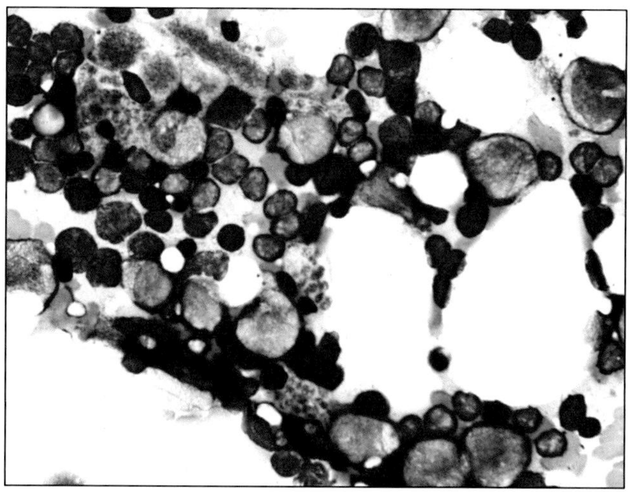

FIGURE 9-36
Granulocytic hypoplasia with maturational arrest of granulocyte precursors in an aspirate smear of bone marrow from a severely neutropenic cat that had been treated with griseofulvin and prednisone for skin lesions. Increased numbers of small lymphocytes are also present. Slight neutrophilia and normal bone marrow cytology were present 3 days later, following cessation of drug treatments. Wright-Giemsa stain.

Neutrophilic hypoplasia occurs in the bone marrow of neutropenic cats and dogs with parvovirus infections.[43,252,255,370] Such infections in pups can also cause a severe erythroid hypoplasia, but animals usually do not become anemic because of the long life span of erythrocytes.[395]

Transient neutrophilic hypoplasia in the marrow with resultant transient peripheral neutropenia occur at 12- to 14-day intervals in gray Collie dogs with inherited cyclic hematopoiesis.[93,284,413] When examined early in the neutropenic phase, myeloblasts and promyelocytes are present, but later stages of neutrophil development are absent and the M:E ratio is low.[413] Over the next few days, later maturational stages increase until the neutrophilic series is complete, the M:E ratio is high, and the number of neutrophils in blood is normal or increased.[284,413] Overall marrow cellularity is fairly constant, because the oscillations of granulopoiesis and erythropoiesis occur in a reciprocal manner.[284] A similar repetitive pattern of neutrophilic hypoplasia followed by neutrophilic hyperplasia has been described in cats with FeLV-induced cyclic hematopoiesis.[453] Cyclic neutropenia has been produced experimentally in dogs using continuous low-dose cyclophosphamide treatment, but bone marrow was not examined.[326]

Familial neutropenia and thrombocytopenia have been reported in eight horses with severe neutrophilic hypoplasia/aplasia and megakaryocytic hypoplasia.[237] Erythroid maturation was orderly, but some degree of erythroid hypoplasia was believed to be present in half of the horses. Chronic (possibly congenital) neutropenia has been described in a young dog with G-CSF deficiency. Bone marrow aspiration biopsy revealed a maturational arrest at the promyelocyte-myelocyte stage.[250]

A decreased M:E ratio may be present when there is an increased demand for neutrophils and depletion of the post-mitotic maturational and storage pool of the bone marrow, as may occur with septicemia and endotoxemia.[58] These alterations may appear as a maturational arrest with cytoplasmic toxicity.

Dysgranulopoiesis

The term *dysgranulopoiesis* refers to various disorders in which abnormal granulocyte maturation and/or morphology is present. Dysgranulopoiesis often results in ineffective granulopoiesis and a peripheral neutropenia. Neutrophilic abnormalities that may be present in bone marrow include increased numbers of myeloblasts (Fig. 9-37); maturational arrest in the neutrophilic series (Fig. 9-38); giant metamyelocytes, bands, and mature neutrophils (Figs. 9-39 and 9-40); multinucleated cells (Fig 9-41,*A,B*); abnormal mitosis (Fig. 9-41, *C*); abnormal granulation; hyposegmented neutrophils (pseudo-Pelger-Huët); hypersegmented neutrophils (Fig. 9-41, *D*); and neutrophils with bizarre nuclear shapes (see Figs. 9-40 and 9-41, *E*).*

*References 39, 88, 167, 185, 208, 319, 382, 507, 528, 530.

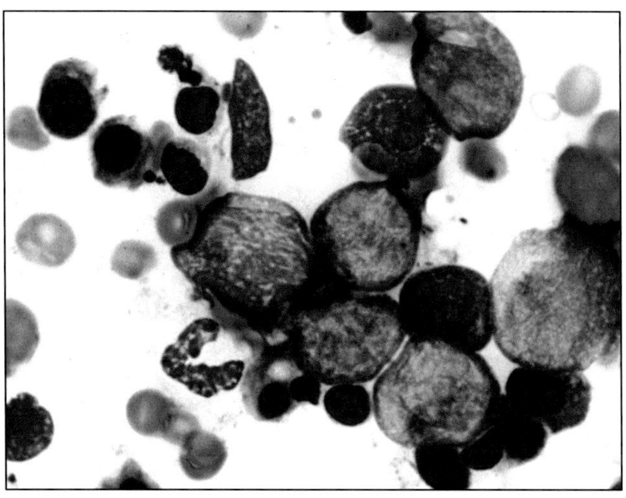

FIGURE 9-37
Increased numbers of myeloblasts (the six largest cells) in an aspirate smear of bone marrow from a horse with MDS. Myeloblasts accounted for 9% of all nucleated cells in the marrow. Wright-Giemsa stain.

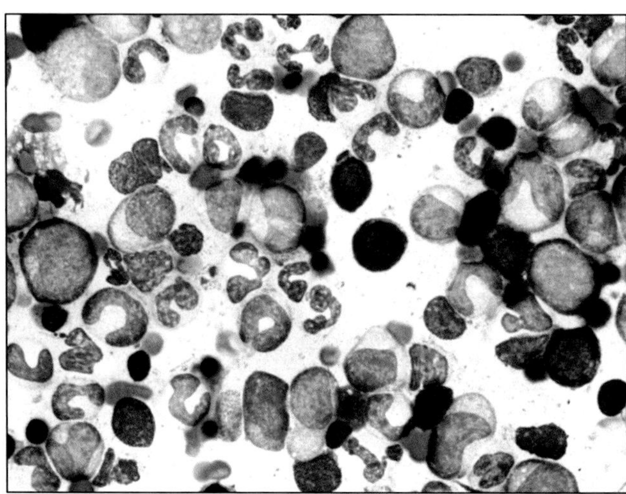

FIGURE 9-39
Giant band neutrophils in an aspirate smear of bone marrow from a cat with MDS. Wright-Giemsa stain.

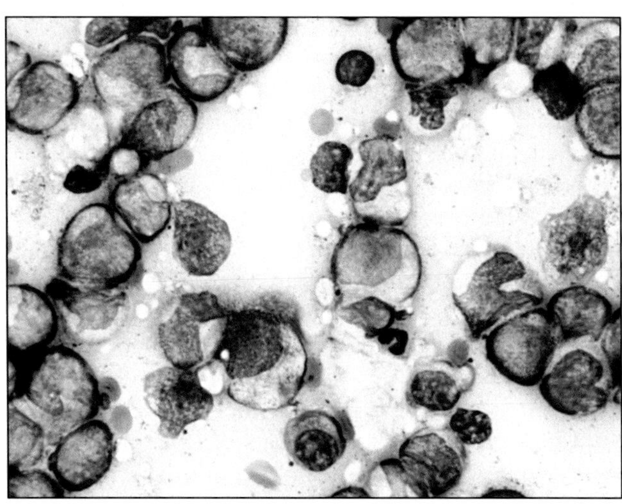

FIGURE 9-38
Maturational arrest in neutrophil development at the myelocyte-metamyelocyte stage in an aspirate smear of bone marrow from a FeLV-negative neutropenic cat with MDS. Erythroid precursors are absent in this field. Wright-Giemsa stain.

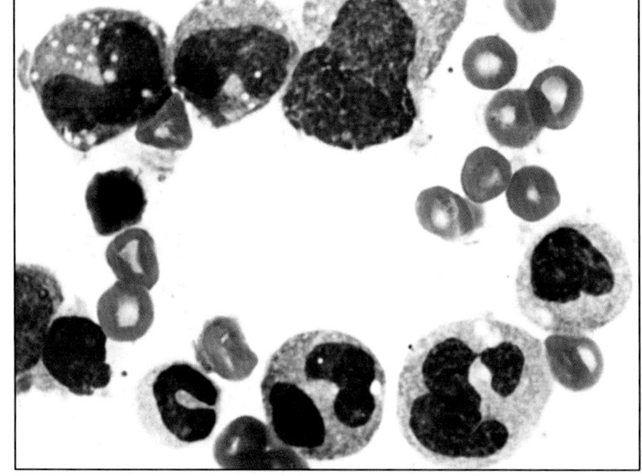

FIGURE 9-40
Idiopathic dysgranulopoiesis with giant neutrophil precursors with abnormal nuclear morphology in some cells and cytoplasmic vacuolation in others in a bone marrow aspirate smear from a dog with pancytopenia. Wright-Giemsa stain.

Dysgranulopoiesis generally occurs in animals with MDS and AML. It is most common in cats with FeLV and/or FIV infections.* Immune-mediated neutropenia can result in increased numbers of neutrophilic precursors in the proliferating pool relative to the number of neutrophilic precursors in the maturational and storage pool.[74] Giant schnauzer dogs with an inherited malabsorption of cobalamin may have neutropenia with hypersegmented neutrophils in the blood and megaloblastic changes in the neutrophilic cell line in the bone marrow.[138,139]

*References 27, 39, 185, 293, 426, 429.

Various drugs may result in dysgranulopoiesis. Experimental studies have shown that lithium treatment causes a neutropenia in cats as a result of a neutrophilic maturational arrest in the bone marrow.[99] Maturational arrests in both the neutrophilic and erythroid series have been reported in the bone marrow of neutropenic anemic dogs treated with a cephalosporin antibiotic.[97] Dysgranulopoiesis and mild erythroid hypoplasia have been reported in the marrow of cats given valacyclovir, an antiviral drug designed for the treatment of herpesvirus infections.[340] Last, an antipsychotic clozapine-related drug resulted in neutropenia with a left shift in myeloid and erythroid cells in the bone marrow of dogs.[274]

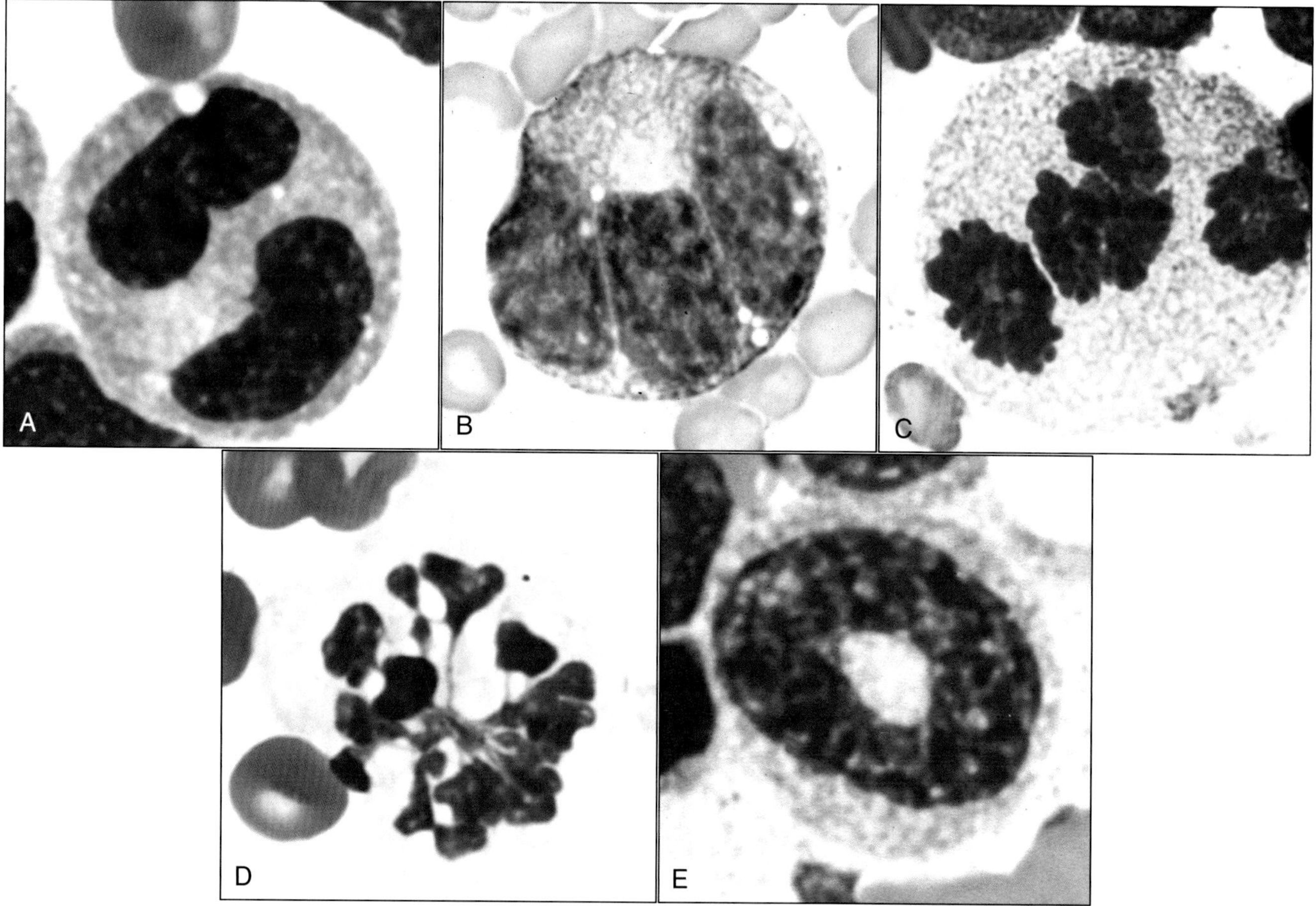

FIGURE 9-41

Dysplastic neutrophilic cells in bone marrow aspirate smears. **A,** Binucleated granulocytic precursor in blood from a dog with idiopathic dysgranulopoiesis. **B,** Trinucleated granulocytic precursor in blood from a cat with MDS. **C,** Abnormal mitotic cell in blood from a cat with MDS. **D,** Hypersegmentation in a dog with idiopathic dysgranulopoiesis. **E,** Doughnut-shaped neutrophil precursor in an aspirate smear of bone marrow from an FIV-infected leukopenic cat. Wright-Giemsa stain.

B, *Courtesy of Rose Raskin.*

The injection of recombinant G-CSF can have profound effects on bone marrow morphology. Recombinant G-CSF shortens the cell cycle in neutrophil precursors, stimulates three to four extra divisions in the mitotic neutrophil pool, and shortens the neutrophil maturational time in the marrow.[273] Hematologic findings in humans treated for neutropenia with G-CSF included a neutrophilia with a prominent left shift, toxic cytoplasm, circulating myeloblasts (less than 2%), dysplastic neutrophils (hyposegmentation, hypersegmentation, and ring nuclei), and a peripheral metarubricytosis. Granulocytic hyperplasia with marked increases in promyelocytes and myelocytes was present early in therapy, but the M:E ratio and the relative distribution of neutrophil stages normalized over time during therapy.[411] Similar findings are expected in dogs and cats treated with recombinant G-CSF (Fig. 9-42).[137]

The early recovery stage from neutrophilic aplasia/hypoplasia can exhibit some of the morphologic abnormalities reported in animals with dysgranulopoiesis.[209] When neutrophils begin to proliferate after a period of neutrophilic aplasia, myeloblasts and promyelocytes predominate early (Fig. 9-43), followed progressively by the appearance of the later stages of development (Fig. 9-44).[93,413,453] When an animal is examined prior to the production of mature neutrophils, the appearance of a maturational arrest is present (see Fig. 9-43). Overwhelming sepsis or endotoxemia with a compensatory premature release of mature neutrophils can also give the impression of a maturational arrest.

Bone marrow toxicity (myelotoxicity) is induced by strong septic and nonseptic inflammatory conditions as well as by some drugs. Although all bone marrow cell lines may be affected, evidence of toxicity is most apparent in neutrophilic precursors.[391] Cytoplasmic basophilia and foaminess can be seen in later stages of neutrophil development in the bone marrow, as is seen in circulating toxic neutrophilic cells. In contrast, discrete cytoplasmic vacuoles may be present in

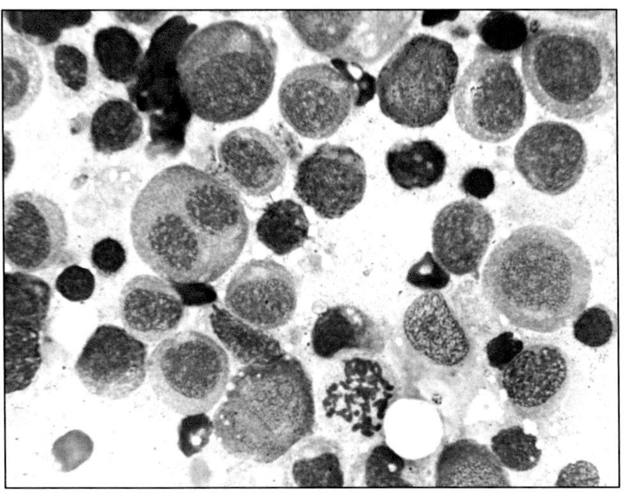

FIGURE 9-42

Increased myeloblasts and promyelocytes in a bone marrow aspirate smear from a persistently neutropenic dog treated with recombinant G-CSF twice (1 and 2 days) before this aspirate was taken. The total leukocyte count and neutrophil count at the time of the bone marrow aspiration were 1.2 and 0.1 × $10^3/\mu L$, respectively. The M:E ratio was 0.8:1, and 41% of all nucleated cells present were myeloblasts and promyelocytes. The absolute neutrophil count was within the reference interval 2 days later.

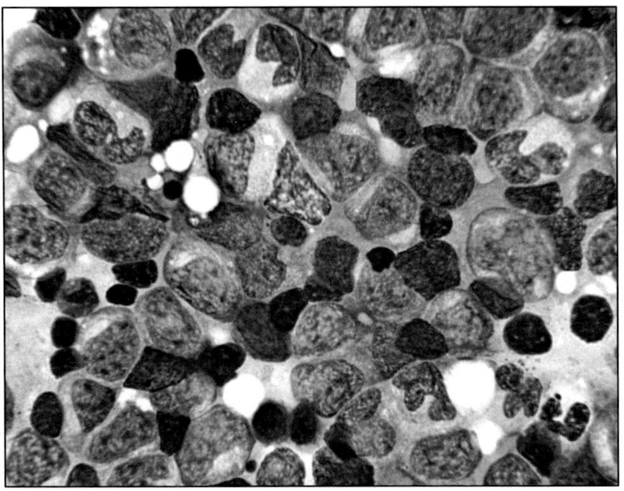

FIGURE 9-43

Marked granulocytic hyperplasia in a bone marrow aspirate smear from a dog recovering from diethylstilbestrol-induced bone marrow toxicosis. Approximately 95% of myeloid cells are early (proliferating) precursors; of these, 85% are type I myeloblasts, 10% are type II myeloblasts, and about 5% are promyelocytes. There are occasional myelocytes. Myeloid cells incapable of division (metamyelocytes, bands and segmented cells) comprise less than 5% of the myeloid cells. The blood neutrophil count was 0.1 × $10^3/\mu L$, and the M:E ratio was 15:1. The blood neutrophil count was 3.0 × $10^3/\mu L$ when rechecked 2 weeks later. Modified Wright stain.

Photograph of a bone marrow smear from a 2009 ASVCP slide review case submitted by C. Mastrorilli, E. Welles, J. Seay, and K. McIlwaine.

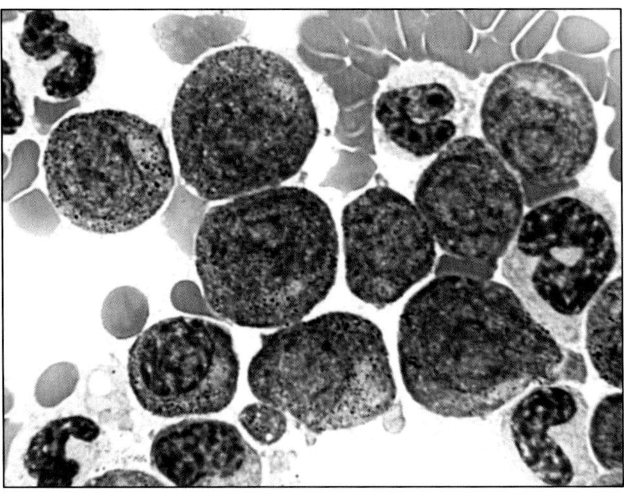

FIGURE 9-44

Intense granulocytic proliferative response with marked left shift in a bone marrow aspirate from a cat responding to an acute bone marrow insult. Nearly half of the nucleated cells present were myeloblasts (especially type II and III myeloblasts with primary granules) and promyelocytes. Megakaryocytic and erythroid hypoplasia was present. The cat presented with a pancytopenia (hematocrit, 8%; neutrophil count, 1.4 × $10^3/\mu L$; total leukocyte count, 2.5 × $10^3/\mu L$; and platelets, 17 × $10^3/\mu L$), toxic degenerative left shift, and life-threatening hemorrhaging, with a markedly prolonged activated partial thromboplastin time. FeLV and FIV tests were negative. The cat was given supportive care, including a blood transfusion. Hematology findings 2 days later included a hematocrit of 21%, neutrophilic cell count and total leukocyte count of 6.5 and 9.7 × $10^3/\mu L$, respectively, and a platelet count of 69 × $10^3/\mu L$. The cause of the bone marrow insult was not determined. A toxin was not identified, but the client had treated the cat for several days with an unknown antihistamine and cefadroxil for respiratory signs prior to presentation.

myeloblasts and promyelocytes. These vacuolated precursors may have lobulated nuclei suggestive of monocyte precursors (Fig. 9-45, *A,B*).[152] Discrete cytoplasmic vacuoles in neutrophilic precursors have also been reported with drugs, including chloramphenicol, metronidazole, and cyclophosphamide.[496,508] The experimental administration of recombinant G-CSF to cats resulted in not only a marked increase in the mitotic granulocytic pool but also in variable vacuolation of granulocytic precursors, large granules in promyelocytes, and visible granules in myelocytes and metamyelocytes.[137] Additional nuclear abnormalities—including hyposegmentation, hypersegmentation, ring-formation, and binucleation—may also be present in myelotoxicity. Giant neutrophils with nuclear abnormalities are most often seen in cats.[209,391]

ABNORMALITIES OF MEGAKARYOCYTES

Megakaryocytic Hyperplasia

Megakaryocyte number, ploidy, and size increase in bone marrow within a few days following a thrombocytopenia resulting from premature destruction or utilization of platelets in blood (Fig. 9-46, *A,B*).[222,225] Although other growth factors

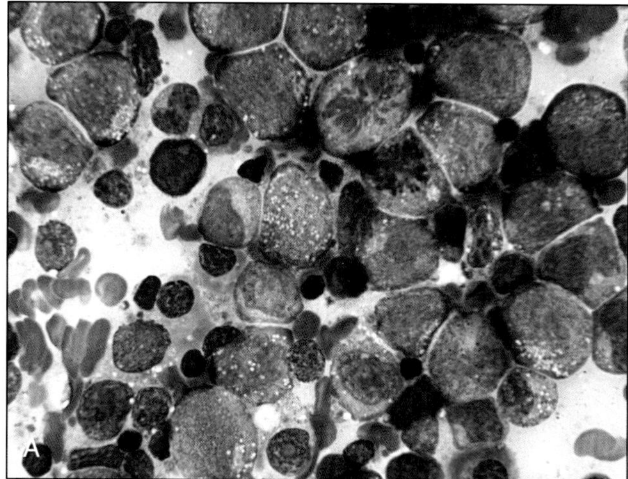

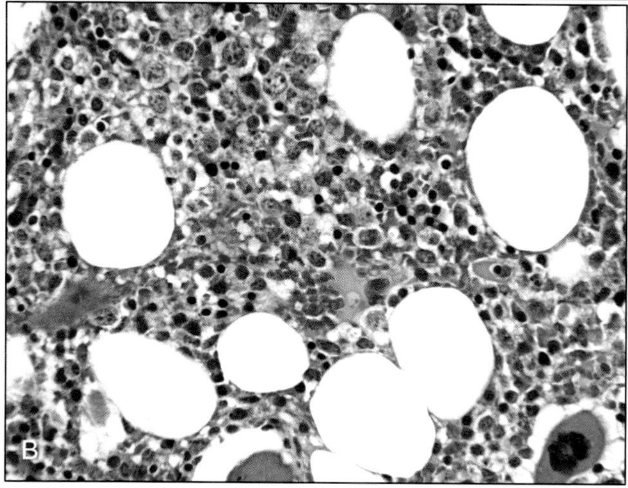

FIGURE 9-45

Apparent maturational arrest in the neutrophilic series in bone marrow from a dog with a severe leukopenia and neutropenia, 1.1 and 0.1 × $10^3/\mu L$, respectively. Marked cytoplasmic toxicity and a degenerative left shift of neutrophilic cells were present in blood. **A,** Toxic neutrophilic precursors in a bone marrow aspirate smear. Discrete cytoplasmic vacuoles were apparent in early neutrophilic precursors. The M:E ratio was about 2:1, but it was difficult to differentiate toxic granulocytic precursors from monocytic precursor cells in bone marrow. Lymphocytes (19%) and plasma cells (15%) were increased. Wright-Giemsa stain. **B,** Vacuolated neutrophilic precursors with marked left shift (few cells more mature than myelocytes) in a core bone marrow biopsy section from the dog presented in **(A).** A megakaryocyte is located at the bottom right. H&E stain. Sepsis was considered likely and antibiotic therapy was initiated. The blood total leukocyte and total neutrophilic cell counts were 17.4 and 12.7 × $10^3/\mu L$, respectively, when measured 2 days later. A regenerative left shift with 3+ cytoplasmic toxicity was present in blood neutrophilic cells at that time.

have synergistic effects, these changes are largely the result of increased thrombopoietin, which also accelerates the rate of megakaryocyte maturation. Most megakaryocytes are mature in animals with megakaryocytic hyperplasia, but increased numbers of promegakaryocytes and basophilic megakaryocytes are often recognized. Thrombocytopenic disorders in which megakaryocytic hyperplasia is expected include primary and secondary IMT, ongoing intravascular coagulation, hypersplenism, and vascular injury. Various viral, rickettsial, bacterial, protozoal, and fungal agents and therapeutic drugs result in platelet destruction or utilization and subsequent megakaryocytic hyperplasia (Fig. 9-47). *E. canis* infection is a common cause of thrombocytopenia in dogs in the southern United States. Although generalized marrow hypoplasia occurs in severe chronic ehrlichiosis, megakaryocytic hyperplasia is present early in the disease when immune-mediated platelet destruction largely accounts for the thrombocytopenia.[166,390] Chapter 7 offers more information about the pathogenesis of thrombocytopenic disorders in animals.

Megakaryocytic hyperplasia is also present in disorders with accompanying thrombocytosis, including iron-deficiency anemia (see Fig. 9-1), some chronic inflammatory conditions, and essential thrombocythemia, which is a myeloproliferative neoplasm characterized by a persistent, markedly increased (greater than $1 \times 10^6/\mu L$) platelet count.[25,106,115,292] Megakaryocyte morphology appears normal when examined by light microscopy (Fig. 9-48, *A,B*).

Selective Megakaryocytic Hypoplasia or Aplasia

Selective amegakaryocytic thrombocytopenia is a rare syndrome in humans, in which it occurs as a congenital defect or an acquired defect in adults. Congenital amegakaryocytic thrombocytopenia generally results from genetic mutations in the thrombopoietin recepter gene.[22] Acquired amegakaryocytic thrombocytopenia in humans appears to be an immune-mediated disorder.[473] Idiopathic amegakaryocytic thrombocytopenia is also rare in adult dogs and cats, in which it is presumed to be immune-mediated (Fig. 9-49).* It has been reported in a quarter horse foal with associated IMHA.[437] Familial neutropenia and thrombocytopenia have been reported in eight horses with severe neutrophilic hypoplasia/aplasia and megakaryocytic hypoplasia.[237]

Various drugs may induce thrombocytopenia as a result of marrow suppression. Usually marrow suppression is generalized, but megakaryocytes may be specifically decreased.[163] For example, dapsone treatment has been associated with amegakaryocytic thrombocytopenia in a dog,[261] and megakaryocytic and/or erythroid hypoplasia were reported to occur in cats treated with ribavirin, a broad-spectrum antiviral agent.[532]

Dysmegakaryocytopoiesis

Dysmegakaryocytopoiesis refers to the presence of maturational and/or morphologic abnormalities in megakaryocytic cells. Apparent maturational arrests with early stages (e.g., promegakaryocytes) predominating may not be reflective of a dysplastic process, but rather may result from immune-mediated reactions against megakaryocyte antigens (see Fig. 9-46, *A*).[220] Dysplastic abnormalities that may be present in bone marrow include asynchronous maturation resulting in the formation of dwarf granular megakaryocytes with single

*References 143, 189, 219, 249, 329, 537, 552.

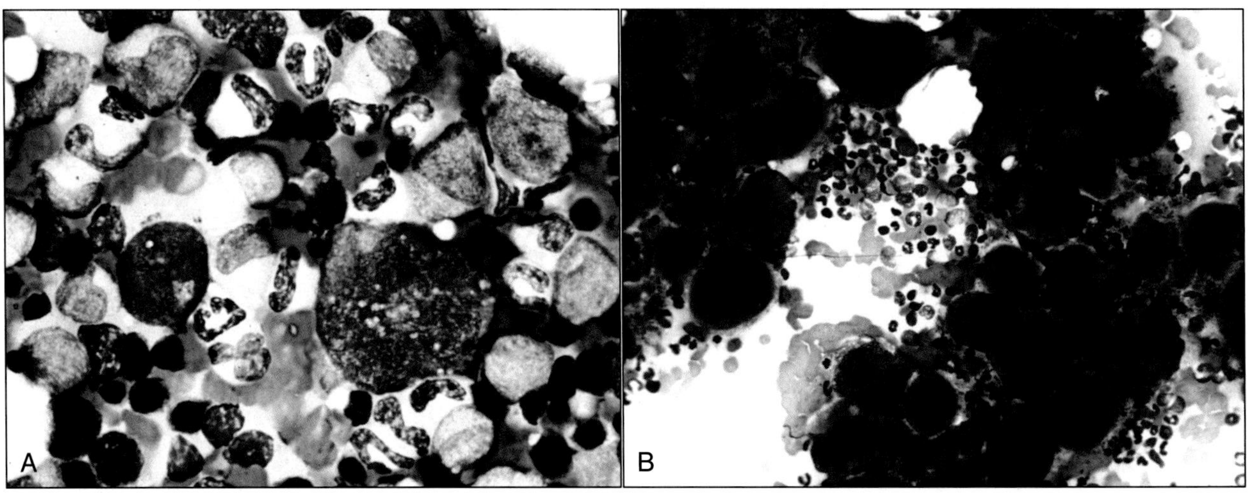

FIGURE 9-46

Megakaryocyte morphology and numbers in bone marrow aspirate smears, before and after therapy, from a dog with immune-mediated thrombocytopenia. **A,** Mature megakaryocytes were absent prior to therapy. Most megakaryocyte precursors present were promegakaryocytes *(binucleated cell at left),* but some basophilic megakaryocytes *(large cell at right)* were observed. **B,** Marked megakaryocytic hyperplasia in bone marrow from the same dog 1 week after prednisone therapy was begun. The image of this second aspirate smear was taken at lower magnification. Wright-Giemsa stain.

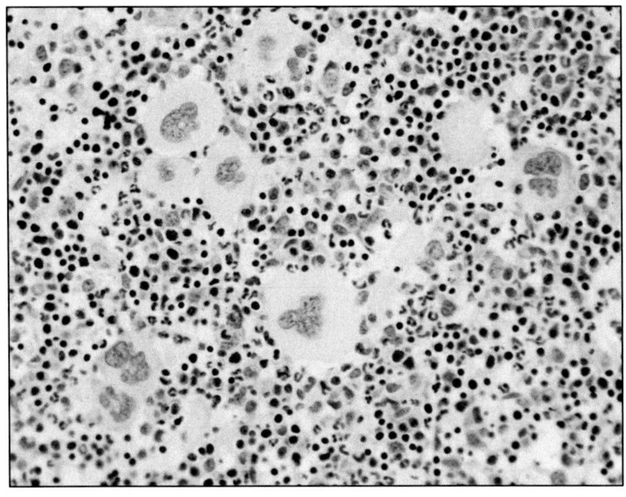

FIGURE 9-47

Megakaryocytic hyperplasia in a bone marrow section from a core biopsy collected from a thrombocytopenic dog with disseminated intravascular coagulation that developed 1.5 weeks after treatment for occult heartworm disease. H&E stain.

or multiple nuclei (Fig. 9-50, *A-C*) and large megakaryocytes with nuclear abnormalities including hypolobulation, hyperlobulation, or multiple round nuclei (Fig. 9-51, *A,B*).[39] Megakaryocytic dysplasia may occur in association with IMT and/or IMHA,[502,518] lymphoma,[502] and following drug administration,[276,532] but it most frequently occurs in MDS and AML.*

*References 39, 167, 309, 466, 502, 507, 530.

Asynchronous maturation and anisokaryosis of megakaryocytes have been reported in a Cavalier King Charles spaniel with inherited macrothrombocytopenia.[518] Chapter 7 offers information about this disorder.

Emperipolesis

Megakaryocytic emperipolesis refers to the movement of blood cells (neutrophils, erythrocytes, and lymphocytes) within megakaryocytes (Fig. 9-52, *A,B*).[412] Emperipolesis differs from phagocytosis in that entering cells exist temporarily within the cell. The mechanism and significance of this finding remain to be defined. Increased emperipolesis has been reported in humans with various conditions including active blood loss, carcinomas, myeloid neoplasms, non-Hodgkin lymphoma, idiopathic thrombocytopenia purpura, and reactive thrombocytosis.[69,109,328,405]

Emperipolesis occurs at low levels in young rats but is common in aged rats, and the incidence is markedly increased in animals with hyperplastic bone marrow secondary to chronic suppurative or neoplastic lesions.[260] Increased emperipolesis has been produced experimentally in animals in which thrombopoiesis is increased by phlebotomy,[463] IL-6 injections,[440] vincristine treatment,[442] and lipopolysaccharide (LPS) injections.[460] Studies with LPS indicate that emperipolesis is at least partly dependent on interactions between adhesion molecules on leukocytes and megakaryocytes.[460] Emperipolesis has been reported in dogs with leishmaniasis and in cats with presumptive IMT.[33,127,141] This may be a nonspecific response to increased thrombopoietin.[103] Internalization of *Histoplasma capsulatum* organisms within megakaryocytes has also been reported in a cat.[373]

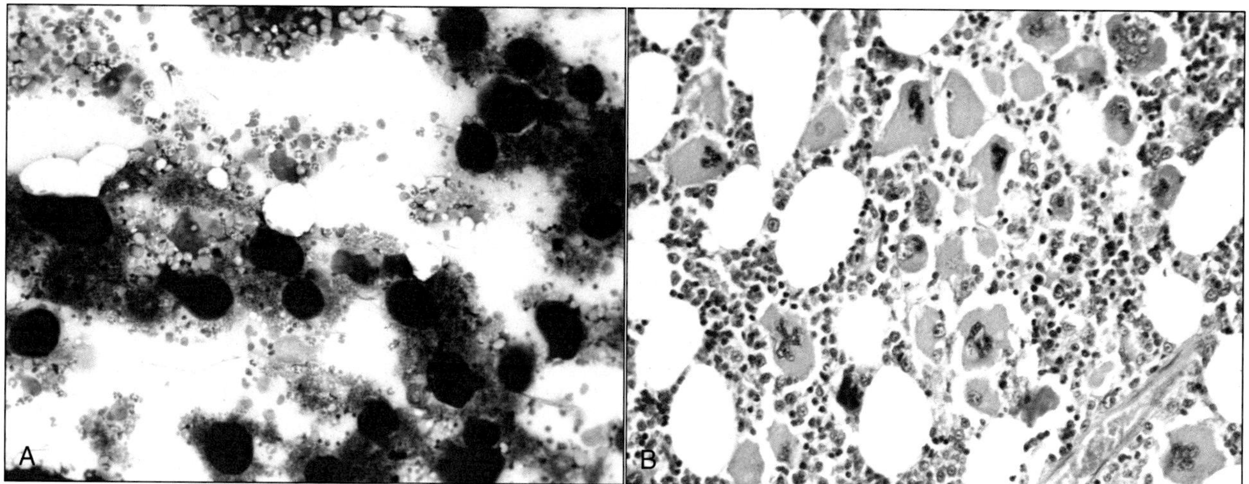

FIGURE 9-48
Megakaryocyte hyperplasia in bone marrow from a cat with essential thrombocythemia and a platelet count of $1.4 \times 10^6/\mu L$. **A,** Aspirate smear with many megakaryocytes. Wright-Giemsa stain. **B,** Section from a core biopsy with many megakaryocytes. H&E stain.

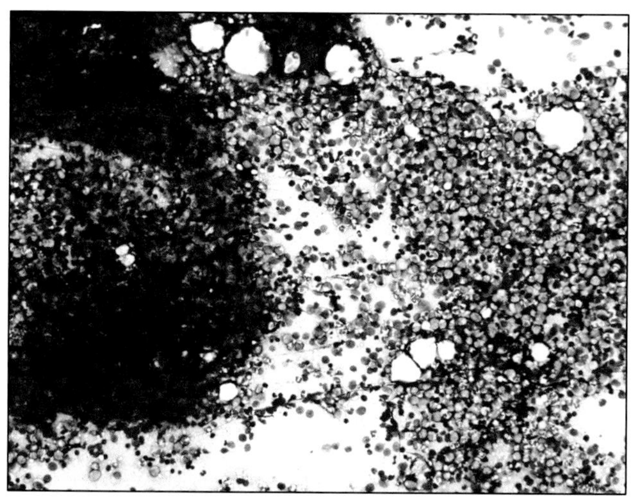

FIGURE 9-49
Megakaryocyte aplasia in a hypercellular aspirate smear of bone marrow from a thrombocytopenic cat with associated immune-mediated hemolytic anemia. Only one megakaryocyte was seen when multiple smears were scanned. Megakaryocytes were not seen in sections of bone marrow collected at necropsy. Wright-Giemsa stain.

ABNORMALITIES OF MONONUCLEAR PHAGOCYTES

Monocytic Hyperplasia

Monocyte precursors are normally present in low numbers in the bone marrow, and they are difficult to differentiate from neutrophilic precursors based on morphology alone. Consequently mild monocytic hyperplasia is difficult to recognize and monocytic hypoplasia is not recognized at all. Monocytic hyperplasia often accompanies granulocytic hyperplasia in response to various inflammatory cytokines and growth factors.[15,38,149,338,477] Monocytic hyperplasia may be appreciated in inflammatory conditions with increased monocyte production and in some myeloid neoplasms.[380] Monocyte precursors are markedly increased in two forms of AML. When myeloblasts as well as monoblasts are increased, the term *acute myelomonocytic leukemia* (AML-M4) may be used. When only monoblasts are increased, the disorder is classified as acute monocytic leukemia (AML-M5).[210]

Reactive Macrophage Hyperplasia

Macrophage hyperplasia occurs in the bone marrow in response to a variety of systemic viral, bacterial, fungal, and protozoal infectious agents (Fig. 9-53,*A,B*).[539] Organisms that may be visualized in bone marrow macrophages include *Mycobacterium* species (Fig. 9-54, *A,B*),[217,347,490] *Histoplasma capsulatum* (Fig. 9-55),[78,79,373] *Leishmania donovani* (Fig. 9-53,*A,B;* Fig. 9-56),[76,127,295,349] *Cytauxzoon felis* schizonts (Fig. 9-57; Fig. 9-58,*A,B;* Fig. 9-59; Fig. 9-60,*A,B*),[132,154,235,431] and *Philemonium obovatum*.[433]

Macrophages may be increased in the marrow and contain phagocytized cellular debris in response to marrow necrosis[195,391,503] or increased apoptosis, as may occur in dyserythropoiesis,[531] immune-mediated destruction of hematopoietic cells (Figs. 9-61, 9-62), or hematopoietic neoplasia (Fig. 9-63).[387,530] Increased numbers of vacuolated macrophages may be seen in some inherited lipid storage diseases (Fig. 9-64).[57,84,164]

Phagocytosis of Blood Cells and Their Precursors

Phagocytosis of blood cells is rare in the bone marrow of normal animals and generally involves only mature erythrocytes. Phagocytosis of blood precursor cells is considered

Text continued on p. 292

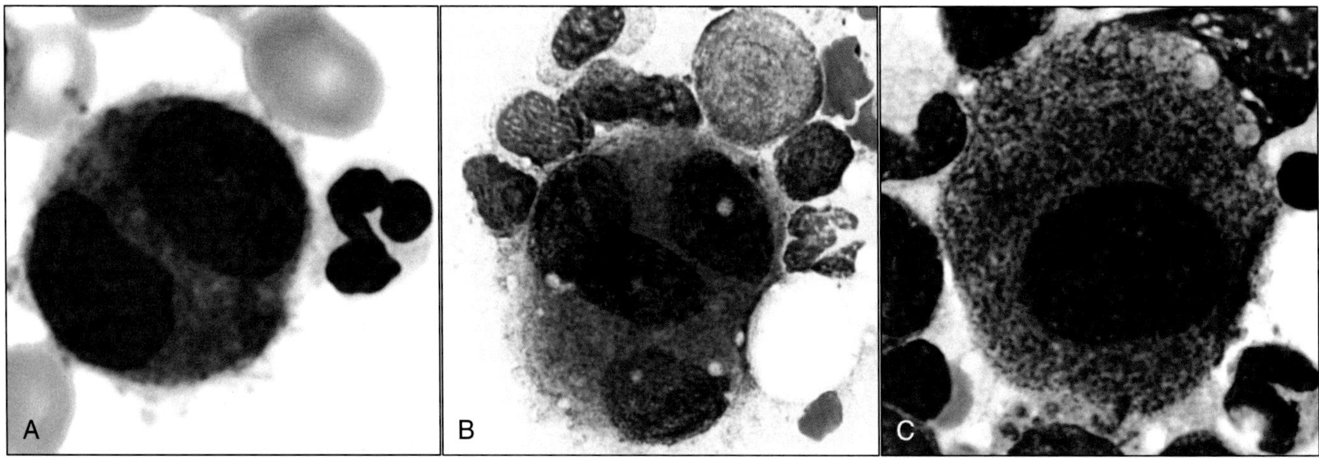

FIGURE 9-50

Dwarf megakaryocytes in bone marrow aspirate smears from animals with myeloid neoplasms. **A,** Binucleated dwarf megakaryocyte from a dog with CML. Magenta-staining granules in the cytoplasm and lack of intense basophilia indicate that it is not a promegakaryocyte. **B,** Dwarf megakaryocyte with four discrete nuclei from a dog with MDS. **C,** Dwarf megakaryocyte from an FeLV-positive, thrombocytopenic cat with MDS. Large numbers of magenta-staining granules are present in the cytoplasm, as is expected for mature megakaryocytes, but the cell has a single nucleus and is much smaller than normal. Wright-Giemsa stain.

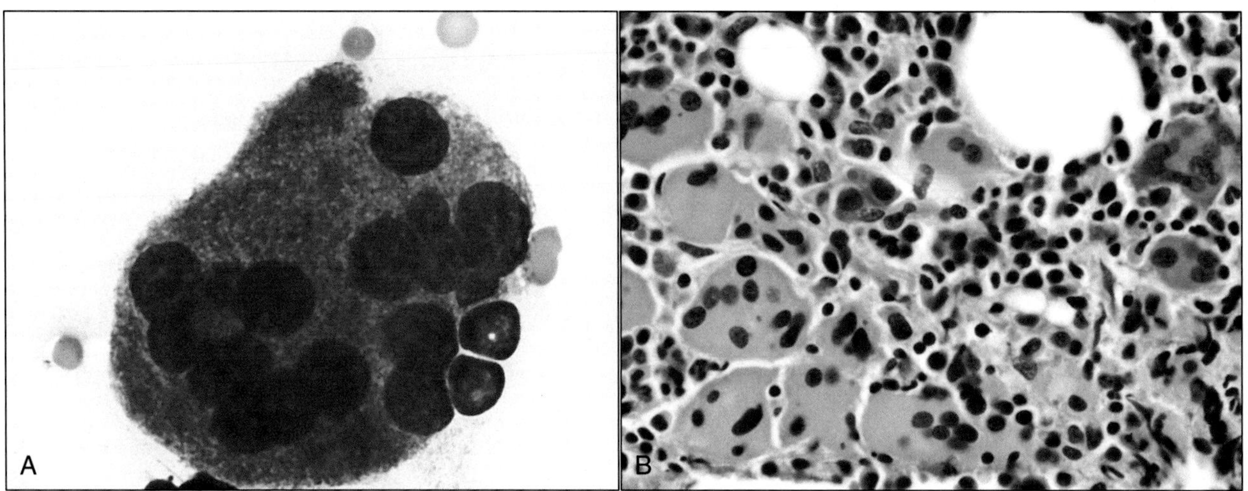

FIGURE 9-51

Dysmegakaryocytopoiesis in bone marrow from a cat with a glucocorticoid-responsive thrombocytopenia. Erythrocyte and leukocyte parameters were normal in blood, and the FeLV test was negative. **A,** Mature megakaryocyte with multiple separate nuclei, rather than a single lobulated nucleus, in an aspirate smear. Dwarf megakaryocytes with separate nuclei were also present *(not shown)*. Wright stain. **B,** Megakaryocytic hyperplasia in a core biopsy section. Megakaryocytes vary considerably in size and have multiple separate nuclei. H&E stain. The thrombocytopenia resolved following glucocorticoid therapy.

Courtesy of Jeff Sirninger.

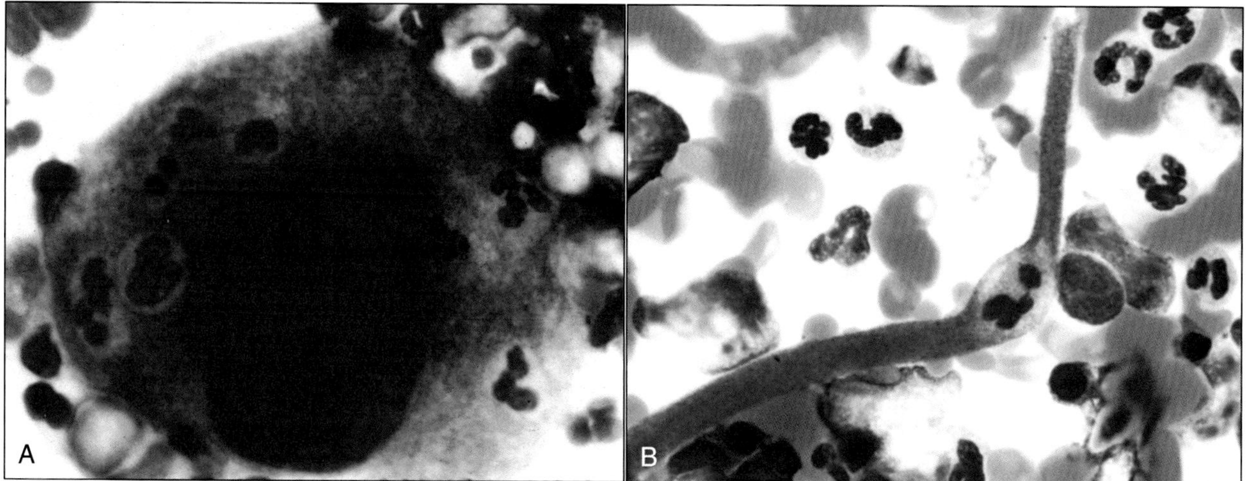

FIGURE 9-52

Megakaryocytic emperipolesis in bone marrow aspirate smears. **A,** Emperipolesis of neutrophils in a megakaryocyte from a cat with essential thrombocythemia. **B,** Emperipolesis of a neutrophil in a megakaryocyte proplatelet process from a dog. Modified Wright stain.

From Scott MA, Friedrichs KR. Megakaryocyte podography. Vet Clin Pathol *2009;38:135.*

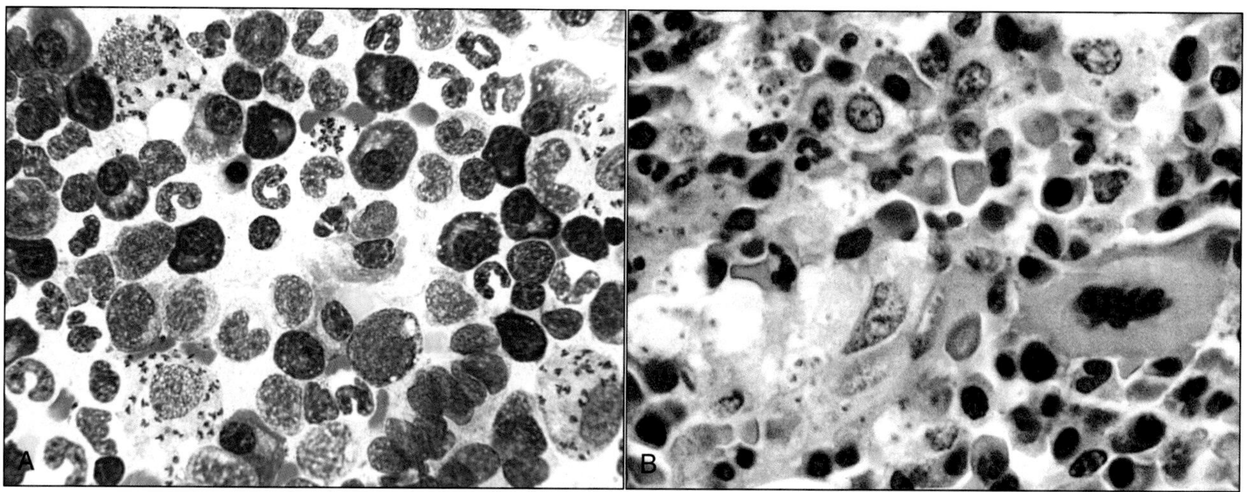

FIGURE 9-53

Increased numbers of macrophages and plasma cells in bone marrow from a dog with disseminated leishmaniasis. **A,** Three intact macrophages are filled with *Leishmania donovani* organisms. Many blue-staining plasma cells are also present in this aspirate smear. Wright-Giemsa stain. **B,** Macrophages containing *L. donovani* organisms *(dark dots)* in a bone marrow section from a core biopsy. A megakaryocyte is present at the right side. H&E stain.

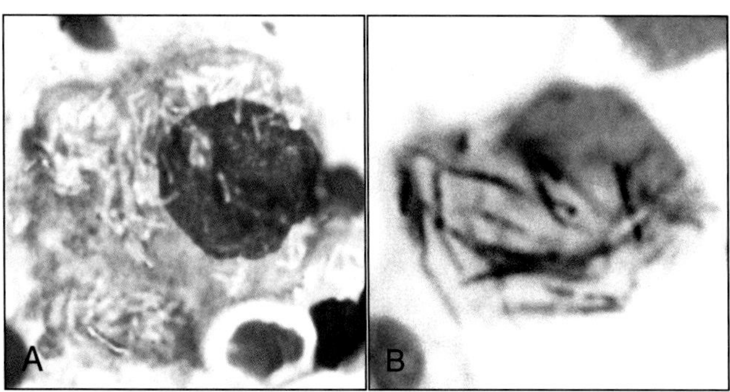

FIGURE 9-54

Macrophages containing *Mycobacterium avium* organisms in bone marrow aspirate smears from cats with disseminated mycobacteriosis. **A,** *M. avium* organisms appear as unstained rods in the cytoplasm of a macrophage. Wright-Giemsa stain. **B,** *M. avium* organisms appear as red-staining rods in the cytoplasm of a macrophage. Modified acid-fast stain.

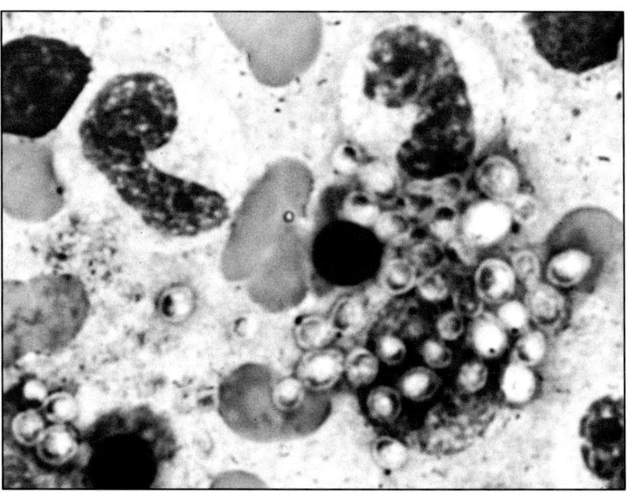

FIGURE 9-55

Macrophage *(right)* containing many *Histoplasma capsulatum* organisms in an aspirate smear of bone marrow from a cat with disseminated histoplasmosis. Free organisms *(left bottom)* may have come from damage to this cell or other macrophages present. Wright-Giemsa stain.

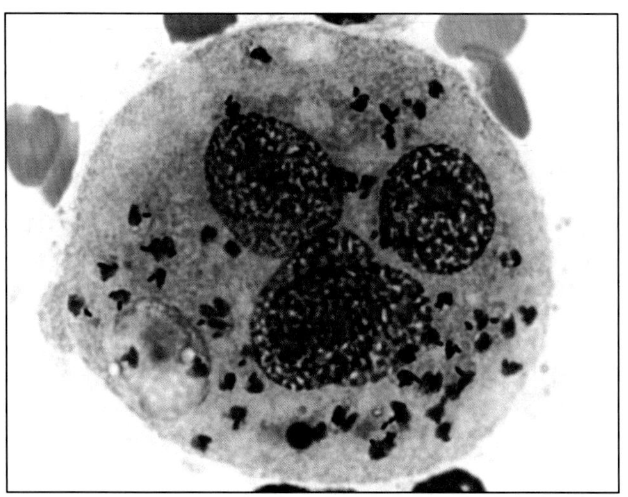

FIGURE 9-56

Multinucleated macrophage containing many *Leishmania donovani* organisms in an aspirate smear of bone marrow from a dog with disseminated leishmaniasis. These protozoal organisms are identified by a distinctive bar-shaped kinetoplast in the cytoplasm which stains similar to the nucleus. Wright-Giemsa stain.

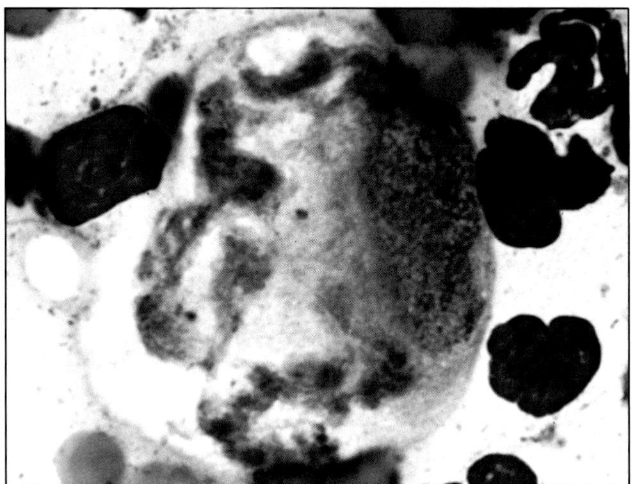

FIGURE 9-57

Early *Cytauxzoon felis* schizont development within a macrophage in an aspirate smear of bone marrow from a cat with cytauxzoonosis. The "ribbons" of darker blue material with reddish inclusions represent protoplasm of the infectious agent without definable nuclei. The macrophage nucleus is eccentrically located on the right side of the cell. Wright-Giemsa stain.

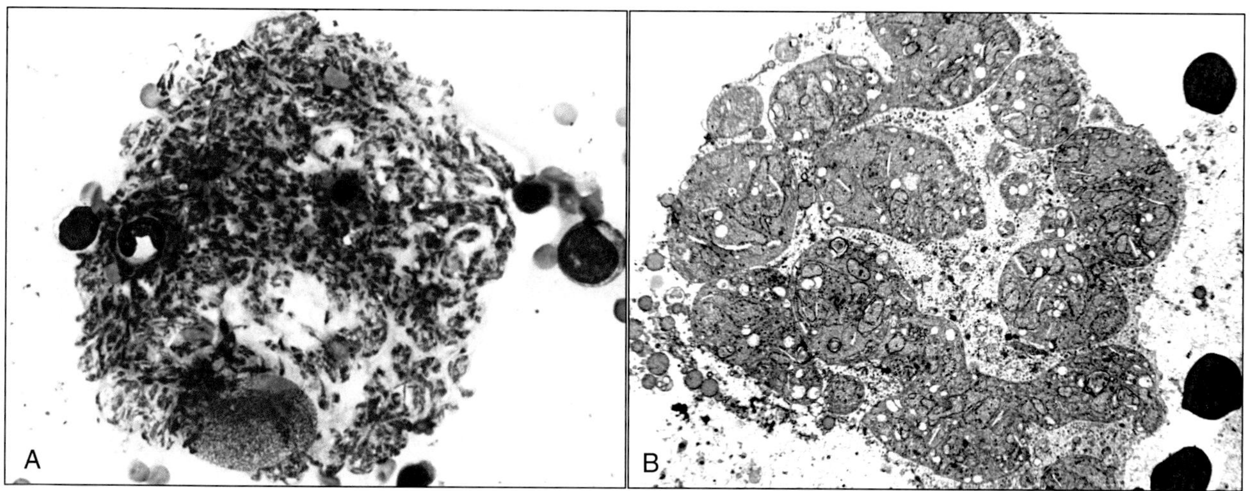

FIGURE 9-58

Intermediate *Cytauxzoon felis* schizont development within macrophages. **A,** A macrophage containing a developing schizont in an aspirate smear of bone marrow from a cat with cytauxzoonosis is shown at a much lower magnification than the macrophage in Figure 9-57. Separation of nuclear and cytoplasmic material has occurred. The nucleus of the macrophage is eccentrically located at the bottom edge of the cell. **B,** Transmission electron microscopy of a macrophage with an intermediate schizont. With development, there has been a progressive branching and elongation of lobules until the enlarged tortuous schizont fills the host cell, which has also become progressively larger. Concentrations of karyoplasm begin to occur beneath the surface membranes of the villous-like elongations of the schizont, and many nuclei can be visualized as concentrated areas of karyoplasm become membrane bound. At this stage, the parasite appears to contain multiple multinucleated structures. These have been called cytomeres in the past; however, they are not separate structures but lobules that are interconnected by numerous small cytoplasmic bridges.

***B,** From Simpson CF, Harvey JW, Lawman MJP, Murray J, Kocan AA, Carlisle JW. Ultrastructure of schizonts in the liver of cats with experimentally induced cytauxzoonosis.* Am J Vet Res. *1985;46:384-390.*

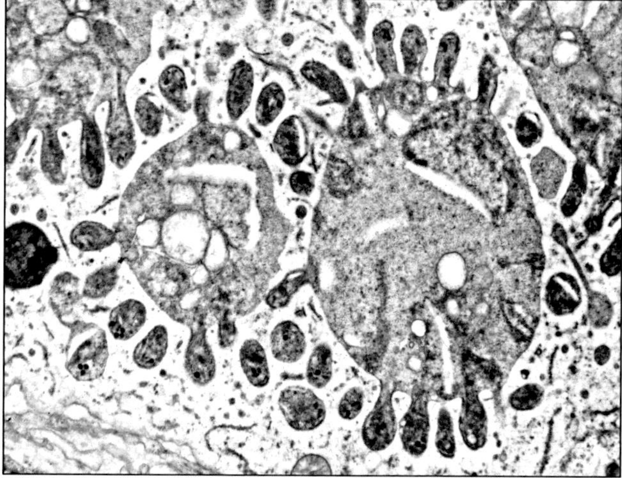

FIGURE 9-59

Transmission electron microscopy of *Cytauxzoon felis* merozoites forming as everted sacculations from schizont lobules in areas of lobule membrane adjacent to schizont nuclei.

From Simpson CF, Harvey JW, Lawman MJP, Murray J, Kocan AA, Carlisle JW. Ultrastructure of schizonts in the liver of cats with experimentally induced cytauxzoonosis. Am J Vet Res. *1985;46:384-390.*

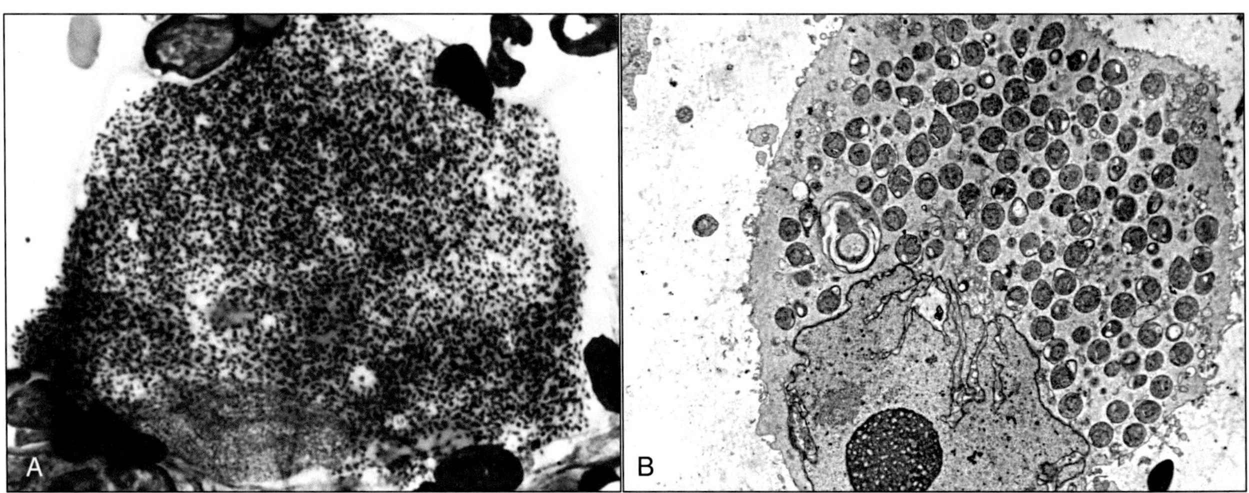

FIGURE 9-60

Completion of *Cytauxzoon felis* schizont development within macrophages. **A,** A macrophage in an aspirate smear of bone marrow from a cat with cytauxzoonosis shown at the same magnification as in Figure 9-58, *A.* Nuclei of hundreds of individual merozoites appear as small dots. The nucleus of the macrophage is eccentrically located at the bottom left edge of the cell. **B,** Transmission electron photomicrograph of a macrophage following completion of schizogony. The cytoplasm of the host macrophage is filled with mature merozoites. The nucleus of the macrophage with a large nucleolus is located at the bottom center of the image. A residual body in the cytoplasm *(slightly left of center)* constitutes the remains of the schizont. Following release by the macrophage, individual merozoites, containing a single mitochondrion and nucleus, enter erythrocytes by endocytosis *(not shown).*

B, *From Simpson CF, Harvey JW, Lawman MJP, Murray J, Kocan AA, Carlisle JW. Ultrastructure of schizonts in the liver of cats with experimentally induced cytauxzoonosis.* Am J Vet Res. *1985;46:384-390.*

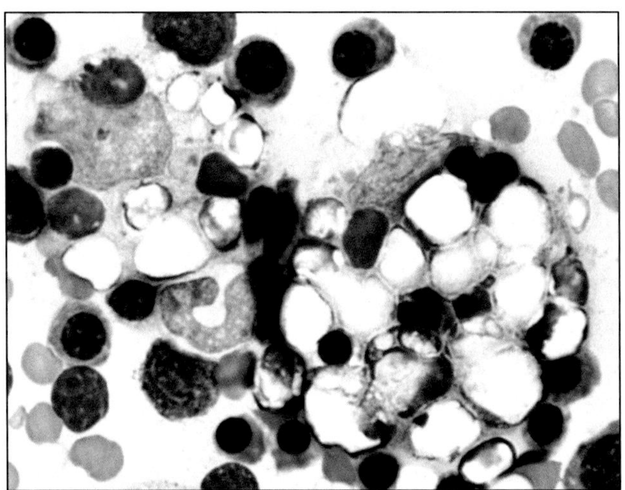

FIGURE 9-61

Two large macrophages filled with phagocytized cellular material and vacuoles in an aspirate smear of bone marrow from an anemic cat with ineffective erythropoiesis. Erythroid hyperplasia was present in bone marrow without accompanying reticulocytosis in blood. Wright-Giemsa stain.

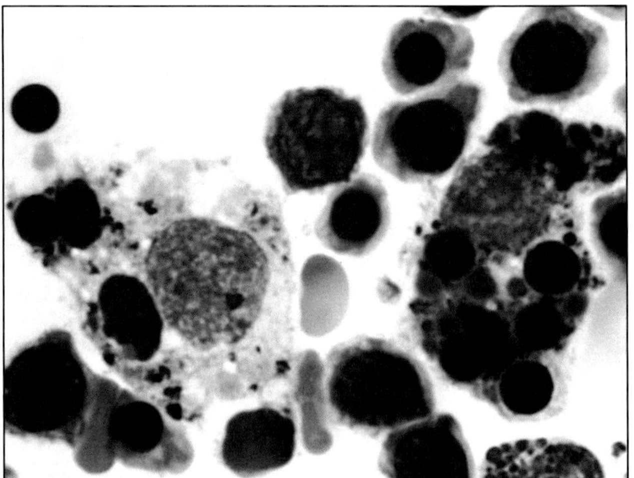

FIGURE 9-62

Two macrophages with phagocytized cellular material (primarily nuclei) in an aspirate smear of bone marrow from a dog with mild nonregenerative anemia and erythroid hyperplasia in the bone marrow. Wright-Giemsa stain.

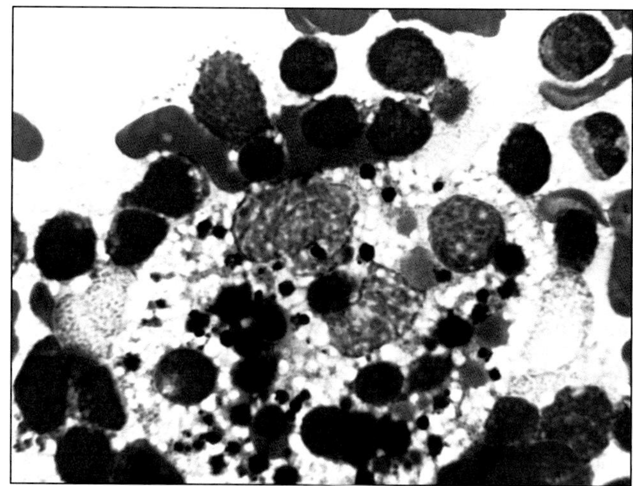

FIGURE 9-63
Binucleated macrophage with phagocytized cells and nuclear debris in a bone marrow aspirate smear form a dog with ALL. Neoplastic cells are also located within and outside the macrophage. Wright-Giemsa stain.

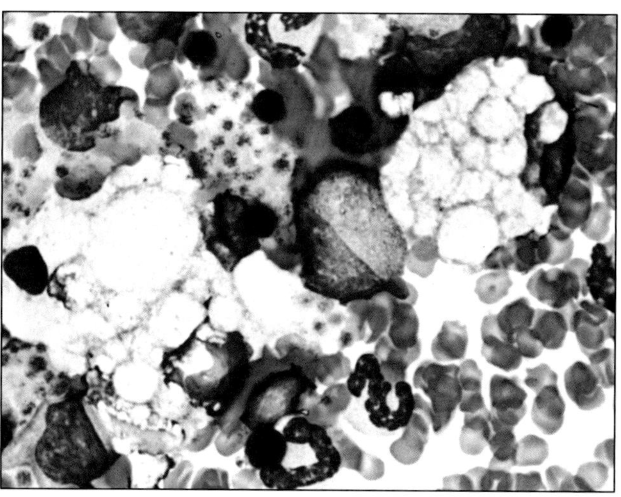

FIGURE 9-64
Two vacuolated macrophages in an aspirate smear of bone marrow from a cat with inherited Niemann-Pick type C disease.

Photograph of a stained bone marrow smear from a 1993 ASVCP slide review case submitted by D. E. Brown and M. A. Thrall.

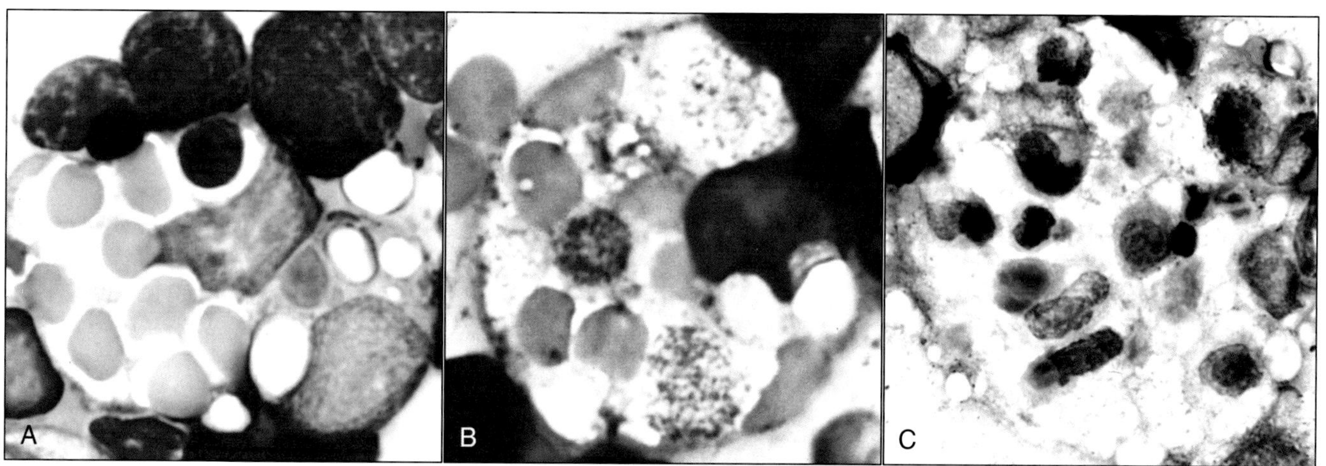

FIGURE 9-65
Macrophages with phagocytized cells in bone marrow aspirate smears. **A,** Macrophage with phagocytized erythrocytes and a nucleus *(left)* from a cat with ineffective erythropoiesis. **B,** Macrophage with phagocytized erythrocytes and platelets from a cat with cytauxzoonosis. **C,** Macrophage with phagocytized leukocytes from a leukopenic cat with MDS.

abnormal and implies increased cell destruction or death within the marrow (Fig. 9-65, *A-C*). Increased phagocytosis of blood cells and/or their precursors, primarily erythroid cells, may be observed in primary or secondary immune-mediated disorders.[270] However, increased phagocytosis of blood cells and/or their precursors may also be observed secondary to various infectious and neoplastic diseases.[43,70,289,491] The production of increased amounts of inflammatory cytokines, especially by excessive T lymphocyte activation, has been proposed as a likely mechanism for increased macrophage activation and increased phagocytosis of blood cells. The production of cytokines—such as IFN-γ, TNF-α, IL-1, IL-12, and/or IL-18—either directly or indirectly through the production of growth factors such as macrophage-CSF (M-CSF) and GM-CSF will stimulate the production and phagocytic activity of macrophages.[254,394,491,539]

Pronounced macrophage activation can result in the hemophagocytic syndrome (macrophage activation syndrome), which is characterized as an acute, severe clinical event in humans, with fever, hepatosplenomegaly, and pancytopenia due to uncontrolled phagocytosis of blood cells and/or their precursors.[98,248] Icterus and diarrhea have also been reported in some dogs with this syndrome.[511] The hemophagocytic syndrome is a secondary phenomenon that can sometimes mask an underlying immune-mediated, infectious, or neoplastic disease.[70,392,474]

Recommended hematologic criteria for classifying an animal as having the hemophagocytic syndrome include pancytopenia or bicytopenia with increased numbers of benign-appearing macrophages in bone marrow (a minimum of 2% of all nucleated cells) that have phagocytized blood cells and/or their precursors.[511] This syndrome has been associated with infections, immune-mediated disorders, and hematopoietic neoplasms, but an underlying disease may not always be found.[135,333,444,491,508] Schistocytes and activated monocytes may also be present in blood.[491]

Histiocytic Sarcoma

The term *histiocyte* is used to describe cells of both the macrophage and dendritic cell series.[77] Canine histiocytic diseases have been classified into the histiocytoma complex, reactive histiocytosis, and the histiocytic sarcoma complex. The histiocytic sarcoma complex includes localized histiocytic sarcoma, disseminated histiocytic sarcoma, and hemophagocytic histiocytic sarcoma. Localized and disseminated histiocytic sarcomas are of interstitial dendritic cell origin, and hemophagocytic histiosarcoma originates from macrophages.[321] Disseminated histiocytic sarcoma and hemophagocytic histiosarcoma have been classified as malignant histiocytosis in the past. The morphology of the neoplastic histiocytes varies from mature histiocytes to anaplastic histiocytes (Fig. 9-66, *A-C*). Anaplastic features which may be present include moderate to marked anisocytosis and anisokaryosis, with moderate to abundant lightly basophilic vacuolated cytoplasm. Nuclei are round, oval, or reniform with prominent nucleoli. Bizarre mitotic figures and multinucleated giant cells may be present. Histiocytic sarcomas are most common in Bernese Mountain dogs, Rottweilers, Golden Retrievers, and Flat-Coat Retrievers.[3,322]

Canine hemophagocytic histiosarcoma is a proliferative disorder of $CD11d^{+}$ macrophages originating in the spleen and possibly bone marrow that spreads rapidly to the liver and lungs. Laboratory findings in most cases of canine hemophagocytic histiosarcoma include a Coombs-negative regenerative anemia, thrombocytopenia, hypoalbuminemia, and hypocholesterolemia. Neoplastic macrophages appear as infiltrates in the spleen, liver, bone marrow, and lungs. The macrophages often contain phagocytized erythrocytes and/or hemosiderin (Fig. 9-67, *A,B*) and are accompanied by areas of extramedullary hematopoiesis in affected tissues. Cellular atypia may be more pronounced in the spleen than it is in the bone marrow.[322]

Nonhemophagocytic disseminated histiocytic sarcoma may originate in the spleen, lymph nodes, lungs, bone marrow, skin (especially of the extremities), or periarticular tissues of the limbs, followed by widespread metastasis. These tumors are more likely to appear as masses, in contrast to the more diffuse infiltrates typically seen in hemophagocytic histiosarcoma. The cell of origin is the interstitial dendritic cell, which expresses leukocyte surface molecules CD1, CD11c/CD18, and major histocompatibility complex class II (MHC-II).[3] Although neoplastic macrophages in hemophagocytic histiocytic sarcoma express MHC-II, they have low and/or inconsistent expression of CD1 and CD11c and express CD11d instead of CD11c.[322] A lack of prominent erythrophagocytosis in a histiocytic tumor suggests that the neoplasm is of dendritic cell origin; however, surface markers may be required to make a definitive diagnosis.

Although much less common than in dogs, histiocytic neoplasms are recognized in cats and a horse.[266] Histiocytic disorders in cats have been classified as feline progressive histiocytosis, feline pulmonary Langerhans cell histiocytosis, and the feline histiocytic sarcoma complex.[61,321] Several cases of histiocytic sarcoma (malignant histiocytosis) have been reported in cats that appear similar to hemophagocytic histiosarcoma in dogs, although the accompanying anemia is most often nonregenerative.[85,87,133,134,239] Like dogs, a macrophage origin of the hemophagocytic neoplastic cells has been demonstrated in cats.[85,134]

INFLAMMATORY DISORDERS OF BONE MARROW

Inflammatory disorders of bone marrow are seldom recognized because inflammatory cells—including neutrophils, eosinophils, monocytes, macrophages, lymphocytes, and plasma cells—are normally present in bone marrow, making recognition of inflammation difficult in aspirate smears. Increased numbers of neutrophils, eosinophils, and monocytes in bone marrow usually represent increased production to meet peripheral demands rather than inflammation within the marrow. Core biopsies are generally needed to make a diagnosis of inflammation in the bone marrow, but it is rarely diagnosed because the multifocal distributions of the lesions are easily missed using a small biopsy needle. Recognition of inflammation within the marrow is increased if biopsies are collected from lesions identified using diagnostic imaging techniques. Inflammation in the bone marrow has been classified into the various categories discussed below.[524]

Acute Inflammation

Lesions are characterized by circumscribed infiltrates of mature neutrophils (Fig. 9-68, *A*). Some of these microabscesses have necrotic material in their centers. Vascular dilatation, fibrin exudate, and hemorrhage may also be present. Acute inflammation is generally associated with bacterial infection.[129,214,524]

Fibrinous Inflammation

Fibrin exudation without accompanying inflammatory cells has been called fibrinous inflammation. Fibrin, which typically appears as small tangled pink fibrils in bone marrow sections stained with hematoxylin and eosin (H&E), must be

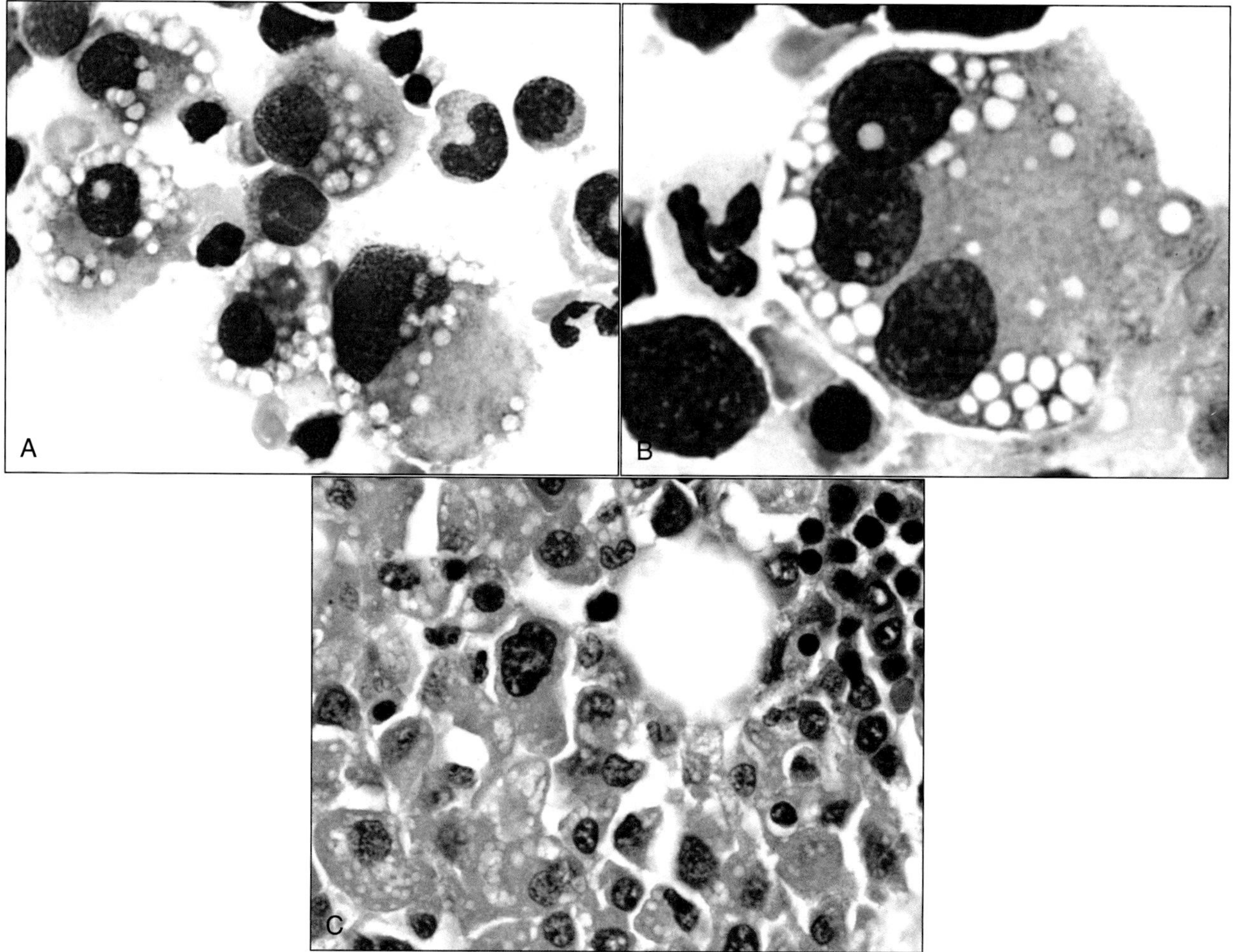

FIGURE 9-66

Bone marrow from a dog with histiocytic sarcoma. Neoplastic cells were also present in the liver and spleen at necropsy. **A,** Histiocytic proliferation with marked anisocytosis and anisokaryosis in an aspirate smear. The cytoplasm of each cell contains prominent vacuolation. Erythrophagocytosis was not a prominent feature in this case. Wright-Giemsa stain. **B,** A large trinucleated histiocyte with prominent cytoplasmic vacuolation in an aspirate smear. Wright-Giemsa stain. **C,** Histiocytic proliferation with marked anisocytosis and anisokaryosis in a bone marrow section from a core biopsy. The cytoplasm of each cell contains prominent vacuolation. A cluster of erythroid precursors is located in the upper right corner. H&E stain.

differentiated from edema and necrotic debris, which appear as pink homogeneous material. Special stains, including the Frazier-Lundrum stain, may be used to identify fibrin.[512] Fibrinous inflammation has been recognized in animals with disseminated intravascular coagulation and systemic vasculitis.[524]

Chronic Inflammation/Hyperplasia

Chronic inflammation consists of proliferations or infiltrations of plasma cells, lymphocytes, and/or mast cells. Proliferations of plasma cells and/or lymphocytes have been reported in the bone marrow of dogs with chronic renal disease and in dogs with myelofibrosis.[524] Plasma cells are increased in bone marrow in response to some infectious agents, including *E. canis* and visceral leishmaniasis in dogs and feline infectious peritonitis in cats.[35,243] Lymphoid aggregates are infrequently recognized in bone marrow sections of dogs and cats; their presence may be the result of chronic immune stimulation (Fig. 9-69).[524]

Increased numbers of small lymphocytes and/or plasma cells may be present in various immune-mediated disorders including immune-mediated neutropenia, IMHA, and IMT.*

Chronic Granulomatous Inflammation

Macrophage infiltrates characterize chronic granulomatous inflammation (see Fig. 9-68, *B*). Both diffuse macrophage infiltrates and focal granulomas have been described.[524]

*References 310, 359, 383, 446, 504, 507, 512, 525.

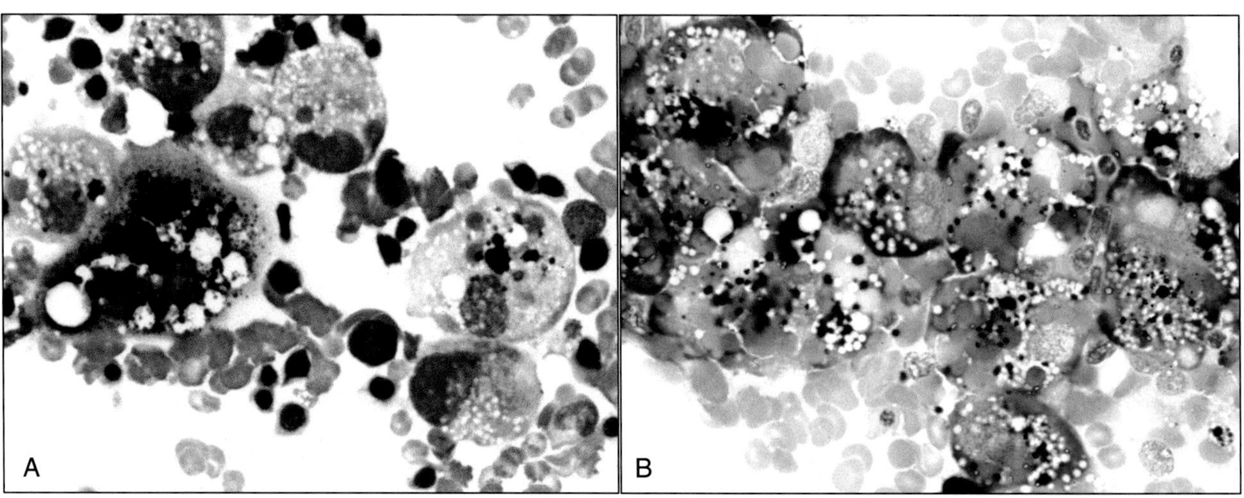

FIGURE 9-67

Aspirate bone marrow smears from a dog with hemophagocytic histiocytic sarcoma. **A,** Macrophage proliferation with moderate anisocytosis and anisokaryosis are present. Vacuoles, phagocytized erythrocytes, and/or gray-black hemosiderin are visible in the cytoplasm of multiple cells. One large macrophage at left center is filled with hemosiderin. Wright-Giemsa stain. **B,** Macrophage proliferation with cells containing large amounts of hemosiderin (diffuse and granular blue-staining cytoplasm). Prussian blue stain.

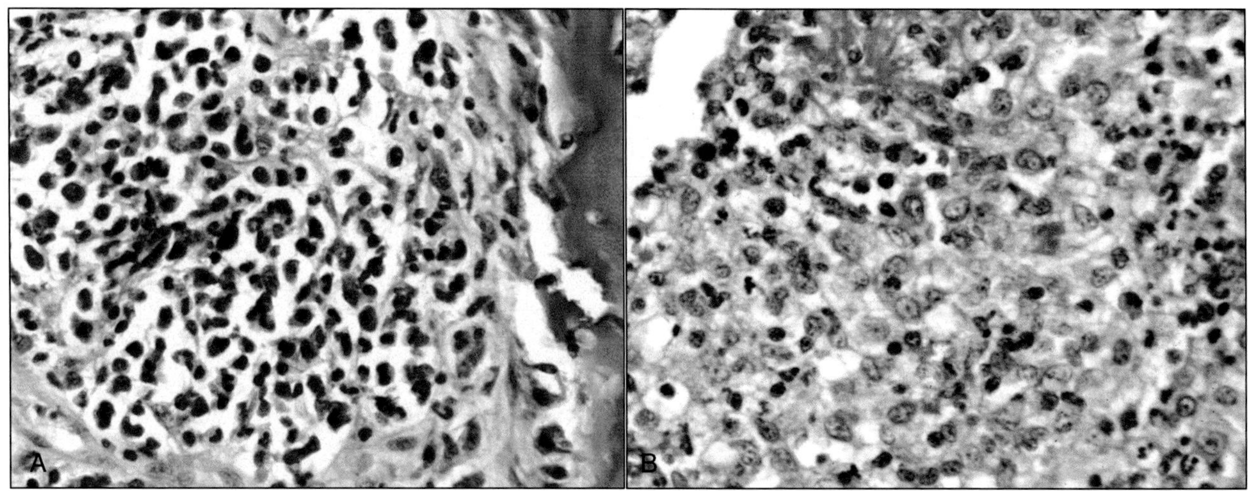

FIGURE 9-68

Pyogranulomatous inflammation in postmortem bone marrow sections from a dog with unknown etiology. **A,** Focal area of neutrophilic inflammation (microabscess). Trabecular bone is located at the right edge of the image. **B,** Macrophages and neutrophils are distributed throughout this section of bone marrow. H&E stain.

Diffuse infiltrates are included in the "Reactive Macrophage Hyperplasia" section in this chapter. A granuloma is a site of chronic inflammation characterized by the presence of various monocytic cells (monocytes, macrophages, epithelioid cells, and multinucleated giant cells) arranged in compact masses. Fibrosis and variable numbers of neutrophils and eosinophils may also be present. When neutrophilic inflammation is also prominent, the term *pyogranulomatous inflammation* is used (see Fig. 9-68, *A,B*). Multifocal granulomatous or pyogranulomatous inflammation involving bone marrow occurs in animals, especially in association with mycobacteriosis (Fig. 9-70, *A,B*) and fungal infections such as coccidiomycosis, penicilliosis (Fig. 9-71, *A,B*), aspergillosis (Fig. 9-72, *A-C*), blastomycosis, cryptococcosis, histoplasmosis, and *Phialemonium obovatum* infections.[48,214,357,433] German Shepherd dogs appear to be more susceptible to systemic *Aspergillus* and *Phialemonium* infections than other dog breeds.[433] A specific etiology cannot always be determined.[65]

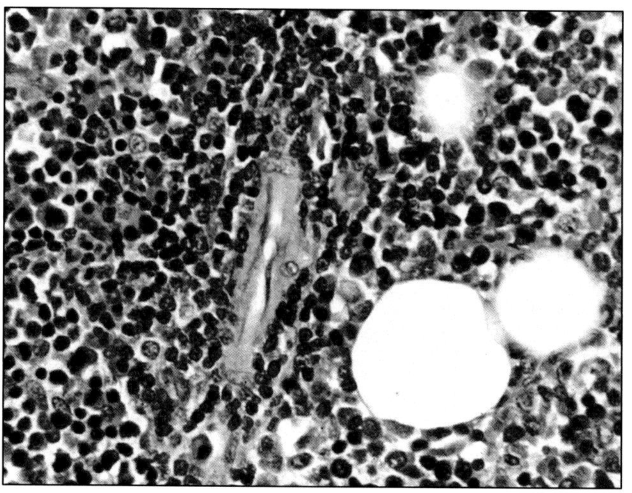

FIGURE 9-69
A small lymphoid follicle around a longitudinal section of a vessel *(left of center)* in a bone marrow section from a core biopsy collected from a dog. H&E stain.

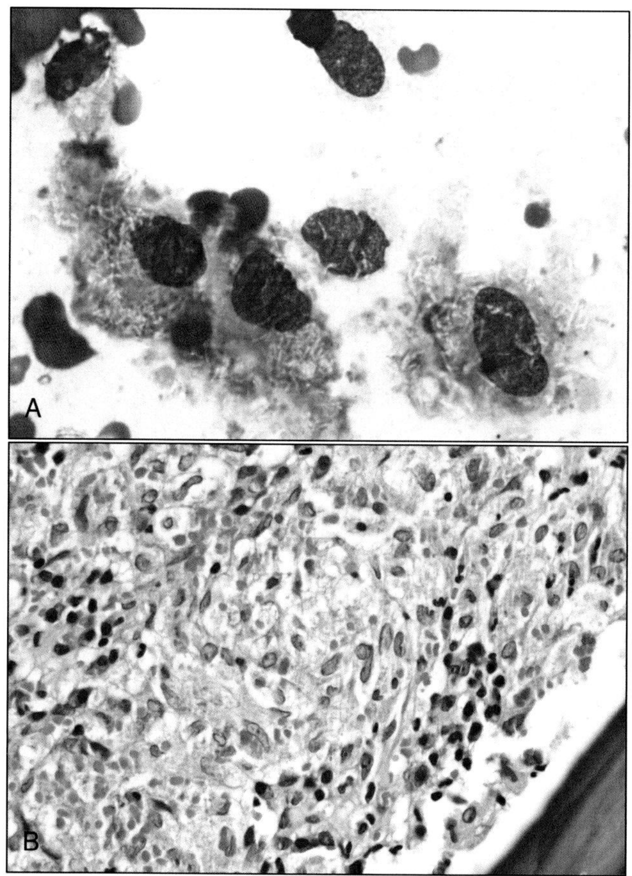

FIGURE 9-70
Bone marrow from a cat with disseminated *Mycobacterium avium* infection. **A,** Bone marrow aspirate smear with three macrophages filled with *Mycobacterium* organisms, which appear as linear unstained structures. Wright-Giemsa stain. **B,** Bone marrow core biopsy containing macrophages filled with unstained *Mycobacterium* organisms. Clusters of plasma cells are present between macrophages. Trabecular bone is present in the bottom right. H&E stain.

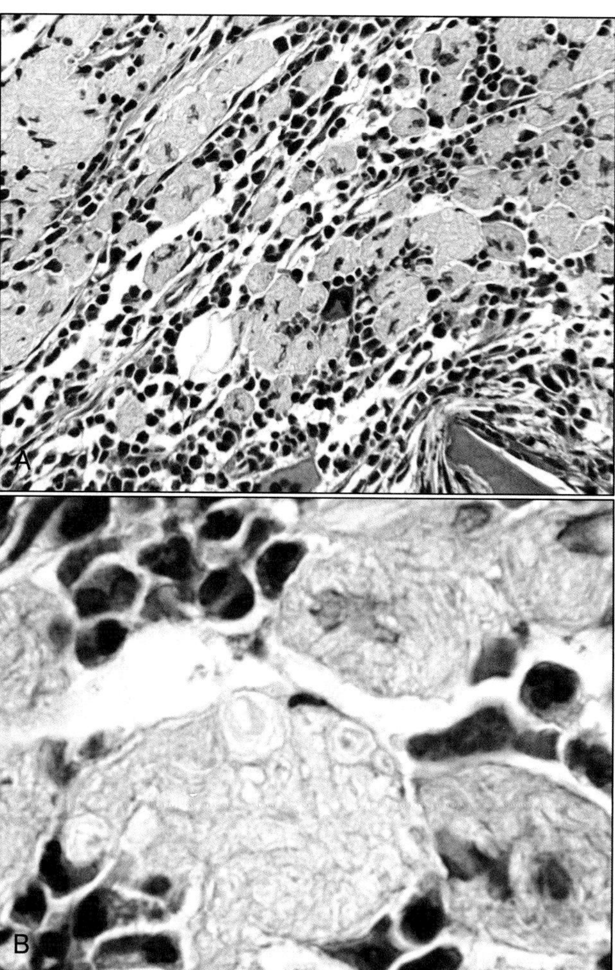

FIGURE 9-71
Core bone marrow biopsy from a lytic/proliferative lesion in the humerus of a Collie dog. **A,** Many large epithelioid macrophages are filled with phagocytized swollen fungal hyphae. Hyphae with clear cell walls and no discernible internal structure predominated. Neutrophils, eosinophils, and fibrocytes are also present. **B,** Higher magnification demonstrating the swollen fungal hyphae in macrophages. A *Penicillium* species was cultured from the lesion. H&E stain.

Photograph of a bone marrow core biopsy from a 2008 ASVCP slide review case submitted by K. Miyakawa, C. Swenson, L. Mendoza, B. Steficek, M. Seavey, F. Gomes, and C. Warzee.

HEMATOPOIETIC NEOPLASMS

Hematopoietic neoplasms arise from the bone marrow, lymph nodes, spleen, or thymus. They are classified as either lymphoid or myeloid neoplasms. The term *leukemia* is used when neoplastic cells are seen in the blood and/or bone marrow. An exception is the neoplastic proliferation of plasma cells in bone marrow (multiple myeloma), which is not referred to as a leukemia. Blood leukocyte counts may be low, normal, or high in animals with leukemia. The term *acute* is used to describe leukemias in which a predominance of blast cells occurs in the bone marrow; the term *chronic* is used for

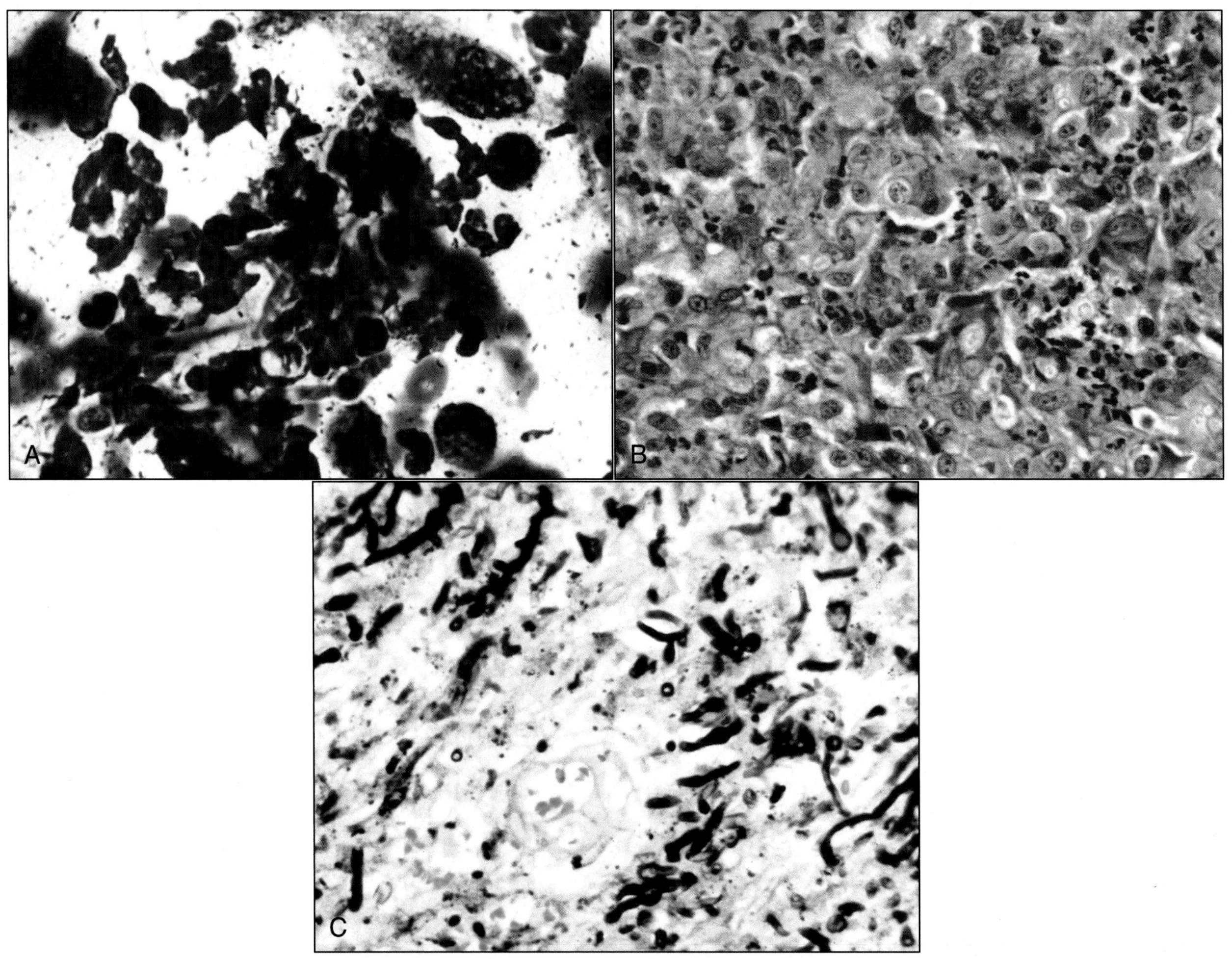

FIGURE 9-72

Pyogranulomatous inflammation from a lytic lesion in the proximal humerus of a dog with aspergillosis. **A,** Aspirate smear containing lysed cells, degenerate neutrophils, macrophages, a reactive fibroblast *(top right),* and septate fungal hyphae *(bottom left quadrant).* Wright-Giemsa stain. **B,** Section of a core biopsy contains numerous macrophages and fewer neutrophils. Vague outlines of fungal hyphae (round to ovoid to bulbous, sharply demarcated clear spaces, often with eosinophilic centers) can also be identified. H&E stain. **C,** Numerous branching septate argyrophilic fungal hyphae visible in a core biopsy section. GMS stain.

leukemias in which there is a predominance of maturing cells in blood and bone marrow. The progression of disease is usually rapid (weeks to months) in acute leukemias and slow (months to years) in chronic leukemias.

Precursor cells for mast cell tumors and histiocytic sarcomas arise from the bone marrow,[126,294,321] but these neoplasms usually develop from more differentiated cells in the peripheral tissues. Consequently they are typically not included with myeloid neoplasms, even though some cases of noncutaneous systemic mastocytosis and hemophagocytic histiocytic sarcomas might qualify as hematopoietic neoplasms.

Although this book focuses on the morphologic appearance of neoplastic hematopoietic cells, it is not possible to differentiate some cell types, especially blast cells and lymphocyte types, using morphology alone.[303] Cytochemical stains have improved the quality of diagnosing hematopoietic neoplasms, especially in recognizing and differentiating myeloid neoplasms.[381] The development of monoclonal antibodies against various cell surface and cytosolic proteins has allowed for the classification of cells using immunophenotype analysis. Many antibodies are available for use in dogs, but limited panels are available in other domestic animals.[303] Antibodies bound to cells are detected using fluorescent or enzymatic labels. Assays may be performed on exfoliative cytology preparations or paraffin-imbedded tissue biopsies, using immunocytochemistry and immunohistochemistry, respectively. Immunophenotyping is also performed in fluid samples using flow cytometry, where it has been especially useful in identifying lymphoid cell types.[18] Antibodies have recently been developed for use in identifying granulocytic and monocytic lines in dogs, but there remains a need for early erythroid markers.[487] Panels of antibodies have been validated for use in the differential diagnosis of acute leukemias in dogs (Table 9-1).[6,487] In addition, clonality assays have been

TABLE 9-1

Antibodies Used to Phenotype Leukemia in Dogs

General Leukocyte Markers	
CD45	All leukocytes
CD11a	All leukocytes
Acute Leukemia Marker	
CD34	Stem cells/early progenitor cells
Lymphoid Markers	
CD3	T lymphocytes
CD4	T_H lymphocytes, neutrophils, monocytes
CD5	T lymphocytes, subset of B lymphocytes
CD8	Cytotoxic T lymphocytes
CD11d	LGLs, macrophages in spleen and marrow
CD21	B lymphocytes at a later stage than CD79a
CD79a	B lymphocytes
Myeloid Markers	
CD11b	Granulocytes, monocytes, macrophages
CD11c	Granulocytes, monocytes, dendritic cells
CD14	Monocytes
CD41/61	Megakaryoblasts
CD61	Megakaryoblasts
MPO	Neutrophils, monocytes
MAC387	Neutrophils, monocytes/macrophages
NSA	Neutrophils

From Villiers E, Baines S, Law AM, et al. Identification of acute myeloid leukemia in dogs using flow cytometry with myeloperoxidase, MAC387, and a canine neutrophil-specific antibody. *Vet Clin Pathol.* 2006;35:55-71.
CD, cluster of differentiation antigen; MPO, myeloperoxidase; NSA, neutrophil specific antibody; LGL, large granular lymphocyte.

developed that can be used to differentiate reactive from neoplastic disorders.[18,183]

LYMPHOID NEOPLASMS

The term *lymphoma* denotes a solid tumor or tumors of neoplastic lymphocytes located outside of the bone marrow. The term lymphoid leukemia indicates a neoplastic condition of lymphocytes present in bone marrow and/or blood that is not associated with a solid tumor. Lymphoid leukemias are further classified as acute or chronic, depending on the maturity of the cells involved. When neoplastic cells are present in the blood of an animal with a lymphoma, the terms *leukemic lymphoma* or *lymphosarcoma cell leukemia* have been used, but the former term is preferred. Metastasis from bone marrow to lymphoid tissues and from lymphoid tissues to bone marrow is common. Consequently it may be difficult to differentiate a true leukemia from a lymphoma with leukemia in animals with advanced stages of disease. The measurement of CD34 on neoplastic cells may help differentiate acute lymphoblastic leukemia (ALL) from leukemic lymphoma in dogs. Neoplastic cells in dogs with ALL are typically positive, and neoplastic cells in the blood of dogs with leukemic lymphoma are usually negative.[2,146,485]

Acute Lymphoblastic Leukemia

Neoplastic lymphoblasts and/or prolymphocytes are present in the bone marrow of animals with ALL (Fig. 9-73, *A,B;* Fig. 9-74, *A,B;* Figs. 9-75, 9-76). Neoplastic cells are also usually present in blood (see Figs. 5-60, 5-61) with or without

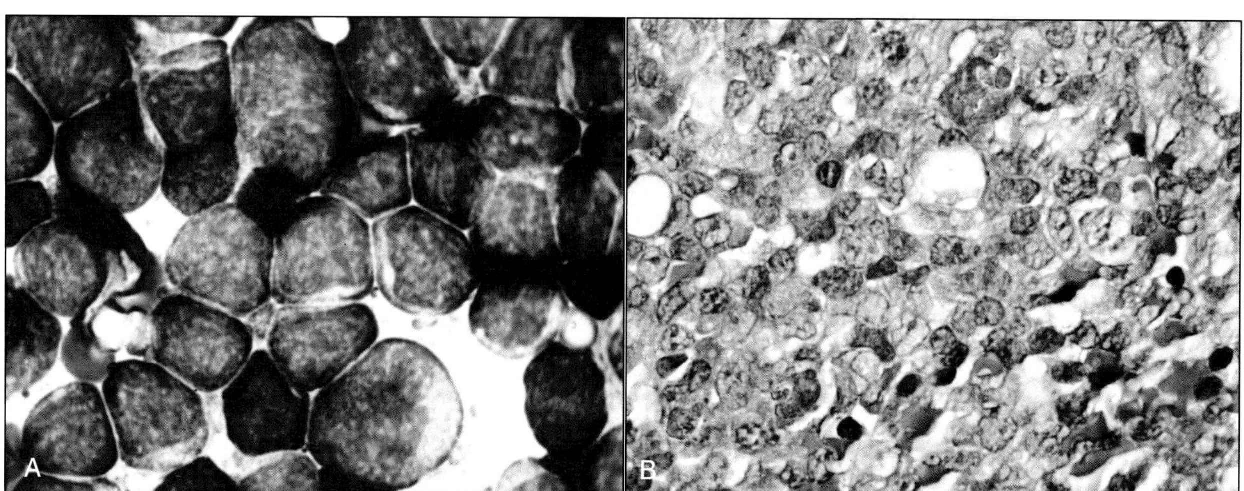

FIGURE 9-73

ALL in bone marrow from a dog. **A,** Lymphoblasts with dark-blue cytoplasm and indistinct nucleoli in an aspirate smear. Wright-Giemsa stain. **B,** Lymphoblasts in a core biopsy section. The orange material present is hemosiderin. H&E stain.

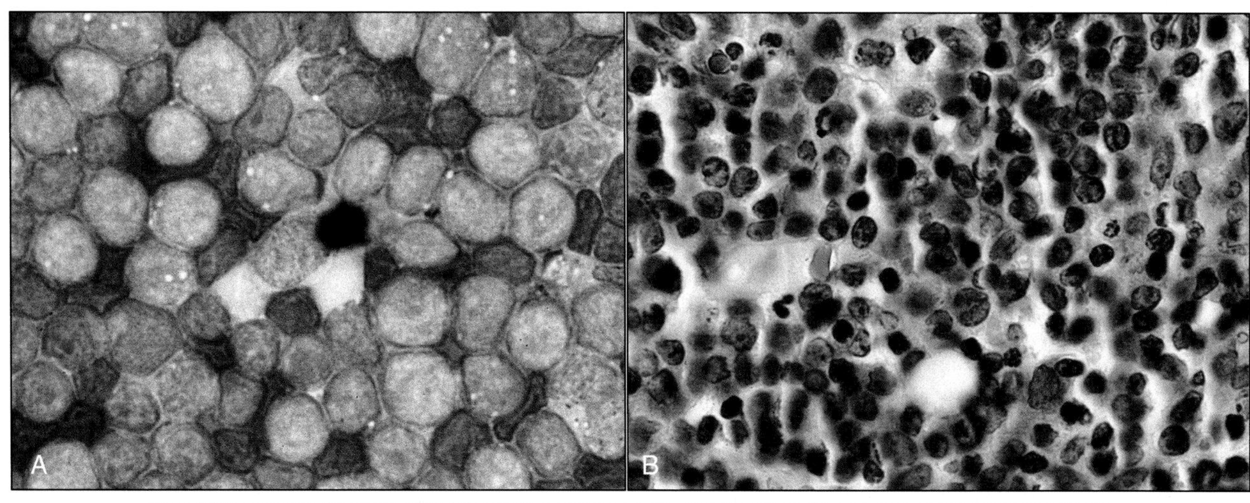

FIGURE 9-74

ALL in bone marrow from a dog. **A,** Lymphoblasts with dark-blue cytoplasm and indistinct nucleoli in an aspirate smear. Lymphoblasts were not visible in blood from this animal. Wright-Giemsa stain. **B,** Lymphoblasts in a bone marrow section from a core biopsy section. The orange material present is hemosiderin. H&E stain.

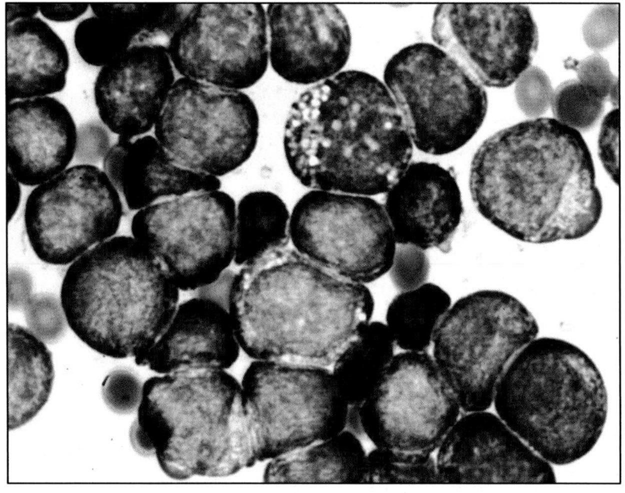

FIGURE 9-75

Lymphoblasts with dark-blue cytoplasm and indistinct nucleoli in an aspirate smear of bone marrow from a cat with ALL. A minority of neoplastic cells had cytoplasmic vacuoles. Wright-Giemsa stain.

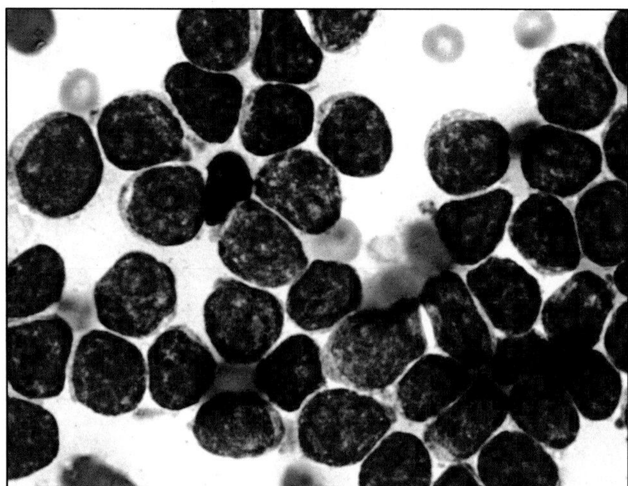

FIGURE 9-76

Lymphoblasts, often with visible nucleoli, in a roll preparation from a core biopsy from a horse with ALL. Wright-Giemsa stain.

an absolute lymphocytosis. A moderate to marked nonregenerative anemia with thrombocytopenia and/or neutropenia is usually present in dogs with ALL.[2,462] Pancytopenia has been recognized in horses and dogs diagnosed with ALL by bone marrow biopsy (see Fig. 9-10).[2,267,523] Neoplastic lymphocytes present in ALL exhibit decreased nuclear chromatin condensation and increased cytoplasmic basophilia compared with normal blood lymphocytes.[279,299] Nucleoli may or may not be visible in the nuclei of these neoplastic cells and, when present, may be difficult to visualize. Other abnormalities—including increased anisocytosis, anisokaryosis, and nuclear pleomorphism—may also be present. Lymphoblasts are generally difficult to differentiate from blast cells of other hematopoietic lineages without the use of special stains and/or surface markers. Compared with myeloblasts, lymphoblasts tend to exhibit more condensed chromatin and less prominent nucleoli.[283]

Most cases of ALL in cats have a T lymphocyte phenotype and most are FeLV positive,[279,507] but FIV positive FeLV negative cats with ALL have been reported.[193,426,439] Neoplastic cells from dogs with ALL may be of the T lymphocyte, B lymphocyte, NK cell, or null cell phenotype.[403,485,508] Canine B lymphocyte ALL ($CD79a^+$ and/or $CD21^+$) has been identified more often than T lymphocyte ALL ($CD3^+$).[2,462,485] Like AML, neoplastic cells in ALL are generally $CD34^+$ in dogs.[2,462] However, neoplastic cells in dogs with acute large granular lymphocytic (LGL) leukemia (see Fig. 5-59) are typically CD34⁻, and the neoplasm appears to originate in the spleen with secondary bone marrow involvement.[305,485] Likewise, CD34 is negative in dogs with leukemic high-grade lymphoma.[462]

Chronic Lymphocytic Leukemia

Chronic lymphocytic leukemia (CLL) is reported most often in older animals.[542] The clinical presentation varies, but dogs and cats with CLL are often asymptomatic when diagnosed. A lymphocytosis ($6 \times 10^3/\mu L$ to over $200 \times 10^3/\mu L$) involving normal-appearing lymphocytes is consistently present in blood (see Figs. 5-56, 5-57, 5-58).[95,263,279,542] Mild to moderate anemia is generally present. Moderate thrombocytopenia may be present at times, but neutropenia is generally not seen.[2,462,542] The nuclear chromatin is more condensed in CLL cells than in those of ALL. In contrast with ALL, most cats with CLL are FeLV-negative.[279]

T lymphocyte CLL is more common than B lymphocyte CLL in dogs and cats.[2,403,542] Of the T lymphocyte subsets, cytotoxic T lymphocytes with granular lymphocyte morphology predominate in dogs.[304,485,534] In contrast, T_H lymphocyte neoplasms appear to be most common in cats with CLL.[504,542] Dogs with CLL of the B lymphocyte type often have an accompanying monoclonal gammopathy that is typically of the immunoglobulin M (IgM) type.[136,263,281,283] An IgG monoclonal gammopathy has also been reported in a horse with CLL.[95]

Non-LGL types of CLL are composed of normal-appearing small to medium-sized lymphocytes with scant amounts of light-blue cytoplasm. Immunophenotyping for CD34 can be performed in cases where there is a question concerning the maturity of the lymphocytes. Lymphocytes from dogs with CLL are negative for CD34, and lymphocytes from dogs with ALL are usually positive.[462,485] Lymphocytes present in the LGL type of CLL have red- or purple-staining (generally focal) granules within light-blue cytoplasm (see Fig. 5-58). These cells also have condensed nuclear chromatin, but they are generally larger, with more cytoplasm and lower nuclear-to-cytoplasmic (N:C) ratios, than cells present in non-LGL types of CLL.[186,360,534] Although most cases of LGL leukemia in dogs behave like CLL and progress slowly over several years, some cases behave like an aggressive form of ALL (see Fig. 5-59).[304,485,533] Nearly all cases of the LGL form of CLL involve neoplastic T lymphocytes in dogs, but cells of the LGL form of ALL in dogs may be of either the T lymphocyte or the NK cell lineage.[304,485]

Bone marrow examination of animals with CLL often reveals increased numbers of normal-appearing lymphocytes (Fig. 9-77, *A,B;* Fig. 9-78, *A,B*; Fig. 9-79); however, the extent of the neoplastic infiltration is generally less than that seen in ALL. Bone marrow may contain some reactive lymphoid follicles consisting primarily of normal-appearing lymphocytes (see Fig. 9-69), which must be differentiated from a neoplastic lymphoid infiltrate. CLL of the B lymphocyte type appears to originate in the bone marrow; consequently lymphocyte infiltrates are consistently present with this type of CLL. In contrast, T lymphocyte development requires processing by the thymus and T lymphocyte CLL appears to develop outside the marrow (i.e., in the spleen) with secondary marrow infiltration.[304,485] Tests for CD antigens are usually needed to identify the cell type involved; however, the coexistence of a monoclonal gammopathy with CLL indicates neoplasia of a B lymphocyte type, while the presence of cytoplasmic granules suggests a cytotoxic T lymphocyte type or, less likely, a NK cell type of neoplasm.[403,485]

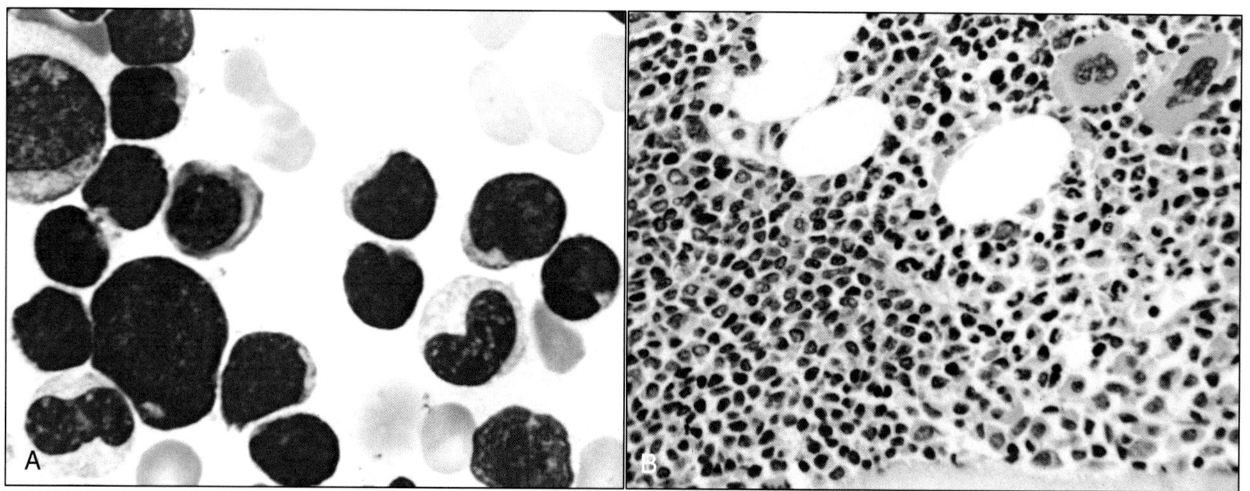

FIGURE 9-77
Bone marrow from a dog with CLL. **A,** Infiltrate of small lymphocytes with condensed nuclear chromatin and minimal cytoplasm in an aspirate smear. Wright-Giemsa stain. **B,** Infiltrate of small lymphocytes *(especially in the left half of the image)* in a bone marrow section from a core biopsy. Two megakaryocytes are present in the upper right corner. H&E stain.

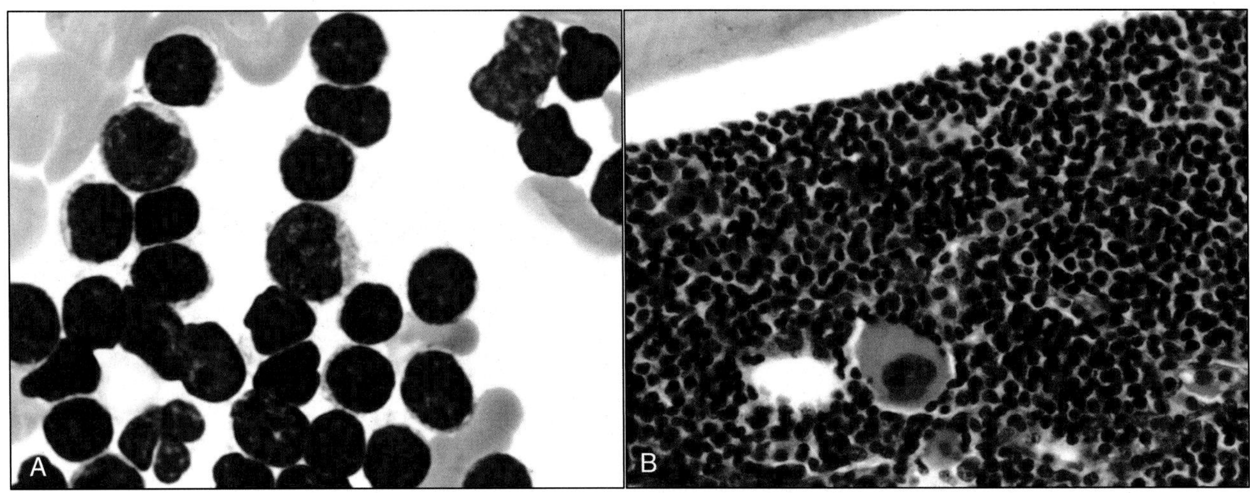

FIGURE 9-78

Bone marrow from a dog with B lymphocyte CLL. **A,** Infiltrate of small lymphocytes with condensed nuclear chromatin and minimal cytoplasm in an aspirate smear. A monoclonal hyperglobulinemia is also present in this dog. Wright-Giemsa stain. **B,** Marked infiltrate of small lymphocytes in a bone marrow section from a core biopsy. Trabecular bone is located at upper left and a megakaryocyte is present at bottom center. H&E stain.

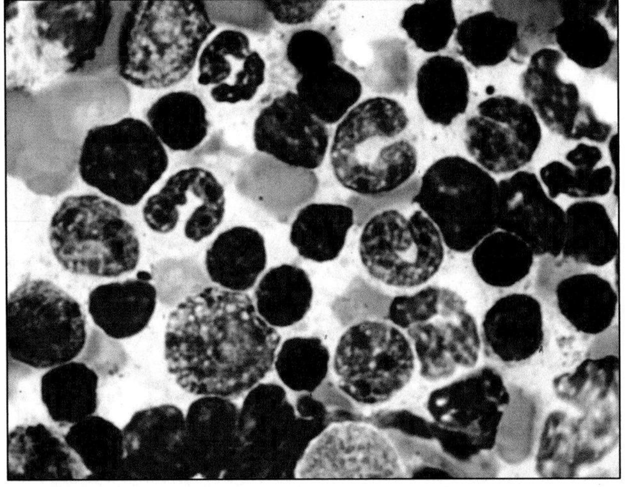

FIGURE 9-79

Infiltrate of normal-appearing small lymphocytes in an aspirate smear of bone marrow from a cat with CLL. Wright-Giemsa stain.

Lymphomas

Lymphomas are solid tumors of neoplastic lymphocytes that develop outside of the bone marrow. They may be classified by the anatomic site involved (e.g., alimentary, thymic, cutaneous, multicentric), by location of neoplastic cells within lymph nodes (e.g., diffuse, follicular, marginal zone, T zone), by cell morphology (e.g., large cell, lymphoblastic, large granular), by cell type (e.g., B lymphocyte, T lymphocyte, NK cell), or combinations of these categories.* The reader is referred to a recent text for a comprehensive discussion of lymphomas in animals.[479]

Based on abnormal morphology, neoplastic cells are recognized in the blood of about one-quarter to one-half of the animals presenting with a lymphoma.[279,285,384,481] In the remaining cases, neoplastic lymphocytes may be absent from blood or may not have sufficiently abnormal morphology to be recognized. Bone marrow infiltrates may sometimes be recognized in animals even when neoplastic cells are not appreciated in blood (Fig. 9-80, *A,B;* Fig. 9-81, *A,B*).[285,383,384] Core biopsies offer the advantage that small infiltrates of lymphoid cells that would be dispersed during bone marrow aspiration and smear preparation can be recognized with histopathology. Lymphoid infiltrates in the bone marrow of dogs with lymphomas are most often paratrabecular in location.[383] Focal infiltrates must be differentiated from benign lymphoid follicles, which have well-defined borders and are composed primarily of small mature lymphocytes (see Fig. 9-69). Neoplastic aggregates are generally larger, with poorly defined borders, and cells within these aggregates are often large and immature in appearance.[383]

Lymphomas involving LGLs have been primarily reported in cats, in which they generally occur as intestinal lymphomas that metastasize to various other organs, including the spleen, liver, lymph nodes, blood, and bone marrow (Fig. 9-82).[94,131,224,396,535] Their granules are generally much larger than those seen in normal LGLs in blood. They appear blue, red, or purple with Wright-Giemsa stain but may not stain well with Diff-Quik stain.[131] In some cases the granules appear eosinophilic in H&E-stained sections; in others, they are difficult to identify with H&E. The neoplastic cells appear to originate from intraepithelial lymphocytes, and most of these tumors appear to be composed of cytotoxic T lymphocytes.[224,396]

*References 63, 314, 479, 480, 484, 486.

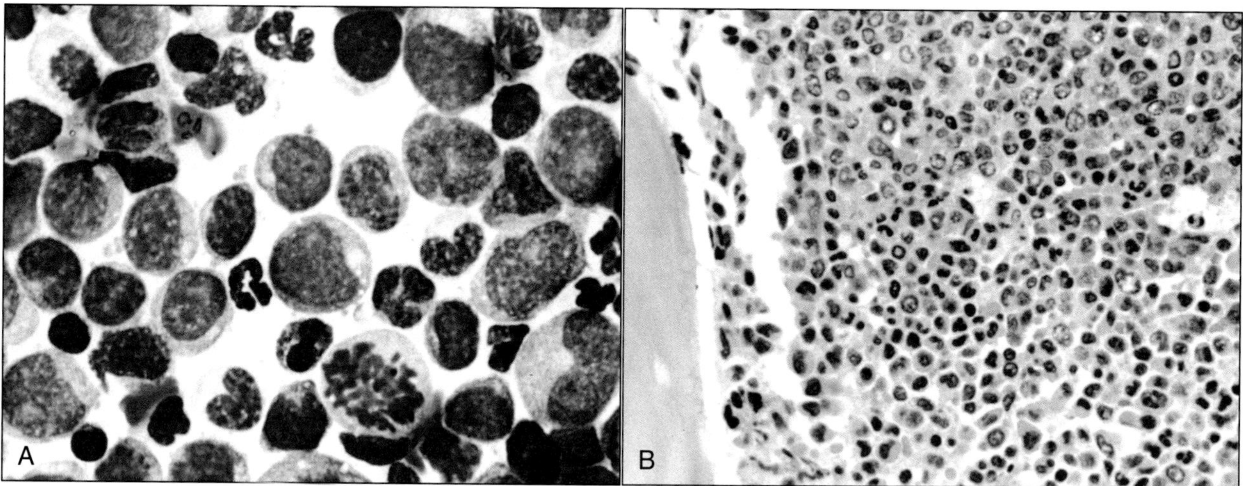

FIGURE 9-80

Metastatic lymphoma in bone marrow from a dog. **A,** Infiltrate of variably sized lymphoblasts in an aspirate smear. A mitotic cell is present at bottom center. Wright-Giemsa stain. **B,** Diffuse infiltrate of variably sized lymphoblasts in a bone marrow section from a core biopsy. Trabecular bone is located along the left edge of the image. H&E stain.

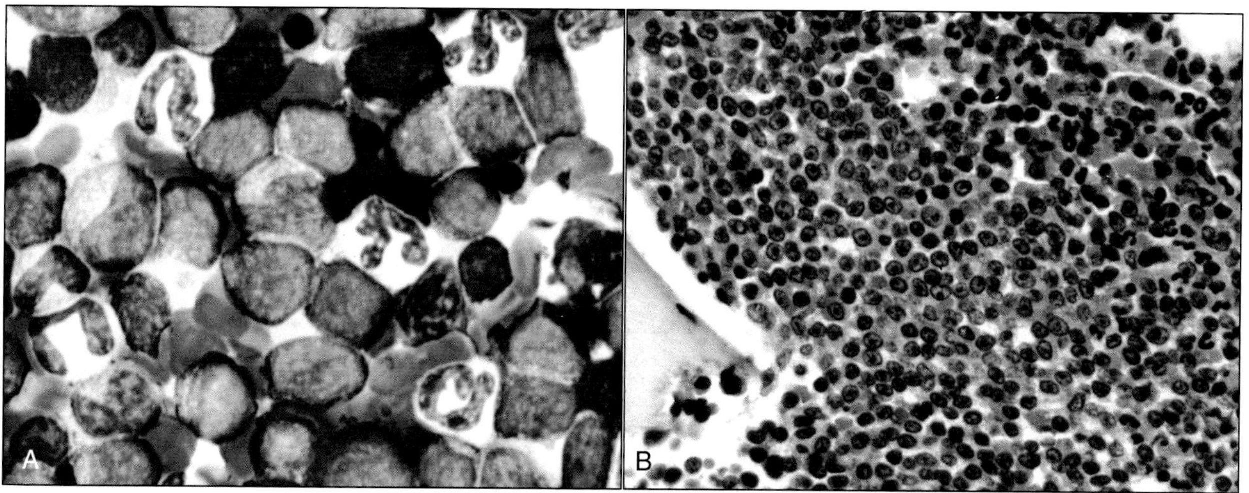

FIGURE 9-81

Metastatic lymphoma in bone marrow from a dog. **A,** Infiltrate of variably sized lymphoblasts in an aspirate smear. The lymphoblasts have round nuclei and scant amounts of cytoplasm. Wright-Giemsa stain. **B,** Focal infiltrate of lymphoblasts near trabecular bone *(lower left)* in a bone marrow section from a core biopsy. H&E stain.

Two cases of LGL lymphoma have been reported in horses.[156,240] Neoplastic cells were recognized in the blood of one horse and in the bone marrow of the other.

Multiple Myeloma and Other Immunoproliferative Neoplasms

Any cell type in the normal B lymphocyte maturational pathway may become neoplastic and produce an immunoglobulin. The nature of a lymphoproliferative disorder is determined by the stage at which B lymphocyte maturation is arrested.

Multiple Myeloma

Multiple myeloma (plasma cell myeloma) is a B lymphocyte tumor of the bone marrow that manifests as a proliferation of plasma cells. It is a rare tumor in dogs,[298,300] cats,[312,356] and horses,[23,110,233,375] occurring primarily in older animals.[44] A monoclonal IgG or IgA immunoglobulin is usually secreted by the tumor, resulting in a monoclonal hyperglobulinemia, which can be recognized using serum protein electrophoresis.[150,300] The type of immunoglobulin produced can be identified using immunoelectrophoresis and quantified using methods such as single radial immunodiffusion. Biclonal proteins may be produced in some cases[150,205,312,356,378] and may be recognized more frequently if capillary zone electrophoresis is used in place of conventional serum protein electrophoresis.[117] Biclonal-appearing proteins during serum protein electrophoresis may result from two plasma cell clones, one plasma cell clone producing two separate immunoglobulins, or spurious peaks of a single protein with dimeric or multimeric forms.[34,356]

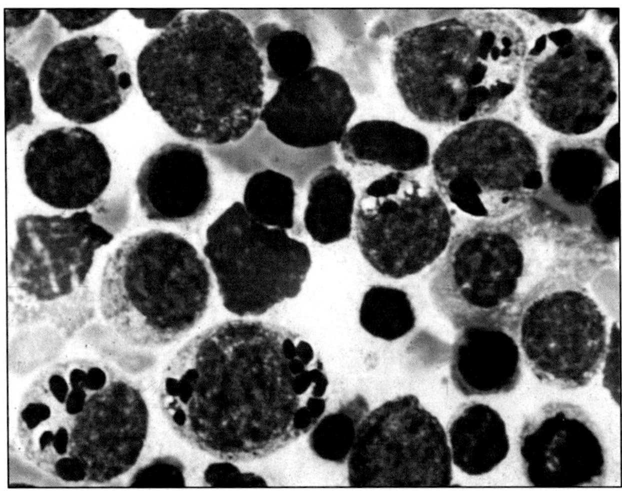

FIGURE 9-82
Infiltrate of large granular lymphocytes in an aspirate smear of bone marrow from a cat with metastatic lymphoma involving large granular lymphocytes. The granules in these cells are larger than those seen in the granular lymphocytes that normally circulate in blood. Wright-Giemsa stain.

Sometimes, only a component of an immunoglobulin molecule (light chains or heavy chains) is produced.[89,187,201,545] Rarely, a multiple myeloma secretes no visible monoclonal protein that is recognizable by conventional serum protein electrophoresis[282,296]; however, monoclonal immunoglobulin proteins may be identifiable using more sensitive methods.[419] Focal lytic or diffuse osteoporotic bone lesions may be recognized using survey radiography, and a Bence Jones proteinuria (immunoglobulin light chains in urine) may be present.

Increased numbers of plasma cells are usually identified in routine bone marrow biopsies of animals with multiple myeloma (Fig. 9-83, *A,B;* Fig. 9-84, *A,B;* Figs. 9-85, 9-86). In some cases, it is necessary to biopsy lytic bone lesions to demonstrate the plasma cell infiltrates. The morphology of the neoplastic cells can vary from normal-appearing mature plasma cells to large immature pleomorphic plasma cells with diffuse chromatin, abundant cytoplasm, and an increased mitotic index. Multiple nuclei may be present. The cytoplasm generally appears light blue to dark blue when Romanowsky-type blood stains are used; but in rare instances the cytoplasm of the neoplastic cells is filled with Russell bodies (Mott cells) or it stains red (flame cells), especially at the periphery of the cell.[8,356,554] The appearance of the flame cells may depend on the blood stain used (Fig. 9-87, *A-C*).

Plasma cell neoplasia presents quite differently in cats than it does in dogs and humans.[312,356] Rather than have bone marrow tumors with limited metastasis (multiple myeloma) or solitary extramedullary tumors with limited metastasis (extramedullary plasmacytoma), as are seen in dogs and humans, plasma cell tumors in cats are much more likely to exhibit metastasis whether they begin within or outside of the bone marrow. As a result, the term *myeloma-related disorders* has been used in regard to these coditions in cats.[312] Cats with

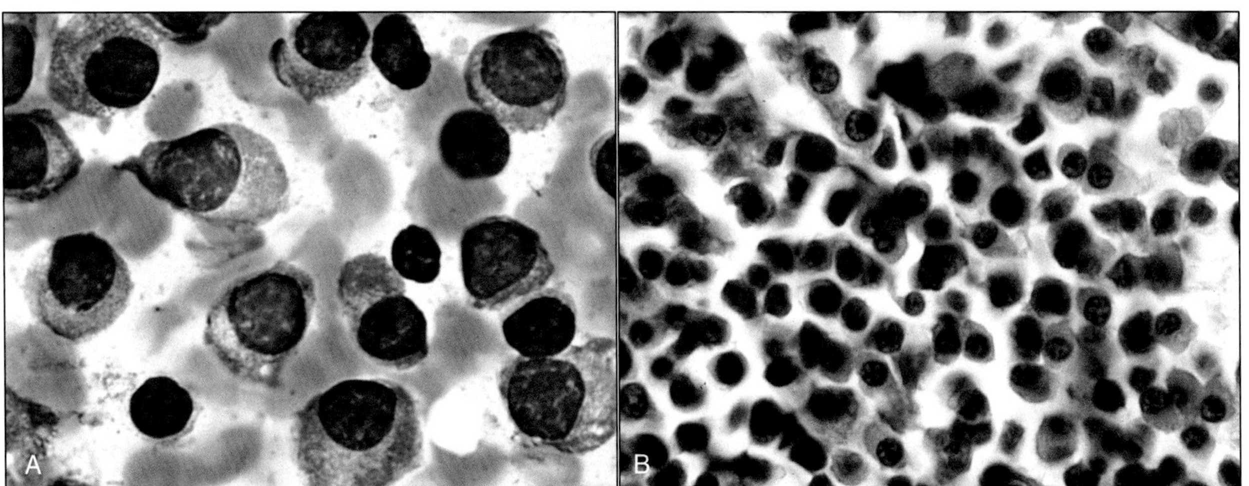

FIGURE 9-83
Multiple myeloma in bone marrow from a dog. **A,** Infiltrate of plasma cells with basophilic cytoplasm and eccentric nuclei in an aspirate smear. Wright-Giemsa stain. **B,** Infiltrate of plasma cells with eccentric nuclei, exhibiting coarsely clumped chromatin in a characteristic mosaic pattern, in a section of bone marrow collected as a core biopsy. H&E stain.

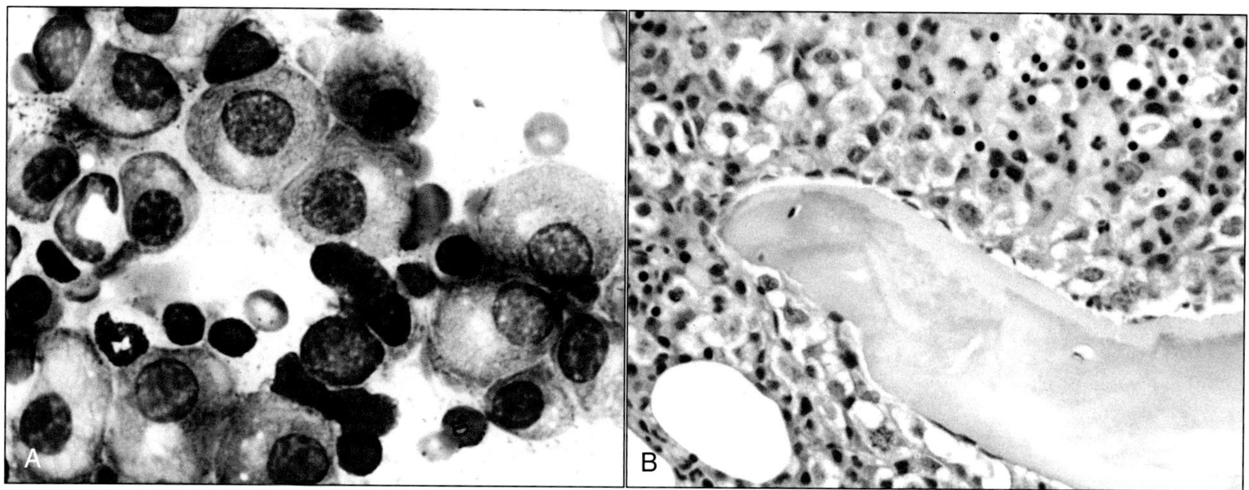

FIGURE 9-84
Multiple myeloma in bone marrow from a dog. **A,** Infiltrate of plasma cells with eccentric nuclei and abundant basophilic cytoplasm containing pale Golgi zones in an aspirate smear. Wright-Giemsa stain. **B,** Infiltrate of plasma cells with abundant cytoplasm near trabecular bone in a core biopsy section. H&E stain.

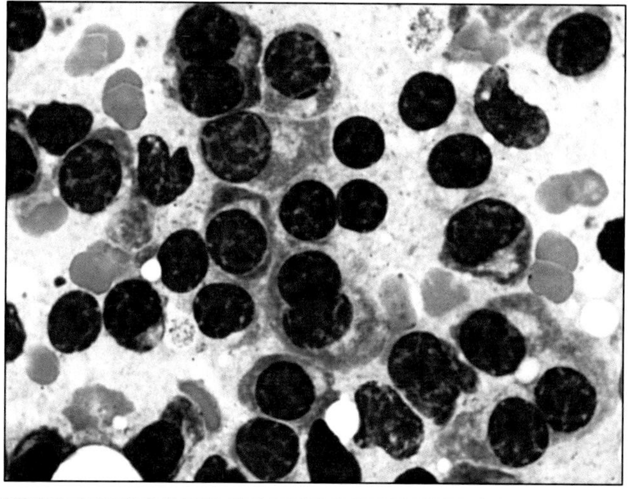

FIGURE 9-85
Infiltrate of plasma cells with eccentric nuclei and basophilic cytoplasm, containing pale Golgi zones, in an aspirate smear of bone marrow from a cat with multiple myeloma. Nuclear chromatin is coarsely clumped in a characteristic mosaic pattern. Two binucleated plasma cells are present. Wright-Giemsa stain.

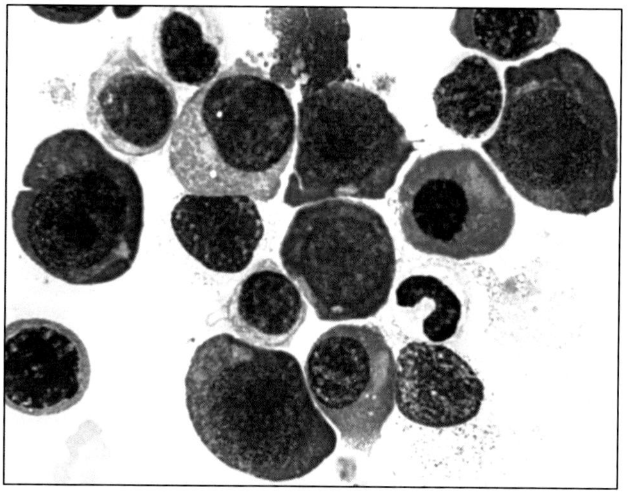

FIGURE 9-86
Infiltrate of five plasmacytoblasts with intensely basophilic cytoplasm in an aspirate smear of bone marrow from a dog with multiple myeloma. Wright-Giemsa stain.

myeloma-related neoplasms are typically FeLV and FIV negative.

Cats with bone marrow plasmacytosis typically have hyperglobulinemia and paraproteinemia, with an IgG paraprotein occurring about twice as often as an IgA paraprotein. Most paraproteinemias appear to be monoclonal by serum protein electrophoresis, but some appear biclonal. Plasma cell infiltrates are generally present in abdominal organs, especially the spleen and liver, when animals are initially diagnosed. Atypical plasma cell morphology, a nonregenerative anemia, and hypocholesterolemia are common, and a moderate number of cases involve light-chain proteinuria and thrombocytopenia. Lytic lesions in bone were reported as common in one study[356] and rare in another study.[312] Low numbers of plasma cells may be found in the blood of some affected cats but rarely in high enough numbers to justify use of the term *plasma cell leukemia.*[356,458]

Cats have been reported to have noncutaneous extramedullary plasma cell tumors with infiltrates of plasma cells in multiple organs, with no detectable bone marrow involvement. These cats have hyperglobulinemia and systemic illness similar to cats with documented bone marrow

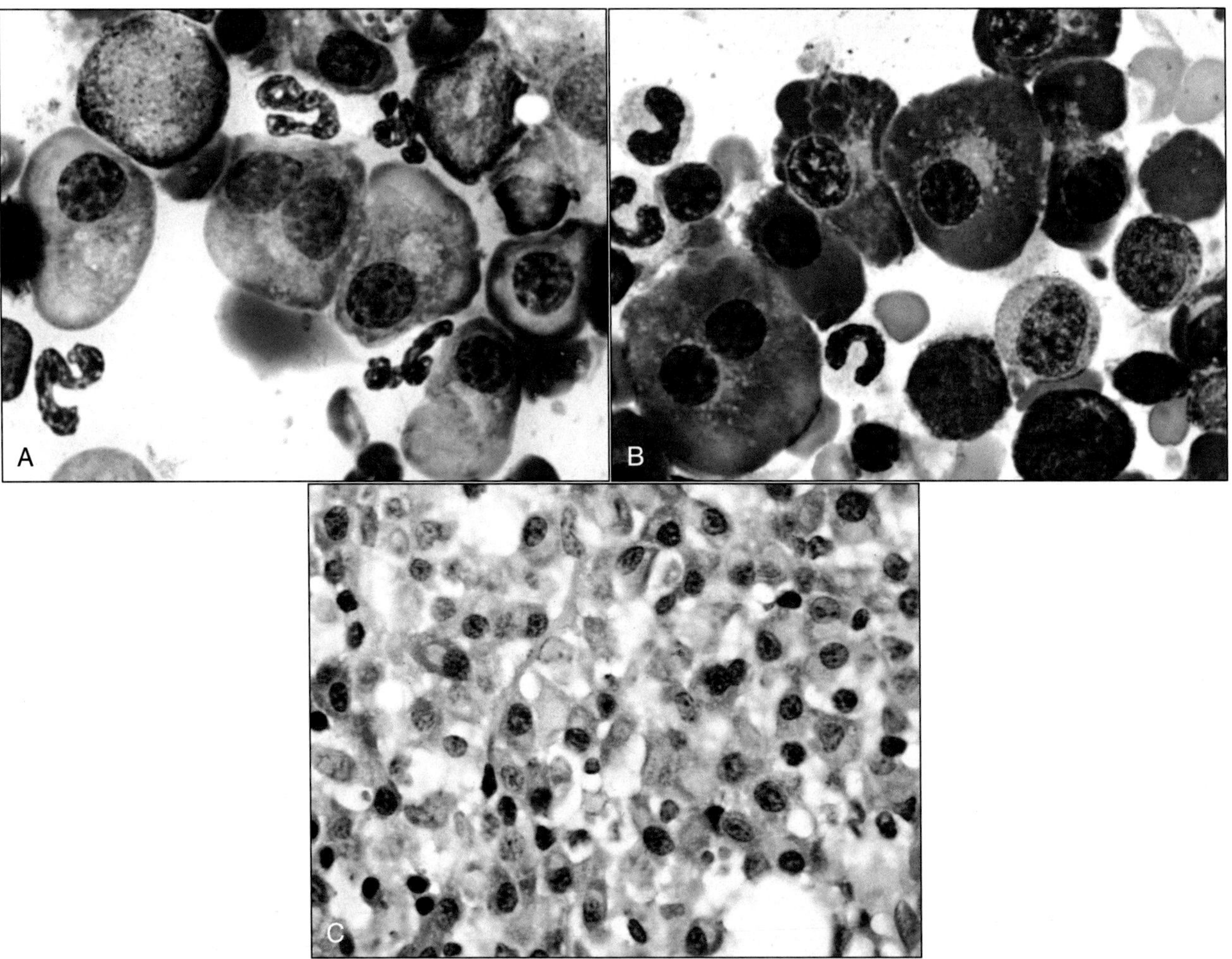

FIGURE 9-87

Bone marrow from a dog with multiple myeloma and a biclonal hyperglobulinemia migrating in the gamma region on serum protein electrophoresis. Red staining cytoplasm is visible with the Diff-Quik. **A,** Infiltrate of plasma cells with eccentric nuclei and abundant basophilic cytoplasm containing pale Golgi zones in an aspirate smear. A binucleated plasma cell is present near the center. Wright-Giemsa stain. **B,** Infiltrate of plasma cells with eccentric nuclei and abundant cytoplasm in an aspirate smear. These cells have been called flame cells because of their red-staining cytoplasm. A binucleated plasma cell is present near the bottom left corner. Diff-Quik stain. **C,** Infiltrate of plasma cells with eccentric nuclei and abundant cytoplasm in a section of bone marrow collected as a core biopsy. H&E stain.

plasmacytosis.[312] It has been proposed that these plasma cell neoplasms develop as primary extramedullary tumors.[313] Cats with mature plasma cell neoplasms survive longer than cats with anaplastic plasma cell neoplasms.[313]

Extramedullary Plasmacytoma

In addition to the metastasis of multiple myeloma from bone marrow, extramedullary plasma cell tumors (plasmacytomas) may arise as primary tumors of soft tissues. They occur most frequently as solitary tumors in the skin or the mouths of dogs but have also been reported in various gastrointestinal sites.[44,246,377,543] They rarely have an associated monoclonal or biclonal hyperglobulinemia[203,472] and in dogs rarely metastasize to distant sites.[268,472] Some cutaneous plasmacytomas in cats behave like those of dogs,[290] but others are much more aggressive, producing a paraprotein and quickly metastasizing (Fig. 9-88, *A,B*).[312]

Other B Lymphocyte Neoplasms

Any cell type in the B lymphocyte maturational pathway may become neoplastic and produce an immunoglobulin. The nature of a lymphoid neoplasm is determined by the stage at which B lymphocyte maturation is arrested. Other B lymphocyte neoplasms—including multicentric lymphomas, B lymphocyte CLL (discussed previously), and primary macroglobulinemia—may produce monoclonal hyperglobulinemias.[298] Lytic bone lesions are generally absent in these disorders, even when bone marrow infiltrates are present. In

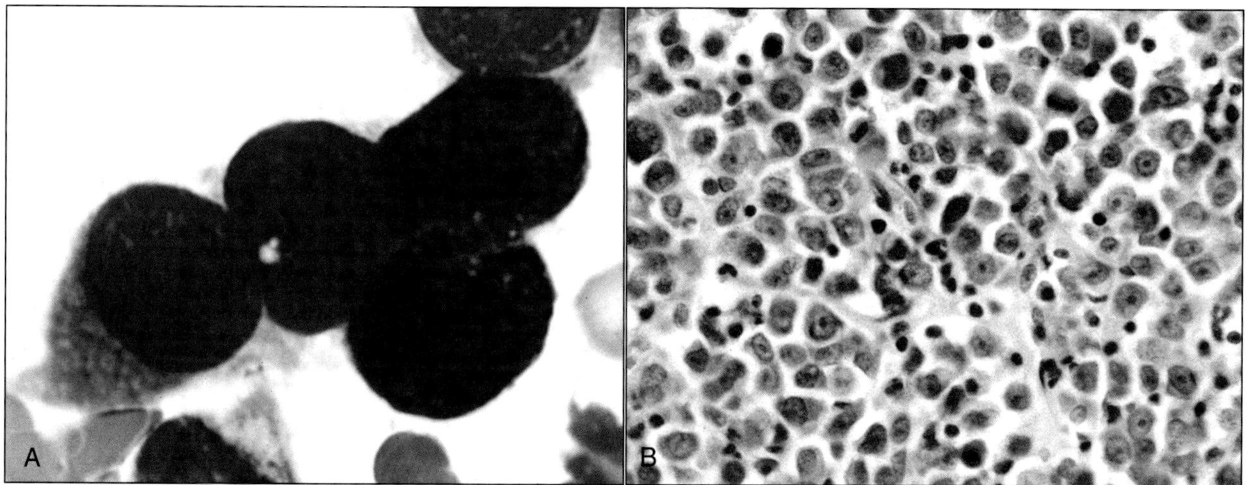

FIGURE 9-88
Anaplastic plasma cell neoplasm in bone marrow from a cat that originally presented as a cutaneous tumor. A monoclonal IgA hyperglobulinemia was also present. **A,** Basophilic plasmacytoid blast cell infiltrate in an aspirate smear. Similar blast cells were present in blood, skin, lungs, and liver. Wright-Giemsa stain. **B,** Marked infiltrate of plasmacytoid blast cells in a postmortem bone marrow section. H&E stain.

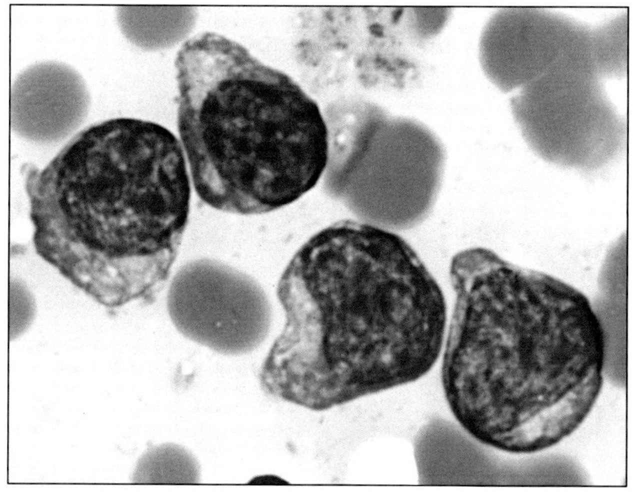

FIGURE 9-89
Infiltrate of basophilic lymphoid cells in an aspirate smear of bone marrow from a dog with macroglobulinemia (IgM hyperglobulinemia). Neoplastic cells were also present in the spleen but not in the lymph nodes. Wright-Giemsa stain.

humans, primary (Waldenström) macroglobulinemia is characterized as a lymphoplasmacytic neoplasm that produces an IgM monoclonal protein. The marrow aspirate is often of low cellularity, but the core biopsy is generally hypercellular and diffusely infiltrated with lymphocytes, plasmacytoid lymphocytes, and some plasma cells.[234] This syndrome is rarely reported in dogs (Fig. 9-89).[147,150,202,257,298] The spleen, liver, and lymphoid tissues rather than the bone marrow may have neoplastic infiltrates.[478]

MYELOID NEOPLASMS

The classification of myeloid neoplasia (formerly termed *myeloproliferative disorders*) is continually changing in human medicine based on expanded phenotype analyses, cytogenetic analyses, and the prognosis and response to therapy of these various neoplasms.[454] Until more molecular tools become available and large studies can be performed, myeloid neoplasms in animals will continue to be largely classified based on morphology, supplemented with some cytochemical staining and phenotype markers to help differentiate primitive cell types.[158,381,462,487]

Myeloid neoplasms are characterized by the clonal proliferation of one or more of the nonlymphoid marrow cell lines (granulocytic, monocytic, erythrocytic, or megakaryocytic).* They are subclassified as MDS, AML, and myeloproliferative neoplasms (MPNs).[176,436,516] AML is characterized by a block in differentiation/maturation, but an ongoing ability of neoplastic cells to survive and proliferate (see Table 9-2). In contrast, MDS is characterized by both impaired survival of neoplastic cells (increased apoptosis) and impaired differentiation/maturation of these cells. Both AML and MDS have been shown to be clonal abnormalities in cats.[182] MPNs exhibit increased proliferation/survival of neoplastic cells and relatively normal differentiation/maturation, at least initially.[343] Myeloid neoplasms have been associated with a variety of genetic mutations in humans. It is suggested that MDS progresses to AML following a second genetic mutation that allows blast cells to survive and proliferate (Table 9-2) and that MPN progresses to AML following a second

*References 39, 167, 208, 210, 223, 380.

TABLE 9-2

Myeloid Neoplasms

	MDS	AML	MPN
Differentiation/maturation	Impaired	Impaired	Normal ←←←
Proliferation/survival	Impaired →→→	Preserved	Increased

Modified from Nimer SD. Myelodysplastic syndromes. *Blood.* 2008;111: 4841-4851.
MDS, myelodysplastic syndrome; AML, acute myeloid leukemia; MPN, myeloproliferative neoplasms. Arrows indicate where a second genetic mutation could result in the progression to AML.

genetic mutation that results in impaired differentiation and maturation of neoplastic cells (see Table 9-2).[343] In addition to further genetic mutations, alterations in the bone marrow microenvironment and abnormalities in the immune system appear to contribute to the pathogenesis of various subtypes of myeloid neoplasms.[206]

Neoplastic transformations in myeloid neoplasms usually occur in hematopoietic stem cells/pluripotent progenitor cells.[308,385] Although the proliferation of one cell type may predominate, a marrow cell line is seldom singly affected. Morphologic or functional disorders of other cell lines can usually be detected. In addition, some myeloid neoplasms appear to evolve into one another. For example, MDS with excessive proliferation of nucleated erythrocytes (MDS-Er) in cats may evolve into erythroleukemia (AML-M6) and eventually AML-M1 or AML-M2,[173,207] and dogs with CML may have a "blast crisis" that develops into AML.[264,368]

Cats with myeloid neoplasms are generally infected with FeLV and/or FIV.[185,425,429,439,471] Irradiation has been experimentally shown to cause myeloid neoplasms in dogs.[417,466] Myeloid neoplasms are rare in domestic animal species other than cats and dogs, and their causes are unknown.

Excluding primary erythrocytosis and essential thrombocythemia, abnormalities that may be present in the blood of animals with myeloid neoplasms include a nonregenerative anemia with erythrocyte macrocytosis, anisocytosis, and/or poikilocytosis, nucleated erythrocytes out of proportion to the number of reticulocytes present and/or nucleated erythrocytes with lobulated or fragmented nuclei, large bizarre and/or hypogranular platelets, and immature granulocytes and/or abnormal granulocyte morphology (large size, hyposegmentation, hypersegmentation). Nonlymphoid blast cells may be present in blood, depending on the type of myeloid neoplasm and stage of development. The platelet count is frequently low but may be normal or high. The total leukocyte counts and absolute neutrophil, monocyte, eosinophil, and basophil counts vary from low to high, depending on the type of myeloid neoplasm that is present. Although a preliminary diagnosis of a myeloid neoplasm can sometimes be made based on hematologic findings, a definitive diagnosis and classification requires bone marrow evaluation.[208]

Myelodysplastic Syndromes

The term *myelodysplasia* is used when more than 10% of the cells in one or more bone marrow cell lines are dysplastic.[509,518] Myelodysplasia may be primary (neoplastic) or secondary (nonneoplastic). The term *MDS* is generally used as a synonym for primary myelodysplasia. MDS consists of a heterogeneous group of neoplastic disorders that are characterized by peripheral cytopenias (especially nonregenerative anemia and thrombocytopenia) with normal or hypercellular, dysplastic-appearing bone marrow.[343] Hypocellular bone marrow is rarely recognized.[547] This ineffective hematopoiesis results from defective maturation and extensive apoptosis of hematopoietic cells.[229,336,387] Apoptosis or physiologic cell death is a mechanism of gene-directed cellular self-destruction in which intracellular endonucleases initially cut DNA into fragments.[196] Recognizable apoptotic cells with fragmented nuclei exist for only 10 to 15 minutes before they are removed by phagocytic cells.[387] In addition to genetic abnormalities in hematopoietic stem cells/progenitor cells, abnormalities in the bone marrow microenvironment (including increased cytokine secretion by macrophages), immune deregulation, and other factors contribute to the appearance and behavior of MDS.[206,229] As in human MDS, a clonal proliferation of hematopoietic cells has been identified in two-thirds of cats with MDS, indicating that MDS may be considered a preleukemic state of AML in cats.[183]

Based on criteria recommended by the Animal Leukemia Study Group in 1991, the percentage of blast cells (myeloblasts, rubriblasts, or megakaryoblasts) in bone marrow should be less than 30% of all nucleated cells in MDS, and a diagnosis of AML should be made when the percentage of nonlymphoid blast cells equals or exceeds 30% of all nucleated cells.[210] This percentage of blast cells was also used as a cutoff value to differentiate MDS from AML in humans at that time. However, the World Health Organization (WHO) has since decreased this cutoff value differentiating MDS and AML from 30% blasts to 20% blasts for humans.[454] This has generated considerable debate concerning how best to treat human patients who have between 20% and 30% blast cells in their bone marrow, because this group appears to include some patients with advanced MDS, some with "smoldering" AML, and some with early stages of classic AML.[343] Nonetheless, there appears to be a consensus among veterinary clinical pathologists to decrease the cutoff value to 20% for animals as well.[223,505]

FeLV and probably FIV infections can produce MDS in cats,* although some cats with MDS have negative tests for these viruses.[128] The experimental infection of cats with a FeLV variant that had three tandem direct 47-bp repeats in the upstream region of the enhancer (URE) in the long terminal repeat (LTR) of the proviral sequence resulted in MDS in some cats and AML in others. In addition, analysis of the proviral sequences obtained from 13 cats with naturally occurring MDS revealed that they also had the characteristic URE repeats in the LTR.[182]

*References 27, 39, 185, 293, 426, 429.

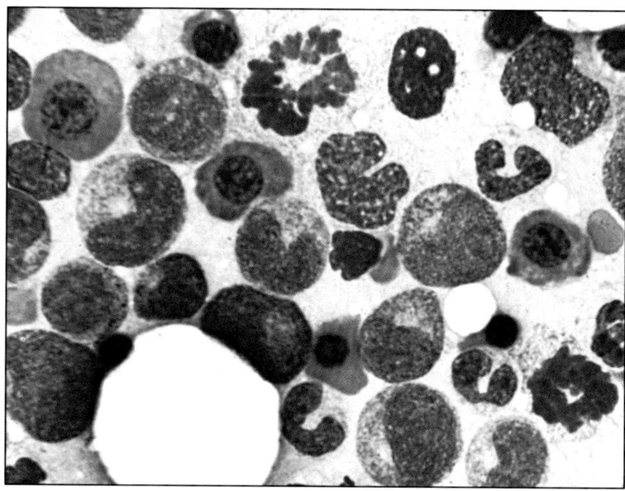

FIGURE 9-90
Bone marrow aspirate from a cat with MDS. Three megaloblastic rubricytes, two mitotic figures, and a left shift in the neutrophilic series is present. Wright-Giemsa stain.

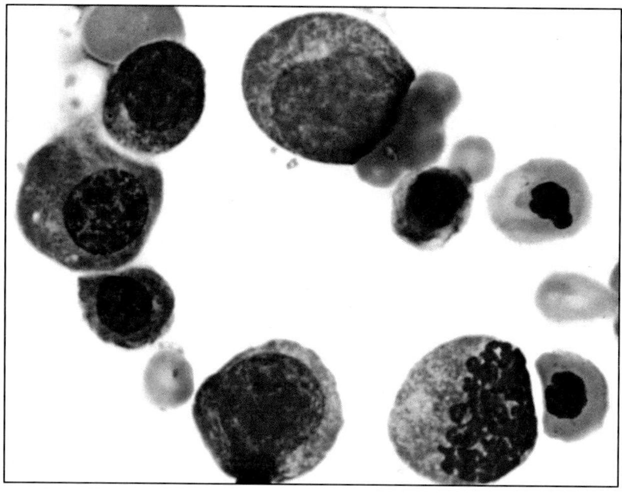

FIGURE 9-91
Dyserythropoiesis in an aspirate smear of bone marrow from a horse with MDS. A megaloblastic rubricyte is present at the far left, and a macrocytic metarubricyte with peanut-shaped nucleus is present at the right center. A mitotic figure is present near the bottom right. Wright-Giemsa stain.

Evidence of dyserythropoiesis, dysgranulopoiesis, and/or dysmegakaryocytopoiesis is present in the marrow of animals with MDS.* Erythroid abnormalities that may be present include increased numbers of rubriblasts, maturational arrest, megaloblastic cells, abnormal nuclear shapes, premature nuclear pyknosis, nuclear fragmentation, multinucleated cells, nuclear and cytoplasmic asynchrony, and siderotic inclusions (Figs. 9-90, 9-91). Neutrophilic abnormalities that may be present include increased numbers of myeloblasts, maturational arrest in the neutrophilic series (Fig. 9-92), giant metamyelocytes, band and mature neutrophils, abnormal granulation such as large primary granules, hyposegmented neutrophils (pseudo-Pelger-Huët), hypersegmented neutrophils, and neutrophils with bizarre nuclear shapes. Increased numbers of eosinophilic cells are also commonly observed with MDS in cats.[208,429] Megakaryocytic abnormalities that may be present include dwarf granular megakaryocytes with single or multiple nuclei and large megakaryocytes with nuclear abnormalities including hypolobulation, hyperlobulation, or multiple round nuclei (see Fig. 9-50, *B, C*). Some cats with MDS have stainable iron in their marrow (see Fig. 8-36, *C*).[37,286]

Additional abnormalities that may be present in blood include a nonregenerative anemia with erythrocyte macrocytosis, anisocytosis, and/or poikilocytosis, nucleated erythrocytes (metarubricytosis) out of proportion to the number of reticulocytes present, nucleated erythrocytes with lobulated or fragmented nuclei, thrombocytopenia, large bizarre platelets, immature granulocytes, and abnormal granulocyte morphology (large size, hyposegmentation, hypersegmentation).† The total leukocyte counts and absolute neutrophil counts vary from low to high.[185,208]

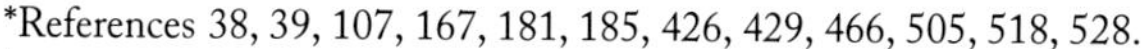

*References 38, 39, 107, 167, 181, 185, 426, 429, 466, 505, 518, 528.
†References 39, 88, 107, 181, 185, 286.

In animals, MDS has been classified into three subtypes based on blood and bone marrow findings.[223,380] MDS with erythroid predominance in the bone marrow (M:E ratio below 1) may be classified as MDS-Er.[88,208,210,530] Cases previously diagnosed as erythremic myelosis would now be placed in this category as long as the number of blast cells in the marrow was less than 20% of all nucleated cells. Cases with refractory anemia and an M:E ratio above 1, with or without other refractory cytopenias, may be described as myelodysplastic syndrome-refractory cytopenia (MDS-RC).[39,286,309] Myeloblasts account for less than 5% of all nucleated cells in this subtype. When myeloblasts are increased (5%-19% of bone marrow nucleated cells), the term *myelodysplastic syndrome-excess blasts* (MDS-EB) may be used.[223]

Dogs and cats with MDS may subsequently develop AML,* and FeLV-positive cats with MDS may also develop lymphoid neoplasms.[287] It is unknown what percentage of MDS cases represents a preleukemic state. Extended and costly supportive care is generally required for the survival of animals with MDS, and many such animals die or are euthanized before sufficient time has elapsed for an acute leukemia to develop. Longitudinal studies of animals with MDS are limited; however, it appears that high blast percentages as well as the presence of multiple cytopenias and marked dysplastic morphology are negative prognostic indicators.[185,505] Although recovery is rare, animals with MDS may recover spontaneously, as occurred in a FeLV-positive cat that became FeLV-negative.[269]

MDS must be differentiated from secondary myelodysplasia, which may be associated with immune-mediated disorders

*References 88, 173, 286, 287, 309, 466, 471, 530.

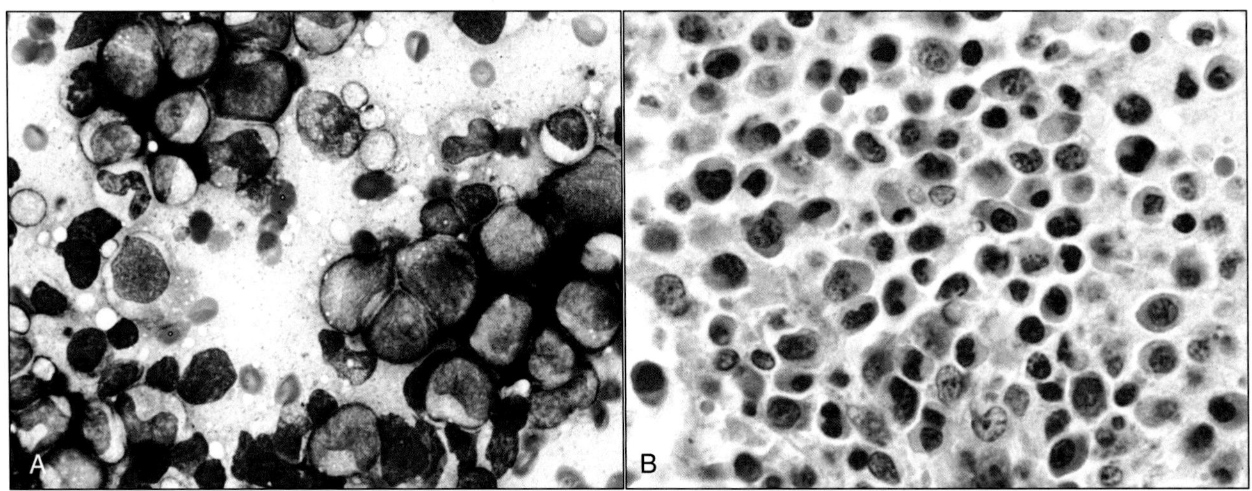

FIGURE 9-92

Maturational arrest in neutrophil development at the myelocyte-metamyelocyte stage in bone marrow from a neutropenic dog with MDS. **A,** No mature neutrophils and only one band neutrophil are present in this aspirate smear. Erythroid precursors are absent in this field. The M:E ratio was 19. Wright-Giemsa stain. **B,** Maturational arrest in neutrophil development in a core biopsy section. H&E stain.

(IMHA and IMT), lymphoid neoplasms (lymphoma, multiple myeloma), myelofibrosis, drugs that interfere with DNA synthesis (antimetabolites, alkylating agents, folate antagonists, and plant alkaloids), heavy metal toxicity (lead and zinc), antibiotics (cephalosporins, chlorampenicol, oxazolidinone), anticonvulant drugs, and hydroxyzine.* Dyserythropoiesis also occurs in association with some idiopathic and hereditary disorders discussed earlier in this chapter. Blast cells rarely exceed 5% of all nucleated cells in the bone marrow in secondary myelodysplasia and often exceed 5% in MDS. Dysplastic features are generally more pronounced and affect more than one cell line in MDS compared to secondary myelodysplasia. However, morphology alone is often not sufficient to differentiate these disorders.[38,505,518]

Acute Myeloid Leukemias

A classification system for AML in dogs and cats has been developed by the American Society for Veterinary Clinical Pathology Animal Leukemia Study Group.[210] It was adapted from the French-American-British (FAB) system established by a National Cancer Institute workshop for use in humans.[71] AML was diagnosed when the percentage of nonlymphoid hematopoietic blast cells in the bone marrow equaled or exceeded 30% of all nucleated cells (ANCs) excluding lymphocytes, macrophages, plasma cells, and mast cells. This percentage has been decreased to 20% for humans in the most recent WHO classification scheme, and there appears to be a consensus to do so in veterinary medicine as well; that change has been accepted for this text.[223]

Dyserythropoiesis, dysgranulopoiesis, and/or dysmegakaryocytopoiesis are also usually present, with megaloblastic nucleated erythroid cells being most commonly observed.[210] If blast cells account for less than 20% of ANCs and dysplastic changes are present, a diagnosis of MDS is made. Some cases of erythroleukemia (AML-M6) are exceptions to these guidelines, as discussed further on. Cytochemistry, immunocytochemistry, and lineage-specific antigens may be used to help identify the type or types of blast cells present. Several subtypes of AML have been recognized in animals.* In addition to quantifying cells as a percentage of ANC, they may also be quantified based on the total nonerythroid cells (NECs), which is determined by subtracting the nucleated erythroid cells from the ANC count.[380]

AML-M1

Myeloblastic leukemia without maturation is designated as AML-M1. Myeloblasts (primarily type I myeloblasts) account for 90% or more of NECs. Type I myeloblasts appear as large round cells with round to oval nuclei that are generally centrally located in the cell. The N:C ratio is high (greater than 1.5) and the nuclear outline is usually regular and smooth. Nuclear chromatin is finely stippled, containing one or more nucleoli or nucleolar rings. The cytoplasm is generally moderately basophilic.[210] Differentiated granulocytes (promyelocytes through mature neutrophils and eosinophils) and monocytes account for the remaining NECs.

AML-M2

Myeloblastic leukemia with maturation is designated AML-M2. Myeloblasts account for 20% to 89% of NECs (Fig. 9-93, *A,B*; Fig. 9-94, *A-C*; Figs. 9-95, 9-96, *A,B*). In addition to type I myeloblasts, variable numbers of type II

*References 38, 97, 174, 276, 512, 518.

*References 208, 210, 223, 308, 374, 380.

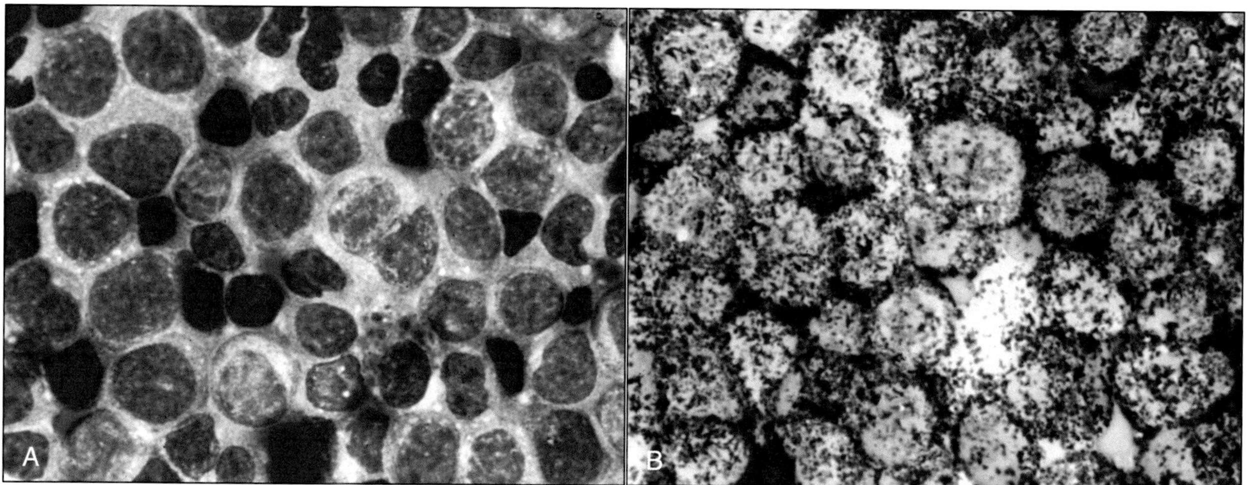

FIGURE 9-93

Bone marrow aspirate smears from a cat with AML-M2. **A,** Proliferation of myeloblasts, promyelocytes, and myelocytes. Approximately 35% of all nucleated cells were myeloblasts. Few band or mature neutrophils were present and rare erythroid precursors were recognized. Wright-Giemsa stain. **B,** Proliferation of myeloblasts, promyelocytes, and myelocytes. The strongly peroxidase-positive nature of the cells present rules out a lymphoproliferative disorder and indicates that these cells are granulocytic precursors. Peroxidase stain.

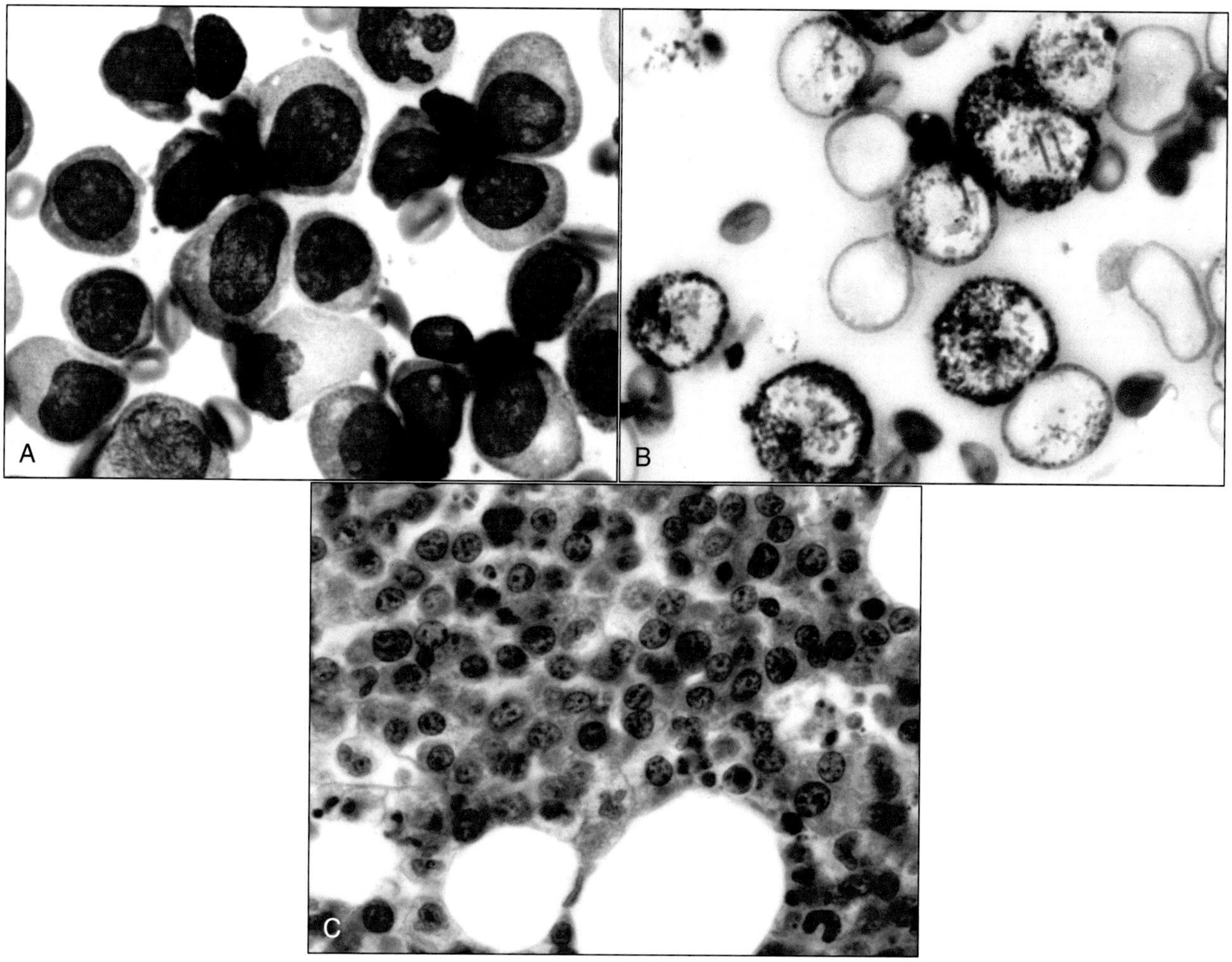

FIGURE 9-94

Bone marrow from a dog with AML-M2. **A,** Proliferation of myeloblasts, with nucleoli easily visible in many cells, in an aspirate smear. Wright-Giemsa stain. **B,** Proliferation of myeloblasts in an aspirate smear. Most of these cells were peroxidase-positive, ruling out a lymphoproliferative disorder. Peroxidase stain. **C,** Proliferation of myeloblasts in a core biopsy section. H&E stain.

myeloblasts containing a few (less than 15) small, magenta-staining granules in the cytoplasm may be present. Differentiated granulocytes account for 10% or more of NECs and monocytic cells account for less than 20% of NECs. Increased marrow basophil and/or eosinophil precursors may be seen in some cats with myeloid neoplasms (see Fig. 9-33), and variants of AML-M2 with basophilic differentiation and eosinophilic differentiation have been reported in cats and classified as M2-B and M2-Eos, respectively.[46,208]

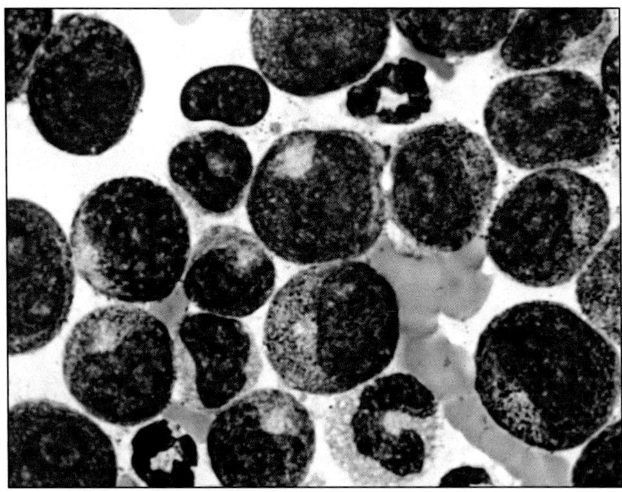

FIGURE 9-95
Proliferation of myeloblasts and promyelocytes in an aspirate smear of bone marrow from a dog with AML-M2. Many of the cells contain primary magenta-staining granules. Wright-Giemsa stain.

AML-M3

Promyelocytic leukemia has not been reported in animals. In humans, the predominant cells involved are abnormal-appearing promyelocytes with folded, reniform, or bilobed nuclei. Type III myeloblasts may also be present in this disorder. These cells have distinct nucleoli and abundant cytoplasm containing many magenta-staining cytoplasmic granules. Type III myeloblasts appear to represent blast cells with asynchronous cytoplasmic maturation. Low numbers of these cells may be present in cats with AML.[208]

AML-M4

Acute myelomonocytic leukemia is diagnosed when combined numbers of myeloblasts and monoblasts equal or exceed 20% of ANCs and differentiated granulocytes and monocytes each account for 20% or more of NECs. Monoblasts resemble myeloblasts except that their nuclear shape is irregularly round to convoluted in appearance (Figs. 9-97, *A,B*). A clear area in the cytoplasm, representing the Golgi zone, is often observed, especially near the site of nuclear indentation. The N:C ratio is high but may be somewhat lower than that in myeloblasts.[153,184,210]

AML-M5

Acute monocytic leukemia is diagnosed when monoblasts are increased but myeloblasts are not (Figs. 9-98, 9-99). It may be separated into subtypes depending on the maturity of the monocytic cells present. Little maturation to monocytes is present in M5a, with monoblasts and promonocytes accounting for 80% or more of all NECs. When 20% to 79% of NECs are monoblasts and promonocytes and maturation to monocytes is prominent, the leukemia is classified as M5b. Granulocytes account for less than 20% of NECs.

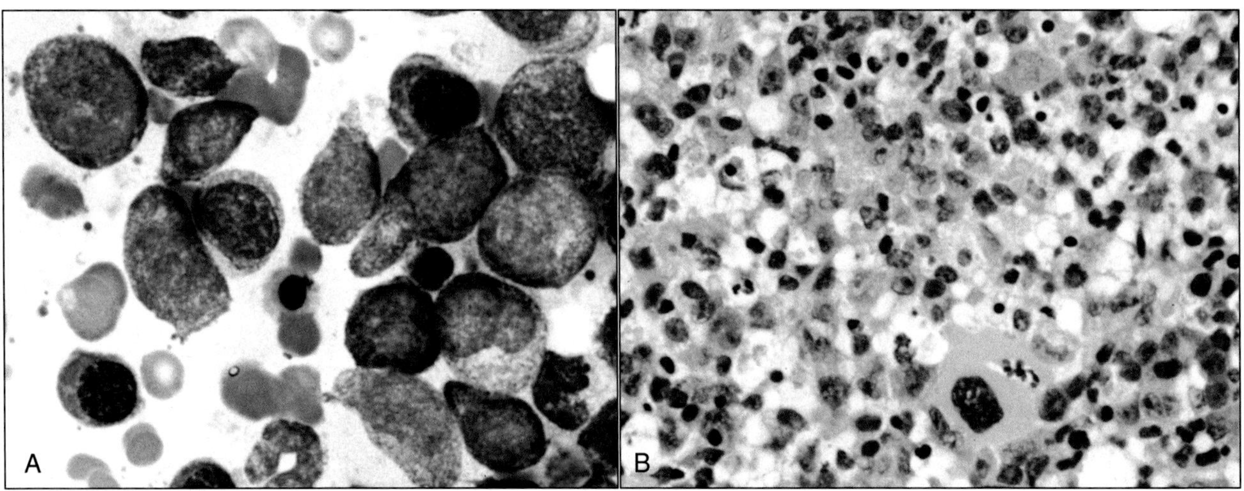

FIGURE 9-96
Bone marrow from a horse with AML-M2. **A,** Increased numbers of myeloblasts (large round cells with medium-blue cytoplasm) in an aspirate smear. The smaller and more darkly staining cells present are erythroid precursors. Wright-Giemsa stain. **B,** Proliferation of myeloblasts in a core biopsy section. Darker cells are erythroid precursors. Several red-staining eosinophils are also present. A megakaryocyte is present at bottom center. H&E stain.

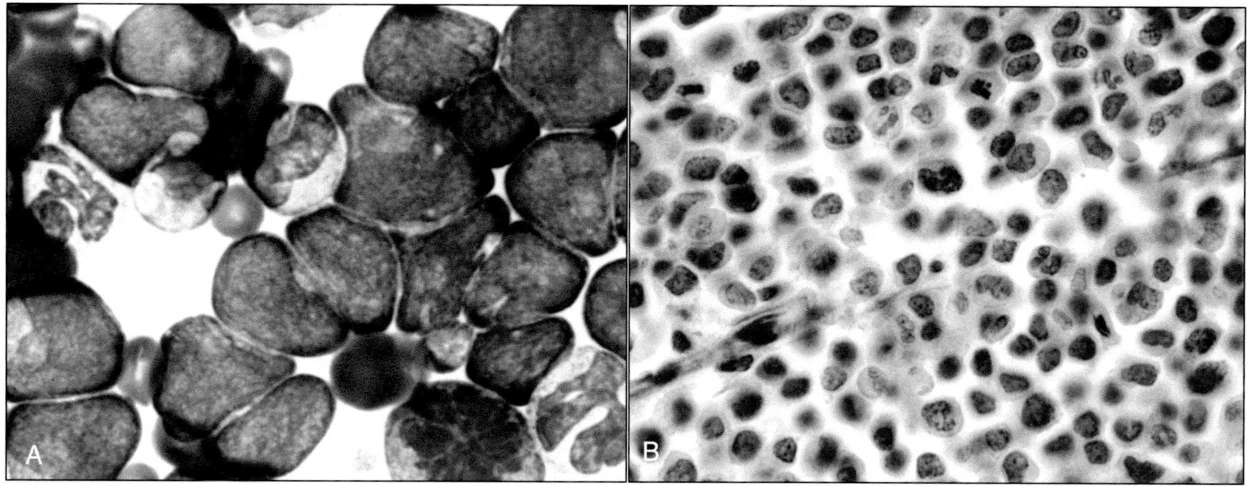

FIGURE 9-97
Bone marrow from a dog with AML-M4. **A,** Proliferation of myeloblasts (generally round nuclei) and monoblasts (frequently indented nuclei) in an aspirate smear. Wright-Giemsa stain. **B,** Proliferation of myeloblasts and monoblasts in a core biopsy section. H&E stain.

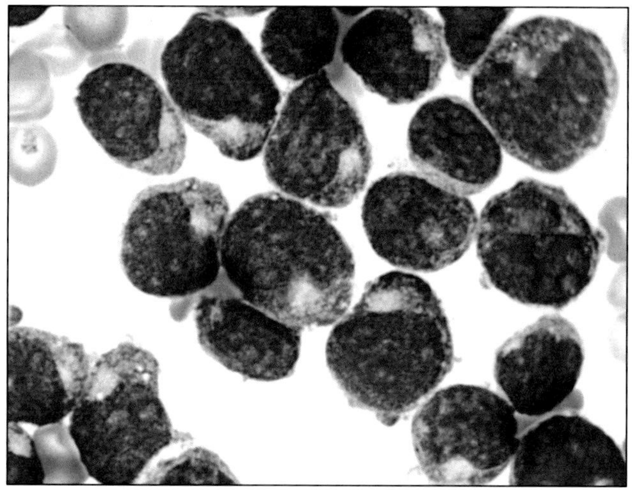

FIGURE 9-98
Proliferation of monoblasts (frequently indented nuclei) in an aspirate smear of bone marrow from a dog with acute monocytic leukemia (AML-M5a). Wright-Giemsa stain.

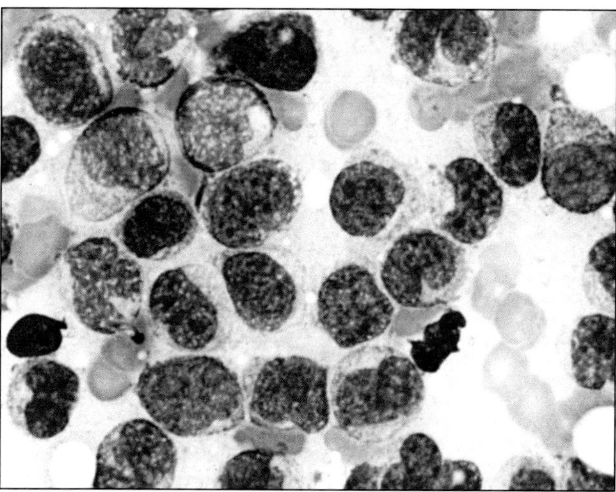

FIGURE 9-99
Proliferation of monoblasts (frequently indented nuclei) in an aspirate smear of bone marrow from a dog with acute monocytic leukemia (AML-M5b). Wright-Giemsa stain.

AML-M6

Erythroleukemia is a term used to describe myeloid neoplasms in which erythroid abnormalities are prominent.[208,210,380] In contrast to the subtypes of AML discussed previously, the M:E ratio is less than 1 in AML-M6, and blast cells (myeloblasts, monoblasts, and megakaryoblasts combined) may not equal or exceed 20% of ANCs, but they will equal or exceed 20% of the NECs (Fig. 9-100). The designation *AML-M6Er* is used when the M:E ratio is less than 1 and rubriblasts are included with myeloblasts, monoblasts, and megakaryoblasts in the blast count to equal or exceed 20% of ANCs. In some cases most of the blasts present appear to be rubriblasts (Figs. 9-101, 9-102). Rubriblasts have deeply basophilic cytoplasm that is devoid of granules. The nucleus of a rubriblast is usually almost perfectly round and has finely stippled chromatin with one or more distinct nucleoli.

AML-M7

Megakaryoblastic leukemia is diagnosed when megakaryoblasts account for 20% or more of ANCs or NECs in bone marrow (Fig. 9-103, *A,B*).* Nuclei of megakaryoblasts are nearly as round as rubriblast nuclei, but their cytoplasm is typically less basophilic. Additional features that are typically

*References 9, 60, 80, 81, 316, 451.

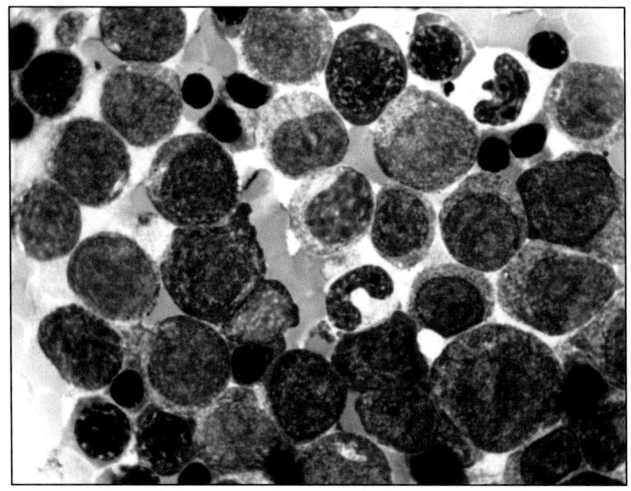

FIGURE 9-100
Increased myeloblasts and rubriblasts in an aspirate smear of bone marrow from a cat with AML-M6. Wright-Giemsa stain.

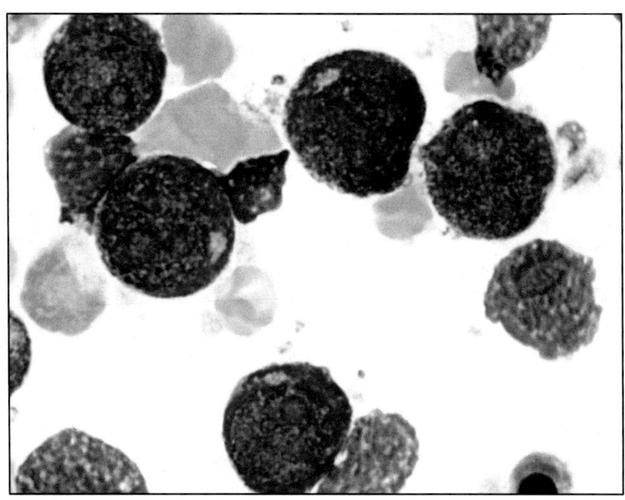

FIGURE 9-101
Rubriblasts in an aspirate smear of bone marrow from a dog with erythroleukemia with erythroid predominance (AML-M6Er). Several free nuclei (basket cells) are also present. Wright-Giemsa stain.

present in some cells include binucleation/multinucleation, multiple discrete cytoplasmic vacuoles, cytoplasmic projections (blebs), cytoplasmic fragments, and sometimes purple granules. Some differentiation with dysplastic multinucleated megakaryocytes is also generally present. Using immunocytochemical staining or flow cytometry, blast cells may be identified as megakaryoblasts. Megarkaryoblasts are generally positive for vWF, CD41 (GPIIb), CD61 (GPIIIa), and CD62P (P selectin).[9,81,259,353,451] Some cases are also positive for CD34.[9,81,451] A severe nonregenerative anemia is consistently present in dogs. Other common hematologic findings include metarubricytosis, thrombocytopenia, and variable numbers of megakaryoblasts in the blood. Metastasis to the spleen and lymph nodes is common.[81]

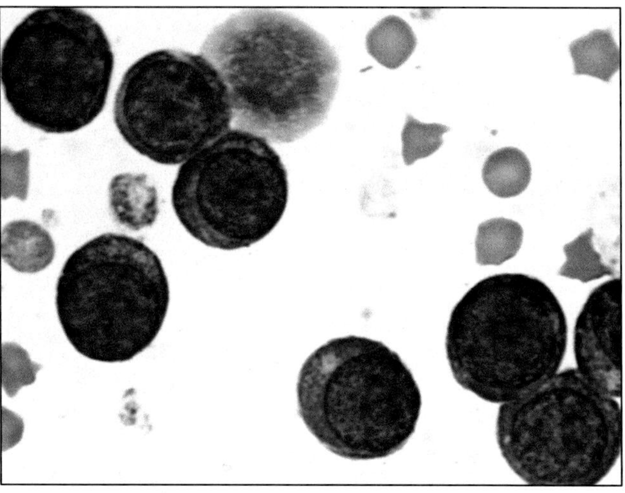

FIGURE 9-102
Rubriblasts in an aspirate smear of bone marrow from a cat with AML-M6Er. Wright-Giemsa stain.

Acute Undifferentiated Leukemia

Acute undifferentiated leukemia (AUL) is diagnosed when the blast cells cannot be identified with certainty using routine blood stains or cytochemical markers (Fig. 9-104). This term may be used as a temporary category in some cases, pending the use of specialized cell markers. As more cellular markers are developed, the percentage of cases classified as AUL will decrease. The hallmark of AUL is the presence of blast cells with broad cytoplasmic pseudopods and/or some magenta-staining cytoplasmic granules.[208] Cats with a myeloid neoplasm previously referred to as reticuloendotheliosis may be included in this category. However, some cases previously diagnosed as reticuloendotheliosis would now be included in AML-M6Er, because the blast cells present had deeply basophilic cytoplasm without granules and nuclei that were characteristic of those present in rubriblasts.[167]

Peripheral Blood Findings

Peripheral blood findings for AML are similar to those described previously for MDS except that blast cells and a leukocytosis are more likely to be present in the circulation in AML. Moderate to severe nonregenerative anemia with thrombocytopenia and/or neutropenia is generally present.[2,462] Leukopenia occurs in nearly one-third of AML-M2 cats.[208] A monocytosis is generally prominent in M4 and M5 types of AML. Additionally, a minority of animals with AML-M7 have a thrombocytosis while most have a thrombocytopenia, as is commonly seen in all other types of AML.[81,208]

Frequency in Animal Species

AML is seen most commonly in cats, with myeloblastic leukemia (M1 and M2 combined) being most common.[208] Myelomonocytic leukemia (AML-M4) and monocytic leukemia (AML-M5) appear to be most common in dogs.[2,158,462] Although rare, most horses reported with AML have had

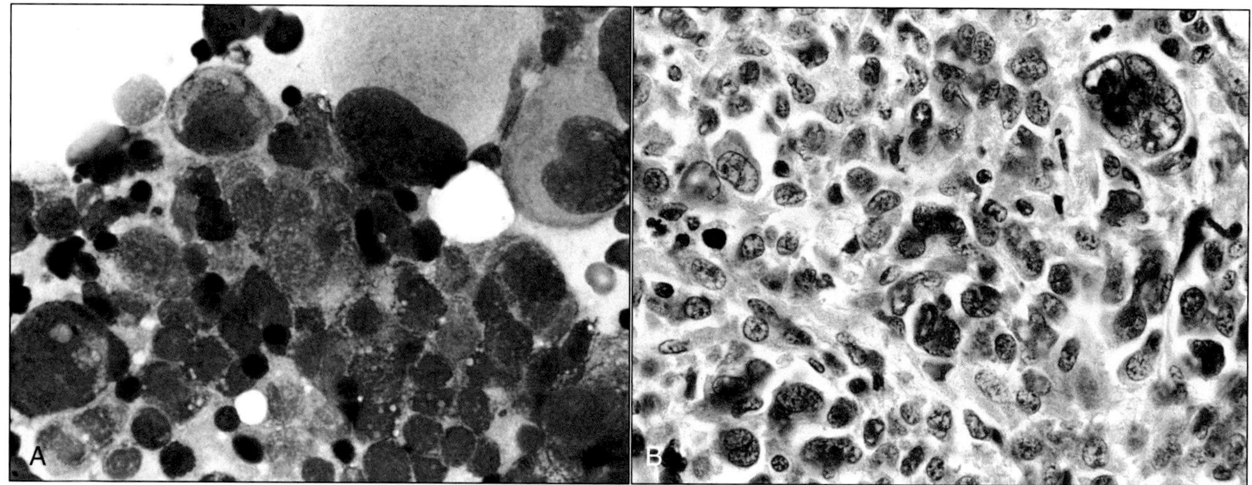

FIGURE 9-103
Megakaryoblastic leukemia (AML-M7) in bone marrow from a dog. **A,** Predominance of megakaryoblasts and abnormal megakaryocytes in an aspirate smear. Wright-Giemsa stain. **B,** Predominance of megakaryoblasts and abnormal megakaryocytes in a core biopsy section. H&E stain.

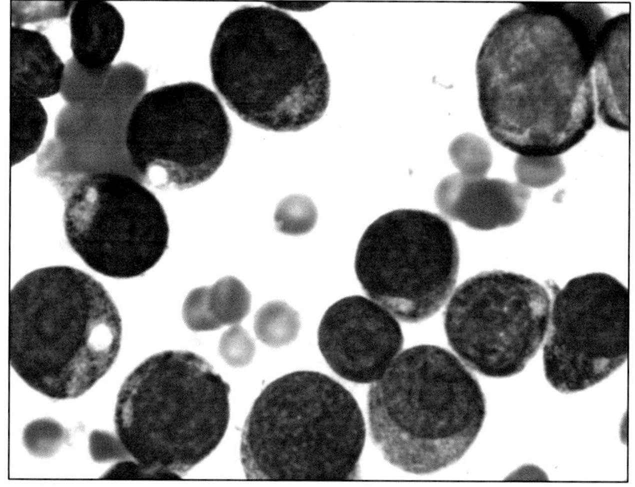

FIGURE 9-104
Predominance of blast cells in an aspirate smear of bone marrow from a cat with an AUL in which the neoplastic cells could not be classified with certainty. Wright-Giemsa stain.

either AML-M4 or AML-M5.[407] Erythroleukemia (AML-M6 and AML-M6Er combined) has been reported primarily in cats.[208] Megakaryoblastic leukemia (AML-M7) is rare, being reported primarily in dogs.[81] AML is rarely reported in cattle.[457,541]

Myeloproliferative Neoplasms

MPNs (formerly termed *chronic myeloproliferative disease*) are neoplastic proliferations of hematopoietic cells resulting in high numbers of differentiated cells in blood. Like those with MDS, animals with MPN have less than 20% blast cells in the bone marrow, with few or no blast cells in the blood. Dysplastic changes may be present in both disorders, but they tend to be more noticeable in MDS. The major difference between these disorders is that high numbers of one or more blood cell types occur in MPNs and cytopenias frequently occur in MDS.

Chronic Myeloid Leukemia

CML is a rare disorder in animals, occurring primarily in dogs.* A BCR-ABL chromosomal abnormality (Raleigh chromosome) has recently been reported in dogs with CML that is similar to the Philadelphia chromosome abnormality found in most human CML.[49] CML presents with a high total leukocyte count (typically greater than 50,000/μL) with a marked neutrophilic left shift in blood. Increased numbers of monocytes, eosinophils, and/or basophils may also be present. Myeloblasts are either absent or present in low numbers in blood. Nucleated erythrocytes are often found in blood in the presence of a nonregenerative anemia. Platelet counts may be low, normal, or increased. If monocytes predominate, a diagnosis of chronic monocytic leukemia or chronic myelomonocytic leukemia may be considered.

Granulocytic hyperplasia is present in bone marrow with or without erythroid and megakaryocytic hypoplasia. The percentage of immature granulocytic cells is increased but the percentage of myeloblasts does not exceed 20% of all nucleated cells (Fig. 9-105). Dysplastic changes are typically also present in one or more marrow cell lines.

CML must be differentiated from severe inflammatory leukemoid reactions. The presence of cytoplasmic toxicity, increased inflammatory plasma proteins, and physical evidence of inflammation suggests that a leukemoid reaction is present. The presence of myelodysplasia suggests that CML is present. In some canine cases, CML has been recognized to terminate in a blast crisis, in which maturation of

*References 157, 167, 215, 264, 368, 461.

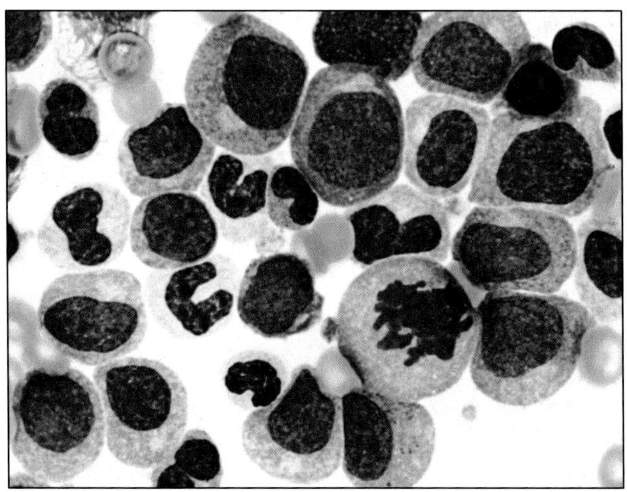

FIGURE 9-105
Granulocytic hyperplasia with a left shift in an aspirate smear of bone marrow from a dog with CML. Wright-Giemsa stain

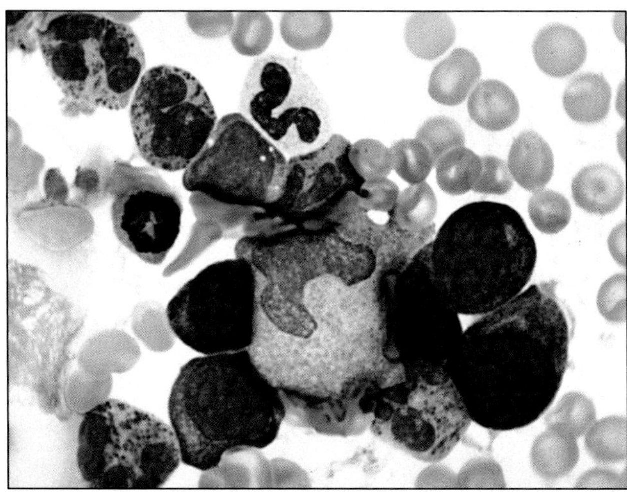

FIGURE 9-106
Increased numbers of basophils and blast cells in an aspirate smear of bone marrow from a dog with basophilic leukemia. Basophils accounted for nearly half and blast cells in this hypercellular marrow preparation.

Courtesy of Rose E. Raskin.

granulocytic cells is greatly diminished and blast cells predominate in blood and bone marrow.[264,368,461]

Chronic granulocytic leukemia,[125,213] chronic myelomonocytic leukemia,[382] and chronic monocytic leukemia may be considered variants of CML.[91,401] It should be noted that a dog diagnosed with chronic monocytic leukemia had a chromosomal translocation producing a BCR-ABL gene hybrid like that previously reported in CML in dogs.[91]

Eosinophilic Leukemia

Eosinophilic leukemia is a variant of CML in which eosinophilic cells predominate in blood and marrow. Differentiation of eosinophilic leukemia and hypereosinophilic syndrome in cats can be difficult. Hypereosinophilic syndrome is characterized by a mature eosinophilia with frequent involvement of the intestines. Prominent eosinophilic left shifts in the bone marrow and blood as well as organ infiltrates are more likely to occur in animals with eosinophilic leukemia[145,200,342,452,470]; however, some left shifting in eosinophil precursors within the bone marrow may occur in reactive disorders.[358]

Basophilic Leukemia

Basophilic leukemia is a variant of CML in which basophilic cells predominate in blood and marrow. It has rarely been reported in dogs.[280,288,311] Early reports of basophilic leukemia in animals represented misdiagnosed cases of systemic mastocytosis with mastocytemia. Basophilic leukemia is characterized by a marked basophilia with many immature basophilic cells in the blood and bone marrow (Fig. 9-106).

Primary Erythrocytosis

Primary erythrocytosis (polycythemia vera) in adult dogs and cats is considered to be a MPN that is characterized by an autonomous (EPO-independent) proliferation of erythroid precursor cells, resulting in high numbers of mature erythrocytes in blood.[231] In contrast to polycythemia vera in humans, granulocyte and platelet numbers are generally not increased.[155,548] The bone marrow is hyperplastic with orderly maturation of cells. Erythroid hyperplasia may be accompanied by megakaryocytic and/or granulocytic hyperplasia in some cases.[362,500] The M:E ratio is often normal but may be decreased secondary to erythroid hyperplasia.[231,306,548] Marrow iron stores may be low, presumably as a result of increased demands for erythrocyte production.[500]

Essential Thrombocythemia

Essential thrombocythemia is a MPN that is characterized by persistent, markedly increased (usually above $1 \times 10^6/\mu L$) platelet counts and megakaryocytic hyperplasia in the bone marrow (Fig. 9-48, *A,B*) in the absence of iron deficiency, recovery from severe hemorrhage, rebound from a thrombocytopenia, splenectomy, an underlying chronic inflammatory condition, or another myeloid neoplasm.[24,161,445] Approximately half of the cases in humans have a somatic point mutation that causes a constitutive activation of the *JAK2* gene.[116] In humans, the HCT is normal, megakaryocytes appear large and mature, stainable iron is present in the marrow, and no myelodysplasia or myelofibrosis is seen. Some of the cases reported as essential thrombocythemia in animals differ from these criteria and may represent other forms of myeloid neoplasms.

NONHEMATOPOIETIC NEOPLASMS

Nonhematopoietic neoplasms of bone marrow develop in other tissues and metastasize to the marrow. A metastasis to bone marrow may be relatively common, but it is rarely

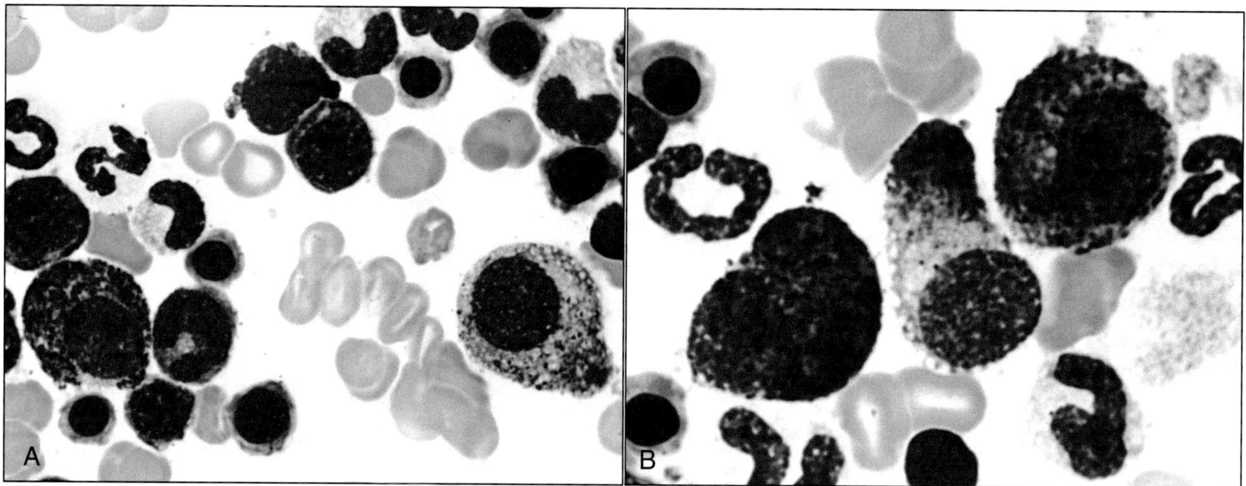

FIGURE 9-107
Mast cell infiltrates in bone marrow aspirate smears from a dog with a metastatic mast cell tumor. **A,** Mast cell infiltrate *(slightly below center at right and left edges).* **B,** Three mast cells with round nuclei and purple granules are located diagonally from top right to bottom left. Wright-Giemsa stain.

diagnosed because the multifocal distributions of neoplastic infiltrates are easily missed when a small biopsy needle is used. Recognition of metastatic neoplasms within the marrow is increased if biopsies are collected from lesions identified with the use of diagnostic imaging techniques.[371]

Mast Cell Tumors

Mast cells are round cells with round nuclei. They typically have large numbers of purple granules in the cytoplasm, although the granules may not stain with Diff-Quik or other water-based Wright stains. Mast cell precursors are produced in the bone marrow but rarely develop into mast cells there.[42] Rather, these precursors leave the marrow, circulate in blood, and migrate into tissue sites, where they develop into mast cells.[126]

Mast cell tumors originating in the skin, spleen, and other peripheral sites may metastasize to bone marrow; consequently bone marrow examination may be a part of staging this neoplasm (Fig. 9-107,*A,B*).[294,345] Bone marrow metastasis (as evaluated using bone marrow aspirate smears) was recognized in less than 5% of 157 dogs with primary cutaneous mast cell tumors.[113] Most dogs with mast cell tumor metastasis to bone marrow have one or more peripheral cytopenias (anemia, leukopenia, thrombocytopenia). Other hematologic abnormalities that may be present include leukocytosis, eosinophilia, and basophilia.[113,294] In addition to bone marrow metastasis, these dogs generally have metastasis to other organs, especially the spleen and liver.[294] Bone marrow involvement is more likely in noncutaneous systemic mastocytosis, as occurs most frequently in cats.[96,140,230,272,345]

Mast cells may occur in the bone marrow of dogs with aplastic anemia of various etiologies.[332,489] They may also be present in some inflammatory conditions.[307,428]

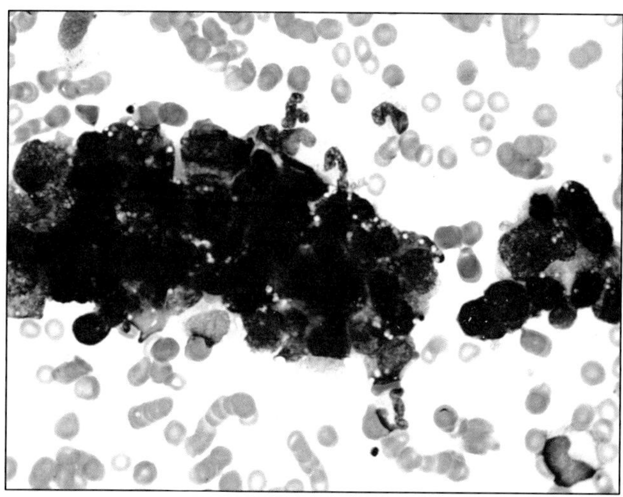

FIGURE 9-108
Metastatic adenocarcinoma in a bone marrow aspirate smear from a dog. Cohesive clusters of basophilic epithelial cells. Wright-Giemsa stain.

Metastatic Neoplasms

Metastatic carcinomas are rarely recognized in routine bone marrow biopsies (Figs. 9-108, 9-109, *A,B*),[179,318] but they are identified more commonly at necropsy or in instances where biopsy needles are directed at bone lesions identified with the help of diagnostic imaging.[82,108,160,371,544] Dogs with skeletal metastasis often present with clinical signs such as pain and lameness attributable to skeletal involvement. Metastasis occurs most frequently in the axial skeletal and proximal long bones, with about 10% of the metastases occurring below the elbow and stifle. Prostate, mammary, and lung are the most frequent sites for the primary tumors that metastasize to the

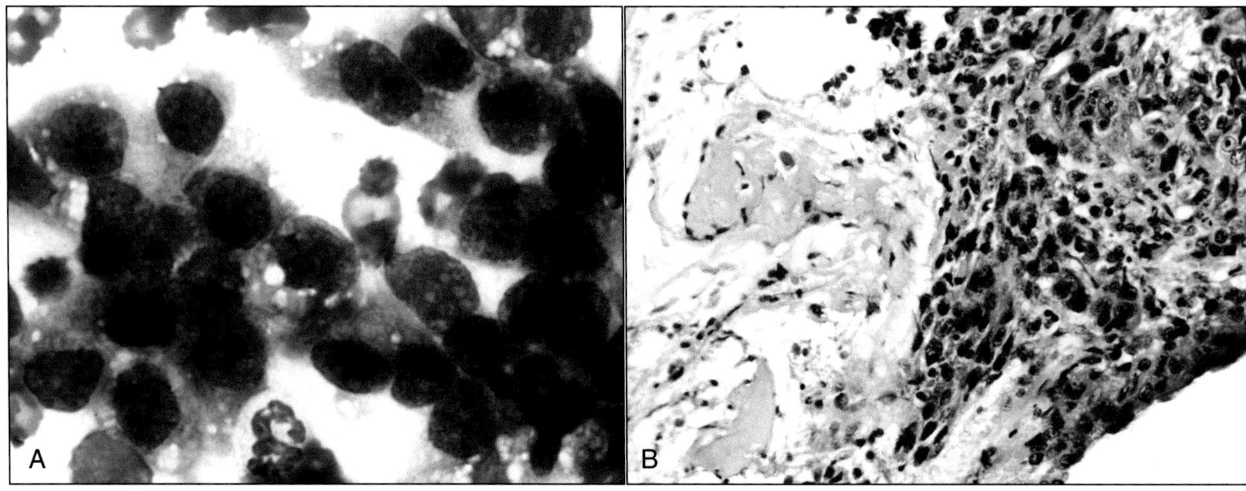

FIGURE 9-109

Metastatic adenocarcinoma in bone marrow from a dog. **A,** Cohesive clusters of basophilic epithelial cells in an aspirate smear. The origin could not be determined even after necropsy examination. Wright-Giemsa stain. **B,** Metastatic foci of neoplastic epithelial cells *(right)* in a core biopsy section. The remaining marrow is hypocellular with myelofibrosis. H&E stain.

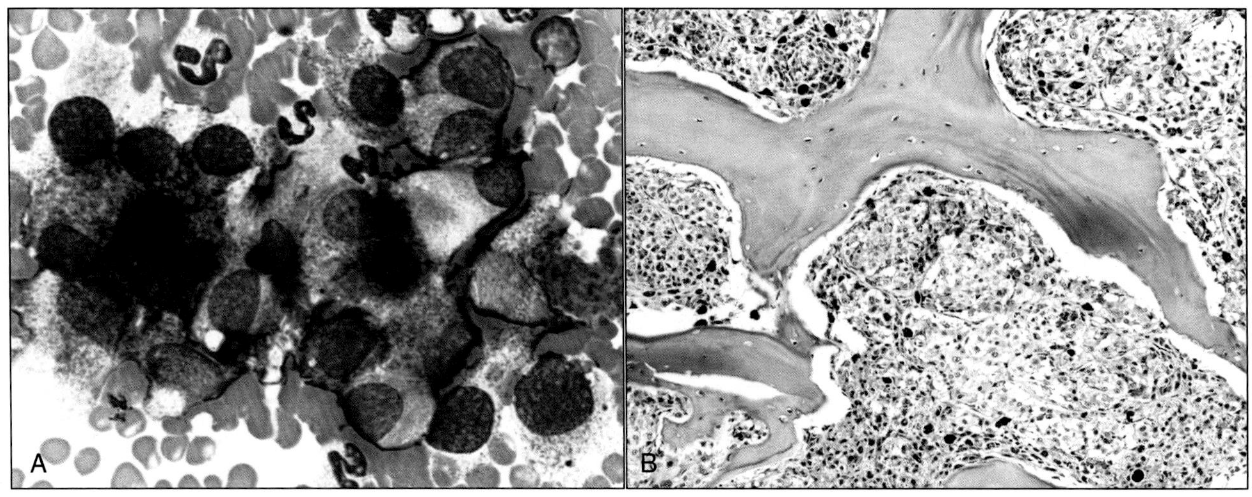

FIGURE 9-110

Metastatic melanoma in bone marrow from a dog. **A,** Cohesive neoplastic melanocytes with moderate anisocytosis and fine dark cytoplasmic granules in an aspirate smear. Wright-Giemsa stain. **B,** Pigmented neoplastic melanocytes infiltrating the bone marrow in a biopsy section. H&E stain.

From Kim DY, Royal AB, Villamil JA. Disseminated melanoma in a dog with involvement of the leptomeninges and bone marrow. Vet Pathol. *2009;46:80-83.*

marrow, but the primary site can be difficult or impossible to identify (carcinoma of unknown origin).[82]

The morphology of cells observed varies with the tumor type present. A disseminated adenocarcinoma, diagnosed in a dog using a routine bone marrow biopsy, appeared as cohesive clusters of epithelial cells exhibiting morphologic abnormalities. Abnormalities that may be present in metastatic adenocarcinomas include anisocytosis, anisokaryosis, high N:C ratios, coarse nuclear chromatin, multiple nucleoli, deeply basophilic cytoplasm, discrete cytoplasmic vacuoles, mitotic figures, and the formation of acini.[179] Histologic sections are preferred to aspirate smears in the diagnosis of metastatic carcinomas in human bone marrow.[397]

A metastatic melanoma to bone marrow was diagnosed in a dog evaluated for lameness (Fig. 9-110, *A,B*). The primary site appeared to be the leptomeninges.[232] Other tumors that have metastasized to bone marrow in dogs include mesothelioma[434] and nephroblastoma.[144]

Sarcomas of Bone

Bone tumors often spread into the marrow space. Osteosarcoma is a common bone tumor of dogs that is easily diagnosed

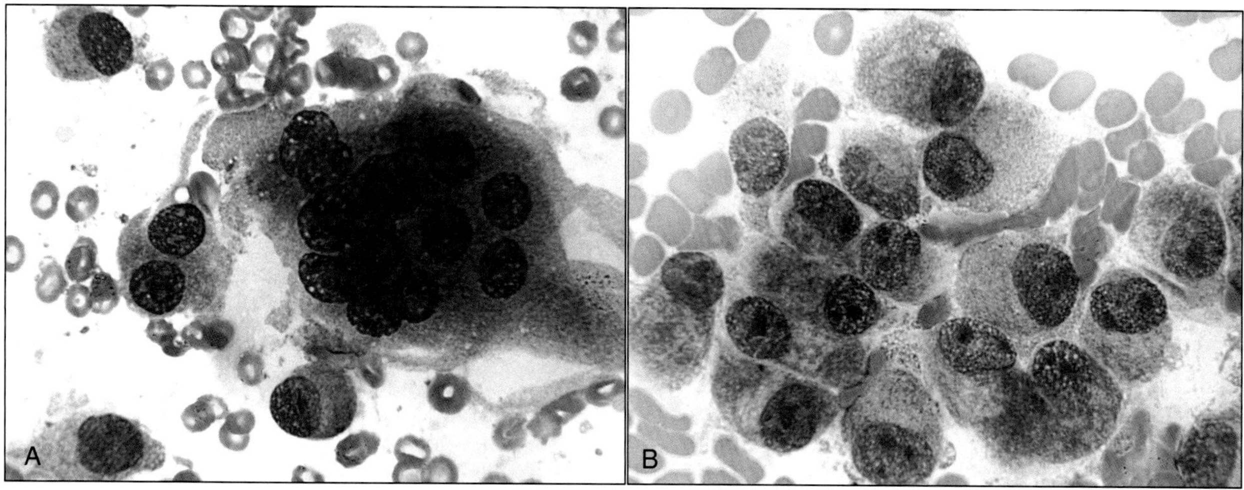

FIGURE 9-111
Aspirate smears from a lytic bone lesion from a dog with osteosarcoma. **A,** A large multinucleated osteoclast *(right)* and osteoblasts with eccentric nuclei. **B,** Cluster of osteoblasts with eccentric round to oval nuclei containing prominent nucleoli. Wright-Giemsa stain.

using exfoliative cytology of biopsy material collected from bone lesions (Fig. 9-111, *A,B*). Malignant osteoblasts are polygonal to fusiform, with abundant foamy basophilic cytoplasm. Nuclei are often eccentrically located and variable in size, exhibiting coarse chromatin patterns and multiple nucleoli. These cells produce osteoid; consequently they may contain reddish granules in the cytoplasm and may be found embedded in an eosinophilic osteoid matrix. Variable numbers of nonneoplastic osteoclasts are also usually present.[122]

Chondrosarcomas of bone appear similar to osteosarcomas on exfoliative cytology except that they are usually associated with more eosinophilic matrix material than are osteosarcomas. Other potential bone tumors that might be diagnosed by aspirate or core biopsy include fibrosarcomas, hemangiosarcomas, liposarcoma, and giant-cell tumors of bone.[122,492]

REFERENCES

1. Abkowitz JL, Holly RD. Cyclic hematopoiesis in dogs: studies of erythroid burst-forming cells confirm an early stem cell defect. *Exp Hematol.* 1988;16:941-945.
2. Adam F, Villiers E, Watson S, et al. Clinical pathological and epidemiological assessment of morphologically and immunologically confirmed canine leukaemia. *Vet Comp Oncol.* 2009;7:181-195.
3. Affolter VK, Moore PF. Localized and disseminated histiocytic sarcoma of dendritic cell origin in dogs. *Vet Pathol.* 2002;39:74-83.
4. Allan GS, Watson AD, Duff BC, et al. Disseminated mastocytoma and mastocytemia in a dog. *J Am Vet Med Assoc.* 1974;165:346-349.
5. Alleman AR, Harvey JW. The morphologic effects of vincristine sulfate on canine bone marrow cells. *Vet Clin Pathol.* 1993;22:36-41.
6. Allison RW, Brunker JD, Breshears MA, et al. Dendritic cell leukemia in a golden retriever. *Vet Clin Pathol.* 2008;37:190-197.
7. Alsaker RD, Laber J, Stevens JB, et al. A comparison of polychromasia and reticulocyte counts in assessing erythrocyte regenerative response in the cat. *J Am Vet Med Assoc.* 1977;170:39-41.
8. Altman DH, Meyer DJ, Thompson JP, et al. Canine IgG_{2c} myeloma with Mott and flame cells. *J Am Anim Hosp Assoc.* 1991;27:419-423.
9. Ameri M, Wilkerson MJ, Stockham SL, et al. Acute megakaryoblastic leukemia in a German Shepherd dog. *Vet Clin Pathol.* 2010;39:39-45.
10. Ammann VJ, Fecteau G, Helie P, et al. Pancytopenia associated with bone marrow aplasia in a Holstein heifer. *Can Vet J.* 1996;37:493-495.
11. Anderson TD. Cytokine-induced changes in the leukon. *Toxicol Pathol.* 1993;21:147-157.
12. Andres E, Federici L, Weitten T, et al. Recognition and management of drug-induced blood cytopenias: the example of drug-induced acute neutropenia and agranulocytosis. *Expert Opin Drug Saf.* 2008;7:481-489.
13. Angel KL, Spano JS, Schumacher J, et al. Myelophthisic pancytopenia in a pony mare. *J Am Vet Med Assoc.* 1991;198:1039-1042.
14. Antognoni MT, Spaterna A, Lepri E, et al. Characteristic clinical, haematological and histopathological findings in feline mastocytoma. *Vet Res Commun.* 2003;27(Suppl 1):727-730.
15. Arai M, Darmen J, Lewis A, et al. The use of human hematopoietic growth factors (rhGM-CSF and rhEPO) as a supportive therapy for FIV-infected cats. *Vet Immunol Immunopathol.* 2000;77:71-92.
16. Aroch I, Perl S, Markovics A. Disseminated eosinophilic disease resembling idiopathic hypereosinophilic syndrome in a dog. *Vet Rec.* 2001;149:386-389.
17. Atkins CE, DeFrancesco TC, Miller MW, et al. Prevalence of heartworm infection in cats with signs of cardiorespiratory abnormalities. *J Am Vet Med Assoc.* 1998;212:517-520.
18. Avery AC. Immunophenotyping and determination of clonality. In: Weiss DJ, Wardrop KJ, eds. *Schalm's Veterinary Hematology,* 6th ed. Ames, IA: Wiley-Blackwell; 2010:1133-1140.
19. Bader R, Bode G, Rebel W, et al. Stimulation of bone marrow by administration of excessive doses of recombinant human erythropoietin. *Pathol Res Pract.* 1992;188:676-679.
20. Bain BJ. Relationship between idiopathic hypereosinophilic syndrome, eosinophilic leukemia, and systemic mastocytosis. *Am J Hematol.* 2004;77:82-85.
21. Bain PJ, Alleman AR, Sheppard BJ, et al. What is your diagnosis? An 18-month old spayed female boxer dog. *Vet Clin Pathol.* 1997;26:55.
22. Ballmaier M, Germeshausen M. Advances in the understanding of congenital amegakaryocytic thrombocytopenia. *Br J Haematol.* 2009;146:3-16.
23. Barton MH, Sharma P, LeRoy BE, et al. Hypercalcemia and high serum parathyroid hormone-related protein concentration in a horse with multiple myeloma. *J Am Vet Med Assoc.* 2004;225:409-413, 376.
24. Bass MC, Schultze AE. Essential thrombocythemia in a dog: case report and literature review. *J Am Anim Hosp Assoc.* 1998;34:197-203.
25. Bass MC, Schultze AE. Essential thrombocythemia in a dog: case report and literature review. *J Am Anim Hosp Assoc.* 1998;34:197-203.
26. Beale KM, Altman D, Clemmons RR, et al. Systemic toxicosis associated with azathioprine administration in domestic cats. *Am J Vet Res.* 1992;53:1236-1240.
27. Beebe AM, Gluckstern TG, George J, et al. Detection of feline immunodeficiency virus infection in bone marrow of cats. *Vet Immunol Immunopathol.* 1992;35:37-49.
28. Beeler-Marfisi J, Menoyo AG, Beck A, et al. Gelatinous marrow transformation and hematopoietic atrophy in a miniature horse stallion. *Vet Pathol.* 2011;48:451-455.

29. Berggren PC. Aplastic anemia in a horse. *J Am Vet Med Assoc.* 1981;179: 1400-1402.
30. Bernard SL, Leathers CW, Brobst DF, et al. Estrogen-induced bone marrow depression in ferrets. *Am J Vet Res.* 1983;44:657-661.
31. Berry CR, House JK, Poulos PP, et al. Radiographic and pathologic features of osteopetrosis in two Peruvian Paso foals. *Veterinary Radiology and Ultrasound.* 1994;35:355-361.
32. Bhatt V, Saleem A. Review: Drug-induced neutropenia–pathophysiology, clinical features, and management. *Ann Clin Lab Sci.* 2004;34:131-137.
33. Bianco D, Armstrong PJ, Washabau RJ. Presumed primary immune-mediated thrombocytopenia in four cats. *J Feline Med Surg.* 2008;10:495-500.
34. Bienzle D, Silverstein DC, Chaffin K. Multiple myeloma in cats: variable presentation with different immunoglobulin isotypes in two cats. *Vet Pathol.* 2000;37:364-369.
35. Binhazim AA, Chapman WL Jr, Latimer KS, et al. Canine leishmaniasis caused by *Leishmania leishmania infantum* in two Labrador retrievers. *J Vet Diagn Invest.* 1992;4:299-305.
36. Bloom JC, Lewis HB, Sellers TS, et al. The hematopathology of cefonicid- and cefazedone-induced blood dyscrasias in the dog. *Toxicol Appl Pharmacol.* 1987;90: 143-155.
37. Blue JT. Myelofibrosis in cats with myelodysplastic syndrome and acute myelogenous leukemia. *Vet Pathol.* 1988;25:154-160.
38. Blue JT. Myelodysplasia: differentiating neoplastic from nonneoplastic syndromes of ineffective hematopoiesis in dogs. *Toxicol Pathol.* 2003;31(Suppl):44-48.
39. Blue JT, French TW, Kranz JS. Non-lymphoid hematopoietic neoplasia in cats: a retrospective study of 60 cases. *Cornell Vet.* 1988;78:21-42.
40. Bohm J. Gelatinous transformation of the bone marrow: the spectrum of underlying diseases. *Am J Surg Pathol.* 2000;24:56-65.
41. Bollen P, Skydsgaard M. Restricted feeding may induce serous fat atrophy in male Gottingen minipigs. *Exp Toxicol Pathol.* 2006;57:347-349.
42. Bookbinder PF, Butt MT, Harvey HJ. Determination of the number of mast cells in lymph node, bone marrow, and buffy coat cytologic specimens from dogs. *J Am Vet Med Assoc.* 1992;200:1648-1650.
43. Boosinger TR, Rebar AH, DeNicola DB, et al. Bone marrow alterations associated with canine parvoviral enteritis. *Vet Pathol.* 1982;19:558-561.
44. Borgatti A. Plasma cell tumors. In: Weiss DJ, Wardrop KJ, eds. *Schalm's Veterinary Hematology*, 6th ed. Ames, IA: Wiley-Blackwell; 2010:511-519.
45. Bortnowski HB, Rosenthal RC. Gastrointestinal mast cell tumors and eosinophilia in two cats. *J Am Anim Hosp Assoc.* 1992;28:271-275.
46. Bounous DI, Latimer KS, Campagnoli RP, et al. Acute myeloid leukemia with basophilic differentiation (AML, M-2B) in a cat. *Vet Clin Pathol.* 1994;23:15-18.
47. Brazzell JL, Weiss DJ. A retrospective study of aplastic pancytopenia in the dog: 9 cases (1996-2003). *Vet Clin Pathol.* 2006;35:413-417.
48. Brearley MJ, Jeffery N. Cryptococcal osteomyelitis in a dog. *J Small Anim Pract.* 1992;33:601-604.
49. Breen M, Modiano JF. Evolutionarily conserved cytogenetic changes in hematological malignancies of dogs and humans–man and his best friend share more than companionship. *Chromosome Res.* 2008;16:145-154.
50. Breitschwerdt EB, Abrams-Ogg AC, Lappin MR, et al. Molecular evidence supporting *Ehrlichia canis*-like infection in cats. *J Vet Intern Med.* 2002;16:642-649.
51. Bremner KC. The reticulocyte response in calves made anaemic by phlebotomy. *Aust J Exp Biol Med Sci.* 1966;44:251-258.
52. Breuer W, Darbès J, Hermanns W, et al. Idiopathic myelofibrosis in a cat and in three dogs. *Comp Haematol Int.* 1999;9:17-24.
53. Breuer W, Stahr K, Majzoub M, et al. Bone-marrow changes in infectious diseases and lymphohaemopoietic neoplasias in dogs and cats–a retrospective study. *J Comp Pathol.* 1998;119:57-66.
54. Brock KV, Jones JB, Shull RM, et al. Effect of canine parvovirus on erythroid progenitors in phenylhydrazine-induced regenerative hemolytic anemia in dogs. *Am J Vet Res.* 1989;50:965-969.
55. Brockus CW. Endogenous estrogen myelotoxicity associated with functional cystic ovaries in a dog. *Vet Clin Pathol.* 1998;27:55-56.
56. Brown CD, Parnell NK, Schulman RL, et al. Evaluation of clinicopathologic features, response to treatment, and risk factors associated with idiopathic neutropenia in dogs: 11 cases (1990-2002). *J Am Vet Med Assoc.* 2006;229:87-91.
57. Brown DE, Thrall MA, Walkley SU, et al. Feline Niemann-Pick disease type C. *Am J Pathol.* 1994;144:1412-1415.
58. Brown MR, Rogers KS. Neutropenia in dogs and cats: a retrospective study of 261 cases. *J Am Anim Hosp Assoc.* 2001;37:131-139.
59. Buhles WC Jr, Huxsoll DL, Hildebrandt PK. Tropical canine pancytopenia: role of aplastic anaemia in the pathogenesis of severe disease. *J Comp Pathol.* 1975;85:511-521.
60. Burton S, Miller L, Horney B, et al. Acute megakaryoblastic leukemia in a cat. *Vet Clin Pathol.* 1996;25:6-9.
61. Busch MD, Reilly CM, Luff JA, et al. Feline pulmonary Langerhans cell histiocytosis with multiorgan involvement. *Vet Pathol.* 2008;45:816-824.
62. Cain GR, East N, Moore PF. Myelofibrosis in young pygmy goats. *Comp Haematol Int.* 1994;4:167-172.
63. Callanan JJ, Jones BA, Irvine J, et al. Histologic classification and immunophenotype of lymphosarcomas in cats with naturally and experimentally acquired feline immunodeficiency virus infections. *Vet Pathol.* 1996;33:264-272.
64. Canfield PJ, Church DB, Russ IG. Myeloproliferative disorder involving the megakaryocytic line. *J Small Anim Pract.* 1993;34:296-301.
65. Canfield PJ, Malik R, Davis PE, et al. Multifocal idiopathic pyogranulomatous bone disease in a dog. *J Small Anim Pract.* 1994;35:370-373.
66. Canfield PJ, Watson ADJ. Investigations of bone marrow dyscrasia in a poodle with macrocytosis. *J Comp Pathol.* 1989;101:269-278.
67. Canfield PJ, Watson ADJ, Ratcliffe RCC. Dyserythropoiesis, sideroblasts/siderocytes and hemoglobin crystallization in a dog. *Vet Clin Pathol.* 1987;16(1):21-28.
68. Capsoni F, Sarzi-Puttini P, Zanella A. Primary and secondary autoimmune neutropenia. *Arthritis Res Ther.* 2005;7:208-214.
69. Cashell AW, Buss DH. The frequency and significance of megakaryocytic emperipolesis in myeloproliferative and reactive states. *Ann Hematol.* 1992;64:273-276.
70. Chang CS, Wang CH, Su IJ, et al. Hematophagic histiocytosis: a clinicopathologic analysis of 23 cases with special reference to the association with peripheral T cell lymphoma. *J Formos Med Assoc.* 1994;93:421-428.
71. Cheson BD, Cassileth PA, Head DR, et al. Report of the National Cancer Institute-sponsored workshop on definitions of diagnosis and response in acute myeloid leukemia. *J Clin Oncol.* 1990;8:813-819.
72. Cheville NF. The gray collie syndrome. *J Am Vet Med Assoc.* 1968;152:620-630.
73. Chiabrando D, Tolosano E. Diamond blackfan anemia at the crossroad between ribosome biogenesis and heme metabolism. *Adv Hematol.* 2010;2010:790632.
74. Chickering WR, Brown J, Prasse KW, et al. Effects of heterologous antineutrophil antibody in the cat. *Am J Vet Res.* 1985;46:1815-1819.
75. Chickering WR, Prasse KW. Immune-mediated neutropenia in man and animals: a review. *Vet Clin Pathol.* 1981;10(1):6-16.
76. Ciaramella P, Oliva G, Luna RD, et al. A retrospective clinical study of canine leishmaniasis in 150 dogs naturally infected by *Leishmania infantum. Vet Rec.* 1997;141:539-543.
77. Cline MJ. Histiocytes and histiocytosis. *Blood.* 1994;84:2840-2853.
78. Clinkenbeard KD, Cowell RL, Tyler RD. Disseminated histoplasmosis in cats: 12 cases (1981-1986). *J Am Vet Med Assoc.* 1987;190:1445-1448.
79. Clinkenbeard KD, Cowell RL, Tyler RD. Disseminated histoplasmosis in dogs: 12 cases (1981-1986). *J Am Vet Med Assoc.* 1988;193:1443-1447.
80. Colbatzky F, Hermanns W. Acute megakaryoblastic leukemia in one cat and two dogs. *Vet Pathol.* 1993;30:186-194.
81. Comazzi S, Gelain ME, Bonfanti U, et al. Acute megakaryoblastic leukemia in dogs: a report of three cases and review of the literature. *J Am Anim Hosp Assoc.* 2010;46:327-335.
82. Cooley DM, Waters DJ. Skeletal metastasis as the initial clinical manifestation of metastatic carcinoma in 19 dogs. *J Vet Intern Med.* 1998;12:288-293.
83. Cooper BJ, Watson ADJ. Myeloid neoplasia in a dog. *Aust Vet J.* 1975;51:150-154.
84. Cork LC, Munnell JF, Lorenz MD. The pathology of feline G_{M2} gangliosidosis. *Am J Pathol.* 1978;90:723-734.
85. Cortese L, Paciello O, Papparella S. Morphological characterisation of malignant histiocytosis in a cat. *Folia Morphol (Warsz).* 2008;67:299-303.
86. Cotter SM. Anemia associated with feline leukemia virus infection. *J Am Vet Med Assoc.* 1979;175:1191-1194.
87. Court EA, Earnest-Koons KA, Barr SC, et al. Malignant histiocytosis in a cat. *J Am Vet Med Assoc.* 1993;203:1300-1302.
88. Couto CG, Kallet AJ. Preleukemic syndrome in a dog. *J Am Vet Med Assoc.* 1984;184:1389-1392.
89. Cowgill ES, Neel JA, Ruslander D. Light-chain myeloma in a dog. *J Vet Intern Med.* 2004;18:119-121.
90. Cowgill LD, James KM, Levy JK, et al. Use of recombinant human erythropoietin for management of anemia in dogs and cats with renal failure. *J Am Vet Med Assoc.* 1998;212:521-528.
91. Cruz Cardona JA, Milner R, Alleman AR, et al. BCR-ABL translocation in a dog with chronic monocytic leukemia. *Vet Clin Pathol* 2011:40:40-47.
92. Cullor JS, Smith W, Zinkl JG, et al. Hematologic and bone marrow changes after short- and long-term administration of two recombinant bovine granulocyte colony-stimulating factors. *Vet Pathol.* 1992;29:521-527.
93. Dale DC, Alling DW, Wolff SM. Cyclic hematopoiesis: the mechanism of cyclic neutropenia in grey collie dogs. *J Clin Invest.* 1972;51:2197-2204.
94. Darbès J, Majzoub M, Breuer W, et al. Large granular lymphocytic leukemia/lymphoma in six cats. *Vet Pathol.* 1998;35:370-379.
95. Dascanio JJ, Zhang CH, Antczak DF, et al. Differentiation of chronic lymphocytic leukemia in the horse. A report of two cases. *J Vet Intern Med.* 1992;6:225-229.

96. Davies AP, Hayden DW, Klausner JS, et al. Noncutaneous systemic mastocytosis and mast cell leukemia in a dog: case report and literature review. *J Am Anim Hosp Assoc.* 1981;17:361-368.
97. Deldar A, Lewis H, Bloom J, et al. Cephalosporin-induced changes in the ultrastructure of canine bone marrow. *Vet Pathol.* 1988;25:211-218.
98. Dhote R, Simon J, Papo T, Detournay B, et al. Reactive hemophagocytic syndrome in adult systemic disease: report of twenty-six cases and literature review. *Arthritis Rheum.* 2003;49:633-639.
99. Dieringer TM, Brown SA, Rogers KS, et al. Effects of lithium carbonate administration to healthy cats. *Am J Vet Res.* 1992;53:721-726.
100. Dodds WJ. Immune-mediated diseases of the blood. *Adv Vet Sci Comp Med.* 1983;27:163-196.
101. Doige CE. Bone and bone marrow necrosis associated with the calf form of sporadic bovine leukosis. *Vet Pathol.* 1987;24:186-188.
102. Dole RS, MacPhail CM, Lappin MR. Paraneoplastic leukocytosis with mature neutrophilia in a cat with pulmonary squamous cell carcinoma. *J Feline Med Surg.* 2004;6:391-395.
103. Douglas VK, Tallman MS, Cripe LD, et al. Thrombopoietin administered during induction chemotherapy to patients with acute myeloid leukemia induces transient morphologic changes that may resemble chronic myeloproliferative disorders. *Am J Clin Pathol.* 2002;117:844-850.
104. Dunavant ML, Murry ES. Clinical evidence of phenylbutazone induced hypoplastic anemia. In: Kitchen H, Krehbiel JD, eds. *Proceedings First International Symposium on Equine Hematology.* Golden, CO: American Association of Equine Practitioners; 1975:383-385.
105. Dunn JK, Doige CE, Searcy GP, et al. Myelofibrosis-osteosclerosis syndrome associated with erythroid hypoplasia in a dog. *J Small Anim Pract.* 1986;27:799-806.
106. Dunn JK, Heath MF, Jefferies AR, et al. Diagnosis and hematologic features of probable essential thrombocythemia in two dogs. *Vet Clin Pathol.* 1999;28:131-138.
107. Durando MM, Alleman AR, Harvey JW. Myelodysplastic syndrome in a quarter horse gelding. *Equine Vet J.* 1994;26:83-85.
108. Durham SK, Dietze AE. Prostatic adenocarcinoma with and without metastasis to bone in dogs. *J Am Vet Med Assoc.* 1986;188:1432-1436.
109. Dzieciol J, Lemancewicz D, Kloczko J, et al. Megakaryocytes emperipolesis in bone marrow of the patients with non-Hodgkin's lymphoma. *Folia Histochem Cytobiol.* 2001;39(Suppl 2):142-143.
110. Edwards DF, Parker JW, Wilkinson JE, et al. Plasma cell myeloma in the horse. A case report and literature review. *J Vet Intern Med.* 1993;7:169-176.
111. Eldor A, Hershko C, Bruchim A. Androgen-responsive aplastic anemia in a dog. *J Am Vet Med Assoc.* 1978;173:304-305.
112. Ellis JA, West KH, Cortese VS, et al. Lesions and distribution of viral antigen following an experimental infection of young seronegative calves with virulent bovine virus diarrhea virus-type II. *Can J Vet Res.* 1998;62:161-169.
113. Endicott MM, Charney SC, McKnight JA, et al. Clinicopathological findings and results of bone marrow aspiration in dogs with cutaneous mast cell tumours: 157 cases (1999-2002). *Vet Comp Oncol.* 2007;5:31-37.
114. English RV, Breitschwerdt EB, Grindem CB, et al. Zollinger-Ellison syndrome and myelofibrosis in a dog. *J Am Vet Med Assoc.* 1988;192:1430-1434.
115. Evans RJ, Jones DRE, Gruffydd-Jones TJ. Essential thrombocythaemia in the dog and cat: a report of four cases. *J Small Anim Pract.* 1982;23:457-467.
116. Fabris F, Randi ML. Essential thrombocythemia: past and present. *Intern Emerg Med.* 2009;4:381-388.
117. Facchini RV, Bertazzolo W, Zuliani D, et al. Detection of biclonal gammopathy by capillary zone electrophoresis in a cat and a dog with plasma cell neoplasia. *Vet Clin Pathol.* 2010;39:440-446.
118. Favier RP, van Leeuwen M, Teske E. Essential thrombocythaemia in two dogs. *Tijdschr Diergeneeskd.* 2004;129:360-364.
119. Felchle LM, McPhee LA, Kerr ME, et al. Systemic lupus erythematosus and bone marrow necrosis in a dog. *Can Vet J.* 1996;37:742-744.
120. Fenger CK, Bertone JJ, Biller D, et al. Generalized medullary infarction of the long bones in a horse. *J Am Vet Med Assoc.* 1993;202:621-623.
121. Fidel JL, Pargass IS, Dark MJ, et al. Granulocytopenia associated with thymoma in a domestic shorthaired cat. *J Am Anim Hosp Assoc.* 2008;44:210-217.
122. Fielder SE, Mahaffey EA. The musculoskeletal system. In: Cowell RL, Tyler RD, Meinkoth JH, DeNicola DB, eds. *Diagnostic Cytology and Hematology of the Dog and Cat,* 3rd ed. St. Louis: Mosby Elsevier; 2008:210-214.
123. Finco DR, Duncan JR, Schall WD, et al. Acetaminophen toxicosis in the cat. *J Am Vet Med Assoc.* 1975;166:469-472.
124. Fine DM, Tvedten H. Chronic granulocytic leukemia in a dog. *J Am Vet Med Assoc.* 1999;214:1809-1812.
125. Fine DM, Tvedten HW. Chronic granulocytic leukemia in a dog. *J Am Vet Med Assoc.* 1999;214:1809-1812, 1791.
126. Födinger M, Fritsch G, Winkler K, et al. Origin of human mast cells: development from transplanted hematopoietic stem cells after allogeneic bone marrow transplantation. *Blood.* 1994;84:2954-2959.
127. Foglia MV, Restucci B, Pagano A, et al. Pathological changes in the bone marrow of dogs with leishmaniosis. *Vet Rec.* 2006;158:690-694.
128. Ford SL, Raskin RE, Snyder, PS. Clinical implications of feline bone marrow dysplasia—a retrospective study of 16 cats (abstract). *J Vet Intern Med.* 1998;12:226.
129. Fossum TW, Hulse DA. Osteomyelitis. *Semin Vet Med Surg Small Anim.* 1992;7:85-97.
130. Fox LE, Ford S, Alleman AR, et al. Aplastic anemia associated with prolonged high-dose trimethoprim-sulfadiazine administration in two dogs. *Vet Clin Pathol.* 1993;22:89-92.
131. Franks PT, Harvey JW, Mays MC, et al. Feline large granular lymphoma. *Vet Pathol.* 1986;23:200-202.
132. Franks PT, Harvey JW, Shields RP, et al. Hematological findings in experimental feline cytauxzoonosis. *J Am Anim Hosp Assoc.* 1988;24:395-401.
133. Freeman L, Stevens J, Loughman C, et al. Malignant histiocytosis in a cat. *J Vet Intern Med.* 1995;9:171-173.
134. Friedrichs KR, Young KM. Histiocytic sarcoma of macrophage origin in a cat: case report with a literature review of feline histiocytic malignancies and comparison with canine hemophagocytic histiocytic sarcoma. *Vet Clin Pathol.* 2008;37:121-128.
135. Fry MM, Vernau W, Pesavento PA, et al. Hepatosplenic lymphoma in a dog. *Vet Pathol.* 2003;40:556-562.
136. Fujino Y, Sawamura S, Kurakawa N, et al. Treatment of chronic lymphocytic leukaemia in three dogs with melphalan and prednisolone. *J Small Anim Pract.* 2004;45:298-303.
137. Fulton R, Gasper PW, Ogilvie GK, et al. Effect of recombinant human granulocyte colony-stimulating factor on hematopoiesis in normal cats. *Exp Hematol.* 1991;19:759-767.
138. Fyfe JC, Giger U, Hall CA, et al. Inherited selective intestinal cobalamin malabsorption and cobalamin deficiency in dogs. *Pediatr Res.* 1991;29:24-31.
139. Fyfe JC, Jezyk PF, Giger U, et al. Inherited selective malabsorption of vitamin B12 in giant schnauzers. *J Am Anim Hosp Assoc.* 1989;25:533-539.
140. Garner FM, Lingeman CH. Mast-cell neoplasms in the domestic cat. *Pathol Vet.* 1970;7:517-530.
141. Garon CL, Scott MA, Selting KA, et al. Idiopathic thrombocytopenic purpura in a cat. *J Am Anim Hosp Assoc.* 1999;35:464-470.
142. Gary AT, Kerl ME, Wiedmeyer CE, et al. Bone marrow hypoplasia associated with fenbendazole administration in a dog. *J Am Anim Hosp Assoc.* 2004;40:224-229.
143. Gaschen FP, Smith Meyer B, Harvey JW. Amegakaryocytic thrombocytopenia and immune-mediated haemolytic anaemia in a cat. *Comp Haematol Int.* 1992;2:175-178.
144. Gasser AM, Bush WW, Smith S, et al. Extradural spinal, bone marrow, and renal nephroblastoma. *J Am Anim Hosp Assoc.* 2003;39:80-85.
145. Gelain ME, Antoniazzi E, Bertazzolo W, et al. Chronic eosinophilic leukemia in a cat: cytochemical and immunophenotypical features. *Vet Clin Pathol.* 2006;35:454-459.
146. Gelain ME, Mazzilli M, Riondato F, et al. Aberrant phenotypes and quantitative antigen expression in different subtypes of canine lymphoma by flow cytometry. *Vet Immunol Immunopathol.* 2008;121:179-188.
147. Gentilini F, Calzolari C, Buonacucina A, et al. Different biological behaviour of Waldenstrom macroglobulinemia in two dogs. *Vet Comp Oncol.* 2005;3:87-97.
148. Giger U, Boxer LA, Simpson PJ, et al. Deficiency of leukocyte surface glycoproteins Mo1, LFA-1, and Leu M5 in a dog with recurrent bacterial infections: an animal model. *Blood.* 1987;69:1622-1630.
149. Gilmore GL, DePasquale DK, Fischer BC, et al. Enhancement of monocytopoiesis by granulocyte colony-stimulating factor: evidence for secondary cytokine effects in vivo. *Exp Hematol.* 1995;23:1319-1323.
150. Giraudel JM, Pages JP, Guelfi JF. Monoclonal gammopathies in the dog: a retrospective study of 18 cases (1986-1999) and literature review. *J Am Anim Hosp Assoc.* 2002;38:135-147.
151. Gold JR, Warren AL, French TW, et al. What is your diagnosis? Biopsy impression smear of a hepatic mass in a yearling Thoroughbred filly. *Vet Clin Pathol.* 2008;37:339-343.
152. Gossett KA, MacWilliams PS, Cleghorn B. Sequential morphological and quantitative changes in blood and bone marrow neutrophils in dogs with acute inflammation. *Can J Comp Med.* 1985;49:291-297.
153. Graves TK, Swenson CL, Scott MA. A potentially misleading presentation and course of acute myelomonocytic leukemia in a dog. *J Am Anim Hosp Assoc.* 1997;33:37-41.
154. Greene CE, Meinkoth J, Kocan AA. Cytauxzoonosis. In: Greene CE, ed. *Infectious Diseases of the Dog and Cat,* 3rd ed. St. Louis: Saunders Elsevier; 2006:716-722.
155. Grindem CB. Classification of myeloproliferative diseases. In: August JR, ed. *Consultations in Feline Medicine 3.* Philadelphia: W.B. Saunders Co.; 1997:499-508.

156. Grindem CB, Roberts MC, McEntee MF, et al. Large granular lymphocyte tumor in a horse. *Vet Pathol.* 1989;26:86-88.
157. Grindem CB, Stevens JB, Brost DR, et al. Chronic myelogenous leukaemia with meningeal infiltration in a dog. *Comp Haematol Int.* 1992;2:170-174.
158. Grindem CB, Stevens JB, Perman V. Cytochemical reactions in cells from leukemic dogs. *Vet Pathol.* 1986;23:103-109.
159. Gruntman A, Nolen-Walston R, Parry N, et al. Presumptive albendazole toxicosis in 12 alpacas. *J Vet Intern Med.* 2009;23:945-949.
160. Hahn KA, Matlock CL. Nasal adenocarcinoma metastatic to bone in two dogs. *J Am Vet Med Assoc.* 1990;197:491-494.
161. Hammer AS, Couto CG, Getzy D, et al. Essential thrombocythemia in a cat. *J Vet Intern Med.* 1990;4:87-91.
162. Hammond WP, Csiba E, Canin A, et al. Chronic neutropenia. A new canine model induced by human granulocyte colony-stimulating factor. *J Clin Invest.* 1991;87:704-710.
163. Handagama PJ, Feldman BF. Drug-induced thrombocytopenia. *Vet Res Commun.* 1986;10:1-20.
164. Hanichen T, Breuer W, Hermanns W. Lipid storage disease. *Lab Anim Sci.* 1997;47:275-279.
165. Harmon DC, Weitzman SA, Stossel TP. The severity of immune neutropenia correlates with the maturational specificity of antineutrophil antibodies. *Br J Haematol.* 1984;58:209-215.
166. Harrus S, Waner T, Weiss DJ, et al. Kinetics of serum antiplatelet antibodies in experimental acute canine ehrlichiosis. *Vet Immunol Immunopathol.* 1996;51:13-20.
167. Harvey JW. Myeloproliferative disorders in dogs and cats. *Vet Clin North Am Small Anim Pract.* 1981;11:349-381.
168. Harvey JW. Canine bone marrow: normal hematopoiesis, biopsy techniques, and cell identification and evaluation. *Comp Cont Ed Pract Vet.* 1984;6:909-926.
169. Harvey JW. Unpublished studies. 2000.
170. Harvey JW. Pathogenesis, laboratory diagnosis, and clinical implications of erythrocyte enzyme deficiencies in dogs, cats, and horses. *Vet Clin Pathol.* 2006;35:144-156.
171. Harvey JW. The erythrocyte: physiology, metabolism and biochemical disorders. In: Kaneko JJ, Harvey JW, Bruss ML, eds. *Clinical Biochemistry of Domestic Animals,* 6th ed. San Diego, CA: Academic Press; 2008:173-240.
172. Harvey JW, Clapp WL, Yao Y, et al. Microcytic hypochromic erythrocytes containing siderotic inclusions, Heinz bodies, and hemoglobin crystals in a dog (abstract). *Vet Clin Pathol.* 2007;36:313-314.
173. Harvey JW, Shields RP, Gaskin JM. Feline myeloproliferative disease. Changing manifestations in the peripheral blood. *Vet Pathol.* 1978;15:437-448.
174. Harvey JW, Wolfsheimer KJ, Simpson CF, et al. Pathologic sideroblasts and siderocytes associated with chloramphenicol therapy in a dog. *Vet Clin Pathol.* 1985;14(1):36-42.
175. Hasler AH, Giger U. Serum erythropoietin values in polycythemic cats. *J Am Anim Hosp Assoc.* 1996;32:294-301.
176. Helfand SC, Kisseberth WC. General features of leukemia and lymphoma. In: Weiss DJ, Wardrop KJ, eds. *Schalm's Veterinary Hematology,* 6th ed. Ames, IA: Wiley-Blackwell; 2010:455-466.
177. Helfand SC, Soergel SA, MacWilliams PS, et al. Clinical and immunological effects of human recombinant interleukin-2 given by repetitive weekly infusion to normal dogs. *Cancer Immunol Immunother.* 1994;39:84-92.
178. Helton KA, Nesbitt GH, Caciolo PL. Griseofulvin toxicity in cats: literature and report of seven cases. *J Am Anim Hosp Assoc.* 1986;22:453-458.
179. Henson KL, Alleman AR, Fox LE, et al. Diagnosis of disseminated adenocarcinoma by bone marrow aspiration in a dog with leukoerythroblastosis and fever of unknown origin. *Vet Clin Pathol.* 1998;27:80-84.
180. Hikasa Y, Morita T, Futaoka Y, et al. Connective tissue-type mast cell leukemia in a dog. *J Vet Med Sci.* 2000;62:187-190.
181. Hirsch V, Dunn J. Megaloblastic anemia in the cat. *J Am Anim Hosp Assoc.* 1983;19:873-880.
182. Hisasue M, Nagashima N, Nishigaki K, et al. Myelodysplastic syndromes and acute myeloid leukemia in cats infected with feline leukemia virus clone33 containing a unique long terminal repeat. *Int J Cancer.* 2009;124:1133-1141.
183. Hisasue M, Nishigaki K, Katae H, et al. Clonality analysis of various hematopoietic disorders in cats naturally infected with feline leukemia virus. *J Vet Med Sci.* 2000;62:1059-1065.
184. Hisasue M, Nishimura T, Neo S, et al. A dog with acute myelomonocytic leukemia. *J Vet Med Sci.* 2008;70:619-621.
185. Hisasue M, Okayama H, Okayama T, et al. Hematologic abnormalities and outcome of 16 cats with myelodysplastic syndromes. *J Vet Intern Med.* 2001;15:471-477.
186. Hodgkins EM, Zinkl JG, Madewell BR. Chronic lymphocytic leukemia in the dog. *J Am Vet Med Assoc.* 1980;177:704-707.
187. Hoenig M. Multiple myeloma associated with the heavy chains of immunoglobulin A in a dog. *J Am Vet Med Assoc.* 1987;190:1191-1192.
188. Hoenig M. Six dogs with features compatible with myelonecrosis and myelofibrosis. *J Am Anim Hosp Assoc.* 1989;25:335-339.
189. Hoff B, Lumsden JH, Valli VE. An appraisal of bone marrow biopsy in assessment of sick dogs. *Can J Comp Med.* 1985;49:34-42.
190. Hoff B, Lumsden JH, Valli VEO, et al. Myelofibrosis: review of clinical and pathological features in fourteen dogs. *Can Vet J.* 1991;32:357-361.
191. Holland CT, Canfield PJ, Watson ADJ, et al. Dyserythropoiesis, polymyopathy, and cardiac disease in three related English springer spaniels. *J Vet Intern Med.* 1991;5:151-159.
192. Hoover EA, Kociba GJ. Bone lesions in cats with anemia induced by feline leukemia virus. *J Natl Cancer Inst.* 1974;53:1277-1284.
193. Hopper CD, Sparkes AH, Gruffydd-Jones TJ, et al. Clinical and laboratory findings in cats infected with feline immunodeficiency virus. *Vet Rec.* 1989;125:341-346.
194. Hopper PE, Mandell CP, Turrel JM, et al. Probable essential thrombocythemia in a dog. *J Vet Intern Med.* 1989;3:79-85.
195. Hoshi H, Weiss L. Rabbit bone marrow after administration of saponin. *Lab Invest.* 1978;38:67-80.
196. Hotchkiss RS, Strasser A, McDunn JE, et al. Cell death. *N Engl J Med.* 2009;361:1570-1583.
197. Hotston Moore A, Day MJ, Graham MWA. Congenital pure red blood cell aplasia (Diamond-Blackfan anaemia) in a dog. *Vet Rec.* 1993;132:414-415.
198. Houston DM, Taylor JA. Acute pancreatitis and bone marrow suppression in a dog given azathioprine. *Can Vet J.* 1991;32:496-497.
199. Hughes K, Scase TJ, Ward C, et al. Vincristine overdose in a cat: clinical management, use of calcium folinate, and pathological lesions. *J Feline Med Surg.* 2009;11:322-325.
200. Huibregtse BA, Turner JL. Hypereosinophilic syndrome and eosinophilic leukemia: a comparison of 22 hypereosinophilic cats. *J Am Anim Hosp Assoc.* 1994;30:591-599.
201. Hurvitz AI, Kehoe JM, Capra JD, et al. Bence Jones proteinemia and proteinuria in a dog. *J Am Vet Med Assoc.* 1971;159:1112-1116.
202. Hurvitz AI, MacEwen EG, Middaugh CR, et al. Monoclonal cryoglobulinemia with macroglobulinemia in a dog. *J Am Vet Med Assoc.* 1977;170:511-513.
203. Jackson MW, Helfand SC, Smedes SL, et al. Primary IgG secreting plasma cell tumor in the gastrointestinal tract of a dog. *J Am Vet Med Assoc.* 1994;204:404-406.
204. Jacobs G, Calvert C, Kaufman A. Neutropenia and thrombocytopenia in three dogs treated with anticonvulsants. *J Am Vet Med Assoc.* 1998;212:681-684.
205. Jacobs RM, Couto CG, Wellman ML. Biclonal gammopathy in a dog with myeloma and cutaneous lymphoma. *Vet Pathol.* 1986;23:211-213.
206. Jadersten M, Hellstrom-Lindberg E. New clues to the molecular pathogenesis of myelodysplastic syndromes. *Exp Cell Res.* 2010;316:1390-1396.
207. Jain NC. *Schalm's Veterinary Hematology,* 4th ed. Philadelphia: Lea & Febiger; 1986.
208. Jain NC. Classification of myeloproliferative disorders in cats using criteria proposed by the Animal Leukaemia Study Group: a retrospective study of 181 cases (1969-1992). *Comp Haematol Int.* 1993;3:125-134.
209. Jain NC. *Essentials of Veterinary Hematology.* Philadelphia: Lea & Febiger; 1993.
210. Jain NC, Blue JT, Grindem CB, et al. Proposed criteria for classification of acute myeloid leukemia in dogs and cats. *Vet Clin Pathol.* 1991;20:63-82.
211. James FE, Mansfield CS. Clinical remission of idiopathic hypereosinophilic syndrome in a Rottweiler. *Aust Vet J.* 2009;87:330-333.
212. Jensen AL, Nielsen OL. Eosinophilic leukaemoid reaction in a dog. *J Small Anim Pract.* 1992;33:337-340.
213. Johansson AM, Skidell J, Lilliehook I, et al. Chronic granulocytic leukemia in a horse. *J Vet Intern Med.* 2007;21:1126-1129.
214. Johnson KA. Osteomyelitis in dogs and cats. *J Am Vet Med Assoc.* 1994;204:1882-1887.
215. Joiner GN, Fraser CJ, Jardine JH, et al. A case of chronic granulocytic leukemia in a dog. *Can J Comp Med.* 1976;40:153-160.
216. Jonas LD, Thrall MA, Weiser MG. Nonregenerative form of immune-mediated hemolytic anemia in dogs. *J Am Anim Hosp Assoc.* 1987;23:201-204.
217. Jordan HL, Cohn LA, Armstrong PJ. Disseminated *Mycobacterium avium* complex infection in three Siamese cats. *J Am Vet Med Assoc.* 1994;204:90-93.
218. Josefsen TD, Sorensen KK, Mork T, et al. Fatal inanition in reindeer (Rangifer tarandus tarandus): pathological findings in completely emaciated carcasses. *Acta Vet Scand.* 2007;49:27.
219. Joshi BC, Jain NC. Detection of antiplatelet antibody in serum and on megakaryocytes in dogs with autoimmune thrombocytopenia. *J Am Vet Med Assoc.* 1976;681-685.
220. Joshi BC, Jain NC. Experimental immunologic thrombocytopenia in dogs: a study of thrombocytopenia and megakaryocytopoiesis. *Res Vet Sci.* 1977;22:11-17.
221. Juliá A, Olona M, Bueno J, Revilla E, et al. Drug-induced agranulocytosis: prognostic factors in a series of 168 episodes. *Br J Haematol.* 1991;79:366-371.

222. Junt T, Schulze H, Chen Z, et al. Dynamic visualization of thrombopoiesis within bone marrow. *Science.* 2007;317:1767-1770.
223. Juopperi TA, Bienzle D, Bernreuter DC, et al. Prognostic markers for myeloid neoplasms: a comparative review of the literature and goals for future investigation. *Vet Pathol.* 2011;48:182-197.
224. Kariya K, Konno A, Ishida T. Perforin-like immunoreactivity in four cases of lymphoma of large granular lymphocytes in the cat. *Vet Pathol.* 1997;34:156-159.
225. Kaushansky K. Historical review: megakaryopoiesis and thrombopoiesis. *Blood.* 2008;111:981-986.
226. Keel SB, Doty RT, Yang Z, et al. A heme export protein is required for red blood cell differentiation and iron homeostasis. *Science.* 2008;319:825-828.
227. Kelton DR, Holbrook TC, Gilliam LL, et al. Bone marrow necrosis and myelophthisis: manifestations of T-cell lymphoma in a horse. *Vet Clin Pathol.* 2008;37:403-408.
228. Keohane EM. Acquired aplastic anemia. *Clin Lab Sci.* 2004;17:165-171.
229. Kerbauy DB, Deeg HJ. Apoptosis and antiapoptotic mechanisms in the progression of myelodysplastic syndrome. *Exp Hematol.* 2007;35:1739-1746.
230. Khan KN, Sagartz JE, Koenig G, et al. Systemic mastocytosis in a goat. *Vet Pathol.* 1995;32:719-721.
231. Khanna C, Bienzle D. Polycythemia vera in a cat: bone marrow culture in erythropoietin-deficient medium. *J Am Anim Hosp Assoc.* 1994;30:45-49.
232. Kim DY, Royal AB, Villamil JA. Disseminated melanoma in a dog with involvement of leptomeninges and bone marrow. *Vet Pathol.* 2009;46:80-83.
233. Kim DY, Taylor HW, Eades SC, et al. Systemic AL amyloidosis associated with multiple myeloma in a horse. *Vet Pathol.* 2005;42:81-84.
234. Kipps TJ. Macroglobulinemia. In: Beutler E, Lichtman MA, Coller BS, Kipps TJ, eds. *Williams Hematology*, 5th ed. New York: McGraw-Hill; 1995:1127-1131.
235. Kocan AA, Kocan KM, Blouin EF, et al. A redescription of schizogony of *Cytauxzoon felis* in the domestic cat. *Ann N Y Acad Sci.* 1992;653:161-167.
236. Kociba GJ, Caputo CA. Aplastic anemia associated with estrus in pet ferrets. *J Am Vet Med Assoc.* 1981;178:1293-1294.
237. Kohn CW, Swardson C, Provost P, et al. Myeloid and megakaryocytic hypoplasia in related standardbreds. *J Vet Intern Med.* 1995;9:315-323.
238. Kouro T, Takatsu K. IL-5- and eosinophil-mediated inflammation: from discovery to therapy. *Int Immunol.* 2009;21:1303-1309.
239. Kraje AC, Patton CS, Edwards DF. Malignant histiocytosis in 3 cats. *J Vet Intern Med.* 2001;15:252-256.
240. Kramer J, Tornquist S, Erfle J, et al. Large granular lymphocyte leukemia in a horse. *Vet Clin Pathol.* 1993;22:126-128.
241. Kramers P, Fluckiger MA, Rahn BA, et al. Osteopetrosis in cats. *J Small Anim Pract.* 1988;29:153-164.
242. Kueck BD, Smith RE, Parkin J, et al. Eosinophilic leukemia: A myeloproliferative disorder distinct from the hypereosinophilic syndrome. *Hematol Pathol.* 1991;5:195-205.
243. Kuehn NF, Gaunt SD. Clinical and hematologic findings in canine ehrlichiosis. *J Am Vet Med Assoc.* 1985;186:355-358.
244. Kuehn NF, Gaunt SD. Hypocellular marrow and extramedullary hematopoiesis in a dog: hematologic recovery after splenectomy. *J Am Vet Med Assoc.* 1986;188:1313-1315.
245. Kunkle GA, Meyer DJ. Toxicity of high doses of griseofulvin in cats. *J Am Vet Med Assoc.* 1987;191:322-323.
246. Kupanoff PA, Popovitch CA, Goldschmidt MH. Colorectal plasmacytomas: a retrospective study of nine dogs. *J Am Anim Hosp Assoc.* 2006;42:37-43.
247. Kuter DJ, Bain B, Mufti G, et al. Bone marrow fibrosis: pathophysiology and clinical significance of increased bone marrow stromal fibres. *Br J Haematol.* 2007;139:351-362.
248. Kuzmanova SI. The macrophage activation syndrome: a new entity, a potentially fatal complication of rheumatic disorders. *Folia Med (Plovdiv).* 2005;47:21-25.
249. Lachowicz JL, Post GS, Moroff SD, et al. Acquired amegakaryocytic thrombocytopenia—four cases and a literature review. *J Small Anim Pract.* 2004;45:507-514.
250. Lanevschi A, Daminet S, Niemeyer GP, et al. Granulocyte colony-stimulating factor deficiency in a rottweiler with chronic idiopathic neutropenia. *J Vet Intern Med.* 1999;13:72-75.
251. Lange RD, Jones JB, Chambers C, et al. Erythropoiesis and erythrocytic survival in dogs with cyclic hematopoiesis. *Am J Vet Res.* 1976;37:331-334.
252. Langheinrich KA, Nielsen SW. Histopathology of feline panleukopenia: a report of 65 cases. *J Am Vet Med Assoc.* 1971;158:863-872.
253. Lappin MR, Latimer KS. Hematuria and extreme neutrophilic leukocytosis in a dog with renal tubular carcinoma. *J Am Vet Med Assoc.* 1988;192:1289-1292.
254. Larroche C, Mouthon L. Pathogenesis of hemophagocytic syndrome (HPS). *Autoimmun Rev.* 2004;3:69-75.
255. Larsen S, Flagstad A, Aalbaek B. Experimental panleukopenia in the conventional cat. *Vet Pathol.* 1976;13:216-240.
256. Latimer KS, Bounous DI, Collatos C, et al. Extreme eosinophilia with disseminated eosinophilic granulomatous disease in a horse. *Vet Clin Pathol.* 1996;25:23-26.
257. Lautzenhiser SJ, Walker MC, Goring RL. Unusual IgM-secreting multiple myeloma in a dog. *J Am Vet Med Assoc.* 2003;223:645-648, 636.
258. Lavoie JP, Morris DD, Zinkl JG, et al. Pancytopenia caused by marrow aplasia in a horse. *J Am Vet Med Assoc.* 1987;191:1462-1464.
259. Ledieu D, Palazzi X, Marchal T, et al. Acute megakaryoblastic leukemia with erythrophagocytosis and thrombosis in a dog. *Vet Clin Pathol.* 2005;34:52-56.
260. Lee KP. Emperipolesis of hematopoietic cells within megakaryocytes in bone marrow of the rat. *Vet Pathol.* 1989;26:473-478.
261. Lees GE, McKeever PJ, Ruth GR. Fatal thrombocytopenic hemorrhagic diathesis associated with dapsone administration to a dog. *J Am Vet Med Assoc.* 1979;175:49-52.
262. Lees GE, Sautter JH. Anemia and osteopetrosis in a dog. *J Am Vet Med Assoc.* 1979;175:820-824.
263. Leifer CE, Matus RE. Chronic lymphocytic leukemia in the dog: 22 cases (1974-1984). *J Am Vet Med Assoc.* 1986;189:214-217.
264. Leifer CE, Matus RE, Patnaik AK, et al. Chronic myelogenous leukemia in the dog. *J Am Vet Med Assoc.* 1983;183:686-689.
265. Leipold HW, Cook JE. Animal model: osteopetrosis in Angus and Hereford calves. *Am J Pathol.* 1977;86:745-748.
266. Lester GD, Alleman AR, Raskin RE, et al. Malignant histiocytosis in an Arabian filly. *Equine Vet J.* 1993;25:471-473.
267. Lester GD, Alleman AR, Raskin RE, et al. Pancytopenia secondary to lymphoid leukemia in three horses. *J Vet Intern Med.* 1993;7:360-363.
268. Lester SJ, Mesfin GM. A solitary plasmacytoma in a dog with progression to a disseminated myeloma. *Can Vet J.* 1980;21:284-286.
269. Lester SJ, Searcy GP. Hematologic abnormalities preceding apparent recovery from feline leukemia virus infection. *J Am Vet Med Assoc.* 1981;178:471-474.
270. Lewis HB, Rebar AH. *Bone Marrow Evaluation in Veterinary Practice.* St. Louis: Ralston Purina Co.; 1979.
271. Lipton JM. Diamond blackfan anemia: new paradigms for a "not so pure" inherited red cell aplasia. *Semin Hematol.* 2006;43:167-177.
272. Liska WD, MacEwen EG, Zaki FA, et al. Feline systemic mastocytosis: a review and results of splenectomy in seven cases. *J Am Anim Hosp Assoc.* 1979;15:589-597.
273. Lord BI. Myeloid cell kinetics in response to haemopoietic growth factors. *Baillieres Clin Haematol.* 1992;5:533-550.
274. Lorenz M, Evering WE, Provencher A, et al. Atypical antipsychotic-induced neutropenia in dogs. *Toxicol Appl Pharmacol.* 1999;155:227-236.
275. Lukaszewska J, Lewandowski K. Cabot rings as a result of severe dyserythropoiesis in a dog. *Vet Clin Pathol.* 2008;37:180-183.
276. Lund JE, Brown PK. Hypersegmented megakaryocytes and megakaryocytes with multiple separate nuclei in dogs treated with PNU-100592, an oxazolidinone antibiotic. *Toxicol Pathol.* 1997;25:339-343.
277. Lutz H, Castelli I, Ehrensperger F, et al. Panleukopenia-like syndrome of FeLV caused by co-infection with FeLV and feline panleukopenia virus. *Vet Immunol Immunopathol.* 1995;46:21-33.
278. Macdonald D, Gordon AA, Kajitani H, et al. Interleukin-2 treatment-associated eosinophilia is mediated by interleukin-5 production. *Br J Haematol.* 1990;76:168-173.
279. MacEwen EG. Feline lymphoma and leukemias. In: Withrow SJ, MacEwen EG, eds. *Small Animal Clinical Oncology.* Philadelphia: W.B. Saunders Co.; 1996:479-495.
280. MacEwen EG, Drazner FH, McClelland AJ, et al. Treatment of basophilic leukemia in a dog. *J Am Vet Med Assoc.* 1975;166:376-380.
281. MacEwen EG, Hurvitz AI, Hayes A. Hyperviscosity syndrome associated with lymphocytic leukemia in three dogs. *J Am Vet Med Assoc.* 1977;170:1309-1312.
282. MacEwen EG, Patnaik AK, Hurvitz AI, et al. Nonsecretory multiple myeloma in two dogs. *J Am Vet Med Assoc.* 1984;184:1283-1286.
283. MacEwen EG, Young KM. Canine lymphoma and lymphoid leukemias. In: Withrow SJ, MacEwen EG, eds. *Small Animal Clinical Oncology.* Philadelphia: W.B. Saunders Co.; 1996:451-479.
284. Machado EA, Jones JB, Aggio MC, et al. Ultrastructural changes of bone marrow in canine cyclic hematopoiesis (CH dog). A sequential study. *Virchows Arch Pathol Anat.* 1981;390:93-108.
285. Madewell BR. Hematologic and bone marrow cytological abnormalities in 75 dogs with malignant lymphoma. *J Am Anim Hosp Assoc.* 1986;22:235-240.
286. Madewell BR, Jain NC, Weller RE. Hematologic abnormalities preceding myeloid leukemia in three cats. *Vet Pathol.* 1979;16:510-519.
287. Maggio L, Hoffman R, Cotter SM, et al. Feline preleukemia: an animal model of human disease. *Yale J Biol Med.* 1978;51:469-476.
288. Mahaffey EA, Brown TP, Duncan JR, et al. Basophilic leukaemia in a dog. *J Comp Pathol.* 1987;97:393-399.
289. Majluf Cruz A, Sosa Camas R, Perez Ramirez O, et al. Hemophagocytic syndrome associated with hematological neoplasias. *Leuk Res.* 1998;22:893-898.
290. Majzoub M, Breuer W, Platz SJ, et al. Histopathologic and immunophenotypic characterization of extramedullary plasmacytomas in nine cats. *Vet Pathol.* 2003;40:249-253.

291. Malka S, Hawkins MG, Zabolotzky SM, et al. Immune-mediated pure red cell aplasia in a domestic ferret. *J Am Vet Med Assoc.* 2010;237:695-700.
292. Mandell CP, Goding B, Degen MA, et al. Spurious elevation of serum potassium in two cases of thrombocythemia. *Vet Clin Pathol.* 1988;17:32-33.
293. Mandell CP, Sparger EE, Pedersen NC, et al. Long-term haematological changes in cats experimentally infected with feline immunodeficiency virus (FIV). *Comp Haematol Int.* 1992;2:8-17.
294. Marconato L, Bettini G, Giacoboni C, et al. Clinicopathological features and outcome for dogs with mast cell tumors and bone marrow involvement. *J Vet Intern Med.* 2008;22:1001-1007.
295. Marcos R, Santos M, Malhao F, et al. Pancytopenia in a cat with visceral leishmaniasis. *Vet Clin Pathol.* 2009;38:201-205.
296. Marks SL, Moore PF, Taylor DW, et al. Nonsecretory multiple myeloma in a dog: immunohistologic and ultrastructural observations. *J Vet Intern Med.* 1995;9:50-54.
297. Marsh JC. Bone marrow failure syndromes. *Clin Med.* 2005;5:332-336.
298. Matus RE, Leifer CE. Immunoglobulin-producing tumors. *Vet Clin North Am Small Anim Pract.* 1985;15:741-753.
299. Matus RE, Leifer CE, MacEwen EG. Acute lymphoblastic leukemia in the dog: a review of 30 cases. *J Am Vet Med Assoc.* 1983;183:859-862.
300. Matus RE, Leifer CE, MacEwen EG, et al. Prognostic factors for multiple myeloma in the dog. *J Am Vet Med Assoc.* 1986;188:1288-1292.
301. Maylin GA, Eckerlin RH, Krook L. Fluoride intoxication in dairy calves. *Cornell Vet.* 1987;77:84-98.
302. McCandlish IAP, Munro CD, Breeze RG, et al. Hormone producing ovarian tumour in the dog. *Vet Rec.* 1979;105:9-11.
303. McClure JT, Young KM, Fiste M, et al. Immunophenotypic classification of leukemia in 3 horses. *J Vet Intern Med.* 2001;15:144-152.
304. McDonough SP, Moore PF. Clinical, hematologic, and immunophenotypic characterization of canine large granular lymphocytosis. *Vet Pathol.* 2000;37:637-646.
305. McDonough SP, Moore PF. Clinical, hematologic, and immunophenotypic characterization of canine large granular lymphocytosis. *Vet Pathol.* 2000;37:637-646.
306. McGrath C. Polycythemia vera in dogs. *J Am Vet Med Assoc.* 1974;164:1117-1122.
307. McManus PM. Frequency and severity of mastocytemia in dogs with and without mast cell tumors: 120 cases (1995-1997). *J Am Vet Med Assoc.* 1999;215:355-357.
308. McManus PM. Classification of myeloid neoplasms: a comparative review. *Vet Clin Pathol.* 2005;34:189-212.
309. McManus PM, Hess RS. Myelodysplastic changes in a dog with subsequent acute myeloid leukemia. *Vet Clin Pathol.* 1998;27:112-115.
310. McManus PM, Litwin C, Barber L. Immune-mediated neutropenia in 2 dogs. *J Vet Intern Med.* 1999;13:372-374.
311. Mears EA, Raskin RE, Legendre AM. Basophilic leukemia in a dog. *J Vet Intern Med.* 1997;11:92-94.
312. Mellor PJ, Haugland S, Murphy S, et al. Myeloma-related disorders in cats commonly present as extramedullary neoplasms in contrast to myeloma in human patients: 24 cases with clinical follow-up. *J Vet Intern Med.* 2006;20:1376-1383.
313. Mellor PJ, Haugland S, Smith KC, et al. Histopathologic, immunohistochemical, and cytologic analysis of feline myeloma-related disorders: further evidence for primary extramedullary development in the cat. *Vet Pathol.* 2008;45:159-173.
314. Meyer J, Delay J, Bienzle D. Clinical, laboratory, and histopathologic features of equine lymphoma. *Vet Pathol.* 2006;43:914-924.
315. Meyers SN, McDaneld TG, Swist SL, et al. A deletion mutation in bovine SLC4A2 is associated with osteopetrosis in Red Angus cattle. *BMC Genomics.* 2010;11:337.
316. Michel RL, O'Handley P, Dade AW. Megakaryocytic myelosis in a cat. *J Am Vet Med Assoc.* 1976;168:1021-1025.
317. Milne EM, Pyrah ITG, Smith KC, et al. Aplastic anemia in a Clydesdale foal: a case report. *J Equine Vet Sci.* 1995;15:129-131.
318. Mischke R, Hoinghaus R, Lutkefels E, et al. Immunocytological confirmation of bone marrow metastases in a dog with cholangiocarcinoma. *J Small Anim Pract.* 2003;44:411-414.
319. Miyamoto T, Horie T, Shimada T, et al. Long-term case study of myelodysplastic syndrome in a dog. *J Am Anim Hosp Assoc.* 1999;35:475-481.
320. Mizukoshi T, Fujino Y, Yasukawa K, et al. Essential thrombocythemia in a dog. *J Vet Med Sci.* 2006;68:1203-1206.
321. Moore PF. Histiocytic proliferative diseases. In: Weiss DJ, Wardrop KJ, eds. *Schalm's Veterinary Hematology*, 6th ed. Ames, IA: Wiley-Blackwell; 2010:540-549.
322. Moore PF, Affolter VK, Vernau W. Canine hemophagocytic histiocytic sarcoma: a proliferative disorder of CD11d+ macrophages. *Vet Pathol.* 2006;43:632-645.
323. Moreb J, Shemesh O, Manor C, et al. Transient methimazole-induced bone marrow aplasia: in vitro evidence of a humoral mechanism of bone marrow suppression. *Acta Haematol.* 1983;69:127-131.
324. Morgan LW, McConnell J. Cobalamin deficiency associated with erythroblastic anemia and methylmalonic aciduria in a border collie. *J Am Anim Hosp Assoc.* 1999;35:392-395.
325. Morgan RV. Blood dyscrasias associated with testicular tumors in the dog. *J Am Anim Hosp Assoc.* 1982;18:970-975.
326. Morley A, Stohlman F. Cyclophosphamide-induced cyclical neutropenia: an animal model of human periodic disease. *N Engl J Med.* 1970;12:643-646.
327. Morris DD, Bloom JC, Roby KA, et al. Eosinophilic myeloproliferative disorder in a horse. *J Am Vet Med Assoc.* 1984;185:993-996.
328. Muhury M, Mathai AM, Rai S, et al. Megakaryocytic alterations in thrombocytopenia: a bone marrow aspiration study. *Indian J Pathol Microbiol.* 2009;52:490-494.
329. Murtaugh RJ, Jacobs RM. Suspected immune-mediated megakaryocytic hypoplasia or aplasia in a dog. *J Am Vet Med Assoc.* 1985;186:1313-1315.
330. Myers S, Wiks K, Giger U. Macrocytic anemia caused by naturally occurring folate-deficiency in the cat (abstract). *Vet Clin Pathol.* 1996;25:30.
331. Mylonakis ME, Day MJ, Siarkou V, et al. Absence of myelofibrosis in dogs with myelosuppression induced by *Ehrlichia canis* infection. *J Comp Pathol.* 2010;142:328-331.
332. Mylonakis ME, Koutinas AF, Leontides LS. Bone marrow mastocytosis in dogs with myelosuppressive monocytic ehrlichiosis *(Ehrlichia canis)*: a retrospective study. *Vet Clin Pathol.* 2006;35:311-314.
333. Naessens J. Bovine trypanotolerance: a natural ability to prevent severe anaemia and haemophagocytic syndrome? *Int J Parasitol.* 2006;36:521-528.
334. Nagahata H, Kehrli ME Jr, Murata H, et al. Neutrophil function and pathologic findings in Holstein calves with leukocyte adhesion deficiency. *Am J Vet Res.* 1994;55:40-48.
335. Nagahata H, Nochi H, Tamoto K, et al. Characterization of functions of neutrophils from bone marrow of cattle with leukocyte adhesion deficiency. *Am J Vet Res.* 1995;56:167-171.
336. Nagashima N, Hisasue M, Higashi K, et al. Bone marrow colony-forming unit assay in cats with naturally occurring myelodysplastic syndromes. *Int J Hematol.* 2001;73:453-456.
337. Naito K, Maruyama M, Dobashi K, et al. Congenital chondrodysplastic dwarfism with dyshematopoiesis in a holstein calf. *J Vet Med Sci.* 2002;64:937-939.
338. Nash RA, Schuening F, Appelbaum F, et al. Molecular cloning and in vivo evaluation of canine granulocyte-macrophage colony-stimulating factor. *Blood.* 1991;78:930-937.
339. Nash RA, Schuening FG, Seidel K, et al. Effect of recombinant canine granulocyte-macrophage colony-stimulating factor on hematopoietic recovery after otherwise lethal total body irradiation. *Blood.* 1994;83:1963-1970.
340. Nasisse MP, Dorman DC, Jamison KC, et al. Effects of valacyclovir in cats infected with feline herpesvirus. *Am J Vet Res.* 1997;58:1141-1144.
341. Nation PN, Klavano GG. Osteopetrosis in two foals. *Can Vet J.* 1986;27:74-77.
342. Ndikuwera J, Smith DA, Obwolo MJ, et al. Chronic granulocytic leukaemia/eosinophilic leukaemia in a dog? *J Small Anim Pract.* 1992;33:553-557.
343. Nimer SD. Myelodysplastic syndromes. *Blood.* 2008;111:4841-4851.
344. O'Brien SE, Riedesel EA, Miller LD. Osteopetrosis in an adult dog. *J Am Anim Hosp Assoc.* 1987;23:213-216.
345. O'Keefe DA, Couto CG, Burke-Schwartz C, et al. Systemic mastocytosis in 16 dogs. *J Vet Intern Med.* 1987;1:75-80.
346. O'Keefe DA, Schaeffer DJ. Hematologic toxicosis associated with doxorubicin administration in cats. *J Vet Intern Med.* 1992;6:276-283.
347. O'Toole D, Tharp S, Thomsen BV, et al. Fatal mycobacteriosis with hepatosplenomegaly in a young dog due to *Mycobacterium avium*. *J Vet Diagn Invest.* 2005;17:200-204.
348. Obradovich JE, Ogilvie GK, Powers BE, et al. Evaluation of recombinant canine granulocyte colony-stimulating factor as an inducer of granulopoiesis. *J Vet Intern Med.* 1991;5:75-79.
349. Ozon C, Marty P, Pratlong F, et al. Disseminated feline leishmaniosis due to *Leishmania infantum* in Southern France. *Vet Parasitol.* 1998;75:273-277.
350. Palmblad J, Papadaki HA. Chronic idiopathic neutropenias and severe congenital neutropenia. *Curr Opin Hematol.* 2008;15:8-14.
351. Pardanani A, Verstovsek S. Hypereosinophilic syndrome, chronic eosinophilic leukemia, and mast cell disease. *Cancer J.* 2007;13:384-391.
352. Pardon B, Steukers L, Dierick J, et al. Haemorrhagic diathesis in neonatal calves: an emerging syndrome in Europe. *Transbound Emerg Dis.* 2010;57:135-146.
353. Park HM, Doster AR, Tashbaeva RE, et al. Clinical, histopathological and immunohistochemical findings in a case of megakaryoblastic leukemia in a dog. *J Vet Diagn Invest.* 2006;18:287-291.
354. Parker WH, McCrea CT. Bracken *(Pteris aquilina)* poisoning of sheep in the North York moors. *Vet Rec.* 1965;77:861-865.
355. Parsons JC, Bowman DD, Grieve RB. Pathological and haematological responses of cats experimentally infected with *Toxocara canis* larvae. *Int J Parasitol.* 1989;19:479-488.

356. Patel RT, Caceres A, French AF, et al. Multiple myeloma in 16 cats: a retrospective study. *Vet Clin Pathol.* 2005;34:341-352.
357. Perdue BD, Collier MA, Dzata GK, et al. Multisystemic granulomatous inflammation in a horse. *J Am Vet Med Assoc.* 1991;198:663-664.
358. Perkins M, Watson A. Successful treatment of hypereosinophilic syndrome in a dog. *Aust Vet J.* 2001;79:686-689.
359. Perkins MC, Canfield P, Churcher RK, et al. Immune-mediated neutropenia suspected in five dogs. *Aust Vet J.* 2004;82:52-57.
360. Peterson JL, Couto CG. Lymphoid leukemias. In: August JR, ed. *Consultations in Feline Internal Medicine 2.* Philadelphia: W.B. Saunders; 1994:509-513.
361. Peterson ME, Kintzer PP, Hurvitz AI. Methimazole treatment of 262 cats with hyperthyroidism. *J Vet Intern Med.* 1988;2:150-157.
362. Peterson ME, Randolph JF. Diagnosis of canine primary polycythemia and management with hydroxyurea. *J Am Vet Med Assoc.* 1982;180:415-418.
363. Phillips B. Severe, prolonged bone marrow hypoplasia secondary to the use of carboplatin in an azotemic dog. *J Am Vet Med Assoc.* 1999;215:1250-1252.
364. Piercy RJ, Swardson CJ, Hinchcliff KW. Erythroid hypoplasia and anemia following administration of recombinant human erythropoietin to two horses. *J Am Vet Med Assoc.* 1998;212:244-247.
365. Plier M. Unpublished studies. 2000.
366. Pohlman LM. Basophils, mast cells, and their disorders. In: Weiss DJ, Wardrop KJ, eds. *Schalm's Veterinary Hematology,* 6th ed. Ames, IA: Wiley-Blackwell; 2010:290-297.
367. Pollack MJ, Flanders JA, Johnson RC. Disseminated malignant mastocytoma in a dog. *J Am Anim Hosp Assoc.* 1991;27:435-440.
368. Pollet L, Van Hove W, Mattheeuws D. Blastic crisis in chronic myelogenous leukaemia in a dog. *J Small Anim Pract.* 1978;19:469-475.
369. Postorino NC, Wheeler SL, Park RD, et al. A syndrome resembling lymphomatoid granulomatosis in the dog. *J Vet Intern Med.* 1989;3:15-19.
370. Potgieter LN, Jones JB, Patton CS, et al. Experimental parvovirus infection in dogs. *Can J Comp Med.* 1981;45:212-216.
371. Powers BE, LaRue SM, Withrow SJ, et al. Jamshidi needle biopsy for diagnosis of bone lesions in small animals. *J Am Vet Med Assoc.* 1988;193:205-210.
372. Prasse KW, Crouser D, Beutler E, et al. Pyruvate kinase deficiency anemia with terminal myelofibrosis and osteosclerosis in a beagle. *J Am Vet Med Assoc.* 1975;166:1170-1175.
373. Prater MR, De Gopegui RR, Burdette K, et al. Bone marrow aspirate from a cat with cutaneous lesions. *Vet Clin Pathol.* 1999;28:52-58.
374. Prihirunkit K, Narkkong NA, Apibal S. Acute monoblastic leukemia in a FeLV-positive cat. *J Vet Sci.* 2008;9:109-111.
375. Pusterla N, Stacy BA, Vernau W, et al. Immunoglobulin A monoclonal gammopathy in two horses with multiple myeloma. *Vet Rec.* 2004;155:19-23.
376. Quigley JG, Yang Z, Worthington MT, et al. Identification of a human heme exporter that is essential for erythropoiesis. *Cell.* 2004;118:757-766.
377. Rakich PM, Latimer KS, Weiss R, et al. Mucocutaneous plasmacytomas in dogs: 75 cases (1980-1987). *J Am Vet Med Assoc.* 1989;194:803-810.
378. Ramaiah SK, Seguin MA, Carwile HF, et al. Biclonal gammopathy associated with immunoglobulin A in a dog with multiple myeloma. *Vet Clin Pathol.* 2002;31:83-89.
379. Randolph JF, Center SA, Kallfelz FA, et al. Familial nonspherocytic hemolytic anemia in poodles. *Am J Vet Res.* 1986;47:687-695.
380. Raskin RE. Myelopoiesis and myeloproliferative disorders. *Vet Clin North Am Small Anim Pract.* 1996;26:1023-1042.
381. Raskin RE. Cytochemical staining. In: Weiss DJ, Wardrop KJ, eds. *Schalm's Veterinary Hematology,* 6th ed. Ames, IA: Wiley-Blackwell; 2010:1141-1156.
382. Raskin RE, Krehbiel JD. Myelodysplastic changes in a cat with myelomonocytic leukemia. *J Am Vet Med Assoc.* 1985;187:171-174.
383. Raskin RE, Krehbiel JD. Histopathology of canine bone marrow in malignant lymphoproliferative disorders. *Vet Pathol.* 1988;25:83-88.
384. Raskin RE, Krehbiel JD. Prevalence of leukemic blood and bone marrow in dogs with multicentric lymphoma. *J Am Vet Med Assoc.* 1989;194:1427-1429.
385. Raskind WH, Steinmann L, Najfeld V. Clonal development of myeloproliferative disorders: clues to hematopoietic differentiation and multistep pathogenesis of cancer. *Leukemia.* 1998;12:108-116.
386. Rawlings CA. Clinical laboratory evaluations of seven heartworm infected beagles: during disease development and following treatment. *Cornell Vet.* 1982;72:49-56.
387. Raza A, Mundle S, Iftikhar A, et al. Simultaneous assessment of cell kinetics and programmed cell death in bone marrow biopsies of myelodysplastics reveals extensive apoptosis as the probable basis for ineffective hematopoiesis. *Am J Hematol.* 1995;48:143-154.
388. Reagan WJ. A review of myelofibrosis in dogs. *Toxicol Pathol.* 1993;21:164-169.
389. Reagan WJ, Murphy D, Battaglino M, et al. Antibodies to canine granulocyte colony-stimulating factor induce persistent neutropenia. *Vet Pathol.* 1995;32:374-378.
390. Reardon MJ, Pierce KR. Acute experimental canine ehrlichiosis. I. Sequential reaction of the hemic and lymphoreticular systems. *Vet Pathol.* 1981;18:48-61.
391. Rebar AH. General responses of the bone marrow to injury. *Toxicol Pathol.* 1993;21:118-129.
392. Reiner AP, Spivak JL. Hematophagic histiocytosis. A report of 23 new patients and a review of the literature. *Medicine (Baltimore).* 1988;67:369-388.
393. Rinkardt NE, Kruth SA. Azathioprine-induced bone marrow toxicity in four dogs. *Can Vet J.* 1996;37:612-613.
394. Risti B, Flury RF, Schaffner A. Fatal hematophagic histiocytosis after granulocyte-macrophage colony-stimulating factor and chemotherapy for high-grade malignant lymphoma. *Clin Invest.* 1994;72:457-461.
395. Robinson WF, Wilcox GE, Fowler RLP. Canine parvoviral disease: experimental reproduction of the enteric form with a parvovirus isolated from a case of myocarditis. *Vet Pathol.* 1980;17:589-599.
396. Roccabianca P, Vernau W, Caniatti M, et al. Feline large granular lymphocyte (LGL) lymphoma with secondary leukemia: primary intestinal origin with predominance of a CD3/CD8(alpha)(alpha) phenotype. *Vet Pathol.* 2006;43:15-28.
397. Roeckel IE. Diagnosis of metastatic carcinoma by bone marrow biopsy versus bone marrow aspiration. *Ann Clin Lab Sci.* 1974;4:193-197.
398. Rojko JL, Hartke JR, Cheney CM, et al. Cytopathic feline leukemia viruses cause apoptosis in hemolymphatic cells. *Prog Mol Subcell Biol.* 1996;16:13-43.
399. Rojko JL, Olsen RG. The immunobiology of the feline leukemia virus. *Vet Immunol Immunopathol.* 1984;6:107-165.
400. Rosenthal RC. Chemotherapy induced myelosuppression. In: Kirk RW, ed. *Current Veterinary Therapy X. Small Animal Practice.* Philadelphia: W.B. Saunders; 1989:494-496.
401. Rossi G, Gelain ME, Foroni S, et al. Extreme monocytosis in a dog with chronic monocytic leukaemia. *Vet Rec.* 2009;165:54-56.
402. Rottman JB, English RV, Breitschwerdt EB, et al. Bone marrow hypoplasia in a cat treated with griseofulvin. *J Am Vet Med Assoc.* 1991;198:429-431.
403. Ruslander DA, Gebhard DH, Tompkins MB, et al. Immunophenotypic characterization of canine lymphoproliferative disorders. *In Vivo.* 1997;11:169-172.
404. Russell KE, Sellon DC, Grindem CB. Bone marrow in horses: indications, sample handling, and complications. *Comp Cont Ed Pract Vet.* 1994;16:1359-1365.
405. Sahebekhtiari HA, Tavassoli M. Marrow cell uptake by megakaryocytes in routine bone marrow smears during blood loss. *Scand J Haematol.* 1976;16:13-17.
406. Sakai N, Johnstone C, Weiss L. Bone marrow cells associated with heightened eosinophilopoiesis: an electron microscope study of murine bone marrow stimulated by *Ascaris suum. Am J Anat.* 1981;161:11-32.
407. Savage CJ. Lymphoproliferative and myeloproliferative disorders. *Vet Clin North Am Equine Pract.* 1998;14:563-578.
408. Sawada K, Hirokawa M, Fujishima N. Diagnosis and management of acquired pure red cell aplasia. *Hematol Oncol Clin North Am.* 2009;23:249-259.
409. Schalm OW. Autoimmune hemolytic anemia in the dog. *Can Pract.* 1975;2:37-45.
410. Schalm OW. Erythrocyte macrocytosis in miniature and toy poodles. *Can Pract.* 1976;3(6):55-57.
411. Schmitz LL, McClure JS, Litz CE, et al. Morphologic and quantitative changes in blood and marrow cells following growth factor therapy. *Am J Clin Pathol.* 1994;101:67-75.
412. Scott MA, Friedrichs KR. Megakaryocyte podography. *Vet Clin Pathol.* 2009;38:135.
413. Scott RE, Dale DC, Rosenthal AS, et al. Cyclic neutropenia in grey collie dogs. Ultrastructural evidence for abnormal neutrophil granulopoiesis. *Lab Invest.* 1973;28:514-525.
414. Scruggs DW, Fleming SA, Maslin WR, et al. Osteopetrosis, anemia, thrombocytopenia, and marrow necrosis in beef calves naturally infected with bovine virus diarrhea virus. *J Vet Diagn Invest.* 1995;7:555-559.
415. Scruggs DW, Fleming SA, Maslin WR,et al. Osteopetrosis, anemia, thrombocytopenia, and marrow necrosis in beef calves naturally infected with bovine virus diarrhea virus. *J Vet Diagn Invest.* 1995;7:555-559.
416. Searcy GP, Tasker JB, Miller DR. Animal model: pyruvate kinase deficiency in dogs. *Am J Physiol.* 1979;94:689-692.
417. Seed TM, Carnes BA, Tolle DV, et al. Blood responses under chronic low daily dose gamma irradiation: I. Differential preclinical responses of irradiated male dogs in progression to either aplastic anemia or myeloproliferative disease. *Leuk Res.* 1989;13:1069-1084.
418. Seed TM, Kaspar LV. Changing patterns of radiosensitivity of hematopoietic progenitors from chronically irradiated dogs prone either to aplastic anemia or to myeloproliferative disease. *Leuk Res.* 1990;14:299-307.
419. Seelig DM, Perry JA, Avery AC, et al. Monoclonal gammopathy without hyperglobulinemia in 2 dogs with IgA secretory neoplasms. *Vet Clin Pathol.* 2010;39:447-453.
420. Sharifi H, Nassiri SM, Esmaelli H, et al. Eosinophilic leukaemia in a cat. *J Feline Med Surg.* 2007;9:514-517.
421. Sharkey LC, Rosol IJ, Gröne A, et al. Production of granulocyte colony-stimulating factor and granulocyte-macrophage colony-stimulating factor by carcinomas in a dog and a cat with paraneoplastic leukocytosis. *J Vet Intern Med.* 1996;10:405-408.

422. Sheikh J, Weller PF. Clinical overview of hypereosinophilic syndromes. *Immunol Allergy Clin North Am.* 2007;27:333-355.
423. Shelly SM. Causes of canine pancytopenia. *Comp Cont Ed Pract Vet.* 1988;10:9-16.
424. Shelton GH, Grant CK, Linenberger ML, et al. Severe neutropenia associated with griseofulvin therapy in cats with feline immunodeficiency virus infection. *J Vet Intern Med.* 1990;4:317-319.
425. Shelton GH, Linenberger ML, Abkowitz JL. Hematologic abnormalities in cats seropositive for feline immunodeficiency virus. *J Am Vet Med Assoc.* 1991;199:1353-1357.
426. Shelton GH, Linenberger ML, Grant CK, et al. Hematologic manifestations of feline immunodeficiency virus infection. *Blood.* 1990;76:1104-1109.
427. Sherding RG, Wilson GP, Kociba GJ. Bone marrow hypoplasia in eight dogs with Sertoli cell tumor. *J Am Vet Med Assoc.* 1981;178:497-501.
428. Sheridan WP, Hunt P, Simonet S, et al. Hematologic effects of cytokines. In: Remick DG, Friedland JS, eds. *Cytokines in Health and Disease*, 2nd ed. New York: Marcel Dekker, Inc.; 1997:487-505.
429. Shimoda T, Shiranaga N, Mashita T, et al. A hematological study on thirteen cats with myelodysplastic syndrome. *J Vet Med Sci.* 2000;62:59-64.
430. Shimoda T, Shiranaga N, Mashita T, et al. Bone marrow necrosis in a cat infected with feline leukemia virus. *J Vet Med Sci.* 2000;62:113-115.
431. Simpson CF, Harvey JW, Lawman MJ, et al. Ultrastructure of schizonts in the liver of cats with experimentally induced cytauxzoonosis. *Am J Vet Res.* 1985;46:384-390.
432. Sippel WL. Bracken fern poisoning. *J Am Vet Med Assoc.* 1952;121:9-13.
433. Smith AN, Spencer JA, Stringfellow JS, et al. Disseminated infection with *Phialemonium obovatum* in a German Shepherd dog. *J Am Vet Med Assoc.* 2000;216: 708-712.
434. Smith DA, Hill FW. Metastatic malignant mesothelioma in a dog. *J Comp Pathol.* 1989;100:97-101.
435. Smith JE, Agar NS. The effect of phlebotomy on canine erythrocyte metabolism. *Res Vet Sci.* 1975;18:231-236.
436. Snyder LA. Acute myeloid leukemia. In: Weiss DJ, Wardrop KJ, eds. *Schalm's Veterinary Hematology*, 6th ed. Ames, IA: Wiley-Blackwell; 2010:475-482.
437. Sockett DC, Traub Dargatz J, Weiser MG. Immune-mediated hemolytic anemia and thrombocytopenia in a foal. *J Am Vet Med Assoc.* 1987;190:308-310.
438. Sontas HB, Dokuzeylu B, Turna O, et al. Estrogen-induced myelotoxicity in dogs: A review. *Can Vet J.* 2009;50:1054-1058.
439. Sparkes AH, Hopper CD, Millard WG, et al. Feline immunodeficiency virus infection. Clinicopathologic findings in 90 naturally occurring cases. *J Vet Intern Med.* 1993;7:85-90.
440. Stahl CP, Zucker Franklin D, Evatt BL, et al. Effects of human interleukin-6 on megakaryocyte development and thrombocytopoiesis in primates. *Blood.* 1991;78:1467-1475.
441. Steffen DJ, Elliott GS, Leipold HW, et al. Congenital dyserythropoiesis and progressive alopecia in Polled Hereford calves: hematologic, biochemical, bone marrow cytologic, electrophoretic, and flow cytometric findings. *J Vet Diagn Invest.* 1992;4:31-37.
442. Stenberg PE, McDonald TP, Jackson CW. Disruption of microtubules in vivo by vincristine induces large membrane complexes and other cytoplasmic abnormalities in megakaryocytes and platelets of normal rats like those in human and Wistar Furth rat hereditary macrothrombocytopenias. *J Cell Physiol.* 1995;162: 86-102.
443. Stockham SL, Ford RB, Weiss DJ. Canine autoimmune hemolytic disease with delayed erythroid regeneration. *J Am Anim Hosp Assoc.* 1980;16:927-931.
444. Stockhaus C, Slappendel RJ. Haemophagocytic syndrome with disseminated intravascular coagulation in a dog. *J Small Anim Pract.* 1998;39:203-206.
445. Stokol T. Essential thrombocythemia and reactive thrombocytosis. In: Weiss DJ, Wardrop KJ, eds. *Schalm's Veterinary Hematology*, 6th ed. Ames, IA: Wiley-Blackwell; 2010:605-611.
446. Stokol T, Blue JT. Pure red cell aplasia in cats: 9 cases (1989-1997). *J Am Vet Med Assoc.* 1999;214:75-79.
447. Stokol T, Blue JT, French TW. Idiopathic pure red cell aplasia and nonregenerative immune-mediated anemia in dogs: 43 cases (1988-1999). *J Am Vet Med Assoc.* 2000;216:1429-1436.
448. Stokol T, Randolph JF, Nachbar S, et al. Development of bone marrow toxicosis after albendazole administration in a dog and cat. *J Am Vet Med Assoc.* 1997;210: 1753-1756.
449. Strafuss AC, Sautter JH. Clinical and general pathologic findings of aplastic anemia associated with S-(dichlorovinyl)-L-cysteine in calves. *Am J Vet Res.* 1967;28: 25-37.
450. Suess RPJ, Barr SC, Sacre BJ, et al. Bone marrow hypoplasia in a feminized dog with an interstitial cell tumor. *J Am Vet Med Assoc.* 1992;200:1346-1348.
451. Suter SE, Vernau W, Fry MM, et al. CD34+, CD41+ acute megakaryoblastic leukemia in a dog. *Vet Clin Pathol.* 2007;36:288-292.
452. Swenson CL, Carothers MA, Wellman ML, et al. Eosinophilic leukemia in a cat with naturally acquired feline leukemia virus infection. *J Am Anim Hosp Assoc.* 1993;29:467-501.
453. Swenson CL, Kociba GJ, O'Keefe DA, et al. Cyclic hematopoiesis associated with feline leukemia virus infection in two cats. *J Am Vet Med Assoc.* 1987;191:93-96.
454. Swerdlow SH, Campo E, Harris NL, et al. *WHO Classification of Tumours of Haematopoietic and Lymphoid Tissues, Lyon.* France: International Agency for Research on Cancer; 2008.
455. Sykes JE, Weiss DJ, Buoen LC, et al. Idiopathic hypereosinophilic syndrome in 3 Rottweilers. *J Vet Intern Med.* 2001;15:162-166.
456. Takahashi T, Kadosawa T, Nagase M, et al. Visceral mast cell tumors in dogs: 10 cases (1982-1997). *J Am Vet Med Assoc.* 2000;216:222-226.
457. Takayama H, Gejima S, Honma A, et al. Acute myeloblastic leukaemia in a cow. *J Comp Pathol.* 1996;115:95-101.
458. Takeuchi Y, Iizuka H, Kanemitsu H, et al. Myeloma-related disorder with leukaemic progression in a cat. *J Feline Med Surg.* 2010;12:982-987.
459. Takeuchi Y, Matsuura S, Fujino Y, et al. Hypereosinophilic syndrome in two cats. *J Vet Med Sci.* 2008;70:1085-1089.
460. Tanaka M, Aze Y, Fujita T. Adhesion molecule LFA-1/ICAM-1 influences on LPS-induced megakaryocytic emperipolesis in the rat bone marrow. *Vet Pathol.* 1997;34:463-466.
461. Tarrant JM, Stokol T, Blue JT, et al. Diagnosis of chronic myelogenous leukemia in a dog using morphologic, cytochemical, and flow cytometric techniques. *Vet Clin Pathol.* 2001;30:19-24.
462. Tasca S, Carli E, Caldin M, et al. Hematologic abnormalities and flow cytometric immunophenotyping results in dogs with hematopoietic neoplasia: 210 cases (2002-2006). *Vet Clin Pathol.* 2009;38:2-12.
463. Tavassoli M. Modulation of megakaryocyte emperipolesis by phlebotomy: megakaryocytes as a component of marrow-blood barrier. *Blood Cells.* 1986;12:205-216.
464. Thenen SW, Rasmussen SD. Megaloblastic erythropoiesis and tissue depletion of folic acid in the cat. *Am J Vet Res.* 1978;39:1205-1207.
465. Thompson JP, Christopher MM, Ellison GW, et al. Paraneoplastic leukocytosis associated with a rectal adenomatous polyp in a dog. *J Am Vet Med Assoc.* 1992;201:737-738.
466. Tolle DV, Cullen SM, Seed TM, et al. Circulating micromegakaryocytes preceding leukemia in three dogs exposed to 2.5 R/day gamma radiation. *Vet Pathol.* 1983;20:111-114.
467. Tompkins MB, Novotney C, Grindem CB, et al. Human recombinant interleukin-2 induces maturation and activation signals for feline eosinophils in vivo. *J Leukoc Biol.* 1990;48:531-540.
468. Toribio RE, Bain FT, Mrad DR, et al. Congenital defects in newborn foals of mares treated for equine protozoal myeloencephalitis during pregnancy. *J Am Vet Med Assoc.* 1998;212:697-701.
469. Tornquist SJ, Crawford TB. Suppression of megakaryocyte colony growth by plasma from foals infected with equine infectious anemia virus. *Blood.* 1997;90: 2357-2363.
470. Toth SR, Nash AS, McEwan AM, et al. Chronic eosinophilic leukaemia in blast crises in a cat negative for feline leukaemia virus. *Vet Rec.* 1985;117:471-472.
471. Toth SR, Onions DE, Jarrett O. Histopathological and hematological findings in myeloid leukemia induced by a new feline leukemia virus isolate. *Vet Pathol.* 1986;23:462-470.
472. Trevor PB, Saunders GK, Waldron DR, et al. Metastatic extramedullary plasmacytoma of the colon and rectum in a dog. *J Am Vet Med Assoc.* 1993;203:406-409.
473. Tristano AG. Acquired amegakaryocytic thrombocytopenic purpura: review of a not very well-defined disorder. *Eur J Intern Med.* 2005;16:477-481.
474. Tristano AG. Macrophage activation syndrome: a frequent but under-diagnosed complication associated with rheumatic diseases. *Med Sci Monit.* 2008;14: RA27-RA36.
475. Trowald-Wigh G, Håkansson L, Johannisson A, et al. Leucocyte adhesion protein deficiency in Irish setter dogs. *Vet Immunol Immunopathol.* 1992;32:261-280.
476. Ulich TR, Del Castillo J, Yin S, et al. The erythropoietic effects of interleukin 6 and erythropoietin in vivo. *Exp Hematol.* 1991;19:29-34.
477. Ulich TR, del Castillo J, Busser K, et al. Acute in vivo effects of IL-3 alone and in combination with IL-6 on the blood cells of the circulation and bone marrow. *Am J Pathol.* 1989;135:663-670.
478. Vail DM. Plasma cell neoplasms. In: Withrow SJ, MacEwen EG, eds. *Small Animal Clinical Oncology.* Philadelphia: W.B. Saunders Co.; 1996:509-520.
479. Valli VE. *Veterinary Comparative Hematopathology.* Ames, IA; Blackwell Publishing; 2007.
480. Valli VE, Myint MS, Barthel A, et al. Classification of canine malignant lymphomas according to the World Health Organization criteria. *Vet Pathol.* 2011;48: 198-211.
481. van den Hoven R, Franken P. Clinical aspects of lymphosarcoma in the horse: a clinical report of 16 cases. *Equine Vet J.* 1983;15:49-53.

482. Vande Berg BC, Malghem J, Lecouvet FE, et al. Distribution of serouslike bone marrow changes in the lower limbs of patients with anorexia nervosa: predominant involvement of the distal extremities. *AJR Am J Roentgenol.* 1996;166:621-625.
483. Vargo CL, Taylor SM, Haines DM. Immune mediated neutropenia and thrombocytopenia in 3 giant schnauzers. *Can Vet J.* 2007;48:1159-1163.
484. Vernau W, Jacobs RM, Valli VEO, et al. The immunophenotypic characterization of bovine lymphomas. *Vet Pathol.* 1997;34:222-225.
485. Vernau W, Moore PF. An immunophenotypic study of canine leukemias and preliminary assessment of clonality by polymerase chain reaction. *Vet Immunol Immunopathol.* 1999;69:145-164.
486. Vernau W, Valli VEO, Dukes TW, et al. Classification of 1,198 cases of bovine lymphoma using the National Cancer Institute Working Formulation for human non-Hodgkin's lymphomas. *Vet Pathol.* 1992;29:183-195.
487. Villiers E, Baines S, Law AM, et al. Identification of acute myeloid leukemia in dogs using flow cytometry with myeloperoxidase, MAC387, and a canine neutrophil-specific antibody. *Vet Clin Pathol.* 2006;35:55-71.
488. Villiers EJ, Dunn JK. Clinicopathological features of seven cases of canine myelofibrosis and the possible relationship between the histological findings and prognosis. *Vet Rec.* 1999;145:222-228.
489. Walker D, Cowell RL, Clinkenbeard KD, et al. Bone marrow mast cell hyperplasia in dogs with aplastic anemia. *Vet Clin Pathol.* 1997;26:106-111.
490. Walsh KM, Losco PE. Canine mycobacteriosis: a case report. *J Am Anim Hosp Assoc.* 1984;20:295-299.
491. Walton RM, Modiano JF, Thrall MA, et al. Bone marrow cytological findings in 4 dogs and a cat with hemophagocytic syndrome. *J Vet Intern Med.* 1996;10:7-14.
492. Wang FI, Liang SL, Eng HL, et al. Disseminated liposarcoma in a dog. *J Vet Diagn Invest.* 2005;17:291-294.
493. Ward MV, Mountan PC, Dodds WJ. Severe idiopathic refractory anemia and leukopenia in a horse. *Calif Vet.* 1980;12:19-22.
494. Waters DJ, Prueter JC. Secondary polycythemia associated with renal disease in the dog: two case reports and review of literature. *J Am Anim Hosp Assoc.* 1988;24:109-114.
495. Watson AD. Chloramphenicol toxicity in dogs. *Res Vet Sci.* 1977;23:66-69.
496. Watson AD. Further observations on chloramphenicol toxicosis in cats. *Am J Vet Res.* 1980;41:293-294.
497. Watson AD, Middleton DJ. Chloramphenicol toxicosis in cats. *Am J Vet Res.* 1978;39:1199-1203.
498. Watson AD, Wilson JT, Turner DM, et al. Phenylbutazone-induced blood dyscrasias suspected in three dogs. *Vet Rec.* 1980;107:239-241.
499. Weiss DJ. Antibody-mediated suppression of erythropoiesis in dogs with red blood cell aplasia. *Am J Vet Res.* 1986;47:2646-2648.
500. Weiss DJ. Histopathology of canine nonneoplastic bone marrow. *Vet Clin Pathol.* 1986;15(2):7-11.
501. Weiss DJ. Leukocyte response to toxic injury. *Toxicol Pathol.* 1993;21:135-140.
502. Weiss DJ. Selective dysmegakaryopoiesis in thrombocytopenic dogs (1996-2002). *Comp Clin Pathol.* 2004;13:24-28.
503. Weiss DJ. Bone marrow necrosis in dogs: 34 cases (1996-2004). *J Am Vet Med Assoc.* 2005;227:263-267.
504. Weiss DJ. Differentiating benign and malignant causes of lymphocytosis in feline bone marrow. *J Vet Intern Med.* 2005;19:855-859.
505. Weiss DJ. Recognition and classification of dysmyelopoiesis in the dog: a review. *J Vet Intern Med.* 2005;19:147-154.
506. Weiss DJ. Sideroblastic anemia in 7 dogs (1996-2002). *J Vet Intern Med.* 2005;19:325-328.
507. Weiss DJ. A retrospective study of the incidence and classification of bone marrow disorders in cats (1996-2004). *Comp Clin Pathol.* 2006;14:179-185.
508. Weiss DJ. A retrospective study of the incidence and the classification of bone marrow disorders in the dog at a veterinary teaching hospital (1996-2004). *J Vet Intern Med.* 2006;20:955-961.
509. Weiss DJ. Evaluation of dysmyelopoiesis in cats: 34 cases (1996-2005). *J Am Vet Med Assoc.* 2006;228:893-897.
510. Weiss DJ. Feline myelonecrosis and myelofibrosis: 22 cases (1996-2006). *Comp Clin Pathol.* 2007;16:181-185.
511. Weiss DJ. Hemophagocytic syndrome in dogs: 24 cases (1996-2005). *J Am Vet Med Assoc.* 2007;230:697-701.
512. Weiss DJ. Bone marrow pathology in dogs and cats with non-regenerative immune-mediated haemolytic anaemia and pure red cell aplasia. *J Comp Pathol.* 2008;138:46-53.
513. Weiss DJ. Chronic inflammation and secondary myelofibrosis. In: Weiss DJ, Wardrop KJ, eds. *Schalm's Veterinary Hematology,* 6th ed. Ames, IA: Wiley-Blackwell; 2010:112-117.
514. Weiss DJ. Congenital dyserythropoiesis. In: Weiss DJ, Wardrop KJ, eds. *Schalm's Veterinary Hematology,* 6th ed. Ames, IA: Wiley-Blackwell; 2010: 196-198.
515. Weiss DJ. Drug-induced blood cell disorders. In: Weiss DJ, Wardrop KJ, eds. *Schalm's Veterinary Hematology,* 6th ed. Ames, IA: Wiley-Blackwell; 2010:98-105.
516. Weiss DJ. Myelodysplastic syndromes. In: Weiss DJ, Wardrop KJ, eds. *Schalm's Veterinary Hematology,* 6th ed. Ames, IA: Wiley-Blackwell; 2010:467-474.
517. Weiss DJ. Myelonecrosis and acute inflammation. In: Weiss DJ, Wardrop KJ, eds. *Schalm's Veterinary Hematology,* 6th ed. Ames, IA: Wiley-Blackwell; 2010:106-111.
518. Weiss DJ, Aird B. Cytologic evaluation of primary and secondary myelodysplastic syndromes in the dog. *Vet Clin Pathol.* 2001;30:67-75.
519. Weiss DJ, Armstrong PJ. Secondary myelofibrosis in three dogs. *J Am Vet Med Assoc.* 1985;187:423-425.
520. Weiss DJ, Armstrong PJ, Reimann K. Bone marrow necrosis in the dog. *J Am Vet Med Assoc.* 1985;187:54-59.
521. Weiss DJ, Christopher MM. Idiopathic aplastic anemia in a dog. *Vet Clin Pathol.* 1985;14(2):23-25.
522. Weiss DJ, Evanson OA. A retrospective study of feline pancytopenia. *Comp Haematol Int.* 2000;10:50-55.
523. Weiss DJ, Evanson OA, Sykes J. A retrospective study of canine pancytopenia. *Vet Clin Pathol.* 1999;28:83-88.
524. Weiss DJ, Greig B, Aird B, et al. Inflammatory disorders of bone marrow. *Vet Clin Pathol.* 1992;21:79-84.
525. Weiss DJ, Henson M. Pure white cell aplasia in a dog. *Vet Clin Pathol.* 2007;36:373-375.
526. Weiss DJ, Henson M. Pure white cell aplasia in a dog. *Vet Clin Pathol.* 2007;36:373-375.
527. Weiss DJ, Klausner JS. Drug-associated aplastic anemia in dogs: eight cases (1984-1988). *J Am Vet Med Assoc.* 1990;196:472-475.
528. Weiss DJ, Lulich J. Myelodysplastic syndrome with sideroblastic differentiation in a dog. *Vet Clin Pathol.* 1999;28:59-63.
529. Weiss DJ, Miller DC. Bone marrow necrosis associated with pancytopenia in a cow. *Vet Pathol.* 1985;22:90-92.
530. Weiss DJ, Raskin RE, Zerbe C. Myelodysplastic syndrome in two dogs. *J Am Vet Med Assoc.* 1985;187:1038-1040.
531. Weiss DJ, Reidarson TH. Idiopathic dyserythropoiesis in a dog. *Vet Clin Pathol.* 1989;18:43-46.
532. Weiss RC, Cox NR, Boudreaux MK. Toxicologic effects of ribavirin in cats. *J Vet Pharmacol Ther.* 1993;16:301-316.
533. Wellman ML. *Lymphoproliferative disorders of large granular lymphocytes.* Lake Buena Vista, FL: Proc 15th ACVIM Forum; 1997:20-21.
534. Wellman ML, Couto CG, Starkey RJ, et al. Lymphocytosis of large granular lymphocytes in three dogs. *Vet Pathol.* 1989;26:158-163.
535. Wellman ML, Hammer AS, DiBartola SP, et al. Lymphoma involving large granular lymphocytes in cats: 11 cases (1982-1991). *J Am Vet Med Assoc.* 1992;201:1265-1269.
536. Whyte MP. Skeletal disorders characterized by osteosclerosis or hyperostosis. In: Avioli LV, Krane SM, eds. *Metabolic Bone Disease and Clinically Related Disorders,* 3rd ed. San Diego, CA: Academic Press; 1998:697-738.
537. Williams DA, Maggio Price L. Canine idiopathic thrombocytopenia: clinical observations and long-term follow-up in 54 cases. *J Am Vet Med Assoc.* 1984;185:660-663.
538. Wilson SC, Thomson-Kerr K, Houston DM. Hypereosinophilic syndrome in a cat. *Can Vet J.* 1996;37:679-680.
539. Woda BA, Sullivan JL. Reactive histiocytic disorders. *Am J Clin Pathol.* 1993;99:459-463.
540. Woods PR, Campbell G, Cowell RL. Nonregenerative anaemia associated with administration of recombinant human erythropoietin to a thoroughbred racehorse. *Equine Vet J.* 1997;29:326-328.
541. Woods PR, Gossett RE, Jain NC, et al. Acute myelomonocytic leukemia in a calf. *J Am Vet Med Assoc.* 1993;203:1579-1582.
542. Workman HC, Vernau W. Chronic lymphocytic leukemia in dogs and cats: the veterinary perspective. *Vet Clin North Am Small Anim Pract.* 2003;33:1379-1399.
543. Wright ZM, Rogers KS, Mansell J. Survival data for canine oral extramedullary plasmacytomas: a retrospective analysis (1996-2006). *J Am Anim Hosp Assoc.* 2008;44:75-81.
544. Wykes PM, Withrow SJ, Powers BE, et al. Closed biopsy for diagnosis of long bone tumors: accuracy and results. *J Am Anim Hosp Assoc.* 1985;21:489-494.
545. Yamada O, Tamura K, Yagihara H, et al. Light-chain multiple myeloma in a cat. *J Vet Diagn Invest.* 2007;19:443-447.
546. Yang Z, Philips JD, Doty RT, et al. Kinetics and specificity of feline leukemia virus subgroup C receptor (FLVCR) export function and its dependence on hemopexin. *J Biol Chem.* 2010;285:28874-28882.
547. Yoshida Y, Oguma S, Uchino H, et al. Refractory myelodysplastic anaemias with hypocellular bone marrow. *J Clin Pathol.* 1988;41:763-767.
548. Young KM, MacEwen EG. Canine myeloproliferative disorders and malignant histiocytosis. In: Withrow SJ, MacEwen EG, eds. *Small Animal Clinical Oncology.* Philadelphia: W.B. Saunders Co.; 1996:495-509.

549. Young KM, Meadows RL. Eosinophils and their disorders. In: Weiss DJ, Wardrop KJ, eds. *Schalm's Veterinary Hematology*, 6th ed. Ames, IA: Wiley-Blackwell; 2010,

550. Young NS, Calado RT, Scheinberg P. Current concepts in the pathophysiology and treatment of aplastic anemia. *Blood.* 2006;108:2509-2519.

551. Zaucha JA, Yu C, Lothrop CDJ, et al. Severe canine hereditary hemolytic anemia treated by nonmyeloablative marrow transplantation. *Biol Blood Marrow Transplant.* 2001;7:14-24.

552. Zini E, Hauser B, Meli ML, et al. Immune-mediated erythroid and megakaryocytic aplasia in a cat. *J Am Vet Med Assoc.* 2007;230:1024-1027.

553. Zinkl JG, Cain G, Jain NC, et al. Haematological response of dogs to canine recombinant granulocyte colony stimulating factor (rcG-CSF). *Comp Haematol Int.* 1992;2:151-156.

554. Zinkl JG, LeCouteur RA, Davis DC, et al. "Flaming" plasma cells in a dog with IgA multiple myeloma. *Vet Clin Pathol.* 1983;12(3):15-19.

APPENDIX

I

TABLES

EXAMPLE OF BONE MARROW EVALUATION AND INTERPRETATION

Patient: A 9-year-old castrated male mixed-breed cat.

History: Decreased appetite, lethargy, and weight loss were recognized 2 weeks ago. The referring veterinarian diagnosed severe periodontal disease. Four teeth were pulled and antibiotic therapy was initiated. The animal had intermittent fever, exhibited variable anorexia, became dehydrated, and was referred to the University of Florida Small Animal Hospital for evaluation.

Clinical Findings: The cat was lethargic, slightly dehydrated, and thin, with a dry hair coat. The gums were hyperemic in association with continuing periodontal disease.

Laboratory Findings: Abnormal hematology findings included a hematocrit of 27% and total leukocyte count of 1300/μL, most of which were lymphocytes. Platelets were not counted but numbers appeared normal during stained blood film examination. Erythrocyte morphology was normal. Urinalysis and clinical chemistry values were within normal limits. The FeLV test was negative but the FIV test was positive.

Evaluation of Bone Marrow Aspirate Smear

13% Immature myeloid cells[a]	4% Immature erythroid cells[b]
63% Mature myeloid cells	13% Mature erythroid cells
1% Eosinophilic cells	4% Lymphocytes
<1% Monocytoid cells	<1% Plasma cells
M:E ratio = 4.5	

Multiple particles were present and their cellularity appeared to be increased. Megakaryocyte numbers appeared normal, and most were mature. The myeloid series was left-shifted, with a depletion of mature neutrophils. The erythroid series was complete, with orderly maturation, but a decreased amount of polychromasia was present. Lymphocytes, plasma cells, and macrophages were present in normal numbers. Hemosiderin was not observed, but this is a normal finding in cats. Erythrophagocytosis and leukophagocytosis were rarely observed.

Interpretation: Granulocytic hyperplasia with abnormal maturation.

Comment: An increased M:E ratio in a severely leukopenic, mildly anemic animal with hypercellular marrow and disordered myeloid maturation is most likely secondary to FIV infection in this cat. This pattern could also be detected transiently during a recovery phase after severe granulocytic depletion, although this is less likely based on the history. If the animal is in a recovery phase from neutropenia, the leukocyte count should increase in the peripheral blood within a few days.

[a]Immature myeloid cells include myeloblasts and promyelocytes. Mature myeloid cells include neutrophilic myelocytes, neutrophilic metamyelocytes, neutrophilic bands, and mature neutrophils.

[b]Immature erythroid cells include rubriblasts and prorubricytes. Mature erythroid cells include basophilic rubricytes, polychromatophilic rubricytes, and metarubricytes.

TABLE 1

Reference Intervals for Hematology Values in Domestic Animals

Test	Units	Dogs[a] ($N = 130$)	Cats[a] ($N = 45$)	Horses[a] ($N = 70$)	Cows[b] (58)	Pigs[c] (99)	Goats[d] (NR)
Hematocrit	%	40-56	34-51	30-44	22-32	34-44	22-38
RBC	$\times 10^6/\mu L$	5.7-8.3	7.4-10.4	6.6-11.0	5.1-7.6	6.4-8.4	8.0-18.0
Hemoglobin	g/dL	14-20	11-16	11-16	8-12	10-14	8-12
MCV	fL	64-74	42-52	38-51	38-50	49-59	16-25
MCH	pg	22-26	13-17	13-19	14-18	NR	5.2-8.0
MCHC	g/dL	33-38	30-33	35-39	36-39	29-33	30-36
RDW	(%)	11-14	13-16	16-21	16-20	15-24	NR
Reticulocytes	$\times 10^3/\mu L$	8-65	8-57	0	0	NR	0
Platelets	$\times 10^3/\mu L$	134-396	160-502	100-308	193-637	211-887	300-600
MPV	fL	10-15	10-22	5.9-9.9	4.5-7.5	NR	NR
Icterus index[e]	Units	<5	<5	5-20	2-15	<5	2-5
Plasma protein[e]	g/dL	6.0-8.0	6.2-8.0	6.0-8.0	7.0-8.5	6.0-8.0	6.0-7.5
Fibrinogen[e]	mg/dL	100-400	100-300	100-400	300-700	100-500	100-400
Total leukocytes	$\times 10^3/\mu L$	5.0-13.0	5.4-15.4	5.6-11.6	4.9-12.0	15.6-38.9	4.0-13.0
Bands	$\times 10^3/\mu L$	0-0.3	0-0.3	0-0.1	Rare	NR	Rare
Neutrophils	$\times 10^3/\mu L$	2.7-8.9	2.3-9.8	2.6-6.7	1.8-6.3	3.0-17.4	1.2-7.2
Lymphocytes	$\times 10^3/\mu L$	0.9-3.4	0.9-5.5	1.1-5.7	1.6-5.6	7.7-20.4	2.0-9.0
Monocytes	$\times 10^3/\mu L$	0.1-0.8	0-0.8	0-0.7	0-0.8	0.6-3.4	0-0.6
Eosinophils	$\times 10^3/\mu L$	0.1-1.3	0-1.8	0-0.6	0-0.9	0.1-2.3	0.1-0.7
Basophils	$\times 10^3/\mu L$	0-0.1	0-0.2	0-0.2	0-0.3	0.1-0.3	0-0.1

RBC, red blood cell count; MCV, mean cell volume; MCH, mean cell hemoglobin; MCHC, mean cell hemoglobin concentration; RDW, red blood cell distribution width; MPV, mean platelet volume; NR, not reported.

[a]Data from adult dogs, cats, and horses were determined at the University of Florida College of Veterinary Medicine. Total leukocyte counts, erythrocyte parameters, and platelet values were measured from healthy adult animals of both sexes and various breeds using an Advia 120 hematology analyzer. Greyhounds and other sighthounds were excluded. Thoroughbred and quarter horses in equal numbers accounted for about 90% of the hot-blooded horses studied. Reticulocyte counts represent the minimum and maximum values measured from 58 dogs and 41 cats. The Advia 120 counts primarily aggregate reticulocytes in cats. These automated platelet counts are lower than reference values reported for manual platelet counts in dogs (200-500 $\times 10^3/\mu L$) and cats (300-800 $\times 10^3/\mu L$). Leukocyte differential counts were performed manually by classifying 200 leukocytes in each stained blood film.

[b]Measurements from bovine leukemia virus-negative adult dairy cows in mid-lactation were performed using an Advia 120 hematology analyzer and manual differential leukocyte counts. (From George JW, Snipes J, Lane VM. Comparison of bovine hematology reference intervals from 1957 to 2006. *Vet Clin Pathol.* 2010;39:138-148.)

[c]Measurements from crossbred grower pigs weighing between 30 and 50 kg were performed using an Advia 2120 hematology analyzer. (From Klem TB, Bleken E, Morberg H, Thoresen SI, Framstad T. Hematologic and biochemical reference intervals for Norwegian crossbred grower pigs. *Vet Clin Pathol.* 2010;39:221-226.)

[d]The goat population sampled and hematology analyzer(s) used were not given. The hematocrits were determined using microhematocrit tubes and leukocyte differential counts were determined by examining stained blood films. (From Jain NC. *Schalm's Veterinary Hematology,* 4th ed. Philadelphia: Lea & Febiger; 1986.)

[e]Total protein, fibrinogen, and icterus index values were determined using manual methods. (From Jain NC. *Schalm's Veterinary Hematology,* 4th ed. Philadelphia: Lea & Febiger; 1986.)

TABLE 2

Variations in Reference Intervals for Hematology Values by Age: Beagle Dogs, 3 to 14 Years Old

Laboratory Test[a]	3 Years	6 Years	9 Years	12 Years	14 Years
RBC ($\times 10^6/\mu L$)	6.6-7.8	6.5-7.6	5.9-7.4	6.1-7.3	5.7-7.1
Hemoglobin (g/dL)	15-18	16-18	14-18	14-17	14-17
PCV (%)	43-50	44-49	38-50	40-49	40-47
Band neutrophils/μL	0	0	0-63	0-68	0-54
Segmented neutrophils/μL	3944-9287	3605-7724	4207-7217	4724-9587	4464-10,255
Lymphocytes/μL	2185-3318	1334-2467	1667-2702	1676-2658	1628-2453
Monocytes/μL	101-769	173-626	149-620	181-521	189-688
Eosinophils/μL	208-1010	217-500	275-711	99-721	201-408
Basophils/μL	0	0-70	0-102	0	0

From Lowseth LA, Gillett NA, Gerlach RF, et al. The effects of aging on hematology and serum chemistry values in the beagle dog. *Vet Clin Pathol.* 1990;19:13-19.
RBC, red blood cell count; PCV, packed cell volume.
[a]Limits represent the 10th and 90th percentile values.

TABLE 3

Erythrocyte Changes during Pregnancy in Beagles, Brittany Spaniels, and Labrador Retrievers

	GESTATION WEEK 1			GESTATION WEEK 8			LACTATION WEEK 8		
	Beagles	Brittany Spaniels	Labrador Retrievers	Beagles	Brittany Spaniels	Labrador Retrievers	Beagles	Brittany Spaniels	Labrador Retrievers
RBC ($\times10^6/\mu L$)									
Mean	7.2	6.2	7.3	5.1	5.0	5.6	7.0	5.6	6.7
Range	6.2-9.2	5.2-7.2	5.5-9.1	4.1-6.1	4.1-6.0	4.4-6.8	5.8-8.2	4.4-6.8	5.7-7.7
PCV (%)									
Mean	47	43.3	50	34.3	33.0	38.2	46.6	40.8	44.1
Range[a]	38.4-54.6	38.5-48.1	42.4-57.6	39.2-50.8	25.2-40.8	30.4-46.0	39.2-54.0	32.8-48.8	36.1-52.1
Hemoglobin (g/dL)									
Mean	17.2	15.9	18.1	12.3	11.8	13.9	16.5	14.7	15.9
Range[a]	15.2-19.2	14.1-17.7	15.3-20.9	10.3-14.3	9.2-14.4	11.7-16.1	13.9-19.1	11.7-17.7	13.1-18.7
MCV (fL)									
Mean	66.6	70.3	69.2	67.3	72.6	67.9	67.3	73.3	65.9
Range[a]	59.2-76	59.7-80.9	50.6-87.8	60.7-73.6	58.6-86.6	52.9-82.9	60.7-73.6	63.1-83.4	55.8-76.0
MCHC (g/dL)									
Mean	36.8	36.6	36.2	36	36.4	36.8	35.5	36	36.1
Range[a]	30.6-43	34.4-38.8	34.2-38.2	31.2-40.8	34.6-38.2	31.8-41.4	31.7-39.4	33.0-39.0	32.7-39.5

From Allard RL, Carlos AD, Faltin EC. Canine hematological changes during gestation and lactation. *Comp Anim Pract.* 1989;19:3-6.
RBC, red blood cell count; PCV, packed cell volume; MCV, mean cell volume; MCHC, mean cell hemoglobin concentration.
[a]Range is ±2 SD.

TABLE 4

Hematology Values for Growing Healthy Beagle Dogs from Birth to 8 Weeks of Age

Hematology Parameter	Birth	1 Week	2 Weeks	3 Weeks	4 Weeks	6 Weeks	8 Weeks
RBC ($\times 10^6/\mu L$)	4.7-5.6 (5.1)[a]	3.6-5.9 (4.6)	3.4-4.4 (3.9)	3.5-4.3 (3.8)	3.6-4.9 (4.1)	4.3-5.1 (4.7)	4.5-5.9 (4.9)
Hemoglobin (g/dL)	14-17 (15.2)	10.4-17.5 (12.9)	9-11 (10.0)	8.6-11.6 (9.7)	8.5-10.3 (9.5)	8.5-11.3 (10.2)	10.3-12.5 (11.2)
PCV (%)	45-52.5 (47.5)	33-52 (40.5)	29-34 (31.8)	27-37 (31.7)	27-33.5 (29.9)	26.5-35.5 (32.5)	31-39 (34.8)
MCV (fL)	93.0	89.0	81.5	83.0	73.0	69.0	72.0
MCH (pg)	30.0	28.0	25.5	25.0	23.0	22.0	22.5
MCHC (g/dL)	32.0	32.0	31.5	31.0	32.0	31.5	32.0
NRBC/100 WBC	0-13 (2.3)	0-11 (4.0)	0-6 (2.0)	0-9 (1.6)	0-4 (1.2)	0	0-1 (0.2)
WBC ($\times 10^3/\mu L$)	6.8-18.4 (12.0)	9-23 (14.1)	8.1-15.1 (11.7)	6.7-15.1 (11.2)	8.5-16.4 (12.9)	12.6-26.7 (16.3)	12.7-17.3 (15)
Band neutrophils ($\times 10^3/\mu L$)	0-1.5 (0.23)	0-4.8 (0.50)	0-1.2 (0.21)	0-0.5 (0.09)	0-0.3 (0.06)	0-0.3 (0.05)	0-0.3 (0.08)
Segmented neutrophils ($\times 10^3/\mu L$)	4.4-15.8 (8.6)	3.8-15.2 (7.4)	3.2-10.4 (5.2)	1.4-9.4 (5.1)	3.7-12.8 (7.2)	4.2-17.6 (9.0)	6.2-11.8 (8.5)
Lymphocytes ($\times 10^3/\mu L$)	0.5-4.2 (1.9)	1.3-9.4 (4.3)	1.5-7.4 (3.8)	2.1-10.1 (5.0)	1.0-8.4 (4.5)	2.8-16.6 (5.7)	3.1-6.9 (5.0)
Monocytes ($\times 10^3/\mu L$)	0.2-2.2 (0.9)	0.3-2.5 (1.1)	0.2-1.4 (0.7)	0.1-1.4 (0.7)	0.3-1.5 (0.8)	0.5-2.7 (1.1)	0.5-2.7 (1.1)
Eosinophils ($\times 10^3/\mu L$)	0-1.3 (0.4)	0.2-2.8 (0.8)	0.08-1.8 (0.6)	0.07-0.9 (0.3)	0-0.7 (0.25)	0.1-1.9 (0.5)	0-1.2 (0.4)
Basophils ($\times 10^3/\mu L$)	0.0	0-0.2 (0.01)	0.0	0-0	0-0.15 (0.01)	0.0	0.0

From Earl FL, Melvegar BA, Wilson RL. The hemogram and bone marrow profile of normal neonatal and weanling beagle dogs. *Lab Anim Sci.* 1973;23:690.

RBC, red blood cell count; PCV, packed cell volume; MCV, mean cell volume; MCH, mean cell hemoglobin; MCHC, mean cell hemoglobin concentration; NRBC, nucleated red blood cell; WBC, white blood cell count.

[a]Values expressed as range and (median).

TABLE 5

Hematology Values for Growing Healthy Kittens from Birth to 17 Weeks of Age

Hematology Parameter	0-2 Weeks	2-4 Weeks	4-6 Weeks	6-8 Weeks	8-9 Weeks	12-13 Weeks	16-17 Weeks
RBC (×10^6/μL)	5.29 (4.81-5.77)*	4.67 (4.47-4.87)	5.89 (5.43-6.35)	6.57 (6.05-7.09)	6.95 (6.77-7.13)	7.43 (6.97-7.89)	8.14 (7.60-8.68)
Hemoglobin (g/dL)	12.1 (10.9-13.3)	8.7 (8.3-9.1)	8.6 (8.0-9.2)	9.1 (8.5-9.7)	9.8 (9.4-10.2)	10.1 (9.5-10.7)	11.0 (10.2-11.9)
PCV (%)	35.3 (31.9-38.7)	26.5 (24.9-28.1)	27.1 (25.5-28.7)	29.8 (27.2-32.4)	33.3 (31.9-34.7)	33.1 (29.9-36.3)	34.9 (32.7-37.1)
MCV (fL)	67.4 (63.6-71.2)	53.9 (51.5-56.3)	45.6 (43.0-48.2)	45.6 (43.6-47.6)	47.8 (46.0-49.6)	44.5 (40.9-48.1)	43.1 (40.1-46.1)
MCH (pg)	23.0 (21.8-24.2)	18.8 (17.2-20.4)	14.8 (13.7-16.0)	13.9 (13.3-14.5)	14.1 (13.7-14.5)	13.7 (12.9-14.5)	13.5 (12.7-14.3)
MCHC (g/dL)	34.5 (32.9-36.1)	33.0 (31.0-34.0)	31.9 (30.7-33.1)	30.9 (29.9-31.9)	29.5 (28.7-30.3)	31.3 (29.5-32.1)	31.6 (30.0-33.2)
WBC (×10^3/μL)	9.67 (8.53-10.81)	15.31 (12.89-17.73)	17.45 (14.71-20.19)	18.07 (14.19-21.95)	23.68 (19.9-27.46)	23.10 (16.48-29.92)	19.7 (17.46-21.94)
Band neutrophils (×10^3/μL)	0.06 (0.02-0.10)	0.11 (0.03-0.19)	0.20 (0.08-0.32)	0.22 (0.06-0.38)	0.12 (0.0-0.30)	0.15 (0.01-0.27)	0.16 (0.020-0.30)
Neutrophils (×10^3/μL)	5.96 (4.60-7.32)	6.92 (5.38-8.46)	9.57 (6.27-12.87)	6.75 (4.69-8.81)	11.0 (8.18-13.82)	11.0 (7.46-14.54)	9.74 (7.90-11.58)
Lymphocytes (×10^3/μL)	3.73 (2.69-4.77)	6.56 (5.38-7.74)	6.41 (4.87-7.95)	9.59 (6.45-12.73)	10.17 (6.75-13.59)	10.46 (5.24-15.68)	8.7 (6.58-10.82)
Monocytes (×10^3/μL)	0.01 (0.0-0.03)	0.02 (0.0-0.06)	0.0	0.01 (0.0-0.03)	0.11 (0.0-0.23)	0.0	0.02 (0.0-0.06)
Eosinophils (×10^3/μL)	0.96 (0.10-1.82)	1.40 (1.08-1.72)	1.47 (0.97-1.97)	1.08 (0.68-1.48)	2.28 (1.66-2.90)	1.55 (0.85-2.25)	1.00 (0.62-1.38)
Basophils (×10^3/μL)	0.02 (0.0-0.04)	0	0	0.02 (0.0-0.06)	0	0.03 (0.0-0.09)	0

From Meyers-Wallen VN, Haskins ME, Patterson DF. Hematologic values in healthy neonatal, weanling and juvenile kittens. *Am J Vet Res.* 1984;45:1322.
RBC, red blood cell count; PCV, packed cell volume; MCV, mean cell volume; MCH, mean cell hemoglobin; MCHC, mean cell hemoglobin concentration; WBC, white blood cell count.
*Values expressed as mean and (range). Range calculated from mean ±2 SD.

TABLE 6

Erythrograms of Foals up to 1 Year of Age

Age	PCV (%)	Hb (g/dL)	RBC ($\times 10^6/\mu L$)	MCV (fL)	MCHC (%)
<12 Hours	43 ± 3	15.4 ± 1.2	10.7 ± 0.8	40 ± 2	36 ± 2
1 day	40 ± 3	14.2 ± 1.1	9.9 ± 0.6	41 ± 3	35 ± 2
3 days	38 ± 3	14.1 ± 1.3	9.6 ± 0.7	39 ± 2	37 ± 1
1 week	35 ± 3	13.3 ± 1.2	8.8 ± 0.6	39 ± 2	38 ± 1
2 weeks	34 ± 3	12.6 ± 1.4	8.9 ± 0.9	38 ± 2	38 ± 1
3 weeks	34 ± 3	12.6 ± 1.1	9.2 ± 0.6	37 ± 2	37 ± 1
1 month	34 ± 4	12.5 ± 1.2	9.3 ± 0.8	36 ± 1	37 ± 1
2 months	37 ± 4	13.6 ± 1.5	10.8 ± 1.7	35 ± 2	37 ± 1
3 months	36 ± 2	13.4 ± 0.9	10.5 ± 0.9	35 ± 1	37 ± 2
4 months	36 ± 3	13.4 ± 1.1	10.4 ± 0.9	34 ± 1	38 ± 2
5 months	35 ± 3	12.7 ± 1.2	10.2 ± 0.6	35 ± 2	37 ± 2
6 months	34 ± 2	12.2 ± 0.8	9.5 ± 0.7	36 ± 2	36 ± 1
9 months	36 ± 3	12.6 ± 1.0	9.4 ± 0.8	39 ± 2	35 ± 1
12 months	36 ± 3	13.3 ± 1.0	9.5 ± 0.7	38 ± 2	37 ± 2

From Harvey JW, Asquith RL, McNulty PK, et al. Haematology of foals up to one year old. *Equine Vet J.* 1984;16:347-353.
Values expressed as mean ±1 SD.
PCV, packed cell volume; Hb, hemoglobin; RBC, red blood cell count; MCV, mean cell volume; MCHC, mean cell hemoglobin concentration.

TABLE 7

Leukograms of Foals up to 1 Year of Age

Age	Total WBC ($\times 10^3/\mu L$)	Neutrophils ($\times 10^3/\mu L$)	Lymphocytes ($\times 10^3/\mu L$)	Monocytes ($\times 10^3/\mu L$)	Eosinophils ($\times 10^3/\mu L$)	Basophils ($\times 10^3/\mu L$)
<12 hours	9.5 ± 2.44	7.94 ± 2.22	1.34 ± 0.60	0.19 ± 0.12	0	0.002 ± 0.007
1 day	8.44 ± 1.77	6.80 ± 1.72	1.43 ± 0.42	0.19 ± 0.10	0.11 ± 0.027	0.003 ± 0.010
3 days	7.55 ± 1.50	5.70 ± 1.44	1.45 ± 0.36	0.32 ± 0.13	0.045 ± 0.062	0.032 ± 0.046
1 week	9.86 ± 1.79	7.45 ± 1.55	2.10 ± 0.63	0.27 ± 0.11	0.028 ± 0.042	0.058 ± 0.069
2 weeks	8.53 ± 1.68	6.00 ± 1.54	2.22 ± 0.45	0.24 ± 0.13	0.063 ± 0.063	0.012 ± 0.021
3 weeks	8.57 ± 1.90	5.66 ± 1.64	2.59 ± 0.63	0.22 ± 0.10	0.078 ± 0.066	0.026 ± 0.032
1 month	8.14 ± 2.02	5.27 ± 2.00	2.46 ± 0.45	0.29 ± 0.17	0.121 ± 0.148	0.016 ± 0.032
2 months	9.65 ± 2.13	5.70 ± 1.88	3.46 ± 0.63	0.31 ± 0.15	0.092 ± 0.092	0.018 ± 0.039
3 months	11.69 ± 2.51	6.43 ± 1.96	4.73 ± 1.21	0.38 ± 0.19	0.184 ± 0.181	0.018 ± 0.028
4 months	10.18 ± 1.99	4.78 ± 1.36	4.70 ± 1.31	0.32 ± 0.17	0.353 ± 0.319	0.018 ± 0.027
5 months	10.07 ± 2.29	4.60 ± 1.90	4.92 ± 1.48	0.27 ± 0.12	0.272 ± 0.152	0.010 ± 0.027
6 months	9.03 ± 1.13	4.00 ± 0.84	4.53 ± 0.74	0.23 ± 0.11	0.247 ± 0.150	0.014 ± 0.024
9 months	8.68 ± 1.19	3.82 ± 0.78	4.39 ± 1.10	0.22 ± 0.10	0.234 ± 0.232	0.021 ± 0.024
12 months	9.19 ± 1.36	4.28 ± 0.81	4.27 ± 1.13	0.20 ± 0.12	0.339 ± 0.221	0.019 ± 0.037

From Harvey JW, Asquith RL, McNulty PK, et al. Haematology of foals up to one year old. *Equine Vet J.* 1984;16:347-353.
Values are expressed as mean ±1 SD.

APPENDIX

II

ALGORITHMS

1. Anemia, regenerative
2. Anemia, poorly regenerative or nonregenerative
3. Erythrocytosis
4. Leukopenia
5. Leukocytosis or normal leukocyte count with abnormal differential
6. Platelet/coagulation factor deficiencies

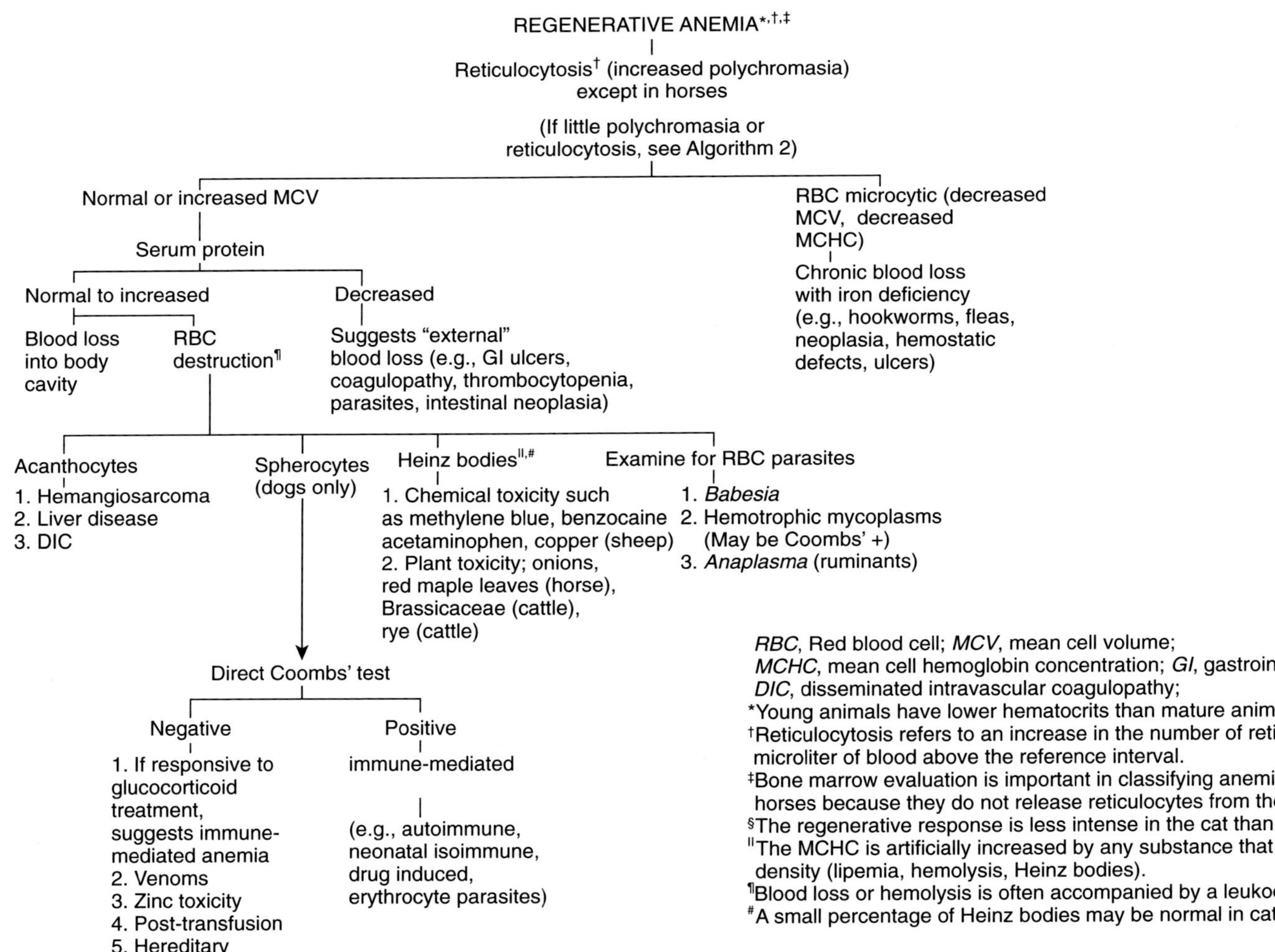

RBC, Red blood cell; *MCV*, mean cell volume; *MCHC*, mean cell hemoglobin concentration; *GI*, gastrointestinal; *DIC*, disseminated intravascular coagulopathy;

*Young animals have lower hematocrits than mature animals.

†Reticulocytosis refers to an increase in the number of reticulocytes per microliter of blood above the reference interval.

‡Bone marrow evaluation is important in classifying anemia in horses because they do not release reticulocytes from the marrow.

§The regenerative response is less intense in the cat than the dog.

‖The MCHC is artificially increased by any substance that increases optical density (lipemia, hemolysis, Heinz bodies).

¶Blood loss or hemolysis is often accompanied by a leukocytosis.

#A small percentage of Heinz bodies may be normal in cats.

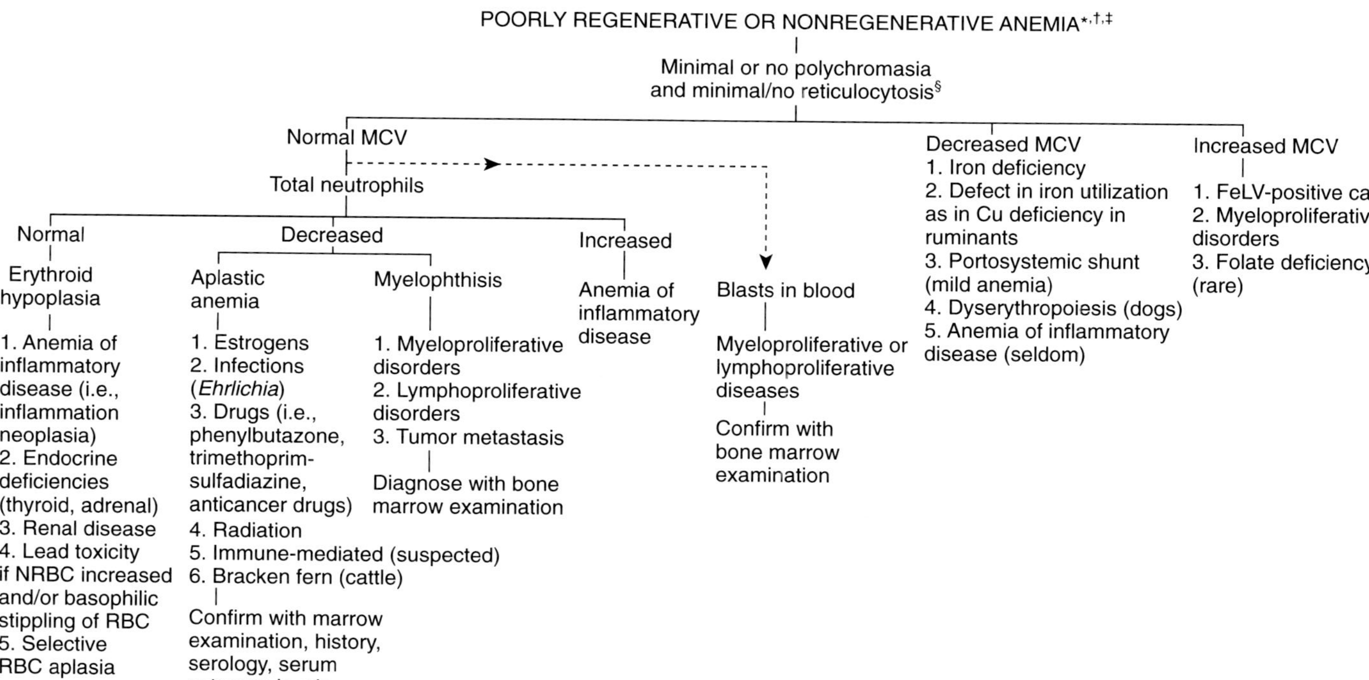

MCV, Mean cell volume; *FeLV*, feline leukemia virus; RBC, red blood cell; *NRBC*, nucleated red blood cell.

*Young animals have lower hematocrits than mature animals.

†Bone marrow evaluation is important in the diagnosis of nonregenerative anemia.

‡All cats with anemias should be tested for FeLV and feline immunodeficiency virus.

§Reticulocytosis refers to an increase in the number of reticulocytes per microliter of blood above the reference interval.

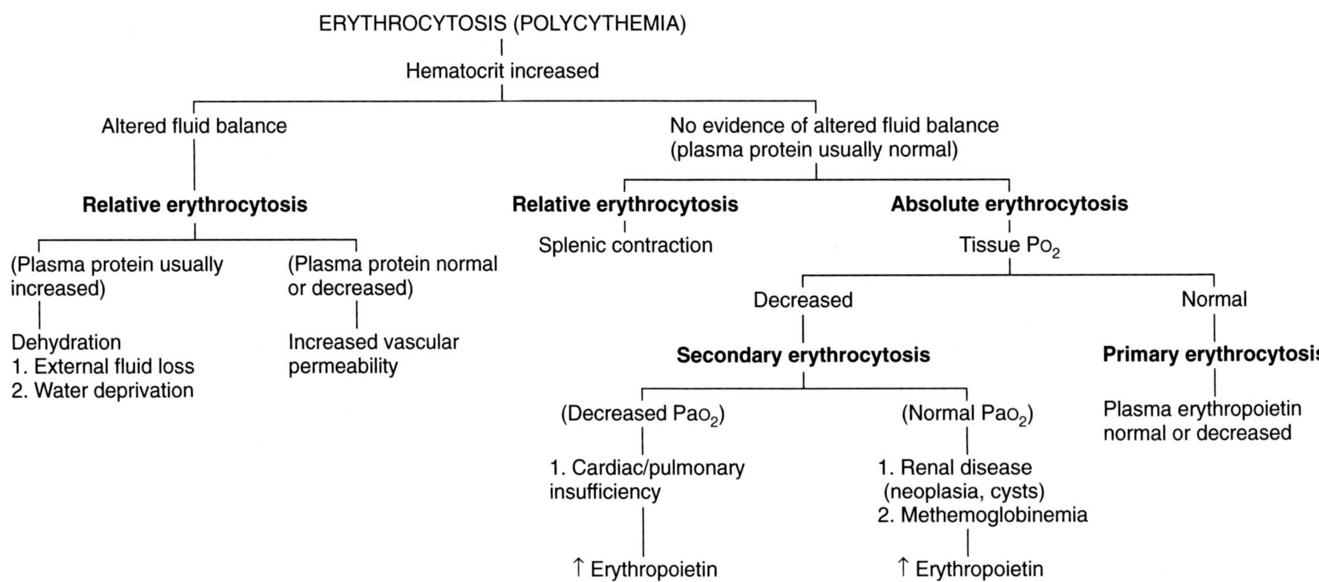
ERYTHROCYTOSIS (POLYCYTHEMIA)
Hematocrit increased
Altered fluid balance
Relative erythrocytosis
(Plasma protein usually increased)
Dehydration
1. External fluid loss
2. Water deprivation
(Plasma protein normal or decreased)
Increased vascular permeability
No evidence of altered fluid balance (plasma protein usually normal)
Relative erythrocytosis
Splenic contraction
Absolute erythrocytosis
Tissue Po_2
Decreased
Secondary erythrocytosis
(Decreased Pao_2)
1. Cardiac/pulmonary insufficiency
↑ Erythropoietin
(Normal Pao_2)
1. Renal disease (neoplasia, cysts)
2. Methemoglobinemia
↑ Erythropoietin
Normal
Primary erythrocytosis
Plasma erythropoietin normal or decreased

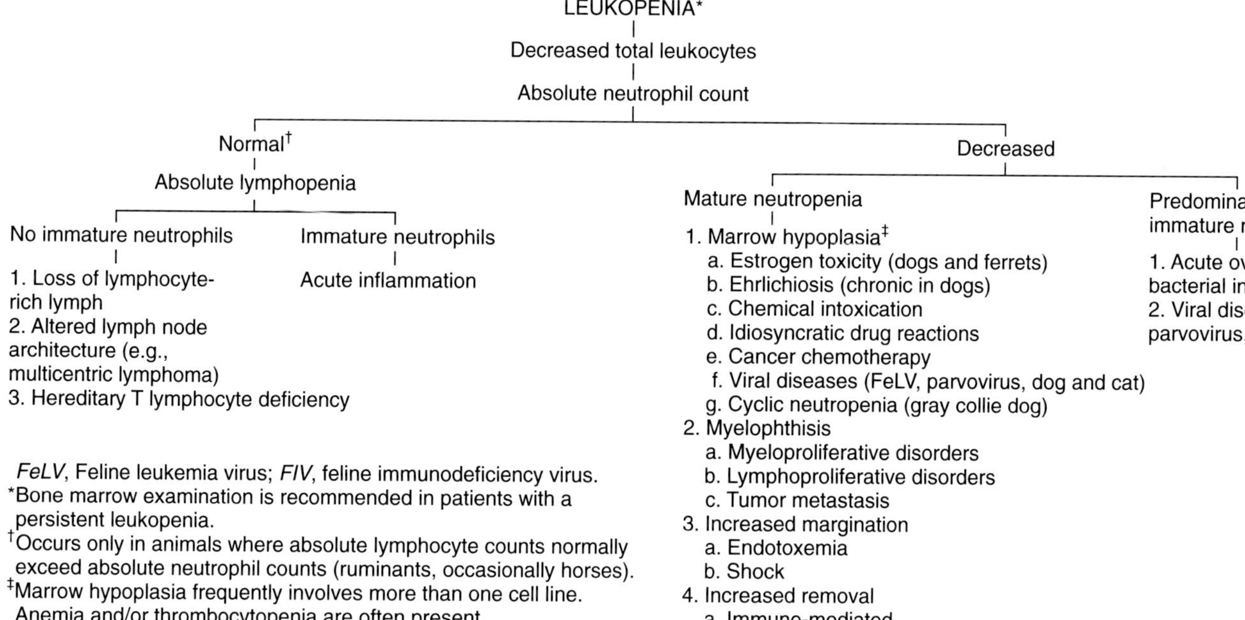

FeLV, Feline leukemia virus; *FIV*, feline immunodeficiency virus.

*Bone marrow examination is recommended in patients with a persistent leukopenia.

†Occurs only in animals where absolute lymphocyte counts normally exceed absolute neutrophil counts (ruminants, occasionally horses).

‡Marrow hypoplasia frequently involves more than one cell line. Anemia and/or thrombocytopenia are often present.

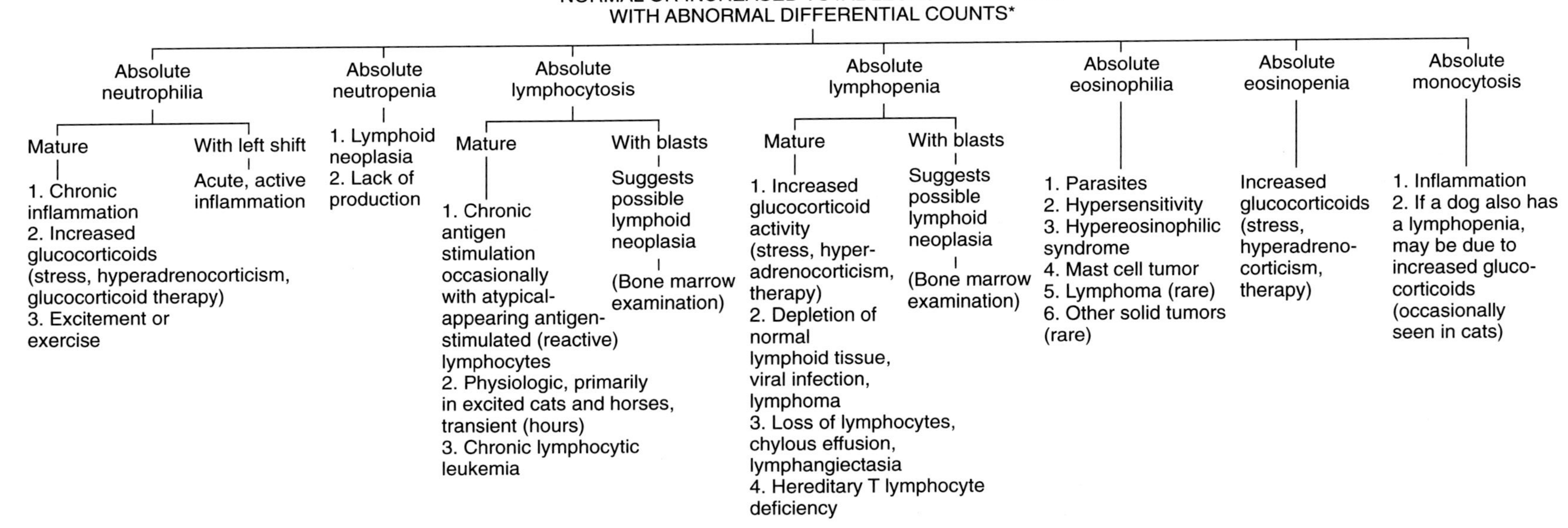

*See Table 1 in the Appendix for hematology values of adult animals.

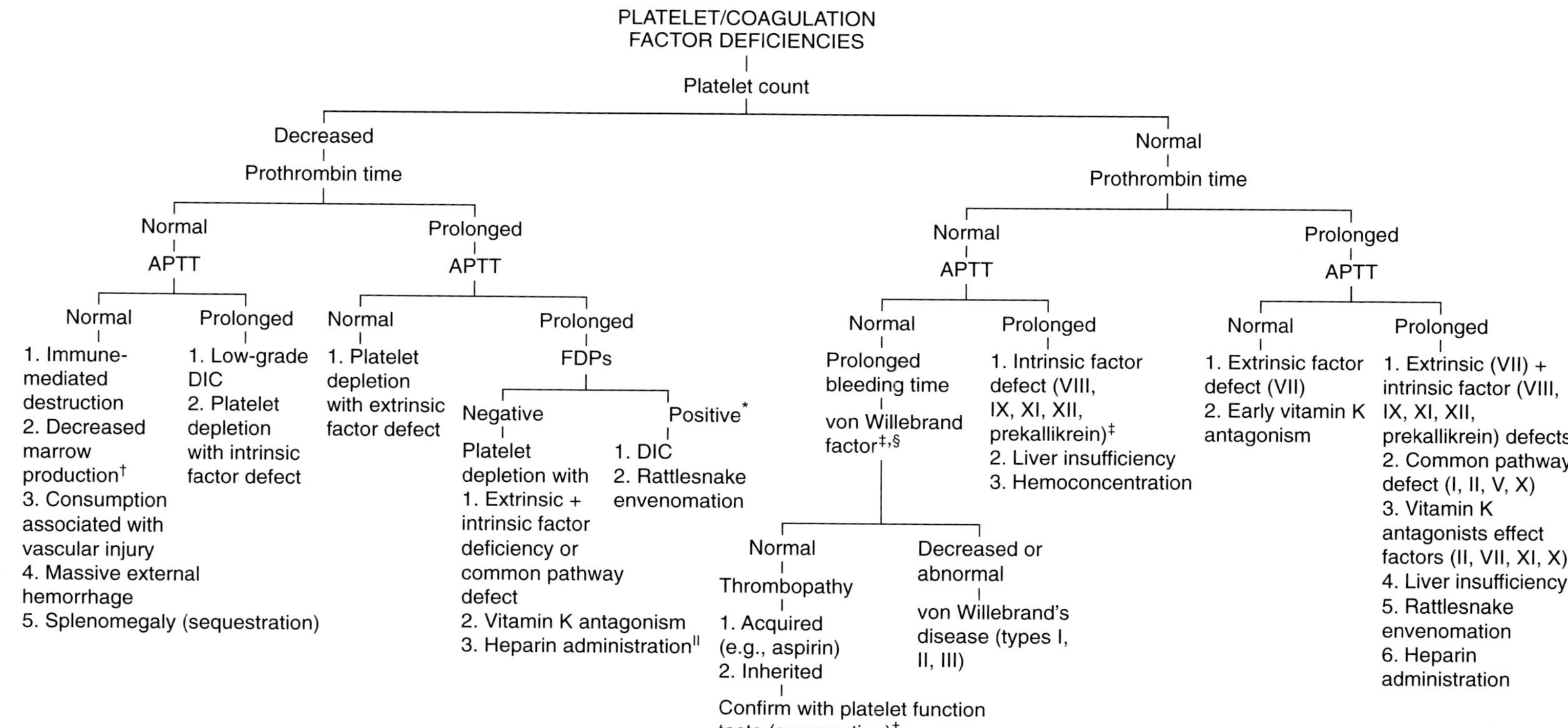

APTT, Activated partial thromboplastin time; *DIC*, disseminated intravascular coagulopathy; *FDPs*, fibrin degradation products.
*Some animals with DIC will have low or undetectable levels of fibrin degradation products.
†Specific tests may be necessary (e.g., *Ehrlichia* and Rocky Mountain spotted fever serologic tests).
‡Tests for these defects should be conducted at a special hemostasis laboratory.
§Formerly called factor VIII–related antigen.
‖Especially if heparin is used to keep an intravenous line open and blood is taken from it.

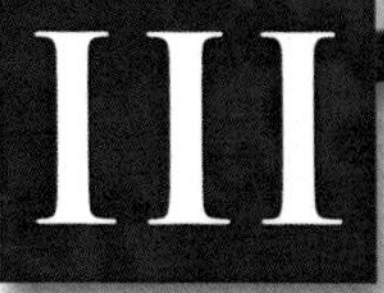

APPENDIX III

Case Studies

CASE 1: ESTROGEN-INDUCED APLASTIC ANEMIA

Patient: German shepherd dog, spayed female, 10 years of age

History: Urinary incontinence began about a month earlier. The referring veterinarian treated the dog with diethylstilbestrol (DES), increasing the dosage to 3 mg orally once each day when the incontinence persisted. A single treatment of estradiol cypionate (ECP) of unknown dose was also given 2½ weeks before referral. The animal was referred with a primary complaint of blood-stained perineal area.

Physical examination: Slightly depressed with normal hydration, mucous membrane color, pulse rate, respiratory rate, and temperature. Moderate dental tartar and gingivitis were present. An open wound was present on the lateral aspect of the left stifle. Isolated ecchymotic hemorrhages were observed on the ventral abdomen.

Notable Laboratory Findings

Hematology: Hematocrit (HCT), 23% with normal erythrocyte indices; platelet count, 6000/μL; neutrophil count, 500/μL; lymphocyte count, 2000/μL; monocyte count, 100/μL; eosinophil count, 0/μL; erythrocyte morphology, 1+ echinocytosis and moderate rouleaux; lymphocyte morphology, frequently reactive

Clinical chemistry: Not done

Bone marrow: Aspirate and core biopsies were markedly hypocellular. The marrow particles present in aspirate smears consisted primarily of reticular cells, macrophages, plasma cells, and mast cells. Low numbers of erythroid precursor cells and even lower numbers of granulocytic precursor cells were present. No megakaryocytes were observed. Large amounts of stainable iron were present.

Assessment

The anemia in this dog was considered nonregenerative because no polychromasia was seen in the stained blood film. The reactive lymphocytes indicated increased antigenic stimulation, probably related to the profound neutropenia and open wound. The subcutaneous hemorrhages resulted from the thrombocytopenia. Bone marrow evaluation revealed that the pancytopenia present resulted from a lack of bone marrow precursor cells. When erythroid precursors, granulocyte precursors, and megakaryocytes are markedly reduced or absent, the term *aplastic anemia* is used. The lymphocyte count was normal because most lymphocytes in blood enter from lymph nodes and spleen rather than from the bone marrow. The reticular cells, macrophages, and plasma cells in the bone marrow were considered to be normal residual cells. Mast cells are rare in bone marrow of normal animals but are sometimes seen in aplastic bone marrow, possibly because microenvironment changes potentiate their development.

Comment

The dog was given a blood transfusion and antibiotic therapy was begun. Epistaxis began 5 days later. The HCT was 27%. A bone marrow aspirate collected at that time was again aplastic. A second blood transfusion was given. Marked hematuria occurred 3 days later and the owner decided to have the dog euthanized. The aplastic anemia in this dog resulted from the prior administration of high doses of estrogens. ECP is much more toxic to canine bone marrow than is DES. Experimental studies have indicated that aplastic anemia develops about 3 weeks after toxic doses of estrogen are given, in agreement with the time course of this case. Only dogs and ferrets have been reported to develop estrogen-induced aplastic anemia. In addition to iatrogenic estrogen toxicity, dogs with endogenous hyperestrogenism (Sertoli cell tumor, interstitial cell tumor, seminoma of the testicle, and granulosa cell tumor of the ovary) can develop aplastic anemia, as can ferrets with protracted estrus.

REFERENCES

Kociba GJ, Caputo CA. Aplastic anemia associated with estrus in pet ferrets. *J Am Vet Med Assoc.* 1981;178:1293-1294.

Miura N, Sasaki N, Ogawa H, et al. Bone marrow hypoplasia induced by administration of estradiol benzoate in male beagle dogs. *Jpn J Vet Sci.* 1985;47:731-739.

Morgan RV. Blood dyscrasias associated with testicular tumors in the dog. *J Am Anim Hosp Assoc.* 1982;18:970-975.

CASE 2: ACUTE LYMPHOBLASTIC LEUKEMIA

Patient: Quarter horse, gelding, 15 years of age
History: Intermittent unilateral epistaxis for 4 months and weight loss for 2 months
Physical examination: Pale mucous membranes, tachycardia, temperature 103.8°F

Notable Laboratory Findings

Hematology: HCT, 12% with normal erythrocyte indices; fibrinogen, 1000 mg/dL; platelets, 142,000/μL; neutrophil count, 400/μL; lymphocyte count, 2200/μL; monocyte count, 100/μL; erythrocyte morphology, 2+ anisocytosis; lymphocyte morphology, 5% of lymphocytes were moderately large with fine nuclear chromatin and scant basophilic cytoplasm
Urinalysis: Normal
Clinical chemistry: Unremarkable
Coggins' test: Negative
Coagulation tests: Prothrombin time (PT) and activated partial thromboplastin (APTT) normal
Platelet function tests: Normal platelet aggregation and normal von Willebrand factor concentration
Bone marrow biopsy: Replacement of normal marrow cells with a monotonous population of moderately large lymphocytes with fine nuclear chromatin and scant basophilic cytoplasm similar to those present in blood. Indistinct nucleoli were visible in some cells. As expected, these neoplastic cells were peroxidase-negative.
Endoscopy: Normal nasopharynx, guttural pouch, and upper trachea

Assessment

In the absence of identifiable peripheral tumors, a presumptive diagnosis of acute lymphoblastic leukemia was made. The severe neutropenia and anemia were explained by the replacement of normal marrow precursor cells with neoplastic cells. The normal platelet count was unexplained, as was the long history of intermittent epistaxis. The increased fibrinogen concentration suggested the presence of concomitant inflammation.

Comment

The horse was euthanized. Multiple submucosal hematomas were present in the maxillary sinuses, and mesenteric and sublumbar lymph nodes were enlarged. As in the antemortem biopsy, the bone marrow was diffusely filled with sheets of neoplastic lymphocytes. Lymphoid infiltrates were present in the spleen, liver, kidney, and lymph nodes. Moderate extramedullary hematopoiesis was present in the spleen; consequently some of the blood platelets may have originated in the spleen. It is also possible that some bone marrow sites, not evaluated during the antemortem biopsy or necropsy, contained megakaryocytes. The necropsy findings were more supportive of a diagnosis of acute lymphoblastic leukemia than of lymphoma with secondary leukemia.

REFERENCE

Lester GD, Alleman AR, Raskin RE, et al. Pancytopenia secondary to lymphoid leukemia in three horses. *J Vet Intern Med.* 1993;7:360-363.

CASE 3: IRON-DEFICIENCY ANEMIA

Patient: Irish setter dog, female, 13 years of age

History: Weakness, anorexia, and weight loss for a week; unable to walk at presentation

Physical examination: The dog was depressed, emaciated, approximately 8% dehydrated, and nonambulatory because of extreme weakness. Pale mucous membranes, ocular and nasal discharges, excessive dental tartar, otitis externa, and large numbers of fleas were present. The rectal temperature was 99.6°F.

Notable Laboratory Findings

Hematology: HCT, 11%; mean cell volume (MCV), 52 fL; mean cell hemoglobin concentration (MCHC), 30 g/dL; red cell distribution width (RDW), 20%; reticulocyte count, 80,000/μL; total plasma protein, 6.8 g/dL; platelet count, 532,000/μL; band count, 3300/μL; neutrophil count, 24,800/μL; lymphocyte count, 500/μL; monocyte count, 3600/μL; eosinophil count, 0; erythrocyte morphology, 1+ polychromasia, 2+ anisocytosis, 2+ hypochromasia

Clinical chemistry: urea nitrogen, 29 mg/dL; creatinine, 1.0 mg/dL

Serum iron assays: Serum iron, 16 μg/dL (reference interval 84 to 233 μg/dL); total iron-binding capacity (TIBC), 462 μg/dL (reference interval 284-572 μg/dL; and ferritin, 140 μg/L (reference interval 80 to 800 μg/L)

Fecal flotation: *Trichuris* eggs

Assessment

The presence of a severe microcytic hypochromic anemia indicates chronic iron deficiency. The low serum iron, normal serum TIBC, and low-normal serum ferritin concentrations support the diagnosis of iron deficiency. Serum ferritin concentration generally correlates well with total body iron content, but ferritin is an acute-phase reactant protein that increases during inflammation. Consequently serum ferritin might have been lower in the absence of the inflammation documented in the physical examination. Iron deficiency is almost always the result of blood loss in adult animals. The massive flea infestation was believed to be the major source of blood loss in this dog. Some blood loss may have also occurred in the feces, but whipworms alone do not cause enough hemorrhage to result in iron-deficiency anemia. The increased RDW indicates that there is increased variation in erythrocyte volumes. In iron-deficiency anemia, this results from a mixture of normocytic erythrocytes and microcytic erythrocytes formed after iron becomes limiting for erythrocyte development. The absolute reticulocyte count was not appropriately increased, indicating that decreased iron availability is limiting the bone marrow response to the anemia. The normal total plasma and serum protein concentrations in a dehydrated animal suggest that the concentration will be low-normal or decreased after rehydration. Serum proteins are synthesized more rapidly than erythrocytes; consequently the total plasma protein concentration may be normal in animals with chronic blood loss. A majority of dogs with iron deficiency anemia have a thrombocytosis, as in this case. The neutrophilia, lymphopenia, monocytosis, and eosinopenia are likely the result of stress (endogenous glucocorticoid release), but the significant left shift and the magnitude of the neutrophilia indicate that a concomitant inflammatory response is also present. The slightly increased urea nitrogen concentration is probably prerenal and secondary to dehydration.

Comment

The dog was given a whole blood transfusion (two units) and treated with intravenous lactated Ringer's solution to correct the dehydration. The following day the HCT was 34%, total plasma protein was 6.2 g/dL, rectal temperature was 101.5°F, and marked clinical improvement was apparent. The animal was also treated for fleas and given an anthelmintic, and the client was instructed on appropriate flea-control measures for the dog's environment. Oral iron therapy was not considered essential because of the amount of iron present in the transfused blood.

REFERENCE

Harvey JW, French TW, Meyer DJ. Chronic iron deficiency anemia in dogs. *J Am Anim Hosp Assoc.* 1982;18:946-960.

CASE 4: *MYCOPLASMA HAEMOFELIS* INFECTION

Patient: Domestic shorthaired cat, castrated male, 2 years of age
History: Presented for evaluation of deformed carpus, which was present when the client acquired the cat as a stray
Physical examination: Deformity of carpus secondary to traumatic luxation, alopecia over pinna secondary to dermatomycosis, slightly depressed and afebrile with marked splenomegaly

Notable Laboratory Findings

Hematology: HCT, 13%; MCV, 86 fL; MCHC, 33% total plasma protein, 8.3 g/dL; platelet count, normal; leukocyte counts, normal; nucleated erythrocytes, 1400/µL; erythrocyte morphology, 1+ anisocytosis, 2+ polychromasia, 4+; *Mycoplasma haemofelis* organisms
Clinical chemistry: Bilirubin, 0.4 mg/dL; alanine aminotransferase (ALT), 143 units/L; globulin, 5.8 g/dL
Serology: Feline leukemia virus (FeLV), negative; feline immunodeficiency virus (FIV), positive

Assessment

The anemia was regenerative based on the degree of polychromasia present. Reticulocyte counts may not be accurate when high numbers of *M. haemofelis* organisms are present. The macrocytosis and nucleated erythrocytes are consistent with the animal's regenerative bone marrow response. The increased total plasma protein concentration is the result of increased globulin concentrations and could represent an inflammatory reaction to the blood parasite. The slightly increased bilirubin concentration is attributable to the increased erythrocyte destruction accompanying these erythrocyte parasites. The slightly increased ALT may reflect hypoxic injury to the liver.

Comment

Doxycycline and glucocorticoid therapy was initiated and the cat was discharged. The client was told that the *M. haemofelis* infection should respond to therapy but that the cat would probably remain FIV-positive, which would likely result in increased susceptibility to bacterial infections at a later date. Concurrent infections of *M. haemofelis* and FeLV generally result in more severe clinical signs and more severe anemia than occurs when a cat is infected with either agent alone. In contrast, concurrent infection with *M. haemofelis* and FIV does not appear to cause more severe anemia than does infection with *M. haemofelis* alone. Consequently the regenerative anemia in this cat is attributable primarily to the *M. haemofelis* infection.

REFERENCE

Harvey JW. Hemotrophic mycoplasmosis (hemobartonellosis). In: Greene CE, ed. *Infectious Diseases of the Dog and Cat*, 3rd ed. Philadelphia: Saunders Elsevier; 2006:252-260.

CASE 5: VAGINAL TEAR

Patient: Standard-bred horse, female, 10 years of age

History: Dystocia resulting in a vaginal tear and displacement of intestines into the vagina. Attempts to repair the laceration on the farm were initially unsuccessful because of hemorrhage and straining. Xylazine was administered as an analgesic and sedative, the intestines were replaced into the abdomen, and the laceration was sutured.

Physical examination: The horse was uncomfortable, exhibiting evidence of pain, but otherwise appeared normal.

Notable Laboratory Findings (Day 1)

Hematology: HCT, 38%; total plasma protein, 6.0 g/dL, fibrinogen, 300 mg/dL; platelet count, normal; metamyelocyte count, 100/μL; band count, 600/μL; neutrophil count, 2400/μL; lymphocyte count, 600/μL; monocyte count, 200/μL; eosinophil count, 0/μL; neutrophilic morphology, 2+ toxicity.

Clinical chemistry: Aspartate aminotransferase (AST), 506 units/L.

Abdominal fluid: HCT, 8%; protein, 4.0 g/dL; nucleated cell count, 13,100/μL; most nucleated cells present were toxic neutrophils.

Microbiology: No bacterial growth was obtained from the abdominal fluid, but antibiotic therapy may have been initiated prior to culture.

Assessment

The abdominal fluid analysis revealed evidence of hemorrhage and inflammation. The toxic left shift with low-normal neutrophil numbers in blood resulted from peritonitis with movement of neutrophils into the abdominal cavity. The absorption of endotoxin, which results in increased margination of neutrophils, may also have contributed to this leukogram. The lymphopenia and eosinopenia probably resulted from the endogenous release of glucocorticoids. The slightly decreased plasma protein concentration probably resulted from the peritonitis with protein movement into the abdominal cavity. The increased serum AST activity was attributed to tissue injury.

Comment

The abdomen was lavaged with large volumes of saline solution containing penicillin and streptomycin and the horse was treated with intravenous penicillin and intravenous fluids. Laboratory analyses were done again on day 3.

Notable Laboratory Findings (Day 3)

Hematology: HCT, 42%; total plasma protein, 7.1 g/dL; fibrinogen, 700 mg/dL; platelet count, normal; band count, 200/μL; neutrophil count, 900/μL; lymphocyte count, 300/μL; monocyte count, 200/μL; eosinophil count, 0/μL; neutrophilic morphology, 2+ toxicity.

Clinical chemistry: AST, 795 units/L.

Abdominal fluid: HCT, 3%; protein; 2.9 g/dL; nucleated cell count, 33,800/μL; most nucleated cells present were toxic neutrophils.

Assessment

The abdominal fluid analysis revealed continued evidence of inflammation. The toxic neutropenia on day 3 resulted from peritonitis with movement of neutrophils into the abdominal cavity. The lymphopenia and eosinopenia resulted from the endogenous release of glucocorticoids. The fibrinogen increased in response to inflammation. The increased serum AST activity was attributed to tissue injury. The horse eventually made a full recovery.

CASE 6: HYPEREOSINOPHILIC SYNDROME

Patient: Himalayan cat, castrated male, 5 years of age

History: Respiratory distress developed 3 days earlier. The referring veterinarian began treatment with an antibiotic, but the condition worsened.

Physical examination: The cat presented with abdominal respiration and tachypnea. Harsh lung sounds were auscultated, the cat was underweight and may have been slightly dehydrated. Enlarged prescapular, axillary, and inguinal lymph nodes and splenomegaly were palpated. Papules and scabs on the head and base of the tail were believed to represent a flea-bite allergy. The rectal temperature was 102.6°F.

Notable Laboratory Findings

Hematology: HCT, 29% with normal erythrocyte indices; total plasma protein, 8.6 g/dL; platelet count, normal; neutrophil count, 15,600/μL; lymphocyte count, 5100/μL; monocyte count, 1200/μL; band eosinophil count, 400/μL; eosinophil count, 22,300/μL; basophil count, 2100/μL; erythrocyte morphology, normal.

Clinical chemistry: Total serum protein, 8.1 g/dL; total globulins, 5.9 g/dL.

Exfoliative cytology: Transthoracic lung aspiration revealed histiocytic eosinophilic inflammation. Increased numbers of eosinophils were also present in splenic and lymph node aspirates that appeared to exceed those present in contaminating blood.

Histopathology: Chronic ulcerative eosinophilic dermatitis.

Parasitology: ELISA heartworm test was negative.

Thoracic radiograph: Patchy interstitial infiltrate.

Abdominal ultrasound: Splenomegaly and slightly thickened loops of bowel.

Assessment

Based on the magnitude of the eosinophilia and evidence of eosinophilic infiltration and injury in multiple organs, a diagnosis of hypereosinophilic syndrome was made. The etiology of this syndrome is unknown. Evidence that the overproduction of IL-5 may be involved in producing this disorder has been presented in humans with hypereosinophilic syndrome. A marked left shift in the eosinophilic series is expected in cats with eosinophilic leukemia. Eosinophilic leukemia was considered unlikely in this cat because most of the eosinophils in blood and tissues were mature. When present in animals, basophilia generally accompanies eosinophilia, possibly because certain growth factors (most notably IL-5) stimulate the production of both cell types. The slight neutrophilia and monocytosis present may be associated with the inflammation recognized in several tissues. The mild nonregenerative anemia is probably the result of the anemia of inflammatory disease. The increased serum protein concentration was the result of increased globulins, further supporting the likelihood of an inflammatory reaction.

Comment

The cat was placed in an oxygen cage and treated with aminophylline (a bronchodilator) and an antibiotic pending the outcome of diagnostic tests. Once a diagnosis of hypereosinophilic syndrome was reached, glucocorticoid therapy was initiated. Clinical signs improved rapidly and the cat was discharged with a plan to taper the glucocorticoid dosage as clinical signs resolved.

REFERENCES

Huibregise BA, Turner JL. Hypereosinophilic syndrome and eosinophilic leukemia: a comparison of 22 hypereosinophilic cats. *J Am Anim Hosp Assoc.* 1994;30:591-599.

Swenson CL, Carothers MA, Wellman ML, et al. Eosinophilic leukemia in a cat with naturally acquired feline leukemia virus infection. *J Am Anim Hosp Assoc.* 1993; 29:467-501.

Weller PF, Bubley GJ. The idiopathic hypereosinophilic syndrome. *Blood.* 1994;83: 2759-2779.

CASE 7: PYOMETRA

Patient: Rottweiler dog, female, 2 years of age

History: Depression, lethargy, fever, and purulent bloody vaginal discharge for several days; vomited the day of admission

Physical examination: Moderately depressed, panting respiration, slightly distended abdomen, dark pink mucous membranes, rectal temperature 102°F

Notable Laboratory Findings (Day 1)

Hematology: HCT, 48%; total plasma protein, 7.5 g/dL; fibrinogen, 200 mg/dL; manual platelet count, 180,000/μL; band neutrophil count, 3700/μL; neutrophil count, 57,400/μL; lymphocyte count, 7700/μL; monocyte count, 3700/μL; eosinophil count, 700/μL; basophil count, 0/μL; erythrocyte morphology, 1+ echinocytes; leukocyte morphology, 1+ toxicity of neutrophilic cells and occasional reactive lymphocytes

Clinical chemistry: Unremarkable

Coagulation tests: PT, 9 seconds (control, 8 seconds); APTT, 20 seconds (control, 10 seconds); activated clotting time (ACT), 105 seconds (reference less than 95 seconds); fibrin degradation products (FDP), positive at 1:20 dilution

Abdominal radiographs: No abnormalities appreciated

Abdominal ultrasound: Large, fluid-filled uterus identified

Assessment

The marked neutrophilia with toxic left shift and monocytosis indicated a severe inflammatory reaction. The presence of a dilated uterus and purulent vaginal discharge indicated that the dog had pyometra. The lymphocytosis may have reflected antigenic stimulation. The slightly decreased manual platelet count, prolonged APTT, slightly prolonged ACT, and positive FDP test indicated the presence of disseminated intravascular coagulation (DIC). Although the PT was normal, this test appears to be less sensitive than the APTT in the diagnosis of DIC. Fibrinogen is an acute-phase protein that tends to increase during inflammation; consequently, the normal fibrinogen value did not rule out DIC.

Comment

Antibiotic and intravenous fluid therapy was begun after the first blood sample was taken. Epistaxis began on the following day and the animal became more depressed.

Notable Laboratory Findings (Day 2)

Hematology: HCT, 32% with normal erythrocyte indices; total plasma protein, 6.4 g/dL; fibrinogen, 400 mg/dL; manual platelet count, 61,000/μL; metamyelocyte count, 800/μL; band neutrophil count, 8400/μL; neutrophil count, 65,900/μL; lymphocyte count, 2100/μL; monocyte count, 7200/μL; eosinophil count, 0/μL; basophil count, 0/μL; erythrocyte morphology, 1+ echinocytes; leukocyte morphology, 1+ toxicity of neutrophilic cells and occasional reactive lymhocytes

Coagulation test: ACT, 150 seconds (reference less than 95 seconds)

Assessment

The neutrophilia with toxic left shift and monocytosis were more pronounced on the second day. The decrease in lymphocyte count and eosinopenia that developed suggested that increased endogenous glucocorticold release occurred as the dog's clinical condition worsened. The decreased HCT on the second day was primarily the result of fluid therapy. The further decrease in the platelet count and the prolonged ACT suggested the continuation of DIC.

Comment

Ovariohysterectomy was performed after the blood sample was collected on the second day and the dog made an uneventful recovery.

REFERENCE

Sevelius E, Tidholm A, Thoren-Tolling K. Pyometra in the dog. *J Am Anim Hosp Assoc.* 1990;26:33-38.

CASE 8: SYSTEMIC LUPUS ERYTHEMATOSUS

Patient: Cocker spaniel dog, male, 4 years of age

History: Rear-leg lameness associated with bilateral hip dysplasia was diagnosed 2 years earlier, and erosive nonseptic arthritis involving the carpal and tarsal joints was recognlzed 4 months previously. The HCT and platelet counts were normal at that time, but the ANA test was positive at 1:100 dilution (reference less than 1:20). The dog has been treated with aspirin for the preceding 4 months.

Physical examination: The dog was depressed with pale mucous membranes. A polyarthropathy was present and all joints were painful. There were multiple raised pigmented skin lesions and small petechial hemorrhages on the penis and abdomen. The rectal temperature was normal.

Notable Laboratory Findings

Hematology: HCT, 23%; MCV, 74 fL; MCHC, 33 g/dL; reticulocyte count, 184,000/μL; total plasma protein, 7.9 g/dL; fibrinogen, 400 mg/dL; manual platelet count, 8000/μL; band neutrophil count, 600/μL; neutrophil count, 12,900/μL; lymphocyte count, 700/μL; monocyte count, 200/μL; eosinophil count, 1000/μL; nucleated erythrocyte count, 500/μL; erythrocyte morphology, 3+ anisocytosis, 2+ polychromasia, 3+ spherocytosis, occasional Howell-Jolly bodies, and autoagglutination of saline washed erythrocytes.

Clinical chemistry: Total serum protein, 8.2 g/dL; the total globulin, 5.6 g/dL.

Urinalysis: Specific gravity, 1.042; moderate bilirubinuria.

Joint fluid: A direct smear from a swollen joint revealed increased numbers of nondegenerate neutrophils and macrophages.

Antinuclear antibody (ANA) test: Positive at 1:320 dilution (reference less than 1:20)

Skin biopsy: Histologic lesions were consistent with pemphigus foliaceous, an immune-mediated skin disorder, but direct immunofluorescence examination for IgG deposits in skin was negative.

Assessment

The presence of autoagglutination of saline-washed RBC-erythrocytes and spherocytosis points to an immune-mediated anemia. The high-normal MCV and low-normal MCHC are consistent with the increased percentage of reticulocytes, and the absolute reticulocytosis indicates an appropriate bone marrow response to the anemia. The low number of nucleated erythrocytes is appropriate for the degree of reticulocytosis. The petechial hemorrhages can be attributed to the severe thrombocytopenia. Based on the presence of an immune-mediated hemolytic anemia and a positive ANA test, the thrombocytopenia was presumed to be immune-mediated. The combined presence of immune-mediated anemia and immune-mediated thrombocytopenia has been termed the Evans syndrome. The presence of high-normal numbers of eosinophils suggests that endogenous glucocorticoid release is not responsible for the neutrophilia, monocytosis, and lymphopenia. The increased total globulins in serum and high-normal plasma fibrinogen concentration are consistent with inflammation, as is the mild neutrophilia with left shift and monocytosis. Bilirubinuria is common in dogs with hemolytic anemia even when bilirubinemia is not present because of the low renal threshold for bilirubin in dogs. A presumptive diagnosis of systemic lupus erythematosus (SLE) was made based on the concomitant occurrence of immune-mediated hemolytic anemia, thrombocytopenia, nonseptic polyarthritis, and positive ANA test. The skin lesion may also have been a component of this syndrome, but an immune-mediated etiology could not be confirmed.

Comment

Therapy consisted of glucocorticoid steroids and cyclophosphamide. When examined 1 week later, the animal appeared to be feeling less pain, skin lesions were resolving, the HCT was 27%, MCV was 77 fL, and platelet count was 1.2×10^6/mL. The resolution of the thrombocytopenia following initiation of immunosuppressive therapy provides retrospective evidence that the thrombocytopenia was immune-mediated. It is assumed that the animal had high plasma thrombopoietin values when thrombocytopenic and that the subsequent thrombocytosis occurred as a rebound phenomenon when premature platelet destruction was reduced or eliminated by immunosuppressive therapy.

REFERENCE

Grindem CB, Johnson KH. Systemic lupus erythematosus: literature review and report of 42 new canine cases. *J Am Anim Hosp Assoc.* 1983;19:489-503.

INDEX

Note: Page numbers followed by f indicate figures; t, tables; b, boxes.

N

Printed in the United States
By Bookmasters

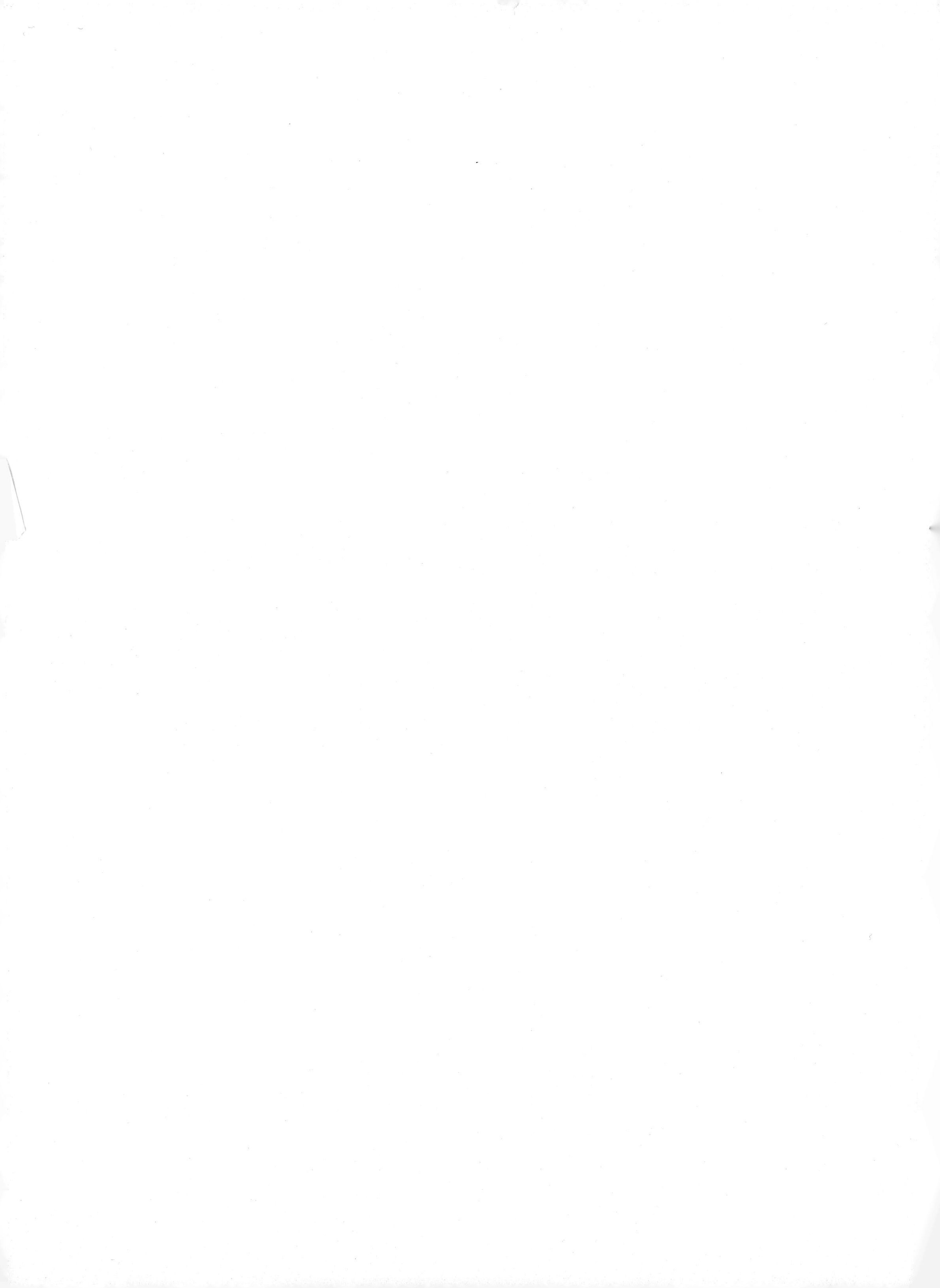